Dinggang Shen · Tianming Liu ·
Terry M. Peters · Lawrence H. Staib ·
Caroline Essert · Sean Zhou ·
Pew-Thian Yap · Ali Khan (Eds.)

Medical Image Computing and Computer Assisted Intervention – MICCAI 2019

22nd International Conference
Shenzhen, China, October 13–17, 2019
Proceedings, Part VI

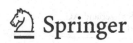

Editors
Dinggang Shen
University of North Carolina
at Chapel Hill
Chapel Hill, NC, USA

Terry M. Peters (iD)
Western University
London, ON, Canada

Caroline Essert (iD)
University of Strasbourg
Illkirch, France

Pew-Thian Yap
University of North Carolina
at Chapel Hill
Chapel Hill, NC, USA

Tianming Liu
University of Georgia
Athens, GA, USA

Lawrence H. Staib (iD)
Yale University
New Haven, CT, USA

Sean Zhou
United Imaging Intelligence
Shanghai, China

Ali Khan
Western University
London, ON, Canada

ISSN 0302-9743   ISSN 1611-3349 (electronic)
Lecture Notes in Computer Science
ISBN 978-3-030-32225-0   ISBN 978-3-030-32226-7 (eBook)
https://doi.org/10.1007/978-3-030-32226-7

LNCS Sublibrary: SL6 – Image Processing, Computer Vision, Pattern Recognition, and Graphics

© Springer Nature Switzerland AG 2019
This work is subject to copyright. All rights are reserved by the Publisher, whether the whole or part of the material is concerned, specifically the rights of translation, reprinting, reuse of illustrations, recitation, broadcasting, reproduction on microfilms or in any other physical way, and transmission or information storage and retrieval, electronic adaptation, computer software, or by similar or dissimilar methodology now known or hereafter developed.
The use of general descriptive names, registered names, trademarks, service marks, etc. in this publication does not imply, even in the absence of a specific statement, that such names are exempt from the relevant protective laws and regulations and therefore free for general use.
The publisher, the authors and the editors are safe to assume that the advice and information in this book are believed to be true and accurate at the date of publication. Neither the publisher nor the authors or the editors give a warranty, expressed or implied, with respect to the material contained herein or for any errors or omissions that may have been made. The publisher remains neutral with regard to jurisdictional claims in published maps and institutional affiliations.

This Springer imprint is published by the registered company Springer Nature Switzerland AG
The registered company address is: Gewerbestrasse 11, 6330 Cham, Switzerland

Lecture Notes in Computer Science 11769

More information about this series at http://www.springer.com/series/7412

Preface

We are pleased to present the proceedings for the 22nd International Conference on Medical Image Computing and Computer-Assisted Intervention (MICCAI), which was held at the InterContinental Hotel, Shenzhen, China, October 13–17, 2019. The conference also featured 34 workshops, 13 tutorials, and 22 challenges held on October 13 or 17. MICCAI 2019 had an approximately 63% increase in submissions and accepted papers compared with MICCAI 2018. These papers, which comprise six volumes of *Lecture Notes in Computer Science* (LNCS) proceedings, were selected after a thorough double-blind peer-review process. Following the example set by the previous program chairs of MICCAI 2018 and 2017, we employed Microsoft's Conference Managing Toolkit (CMT) for paper submissions and double-blind peer-reviews, and the Toronto Paper Matching System (TPMS) to assist with automatic paper assignment to area chairs and reviewers.

From 2625 original intentions to submit, 1809 full submissions were received and sent out to peer-review. Of these, 63% were considered as pure Medical Image Computing (MIC), 5% as pure Computer-Assisted Interventions (CAI), and 32% as both MIC and CAI. The MICCAI 2019 Program Committee (PC) comprised 69 area chairs, with 25 from the Americas, 21 from Europe, and 23 from Asia/Pacific/Middle East. Each area chair was assigned ∼25 manuscripts, with up to 15 suggested potential reviewers using TPMS scoring and self-declared research areas. Subsequently, over 1200 invited reviewers were asked to bid for the papers for which they had been suggested. Final reviewer allocations via CMT took account of PC suggestions, reviewer bidding, and TPMS scores, finally allocating 5–6 papers per reviewer. Based on the double-blinded reviews, 306 papers (17%) were accepted immediately, and 920 papers (51%) were rejected, with the remainder being sent for rebuttal. These decisions were confirmed by the area chairs. During the rebuttal phase, two additional area chairs were assigned to each rebuttal paper using CMT and TPMS scores, who then independently scored them to accept or reject, based on the reviews, rebuttal, and manuscript, resulting in clear paper decisions using majority voting. This process resulted in the acceptance of further 234 papers for an overall acceptance rate of 30%. Regional PC teleconferences were held in late June to confirm the final results and collect PC feedback on the peer-review process.

For the MICCAI 2019 proceedings, 538 accepted papers have been organized in six volumes as follows:

Part I, LNCS Volume 11764: Optical Imaging; Endoscopy; Microscopy

Part II, LNCS Volume 11765: Image Segmentation; Image Registration; Cardiovascular Imaging; Growth, Development, Atrophy, and Progression

Part III, LNCS Volume 11766: Neuroimage Reconstruction and Synthesis; Neuroimage Segmentation; Diffusion-Weighted Magnetic Resonance Imaging; Functional Neuroimaging (fMRI); Miscellaneous Neuroimaging

Part IV, LNCS Volume 11767: Shape; Prediction; Detection and Localization; Machine Learning; Computer-Aided Diagnosis; Image Reconstruction and Synthesis
Part V, LNCS Volume 11768: Computer-Assisted Interventions; MIC Meets CAI
Part VI, LNCS Volume 11769: Computed Tomography; X-ray Imaging

We would like to thank everyone who contributed to the success of MICCAI 2019 and the quality of its proceedings, particularly the MICCAI Society for support, insightful comments, and providing funding for Kitty Wong to be the ongoing Conference System Manager. Given the increase in workload for this year's meeting, the Program Committee simply could not have functioned effectively without her, and she will provide ongoing oversight of the review process for future MICCAI conferences. Without the dedication and support of all of the organizers of the workshops, tutorials, and challenges, under the guidance of Kenji Suzuki, together with satellite event chairs Hongen Liao, Qian Wang, Luping Zhou, Hayit Greenspan, and Bram van Ginneken, none of these peripheral events would have been feasible.

Also, the Industry Forum (led by Xiaodong Tao and Yiqiang Zhan), the Industry Session (led by Sean Zhou), as well as the Doctoral Symposium (led by Junzhou Huang and Dajiang Zhu) brought new events to MICCAI 2019. The publication chairs, Li Wang and Gang Li, undertook the onerous task of assembling the camera-ready proceedings for publication by Springer.

Behind the scenes, MICCAI secretariat personnel, Janette Wallace and Johanne Langford, kept a close eye on logistics and budgets, while Doris Lam and her team from Momentous Asia, this year's Professional Conference Organization, along with the Local Organizing Committee chair, Dong Ni (together with Jing Qin, Qianjin Feng, Dong Liang, Xiaoying Tang), handled the website and local organization. The Student Travel Award Committee chaired by Huiguang He, Jun Shi, and Xi Jiang evaluated numerous applications, including awards for undergraduate students, which is new in the history of MICCAI. We also thank our sponsors for their financial support and presence on site. We are especially grateful to all members of the Program Committee for their diligent work in the reviewer assignments and final paper selection, as well as the reviewers for their support during the entire process. Finally, and most importantly, we thank all authors, co-authors, students/postdocs, and supervisors, for submitting and presenting their high-quality work that made MICCAI 2019 a greatly enjoyable, informative, and successful event. We are indebted to those reviewers and PC members who helped us resolve issues relating to last-minute missing reviews. Overall, we thank all of the authors and attendees for making MICCAI 2019 a spectacular success. We look forward to seeing you in Lima, Peru at MICCAI 2020!

October 2019

Dinggang Shen
Tianming Liu
Terry M. Peters
Lawrence H. Staib
Caroline Essert
Sean Zhou
Pew-Thian Yap
Ali Khan

Organization

General Chairs

Dinggang Shen	The University of North Carolina at Chapel Hill, USA
Tianming Liu	The University of Georgia, USA

Program Executive

Terry Peters	Robarts Research Institute, Western University, Canada
Lawrence H. Staib	Yale University, USA
Sean Zhou	United Imaging Intelligence (UII), China
Caroline Essert	University of Strasbourg, France
Pew-Thian Yap	The University of North Carolina at Chapel Hill, USA
Ali Khan	Robarts Research Institute, Western University, Canada

Submissions Manager

Kitty Wong	Robarts Research Institute, Western University, Canada

Workshops/Challenges/Tutorial Chairs

Kenji Suzuki	Illinois Institute of Technology, USA
Hayit Greenspan	Tel Aviv University, Israel
Bram van Ginneken	Radboud University Medical Center, The Netherlands
Qian Wang	Shanghai Jiao Tong University, China
Luping Zhou	The University of Sydney, Australia
Hongen Liao	Tsinghua University, China

MICCAI Society, Board of Directors

Leo Joskowicz (President)	The Hebrew University of Jerusalem, Israel
Stephen Aylward (Treasurer)	Kitware, Inc., NY, USA
Josien Pluim (Secretary)	Eindhoven University of Technology, The Netherlands
Wiro Niessen (Past President)	Erasmus Medical Centre, The Netherlands
Marleen de Bruijne	Erasmus Medical Centre, The Netherlands and University of Copenhagen, Denmark
Hervé Delinguette	Inria, Sophia Antipolis, France
Caroline Essert	University of Strasbourg, France
Alejandro Frangi	University of Leeds, UK
Lena Maier-Hein	German Cancer Research Center, Germany

Shuo Li   Western University, London, Canada
Tianming Liu   University of Georgia, USA
Anne Martel   University of Toronto, Canada
Daniel Racoceanu   Pontifical Catholic University of Peru, Peru
Julia Schnabel   King's College, London, UK
Guoyan Zheng   Institute for Surgical Technology & Biomechanics,
                                 Switzerland
Kevin Zhou   Chinese Academy of Sciences, China

Industry Forum

Xiaodong Tao   iFLYTEK Health, China
Yiqiang Zhan   United Imaging Intelligence (UII), China

Publication Committee

Gang Li   The University of North Carolina at Chapel Hill, USA
Li Wang   The University of North Carolina at Chapel Hill, USA

Finance Committee

Dong Ni   Shenzhen University, China
Janette Wallace   Robarts Research Institute, Western University, Canada
Stephen Aylward   Kitware, Inc., USA

Local Organization Chairs

Dong Ni   Shenzhen University, China
Jing Qin   The Hong Kong Polytechnic University, SAR China
Qianjin Feng   Southern Medical University, China
Dong Liang   Shenzhen Institutes of Advanced Technology,
                                 Chinese Academy of Sciences, China
Xiaoying Tang   Southern University of Science and Technology, China

Sponsors and Publicity Liaison

Kevin Zhou   Institute of Computing Technology, Chinese Academy
                                 of Sciences, China
Hongen Liao   Tsinghua University, China
Wenjian Qin   Shenzhen Institutes of Advanced Technology,
                                 Chinese Academy of Sciences, China

Keynote Lectures Chairs

Max Viergever	University Medical Center Utrecht, The Netherlands
Kensaku Mori	Nagoya University, Japan
Gözde Ünal	Istanbul Technical University, Turkey

Student Travel Award Committee

Huiguang He	Institute of Automation, Chinese Academy of Sciences, China
Jun Shi	Shanghai University, China
Xi Jiang	University of Electronic Science and Technology of China, China

Student Activities Liaison

Julia Schnabel	King's College London, UK
Caroline Essert	University of Strasbourg, France
Dimitris Metaxas	Rutgers University, USA
MICCAI Student Board Members	

Area Chairs

Purang Abolmaesumi	The University of British Columbia, Canada
Shadi Albarqouni	The Technical University of Munich (TUM), Germany
Elsa Angelini	Imperial College London, UK
Suyash Awate	Indian Institute of Technology (IIT) Bombay, India
Ulas Bagci	University of Central Florida (UCF), USA
Kayhan Batmanghelich	University of Pittsburgh, USA
Christian Baumgartner	Swiss Federal Institute of Technology Zurich, Switzerland
Ismail Ben Ayed	Ecole de Technologie Superieure (ETS), Canada
Weidong Cai	The University of Sydney, Australia
Xiaohuan Cao	United Imaging Intelligence (UII), China
Elvis Chen	Robarts Research Institute, Western University, Canada
Xinjian Chen	Soochow University, China
Jian Cheng	Beihang University, China
Jun Cheng	Cixi Institute of Biomedical Engineering, Chinese Academy of Sciences, China
Veronika Cheplygina	Eindhoven University of Technology, The Netherlands
Elena De Momi	Politecnico di Milano, Italy
Ayman El-Baz	University of Louisville, USA
Aaron Fenster	Robarts Research Institute, Western University, USA
Moti Freiman	Philips Healthcare, The Netherlands
Yue Gao	Tsinghua University, China

Xiujuan Geng	Chinese University of Hong Kong, SAR China
Stamatia Giannarou	Imperial College London, UK
Orcun Goksel	Swiss Federal Institute of Technology Zurich, Switzerland
Xiao Han	AI Healthcare Center, Tencent Inc., China
Huiguang He	Institute of Automation, Chinese Academy of Sciences, China
Yi Hong	The University of Georgia, USA
Junzhou Huang	The University of Texas at Arlington, USA
Xiaolei Huang	The Pennsylvania State University, USA
Juan Eugenio Iglesias	University College London, UK
Pierre Jannin	The University of Rennes, France
Bernhard Kainz	Imperial College London, UK
Ali Kamen	Siemens Healthcare, USA
Jaeil Kim	Kyungpook National University, South Korea
Andrew King	King's College London, UK
Karim Lekadir	Universitat Pompeu Fabra, Spain
Cristian Linte	Rochester Institute of Technology, USA
Mingxia Liu	The University of North Carolina at Chapel Hill, USA
Klaus Maier-Hein	German Cancer Research Center, Germany
Anne Martel	Sunnybrook Research Institute, USA
Andrew Melbourne	University College London, UK
Anirban Mukhopadhyay	Technische Universität Darmstadt, Germany
Anqi Qiu	National University of Singapore, Singapore
Islem Rekik	Istanbul Technical University, Turkey
Hassan Rivaz	Concordia University, USA
Feng Shi	United Imaging Intelligence (UII), China
Amber Simpson	Memorial Sloan Kettering Cancer Center, USA
Marius Staring	Leiden University Medical Center, The Netherlands
Heung-Il Suk	Korea University, South Korea
Tanveer Syeda-Mahmood	University Medical Center Utrecht, The Netherlands
Xiaoying Tang	Southern University of Science and Technology, China
Pallavi Tiwari	Case Western Reserve University, USA
Emanuele Trucco	University of Dundee, UK
Martin Urschler	Graz University of Technology, Austria
Hien Van Nguyen	University of Houston, USA
Archana Venkataraman	Johns Hopkins University, USA
Christian Wachinger	Ludwig Maximilian University of Munich, Germany
Linwei Wang	Rochester Institute of Technology, USA
Yong Xia	Northwestern Polytechnical University, China
Yanwu Xu	Baidu Inc., China
Zhong Xue	United Imaging Intelligence (UII), China
Pingkun Yan	Rensselaer Polytechnic Institute, USA
Xin Yang	Huazhong University of Science and Technology, China
Yixuan Yuan	City University of Hong Kong, SAR China

Daoqiang Zhang   Nanjing University of Aeronautics and Astronautics,
                            China
Miaomiao Zhang   Washington University in St. Louis, USA
Tuo Zhang   Northwestern Polytechnical University, China
Guoyan Zheng   Shanghai Jiao Tong University, China
S. Kevin Zhou   Institute of Computing Technology, Chinese Academy
                            of Sciences, China
Dajiang Zhu   The University of Texas at Arlington, USA

Reviewers

Abdi, Amir	Barbu, Adrian
Abduljabbar, Khalid	Bardosi, Zoltan
Adeli, Ehsan	Bateson, Mathilde
Aganj, Iman	Bathula, Deepti
Aggarwal, Priya	Batmanghelich, Kayhan
Agrawal, Praful	Baumgartner, Christian
Ahmad, Ola	Baur, Christoph
Ahmad, Sahar	Baxter, John
Ahn, Euijoon	Bayramoglu, Neslihan
Akbar, Shazia	Becker, Benjamin
Akhondi-Asl, Alireza	Behnami, Delaram
Akram, Saad	Beig, Niha
Al-Kadi, Omar	Belyaev, Mikhail
Alansary, Amir	Benkarim, Oualid
Alghamdi, Hanan	Bentaieb, Aicha
Ali, Sharib	Bernal, Jose
Allan, Maximilian	Beyeler, Michael
Amiri, Mina	Bhatia, Parmeet
Anton, Esther	Bhole, Chetan
Anwar, Syed	Bhushan, Chitresh
Armin, Mohammad	Bi, Lei
Audigier, Chloe	Bian, Cheng
Aviles-Rivero, Angelica	Bilinski, Piotr
Awan, Ruqayya	Bise, Ryoma
Awate, Suyash	Bnouni, Nesrine
Aydogan, Dogu	Bo, Wang
Azizi, Shekoofeh	Bodenstedt, Sebastian
Bai, Junjie	Bogunovic, Hrvoje
Bai, Wenjia	Bozorgtabar, Behzad
Balbastre, Yaël	Bragman, Felix
Balsiger, Fabian	Braman, Nathaniel
Banerjee, Abhirup	Bridge, Christopher
Bano, Sophia	Broaddus, Coleman

Bron, Esther
Brooks, Rupert
Bruijne, Marleen
Bühler, Katja
Bui, Duc
Burlutskiy, Nikolay
Burwinkel, Hendrik
Bustin, Aurelien
Cabeen, Ryan
Cai, Hongmin
Cai, Jinzheng
Cai, Yunliang
Camino, Acner
Cao, Jiezhang
Cao, Qing
Cao, Tian
Carapella, Valentina
Cardenes, Ruben
Cardoso, M.
Carolus, Heike
Castro, Daniel
Cattin, Philippe
Chabanas, Matthieu
Chaddad, Ahmad
Chaitanya, Krishna
Chakraborty, Jayasree
Chakraborty, Rudrasis
Chang, Ken
Chang, Violeta
Charaborty, Tapabrata
Chatelain, Pierre
Chatterjee, Sudhanya
Chen, Alvin
Chen, Antong
Chen, Cameron
Chen, Chao
Chen, Chen
Chen, Elvis
Chen, Fang
Chen, Fei
Chen, Geng
Chen, Hanbo
Chen, Hao
Chen, Jia-Wei
Chen, Jialei
Chen, Jianxu

Chen, Jie
Chen, Jingyun
Chen, Lei
Chen, Liang
Chen, Min
Chen, Pingjun
Chen, Qingchao
Chen, Xiao
Chen, Xiaoran
Chen, Xin
Chen, Xuejin
Chen, Yang
Chen, Yuanyuan
Chen, Yuncong
Chen, Zhiqiang
Chen, Zhixiang
Cheng, Jun
Cheng, Li
Cheng, Yuan
Cheng, Yupeng
Cheriet, Farida
Chong, Minqi
Choo, Jaegul
Christiaens, Daan
Christodoulidis, Argyrios
Christodoulidis, Stergios
Chung, Ai
Çiçek, Özgün
Cid, Yashin
Clarkson, Matthew
Clough, James
Collins, Toby
Commowick, Olivier
Conze, Pierre-Henri
Cootes, Timothy
Correia, Teresa
Coulon, Olivier
Coupé, Pierrick
Courtecuisse, Hadrien
Craley, Jeffrey
Crimi, Alessandro
Cury, Claire
D'souza, Niharika
Dai, Hang
Dalca, Adrian
Das, Abhijit

Das, Dhritiman
Deeba, Farah
Dekhil, Omar
Demiray, Beatrice
Deniz, Cem
Depeursinge, Adrien
Desrosiers, Christian
Dewey, Blake
Dey, Raunak
Dhamala, Jwala
Ding, Meng
Distergoft, Alexander
Dobrenkii, Anton
Dolz, Jose
Dong, Liang
Dong, Mengjin
Dong, Nanqing
Dong, Xiao
Dong, Yanni
Dou, Qi
Du, Changde
Du, Lei
Du, Shaoyi
Duan, Dingna
Duan, Lixin
Dubost, Florian
Duchateau, Nicolas
Duncan, James
Duong, Luc
Dvornek, Nicha
Dzyubachyk, Oleh
Eaton-Rosen, Zach
Ebner, Michael
Ebrahimi, Mehran
Edwards, Philip
Egger, Bernhard
Eguizabal, Alma
Einarsson, Gudmundur
Ekin, Ahmet
Elazab, Ahmed
Elhabian, Shireen
Elmogy, Mohammed
Eltanboly, Ahmed
Erdt, Marius
Ernst, Floris
Esposito, Marco

Esteban, Oscar
Fan, Jingfan
Fan, Xin
Fan, Yong
Fan, Yonghui
Fang, Xi
Farag, Aly
Farzi, Mohsen
Fauser, Johannes
Fawaz, Hassan
Fedorov, Andrey
Fehri, Hamid
Feng, Chiyu
Feng, Jun
Feng, Xinyang
Feng, Yuan
Fenster, Aaron
Ferrante, Enzo
Feydy, Jean
Fischer, Lukas
Fischer, Peter
Fishbaugh, James
Fletcher, Tom
Flores, Kevin
Forestier, Germain
Forkert, Nils
Fotouhi, Javad
Fountoukidou, Tatiana
Franz, Alfred
Frau-Pascual, Aina
Freysinger, Wolfgang
Fripp, Jurgen
Fu, Huazhu
Funka-Lea, Gareth
Funke, Isabel
Funke, Jan
Fürnstahl, Philipp
Furukawa, Ryo
Gahm, Jin
Galassi, Francesca
Galdran, Adrian
Gan, Yu
Gao, Fei
Gao, Mingchen
Gao, Siyuan
Gao, Zhifan

Gardezi, Syed
Ge, Bao
Gerber, Samuel
Gerig, Guido
Gessert, Nils
Gevaert, Olivier
Gharabaghi, Sara
Ghesu, Florin
Ghimire, Sandesh
Gholipour, Ali
Ghosal, Sayan
Giraud, Rémi
Glocker, Ben
Goceri, Evgin
Goetz, Michael
Gomez, Alberto
Gong, Kuang
Gong, Mingming
Gonzalez, German
Gopal, Sharath
Gopinath, Karthik
Gordon, Shiri
Gori, Pietro
Gou, Shuiping
Granados, Alejandro
Grau, Vicente
Green, Michael
Gritsenko, Andrey
Grupp, Robert
Gu, Lin
Gu, Yun
Gu, Zaiwang
Gueziri, Houssem-Eddine
Guo, Hengtao
Guo, Jixiang
Guo, Xiaoqing
Guo, Yanrong
Guo, Yong
Gupta, Kratika
Gupta, Vikash
Gutman, Boris
Gyawali, Prashnna
Hacihaliloglu, Ilker
Hadjidemetriou, Stathis
Haldar, Justin
Hamarneh, Ghassan

Hamze, Noura
Han, Hu
Han, Jungong
Han, Xiaoguang
Han, Xu
Han, Zhi
Hancox, Jonny
Hanson, Erik
Hao, Xiaoke
Haq, Rabia
Harders, Matthias
Harrison, Adam
Haskins, Grant
Hatamizadeh, Ali
Hatt, Charles
Hauptmann, Andreas
Havaei, Mohammad
He, Tiancheng
He, Yufan
Heimann, Tobias
Heldmann, Stefan
Heller, Nicholas
Hernandez-Matas, Carlos
Hernandez, Monica
Hett, Kilian
Higger, Matt
Hinkle, Jacob
Ho, Tsung-Ying
Hoffmann, Nico
Holden, Matthew
Hong, Song
Hong, Sungmin
Hou, Benjamin
Hsu, Li-Ming
Hu, Dan
Hu, Kai
Hu, Xiaowei
Hu, Xintao
Hu, Yan
Hu, Yipeng
Huang, Heng
Huang, Huifang
Huang, Jiashuang
Huang, Kevin
Huang, Ruobing
Huang, Shih-Gu

Huang, Weilin
Huang, Xiaolei
Huang, Yawen
Huang, Yixing
Huang, Yufang
Huang, Zhongwei
Huaulmé, Arnaud
Huisman, Henkjan
Huo, Xing
Huo, Yuankai
Husch, Andreas
Hussein, Sarfaraz
Hutter, Jana
Hwang, Seong
Icke, Ilknur
Igwe, Kay
Ingalhalikar, Madhura
Irmakci, Ismail
Ivashchenko, Oleksandra
Izadyyazdanabadi, Mohammadhassan
Jafari, Mohammad
Jäger, Paul
Jamaludin, Amir
Janatka, Mirek
Jaouen, Vincent
Jarayathne, Uditha
Javadi, Golara
Javer, Avelino
Jensen, Todd
Ji, Zexuan
Jia, Haozhe
Jiang, Jue
Jiang, Steve
Jiang, Tingting
Jiang, Weixiong
Jiang, Xi
Jiao, Jianbo
Jiao, Jieqing
Jiao, Zhicheng
Jie, Biao
Jin, Dakai
Jin, Taisong
Jin, Yueming
John, Rogers
Joshi, Anand
Joshi, Shantanu

Jud, Christoph
Jung, Kyu-Hwan
Jungo, Alain
Kadkhodamohammadi, Abdolrahim
Kakileti, Siva
Kamnitsas, Konstantinos
Kang, Eunsong
Kao, Po-Yu
Kapoor, Ankur
Karani, Neerav
Karayumak, Suheyla
Kazi, Anees
Kerrien, Erwan
Kervadec, Hoel
Khalifa, Fahmi
Khalili, Nadieh
Khallaghi, Siavash
Khalvati, Farzad
Khan, Hassan
Khanal, Bishesh
Khansari, Maziyar
Khosravan, Naji
Kia, Seyed
Kikinis, Ron
Kim, Geena
Kim, Hosung
Kim, Hyo-Eun
Kim, Jae-Hun
Kim, Jinman
Kim, Jinyoung
Kim, Minjeong
Kim, Namkug
Kim, Seong
Kim, Young-Ho
Kitasaka, Takayuki
Klein, Stefan
Klinder, Tobias
Kolli, Kranthi
Kong, Bin
Kong, Xiang-Zhen
Konukoglu, Ender
Koo, Bongjin
Koohbanani, Navid
Kopriva, Ivica
Kose, Kivanc
Koutsoumpa, Christina

Kozinski, Mateusz
Krebs, Julian
Krishnan, Anithapriya
Krishnaswamy, Pavitra
Krivov, Egor
Kruggel, Frithjof
Krupinski, Elizabeth
Kuang, Hulin
Kügler, David
Kuijper, Arjan
Kulkarni, Prachi
Kumar, Arun
Kumar, Ashnil
Kumar, Kuldeep
Kumar, Neeraj
Kumar, Nitin
Kumaradevan, Punithakumar
Kunz, Manuela
Kunze, Holger
Kuo, Weicheng
Kurc, Tahsin
Kurmann, Thomas
Kwak, Jin
Kwon, Yongchan
Laadhari, Aymen
Ladikos, Alexander
Lalonde, Rodney
Lamata, Pablo
Langs, Georg
Lartizien, Carole
Lasso, Andras
Lau, Felix
Laura, Cristina
Le, Ngan
Ledig, Christian
Lee, Hansang
Lee, Hyekyoung
Lee, Jong-Hwan
Lee, Kyong
Lee, Minho
Lee, Soochahn
Léger, Étienne
Leger, Stefan
Lei, Baiying
Lekadir, Karim
Lenga, Matthias

Leow, Wee
Lessmann, Nikolas
Li, Annan
Li, Bin
Li, Fuhai
Li, Gang
Li, Guoshi
Li, Hongwei
Li, Hongying
Li, Huiqi
Li, Jian
Li, Jianning
Li, Ke
Li, Minli
Li, Quanzheng
Li, Rongjian
Li, Shaohua
Li, Shulong
Li, Shuyu
Li, Wenqi
Li, Xiang
Li, Xianjun
Li, Xiaojie
Li, Xiaomeng
Li, Xiaoxiao
Li, Xiuli
Li, Yang
Li, Yuexiang
Li, Zhang
Li, Zhi-Cheng
Li, Zhiyuan
Li, Zhjin
Lian, Chunfeng
Liang, Jianming
Liang, Shanshan
Liang, Yudong
Liao, Ruizhi
Liao, Xiangyun
Licandro, Roxane
Lin, Hongxiang
Lin, Lanfen
Lin, Muqing
Lindner, Claudia
Lippert, Christoph
Lisowska, Aneta
Litjens, Geert

Liu, Bin
Liu, Daochang
Liu, Dong
Liu, Dongnan
Liu, Fang
Liu, Feihong
Liu, Feng
Liu, Hong
Liu, Hui
Liu, Jianfei
Liu, Jiang
Liu, Jin
Liu, Jing
Liu, Jundong
Liu, Kefei
Liu, Li
Liu, Mingxia
Liu, Na
Liu, Peng
Liu, Shenghua
Liu, Siqi
Liu, Siyuan
Liu, Tianming
Liu, Tiffany
Liu, Xianglong
Liu, Yixun
Liu, Yong
Liu, Yue
Liu, Zhe
Loddo, Andrea
Lopes, Daniel
Lorenzi, Marco
Lou, Bin
Lu, Allen
Lu, Donghuan
Lu, Jiwen
Lu, Le
Lu, Weijia
Lu, Yao
Lu, Yueh-Hsun
Luo, Gongning
Luo, Jie
Lv, Jinglei
Lyu, Ilwoo
Lyu, Junyan
Ma, Benteng

Ma, Burton
Ma, Da
Ma, Kai
Ma, Xuelin
Mahapatra, Dwarikanath
Mahdavi, Sara
Mahmoud, Ali
Maicas, Gabriel
Maier-Hein, Klaus
Maier, Andreas
Makrogiannis, Sokratis
Malandain, Grégoire
Malik, Bilal
Malpani, Anand
Mancini, Matteo
Manhart, Michael
Manjon, Jose
Mansoor, Awais
Mao, Yunxiang
Martel, Anne
Martinez-Torteya, Antonio
Mathai, Tejas
Mato, David
Mcclelland, Jamie
Mcleod, Jonathan
Medrano-Gracia, Pau
Mehta, Ronak
Meier, Raphael
Melbourne, Andrew
Meng, Qingjie
Meng, Xianjing
Meng, Yu
Menze, Bjoern
Mi, Liang
Miao, Shun
Michielse, Stijn
Midya, Abhishek
Milchenko, Mikhail
Min, Zhe
Miyamoto, Tadashi
Mo, Yuanhan
Molina, Rafael
Montillo, Albert
Moradi, Mehdi
Moreno, Rodrigo
Mortazi, Aliasghar

Mozaffari, Mohammad
Muetzel, Ryan
Müller, Henning
Muñoz-Barrutia, Arrate
Munsell, Brent
Nadeem, Saad
Nahlawi, Layan
Nandakumar, Naresh
Nardi, Giacomo
Neila, Pablo
Ni, Dong
Nichols, Thomas
Nickisch, Hannes
Nie, Dong
Nie, Jingxin
Nie, Weizhi
Niethammer, Marc
Nigam, Aditya
Ning, Lipeng
Niu, Shuaicheng
Niu, Sijie
Noble, Jack
Noblet, Vincent
Novo, Jorge
O'donnell, Thomas
Obeid, Mohammad
Oda, Hirohisa
Oda, Masahiro
Odry, Benjamin
Oeltze-Jafra, Steffen
Oksuz, Ilkay
Oliveira, Marcelo
Oliver, Arnau
Oñativia, Jon
Onofrey, John
Orasanu, Eliza
Orihuela-Espina, Felipe
Orlando, Jose
Osmanlioglu, Yusuf
Otalora, Sebastian
Pace, Danielle
Pagador, J.
Pai, Akshay
Pan, Yongsheng
Pang, Shumao
Papiez, Bartlomiej

Parajuli, Nripesh
Park, Hyunjin
Park, Jongchan
Park, Sanghyun
Park, Seung-Jong
Paschali, Magdalini
Paul, Angshuman
Payer, Christian
Pei, Yuru
Peng, Jialin
Peng, Tingying
Pennec, Xavier
Perdomo, Oscar
Pereira, Sérgio
Pérez-Carrasco, Jose-Antonio
Pesteie, Mehran
Peter, Loic
Peters, Jorg
Petitjean, Caroline
Pezold, Simon
Pfeiffer, Micha
Phellan, Renzo
Phophalia, Ashish
Pisharady, Pramod
Playout, Clement
Pluim, Josien
Pohl, Kilian
Portenier, Tiziano
Pouch, Alison
Prasanna, Prateek
Prevost, Raphael
Ps, Viswanath
Pujades, Sergi
Qi, Xin
Qian, Zhen
Qiang, Yan
Qiao, Lishan
Qiao, Yuchuan
Qin, Chen
Qin, Wenjian
Qirong, Bu
Qiu, Wu
Qu, Liangqiong
Raamana, Pradeep
Rabbani, Hossein
Rackerseder, Julia

Rad, Reza
Rafii-Tari, Hedyeh
Rajpoot, Kashif
Ramachandram, Dhanesh
Ran, Lingyan
Raniga, Parnesh
Rashwan, Hatem
Rathore, Saima
Ratnarajah, Nagulan
Raval, Mehul
Ravikumar, Nishant
Raviprakash, Harish
Raza, Shan
Reaungamornrat, Surreerat
Rekik, Islem
Remeseiro, Beatriz
Rempfler, Markus
Ren, Jian
Ren, Xuhua
Ren, Yudan
Reyes-Aldasoro, Constantino
Reyes, Mauricio
Riedel, Brandalyn
Rieke, Nicola
Risser, Laurent
Rittner, Leticia
Rivera, Diego
Ro, Yong
Robinson, Emma
Robinson, Robert
Rodas, Nicolas
Rodrigues, Rafael
Rohr, Karl
Roohani, Yusuf
Roszkowiak, Lukasz
Roth, Holger
Rouco, José
Roy, Abhijit
Ruijters, Danny
Rusu, Mirabela
Rutter, Erica
S., Sharath
Sabuncu, Mert
Sachse, Frank
Safta, Wiem
Saha, Monjoy

Saha, Pramit
Sahu, Manish
Samani, Abbas
Samek, Wojciech
Sánchez-Margallo, Francisco
Sánchez-Margallo, Juan
Sankaran, Sethuraman
Sanroma, Gerard
Sao, Anil
Sarhan, Mhd
Sarikaya, Duygu
Sarker, Md.
Sato, Imari
Saut, Olivier
Savardi, Mattia
Savitha, Ramasamy
Scarpa, Fabio
Scheinost, Dustin
Scherf, Nico
Schirmer, Markus
Schlaefer, Alexander
Schmid, Jerome
Schnabel, Julia
Schultz, Thomas
Schwartz, Ernst
Sdika, Michael
Sedai, Suman
Sekou, Taibou
Sekuboyina, Anjany
Selvan, Raghavendra
Semedo, Carla
Senouf, Ortal
Seoud, Lama
Sermesant, Maxime
Serrano, Carmen
Sethi, Amit
Shaban, Muhammad
Shaffie, Ahmed
Shah, Meet
Shalaby, Ahmed
Shamir, Reuben
Shan, Hongming
Shao, Yeqin
Sharma, Harshita
Shehata, Mohamed
Shen, Haocheng

Shen, Li
Shen, Mali
Shen, Yiru
Sheng, Ke
Shi, Bibo
Shi, Jun
Shi, Kuangyu
Shi, Xiaoshuang
Shi, Yonggang
Shi, Yonghong
Shigwan, Saurabh
Shin, Hoo-Chang
Shin, Jitae
Shontz, Suzanne
Signoroni, Alberto
Siless, Viviana
Silva, Carlos
Silva, Wilson
Simonovsky, Martin
Simson, Walter
Sinclair, Matthew
Singh, Vivek
Soans, Rajath
Sohel, Ferdous
Sokooti, Hessam
Soliman, Ahmed
Sommen, Fons
Sommer, Stefan
Song, Ming
Song, Yang
Sotiras, Aristeidis
Sparks, Rachel
Spiclin, Ziga
St-Jean, Samuel
Steinbach, Peter
Stern, Darko
Stimpel, Bernhard
Strait, Justin
Studholme, Colin
Styner, Martin
Su, Hai
Su, Yun-Hsuan
Subramanian, Vaishnavi
Subsol, Gérard
Sudre, Carole
Suk, Heung-Il

Sun, Jian
Sun, Li
Sun, Tao
Sung, Kyunghyun
Suter, Yannick
Tajbakhsh, Nima
Tan, Chaowei
Tan, Jiaxing
Tan, Wenjun
Tang, Min
Tang, Sheng
Tang, Thomas
Tang, Xiaoying
Tang, Youbao
Tang, Yuxing
Tang, Zhenyu
Tanner, Christine
Tanno, Ryutaro
Tao, Qian
Tarroni, Giacomo
Tasdizen, Tolga
Thung, Kim
Tian, Jiang
Tian, Yun
Toews, Matthew
Tong, Yubing
Topsakal, Oguzhan
Torosdagli, Neslisah
Toussaint, Nicolas
Troccaz, Jocelyne
Trzcinski, Tomasz
Tulder, Gijs
Tustison, Nick
Tuysuzoglu, Ahmet
Ukwatta, Eranga
Unberath, Mathias
Ungi, Tamas
Upadhyay, Uddeshya
Urschler, Martin
Uslu, Fatmatulzehra
Uyanik, Ilyas
Vaillant, Régis
Vakalopoulou, Maria
Valindria, Vanya
Varela, Marta
Varsavsky, Thomas

Vedula, S.
Vedula, Sanketh
Veeraraghavan, Harini
Vega, Roberto
Veni, Gopalkrishna
Verma, Ujjwal
Vetter, Thomas
Vialard, Francois-Xavier
Villard, Pierre-Frederic
Villarini, Barbara
Virga, Salvatore
Vishnevskiy, Valery
Viswanath, Satish
Vlontzos, Athanasios
Vogl, Wolf-Dieter
Voigt, Ingmar
Vos, Bob
Vrtovec, Tomaz
Wang, Bo
Wang, Changmiao
Wang, Chengjia
Wang, Chunliang
Wang, Dadong
Wang, Guotai
Wang, Haifeng
Wang, Haoqian
Wang, Hongkai
Wang, Hongzhi
Wang, Hua
Wang, Huan
Wang, Jiazhuo
Wang, Jingwen
Wang, Jun
Wang, Junyan
Wang, Kuanquan
Wang, Kun
Wang, Lei
Wang, Li
Wang, Liansheng
Wang, Manning
Wang, Mingliang
Wang, Nizhuan
Wang, Pei
Wang, Puyang
Wang, Ruixuan
Wang, Shanshan

Wang, Sheng
Wang, Shuai
Wang, Wenzhe
Wang, Xiangxue
Wang, Xiaosong
Wang, Xuchu
Wang, Yalin
Wang, Yan
Wang, Yaping
Wang, Yuanjun
Wang, Ze
Wang, Zhe
Wang, Zhinuo
Wang, Zhiwei
Wang, Zilei
Weber, Jonathan
Wee, Chong-Yaw
Weese, Jürgen
Wei, Benzheng
Wei, Dong
Wei, Donglai
Wei, Dongming
Weigert, Martin
Wein, Wolfgang
Wels, Michael
Wemmert, Cédric
Werner, Rene
Wesierski, Daniel
Williams, Bryan
Williams, Jacqueline
Williams, Travis
Williamson, Tom
Wilms, Matthias
Wiskin, James
Wittek, Adam
Wollmann, Thomas
Wolterink, Jelmer
Wong, Ken
Woo, Jonghye
Wu, Guoqing
Wu, Ji
Wu, Jian
Wu, Jiong
Wu, Pengxiang
Wu, Xi
Wu, Ye

Wu, Yicheng
Wuerfl, Tobias
Xi, Xiaoming
Xia, Jing
Xia, Wenfeng
Xiao, Deqiang
Xiao, Yiming
Xie, Hai
Xie, Hongtao
Xie, Jianyang
Xie, Long
Xie, Weidi
Xie, Yiting
Xie, Yuanpu
Xie, Yutong
Xing, Fuyong
Xiong, Tao
Xu, Chenchu
Xu, Jiaofeng
Xu, Jun
Xu, Kele
Xu, Rui
Xu, Ting
Xu, Yan
Xu, Yongchao
Xu, Zheng
Xu, Zhenlin
Xu, Zhoubing
Xu, Ziyue
Xue, Jie
Xue, Wufeng
Xue, Yuan
Yahya, Faridah
Yan, Chenggang
Yan, Ke
Yan, Weizheng
Yan, Yu
Yan, Yuguang
Yan, Zhennan
Yang, Guang
Yang, Guanyu
Yang, Hao-Yu
Yang, Jie
Yang, Lin
Yang, Shan
Yang, Xiao

Yang, Xiaohui
Yang, Xin
Yao, Dongren
Yao, Jianhua
Yao, Jiawen
Ye, Chuyang
Ye, Jong
Ye, Menglong
Ye, Xujiong
Yi, Jingru
Yi, Xin
Ying, Shihui
Yoo, Youngjin
Yousefi, Bardia
Yousefi, Sahar
Yu, Jinhua
Yu, Kai
Yu, Lequan
Yu, Renping
Yu, Weichuan
Yushkevich, Paul
Zanjani, Farhad
Zenati, Marco
Zeng, Dong
Zeng, Guodong
Zettinig, Oliver
Zhan, Liang
Zhang, Baochang
Zhang, Chuncheng
Zhang, Dongqing
Zhang, Fan
Zhang, Haichong
Zhang, Han
Zhang, Haopeng
Zhang, Heye
Zhang, Jianpeng
Zhang, Jiong
Zhang, Jun
Zhang, Le
Zhang, Lichi
Zhang, Mingli
Zhang, Pengyue
Zhang, Pin
Zhang, Qiang
Zhang, Rongzhao
Zhang, Shengping

Zhang, Shu
Zhang, Songze
Zhang, Tianyang
Zhang, Tong
Zhang, Wei
Zhang, Wen
Zhang, Wenlu
Zhang, Xiang
Zhang, Xin
Zhang, Yi
Zhang, Yifan
Zhang, Yizhe
Zhang, Yong
Zhang, Yongqin
Zhang, You
Zhang, Yu
Zhang, Yue
Zhang, Yueyi
Zhang, Yungeng
Zhang, Yunyan
Zhang, Yuyao
Zhang, Zizhao
Zhao, Haifeng
Zhao, Jun
Zhao, Qingyu
Zhao, Rongchang
Zhao, Shijie
Zhao, Shiwan
Zhao, Tengda
Zhao, Wei
Zhao, Yitian
Zhao, Yiyuan

Zhao, Yu
Zhao, Zijian
Zheng, Shenhai
Zheng, Yalin
Zheng, Yinqiang
Zhong, Zichun
Zhou, Bo
Zhou, Jianlong
Zhou, Luping
Zhou, Niyun
Zhou, S.
Zhou, Shoujun
Zhou, Tao
Zhou, Wenjin
Zhou, Yuyin
Zhou, Zhiguo
Zhu, Hancan
Zhu, Junjie
Zhu, Qikui
Zhu, Weifang
Zhu, Wentao
Zhu, Xiaofeng
Zhu, Xinliang
Zhu, Yingying
Zhu, Yuemin
Zhu, Zhuotun
Zhuang, Xiahai
Zia, Aneeq
Zimmer, Veronika
Zolgharni, Massoud
Zou, Ju
Zuluaga, Maria

Accepted MICCAI 2019 Papers

By Region of First Author

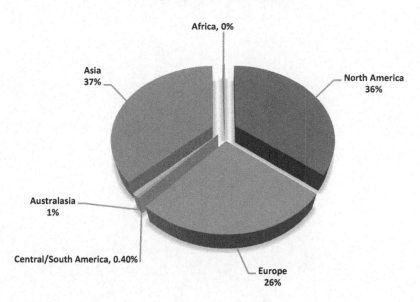

Africa, 0%

Asia
37%

North America
36%

Australasia
1%

Central/South America, 0.40%

Europe
26%

By Technical Keyword

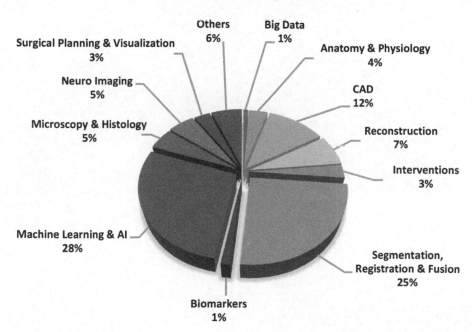

Others
6%

Big Data
1%

Surgical Planning & Visualization
3%

Anatomy & Physiology
4%

Neuro Imaging
5%

CAD
12%

Microscopy & Histology
5%

Reconstruction
7%

Interventions
3%

Machine Learning & AI
28%

Segmentation,
Registration & Fusion
25%

Biomarkers
1%

Awards Presented at MICCAI 2018, Granada, Spain

MICCAI Society Enduring Impact Award: The Enduring Impact Award is the highest award of the MICCAI Society. It is a career award for continued excellence in the MICCAI research field. The 2018 Enduring Impact Award was presented to Sandy Wells, Brigham and Women's Hospital/Harvard Medical School, USA.

MICCAI Society Fellowships: MICCAI Fellowships are bestowed annually on a small number of senior members of the society in recognition of substantial scientific contributions to the MICCAI research field and service to the MICCAI community. In 2018, fellowships were awarded to:

- Pierre Jannin (Université de Rennes, France)
- Anne Martel (University of Toronto, Canada)
- Julia Schnabel (King's College London, UK)

Medical Image Analysis Journal Award Sponsored by Elsevier: Jianyu Lin, for his paper entitled "Dual-modality Endoscopic Probe for Tissue Surface Shape Reconstruction and Hyperspectral Imaging Enabled by Deep Neural Networks," authored by Jianyu Lin, Neil T. Clancy, Ji Qi, Yang Hu, Taran Tatla, Danail Stoyanov, Lena Maier-Hein, and Daniel S. Elson.

Best Paper in *International Journal of Computer-Assisted Radiology and Surgery* (IJCARS) journal: Arash Pourtaherian for his paper entitled "Robust and Semantic Needle Detection in 3D Ultrasound Using Orthogonal-Plane Convolutional Neural Networks," authored by Arash Pourtaherian, Farhad Ghazvinian Zanjani, Svitlana Zinger, Nenad Mihajlovic, Gary C. Ng, Hendrikus H. M. Korsten, and Peter H. N. de With.

Young Scientist Publication Impact Award: MICCAI papers by a young scientist from the past 5 years were eligible for this award. It is made to a researcher whose work had an impact on the MICCAI field in terms of citations, secondary citations, subsequent publications, h-index. The 2018 Young Scientist Publication Impact Award was given to Holger R Roth: "A New 2.5D Representation for Lymph Node Detection Using Random Sets of Deep Convolutional Neural Network Observations" authored by Holger R. Roth, Le Lu, Ari Seff, Kevin M. Cherry, Joanne Hoffman, Shijun Wang, Jiamin Liu, Evrim Turkbey, and Ronald M. Summers.

MICCAI Young Scientist Awards: The Young Scientist Awards are stimulation prizes awarded for the best first authors of MICCAI contributions in distinct subject areas. The nominees had to be full-time students at a recognized university at, or within, two years prior to submission. The 2018 MICCAI Young Scientist Awards were given to:

- Erik J. Bekkers for the paper entitled: "Roto-Translation Covariant Convolutional Networks for Medical Image Analysis"
- Bastian Bier for the paper entitled: "X-ray-transform Invariant Anatomical Landmark Detection for Pelvic Trauma Surgery"

- Yuanhan Mo for his paper entitled: "The Deep Poincaré Map: A Novel Approach for Left Ventricle Segmentation"
- Tanya Nair for the paper entitled: "Exploring Uncertainty Measures in Deep Networks for Multiple Sclerosis Lesion Detection and Segmentation"
- Yue Zhang for the paper entitled: "Task-Driven Generative Modeling for Unsupervised Domain Adaptation: Application to X-ray Image Segmentation"

Contents – Part VI

Computed Tomography

Multi-scale Coarse-to-Fine Segmentation for Screening Pancreatic Ductal Adenocarcinoma

Zhuotun Zhu[1]([envelope]), Yingda Xia[1]([envelope]), Lingxi Xie[1], Elliot K. Fishman[2],
and Alan L. Yuille[1]

[1] The Johns Hopkins University, Baltimore, MD 21218, USA
zhuotun@gmail.com, philyingdaxia@gmail.com, 198808xc@gmail.com,
alan.l.yuille@gmail.com
[2] The Johns Hopkins University School of Medicine, Baltimore, MD 21287, USA
efishman@jhmi.edu

Abstract. We propose an intuitive approach of detecting pancreatic ductal adenocarcinoma (PDAC), the most common type of pancreatic cancer, by checking abdominal CT scans. Our idea is named **multi-scale segmentation-for-classification**, which classifies volumes by checking if at least a sufficient number of voxels is segmented as tumors, by which we can provide radiologists with tumor locations. In order to deal with tumors with different scales, we train and test our volumetric segmentation networks with multi-scale inputs in a coarse-to-fine flowchart. A post-processing module is used to filter out outliers and reduce false alarms. We collect a new dataset containing 439 CT scans, in which 136 cases were diagnosed with PDAC and 303 cases are normal, which is the largest set for PDAC tumors to the best of our knowledge. To offer the best trade-off between sensitivity and specificity, our proposed framework reports a sensitivity of 94.1% at a specificity of 98.5%, which demonstrates the potential to make a clinical impact.

Keywords: PDAC · Pancreas segmentation · CT scan

1 Introduction

Pancreatic cancer is one of the most dangerous killers to human lives, causing more than 330,000 deaths globally in 2014 [11]. Pancreatic ductal adenocarcinoma (PDAC) is the most common type of pancreatic cancer, accounting for about 85% of cancer cases. In early stages, this disease often has few symptoms and is very difficult to discover. By the time of diagnosis, the cancer has often spread to other parts of the body, leading to a very poor prognosis (*e.g.*, a five-year survival rate of 5% [11]). But, for cases diagnosed early, the survival rate rises to about 20% [7]. Hence, it is very important to study the possibility of detecting PDAC in common examinations, *e.g.*, the abdominal CT scan.

Z. Zhu and Y. Xia—Equally contributed to the work.

© Springer Nature Switzerland AG 2019
D. Shen et al. (Eds.): MICCAI 2019, LNCS 11769, pp. 3–12, 2019.
https://doi.org/10.1007/978-3-030-32226-7_1

4   Z. Zhu et al.

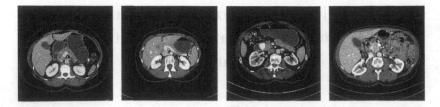

Fig. 1. Examples of normal and abnormal (PDAC) pancreases (best viewed in color). Blue and red region mark the normal pancreas and tumor regions, respectively. (Color figure online)

The early diagnosis of pancreatic cancer requires much expertise in reading the scanned images and making decisions, but the increasing number of cases makes it impossible for a limited number of experienced radiologists to check all CT scans manually. Therefore, an artificial intelligence system for this purpose is in need. In particular, the radiologists in our team are interested in a system working on abdominal CT scans, which filters out a large fraction of normal cases, but preserves almost all abnormal cases for further investigation. To the best of our knowledge, there is no existing work on this task.

With the development of deep learning [5], it is possible to construct a system which learns from professional knowledge in data annotation, and apply it to helping doctors in various clinical purposes. The pancreas is one of the most challenging organs in CT segmentation [9]. The difficulty mainly lies in its irregular shape and low contrast around the boundary. Powered by the recent progress in deep learning for 2D [1,8] and 3D [6,12] image segmentation, researchers designed various approaches [10,15] towards accurate pancreas segmentation. In the pathological cases, the morphology of the pancreas can be largely impacted by the difference in the pancreatic cancer stage [13,14].

Our work is aimed to detect PDAC from a mixture of normal and abnormal CT scans. This is not a simple classification since radiologists also want to know the location of PDAC, we suggest a solution named **segmentation-for-classification**, which trains segmentation models and uses their outputs for classification. To deal with tumors of various sizes (Fig. 1), we adopt a segmentation network with multiple input scales, *i.e.*, 64^3, 32^3 and 16^3 volumes. But, voting that small input regions lead to a high false alarm rate, we adopt a **coarse-to-fine** testing strategy, which uses the 64^3 network for a coarse scan, and then the 32^3&16^3 networks inside the bounding box to detect small tumors that are possibly ignored in the previous stage. A non-parameterized post-processing algorithm is designed to remove outliers.

Our contributions are three folds: (1) we voxelwisely annotate an abdominal CT dataset with 439 cases in total, in which 136 cases are diagnosed with PDAC while the remaining 303 cases are normal, which is currently the largest PDAC dataset to the best of our knowledge; (2) we adopt a **multi-scale segmentation-for-classification** framework to conduct an **interpretable** abnormality detection, which provides radiologists with suspicious regions for further diagnosis; (3) our framework achieves a sensitivity of 94.1% at a specificity of 98.5%, which shows a promising direction to make a potential significant clinical impact.

2 The Segmentation-for-Classification Approach

2.1 The Overall Framework

Let a dataset be $\mathbf{S} = \{(\mathbf{X}_1, y_1^\star), \ldots, (\mathbf{X}_N, y_N^\star)\}$, where N is the number of CT scans, $\mathbf{X}_n \in \mathbb{R}^{W_n \times H_n \times L_n}$ is the 3D volume with each element indicating the Hounsfield unit (HU) of a voxel, and $y_n \in \{0, 1\}$ is the label (0 for a normal case, 1 for an abnormal case). Throughout this paper, by *abnormal* we refer to the cases diagnosed as PDAC. The goal is to design a model $\mathbb{M} : y = f(\mathbf{X})$ to predict the label for each testing volume. We evaluate our approach by ranking all volumes by the probability of being a PDAC, computing the sensitivity and specificity at a given threshold, and plotting the ROC curve indicating the relationship between the sensitivity and specificity at different thresholds. For clinical purposes, we shall guarantee a high sensitivity with a reasonable specificity.

Although some previous work suggested to classify CT or MRI volumes directly using 3D networks [3,4], we argue that a better solution is to perform tumor segmentation at the same time of classification. This makes the classification results **interpretable** by segmentation cues, by which radiologists can take a further investigation of the suspicious abnormal regions. In addition, this integrates voxel-wise annotations into the classification model as deep supervision, so that the entire network is better trained [14]. Therefore, we propose a two-stage framework named *segmentation-for-classification*, in which a segmentation stage first extracts voxel-wise cues from the input CT scan, and a classification stage follows to summarize this information into the final prediction. Our multi-scale segmentation strategy is different from [15], which applied another network of the same scale in the fine stage. **Tumor detection requires multiple scales.**

Mathematically, let each training data be augmented by a segmentation mask $\mathbf{M}_n^\star$ of the same dimensionality as $\mathbf{X}$, so that $m_{n,i}^\star \in \{0, 1, 2\}$ indicates the category of the i-th voxel, *i.e.*, in the tumor ($m_{n,i} = 2$), outside the tumor but inside the pancreas ($m_{n,i} = 1$), or outside the pancreas ($m_{n,i} = 0$). Note that the tumor voxel set is a subset of the pancreas voxel set. The segmentation module is a high-dimensional function $\mathbf{M} = \mathbf{s}(\mathbf{X})$, which is implemented by a deep encoder-decoder network. The classification module is a binary function $y = c(\mathbf{M})$. The overall framework is thus written as:

$$y = f(\mathbf{X}) = c \circ \mathbf{s}(\mathbf{X}). \tag{1}$$

2.2 Training: Multi-scale Deeply-Supervised Segmentation

We start with describing the segmentation stage. The tumor region in a pancreas, as shown in Fig. 1, can vary in scale, appearance and geometric properties.

In particular, the largest tumor in our dataset occupies over one million voxels, but the smallest one has only thousands. This motivates us to train multi-scale networks to deal with such a large variation in scale.

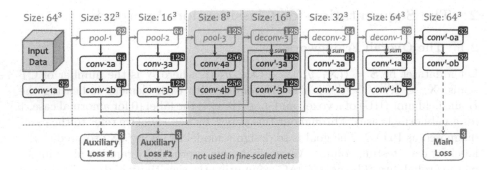

Fig. 2. The architecture of our segmentation backbone (best viewed in color). Each rectangle is a layer, green arrows indicate operations changing spatial resolution, and red arrows mean residual connections. We illustrate the situation when the input volume size is 64^3. If it is 32^3 or 16^3, all volumes are shrunk accordingly (to $1/2^3$ or $1/4^3$ of the displayed size). The number at the upper-right corner of each cube is the number of channels. Each convolution uses $3 \times 3 \times 3$ kernels with 1 as stride, each pooling $2 \times 2 \times 2$ with 2 as stride, and each deconvolution $4 \times 4 \times 4$ with 2 as stride. The weight ratio for auxiliary losses #1, #2 and main loss is $1 : 2 : 5$ for the 64^3 network, and $1 : 3$ for the auxiliary loss #1 and the main loss for the 32^3 and 16^3 networks. (Color figure online)

In practice, we train three networks, taking input volumes of 64^3, 32^3 and 16^3 voxels, respectively. Each segmentation network follows an encoder-decoder flowchart shown in Fig. 2. It has a series of convolutional layers to learn 3D patterns from training data. Down-sampling and up-sampling are implemented by max pooling and deconvolutional layers, respectively. Following [15], we introduce deep supervision in the training process, which is implemented by adding several auxiliary losses to intermediate layers, which delivers better performance for the normal and cystic pancreas segmentation in [15]. Deep supervision is considered as a way of incorporating multi-stage visual cues, which constrains intermediate layers and improves the stability of training deep networks. Multi-scale segmentation is complementary to deep supervision, which aims at capturing visual patterns of various scales. As can be seen in experiments, multi-scale segmentation can take advantage of different scales, *i.e.*, a large network produces a high specificity, and a small network gives a high sensitivity.

The training process starts with sampling patches of a specified size. Since the pancreas and the tumor only occupy a small fraction of the entire volume, a random sampling strategy may lead to that only few patches contain pancreas or tumor voxels, and thus the segmentation models are biased towards the background class. To deal with the issue, we sample lots of foreground patches for training the 32^3 and 16^3 networks. We first compute the region-of-interest (ROI) by padding a 32-voxel margin around the minimal 3D bounding box covering the entire pancreas. Within it, we categorize the randomly sampled patches into three types (*i.e.*, *background*, *tumor* and *pancreas*) according to the fraction of pancreas and tumor voxels, and make the numbers of training patches of these types o be approximately the same. Data augmentation is performed by randomly flipping patches and rotating by 90°, 180° and 270° over three axes.

We use the same configuration for training these networks. The base learning rate is 0.01 and decayed polynomially (the power is 0.9) in a total of 80,000 iterations (the mini-batch size is 16, 32 and 128 for 64^3, 32^3 and 16^3, respectively). The weight decay and momentum are set to be 0.0005 and 0.9, respectively.

2.3 Testing: Coarse-to-Fine Segmentation with Post-processing

The first goal is to perform the pancreas and tumor segmentation. We first slide a 64^3 window in the entire CT volume. The spatial stride is 20 along three axes, which is chosen to have the average testing time for each case within 11 min on a TITAN Xp GPU. Based on the *coarse* segmentation, we compute the ROI, *i.e.*, the smallest box covering all pancreas and tumor voxels padded by 32, and crop the CT image accordingly. Then, we scan the ROI with sliding windows of 32^3 and 16^3 voxels, and the strides are set to be 10 and 5, respectively. We do not run the two small networks on the entire volume because it can easily hallucinate tumors in the background regions. In addition, shrinking the scanning region for the 32^3 and 16^3 networks leads to a significant speedup in the testing process. The predictions of three networks are averaged into final segmentation.

Then, based on the segmentation mask, we classify each volume as normal or abnormal. Advised by the radiologists who desire the classification result to be explainable, we do not formulate the classifier $c(\cdot)$ as another deep network, but use a simple, non-parametrized approach to filter out the outliers. We construct a graph on all voxels predicted as *normal pancreas* or *tumor*. Each voxel is a node, and there exists an edge between the adjacent voxels (each voxel is adjacent to 6 neighbors). We compute all connected component in the graph. A component is preserved if it is larger than 20% of the maximal connected component, otherwise it is removed, *i.e.*, all voxels within this component are predicted as *background*. To obtain our final goal, a volume is predicted as PDAC if at least K voxels are predicted as tumor. In practice, we empirically set $K = 50$.

3   Experiments

3.1   Dataset and Settings

We collected a dataset with 303 normal cases from potential renal donors, as well as 136 biopsy-proven PDAC cases. Four experts in abdominal anatomy annotated the pancreas and tumor voxels on these data using the Varian Velocity software, and each case was checked by an experienced board-certified Abdominal Radiologist. For a radiologist, an average normal case took 20 min, and an

8   Z. Zhu et al.

average abnormal case 40 min to segment. Since the abnormal cases are much harder to obtain and annotate than the normal cases, we adopt a 4-fold cross-validation on our 136 PDAC scans to have testing results on every abnormal case while we use a hard split of training and testing on our 303 normal cases. All in all, each training set contains 103 normal and 102 abnormal cases where the normal-to-abnormal ratio is close to 1, and each testing set contains 34 abnormal and 200 normal cases. The average size of CT scans is $512 \times 512 \times 667$.

Table 1. Comparison of segmentation and classification results by networks of different scales and their combination. From left to right: normal/abnormal pancreas and tumor segmentation accuracy (DSC, %), the number of missing tumors (*i.e.*, DSC is 0%), and the sensitivity (= 1 − miss rate) and specificity.

Scale	N. Pancreas	A. Pancreas	Tumor	Misses	Sensitivity	Specificity
64^3	**86.9 ± 8.6%**	**81.0 ± 10.8%**	**57.3 ± 28.1%**	10/136	92.7%	**99.0%**
32^3	82.0 ± 12.2%	75.7 ± 14.9%	53.8 ± 26.1%	7/136	94.9%	96.0%
16^3	61.5 ± 20.6%	64.1 ± 20.2%	42.5 ± 25.6%	4/136	**97.1%**	86.5%
Multi	84.5 ± 11.1%	78.6 ± 13.3%	56.5 ± 27.2%	8/136	94.1%	98.5%

One goal is to measure the segmentation accuracy by the Dice-Sørensen Coefficient (DSC) between the predicted and the ground-truth tumor sets $\mathcal{Y}$ and $\mathcal{Y}^*$, *i.e.*, DSC $(\mathcal{Y}, \mathcal{Y}^*) = 2 \times |\mathcal{Y} \cap \mathcal{Y}^*|/(|\mathcal{Y}| + |\mathcal{Y}^*|)$. Our main goal is the tumor classification, which involves a tradeoff between sensitivity and specificity.

3.2   Segmentation Results

We first summarize the segmentation results in Table 1, which makes the normal v.s. abnormal classification to be interpretable by segmentation cues. The 64^3 network achieves reasonable pancreas and tumor segmentation accuracies. The segmentation result of normal pancreas is as high as 86.9%, which means that the normal pancreases are easier to segment, as there are often unpredicted changes in shape and geometry in the abnormal cases. As a side comment, the lowest DSC of an abnormal pancreas is 38.4%, lower than the number (44.0%) of a normal pancreas. In tumor segmentation, we observe a lower accuracy and a higher standard deviation (57.3 ± 28.1%). Except for the 10 missing cases, we find 20 more cases with a tumor DSC lower than 30%. All these evidences imply the challenging of finding tumors considering their various size, shape and locations. Note that a recent work on the pancreatic cyst segmentation achieves a DSC of 63.4 ± 27.7% [14], which is not as hard as the tumor segmentation.

Going to smaller scales, fewer tumors are missed, though segmentation accuracies become lower. This is the tradeoff between sensitivity and specificity: a network with a smaller input region has the ability to detect tiny regions, but without seeing contexts, it can be easily confused by false positives. Thus, combining multi-scale predictions achieves a balance between sensitivity and specificity. Figure 3 shows two examples that benefit from multi-scale segmentation.

We replace our backbone with 3D UNet [2] and VNet [6] at the 64^3 scale setting and report their results in Table 2 for comparison. We can find that the three backbones perform roughly similar in terms of the segmentation results. However, our backbone achieves the best results for the sensitivity and specificity.

Table 2. Comparison of different networks as backbone at the 64^3 setting.

Scale	N. Pancreas	A. Pancreas	Tumor	Misses	Sensitivity	Specificity
Ours	$86.9 \pm 8.6\%$	$81.0 \pm 10.8\%$	$57.3 \pm 28.1\%$	**10/136**	**92.7%**	**99.0%**
UNet	**$87.0 \pm 8.4\%$**	**$81.6 \pm 10.2\%$**	$57.6 \pm 27.8\%$	11/136	91.9%	99.0%
VNet	$86.7 \pm 8.8\%$	$80.6 \pm 11.4\%$	**$58.7 \pm 28.0\%$**	10/136	92.7%	98.0%

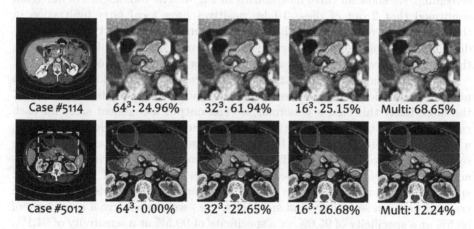

Case #5114 64^3: 24.96% 32^3: 61.94% 16^3: 25.15%   Multi: 68.65%

Case #5012 64^3: 0.00% 32^3: 22.65% 16^3: 26.68%   Multi: 12.24%

Fig. 3. Multi-scale segmentation examples (best viewed in color). Top: a case that all three scales work well, and multi-scale combines them to achieve a higher DSC. Bottom: a failure case in the 64^3 network, but found by the 32^3 and 16^3 networks. The yellow frames indicate the zoomed-in regions, the blue and red contours mark the annotated pancreas and tumor respectively, and the masked regions mark segmentation results. (Color figure online)

3.3 Classification Results

Finally, we summarize classification results in Table 1, which is the crucial goal of making earlier diagnosis possible for doctors. Radiologists care more about a high sensitivity since they don't want to miss a patient who has an abnormal pancreas, which inspires us to adopt a multi-scale strategy to improve the sensitivity while keeping a reasonable specificity. The model with multi-scale information achieves the best overall performance, *i.e.*, a sensitivity of 94.1% at a specificity of 98.5%.

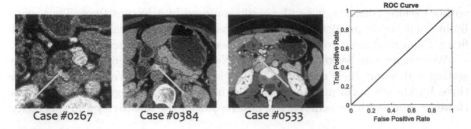

Fig. 4. Left: three false alarm examples, in which the blue contour marks the annotated pancreas, and the blue and red regions mark the predicted pancreas and tumor,
respectively. We use yellow arrows to indicate the detected tiny "tumors". Right: the
ROC curve of multi-scale classification. This figure is best viewed in color. (Color figure
online)

These high scores imply that tumor segmentation provide strong cues for PDAC
screening. We show all three false alarms in Fig. 4. The radiologists of our team
confirmed that 2 out of these 3 false positives have focal fatty infiltration in
the pancreas corresponding to the detected "tumors". Focal fatty infiltration is
difficult for radiologists to distinguish from tumor in current clinical practice. In
this case, the predicted "false alarm" was not normal in view of our radiologists.

By augmenting our segmentation for classification framework with cues from
number of predicted tumor voxels since the more voxels predicted as PDAC
the more likely this case is abnormal, we can output a confident score for each
case, indicating the possibility that this case suffers PDAC. More specifically,
a confidence score is computed by a weighted sum of the volume size and the
segmentation probability of predicted tumor voxels. By sorting all testing cases
according to their confident scores, we obtain a ROC curve of sensitivity and
specificity. From the ROC curve, we can make different emphasis to change the
tradeoff between sensitivity and specificity, *e.g.*, we can achieve a sensitivity of
98.5% at a specificity of 95.6%, or a specificity of 99.5% at a sensitivity of 94.1%.

4   Conclusion

In this paper, we study an important and challenging task, *i.e.*, detecting pancreases diagnosed with PDAC in abdominal CT scans. This topic is crucial in
saving lives from pancreatic cancer yet few studied before, possibly due to the
lack of data. We propose a **segmentation-for-classification** framework which
trains a segmentation network and performs **interpretable** abnormality classification by simply checking the existence of tumor voxels in each testing volume.
There are two key points to improve classification accuracy, known as **multi-
scale** network training and **coarse-to-fine** testing. To offer a best trade-off
between sensitivity and specificity on our own collected dataset containing 303
normal and 136 PDAC cases, we achieve a sensitivity of 94.1% at a specificity of
98.5%. The strong numbers show the promising direction to make a significant
impact in clinics for early detection of pancreatic cancer, which would save lives.

Acknowledgements. This work was supported by the Lustgarten Foundation for Pancreatic Cancer Research.

References

1. Chen, L.C., Papandreou, G., Kokkinos, I., Murphy, K., Yuille, A.L.: Deeplab: semantic image segmentation with deep convolutional nets, atrous convolution, and fully connected CRFs. In: ICLR (2016)
2. Çiçek, Ö., Abdulkadir, A., Lienkamp, S.S., Brox, T., Ronneberger, O.: 3D U-net: learning dense volumetric segmentation from sparse annotation. In: Ourselin, S., Joskowicz, L., Sabuncu, M.R., Unal, G., Wells, W. (eds.) MICCAI 2016. LNCS, vol. 9901, pp. 424–432. Springer, Cham (2016). https://doi.org/10.1007/978-3-319-46723-8_49
3. Dou, Q., Chen, H., Yu, L., Qin, J., Heng, P.A.: Multilevel contextual 3-D CNNs for false positive reduction in pulmonary nodule detection. IEEE TBE **64**, 1558–1567 (2017)
4. Hussein, S., Chuquicusma, M.M., Kandel, P., Bolan, C.W., Wallace, M.B., Bagci, U.: Supervised and unsupervised tumor characterization in the deep learning era. arXiv:1801.03230 (2018)
5. Krizhevsky, A., Sutskever, I., Hinton, G.E.: Imagenet classification with deep convolutional neural networks. In: NIPS (2012)
6. Milletari, F., Navab, N., Ahmadi, S.A.: V-net: fully convolutional neural networks for volumetric medical image segmentation. In: 3DV (2016)
7. PDQ Adult Treatment Editorial Board: Pancreatic cancer treatment (PDQ®)
8. Ronneberger, O., Fischer, P., Brox, T.: U-net: convolutional networks for biomedical image segmentation. In: Navab, N., Hornegger, J., Wells, W.M., Frangi, A.F. (eds.) MICCAI 2015. LNCS, vol. 9351, pp. 234–241. Springer, Cham (2015). https://doi.org/10.1007/978-3-319-24574-4_28
9. Roth, H.R., et al.: DeepOrgan: multi-level deep convolutional networks for automated pancreas segmentation. In: Navab, N., Hornegger, J., Wells, W.M., Frangi, A.F. (eds.) MICCAI 2015. LNCS, vol. 9349, pp. 556–564. Springer, Cham (2015). https://doi.org/10.1007/978-3-319-24553-9_68
10. Roth, H.R., Lu, L., Farag, A., Sohn, A., Summers, R.M.: Spatial aggregation of holistically-nested networks for automated pancreas segmentation. In: Ourselin, S., Joskowicz, L., Sabuncu, M.R., Unal, G., Wells, W. (eds.) MICCAI 2016. LNCS, vol. 9901, pp. 451–459. Springer, Cham (2016). https://doi.org/10.1007/978-3-319-46723-8_52
11. Stewart, B.W.K.P., Wild, C.P., et al.: World cancer report 2014. Health (2017)
12. Xia, Y., Xie, L., Liu, F., Zhu, Z., Fishman, E.K., Yuille, A.L.: Bridging the gap between 2D and 3D organ segmentation with volumetric fusion net. In: Frangi, A.F., Schnabel, J.A., Davatzikos, C., Alberola-López, C., Fichtinger, G. (eds.) MICCAI 2018. LNCS, vol. 11073, pp. 445–453. Springer, Cham (2018). https://doi.org/10.1007/978-3-030-00937-3_51
13. Zhang, L., Lu, L., Summers, R.M., Kebebew, E., Yao, J.: Personalized pancreatic tumor growth prediction via group learning. In: Descoteaux, M., Maier-Hein, L., Franz, A., Jannin, P., Collins, D.L., Duchesne, S. (eds.) MICCAI 2017. LNCS, vol. 10434, pp. 424–432. Springer, Cham (2017). https://doi.org/10.1007/978-3-319-66185-8_48

14. Zhou, Y., Xie, L., Fishman, E.K., Yuille, A.L.: Deep supervision for pancreatic cyst segmentation in abdominal CT scans. In: Descoteaux, M., Maier-Hein, L., Franz, A., Jannin, P., Collins, D.L., Duchesne, S. (eds.) MICCAI 2017. LNCS, vol. 10435, pp. 222–230. Springer, Cham (2017). https://doi.org/10.1007/978-3-319-66179-7_26
15. Zhu, Z., Xia, Y., Shen, W., Fishman, E.K., Yuille, A.L.: A 3D coarse-to-fine framework for volumetric medical image segmentation. In: 3DV (2018)

MVP-Net: Multi-view FPN with Position-Aware Attention for Deep Universal Lesion Detection

Zihao Li[1,2], Shu Zhang[3], Junge Zhang[1], Kaiqi Huang[1], Yizhou Wang[2,3,4], and Yizhou Yu[2(✉)]

[1] Institute of Automation, Chinese Academy of Sciences, Beijing, China
[2] Deepwise AI Lab, Beijing, China
yuyizhou@deepwise.com
[3] Department of Computer Science, Peking University, Haidian District, China
[4] Peng Cheng Laboratory, Shenzhen, China

Abstract. Universal lesion detection (ULD) on computed tomography (CT) images is an important but underdeveloped problem. Recently, deep learning-based approaches have been proposed for ULD, aiming to learn representative features from annotated CT data. However, the hunger for data of deep learning models and the scarcity of medical annotation hinders these approaches to advance further. In this paper, we propose to incorporate domain knowledge in clinical practice into the model design of universal lesion detectors. Specifically, as radiologists tend to inspect multiple windows for an accurate diagnosis, we explicitly model this process and propose a multi-view feature pyramid network (FPN), where multi-view features are extracted from images rendered with varied window widths and window levels; to effectively combine this multi-view information, we further propose a position-aware attention module. With the proposed model design, the data-hunger problem is relieved as the learning task is made easier with the correctly induced clinical practice prior. We show promising results with the proposed model, achieving an absolute gain of **5.65%** (in the sensitivity of FPs@4.0) over the previous state-of-the-art on the NIH DeepLesion dataset.

Keywords: Universal lesion detection · Multi-view · Position-aware · Attention

1 Introduction

Automated detection of lesions from computed tomography (CT) scans can significantly boost the accuracy and efficiency of clinical diagnosis and disease screening. However, existing computer aided diagnosis (CAD) systems usually focus on certain types of lesions, e.g. lung nodules [1], focal liver lesions [2], thus

---

Z. Li and S. Zhang—Equal contribution. This work is done when Zihao Li is an intern at Deepwise AI Lab.

© Springer Nature Switzerland AG 2019
D. Shen et al. (Eds.): MICCAI 2019, LNCS 11769, pp. 13–21, 2019.
https://doi.org/10.1007/978-3-030-32226-7_2

their clinical usage is limited. Therefore, a Universal Lesion Detector which can identify and localize different types of lesions across the whole body all at once is in urgent need.

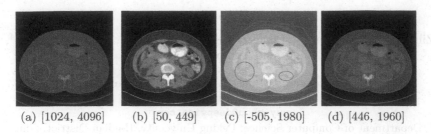

(a) [1024, 4096]   (b) [50, 449]   (c) [-505, 1980]   (d) [446, 1960]

Fig. 1. CT images under different window level and window width. (a) is the image used in 3DCE. (b), (c), (d) are the multi-view images used in our MVP-Net.

Previous methods for ULD are largely inspired by the successful deep models in the field of natural images. For instance, Tang *et al.* [5] adapted a Mask-RCNN [3] based approach to exploit the auxiliary supervision from manually generated pseudo mask. On the other hand, Yan *et al.* proposed a 3D Context Enhanced (3DCE) RCNN model [6] which harness ImageNet pre-trained models for 3D context modeling. Due to a certain degree of resemblance between natural images and CT images, these advanced deep architectures also demonstrated impressive results on ULD.

Nonetheless, the intrinsic quality of medical images should not be overlooked. Beyond that, the inspection of medical images also exhibits different characteristics compared with recognition and detection of natural images. Therefore, it would be helpful if we can efficiently exploit proper domain knowledge to develop deep learning based diagnosis systems. We will try to analyze two aspects of such domain knowledge, and explore how to formulate these human expertise into a unified deep learning framework.

To accommodate for network input, previous studies [5,6] use a significantly wide window[1] to compress CT's 12bit Hounsfield Unit (HU). However, this would severely deteriorate the visibility of lesions as a result of degenerated image contrast, as shown in Fig. 1(a). In the clinical practice, fusing information from multiple windows are effective in improving the accuracy of detecting subtle lesions and reducing false positives (FPs). During visual inspection of the CT images, radiologists would combine complex information of different inner structures and tissues from multiple reconstructions under different window widths and window levels to locate possible lesions. To imitate this process, we propose to extract prominent features from three frequently examined window widths and window levels and capture complementary information across different windows with an attention based feature aggregation module.

---

[1] Windowing, also known as gray-level mapping, is used to change the appearance of the picture to highlight particular structures.

During the inspection of whole body CT, body position of a slice (i.e. the z-axis position of a certain slice), is also a frequently consulted prior knowledge. Experienced specialists often rely on the underlying correspondence between body position and lesion types to conduct lesion diagnosis. Moreover, radiologists would use the position cue as an indicator for choosing proper window width and window level. For instance, radiologists will mainly refer to the lung, bone and mediastinal window when inspecting a chest CT. Therefore, it would be very beneficial if we can exploit the position information to conduct lesion diagnosis and window selection in designing our deep detector.

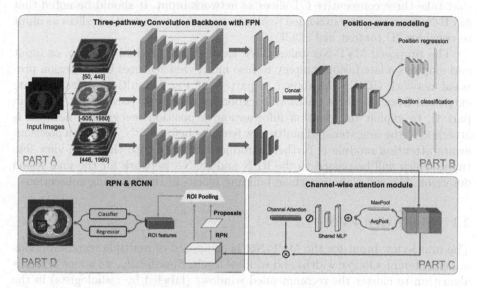

Fig. 2. Overview of our proposed MVP-Net. Coarser feature maps of FPN are omitted in part C and D for clarity, they use the same attention module with shared parameters for feature aggregation.

In order to model the aforementioned domain knowledge and human expertise, we develop a MVP-Net (Multi-View FPN with Position-aware attention) for universal lesion detection. FPN [4] is used as a building block to improve detection performance for small lesions. To leverage information from multiple window reconstructions, we build a multi-view FPN to extract multi-view[2] features using a three-pathway architecture. Then, an channel-wise attention module is employed to capture complementary information across different views. To further consider the position cues, we develop a multi-task learning scheme to embed the position information onto the appearance features. Thus, we can explicitly condition the lesion finding problem on the entangled appearance and position features. Moreover, by connecting the proposed attention module to

---

[2] As a common practice in machine learning, we refer to reconstruction under a certain window width and window level as a view of that CT.

such an entangled feature, we are able to conduct position-aware feature aggregations. Extensive experiments on the DeepLesion Dataset validate the effectiveness of our proposed MVP-Net. We can achieve an absolute gain of **5.65%** over the previous state-of-the-arts (3DCE with 27 slices) while considering 3D context from only 9 slices.

2   Methodology

Figure 2 gives an overview of the MVP-Net. For simplicity, we illustrate the case that take three consecutive CT slices as network input. It should be noted that MVP-Net can be easily extended to alternatives that take multiple slices as input to consider 3D context like 3DCE [6].

The proposed MVP-Net takes three views of the original CT scan as input and employs a late fusion strategy to fuse multi-view features before region proposal network (RPN). As shown in part A of Fig. 2, multi-view features are extracted from the three pathway backbone with shared parameters. Then, in part B, to exploit the position information, a position recognition network is attached to the concatenated multi-view features before RPN. Finally, a position-aware attention module is further introduced to aggregate the multi-view features, which will be passed to the RPN and RCNN network for the final lesion detection. We will elaborate these building blocks in the following subsections.

2.1   Multi-view FPN

The multi-view input for the MVP-Net is composed of multiple reconstructions under different window widths and window levels. Specifically, we adopt k-means algorithm to cluster the recommended windows (labeled by radiologists) in the DeepLesion dataset and obtain three most frequently inspected windows, whose window levels and window widths are $[50, 449]$, $[-505, 1980]$ and $[446, 1960]$ respectively. As shown in Fig. 1, these clustered windows approximately correspond to the soft-tissue window, lung window, and the union of bone, brain, and mediastinal windows respectively.

As shown in Fig. 2, we adopt a three pathway architecture to extract the most prominent features from each representative view. FPN [4] is used as the backbone network of each pathway. It takes in three consecutive slices as input to model 3D context.

2.2   Attention Based Feature Aggregation

Features extracted from different views (windows) need to be properly aggregated for accurate diagnosis. A naive implementation for feature aggregation could be concatenating them along the channel dimension. However, such an implementation would have to rely on the following convolution layers for effective feature fusion.

In the proposed MVP-Net, we employ a channel-wise attention based feature aggregation mechanism to adaptively reweight the feature maps of different views, imitating the process that radiologists put different weights on multiple windows for lesion identification. We adopt an implementation similar to the Convolutional Block Attention Module (CBAM) [9] to realize the channel-wise attention. Details for the attention module is shown in Fig. 2. Denoting F as input feature map, we firstly aggregate the features with average pooling P_{avg} and max pooling P_{max} separately to extract representative descriptions, then a fully-connected bottleneck module $\theta(\cdot)$ and a sigmoid layer $\sigma(\cdot)$ are sequentially applied to the aggregated features to generate combinational weights of different channels. Multiplying F by the weights, the output F_c of the feature aggregation module is can be described as Eq. 1:

$$F_c = F \cdot \sigma(\theta(P_{avg}(F) + P_{max}(F))). \tag{1}$$

2.3 Position-Aware Modeling

Due to FPN's large receptive field, the position information in the xy plane (or context information) has already been inherently modeled. Therefore, we mainly focus on the modeling of the position information along the z-axis. Specifically, we propose to learn position-aware appearance features by introducing a position prediction task during training. Entangled position and appearance features are learned through the multi-task design in the MVP-Net that jointly predicts the position and the detection bounding box.

$$\mathcal{L}_{\text{pos}} = -\frac{1}{n} \sum_i^n y_i \log \phi(x_i) + \frac{1}{n} \sum_i^n (p_i - \psi(x_i))^2 \tag{2}$$

As shown in Fig. 2, our position prediction module is supervised by two losses: a regression loss and a classification loss. The regression loss is applied after the continuous position regressor, whose learning target are generated by a self-supervised body-part regressor [8] in the DeepLesion Dataset[7]. Due to noise in the continuous labels, we further divide position values into three classes (chest, abdomen, and pelvis) according to the distribution of the position values on the z-axis, and use a classification loss to learn this discrete position, as it is more robust to noise and improves training stability.

Let y, p denote the ground-truth of discrete and continuous position values, given the bottleneck feature x of FPN, we use two subnets $\phi(\cdot)$, $\psi(\cdot)$ of several CNN layers to obtain the corresponding predictions. The overall loss function of the position module is described in Eq. 2.

3 Experiments

3.1 Experimental Setup

Dataset and Metric. The NIH DeepLesion [7] is a large-scale CT dataset, consisting of 32,735 lesion instances on 32,120 axial CT slices. Algorithm evaluation is conducted on the official testing set (15%), and we report sensitivity at various FPs per image levels as the evaluation metric. For simplicity, we mainly compare the sensitivity at 4 FPs per image in the text of the following subsections.

Table 1. Sensitivity (%) at various FPs per image on the testing set of DeepLesion. We don't provide results with 27 slices due to memory limitation. * indicates re-implementation of 3DCE with FPN as backbone.

FPs per image	0.5	1	2	3	4
ULDOR [5]	52.86	64.80	74.84	-	84.38
3DCE, 3 slices [6]	55.70	67.26	75.37	-	82.21
3DCE, 9 slices [6]	59.32	70.68	79.09	-	84.34
3DCE, 27 slices [6]	62.48	73.37	80.70	-	85.65
FPN+3DCE, 3 slices*	58.06	68.85	77.48	81.03	83.27
FPN+3DCE, 9 slices*	64.25	74.41	81.90	85.02	87.21
FPN+3DCE, 27 slices*	67.32	76.34	82.90	85.67	87.60
Ours, 3 slices	**70.01**	**78.77**	**84.71**	**87.58**	**89.03**
Ours, 9 slices	**73.83**	**81.82**	**87.60**	**89.57**	**91.30**
Imp over 3DCE, 27slices [6]	↑ **11.35**	↑8.45	↑6.90	-	↑5.65

Baselines. We compare our proposed MVP-Net with two state-of-the-art methods, i.e. 3DCE [6] and ULDOR [5]. ULDOR adopts Mask-RCNN for improved detection performance, while 3DCE exploits 3D context to obtain superior lesion detection results. Previous best results are achieved by 3DCE when using 27 slices to model the 3D context.

Implementation Details. We use FPN with ResNet-50 for all experiments. Parameters of the backbone are initialized from the ImageNet pre-trained models, and all other layers are randomly initialized. Anchor scales in FPN are set to (16, 32, 64, 128, 256). We normalize the CT slices in the z-axis to a slice interval of 2 mm, and then resize them to 800 pixels in the xy-plane for both training and testing. We augment training data with horizontal flip, and no other data augmentation strategies are employed. The models are trained using stochastic gradient descent for 13 epochs. The base learning rate is 0.002, and it is reduced by a factor of 10 after the 10-th and 12-th epoch.

3.2   Comparison with State-of-the-Arts

The comparison between our proposed model and the previous state-of-the-art methods are shown in Table 1. As the original implementation of 3DCE is based on the R-FCN [10], we re-implement 3DCE with the FPN backbone for fair comparison. The result show that with FPN as backbone, the 3DCE model achieves a performance boost of over 2% compared to the RFCN based model. This validates the effectiveness of our choice of using FPN as the base network.

More importantly, even using far less 3D context, our model with 3 slices for context modeling has already achieved SOTA detection results, outperforming 27-slices based RFCN and FPN 3DCE models by 3.38% and 1.43% respectively. When compared with 3-slices based counterpart, our model shows a superior performance gain of 6.82% and 5.76%. This demonstrates the effectiveness of the proposed multi-view learning strategy as well as the position-aware attention module. Finally, by incorporating more 3D context, our model with 9 slices get a further performance boost and surpasses the previous SOTA by a large margin (**5.65%** for FPs@4.0 and **11.35%** for FPs@0.5).

3.3 Ablation Study

Table 2. Ablation study of our approach on the DeepLesion dataset.

FPN	Multi-view	Attention	Position	9 slices	FPs@2.0	FPs@4.0
✓					77.48	83.27
✓	✓				81.29	86.18
✓	✓	✓			84.18	87.89
✓	✓	✓	✓		84.71	89.03
✓	✓	✓	✓	✓	**87.60**	**91.30**

We perform ablation study on four major components: multi-view modeling, attention based feature aggregation, position-aware modeling, and 3D context enhanced modeling. As shown in Table 2, using simple feature concatenation for feature aggregation, the multi-view FPN obtains a 2.91% improvement over the FPN baseline. Further modifying the aggregation strategy to channel-wise attention accounts for another 1.71% improvement. Then learning the entangled position and appearance features with position-aware modeling further brings 1.14% boost on the sensitivity. Combining our proposed approach with 3D context modeling gives the best performance.

We also perform a case study to analyze the importance of multi-view modeling. As shown in Fig. 3, the model indeed benefits from the multi-view modeling: the lesions that are originally indistinguishable in the view of 3DCE due to the wide window range and lack of contrast, now becomes distinguishable under the view of appropriate windows. Thus our model presents better identification and localization performance.

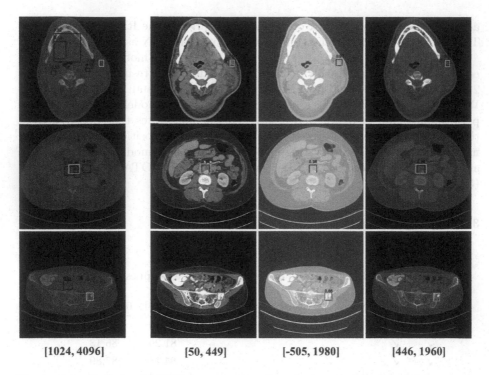

| [1024, 4096] | [50, 449] | [-505, 1980] | [446, 1960] |

Fig. 3. Case study for 3DCE (left-most column) and attention based multi-view modeling (the other three columns). Green and red boxes correspond to ground-truths and predictions respectively. (Color figure online)

4   Conclusion

In this paper, we address the universal lesion detection problem by incorporating human expertise into the design of deep architecture. Specifically, we propose a multi-view FPN with position-aware attention (MVP-Net) to incorporate the clinical practice of multi-window inspection and position-aware diagnosis to the deep detector. Without bells and whistles, our proposed model, which is intuitive and simple to implement, improves current state-of-the-art by a large margin. The MVP-Net reduces the FPs to reach a sensitivity of 91% by over three quarters (from 16 to 4) and reaches a sensitivity of 87.60% with only 2 FPs per image, making it more applicable to serve as an initial screening tool on daily clinical practice.

Acknowledgement. This work is funded by the National Natural Science Foundation of China (Grant No. 61876181, 61721004, 61403383, 61625201, 61527804) and the Projects of Chinese Academy of Sciences (Grant QYZDB-SSW-JSC006 and Grant 173211KYSB20160008). We would like to thank Feng Liu for valuable discussions.

References

1. Wang, B., Qi, G., Tang, S., Zhang, L., Deng, L., Zhang, Y.: Automated pulmonary nodule detection: high sensitivity with few candidates. In: Frangi, A.F., Schnabel, J.A., Davatzikos, C., Alberola-López, C., Fichtinger, G. (eds.) MICCAI 2018. LNCS, vol. 11071, pp. 759–767. Springer, Cham (2018). https://doi.org/10.1007/978-3-030-00934-2_84
2. Lee, S., Bae, J.S., Kim, H., Kim, J.H., Yoon, S.: Liver lesion detection from weakly-labeled multi-phase CT volumes with a grouped single shot multibox detector. In: Frangi, A.F., Schnabel, J.A., Davatzikos, C., Alberola-López, C., Fichtinger, G. (eds.) MICCAI 2018. LNCS, vol. 11071, pp. 693–701. Springer, Cham (2018). https://doi.org/10.1007/978-3-030-00934-2_77
3. He, K., Gkioxari, G., Dollr, P., Girshick, R.: Mask R-CNN. In: ICCV, pp. 2961–2969 (2017)
4. Lin, T.-Y., Dollr, P., Girshick, R., He, K., Hariharan, B., Belongie, S.: Feature pyramid networks for object detection. In: ICCV, pp. 2117–2125 (2017)
5. Tang, Y., Yan, K., Tang, Y., Liu, J., Xiao, J., Summers, R.M.: ULDor: a universal lesion detector for CT scans with pseudo masks and hard negative example mining. arXiv preprint arXiv:1901.06359 (2019)
6. Yan, K., Bagheri, M., Summers, R.M.: 3D context enhanced region-based convolutional neural network for end-to-end lesion detection. In: Frangi, A.F., Schnabel, J.A., Davatzikos, C., Alberola-López, C., Fichtinger, G. (eds.) MICCAI 2018. LNCS, vol. 11070, pp. 511–519. Springer, Cham (2018). https://doi.org/10.1007/978-3-030-00928-1_58
7. Yan, K., et al.: Deep lesion graphs in the wild: relationship learning and organization of significant radiology image findings in a diverse large-scale lesion database. In: CVPR, pp. 9261–9270 (2018)
8. Yan, K., Lu, L., Summers, R.M.: Unsupervised body part regression via spatially self-ordering convolutional neural networks. In: ISBI, pp. 1022–1025 (2018)
9. Woo, S., Park, J., Lee, J.-Y., Kweon, I.S.: CBAM: convolutional block attention module. In: Ferrari, V., Hebert, M., Sminchisescu, C., Weiss, Y. (eds.) ECCV 2018. LNCS, vol. 11211, pp. 3–19. Springer, Cham (2018). https://doi.org/10.1007/978-3-030-01234-2_1
10. Dai, J., Yi, L., He, K., Sun, J.: R-FCN: object detection via region-based fully convolutional networks. In: NIPS, pp. 379–387 (2016)

Spatial-Frequency Non-local Convolutional LSTM Network for pRCC Classification

Yu Zhao[1], Yuan Liu[1], Yansheng Kan[2], Anjany Sekuboyina[1],
Diana Waldmannstetter[1], Hongwei Li[1], Xiaobin Hu[1(✉)], Xiaozhi Zhao[2],
Kuangyu Shi[3], and Bjoern Menze[1]

[1] Department of Computer Science, Technische Universität München,
Munich, Germany
xiaobin.hu@tum.de
[2] Urology Department, The Affiliated Nanjing Drum Tower Hospital,
Nanjing University Medical School, Nanjing, Jiangsu, China
[3] Department of Nuclear Medicine, University of Bern, Bern, Switzerland

Abstract. The accurate classification of 3D medical images is a challenging task for current deep learning methods. Deep learning models struggle to extract features when the data size is small and the data dimension is large. To solve this problem, we develop a spatial-frequency non-local convolutional LSTM network for 3D image classification. Compared to traditional networks, the proposed model has the ability to extract features from both the spatial and frequency domains, which allows the frequency-domain features to contribute to the classification. Furthermore, the non-local blocks in our architecture enable it to capture the long-range dependencies directly in the feature space. Finally, to simplify the classification task and improve the performance, we utilize a two-stage framework that localizes lesions in the first step, and classifies them in the second. We evaluate our method on a challenging and important clinical task, i.e, the differentiation of papillary renal cell carcinoma (pRCC) into subtype 1 and subtype 2. To the best of our knowledge, this is the first time that the advantage of synthesizing spatial- and frequency-domain features by deep learning networks for medical image classification has been demonstrated. Experimental results demonstrate that the proposed method achieves competitive and often superior performance compared to state-of-the-art networks and three clinical experts.

Keywords: Deep neural network · Convolutional LSTM · Non-local network · Spatial domain · Frequency domain · Papillary renal cell carcinoma

Y. Zhao and Y. Liu—Contributed equally.

D. Shen et al. (Eds.): MICCAI 2019, LNCS 11769, pp. 22–30, 2019.
https://doi.org/10.1007/978-3-030-32226-7_3

1   Introduction

As one of the most common malignant diseases of the urinary tract, renal cell carcinoma (RCC) accounts for approximately 85%–90% of all renal malignancies [1]. The papillary RCC (pRCC) is the second most frequent RCC subtype which can be further divided into pRCC-Type 1 and pRCC-Type 2 depending on the histology. Distinguishing between the two subtypes is essential for the treatment decision since these two subtypes show different clinicopathologic behaviour. Furthermore, the pRCC-Type 2 is more likely to metastasize and usually has a worse prognosis than pRCC-Type 1 [5]. Several clinical studies have tried to classify the subtypes based on features like tumor size, margins, heterogeneity, attenuation values, etc. However, there is no successful method to solve this issue until now. Deep neural networks have the advantage of learning salient feature representations automatically and effectively [6]. Therefore, in this paper, we aim at developing a fully automatic method based on deep neural networks for the differentiation of pRCC subtypes.

Recently, various convolutional neural networks (CNNs) such as GoogleNet [12], ResNet [3] and DenseNet [4] have been proposed for the classification of natural images. Simultaneously, CNNs have also been widely used on medical images for computer-aided diagnosis, such as differential diagnosis [11], abnormality detection [9], and prognosis [2]. However, most of the existing classification networks work on the spatial domain of the image and have seldom paid attention to extracting features from the frequency domain. Intuitively, there is potential to further improve the classification performance of the network by employing features from both the spatial and frequency domains. Moreover, recent works [10,16] have used the frequency domain (k-space) for magnetic resonance image reconstruction and segmentation. Additionally, hand-crafted features extracted from the frequency domain have already been utilized to distinguish the pRCC subtypes in clinical research [14]. To this end, we propose a network that automatically learns features from both the spatial and frequency domains for classification. Given that, medical images are generally 3D volumetric data. The 3D CNN is more suitable for feature extraction compared to the 2D network, which can not exploit 3D context. However, current 3D networks usually face following implementation challenges: first, they are computationally expensive yet less stable when trained from scratch; second, the volume needs to be adjusted to a lower resolution reference size or divided into patches, and the capacity is very limited due to memory limitations. To overcome these problems, we develop our network with bidirectional Convolutional Long Short-Term memory (C-LSTM), which makes our network able to learn the 3D context of slices sequentially and alleviate the demand of the memory [7]. Additionally, the recently introduced non-local block [15], which extends self-attention to a general non-local filtering operation, is included in our proposed architecture to increase the ability of the network to capture long-range dependencies in the feature space.

The detailed contributions are as follows: (1) We propose to extract features from both the spatial and frequency domains to enhance the performance of the classification network. (2) We develop a spatial-frequency non-local convolutional LSTM network which can incorporate inter-slice 3D context information and capture long-range dependencies. (3) We make use of a two-stage procedure leveraging the transfer learning idea for localization followed by a classification stage. (4) The proposed method is evaluated on a real clinical dataset consisting of 80 patients, which achieves 84.2% accuracy under a clinically suitable run-time of one second, showing superior performance compared to state-of-the-art networks and three clinical experts.

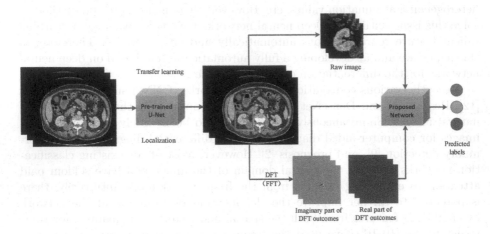

Fig. 1. The overall framework of the proposed approach. It consists of a localization step and a classification step. The localization stage leverages the idea of transfer learning to propose the ROI for the following classification stage. While, in the classification stage, the proposed network synthesizes features from both the spatial and frequency domains for classification.

2 Methodology

2.1 Overview

As illustrated in Fig. 1, the proposed framework consists of a localization and a classification stage. We leverage the idea of transfer learning in the localization stage. First, a 2D U-Net [8] is trained on the VISCERAL challenge dataset [13] and then utilized for predicting the kidney region on our collected clinical data. The VISCERAL dataset contains twenty non-contrast-enhanced whole-body CT (CTwb) and twenty contrast-enhanced CT (CTce) scans with manual annotations of different organs, including kidneys. After obtaining the segmentation map of each slice of one sample, a 3D bounding box covering all the kidney voxels is defined as the proposed ROI. In order to make the

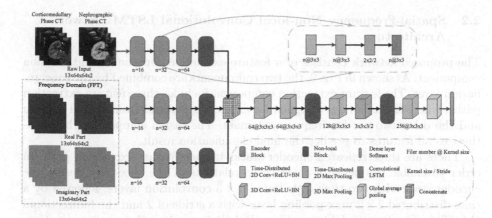

Fig. 2. Proposed spatial-frequency non-local convolutional LSTM network. It consists of a feature-extraction component and a fusion component, which are combined by the concatenation layer. Different operations are denoted by different colors. The details of each operation such as kernel size and filter number are shown below the graph (Conv: Convolutional layer, BN: batch normalization, ReLU: Rectified Linear Unit). (Color figure online)

location robust, a security margin is added to the obtained bounding box. In the classification stage, the proposed spatial-frequency non-local convolutional LSTM network (details in (Sect. 2.2)) is employed to predict the pRCC sub-type in the ROI. Assuming $\mathbf{I}$ is the volumetric ROI, it is composed of a set of slices donated as $\mathbf{I} = \{\mathbf{I}_1, \cdots, \mathbf{I}_N\}$. The proposed network extracts 3D context of slices in a sequential manner, and therefore, alleviates the memory consumption and avoids the downsampling operation. Let o, p, and q represent the sequence length, stepsize and the padding number respectively, $\mathbf{I}$ can be rebuilt into a set of $K = (N - o + 2q)/p + 1$ slice sequences denoted as $\mathbb{S} = \{\mathbb{S}_1, \cdots, \mathbb{S}_K\}$, each sequence contains a slice $\mathbf{I}_n$ and its $(o-1)/2$ neighbouring slices in both sides. In the meanwhile, we transform each slice in $\mathbf{I} = \{\mathbf{I}_1, \cdots, \mathbf{I}_N\}$ into frequency domain with Fast Fourier Transform (FFT) and obtain the set $\mathbf{F} = \{\mathbf{F}_1, \cdots, \mathbf{F}_N\}$. Since the frequency map $\mathbf{F}_n$ is complex-valued, we then built a set $\mathbf{F}^{re} = \{\mathbf{F}_1^{re}, \cdots, \mathbf{F}_N^{re}\}$ and a set $\mathbf{F}^{im} = \{\mathbf{F}_1^{im}, \cdots, \mathbf{F}_N^{im}\}$ with the real and the imaginary part of $\{\mathbf{F}_1, \cdots, \mathbf{F}_N\}$ respectively. Subsequently, based on $\mathbf{F}^{re}$ and $\mathbf{F}^{im}$, we employ the aforementioned sequence building strategy and obtain the corresponding frequency-domain sequences represented as $\mathbb{F}^{re} = \{\mathbb{F}_1^{re}, \cdots, \mathbb{F}_K^{re}\}$ and $\mathbb{F}^{im} = \{\mathbb{F}_1^{im}, \cdots, \mathbb{F}_K^{im}\}$. In the prediction phase, sequence $\mathbb{S}_k$ as well as its counterparts in frequency domain $\mathbb{F}_k^{re}$ and $\mathbb{F}_k^{im}$, are input into the network to predict the classification label of this sequence c_k. Finally, the overall classification label of each patient C is calculated using the majority voting strategy on $\{c_1, \cdots, c_k\}$.

2.2 Spatial-Frequency Non-local Convolutional LSTM Network Architecture

The proposed network consists of a feature-extraction component and a fusion component. As shown in Fig. 2, the two components are combined by the concatenation layer. The feature-extraction component includes three feature-extraction paths, where the top one is designed for extracting features from spatial domain and the other two are for frequency domain. The fusion component then synthesizes all features to predict the final classification result.

There are three repeated encoder stacks in each feature-extraction path. In order to enable the network to learn correlations of the slices, we design the encoder stack with two time-distributed 3×3 convolution layers, followed by a time-distributed 2×2 max-pooling layer with a stride of 2 and the bidirectional C-LSTM. The Rectified Linear Unit (ReLU) is used as the nonlinear activation function for the convolutional layers and Batch Normalization is applied immediately after each convolutional layer. These time-distributed layers are 2D layers enclosed into the time-distributed wrapper, which applies each layer to every temporal frame of the input independently. In this work, the slices of extracted sequences correspond to the temporal frames. The main idea behind this design is that the features of correlated slices should also be correlated. We use the LSTM variant [7] without connections from the cell to the gates to reduce the parameter number and accelerate the training. At the end of each feature-extraction path, there is a non-local block [15]. The non-local block can capture long-range dependencies in the feature space, which is a more general extension of the self-attention mechanism. The feature map after the non-local block has the same size as the input. Similar as the fully connected layer, each obtained feature contains the information of the entire input feature map. We apply the embedded Gaussian version of the non-local block [15].

Assuming the size of the input slice is $W \times H$, the size of the feature map after the feature-extraction component and the concatenation is $o \times round(W/8) \times round(H/8)$. Considering that the size of the feature map is relatively small, we use 3D layers in the fusion component to extract the 3D context information directly. Moreover, since the training samples are usually limited in medical tasks, the fusion component is designed as a simple architecture to reduce the complexity of the overall network and to avoid overfitting to the training dataset despite regularization. The fusion component begins with $3 \times 3 \times 3$ convolutional layers with ReLU, non-local blocks [15], and the 3D max-pooling operations and ends with a global average pooling operation and a fully-connected layer with softmax activation function.

3 Experiments and Results

3.1 Dataset

This study included a total of 80 patients who had taken contrast-enhanced CT before the operation or treatment at Nanjing Drum Tower Hospital. All patients had undergone nephrectomy or biopsy and were pathologically proven to be pRCC-Type 1 and pRCC-Type 2. The contrast-enhanced CT images were performed using 16- or 64-slice multidetector spiral CT (Light Speed Pro 16, VCT, or Discovery HD 750, GE Healthcare, Milwaukee, WI, USA). The obtained CT images include non-contrast, corticomedullary, nephrographic, and excretory phases. Since radiologists usually classify the RCC based on the corticomedullary-phase and nephrographic-phase scans, we use scans of these two phases in this work. Image samples of these two kinds of CT scans are shown in Fig. 3(a) and (b).

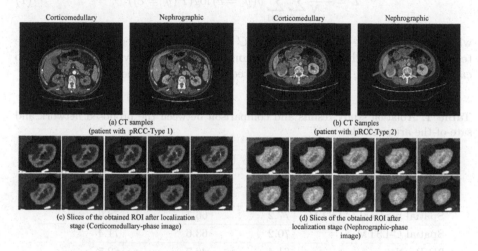

Fig. 3. Examples illustrating the raw CT images (corticomedullary phase and nephrographic phase) as well as the obtained ROIs after localization stage.

3.2 Pre-processing

We windowed the raw axial slices to $[0, 300]$ Hounsfield unit (HU) to emphasize renal area and remove interference information. Then, the results were zero-centred by subtracting mean of individual slices and then additionally normalized by scaling, using the case-wise standard deviation. After the localization stage, b-spline interpolation was leveraged to re-sample the obtained ROIs to uniform 64×64 imaging resolution in the axial plane.

3.3 Implementation Details

The evaluation was performed with five-fold cross-validation. The dataset was randomly split into a training set and a test set and the training set was further split into a training subset and validation subset in a ratio of 4:1 (where the validation set was used for parameter tuning purpose). In the localization step, the security margins were 5% length of each side of the bounding box.

To enlarge the dataset and alleviate the overfitting of our model, we applied data augmentation in slice manner in the classification stage, including random rotation, random zoom and horizontal and vertical flips. We applied mini-batches of size 10. ADAM optimizer was used during training with an initial learning rate $lr_{init} = 10^{-4}$. To regularize the network, we utilized the early stopping strategy with patience of 20 epochs, which is a method employed to detect the convergence of training thereby avoiding overfitting. In this work, the categorical cross-entropy loss was used, which is defined as:

$$L = -\frac{1}{N} \sum_{i=1}^{N} \sum_{c=1}^{C} \delta(y_i = c) \log(P(y_i = c)) \tag{1}$$

where N denotes the data number and C represents the categories number. The term $\delta(y_i = c)$ is the indicator function of the ith observation belonging to category c. The $P(y_i = c)$ is the predicted probability by the model.

Table 1. Ablation study results and comparison between the proposed network and sate-of-the-art methods

Method	Accuracy (%)	Sensitivity (%)	Specificity (%)
Our	**84.2**	**80.3**	**85.7**
Spatial-Frequency C-LSTM	80.7	71.2	81.6
Spatial nonlocal C-LSTM	77.2	66.7	78.6
Spatial C-LSTM	70.2	63.6	71.4
3D ResNet	61.4	46.7	62.5
3D DenseNet	66.7	60.3	69.0

3.4 Results

By leveraging the idea of transfer learning, the localization step proposes the ROI for classification using a pre-trained U-Net. This strategy is beneficial for removing the irrelevant area and simplifying the classification task. In Fig. 3(c) and (d), we show the samples of the obtained ROIs. Classification results of the proposed network for the differentiation of the pRCC subtypes are illustrated in Table 1. The proposed framework achieved 84.2% accuracy, 80.3% sensitivity and 85.7% specificity. We also conduct ablation studies. The proposed network without non-local blocks is denoted as Spatial-Frequency C-LSTM and the one without frequency-domain feature extracting paths is denoted as Spatial Non-Local C-LSTM. Spatial C-LSTM represents the architecture with a spatial-domain feature extracting path and without non-local blocks. Experimental results show that our proposed network outperforms the Spatial-Frequency C-LSTM, the Spatial Non-Local C-LSTM, and the Spatial C-LSTM. This demonstrates that the network can benefit from our proposed strategies including extracting features from both the spatial and frequency domains as well as employing non-local block to capture the long-range dependencies. In Table 1, the comparison between our proposed method and state-of-art methods such as ResNet [3] and DenseNet [4] is illustrated. We can find that the proposed method achieves superior accuracy in comparison to these methods. Due to the relatively small sample size, we deployed a shallow version of ResNet (18 layers) and DenseNet (22 layers, containing 3 dense blocks and each block consists of 6 convolutional layers) to avoid overfitting for a fair comparison. We further evaluated the performance of three radiologists who have more than 8-year experience. The results show that the proposed method exceeds practising radiologists when only referring the CT scans, with average accuracy 84.2% compared to 72.5%.

Runtime: With the application of the GPU, our trained model can predict the subtype of one unseen sample in 1 s, which is suitable in clinical practice. The experiments were conducted on a GNU/Linux server running Ubuntu 16.04, with Intel Core i7-6700 CPU and 32 GB RAM. The networks were trained on a single NVIDIA Titan-Xp GPU with 12 GB RAM.

4 Conclusion

In this paper, we develop a spatial-frequency non-local convolutional LSTM network for the automated differential diagnosis of pRCC subtypes and evaluate the network on a real clinical dataset. Experimental results demonstrate the network benefits from our proposed strategies including extracting features from both the spatial and frequency domains and employing the non-local block to capture the long-range dependencies. Our network shows competitive and often superior performance compared to state-of-the-art classification networks and even clinical experts. Currently, more data is being in collected and annotated. In the future, increasing the amount of training data may further enhance the performance of the method.

References

1. Gupta, K., et al.: Epidemiologic and socioeconomic burden of metastatic renal cell carcinoma (mRCC): a literature review. Cancer Treat. Rev. 34(3), 193–205 (2008)
2. Hazlett, H.C., et al.: Early brain development in infants at high risk for autism spectrum disorder. Nature 542(7641), 348 (2017)
3. He, K., et al.: Deep residual learning for image recognition. In: Proceedings of the IEEE Conference on Computer Vision and Pattern Recognition, pp. 770–778 (2016)
4. Huang, G., et al.: Densely connected convolutional networks. In: Proceedings of the IEEE Conference on Computer Vision and Pattern Recognition, pp. 4700–4708 (2017)
5. Klatte, T., et al.: Cytogenetic and molecular tumor profiling for type 1 and type 2 papillary renal cell carcinoma. Clin. Cancer Res. 15(4), 1162–1169 (2009)

6. LeCun, Y., Bengio, Y., Hinton, G.: Deep learning. Nature **521**(7553), 436 (2015)
7. Novikov, A.A., et al.: Deep sequential segmentation of organs in volumetric medical scans. IEEE Trans. Med. Imaging **36**, 1359–1371 (2018)
8. Ronneberger, O., Fischer, P., Brox, T.: U-net: convolutional networks for biomedical image segmentation. In: Navab, N., Hornegger, J., Wells, W.M., Frangi, A.F. (eds.) MICCAI 2015. LNCS, vol. 9351, pp. 234–241. Springer, Cham (2015). https://doi.org/10.1007/978-3-319-24574-4_28
9. Roth, H.R., et al.: Improving computer-aided detection using convolutional neural networks and random view aggregation. IEEE Trans. Med. Imaging **35**(5), 1170–1181 (2016)
10. Schlemper, J., et al.: Cardiac MR segmentation from undersampled k-space using deep latent representation learning. In: Frangi, A.F., Schnabel, J.A., Davatzikos, C., Alberola-López, C., Fichtinger, G. (eds.) MICCAI 2018. LNCS, vol. 11070, pp. 259–267. Springer, Cham (2018). https://doi.org/10.1007/978-3-030-00928-1_30
11. Suk, H.I., et al.: Latent feature representation with stacked auto-encoder for AD/MCI diagnosis. Brain Struct. Func. **220**(2), 841–859 (2015)
12. Szegedy, C., et al.: Going deeper with convolutions. In: Proceedings of the IEEE Conference on Computer Vision and Pattern Recognition, pp. 1–9 (2015)
13. Jimenez-del Toro, O., et al.: Cloud-based evaluation of anatomical structure segmentation and landmark detection algorithms: visceral anatomy benchmarks. IEEE Trans. Med. Imaging **35**(11), 2459–2475 (2016)
14. Varghese, B.A., et al.: Differentiation of predominantly solid enhancing lipid-poor renal cell masses by use of contrast-enhanced CT: evaluating the role of texture in tumor subtyping. Am. J. Roentgenol. **211**(6), W288–W296 (2018)
15. Wang, X., et al.: Non-local neural networks. In: Proceedings of the IEEE Conference on Computer Vision and Pattern Recognition, pp. 7794–7803 (2018)
16. Zhu, B., et al.: Image reconstruction by domain-transform manifold learning. Nature **555**(7697), 487 (2018)

BCD-Net for Low-Dose CT Reconstruction: Acceleration, Convergence, and Generalization

Il Yong Chun[1], Xuehang Zheng[2], Yong Long[2(✉)], and Jeffrey A. Fessler[1]

[1] Department of Electrical Engineering and Computer Science,
University of Michigan, Ann Arbor, MI, USA
[2] University of Michigan - Shanghai Jiao Tong University Joint Institute,
Shanghai Jiao Tong University, Shanghai, China
yong.long@sjtu.edu.cn

Abstract. Obtaining accurate and reliable images from low-dose computed tomography (CT) is challenging. Regression convolutional neural network (CNN) models that are learned from training data are increasingly gaining attention in low-dose CT reconstruction. This paper modifies the architecture of an iterative regression CNN, *BCD-Net*, for fast, stable, and accurate low-dose CT reconstruction, and presents the convergence property of the modified BCD-Net. Numerical results with phantom data show that applying faster numerical solvers to model-based image reconstruction (MBIR) modules of BCD-Net leads to faster and more accurate BCD-Net; BCD-Net significantly improves the reconstruction accuracy, compared to the state-of-the-art MBIR method using learned transforms; BCD-Net achieves better image quality, compared to a state-of-the-art iterative NN architecture, ADMM-Net. Numerical results with clinical data show that BCD-Net generalizes significantly better than a state-of-the-art deep (non-iterative) regression NN, FBP-ConvNet, that lacks MBIR modules.

1 Introduction

Low-dose computed tomography (CT) reconstruction requires careful regularization design to control noise while preserving crucial image features. Traditional regularizers have been based on mathematical models like total variation, whereas newer methods are based on models that are learned from training data, especially regression neural network (NN) models. Deep convolutional NN

I. Y. Chun and X. Zheng—Equally contributed to this work.
This paper has supplementary document. The prefix "S" indicates the numbers in figure and section in the supplementary document.

Electronic supplementary material The online version of this chapter (https://doi.org/10.1007/978-3-030-32226-7_4) contains supplementary material, which is available to authorized users.

(CNN) methods in an early stage map low- to high-quality images: specifically, they "denoise" the artifacts in the low-quality images obtained by applying some basic solvers to raw data or measurements. However, the greater mapping capability (i.e., higher the NN complexity) can increase the overfitting risks [15]. There exist several ways to prevent NNs from overfitting, e.g., increasing the dataset size, reducing the neural network complexity, and dropout. However, in solving large-scale inverse problems in imaging, the first scheme is limited in training CNNs from large-scale images; the second scheme does not effectively remove complicated noise features; and the third scheme has limited benefits when applied to convolutional layers.

An alternative way to regulate overfitting of regression CNNs in inverse imaging problems is combining them with model-based image reconstruction (MBIR) that considers imaging physics or image formation models, and noise statistics in measurements. BCD-Net [4] is an iterative regression CNN that generalizes a block coordinate descent (BCD) MBIR method using learned convolutional regularizers [5]. Each layer (or iteration) of BCD-Net consists of image denoising and MBIR modules. In particular, the denoising modules use layer-wise regression CNNs to effectively remove layer-dependent noise features. Many existing works can be viewed as a special case of BCD-Net. For example, RED [11] and MoDL [1] are special cases of BCD-Net, because they use identical image denoising modules across layers or only consider quadratic data-fidelity terms (e.g., the first term in (P1)) in their MBIR modules.

This paper modifies BCD-Net that uses convolutional autoencoders in its denoising modules [4], and applies the modified BCD-Net to low-dose CT reconstruction. First, for fast CT reconstruction, we apply the Accelerated Proximal Gradient method using a Majorizer (APG-M), e.g., FISTA [2], to MBIR modules using the statistical CT data-fidelity term. Second, this paper provides the sequence convergence guarantee of BCD-Net when applied to low-dose CT reconstruction. Third, it investigates the generalization capability of BCD-Net for low-dose CT reconstruction, compared to a state-of-the-art deep (non-iterative) regression NN, FBPConvNet [8]. Numerical results with the extended cardiac-torso (XCAT) phantom show that applying faster numerical solvers (e.g., APG-M) to MBIR modules leads to faster and more accurate BCD-Net; regardless of numerical solvers of MBIR modules, BCD-Net significantly improves the reconstruction accuracy, compared to the state-of-the-art MBIR method using learned transforms [15]; given identical denoising CNN architectures, BCD-Net achieves better image quality, compared to a state-of-the-art iterative NN architecture, ADMM-Net [14]. Numerical results with clinical data show that BCD-Net generalizes significantly better than FBPConvNet [8] that lacks MBIR modules.

2   BCD-Net for Low-Dose CT Reconstruction

2.1   Architecture

This section modifies the architecture of BCD-Net in [4] for CT reconstruction. For the image denoising modules, we use layer-wise autoencoding CNNs that apply exponential function to trainable thresholding parameters. (The trainable thresholding parameters replace the bias terms, since biases can differ greatly for

---
Algo. 1. BCD-Net for CT reconstruction

Require: $\{\mathcal{D}_{\theta^{(l)}} : \forall l\}, \mathbf{x}^{(0)}, \mathbf{y}, \mathbf{A}, \mathbf{W}, \beta$
 for $l = 0, \ldots, L - 1$ **do**
  Denoising: $\mathbf{z}^{(l+1)} = \mathcal{D}_{\theta^{(l+1)}}(\mathbf{x}^{(l)})$
  MBIR: $\mathbf{x}^{(l+1)} = \underset{\mathbf{x} \geq 0}{\operatorname{argmin}}\, F(\mathbf{x}; \mathbf{y}, \mathbf{z}^{(l+1)})^{\dagger}$
 end for
$^{\dagger}F(\mathbf{x}; \mathbf{y}, \mathbf{z}^{(l+1)})$ is defined in (P1).

---

different objects in imaging problems.) The layer-wise denoising CNNs are particularly useful to remove layer-dependent artifacts in reconstructed images at the previous layers, without greatly increasing their parameter dimensions. In low-dose CT reconstruction, for example, the CNNs at the early and later layers remove streak artifacts and Gaussian-like noise, respectively. MBIR modules aim to regularize overfitting artifacts by combining information drawn from the data-fidelity term and output of denoising modules. Different from the image denoising and single-coil magnetic resonance imaging applications in [4], the MBIR modules of CT reconstruction BCD-Net involve iterative solvers. For fast CT reconstruction in particular, we apply a fast numerical solver, APG-M, to the MBIR modules. Algorithm 1 shows the architecture of the modified BCD-Net for CT reconstruction.

Image Denoising Module. For the lth layer image denoising module, we use a convolutional autoencoder in the following form:

$$\mathcal{D}_{\theta^{(l+1)}}(\cdot) = \frac{1}{R} \sum_{k=1}^{K} \mathbf{d}_k^{(l+1)} \circledast \mathcal{T}_{\exp(\alpha_k^{(l+1)})}\left(\mathbf{e}_k^{(l+1)} \circledast (\cdot)\right), \qquad (1)$$

where $\theta^{(l+1)} := \{\mathbf{d}_k^{(l+1)}, \mathbf{e}_k^{(l+1)}, \alpha_k^{(l+1)} : k = 1, \ldots, K, l = 1, \ldots, L\}$ is a parameter set of the lth convolutional autoencoder, $\mathbf{d}_k^{(l+1)} \in \mathbb{R}^R$, $\mathbf{e}_k^{(l+1)} \in \mathbb{R}^R$, and $\exp(\alpha_k^{(l+1)})$ are the kth decoding and encoding filters, and thresholding value at the lth layer, respectively, the convolution operator $\circledast$ uses the circulant boundary condition without the filter flip, $\mathcal{T}_a(\cdot)$ is the soft-thresholding operator with the thresholding parameter a, R and K are the size and number of the filters, respectively, and L is the number of layers in BCD-Net. Different from the original convolutional autoencoder in [4], we included the exponential function $\exp(\cdot)$ to prevent the thresholding parameters $\{\alpha_k\}$ from becoming zero during training [6]. The factor $1/R$ comes from the relation between convolution-perspective and patch-based trainings [6]. By applying the trained convolutional autoencoder in (1) to the lth layer input $\mathbf{x}^{(l)}$ (i.e., reconstructed image at the $(l-1)$th layer), we obtain the "denoised" image $\mathbf{z}^{(l+1)} = \mathcal{D}_{\boldsymbol{\theta}^{(l+1)}}(\mathbf{x}^{(l)})$. We next feed $\mathbf{z}^{(l+1)}$ into the lth layer MBIR module.

MBIR Module. The lth layer MBIR module uses the lth layer denoised image $\mathbf{z}^{(l+1)}$, and reconstructs an image $\mathbf{x} \in \mathbb{R}^N$ from post-log measurement $\mathbf{y} \in \mathbb{R}^M$ by solving the following statistical MBIR problem:

$$\mathbf{x}^{(l+1)} = \operatorname*{argmin}_{\mathbf{x} \geq 0} F(\mathbf{x}; \mathbf{y}, \mathbf{z}^{(l+1)}) := \frac{1}{2}\|\mathbf{y} - \mathbf{A}\mathbf{x}\|_{\mathbf{W}}^2 + \frac{\beta}{2}\|\mathbf{x} - \mathbf{z}^{(l+1)}\|_2^2, \quad \text{(P1)}$$

where $\mathbf{A} \in \mathbb{R}^{M \times N}$ is a CT scan system matrix, $\mathbf{W} \in \mathbb{R}^{M \times M}$ is a diagonal weighting matrix with elements $\{W_{m,m} = \rho_m^2/(\rho_m + \sigma^2) : \forall m\}$ based on a Poisson-Gaussian model for the pre-log measurements $\boldsymbol{\rho} \in \mathbb{R}^M$ with electronic readout noise variance σ^2 [15], and $\beta > 0$ is a regularization parameter. To rapidly solve (P1), we apply APG-M, a generalized version of APG (e.g., FISTA [2]) that uses M-Lipschitz continuous gradients [5]. Initialized with $\mathbf{v}^{(0)} = \bar{\mathbf{x}}^{(0)} = \mathbf{x}^{(l)}$ and $t_0 = 1$, the APG-M updates are

$$\bar{\mathbf{x}}^{(j+1)} = \left[\mathbf{v}^{(j)} + \mathbf{M}^{-1}(\mathbf{A}^T\mathbf{W}(\mathbf{y} - \mathbf{A}\mathbf{v}^{(j)}) - \beta(\mathbf{v}^{(j)} - \mathbf{z}^{(l+1)}))\right]_+, \quad \text{(2)}$$

$$\mathbf{v}^{(j+1)} = \bar{\mathbf{x}}^{(j+1)} + \frac{t_j - 1}{t_{j+1}}(\bar{\mathbf{x}}^{(j+1)} - \bar{\mathbf{x}}^{(j)}), \quad \text{where } t_{j+1} = (1 + \sqrt{1 + 4t_j^2})/2, \quad \text{(3)}$$

for $j = 0, \ldots, J-1$, where the operator $[\cdot]_+$ is the proximal operator obtained by considering the non-negativity constraint in (P1) and clips the negative values, and J is the number of APG-M iterations. We design the diagonal majorizer $\mathbf{M} \in \mathbb{R}^{N \times N}$ in (2) as follows [5]: $\mathbf{M} = \operatorname{diag}(\mathbf{A}^T\mathbf{W}\mathbf{A}\mathbf{1}) + \beta\mathbf{I} \succeq \nabla^2 F(\mathbf{x}; \mathbf{y}, \mathbf{z}^{(l+1)}) = \mathbf{A}^T\mathbf{W}\mathbf{A} + \beta\mathbf{I}$, where $\operatorname{diag}(\cdot)$ converts a vector into a diagonal matrix. The lth layer reconstructed image $\mathbf{x}^{(l+1)}$ is given by the Jth APG-M update, i.e., $\mathbf{x}^{(l+1)} = \bar{\mathbf{x}}^{(J)}$, and fed into the next BCD-Net layer as an input.

2.2 Training BCD-Net

This section proposes a BCD-Net training framework for CT reconstruction, based on the image denoising and MBIR modules defined in the previous section. The training process requires I high-quality training images, $\{\mathbf{x}_i : i = 1, \ldots, I\}$, and I training measurements simulated via CT physics, $\{\mathbf{y}_i : i = 1, \ldots, I\}$. Algorithm 2 summarizes the training framework.

Algo. 2. Training BCD-Net for CT recon.

Require: $\{\mathbf{x}_i, \mathbf{x}_i^{(0)}, \mathbf{y}_i, \mathbf{A}, \mathbf{W}_i, \beta : \forall i\}$
  for $l = 0, \ldots, L-1$ **do**
    Train $\boldsymbol{\theta}^{(l+1)}$: Solve (P2) using $\{\mathbf{x}_i, \mathbf{x}_i^{(l)} : \forall i\}$
    for $i = 1, \ldots, I$ **do**
      Denoising: $\mathbf{z}_i^{(l+1)} = \mathcal{D}_{\boldsymbol{\theta}^{(l+1)}}(\mathbf{x}_i^{(l)})$
      MBIR: $\mathbf{x}_i^{(l+1)} = \operatorname*{argmin}_{\mathbf{x} \geq 0} F_i(\mathbf{x}; \mathbf{y}_i, \mathbf{z}_i^{(l+1)})^\dagger$
    end for
  end for
$^\dagger F(\mathbf{x}; \mathbf{y}, \mathbf{z}^{(l+1)})$ is defined in (P1).

At the lth layer, we optimize the parameters $\boldsymbol{\theta}^{(l+1)}$ of the lth convolutional autoencoder in (1) from I training pairs $(\mathbf{x}_i, \mathbf{x}_i^{(l)})$, where $\mathbf{x}_i^{(l)}$ is the ith reconstructed training image at the $(l-1)$th layer. Our patch-based training loss function at the lth layer is

$$\boldsymbol{\theta}^{(l+1)} = \underset{\{\mathbf{D},\boldsymbol{\alpha},\mathbf{E}\}}{\mathrm{argmin}} \frac{1}{R\tilde{P}} \|\widetilde{\mathbf{X}} - \mathbf{D}\mathcal{T}_{\exp(\boldsymbol{\alpha})}(\mathbf{E}^T \widetilde{\mathbf{X}}^{(l)})\|_F^2, \qquad (\mathrm{P2})$$

where encoding and decoding filter matrices $\mathbf{D} \in \mathbb{R}^{R \times K}$ and $\mathbf{E} \in \mathbb{R}^{R \times K}$ are formed by grouping K filters as $\mathbf{D} := [\mathbf{d}_1, \ldots, \mathbf{d}_K]$ and $\mathbf{E} := [\mathbf{e}_1, \ldots, \mathbf{e}_K]$, respectively, $\boldsymbol{\alpha} \in \mathbb{R}^K$ is a vector containing K thresholding values, $\tilde{P}$ is the number of patches extracted from all training images, and $\widetilde{\mathbf{X}} \in \mathbb{R}^{R \times \tilde{P}}$ and $\widetilde{\mathbf{X}}^{(l)} \in \mathbb{R}^{R \times \tilde{P}}$ are paired training matrices whose columns are vectorized patches extracted from $\{\mathbf{x}_i : \forall i\}$ and $\{\mathbf{x}_i^{(l)} : \forall i\}$, respectively. The soft thresholding operator $\mathcal{T}_{\mathbf{a}}(\mathbf{u}) : \mathbb{R}^K \to \mathbb{R}^K$ is defined as follows: $(\mathcal{T}_{\mathbf{a}}(\mathbf{u}))_k$ equals to $u_k - a_k \mathrm{sign}(u_k)$ for $|u_k| > a_k$, and 0 otherwise, $\forall k$. We optimize (P2) via a mini-batch stochastic gradient method.

2.3   Convergence Analysis

There exist two key challenges in understanding the convergence behavior of BCD-Net in Algorithm 1: *(1)* (general) denoising NNs $\{\mathcal{D}_{\boldsymbol{\theta}^{(l+1)}}\}$ change across layers; *(2)* even if they are identical across layers, they are not necessarily non-expansive operators [10] in practice. To moderate these issues, we introduce a new definition:

Definition 1 (Asymptotically nonexpansive paired operators [6]**).**
Paired operators $\{\mathcal{D}_{\boldsymbol{\theta}^{(l)}}, \mathcal{D}_{\boldsymbol{\theta}^{(l+1)}}\}$ *are asymptotically nonexpansive if there exist a summable sequence* $\{\epsilon^{(l+1)} \in [0, \infty) : \sum_{l=0}^{\infty} \epsilon^{(l+1)} < \infty\}$ *such that*

$$\|\mathcal{D}_{\boldsymbol{\theta}^{(l+1)}}(\mathbf{u}) - \mathcal{D}_{\boldsymbol{\theta}^{(l)}}(\mathbf{v})\|_2^2 \le \|\mathbf{u} - \mathbf{v}\|_2^2 + \epsilon^{(l+1)}, \qquad \forall \mathbf{u}, \mathbf{v} \text{ and } \forall l.$$

Based on Definition 1, we obtain the following convergence result for Algorithm 1:

Theorem 2 (Sequence convergence). *Assume that paired denoising neural networks* $\{\mathcal{D}_{\boldsymbol{\theta}^{(l)}}, \mathcal{D}_{\boldsymbol{\theta}^{(l+1)}}\}$ *are asymptotically nonexpansive with the summable sequence* $\{\epsilon^{(l+1)} \in [0, \infty) : \sum_{l=1}^{\infty} \epsilon^{(l+1)} < \infty\}$ *and* $\mathbf{A}^T \mathbf{W} \mathbf{A} \succ 0$. *Then the sequence* $\{\mathbf{x}^{(l+1)} : l \ge 0\}$ *generated by Algorithm 1 (disregarding the non-negativity constraints in the MBIR optimization problems (P1)) is convergent.*

Theorem 2 implies that if denoising neural networks $\{\mathcal{D}_{\boldsymbol{\theta}^{(l)}} : l \ge 1\}$ converge to a nonexpansive one, BCD-Net guarantees the sequence convergence. Figure S.1 shows the convergence behaviors of $\{\mathcal{D}_{\boldsymbol{\theta}^{(l+1)}}\}$ and their Lipschitz constants.

2.4   Computational Complexity

The computational cost of the proposed BCD-Net is $O((MJ + RK)NL)$. Since $MJ \gg RK$, the computational complexity of BCD-Net is dominated by forward and back projections performed in the MBIR modules. To reduce the MJ factor, one can investigate faster optimization methods (e.g., proximal optimized gradient method (POGM) [13]) with ordered subsets. Applying these techniques can reduce the MJ factor to $(M/G)J'$, where G is the number of subsets and the number of POGM iterations $J' < J$ (e.g., $J' = (1/\sqrt{2})J$) due to faster convergence rates of POGM over APG.

3   Experimental Results and Discussion

3.1   Experimental Setup

Imaging. For XCAT phantom images [12] and reconstructed clinical images in [15], we simulated sinograms of size 888×984 (detectors $\times$ projection views) with GE LightSpeed fan-beam geometry corresponding to a monoenergetic source with $\rho_0 = 10^4$ incident photons per ray and electronic noise variance $\sigma^2 = 5^2$ [15] (while avoiding inverse crimes). We reconstructed 420×420 images with pixel-size $\Delta_x = \Delta_y = 0.9766$ mm. For the clinical data collected from the GE scanner using the CT geometry above, and tube voltage 120 kVp and current 160 mA, we reconstructed a 716×716 image (shown in the third row of Fig. 2) with $\Delta_x = \Delta_y = 0.9777$ mm.

Training BCD-Net, ADMM-Net, and FBPConvNet. Based on the proposed framework in Sect. 2.2, we trained 100-layer BCD-Nets with the two parameter sets, $\{K = R = 8^2\}$ and $\{K = 10^2, R = 8^2\}$, and the regularization parameter $\beta = 4 \times 10^6$. In particular, we solved (P2) with Adam [9] and $\tilde{P} \approx 1.7 \times 10^6$ training patches that were extracted from ten training images of the XCAT phantom [12]. We used the mini-batch size 512, 200 epochs, initial learning rates 10^{-3}, and 10^{-2} for $\{\mathbf{D}^{(l)}, \mathbf{E}^{(l)} : \forall l\}$ and $\{\boldsymbol{\alpha}^{(l)} : \forall l\}$, and random i.i.d. Gaussian filter initialization. We decayed the learning rates by a factor of 0.9 every 10 epochs. We trained a 100-layer ADMM-Net that uses the layer-wise denoising NNs (1) with $K = R = 8^2$, with the identical training setup above. We chose the ADMM penalty parameter as 1×10^6, by matching the spatial resolution in the heart region of test sample #1 to that reconstructed by BCD-Net. We trained FBPConvNet with 500 2D XCAT phantom images and the similar parameters suggested in [8].

Image Reconstruction. We compared trained BCD-Nets with the conventional MBIR method using an edge-preserving (EP) regularizer, the state-of-the-art MBIR method using ℓ_2 prior with a learned square transform [15], a state-of-the-art iterative NN architecture, ADMM-Net [14] (i.e., plug-and-play ADMM [3] using denoising NNs), and/or a state-of-the-art (non-iterative) deep regression NN, FBPConvNet [8]. For the first two MBIR methods, we finely tuned their parameters to give the lowest root-mean-square-error (RMSE) values [5]. (See their parameter details in Section S.2). We tested the aforementioned methods to two sets of three representative chest CT images that are selected from the XCAT phantom and clinical data provided by GE. (Note that the testing phantom images are sufficiently different from training phantom images; specifically, they are ≈2 cm away from training images.) We quantitatively evaluated the quality of phantom reconstructions by RMSE (in Hounsfield units, HU) in a region of interest [15].

3.2 Results and Discussion

Convergence of BCD-Net with Different MBIR Modules. Applying faster iterative solvers to MBIR modules leads to faster and more accurate BCD-Net. This assertion is supported by comparing the APG-M and PG-M results in Fig. 1 (given the identical iteration numbers), and noting that APG-M is faster than PG-M (i.e., APG-M using no "momentum", $\bar{\mathbf{x}}^{(j+1)} - \bar{\mathbf{x}}^{(j)}$ in (3)). In addition, Fig. 1 shows that increasing the number of iterations in numerical MBIR solvers leads more accurate BCD-Net, given the identical numbers of BCD-Net layers. This implies that numerical MBIR

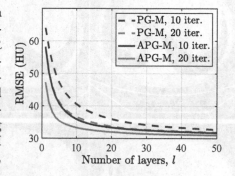

Fig. 1. RMSE convergence of BCD-Nets using different MBIR modules for low-dose CT reconstruction (for the first testing image in Table 1).

solvers using insufficient number of iterations do not fully extract "desired" information from CT data-fidelity (i.e., the first term in (P1)). The importance of using rapidly converging MBIR solvers is underestimated in existing literature: existing literature often considers some applications that have practical and closed-form MBIR solution [4].

Reconstruction Quality Comparisons. For all the testing phantom and clinical images, the proposed BCD-Nets significantly improve the low-dose CT reconstruction accuracy, compared to the conventional MBIR method using EP and/or the state-of-the-art MBIR method using ℓ_2 prior with a learned transform [15]. For all the testing phantom images, BCD-Net consistently achieves better reconstruction quality than ADMM-Net. See Table 1, Fig. 2 & S.2, and Section S.3. In particular, BCD-Net accomplishes the both benefits of EP and image denoising (see Fig. S.2); and increasing the number of filters and thresholding parameters improves its reconstruction performance (see Table 1).

Table 1. RMSE (HU) of three reconstructed XCAT phantom images with different MBIR methods for low-dose CT[a] ($\rho_0 = 10^4$ incident photons)

	EP	Learned trans. $(K = R = 8^2)$ [15]	ADMM-Net $(K = R = 8^2)$ [14]	BCD-Net $(K = R = 8^2)$	**BCD-Net** $(K = 10^2, R = 8^2)$
Test #1	39.4	36.5	31.6	30.7	**27.5**
Test #2	39.6	37.8	32.0	31.4	**29.2**
Test #3	37.1	34.0	32.0	30.6	**27.7**

[a] See reconstructed images and error images in Fig. S.2 and Fig. S.3, respectively.

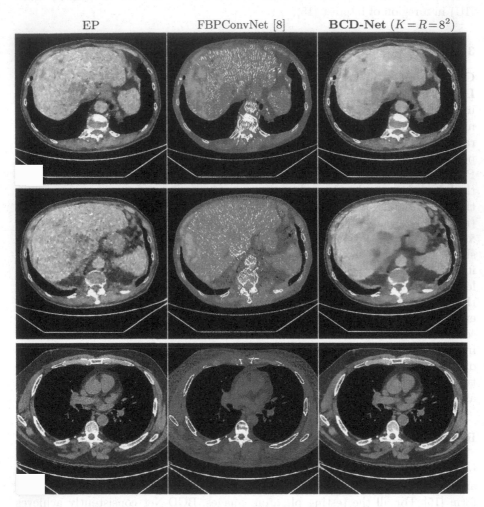

Fig. 2. Comparison of three reconstructed clinical images from different reconstruction methods for low-dose CT (images are magnified to better show differences; display window [800, 1200] HU).

Generalization Capability Comparisons. The proposed BCD-Net has significantly better generalization capability than a state-of-the-art (non-iterative) deep regression NN, FBPConvNet [8]. Clinical scan experiments in Fig. 2 indicate that deep regression NNs, e.g., FBPConvNet, can have high overfitting risks, while our proposed BCD-Net has low overfitting risks, and gives more stable reconstruction. These show that MBIR modules benefit regularizing overfitting artifacts of regression NNs.

The BCD-Net result in the second row of Fig. 2 shows non-uniform spatial resolution or noise; see blurry artifacts particularly around the center of the reconstructed image. One can reduce such blurs by including the technique of controlling local spatial resolution or noise in the reconstructed images [7] to MBIR modules.

4   Conclusions

The proposed BCD-Net uses layer-wise autoencoding CNNs and achieves significantly more accurate low-dose CT reconstruction, compared to the state-of-the-art MBIR method using a learned transform [15]. BCD-Net provides better reconstruction quality, compared to a state-of-the-art iterative NN, ADMM-Net [14]. Taking both benefits of MBIR and low-complexity CNN (i.e., convolutional autoencoder), BCD-Net significantly improves the generalization capability, compared to a state-of-the-art (non-iterative) deep regression NN, FBPConvNet [8]. In addition, applying faster numerical solvers, e.g., APG-M, to MBIR modules leads to faster and more accurate BCD-Net, and those with sufficient iterations can lead to the sequence convergence. Future work will explore BCD-Net with local spatial resolution controls [7], to reduce blur around the center of reconstructed images.

Acknowledgments. This work is supported in part by NSFC 61501292 and NIH U01 EB018753. The authors thank GE Healthcare for supplying the clinical data. The authors thank Zhipeng Li for his help with debugging the codes.

References

1. Aggarwal, H.K., Mani, M.P., Jacob, M.: MoDL: model based deep learning architecture for inverse problems. IEEE Trans. Med. Imag. **38**(2), 394–405 (2019)
2. Beck, A., Teboulle, M.: A fast iterative shrinkage-thresholding algorithm for linear inverse problems. SIAM J. Imaging Sci. **2**(1), 183–202 (2009)
3. Chan, S.H., Wang, X., Elgendy, O.A.: Plug-and-play ADMM for image restoration: fixed-point convergence and applications. IEEE Trans. Comput. Imag. **3**(1), 84–98 (2017)
4. Chun, I.Y., Fessler, J.A.: Deep BCD-net using identical encoding-decoding CNN structures for iterative image recovery. In: Proceedings of IEEE IVMSP Workshop, Zagori, Greece, pp. 1–5, June 2018
5. Chun, I.Y., Fessler, J.A.: Convolutional analysis operator learning: acceleration and convergence. IEEE Trans. Image Process. (2019, to appear). https://arxiv.org/abs/1802.05584

6. Chun, I.Y., Huang, Z., Lim, H., Fessler, J.A.: Momentum-Net: fast and convergent recurrent neural network for inverse problems (2019, submitted). http://arxiv.org/abs/1907.11818
7. Fessler, J.A., Rogers, W.L.: Spatial resolution properties of penalized-likelihood image reconstruction methods: space-invariant tomographs. IEEE Trans. Image Process. **5**(9), 1346–1358 (1996)
8. Jin, K.H., McCann, M.T., Froustey, E., Unser, M.: Deep convolutional neural network for inverse problems in imaging. IEEE Trans. Image Process. **26**(9), 4509–4522 (2017)
9. Kingma, D.P., Ba, J.L.: Adam: a method for stochastic optimization. In: Proceedings of ICLR 2015, San Diego, CA, pp. 1–15, May 2015
10. Rockafellar, R.T.: Monotone operators and the proximal point algorithm. SIAM J. Control Optm. **14**(5), 877–898 (1976)
11. Romano, Y., Elad, M., Milanfar, P.: The little engine that could: regularization by denoising (RED). SIAM J. Imaging Sci. **10**(4), 1804–1844 (2017)
12. Segars, W.P., Mahesh, M., Beck, T.J., Frey, E.C., Tsui, B.M.: Realistic CT simulation using the 4D XCAT phantom. Med. Phys. **35**(8), 3800–3808 (2008)
13. Taylor, A.B., Hendrickx, J.M., Glineur, F.: Exact worst-case performance of first-order methods for composite convex optimization. SIAM J. Optim. **27**(3), 1283–1313 (2017)
14. Yang, Y., Sun, J., Li, H., Xu, Z.: Deep ADMM-Net for compressive sensing MRI. In: Proceedings of NIPS 29, Long Beach, CA, pp. 10–18, December 2016
15. Zheng, X., Chun, I.Y., Li, Z., Long, Y., Fessler, J.A.: Sparse-view X-ray CT reconstruction using ℓ_1 prior with learned transform. Submitted, February 2019. http://arxiv.org/abs/1711.00905

Abdominal Adipose Tissue Segmentation in MRI with Double Loss Function Collaborative Learning

Siyuan Pan[1], Xuhong Hou[2], Huating Li[2(✉)], Bin Sheng[1(✉)], Ruogu Fang[3(✉)], Yuxin Xue[1], Weiping Jia[2], and Jing Qin[4]

[1] Department of Computer Science and Engineering, Shanghai Jiao Tong University, Shanghai, China
shengbin@sjtu.edu.cn

[2] Shanghai Jiao Tong University Affiliated Sixth People's Hospital, Shanghai, China
huarting99@sjtu.edu.cn

[3] Department of Biomedical Engineering, University of Florida, Gainesville, USA
Ruogu.Fang@bme.ufl.edu

[4] Centre for Smart Health, School of Nursing, The Hong Kong Polytechnic University, Hong Kong, China

Abstract. Deep learning has shown promising progress in computer-aided medical image diagnosis in recent years, such adipose tissue segmentation. Generally, training a high-performance deep segmentation model requires a large amount of labeled images. However, in clinical practice many labels are saved in numerical forms rather than image forms while relabelling images with manual segmentation is extremely time-consuming and laborious. To fill in this gap between numerical labels and image-based labels, we propose a novel double loss function to train an adipose segmentation model through collaborative learning. Specifically, the double loss function leverages a large volume of numerical labels available and a small volume of images labels. To validate our collaborative learning model, we collect one dataset of 300 high quality MR images with pixel-level segmentation labels and another dataset of 9000 clinical quantitative MR images with numerical labels of the number of pixels in subcutaneous adipose tissue (SAT), visceral adipose tissue (VAT), and Non-adipose tissues. Our approach achieves 94.3% and 90.8% segmentation accuracy for SAT and VAT respectively in the dataset with image labels, and 93.6% and 88.7% segmentation accuracy for the dataset with only numerical labels. The proposed approach can be generalize to a broad range of clinical problems with different types of ground truth labels.

Keywords: Segmentation · Adipose · Weak supervised data · Deep learning · Multi-correlation data

© Springer Nature Switzerland AG 2019
D. Shen et al. (Eds.): MICCAI 2019, LNCS 11769, pp. 41–49, 2019.
https://doi.org/10.1007/978-3-030-32226-7_5

1   Introduction

Obesity is a significant risk factor of metabolic and cardiovascular disorders, such as type 2 diabetes mellitus, atherosclerosis and hypertension [4]. Numerous studies [7] have shown that the accumulation of visceral adipose tissue (VAT) and subcutaneous adipose tissue (SAT) have substantial correlations with obesity-related diseases. Herein, accurate and rapid quantification through segmenting VAT and SAT in abdominal nuclear magnetic images (MRIs) is critical for clinical assessment and prediction of obesity-related syndromes.

Researchers have made numerous efforts in segmenting adipose tissues from MRI images, mainly in two categories: image processing based [9,12] and machine learning based methods [6]. For image processing based methods, it is challenging to segment adipose tissues from MRI scans due to their inhomogeneous intensities, low contrast, shape variation, and structural complexity. For machine learning methods, a large amount of high quality MRIs with manual segmentation labels are needed. While manual labeling is costly, laborious, subjective, and time-consuming, the numerical labels reflecting the volume of VAT and SAT are more easily available from commercial software and can be collected at patient admission. However these numerical labels are not commonly used for model training due to the lack of pixel-level segmentation information and low precision in the number of pixels for each tissue type.

To address the above challenges, in this paper, we propose a hybrid deep learning based framework which utilizes both high quality MRIs with pixel-level segmentation labels and numerical labels collected at admission time. As shown in Fig. 1, our proposed framework uses two types of input data: MR images with manual segmented SAT and VAT at pixel level (a.k.a. strongly supervised data); MR images with pixels count of SAT and VAT (weakly supervised data). We designed a new loss function L_{value} and a cooperative training method to train on both types of data.

The main contributions of our work are:

1. A general framework to integrate pixel-level and image-level numerical labels is proposed for image segmentation through collaborative learning.
2. A new loss function to utilize weekly supervised data is designed to fill the gap between pixel-level segmentation labels and image-level pixel counts for each class.
3. We demonstrate that the proposed cooperative training method with the double loss function outperforms traditional semi-supervised methods on clinical datasets for abdominal adipose tissue segmentation.

2   Methods

2.1   Dataset

Our development dataset was acquired from 9,300 subjects, including 4230 subjects with normal weights, 3,164 overweight, and 1,906 obese subjects. The

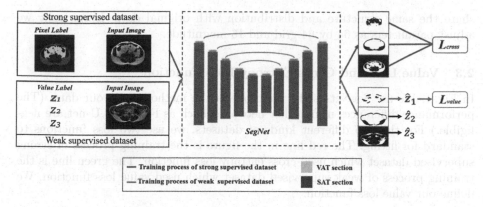

Fig. 1. Overview of proposed method (Color figure online)

statistics of the data are presented in Table 1. The abdominal MR images data were obtained from T1 weighted MR scanner (GE Healthcare, Waukesha, WI). 8–10 contiguous axial slices centered at the L4-L5 level of the abdomen were acquired from each subject, and the representative slice at the umbilicus level was used in our experiments. Each image has 512×512 pixels and each pixel is $0.86 \times 0.86\,\text{mm}^2$. Two radiologists with more than ten years of experiences delineated 300 images of umbilicus using the SliceOmatic software (TomoVision, Canada) to label SAT and VAT, which are used as the ground truth. The other 9,000 images were delineated by two radiologists but only pixel counts of SAT and VAT were recorded. All the images in our datasets are divided into training, validation, testing with a ratio of 7:2:1 randomly using stratified sampling.

Table 1. Data statistics of volunteers

Body type	BMI(kg/m^2)	Age	Numbers
Normal	18.50–23.99	44–70	4230
Overweight	24.00–27.99	44–70	3164
Obese	≥28.00	44–70	1906

Our two datasets include the strongly $S_1 = \{x, y, z\}$ and the weakly $S_2 = \{x, z\}$ supervised data. $z = \{z_1, z_2, z_3 \mid z_1 + z_2 + z_3 = N \times N\}$, where x denotes the source image, y is the pixel-to-pixel labeling, and z is the number of pixels belonging to three categories: (z_1 for VAT, z_2 for SAT, and z_3 for the other tissue types). N denotes the height and width of our image.

2.2 Data Augmentation

We use elastic transform technique [8] to increase volume of strong training data to 3000. This augment processing can produce a mass of synthetic images which share the same structure and distribution with original data. Empirically we adjust parameters as 64 by 64 grid and 16 magnitude.

2.3   Value Loss and Cross Entropy Loss Function

In Fig. 1, We use SegNet as the backbone of the method to fit our data. (The performance differences using other networks, such as FCN and U-net are negligible.) For the two different kinds of datasets, we use two loss functions to standard for fitting. The red line in the figure is the training process of strong supervised dataset which used cross entropy loss function. The green line is the training process of weak supervised dataset which used value loss function. We define our value loss function:

$$L_k = \frac{1}{N \times N}(\hat{z}_k - z_k)^2, k \in (1, 2, 3) \tag{1}$$

where $\hat{z}_k = \sum_{i=1}^{N} \sum_{j=1}^{N} p_{i,j,k}$ and $p_{i,j,k}$ denotes the output probability of the k channel of the (i,j) pixel in the image. The softmax function is $p_{i,j,k} = \frac{e^{f_{i,j,k}(x)}}{\sum_{l=1}^{C} e^{f_{i,l,k}(x)}}$, C denotes the number of output channels (3 in our task), $f_{i,j,k}(x)$ denotes the output value of the k channel of the (i,j) pixel from the network. The gradient of this loss is:

$$\frac{\partial L_k}{\partial f_{i,j,k}(x)} = \frac{\partial L_k}{\partial p_{i,j,k}} \cdot \frac{\partial p_{i,j,k}}{\partial f_{i,j,k}(x)} \tag{2}$$

$$\frac{\partial L_k}{\partial p_{i,j,k}} = \frac{2}{N \times N}\left(\sum_{i=1}^{N} \sum_{j=1}^{N} p_{i,j,k} - z_k\right) \tag{3}$$

Here we give the result of derivation of softmax function.

$$\frac{\partial p_{i,j,k}}{\partial f_{i,j,k}(x)} = \begin{cases} p_{i,j,k} \cdot (1 - p_{i,j,k}) & l = k \\ -p_{i,j,k} \cdot p_{i,j,l} & l \neq k \end{cases} \tag{4}$$

Then we can calculate the output gradient $\frac{\partial L_k}{\partial f_{i,j,k}(x)} = \frac{2}{N \times N}(\sum_{i=1}^{N} \sum_{j=1}^{N} p_{i,j,k} - z_k) \cdot p_{i,j,k} \cdot (1 - p_{i,j,k})$, We can find two points:

- $L_1 + L_2 + L_3 = \frac{2}{N \times N} \sum_{k=1}^{3} (\sum_{i=1}^{N} \sum_{i=1}^{N} p_{i,j,k} - z_k) = 0$, if we consider these three loss together, then whatever the final predicted value, the whole network will not get any gradient.
- Weak supervise data itself can only play a regulatory role in macro-level. For example, if the final value of VAT is not up to the standard value, then each pixel will obtain positive gradient on VAT channel. Although this large amount of data can provide macro information, it lacks semantic information in semantic segmentation. The intuitive representation of neural networks is that some semantically easy pixels will be misclassified. The results are showed in experiment Sect. 3.3. Then we set cross entropy Loss function to train the strong supervised data can limit this negative effect.

$$L_{cross1} = -\frac{1}{N \times N} \cdot \frac{1}{C} \cdot \sum_{i=1}^{N} \cdot \sum_{j=1}^{N} \sum_{k=1}^{C} y_{i,j,k} \log(p_{i,j,k}) \qquad (5)$$

$$L_{cross2} = -\frac{1}{N \times N \times C} \cdot \sum_{i,j,k=1}^{N \times N \times C} (y_{i,j,k} \log(p_{i,j,k}) + (1 - y_{i,j,k}) \log(1 - p_{i,j,k})) \qquad (6)$$

There are two kinds of cross entropy functions, we choose the second loss because it will use the channel probability of scattered errors to correct the errors brought from value loss function. In this task, we just use the VAT loss as our value loss function for two reasons: (1) We mainly segment the SAT and VAT parts. (2) If value loss of VAT is higher means SAT part is low and the converse is also true. So our loss function is:

$$L_{all} = L_{cross2} + \lambda L_1 \qquad (7)$$

λ is used to balance the gap between the two loss. We have tried 0,1,0.3,0.5 and 1.0 as the value of λ and 0.1 is the best one.

3 Experiments and Results

3.1 Evaluation Metrics

We used the Dice Ratio (DR) to assess the agreement between the manual annotations (or ground truth) and the output of the segmentation algorithm. We let A and B denote the binary segmentation labels generated manually and computationally, respectively, and $DR = \frac{2|A \cap B|}{|A|+|B|}$, where $|.|$ represents the number of positive elements in the binary segmentation and $|A \cap B|$ is the number of positive elements shared by A and B. The DR ranges from 0 (no agreement) to 1 (perfect agreement). The modified Hausdorff distance (MHD) is another metric used to evaluate segmentation results. Supposing that C and D are two sets of positive pixels identified manually and computationally, we define $MHD(C, D) = max(d(C, D), d(D, C))$, where $d(C, D) = max_{c \in C} d(c, D)$, and $d(c, D) = min_{d \in D} \|c - d\|$. Small values indicate a high degree of proximity between two sets, which implies a greater accuracy in the segmentation. The weakly-supervised data have no pixel labels. We calculated the accuracy intuitively as $acc = \frac{1}{k} \sum_{i=0}^{k} (1.0 - \frac{|z_i - \hat{z}_i|}{z_i})$ where $\hat{z}_i$ represents the predicted number of pixels for each category.

3.2 Semi-supervised Algorithm

Semi-supervised learning is a universal approach well suited to performing repeated tasks. To verify that our proposed joint-learning scheme is better suited and more effective than semi-supervised learning, we set up a comparison experiment. Our model was trained using the set of strong supervised data. After each iteration, we tested the model with the weak supervised data. If the accuracy of the SAT and VAT results were both higher than the set threshold, the data were then transferred to the training set, and the results of these images will transfer together as their labels. The algorithm terminated when no data was transferred during more than 10 iterations. The results are shown in Table 3.

3.3 Double Loss Function Collaborative Training

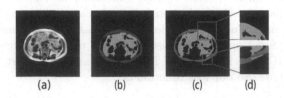

(a)   (b)   (c)   (d)

Fig. 2. (a) is the source image, (b) ground truth, (c) is the result from the network trained by weakly supervised data after pretrained by strong supervised data. (d) enlarged the selection part from c.

We leveraged SegNet [2] to train our segmentation network. We used the network pretrained with the strong supervised data to train the weak supervised data. We found that all pixel values approached the average of three numerical proportions. This can be explained intuitively by supposing that some pixels that are obviously not VAT become misclassified as SAT from the network in Fig. 2. The experiment demonstrates that the loss function for the weak supervised data depends not on the probability distribution but on the probability itself.

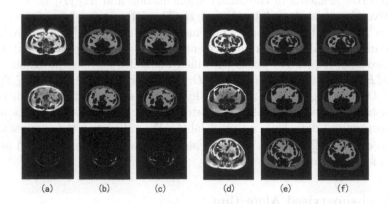

(a)   (b)   (c)   (d)   (e)   (f)

Fig. 3. The result of the test images segmented by double loss function collaborative training network. a and d are the source images, b and e are the results, c and f are the groundtruth

We implement our algorithm proposed in method Sect. 2.3. In the Eq. 7, the λ is used to balance the gap between the two losses preventing the gradient from the value loss bigger orders of magnitude than the gradient from the cross entropy loss, we set 0.1 in our task.

The value loss function will lead to the result that the probabilities in final output channels gradually tend to (move toward) the ratio of VAT, SAT and non-adipose part. Thus we utilize two methods to restrict this phenomenon. First, reduce the proportion of weak supervised data. According to empirical analysis in experiment process, we define the ratio of two dataset S_1 and S_2 as 7:1. Second, the problem illustrated in Fig. 2 still remains in the results of trained models, which is shown in column b and e of Fig. 3. Therefore the DenseCRF which presented in [11] is used for post-processing. With DenseCRF, The MAP (maximum a posteriori) is used to estimate the label of each pixel. The potential energy function takes the position of pixels into account to correct the errors mentioned above. 3000 training images were generated from the training set S_1 using data argumentation algorithm. The results are shown in Tables 2 and 3.

Table 2. Segmentation performance achieved by MSDNN, SVM, RF, Sadananthan and our method. The best performance was highlighted.

Algorithms	Dice Ratio (%)			MHD		
	Normal	Over weight	Obese	Normal	Over weight	Obese
SAT						
Sadananthan [1]	89.84 ± 4.13	88.18 ± 4.09	86.52 ± 3.96	1.84 ± 2.47	1.07 ± 0.49	2.38 ± 1.11
SVM [10]	82.24 ± 7.21	82.13 ± 5.02	83.42 ± 4.77	7.84 ± 3.00	8.03 ± 3.27	7.28 ± 2.95
RF [3]	93.58 ± 4.56	93.73 ± 3.05	93.62 ± 4.18	2.06 ± 1.14	6.27 ± 0.54	2.01 ± 2.47
MSDNN [5]	95.02 ± 3.06	95.59 ± 1.97	96.53 ± 1.36	**0.51 ± 0.61**	0.50 ± 0.39	0.68 ± 0.75
our method	**95.77 ± 1.01**	**96.30 ± 3.11**	96.60 ± 2.06	0.60 ± 0.36	**0.44 ± 0.17**	**0.46 ± 0.4**
VAT						
Sadananthan [1]	73.31 ± 4.09	75.76 ± 5.37	77.94 ± 5.23	5.19 ± 2.48	5.59 ± 1.72	6.25 ± 2.00
SVM [10]	64.18 ± 9.42	65.34 ± 7.84	70.01 ± 8.10	6.90 ± 2.91	6.89 ± 2.70	6.02 ± 1.98
RF [3]	80.40 ± 9.13	82.92 ± 4.22	83.80 ± 9.50	2.67 ± 1.78	3.00 ± 1.49	2.49 ± 1.19
MSDNN [5]	83.56 ± 5.14	86.03 ± 3.6	87.82 ± 3.61	1.48 ± 1.17	1.25 ± 0.79	0.92 ± 0.95
our method	**89.17 ± 2.11**	**91.30 ± 2.37**	**90.13 ± 2.36**	0.83 ± 0.42	0.74 ± 0.37	0.66 ± 0.38

Table 3. Accuracy of the dataset tested by the network trained using only the strong supervised data, the network trained by both kinds of data, and the semi-supervised algorithm. The best performance is highlighted in each case.

Algorithms	Strongly supervised data		Weakly supervised data	
	SAT	VAT	SAT	VAT
The network trained by only strong supervised data	94.3	91.0	88.7	83.6
Semi-supervised algorithm	94.1	**91.3**	92.0	86.6
The network trained by both two kinds of data	94.3	90.8	**93.6**	**88.7**

4   Conclusion and Discussion

Our method performs significantly better than the other algorithms, as confirmed by the comparison in Table 2. As shown in Table 3, a model trained only with the strongly supervised data cannot fit the weakly supervised data well, indicating that the network has been overfitted and is incapable of generalization. The semi-supervised algorithm performs better. However, when the loss function is decreased to a low score, many images will get a higher value than the set threshold; if they transfer into the training set, the loss function will again increase. It is therefore difficult to adjust the learning rate and the sequence of pictures afferent of neural network.

As suggested from Fig. 3, our model performs unsatisfactorily when the image quality is poor (for example, when MRI images are blurred, corresponding to group c). Occasionally, pixels belonging to VAT are incorrectly segmented as SAT. This shortcoming is due to the second contribution to loss in our algorithm being based on probability, as explained in Sect. 3.3. According to Table 3, this problem does not occur with the first two algorithms. DenseCRF, presented by [11] can solve the problem. The original results still put just for easy to discuss.

To conclude, the present study aimed to segment MR images of abdominal adipose tissues. The quality and quantity of data are notoriously essential for training neural networks. Within this context, vast amounts of existing clinical data can be exploited, even dating from a time long before the relevance of labels to deep learning was realized. In fact, collecting large amount of fine-grained data requires long time. As a result, it's very common in medical practice field to preserve labels in format of values instead of pixel-level images. Compared with spending time relabeling these data, it's efficient to use existing data to train the model. To this end, we proposed a collaborative training algorithm based on a double loss function to fit two different kinds of data. This method is accurate and suitable for the task of abdominal fat segmentation.

Acknowledgments. This work was supported in part by the National Natural Science Foundation of China under Grant 61872241 and Grant 61572316, in part by the National Key Research and Development Program of China under Grant 2017YFE0104000 and Grant 2016YFC1300302, in part by the Hong Kong Research Grants Council (No. PolyU 152035/17E), in part by the Science and Technology Commission of Shanghai Municipality One Belt And One Road International Joint Laboratory Construction Project under Grant 18410750700 and in part by the Science and Technology Commission of Shanghai Municipality under Grant 17411952600 and Grant 16DZ0501100.

References

1. Anand, S.S., KN, P.B., et al.: Automated segmentation of visceral and subcutaneous (deep and superficial) adipose tissues in normal and overweight men. J. Magn. Reson. Imaging **41**(4), 924–934 (2015)

2. Badrinarayanan, V., Kendall, A., Cipolla, R.: Segnet: a deep convolutional encoder-decoder architecture for image segmentation. IEEE Trans. Pattern Anal. Mach. Intell. **39**(12), 2481–2495 (2017)
3. Criminisi, A., Shotton, J., Konukoglu, E., et al.: Decision forests: a unified framework for classification, regression, density estimation, manifold learning and semi-supervised learning. Found. Trends® Comput. Graph. Vis. **7**(2–3), 81–227 (2012)
4. Després, J.P., Lemieux, I.: Abdominal obesity and metabolic syndrome. Nature **444**(7121), 881 (2006)
5. Jiang, F., et al.: Abdominal adipose tissues extraction using multi-scale deep neural network. Neurocomputing **229**(C), 23–33 (2017)
6. Langner, T., et al.: Fully convolutional networks for automated segmentation of abdominal adipose tissue depots in multicenter water-fat MRI. Magn. Reson. Med. **81**(4), 2736–2745 (2019)
7. Matsushita, Y., et al.: Associations of visceral and subcutaneous fat areas with the prevalence of metabolic risk factor clustering in 6,292 Japanese individuals: the hitachi health study. Diab. Care **33**(9), 2117–2119 (2010)
8. Ronneberger, O., Fischer, P., Brox, T.: U-net: convolutional networks for biomedical image segmentation. In: Navab, N., Hornegger, J., Wells, W.M., Frangi, A.F. (eds.) MICCAI 2015. LNCS, vol. 9351, pp. 234–241. Springer, Cham (2015). https://doi.org/10.1007/978-3-319-24574-4_28
9. Thörmer, G., et al.: Software for automated MRI-based quantification of abdominal fat and preliminary evaluation in morbidly obese patients. J. Magn. Reson. Imaging **37**(5), 1144–1150 (2013)
10. Tsai, C.H., Lin, C.Y., Lin, C.J.: Incremental and decremental training for linear classification. In: Proceedings of the 20th ACM SIGKDD International Conference on Knowledge Discovery and Data Mining, pp. 343–352. ACM (2014)
11. Wu, X.: Fully convolutional networks for semantic segmentation. Comput. Sci. (2015)
12. Zhou, A., Murillo, H., Peng, Q.: Novel segmentation method for abdominal fat quantification by MRI. J. Magn. Reson. Imaging **34**(4), 852–860 (2011)

Closing the Gap Between Deep and Conventional Image Registration Using Probabilistic Dense Displacement Networks

Mattias P. Heinrich$^{(\boxtimes)}$ (iD)

Institute of Medical Informatics, Universität zu Lübeck, Lübeck, Germany
heinrich@imi.uni-luebeck.de
https://github.com/multimodallearning/pdd_net

Abstract. Nonlinear image registration continues to be a fundamentally important tool in medical image analysis. Diagnostic tasks, image-guided surgery and radiotherapy as well as motion analysis all rely heavily on accurate intra-patient alignment. Furthermore, inter-patient registration enables atlas-based segmentation or landmark localisation and shape analysis. When labelled scans are scarce and anatomical differences large, conventional registration has often remained superior to deep learning methods that have so far mainly dealt with relatively small or low-complexity deformations. We address this shortcoming by leveraging ideas from probabilistic dense displacement optimisation that has excelled in many registration tasks with large deformations. We propose to design a network with approximate min-convolutions and mean field inference for differentiable displacement regularisation within a discrete weakly-supervised registration setting. By employing these meaningful and theoretically proven constraints, our learnable registration algorithm contains very few trainable weights (primarily for feature extraction) and is easier to train with few labelled scans. It is very fast in training and inference and achieves state-of-the-art accuracies for the challenging inter-patient registration of abdominal CT outperforming previous deep learning approaches by 15% Dice overlap.

Keywords: Registration · Deep learning · Probabilistic · Abdominal

1 Introduction and Related Work

Conventional medical image registration mostly relies on iterative and multi-scale warping of a moving towards a fixed scan by minimising a dissimilarity metric together with a regularisation penalty. Deep learning based image registration (DLIR) aims to mimic this process by training a convolutional network

Electronic supplementary material The online version of this chapter (https://doi.org/10.1007/978-3-030-32226-7_6) contains supplementary material, which is available to authorized users.

© Springer Nature Switzerland AG 2019
D. Shen et al. (Eds.): MICCAI 2019, LNCS 11769, pp. 50–58, 2019.
https://doi.org/10.1007/978-3-030-32226-7_6

that can predict the non-linear alignment function given two new unseen scans. Thus instead of multiple warping steps a single feed-forward transfer function has to be found using many convolution layers. The supervision for DLIR can be based on automatic or manual correspondences, semantic labels or intrinsic cost functions. It has immense potential for time-sensitive applications such as image-guidance, fusion, tracking and shape analysis through multi-atlas registration. However, due to the large space of potential deformations that can map two corresponding anatomies onto one another, the problem is much less constrained than image segmentation and therefore remains an open challenge.

A number of approaches has been applied to brain registration [1,17], which usually deals with localised deformations of few millimetres and for which huge labelled datasets ($\gg$100 scans) exist. For other anatomies in the abdomen, the prostate or lungs, with shape variations of several centimetres, DLIR was mainly applied to less complex cases of intra-patient registration [6,9]. For inhale-exhale lung registration the accuracy of DLIR is still inferior to conventional approaches: $\approx$ 2.5 mm in [13,15] compared to <1 mm in [12]. When training the state-of-the-art weakly-supervised DLIR approach Label-Reg [6] on abdominal CT [14] for inter-patient alignment, we reached an average Dice of only 42.7%, which is still substantially worse than the conventional NiftyReg algorithm [10] with a Dice of 56.1% and justifies further research.

Our hypothesis is that large and highly deformable transformations across different patients are difficult to model with a deep continuous regression network without resorting to complex multi-stage warping pipelines. Instead the use of discrete registration, which explores a large space of quantised displacements simultaneously, has been shown to capture abdominal and chest deformations more effectively [5,12,16] and can be realised with few or a single warping step. Unsurprisingly, discrete displacement settings have been explored in 2D vision for DLIR: namely the FlowNet-C [2]. A *correlation layer* (see Eq. 1 in [2]) is proposed that contains no trainable weights and computes a similarity metric of features from two images by shifting the moving image with a densely quantised displacement space (21×21 pixel offsets) yielding a 441-channel joint feature map. Next, a very large $441(+32) \times 256 \times 3 \times 3$ kernel is learned (followed by further convolutions) that disregards the explicit 4D geometry of the displacement space. Hence, the large number of optimisable parameters results in huge requirements of supervised training data. Extending this idea to 3D is very difficult as the dimensionality increases to 6D after dense correlation and has not been yet considered despite its benefits. Probabilistic and uncertainty modelling has been studied in DLIR, cf. [9,17], but not in a discrete setting.

Contributions. We propose a new learning model for DLIR that better leverages the advantages of probabilistic dense displacement sampling by introducing strong regularisation with differentiable constraints that explicitly considers the 6D nature of the problem. We hence decouple convolutional feature learning from the fitting of a spatial transformation using mean-field inference for regularisation [8,18] and approximate min-convolutions [3] for computing inter-label compatibilities. Our feature extractor uses 3D deformable convolutions [4] and is very lightweight. To our knowledge this is the first approach that combines discrete DLIR with the differentiable use of mean-field regularisation. In contrast to previous work, our model requires fewer trainable weights, captures larger deformations and can be trained from few labelled scans to high accuracy. We also introduce a new non-local label loss for improved guidance instead of the more widely used spatial transformer based loss.

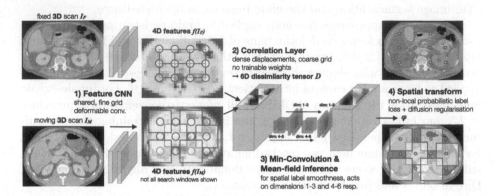

Fig. 1. Concept of probabilistic dense displacement network: (1) deformable convolution layers extract features for both fixed and moving image. (2) the correlation layer evaluates for each 3D grid point a dense displacement space yielding a 6D dissimilarity map. (3) spatial filters that promote smoothness act on dimensions 4–6 (minconvolutions) and dim. 1–3 (mean-field inference) in alternation. (4) the probabilistic transform distribution obtained using a softmax (over dim. 4–6) is used in a non-local label loss and converted to 3D displacements for a diffusion regularisation and to warp images

2   Methods

We aim to align a fixed I_F and moving I_M 3D scan by finding a spatial transformation φ based on a learned feature mapping f of I_F and I_M subject to constraints on the regularity of φ. In order to learn a suitable feature extraction that is invariant to noise and uninformative contrast-variations, we provide a supervisory label during training for both volumes ℓ_F and ℓ_M, for which $\ell_F \approx \varphi \circ \ell_M$ should hold after registration. We define spatial coordinates as continuous variables $\mathbf{x} \in (-1, +1)^3$ and use trilinear interpolation to sample from discrete grids. φ is parameterised with a set of $\mathbf{k} \in |K| \in \mathbb{R}^3$ (a few thousands) control points on a coarser grid. The range of displacements $\mathbf{d}$ is constrained to a discrete displacement space, with linear spacing e.g. $\mathcal{L} = q \cdot \{-1, -\frac{6}{7}, -\frac{5}{7}, \ldots, +\frac{5}{7}, +\frac{6}{7}, +1\}^3$, where q is a scalar that defines the capture range and in our case $|\mathcal{L}|$ is 3375. The network model should predict a 6D tensor of displacement probabilities $K \in \mathbb{R}^3 \times \mathcal{L} \in \mathbb{R}^3$, where the sum over the dimensions 4-6 of $\mathcal{L}$ for each control point is 1. The (inner) product of the probabilities with the displacements $\mathcal{L}$ yields the weighted average of these probabilistic estimates to obtain 3D displacements for φ during inference.

(1) **Convolutional feature learning network:** To learn a meaningful nonlinear mapping from input intensities to a dense feature volume (with $|c| = 16$ channels and a stride of 3), we employ the Obelisk approach [4], which comprises a 3D deformable convolution with trainable offsets followed by a simple 1×1 MLP and captures spatial context very effectively. We extend the authors' implementation by adding a normal $5 \times 5 \times 5$ convolution kernel with 4 channels prior to the Obelisk layer to also learn edge-like features. The network has 64 spatial filter offsets and in total 120k trainable parameters, shared for fixed and moving scan to yield $f(I_F)$ and $f(I_M)$.

(2) **Correlation layer for dense displacement dissimilarity:** Given the feature representation of the first part, we aim to find a regularised displacement field that assigns a vector $\mathbf{d}$ to every control point for a nonlinear transform $\varphi(\mathbf{k}) \leftarrow \mathbf{d}$ that maximises the (label) similarity between fixed and warped moving scan. As done in conventional discrete registration [5] and the correlation layer of [2], we perform a dense evaluation of a similarity metric over the displacement search space $\mathbf{d} \in \mathcal{L}$. The negated mean squared error (MSE) across the feature dimension c of learned descriptors is used to obtain the 6D tensor of dissimilarities $\mathcal{D}(\mathbf{k}, \mathbf{d}) = -\frac{1}{|c|} \sum_c (f_c(I_F)_\mathbf{k} - f_c(I_M)_{\mathbf{k}+\mathbf{d}})^2$. Different metrics such as the correlation coefficient could be employed. Due to the sparsity of the control points the displacement similarity evaluation requires less than 2 GFlops in our experiments. The capture range of displacements q is set to 0.4.

3) **Regularisation using min-convolutions and mean-field inference:** Since nonlinear registration is usually ill-posed, additional priors are used to keep deformations spatially smooth. In contrast to other work on DLIR, which in principle learn an unconstrained deformation and only enforce spatial smoothness as loss term, we propose to model regularisation constraints as part of the network architecture. A diffusion-like regularisation penalty for displacements based on their squared difference $\mathcal{R}(\mathbf{d}_i, \mathbf{d}_j) = ||\mathbf{d}_i - \mathbf{d}_j||^2$ is often used in Markov random field (MRF) registration [3] and e.g. optimised with loopy belief propagation (LBP). [7] and [18] integrated smoothness constraints of graphical models into end-to-end learned segmentation networks. Since, LBP requires many iterations to yield an optimum and is hence not well suited as unrolled network layers, we use the fast mean-field inference (two iterations) used for discrete optimisation in [8] (in [18] 5 iterations were used). It consists of two alternating steps: a label-compatibility transform that acts on spatial control points independently and a filter-based message passing implemented using average pooling layers with a stride of 1.

As noted in [3] the diffusion regularisation for a dense displacement space can be computed using min-convolutions with a lower envelope of parabolas rooted at the (3D) displacement offsets with heights equaling to the sum of dissimilarity term and the previous iteration of the mean-field inference. This lower envelope is not directly differentiable, but we can obtain a very accurate approximation using first, a min-pooling (with stride $= 1$) that finds local minima in the cost tensor followed by two average pooling operations (with stride $= 1$) that provide a quadratic smoothing. As shown with blue blocks in Fig. 1, the novel regularisation part of our approach comprises min- and average-pooling layers that act on the 3 displacement dimensions (min-convolution) followed by average filtering on the 3 spatial dimensions (mean-field inference). Before each operation, scaling and bias factors $\alpha_1 - \alpha_6$ are introduced and optimised together with the feature layers during end-to-end training.

Probabilistic Transform Losses and Label Supervision: We can make further use of the probabilistic nature of our displacement sampling and specify our supervised label loss term based on a non-local means weighting [11]. I.e., we first convert the negated output of the regularisation part (scaled by α_6) into pseudo-probabilities using a softmax computed over the displacements. Next, one-hot representations of the moving segmentation are sampled at the same spatially displaced locations and these vectors are multiplied by the estimated probabilities to compute the label loss as MSE w.r.t. the ground truth (one-hot) segmentation. The continuous valued 3D displacement field φ is obtained by a weighted average of the probabilistic estimates multiplied with the displacement labels and followed by trilinear interpolation to the image resolution. A diffusion regularisation penalty over all 3 spatial gradients $\lambda \cdot (|\nabla\varphi_1|^2 + |\nabla\varphi_2|^2 + |\nabla\varphi_3|^3)$ of the displacement field is employed to enable a user-defined balancing between a smooth transform (with low standard deviation of Jacobians) and accurate structural alignment.

3   Experimental Validation

To demonstrate the ability of our method to capture very large deformations across different patients within the human abdomen, we performed experiments with a 3-fold cross validation on 10 contrast-enhanced 3D CT scans of the VIS-CERAL3 training data [14] with each nine anatomical structures manually segmented: ■ liver, ■ spleen, ■ pancreas, ▨ gallbladder, ▨ unary bladder, ■ right kidney, ■ left kidney, ▨ right psoas major muscle (psoas) and ■ left psoas (see Fig. 2). The images were resampled to isotropic voxel sizes of 1.5 mm^3 with dimensions of $233 \times 168 \times 286$ voxels and without any manual pre-alignment.

We compare our **probabilistic dense displacement network (pdd-net)**[1] with the two conventional algorithms **NiftyReg** [10] and **deeds** [5] that performed best in the inter-patient abdominal CT registration study of [16], a task not yet tackled by DLIR. NiftyReg was used with mutual information and a 5-level multi-resolution scheme to capture large deformations and has a run-time of 40–50 s. Deeds was considered with a single scale dense displacement space (which takes about 4–6 s) and then extended to three-levels of discrete optimisation (25–35 s run-time). Next, we trained the weakly-supervised DLIR method

---

[1] Our code with all implementation details will be made publicly available.

Label-Reg [6] on our data (in >24 h per fold). To reduce memory requirements below 32 GBytes, the resolution was reduced to 2.2 mm and the base channel number halved to 16. Further small adjustments were made to optimise for inter-patient training. We implemented a 3D extension of **FlowNet-C** [2] in pytorch with Obelisk feature extraction, a dense correlation layer and a regularisation network that has $|\mathcal{L}| = 3375$ input channels, comprises five 3D conv. layers with batch-norm and PReLU. It has 2 million weights and outputs a (non-probabilistic) 3D displacement field. In order to obtain meaningful results it was necessary to add a semantic segmentation loss to the intermediate output of the Obelisk layers. Our proposed method employs the same feature learning part (with 200k parameters) but now uses min-convolutions, mean-field inference (no semantic guidance) and the non-local label loss, which adds only 6 trainable weights (and not 2 million). The influence of these three choices is analysed with an ablation study, where a replacement of Obelisk feature learning with handcraft self-similarity context features [5] is also considered. We use a diffusion regularisation weight of $\lambda = 1.5$ for control grids of size 32^3 and affine augmentation of fixed scans throughout and trained our networks with Adam (learning rate of 0.01) for 1500 iterations in $\approx$90 min and $\approx$16 GByte of GPU memory with checkpointing. We implemented an instance-wise gradient descent optimiser that refines the feed-forward predictions. [1] also used this idea, but in our case it is a hundred times faster (0.24 s vs 24 s), since we can directly operate on the pre-computed displacement probabilities and require no iterative back-propagation through the network.

Table 1. Quantitative comparative evaluation of cross-validation for 10 scans of the VISCERAL anatomy 3 dataset, based on 24 combinations of test scans not seen in training (numbers are Dice scores). Our method **pdd-net** outperforms the considered DLIR methods, Label-Reg and FlowNet-C, by a margin of about 15% and closes the gap to conventional methods, NiftyReg and deeds, for this task. Our ablation study shows the benefits of (1) the use of learned Obelisk features vs handcrafted self-similarity context (SSC) descriptors, (2) employing mean-field inference and (3) the use of our new non-local label loss. °Additionally a fast instance level optimisation was implemented for **pdd-net+inst.**. *FlowNet-C is our 3D extension of [2] with Obelisk features and a trainable regularisation network. To compare: the Dice before registration was 30.0% on average.

Method	(1)	(2)	(3)	■	■	■	■	■	■	■	■	■	Average	std(Jac)	Runtime
Label-Reg				71	51	7	5	38	53	59	45	55	42.7±5.5	0.58	4 s
FlowNet-C*	✔		✔	73	45	9	7	40	48	53	49	52	41.8±7.2	0.34	0.13 s
pdd+SSC	✘	✔	✔	69	47	8	6	49	56	56	59	57	45.2±5.4	0.54	1.38 s
pdd w/o MF	✔	✘	✔	74	53	7	8	49	65	63	56	60	48.2±4.8	0.38	0.45 s
pdd w/o NL	✔	✔	✘	83	62	11	8	47	69	68	60	60	51.9±7.1	0.39	0.57 s
pdd-net	✔	✔	✔	84	62	13	12	57	76	70	69	68	**56.7±6.0**	0.40	0.57 s
pdd+inst.°	✔	✔	✔	83	66	18	14	58	77	74	68	68	**58.4±5.9**	0.26	0.71 s
deeds+SSC	1 level			72	50	14	13	51	54	58	62	60	48.0±6.8	0.67	4 s
deeds+SSC	3 level			78	62	18	19	60	71	67	70	69	57.0±8.2	0.27	25 s
NiftyReg NMI	5 level			77	58	19	27	56	70	65	67	66	56.1±18	1.30	42 s

4   Results and Discussions

The inference time of **pdd-net** is only 0.57 s, yielding plausible displacement fields with a standard deviation of the Jacobian determinants of 0.40 and <1% folding voxels (negative Jacobians). Table 1 shows the average Dice scores across 24 registrations of the cross-validation, where no labelled training scan was used for any evaluated test registration. Our method outperforms the two compared DL approaches, **Label-Reg** and **FlowNet-C**, by a margin of about 15% points and achieves 56.7% Dice for this challenging inter-patient task with an initial alignment of only 30%. It is 10% better than a comparable setting of the conventional discrete registration **deeds** with one grid-level. In particular the labels ■, ■, ■, ■, ■, ■ and ■ are very well aligned. Our instance-wise (per scan-pair) optimisation requires 0.24 s, reduces foldings (to less than 0.6%) and further increases the accuracy to 58.4%, which is above the level of the conventional multi-level registrations **deeds** and **NiftyReg**.

Comparing deeds+SSC with one grid-level to our variant pdd+SSC, which uses the same self-similarity features and only adapts the α parameters of the regularisation part, we get a similar accuracy and deformation complexity. This suggests that the proposed regularisation layers with min-convolutions and two mean-field inference steps can nearly match the capabilities of the full sequential MRF optimisation in [5]. Using weak supervision to learn features results in more than 20% increased Dice. The non-local loss term and our instance-wise fine-tuning, contribute further gains of 5% and 2% Dice overlap, respectively. The importance of the mean-field inference is clear, given the inferior quality of an unconstrained FlowNet-C with more trainable weights or our variant that only uses min-convolutions but no filtering in spatial domain. We achieve a more robust alignment quality (lower std.dev. of Dice) than conventional registration. Visual registration examples are shown in Fig. 2 and as surface-rendered video files in the supplementary material.

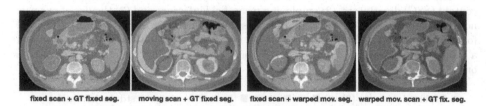

fixed scan + GT fixed seg.   moving scan + GT fixed seg.   fixed scan + warped mov. seg.   warped mov. scan + GT fix. seg.

Fig. 2. Visual outcome of proposed **pdd-net** method to register two patients and transfer a segmentation (moderate example). Most organs have been very well aligned and also anatomies that are not labelled in training (stomach, vertebras) can be registered.

5   Conclusion

Our novel **pdd-net** combines probabilistic dense displacements with differentiable mean-field regularisation to achieve one-to-one accuracies of over 70%

Dice for 7 larger anatomies for inter-patient abdominal CT registration. It outperforms the previous deep learning-based image registration (DLIR) methods, Label-Reg and FlowNet-C, by a margin of 15% points and can be robustly trained with few labelled scans. It closes the quality gap of DLIR (with small training datasets) to state-of-the-art conventional methods, exemplified by NiftyReg and deeds, while being extremely fast (0.5 s). Our concept offers a clear new potential to enable the use of DLIR in image-guided interventions, diagnostics and atlas-based shape analysis beyond the currently used pixel segmentation networks that lack geometric interpretability. Future work could yield further gains by using multiple alignment stages and a more adaptive sampling of control points. A more elaborate evaluation on larger datasets with additional evaluation metrics (surface distances) could provide more insights into the method's strengths and weaknesses.

References

1. Balakrishnan, G., Zhao, A., Sabuncu, M.R., Guttag, J., Dalca, A.V.: Voxelmorph: a learning framework for deformable medical image registration. IEEE Trans. Med. Imaging (2019)
2. Dosovitskiy, A., et al.: Flownet: learning optical flow with convolutional networks. In: Proceedings of ICCV, pp. 2758–2766 (2015)
3. Felzenszwalb, P.F., Huttenlocher, D.P.: Efficient belief propagation for early vision. Int. J. Comput. Vis. **70**(1), 41–54 (2006)
4. Heinrich, M.P., Oktay, O., Bouteldja, N.: Obelisk-net: fewer layers to solve 3D multi-organ segmentation with sparse deformable convolutions. Med. Image Anal. **54**, 1–9 (2019)
5. Heinrich, M.P., Jenkinson, M., Papież, B.W., Brady, S.M., Schnabel, J.A.: Towards realtime multimodal fusion for image-guided interventions using self-similarities. In: Mori, K., Sakuma, I., Sato, Y., Barillot, C., Navab, N. (eds.) MICCAI 2013. LNCS, vol. 8149, pp. 187–194. Springer, Heidelberg (2013). https://doi.org/10.1007/978-3-642-40811-3_24
6. Hu, Y., et al.: Weakly-supervised convolutional neural networks for multimodal image registration. Med. Image Anal. **49**, 1–13 (2018)
7. Kamnitsas, K., et al.: Efficient multi-scale 3D CNN with fully connected CRF for accurate brain lesion segmentation. Med. Image Anal. **36**, 61–78 (2017)
8. Krähenbühl, P., Koltun, V.: Efficient inference in fully connected CRFs with Gaussian edge potentials. In: NeurIPS, pp. 109–117 (2011)
9. Krebs, J., Mansi, T., Mailhé, B., Ayache, N., Delingette, H.: Unsupervised probabilistic deformation modeling for robust diffeomorphic registration. In: Stoyanov, D., et al. (eds.) DLMIA 2018, ML-CDS 2018. LNCS, vol. 11045, pp. 101–109. Springer, Heidelberg (2018). https://doi.org/10.1007/978-3-030-00889-5_12
10. Modat, M., et al.: Fast free-form deformation using graphics processing units. Comput. Methods Programs Biomed. **98**(3), 278–284 (2010)
11. Rousseau, F., Habas, P.A., Studholme, C.: A supervised patch-based approach for human brain labeling. IEEE Trans. Med. Imaging **30**(10), 1852–1862 (2011)
12. Rühaak, J., et al.: Estimation of large motion in lung CT by integrating regularized keypoint correspondences into dense deformable registration. IEEE Trans. Med. Imaging **36**(8), 1746–1757 (2017)

13. Sentker, T., Madesta, F., Werner, R.: GDL-FIRE^{4D}: deep learning-based fast 4D CT image registration. In: Frangi, A.F., Schnabel, J.A., Davatzikos, C., Alberola-López, C., Fichtinger, G. (eds.) MICCAI 2018. LNCS, vol. 11070, pp. 765–773. Springer, Cham (2018). https://doi.org/10.1007/978-3-030-00928-1_86
14. Jimenez-del Toro, O., Müller, H., Krenn, M., et al.: Cloud-based evaluation of anatomical structure segmentation and landmark detection algorithms: visceral anatomy benchmarks. IEEE Trans. Med. Imaging **35**(11), 2459–2475 (2016)
15. de Vos, B.D., Berendsen, F.F., Viergever, M.A., Sokooti, H., Staring, M., Išgum, I.: A deep learning framework for unsupervised affine and deformable image registration. Med. Image Anal. **52**, 128–143 (2019)
16. Xu, Z., et al.: Evaluation of 6 registration methods for the human abdomen on clinically acquired CT. IEEE Trans. Biomed. Eng. **63**(8), 1563–1572 (2016)
17. Yang, X., Kwitt, R., Styner, M., Niethammer, M.: Quicksilver: fast predictive image registration-a deep learning approach. NeuroImage **158**, 378–396 (2017)
18. Zheng, S., et al.: Conditional random fields as recurrent neural networks. In: Proceedings of ICCV, pp. 1529–1537 (2015)

Generating Pareto Optimal Dose Distributions for Radiation Therapy Treatment Planning

Dan Nguyen[✉], Azar Sadeghnejad Barkousaraie, Chenyang Shen, Xun Jia, and Steve Jiang

Medical Artificial Intelligence and Automation (MAIA) Laboratory,
Department of Radiation Oncology,
UT Southwestern Medical Center, Dallas, TX, USA
Dan.Nguyen@UTSouthwestern.edu

Abstract. Radiotherapy treatment planning currently requires many trial-and-error iterations between the planner and treatment planning system, as well as between the planner and physician for discussion/consultation. The physician's preferences for a particular patient cannot be easily quantified and precisely conveyed to the planner. In this study we present a real-time volumetric Pareto surface dose generation deep learning neural network that can be used after segmentation by the physician, adding a tangible and quantifiable endpoint to portray to the planner. From 70 prostate patients, we first generated 84,000 intensity modulated radiation therapy plans (1,200 plans per patient) sampling the Pareto surface, representing various tradeoffs between the planning target volume (PTV) and the organs-at-risk (OAR), including bladder, rectum, left femur, right femur, and body. We divided the data to 10 test patients and 60 training/validation patients. We then trained a hierarchically densely connected convolutional U-net (HD U-net), to take the PTV and avoidance map representing OARs masks and weights, and predict the optimized plan. The HD U-net is capable of accurately predicting the 3D Pareto optimal dose distributions, with average [mean, max] dose errors of [3.4%, 7.7%](PTV), [1.6%, 5.6%] (bladder), [3.7%, 4.2%](rectum), [3.2%, 8.0%](left femur), [2.9%, 7.7%](right femur), and [0.04%, 5.4%](body) of the prescription dose. The PTV dose coverage prediction was also very similar, with errors of 1.3% (D98) and 2.0% (D99). Homogeneity was also similar, differing by 0.06 on average. The neural network can predict the dose within 1.7 s. Clinically, the optimization and dose calculation is much slower, taking 5–10 min.

Keywords: Radiation therapy treatment planning · Intensity modulation · Pareto surface · Dose distribution · Deep learning · U-net · Neural network

1 Introduction

Radiation therapy is one of the major cancer therapy modalities, accounting for two-thirds of cancer patients in the US, either standalone or in conjunction with surgery, chemotherapy, immunotherapy, etc. In the typical current treatment planning work-flow, a treatment planner interacts with a commercial treatment planning system to solve an inverse optimization problem, either in an intensity modulated radiation

© Springer Nature Switzerland AG 2019
D. Shen et al. (Eds.): MICCAI 2019, LNCS 11769, pp. 59–67, 2019.
https://doi.org/10.1007/978-3-030-32226-7_7

therapy (IMRT) [1–3] or volumetric modulated arc therapy (VMAT) [4–7] setting. The planner manually tunes many hyperparameters, such as dose-volume constraints and weightings, to control the tradeoff between multiple clinical objectives. These hyperparameters are meticulously tuned in a time-consuming trial-and-error fashion to reach a suitable clinical solution. In addition, many rounds feedback from the physician is needed for the physician to discuss the plan quality with the planner and to properly portray their desired tradeoffs. This is largely due to the fact that the physician's preferences for a particular patient cannot be fully quantified and precisely conveyed to the planner. This trial-and-error process results in hours of planning time, and the many iterations of physician feedback may extend the time to several days until the plan is accepted.

Recently, deep learning with multi-layered neural networks has exploded in progress, particularly in computer vision. We realize that these new developments can be utilized to solve aspects of the treatment planning problem. Specifically, deep learning can be utilized to quickly realize the physician's preferences in a tangible and quantifiable manner that can be presented to the treatment planner prior to treatment planning. In this study we present a real-time Pareto surface dose generation deep learning neural network that can be used immediately after segmentation by the physician. Pareto optimal plans are the solutions to a multicriteria problem with various tradeoffs. In particular, the tradeoff lies with the dose coverage of the tumor and the dose sparing of the various critical structures. The benefit of such a model is two-fold. First, the physician can interact with the model to immediately view a dose distribution, and then adjust some parameters to push the dose towards their desired tradeoff in real time. This also allows for the physician to quickly comprehend the kinds of the tradeoffs that are feasible for the patient. Second, the treatment planner, upon receiving the physician's desired dose distribution, can quickly generate a fully deliverable plan that matches this dose distribution, saving time in tuning the optimization hyperparameters and discussing with the physician. We developed, trained, and tested the feasibility of the model on prostate cancer patients planned with 7 beam IMRT.

2   Methods

2.1   Prostate Patient Data and Pareto Plan Generation

We acquired the anatomical data for 70 prostate patients, in terms of the segmentation of the planning target volume (PTV) and the organs-at-risk, including bladder, rectum, left femur, right femur, and body. Ring and skin structures were added as tuning structures. The patient contours and dose arrays were formatted into $192 \times 192 \times 64$ arrays at 2.5 mm^3 voxel size. We then calculated the dose influence arrays for these 70 patients, for a 7 equidistant coplanar beam plan IMRT, with 2.5 mm^2 beamlets at 100 cm isocenter—a typical setup for prostate IMRT. Using this dose calculation data, we generated IMRT plans that sampled the Pareto surface, representing various tradeoffs between the PTV and OARs. The multicriteria objective can be written as

$$\underset{x}{minimize} \quad \{f_{PTV}(x), f_{OAR_1}(x), f_{OAR_2}(x), \ldots, f_{OAR_n}(x)\} \tag{1}$$
$$subject\ to \quad x \geq 0,$$

where x is the fluence map intensities to be optimized. There exists individual objectives, $f_s(x)\forall s \in PTV, OAR$, for the PTV and each of the OARs. Typically, the objective function is designed such that the goal is to deliver the prescribed dose to the PTV, while minimizing the dose to each OAR. Due to the physical aspects of external beam radiation, it is impossible to give the PTV exactly the prescription dose without irradiating normal tissue. Thus, we arrive at a multicriteria objective, where there does not exist a single optimal x^* that would minimize all $f_s(x)\forall s \in PTV, OAR$. For a proof of concept in this study, we choose to use the L2-norm to represent the objective, $f_s(x) = \frac{1}{2}\|A_s x - p_s\|_2^2$. Here, A_s is the dose influence matrix for a given structure, and p_s is the desired dose for a given structure, assigned as the prescription dose if s is the PTV, and 0 otherwise. This allows for us to linearly scalarize [8] the multicriteria optimization problem into a single-objective, convex optimization problem,

$$\underset{x}{minimize} \quad \frac{1}{2}\sum_{s \in S} w_s^2 \|D_s x - p_s\|_2^2 \tag{2}$$
$$subject\ to \quad x \geq 0.$$

The key to scalarizing the problem is the addition of w_s, which are the tradeoff weights for each objective function, $f_s(x)\forall s \in PTV, OAR$. With different values of w_s, different Pareto optimal solutions are generated. Using an in-house GPU-based proximal-class first-order primal-dual algorithm, Chambolle-Pock [9], we generated 1,200 pseudo-random plans per patient, totaling to 84,000 plans.

The generation of each plan entailed assigning pseudo-random weights to the organs-at-risk. The weight for the PTV was kept at 1. The weight assignment fell into 1 of 6 categories as shown in Table 1. For each patient, 100 plans for each organ-at-risk used the single organ spare category (bladder, rectum, left femoral head, right femoral head, shell, skin), totaling to 600 single organ spare plans for each patient. To ensure a larger sampling of weights, another 100 plans of the high, medium, low, and extra low weights were generated, as well as 200 plans of the controlled weights category. The bounds for the controlled weights were chosen through trial and error such that the final plan generated had a high likelihood of being in acceptable clinical bounds for an inexperienced human operator, but not necessarily acceptable for an experienced physician. In total 1,200 plans were generated per patient. With 70 patients, the total number of plans generated was 84,000 plans.

2.2 Deep Learning Architecture

We utilized a volumetric Hierarchically Dense U-net (HD U-net) architecture [10], as shown in Fig. 1, which adds in the densely connected convolutional layers [11] into the U-net architecture [12]. The HD U-net was trained to take as input the PTV contour, the body contour, and an avoidance map representing OARs masks assigned their respective w_s, and to predict the optimized 3D dose distribution.

62   D. Nguyen et al.

Table 1. Weight assignment categories. The function *rand*(*lb*, *ub*) represents a uniform random number between a lower bound, *lb*, and an upper bound, *ub*.

Category	Description
Single organ spare	$w_{s_i} = rand(0,1)$
	$w_{OAR\backslash s_i} = rand(0,0.1)$
High weights	$w_s = rand(0,1) \forall s \in OAR$
Medium weights	$w_s = rand(0,0.5) \forall s \in OAR$
Low weights	$w_s = rand(0,0.1) \forall s \in OAR$
Extra low weights	$w_s = rand(0,0.05) \forall s \in OAR$
Controlled weights	$w_{bladder} = rand(0,0.2)$
	$w_{rectum} = rand(0,0.2)$
	$w_{ltfemhead} = rand(0,0.1)$
	$w_{rtfemhead} = rand(0,0.1)$
	$w_{shell} = rand(0,0.1)$
	$w_{skin} = rand(0,0.3)$

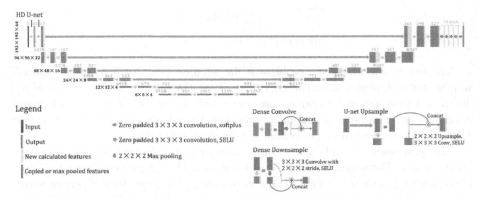

Fig. 1. Specific HD U-net architecture used in this study. Black numbers to the left of the model represents the current dimensions of the 3D data at each hierarchy. -The red numbers indicate the number of feature maps present at the current layer in the neural network. The large number of features maps are due to the densely connected convolutional layers. (Color figure online)

Specifically, our HD U-net architecture has 5 max pooling and 5 upsampling operations, ultimately reducing our image size from 192 × 192 × 64 voxels to 6 × 6 × 4 voxels (the lowest level max pooling/upsampling layer reduces/expands leaves the slice dimension untouched), and back to 192 × 192 × 64 voxels. Skip connections are added between the first half and second half of the network, to allow for the propagation of local information with the global information. Densely connected convolutional connections are added in each block of the network, allowing for efficient information flow of features. The non-linearity used after each convolution was the scaled exponential linear unit (SELU) as presented by Klambauer et al. for self-normalizing neural networks [13]. The study proved, using the Banach fixed-point theorem, that by having the SELU nonlinear activation, the neuron activations automatically converge towards zero mean and unit variance. Also, by the paper suggestion, we did not include batch normalization, as that disrupts the self-normalizing property of SELU-based networks. Since the densely connection convolutional layers allows for less trainable parameters to be used, instead of doubling the number of kernels after every max pooling, we increased number of kernels by 1.25 fold, to the nearest integer. We chose our final activation layer as the softplus activation, as our output data is non-negative and we had found that it is much more stable for training than linear and the rectified linear unit (ReLU) when using SELU as the hidden layer activation.

2.3 Training and Evaluation

We randomly divided the data to 10 test patients and 60 model development (training and validation) patients. The 10 test patients were held out during the entire model development phase, and only used during evaluation. Five instances of the model were trained and validated, using 54 training patients and 6 validation patients, according the schematic outlined in Fig. 2.

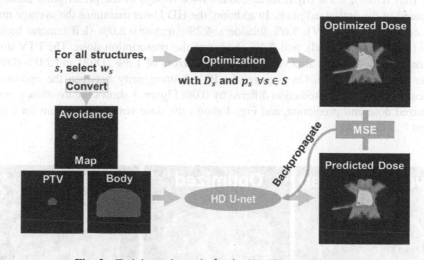

Fig. 2. Training schematic for the HD U-net architecture

At each training iteration, first a patient is selected and then set of w_s is selected from one of the 1,200 plans. These set of weights are then converted into an avoidance map, which is a single channel of the input that represents the OAR masks assigned their corresponding w_s. In addition, the binary mask of the PTV and body are included as input. The HD U-net then makes a prediction using these inputs. The optimized dose, that was generated using the dose influence array and Chambolle-Pock algorithm, is used to minimize against the predicted dose distribution with a mean squared error loss. Alternatively, a plan can be generated on the fly from a given set of w_s, but is less efficient for training on a single GPU. During training the model was assessed on the validation data every 200 iterations of training. Each instance of the model used a different set of validation patients for determining which iteration the lowest validation score was obtained. Using all 1,200 plans per training patient—64,800 training plans total—we trained the model for 100,000 iterations using the Adam optimizer, with a learning rate of 1×10^{-4}, using an NVIDIA V100 GPU. The 10 test patients were then evaluated using the trained models.

To equally compare across patients, the test plans were first normalized such that the dose to 95% of the PTV (D95) was equal to the prescription dose. For evaluation criteria, the PTV coverage (D98, D99), PTV max dose (defined as D2 by the ICRU-83 report [14]), homogeneity $\left(\frac{D2-D98}{D50}\right)$, and the structure max and mean doses (D_{max} and D_{mean}) were evaluated.

3   Results

The HD U-net is capable of accurately predicting the Pareto optimal 3D dose distributions, with average mean dose errors of 3.4% (PTV), 1.6% (bladder), 3.7% (rectum), 3.2% (left femur), 2.9% (right femur), and 0.04% (body) of the prescription dose, as compared to the optimized plans. In addition, the HD U-net maintains the average max dose error of 7.7% (PTV), 5.6% (bladder), 4.2% (rectum), 8.0% (left femoral head), 7.7% (right femoral head), and 5.4% (body) of the prescription dose. The PTV dose coverage prediction was also very similar, with errors of 1.3% (D98) and 2.0% (D99) of the prescription dose. On average, the PTV homogeneity between the optimized reference dose and the prediction differed by 0.06. Figure 3 shows the avoidance map, optimized dose and prediction, and Fig. 4 shows the dose volume histogram for a test patient.

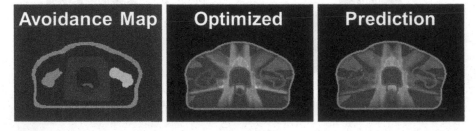

Fig. 3. Example avoidance map, optimized dose, and prediction for a test patient. The avoidance map represents the structure masks assigned their respective optimization structure weights, w_s.

It took approximately 15 days to train each instance of the model for 100,000 iterations. Figure 5 represents the mean training and validation loss for the HD U-net over the 100,000 iterations of training. The validation curve begins to flatten out at around 80,000 iterations while the training loss continues to decrease. The small

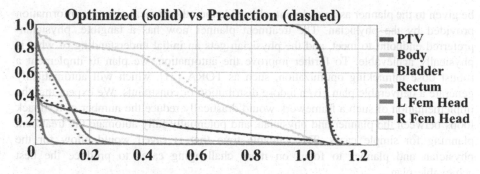

Fig. 4. Example dose volume histogram for a test patient.

standard deviation in validation loss between the model instances indicate the stability and reproducibility of the overall model framework and choice of hyperparameters.

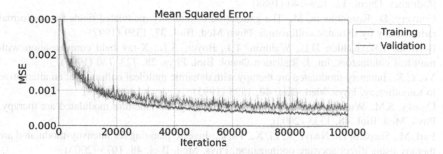

Fig. 5. Training and validation loss. Solid line represents the mean loss of the 5 model instances trained on different training/validation sets. Error represents one standard deviation.

Given any structure weights set and anatomy, the neural network is capable of predicting the dose distribution in 1.7 s. Clinically, the optimization and dose calculation for IMRT takes approximately 5–10 min to complete. This makes it feasible for the model to be used in a real-time setting with a human operator.

4 Discussion and Conclusion

While other deep learning models designed to learn and predict the dose distribution of a patient plans, based either on historical clinical data or optimized plans to meet standardized clinical criteria, were developed in recent years [10, 15–20], this Pareto dose distribution model, to our knowledge, is the first deep learning model to able to generate any optimized plan from just the anatomy and structure weights. Although the model does not generate the final plan in terms of deliverability, its real-time prediction capabilities allow for it to be used as a tool for the physician quickly generate a dose distribution with realistic tradeoffs between the PTV and various OARs. This can then be given to the planner as an endpoint, alongside the other typical planning information provided by the physician. The treatment planner now has a tangible, physician-preferred endpoint to meet, and the physician gets an initial understanding of what is physically achievable. To further improve the automation, we plan to implement a robust dose mimicking optimization, such as TORA [21], which will automatically generate a deliverable plan given a dose distribution or constraints. We expect that the implementation of such a framework would drastically reduce the number of feedback loops between the planner and physician, and potentially fully automate the treatment planning for simple cases. The valuable time that is saved would allow for the physician and planner to focus on more challenging cases to produce the best achievable plan.

References

1. Brahme, A.: Optimization of stationary and moving beam radiation therapy techniques. Radiother. Oncol. **12**, 129–140 (1988)
2. Convery, D., Rosenbloom, M.: The generation of intensity-modulated fields for conformal radiotherapy by dynamic collimation. Phys. Med. Biol. **37**, 1359 (1992)
3. Bortfeld, T.R., Kahler, D.L., Waldron, T.J., Boyer, A.L.: X-ray field compensation with multileaf collimators. Int. J. Radiation Oncol. Biol. Phys. **28**, 723–730 (1994)
4. Yu, C.X.: Intensity-modulated arc therapy with dynamic multileaf collimation: an alternative to tomotherapy. Phys. Med. Biol. **40**, 1435 (1995)
5. Crooks, S.M., Wu, X., Takita, C., Watzich, M., Xing, L.: Aperture modulated arc therapy. Phys. Med. Biol. **48**, 1333 (2003)
6. Earl, M., Shepard, D., Naqvi, S., Li, X., Yu, C.: Inverse planning for intensity-modulated arc therapy using direct aperture optimization. Phys. Med. Biol. **48**, 1075 (2003)
7. Otto, K.: Volumetric modulated arc therapy: IMRT in a single gantry arc. Med. Phys. **35**, 310–317 (2008)
8. Jahn, J.: Scalarization in multi objective optimization. In: Serafini, P. (ed.) Mathematics of Multi Objective Optimization. ICMS, vol. 289, pp. 45–88. Springer, Vienna (1985). https://doi.org/10.1007/978-3-7091-2822-0_3
9. Chambolle, A., Pock, T.: A first-order primal-dual algorithm for convex problems with applications to imaging. J. Math. Imaging Vis. **40**, 120–145 (2011)
10. Nguyen, D., et al.: 3D radiotherapy dose prediction on head and neck cancer patients with a hierarchically densely connected U-net deep learning architecture. Phys. Med. Biol. **64**, 065020 (2019)
11. Huang, G., Liu, Z., van der Maaten, L., Weinberger, K.Q.: Densely connected convolutional networks. In: 30th IEEE Conference on Computer Vision and Pattern Recognition, (CVPR 2017), vol. 1, pp. 2261–2269 (2017)
12. Ronneberger, O., Fischer, P., Brox, T.: U-net: convolutional networks for biomedical image segmentation. In: Navab, N., Hornegger, J., Wells, W.M., Frangi, A.F. (eds.) MICCAI 2015. LNCS, vol. 9351, pp. 234–241. Springer, Cham (2015). https://doi.org/10.1007/978-3-319-24574-4_28
13. Klambauer, G., Unterthiner, T., Mayr, A., Hochreiter, S.: Self-normalizing neural networks. In: Advances in Neural Information Processing Systems, pp. 971–980. (2017)

14. Grégoire, V., Mackie, T.R.: State of the art on dose prescription, reporting and recording in Intensity-Modulated Radiation Therapy (ICRU report No. 83). Cancer/Radiothérapie **15**, 555–559 (2011)
15. Nguyen, D., et al.: A feasibility study for predicting optimal radiation therapy dose distributions of prostate cancer patients from patient anatomy using deep learning. Sci. Rep. **9**, 1076 (2019)
16. Chen, X., Men, K., Li, Y., Yi, J., Dai, J.: A feasibility study on an automated method to generate patient-specific dose distributions for radiotherapy using deep learning. Med. Phys. **46**, 56–64 (2019)
17. Fan, J., Wang, J., Chen, Z., Hu, C., Zhang, Z., Hu, W.: Automatic treatment planning based on three-dimensional dose distribution predicted from deep learning technique. Med. Phys. **46**, 370–381 (2019)
18. Shiraishi, S., Moore, K.L.: Knowledge-based prediction of three-dimensional dose distributions for external beam radiotherapy. Med. Phys. **43**, 378–387 (2016)
19. Mahmood, R., Babier, A., McNiven, A., Diamant, A., Chan, T.C.: Automated treatment planning in radiation therapy using generative adversarial networks. arXiv preprint arXiv:1807.06489 (2018)
20. Babier, A., Mahmood, R., McNiven, A.L., Diamant, A., Chan, T.C.: Knowledge-based automated planning with three-dimensional generative adversarial networks. arXiv preprint arXiv:1812.09309 (2018)
21. Long, T., Chen, M., Jiang, S.B., Lu, W.: Threshold-driven optimization for reference-based auto-planning. Phys. Med. Biol. **63**, 04NT01 (2018)

PAN: Projective Adversarial Network for Medical Image Segmentation

Naji Khosravan[2], Aliasghar Mortazi[2], Michael Wallace[1], and Ulas Bagci[2(✉)]

[1] Mayo Clinic Cancer Center, Jacksonville, FL, USA
[2] Center for Research in Computer Vision (CRCV), School of Computer Science, University of Central Florida, Orlando, FL, USA
bagci@ucf.edu

Abstract. Adversarial learning has been proven to be effective for capturing long-range and high-level label consistencies in semantic segmentation. Unique to medical imaging, capturing 3D semantics in an effective yet computationally efficient way remains an open problem. In this study, we address this computational burden by proposing a novel projective adversarial network, called PAN, which incorporates high-level 3D information through 2D projections. Furthermore, we introduce an attention module into our framework that helps for a selective integration of global information directly from our *segmentor* to our adversarial network. For the clinical application we chose pancreas segmentation from CT scans. Our proposed framework achieved state-of-the-art performance without adding to the complexity of the segmentor.

Keywords: Object segmentation · Deep learning ·
Adversarial learning · Attention · Projective · Pancreas

1 Introduction

Segmentation has been a major area of interest within the fields of computer vision and medical imaging for years. Owing to their success, deep learning based algorithms have become the standard choice for semantic segmentation in the literature. Most state-of-the-art studies model segmentation as a pixel-level classification problem [2–4]. Pixel-level loss is a promising direction but, it fails to incorporate global semantics and relations. To address this issue researchers have proposed a variety of strategies. A great deal of previous research uses a post-processing step to capture pairwise or higher level relations. Conditional Random Field (CRF) was used in [2] as an offline post-processing step to modify edges of objects and remove false positives in CNN output. In other studies, to avoid offline post-processing and provide an end-to-end framework for segmentation, mean-field approximate inference for CRF with Gaussian pairwise potentials was modeled through Recurrent Neural Network (RNN) [17].

In parallel to post processing attempts, another branch of research tried to capture this global context through multi-scale or pyramid frameworks. In [2–4], several spatial pyramid pooling at different scales with both conventional

© Springer Nature Switzerland AG 2019
D. Shen et al. (Eds.): MICCAI 2019, LNCS 11769, pp. 68–76, 2019.
https://doi.org/10.1007/978-3-030-32226-7_8

convolution layers and *Atrous* convolution layers were used to keep both contextual and pixel-level information. Despite such efforts, combining local and global information in an optimal manner is not a solved problem, yet.

Following by the seminal work by Goodfellow et al. in [7] a great deal of research has been done on adversarial learning [8,10,14,15]. Specific to segmentation, for the first time, Luc et al. [8] proposed the use of a discriminator along with a segmentor in an adversarial min-max game to capture long-range label consistencies. In another study *SegAN* was introduced, in which the segmentor plays the role of generator being in a min-max game with a discriminator with a multi-scale *L1* loss [14]. A similar approach was taken for structure correction in chest X-rays segmentation in [5]. A conditional GAN approach was taken in [10] for brain tumor segmentation.

In this paper, we focused on the challenging problem of pancreas segmentation from CT images, although our framework is generic and can be applied to any 3D object segmentation problem. This particular application has unique challenges due to the complex shape and orientation of pancreas, having low contrast with neighbouring tissues and relatively small and varying size. Pancreas segmentation were studied widely in the literature. Yu et al. introduced a recurrence saliency transformation network, which uses the information from previous iteration as a spatial weight for current iteration [16]. In another attempt, U-Net with an attention gate was proposed in [9]. Similarly, a two-cascaded-stage based method was used to localize and segment pancreas from CT scans in [13]. A prediction-segmentation mask was used in [18] for constraining the segmentation with a coarse-to-fine strategy. Furthermore, a segmentation network with RNN was proposed in [1] to capture the spatial information among slices. The unique challenges of pancreas segmentation (complex shape and small organ) shifted the literature towards methods with coarse-to-fine and multi-stage frameworks, promising but computationally expensive.

Summary of Our Contributions: The current literature on segmentation fails to capture 3D high-level shape and semantics with a low-computation and effective framework. In this paper, for the fist time in the literature, we propose a projective adversarial network (PAN) for segmentation to fill this research gap. Our method is able to capture 3D relations through 2D projections of objects, without relying on 3D images or adding to the complexity of the segmentor. Furthermore, we introduce an attention module to selectively integrate high-level, whole-image features from the *segmentor* into our adversarial network. With comprehensive evaluations, we showed that our proposed framework achieves the state-of-the-art performance on publicly available CT pancreas segmentation dataset [11] even with a very simple encoder-decoder network as *segmentor*.

2   Method

Our proposed method is built upon the adversarial networks. The proposed framework's overview is illustrated in Fig. 1. We have three networks: a segmentor (S in Fig. 1), which is the only network being used during the test phase,

70   N. Khosravan et al.

and two adversarial networks (D_s and D_p in Fig. 1), each with a specific task to
guide the training of S. The first adversarial network (D_s) captures high-level
spatial label contiguity while the second adversarial network (D_p) enforces the
3D semantics through a 2D projection learning strategy. The adversarial networks were used only during the training phase to boost the performance of the
segmentor without adding to its complexity.

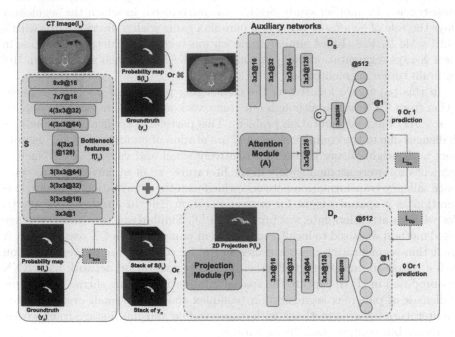

Fig. 1. The proposed framework consists of a segmentor S and two adversarial networks, D_s and D_p. S was trained with a hybrid loss from D_s, D_p and the ground-truth.

2.1 Adversarial Training

To train our framework, we use a hybrid loss function, which is a weighted sum
of three terms. For a dataset of N training samples of images and ground truths
(I_n, y_n), we define our hybrid loss function as:

$$l_{hybrid} = \sum_{n=1}^{N} l_{bce}(S(I_n), y_n) - \lambda l_{D_s} - \beta l_{D_p},\qquad(1)$$

where l_{D_s} and l_{D_p} are the losses corresponding to D_s and D_p and $S(I_n)$ is the
segmentor's prediction. The first term in Eq. 1 is a weighted binary cross-entropy
loss. This loss is the state-of-the-art loss function for semantic segmentation and
for a grey-scale image I with size $H \times W \times 1$ is defined as:

$$l_{bce}(\hat{y}, y) = - \sum_{i=1}^{H \times W} (wy_i \log \hat{y}_i + (1 - y_i) \log(1 - \hat{y}_i)), \qquad (2)$$

where w is the weight for positive samples, y is the ground-truth label and $\hat{y}$ is the network's prediction. Equation 2 encourages S to produce predictions similar to ground-truth and penalizes each pixel *independently*. High-order relations and semantics cannot be captured by this term.

To account for this drawback, the second and third terms are added to train our auxiliary networks. l_{D_s} and l_{D_p} are defined below, respectively:

$$l_{D_s} = l_{bce}(D_s(I_n, y_n), 1) + l_{bce}(D_s(I_n, S(I_n)), 0), \qquad (3)$$

$$l_{D_p} = l_{bce}(D_p(P_{I_n}, P_{y_n}), 1) + l_{bce}(D_p(P_{I_n}, P_{S(I_n)}), 0). \qquad (4)$$

Here P is the projection module, l_{bce} is the binary cross-entropy loss with $w = 1$ in Eq. 2 corresponding to a single number (0 or 1) as the output. Minimizing Eq. 1 while training D_s and D_p with l_{D_s} and l_{D_p} will put the whole framework into a min-max adversarial game.

2.2   Segmentor (S)

Our base network is a simple fully convolutional network with an encoder-decoder architecture. The input to the segmentor is a 2D grey-scale image and the output is a pixel-level probability map. The probability map shows probability of presence of the object at each pixel. We use a hybrid loss function (explained in details in Sect. 2.1) to update the parameters our segmentor (S). This loss function is composed of three terms enforcing: (1) pixel-level high-resolution details, (2) spatial and high-range label continuity, (3) 3D shape and semantics, through our novel projective learning strategy.

As can be seen in Fig. 1, the segmentor contains 10 conv layers in the encoder, 10 conv layers in the decoder and 4 conv layers as the bottleneck. The last conv layer is a 1×1 conv layer with the channel output of 1, combining channel-wise information in the highest scale. This layer is followed by a sigmoid function to create the notion of probability.

2.3   Adversarial Networks

Our adversarial networks are designed with the goal of compensating for the missing global relations and correcting higher-order inconsistencies, produced by a single pixel-level loss. Each of these networks produces an adversarial signal and apply it to the segmentor as a term in the overall loss function (Eq. 1). The details of each network is described below:

Spatial Semantics Network (D_s): This network is designed to capture spatial consistencies within each frame. The input to this network is either the segmented object by the ground-truth or by the segmentor's prediction. The Spatial semantics network (D_s) is trained to discriminate between these two inputs with a binary cross-entropy loss, formulated as in Eq. 3. The adversarial signal produced by the negative loss of D_s to S forces S to produce predictions closer to ground-truth in terms of spatial semantics.

As illustrated in Fig. 1 top right, D_s has a two-branch architecture with a late fusion. The top branch processes the segmented objects by ground-truth or segmentor's prediction. We propose an extra branch of processing, getting the bottleneck features corresponding to the original gray-scale input image, and passing them to an attention module for an information selection. The processed features are then concatenated with the first branch and passed through the shared layers. We believe that having the high-level features of whole image along with the segmentations improves the performance of D_s.

Our attention module learns where to attend in the feature space to have a more discriminative information selection and processing. The details of the attention module are described in the following.

Attention Module (A): We feed the high-level features form the segmentor's bottleneck to D_s. These features contain global information about the whole frame. We use a soft-attention mechanism, in which our attention module assigns a weight to each feature based on its importance for discrimination. The attention module gets the features with shape $w \times h \times c$, as input, and outputs a

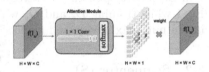

Fig. 2. Attention module assigns a weight to each feature allowing for a soft selection of information.

weight set with a shape of $w \times h \times 1$. A is composed of two 1×1 convolution layers followed by a softmax layer (Fig. 2). The softmax layer introduces the notion of *soft selection* to this module. The output of A is then multiplied to the features before being passed to the rest of the network.

Projective Network (D$_p$): Any 3D object can be projected into 2D planes from specific viewpoints, resulting in multiple 2D images. The 2D projection contains 3D semantics information, to be retrieved. In this section, we introduce our projective network (D_p). The main task of D_p is to capture 3D semantics without relying on 3D data and from the 2D projections. Inducing 3D shapes form 2D images has previously been done for 3D shape generation [6]. Unlike existing notions, however, in this paper we propose 3D semantics induction from 2D projections, to benefit segmentation for the first time in the literature.

The projection module (P) projects any 3D volume (V) on a 2D plane as:

$$P((i,j),V) = 1 - \exp^{-\Sigma_k V(i,j,k)}, \tag{5}$$

where each pixel in the 2D projection $P((i,j),V)$ gets a value in the range of $[0,1]$ based on the number of voxel occupancy in the third dimension of corresponding $3D$ volume (V). For the sake of simplicity, we refer to the projection of a 3D volume V as $P(V)$. We pass each 3D image through our segmentor (S) slice by slice and stack the corresponding prediction maps. Then, these maps are fed to the projection module (P) and are projected in the axial view.

The input to D_p is either the projected ground-truth or projected prediction map produced by S. D_p is trained to discriminate these inputs using the loss function defined in Eq. 4. The adversarial term produced by D_p in Eq. 1 forces S to create predictions which are closer to ground-truth in terms of 3D semantics. Incorporating D_p as an adversarial network to our segmentation framework helps S to capture 3D information through a very simple 2D architecture and without adding to its complexity in the test time.

3   Experiments and Results

We evaluated the efficacy of our proposed system with the challenging problem of pancreas segmentation. This particular problem was selected due to the complex and varying shape of pancreas and relatively more difficult nature of the segmentation problem compared to other abdominal organs. In our experiments we show that our proposed framework outperforms other state-of-the-art methods and captures the complex 3D semantics with a simple encoder-decoder. Furthermore, we have created an extensive comparison to some baselines, designed specifically to show the effects of each block of our framework.

Data and Evaluation: We used the publicly available TCIA CT dataset from NIH [11]. This dataset contains a total of 82 CT scans. The resolution of scans is $512 \times 512 \times Z$, $Z \in [181, 466]$ is the number of slices in the axial plane. The voxels spacing ranges from 0.5 mm to 1.0 mm. We used a randomly selected set of 62 images for training and 20 for testing to perform a 4-fold cross-validation. Dice Similarity Coefficient (DSC) is used as the metric of evaluation.

Comparison to Baselines: To show the effect of each building block of our framework we designed an extensive set of experiments. In our experiments we start from only training a single segmentor (S) and go to our final proposed framework. Furthermore, we show comparison of encoder-decoder architecture with other state-of-the-art semantic segmentation architectures.

Table 1 shows the results adding of each

Table 1. Comparison with baselines.

	Model	DSC%
1-fold	Encoder-decoder (S)	57.7
	Atrous pyramid	48.2
	$S + D_s$	85.0
	$S + D_s + A$	85.9
	$S + D_s + A + D_p$	**86.8**

building block of our framework. The encoder-decoder architecture is the one showed in Fig. 1 as S, while the Atrous pyramid architecture is similar to the recent work of [4]. This architecture is currently state-of-the-art for semantic segmentation. In which an Atrous pyramid is used to capture global context. We added an Atrous pyramid with 5 different scales: 4 Atrous convolutions at rates of $1, 2, 6, 12$, with the global image pooling. We also replaced the decoder with 2 simple upsampling and conv layers similar to the main paper [4]. We refer the readers to the main paper for more details about this architecture due to space limitations [4]. We found out having an extensive processing in the decoder improves the results compared to the Atrous pyramid architecture (possibly a better choice for segmentation of objects at multiple scales). This is because our object of interest is relatively small.

Moreover, we showed that adding a spatial adversarial notwork (D_s) can boost the performance of S dramatically, in our task. Introducing attention (A) helps for a better information selection (as described in Sect. 2.3) and boosts the performance further. Finally, our best results is achieved by adding the projective adversarial network (D_p), which adds integration of 3D semantics into the framework. This supports our hypothesis that our segmentor has enough capacity in terms of parameters to capture all this information and with proper and explicit supervision can achieve state-of-the-art results.

Comparison to the State-of-the-Art: We provide the comparison of our method's performance with current state-of-the-art literature on the same TCIA CT dataset for pancreas segmentation. As can be seen from experimental validation, our method outperforms the state-of-the-art with dice scores, provides better efficiency (less computational burden). Of a note, the proposed algorithm's least achievement is consistently higher than the state of the art methods (Table 2).

Table 2. Comparison with state-of-the-art on TCIA dataset.

	Approach	Average DSC%	Max DSC%	Min DSC%
4-fold cross validation	Roth et al. [11]	71.42 ± 10.11	86.29	23.99
	Roth et al. [12]	78.01 ± 8.20	88.65	34.11
	Roth et al. [13]	81.27 ± 6.27	88.96	50.69
	Zhou et al. [18]	82.37 ± 5.68	90.85	62.43
	Cai et al. [1]	82.40 ± 6.70	90.10	60.00
	Yu et al. [16]	84.50 ± 4.97	**91.02**	62.81
	Ours	**85.53 ± 1.23**	88.71	**83.20**

4   Conclusion

In this paper we proposed a novel adversarial framework for 3D object segmentation. We introduced a novel projective adversarial network, inferring 3D shape and semantics form 2D projections. The motivation behind our idea is that integration of 3D information through a fully 3D network, having all slices as input, is computationally infeasible. Possible workarounds are: (1) down-sampling the data or (2) sacrificing number of parameters, which are sacrificing information or computational capacity, respectively. We also introduced an attention module to selectively pass whole-frame high-level feature from the segmentor's bottleneck to the adversarial network, for a better information processing. We showed that with proper and guided supervision through adversarial signals a simple encoder-decoder architecture, with enough parameters, achieves state-of-the-art performance on the challenging problem of pancreas segmentation. We achieved a dice score of **85.53%**, which is state-of-the art performance on pancreas segmentation task, outperforming previous methods. Furthermore, we argue that our framework is general and can be applied to any 3D object segmentation problem and is not specific to a single application.

References

1. Cai, J., Lu, L., Xie, Y., Xing, F., Yang, L.: Improving deep pancreas segmentation in ct and mri images via recurrent neural contextual learning and direct loss function. arXiv preprint arXiv:1707.04912 (2017)
2. Chen, L.C., Papandreou, G., Kokkinos, I., Murphy, K., Yuille, A.L.: Deeplab: semantic image segmentation with deep convolutional nets, atrous convolution, and fully connected CRFs. IEEE Trans. Pattern Anal. Mach. Intell. **40**(4), 834–848 (2018)
3. Chen, L.C., Papandreou, G., Schroff, F., Adam, H.: Rethinking atrous convolution for semantic image segmentation. arXiv preprint arXiv:1706.05587 (2017)
4. Chen, L.-C., Zhu, Y., Papandreou, G., Schroff, F., Adam, H.: Encoder-decoder with atrous separable convolution for semantic image segmentation. In: Ferrari, V., Hebert, M., Sminchisescu, C., Weiss, Y. (eds.) ECCV 2018. LNCS, vol. 11211, pp. 833–851. Springer, Cham (2018). https://doi.org/10.1007/978-3-030-01234-2_49
5. Dai, W., Dong, N., Wang, Z., Liang, X., Zhang, H., Xing, E.P.: SCAN: structure correcting adversarial network for organ segmentation in chest X-rays. In: Stoyanov, D., et al. (eds.) DLMIA/ML-CDS -2018. LNCS, vol. 11045, pp. 263–273. Springer, Cham (2018). https://doi.org/10.1007/978-3-030-00889-5_30
6. Gadelha, M., Maji, S., Wang, R.: 3D shape induction from 2D views of multiple objects. In: 2017 International Conference on 3D Vision (3DV), pp. 402–411. IEEE (2017)
7. Goodfellow, I., et al.: Generative adversarial nets. In: Advances in Neural Information Processing Systems, pp. 2672–2680 (2014)
8. Luc, P., Couprie, C., Chintala, S., Verbeek, J.: Semantic segmentation using adversarial networks. arXiv preprint arXiv:1611.08408 (2016)
9. Oktay, O., et al.: Attention U-net: learning where to look for the pancreas. arXiv preprint arXiv:1804.03999 (2018)
10. Rezaei, M., et al.: A conditional adversarial network for semantic segmentation of brain tumor. In: Crimi, A., Bakas, S., Kuijf, H., Menze, B., Reyes, M. (eds.) BrainLes 2017. LNCS, vol. 10670, pp. 241–252. Springer, Cham (2018). https://doi.org/10.1007/978-3-319-75238-9_21
11. Roth, H.R., et al.: DeepOrgan: multi-level deep convolutional networks for automated pancreas segmentation. In: Navab, N., Hornegger, J., Wells, W.M., Frangi, A.F. (eds.) MICCAI 2015. LNCS, vol. 9349, pp. 556–564. Springer, Cham (2015). https://doi.org/10.1007/978-3-319-24553-9_68
12. Roth, H.R., Lu, L., Farag, A., Sohn, A., Summers, R.M.: Spatial aggregation of holistically-nested networks for automated pancreas segmentation. In: Ourselin, S., Joskowicz, L., Sabuncu, M.R., Unal, G., Wells, W. (eds.) MICCAI 2016. LNCS, vol. 9901, pp. 451–459. Springer, Cham (2016). https://doi.org/10.1007/978-3-319-46723-8_52

13. Roth, H.R., et al.: Spatial aggregation of holistically-nested convolutional neural networks for automated pancreas localization and segmentation. Med. Image Anal. **45**, 94–107 (2018)
14. Xue, Y., Xu, T., Zhang, H., Long, L.R., Huang, X.: Segan: adversarial network with multi-scale L_1 loss for medical image segmentation. Neuroinformatics **16**(3–4), 383–392 (2018)
15. Yi, X., Walia, E., Babyn, P.: Generative adversarial network in medical imaging: A review. arXiv preprint arXiv:1809.07294 (2018)
16. Yu, Q., Xie, L., Wang, Y., Zhou, Y., Fishman, E.K., Yuille, A.L.: Recurrent saliency transformation network: incorporating multi-stage visual cues for small organ segmentation. In: Proceedings of the IEEE Conference on Computer Vision and Pattern Recognition, pp. 8280–8289 (2018)
17. Zheng, S., et al.: Conditional random fields as recurrent neural networks. In: Proceedings of the IEEE International Conference on Computer Vision, pp. 1529–1537 (2015)
18. Zhou, Y., Xie, L., Shen, W., Wang, Y., Fishman, E.K., Yuille, A.L.: A fixed-point model for pancreas segmentation in abdominal CT scans. In: Descoteaux, M., Maier-Hein, L., Franz, A., Jannin, P., Collins, D.L., Duchesne, S. (eds.) MICCAI 2017. LNCS, vol. 10433, pp. 693–701. Springer, Cham (2017). https://doi.org/10.1007/978-3-319-66182-7_79

Generative Mask Pyramid Network for CT/CBCT Metal Artifact Reduction with Joint Projection-Sinogram Correction

Haofu Liao[1]([✉]), Wei-An Lin[2], Zhimin Huo[4], Levon Vogelsang[4],
William J. Sehnert[4], S. Kevin Zhou[3,5], and Jiebo Luo[1]

[1] Department of Computer Science, University of Rochester, Rochester, NY, USA
haofu.liao@rochester.edu
[2] Department of ECE, University of Maryland, College Park, MD, USA
[3] Institute of Computing Technology, Chinese Academy of Sciences, Beijing, China
[4] Carestream Health, Inc., Rochester, NY, USA
[5] Peng Cheng Laboratory, Shenzhen, China

Abstract. A conventional approach to computed tomography (CT) or cone beam CT (CBCT) metal artifact reduction is to replace the X-ray projection data within the metal trace with synthesized data. However, existing projection or sinogram completion methods cannot always produce anatomically consistent information to fill the metal trace, and thus, when the metallic implant is large, significant secondary artifacts are often introduced. In this work, we propose to replace metal artifact affected regions with anatomically consistent content through *joint projection-sinogram correction* as well as *adversarial learning*. To handle the metallic implants of diverse shapes and large sizes, we also propose a novel *mask pyramid network* that enforces the mask information across the network's encoding layers and a *mask fusion loss* that reduces early saturation of adversarial training. Our experimental results show that the proposed projection-sinogram correction designs are effective and our method recovers information from the metal traces better than the state-of-the-art methods.

1 Introduction

Metal artifact is one of the most prominent artifacts which impede reliable computed tomography (CT) or cone beam CT (CBCT) image interpretation. It is commonly addressed in the *sinogram domain* where the metal-affected regions in the sinograms are segmented and replaced with synthesized values so that metal-free CT images can be ideally reconstructed from the corrected sinograms. Early sinogram domain approaches fill the metal-affected regions by interpolation [4]

Electronic supplementary material The online version of this chapter (https://doi.org/10.1007/978-3-030-32226-7_9) contains supplementary material, which is available to authorized users.

or from prior images [6]. These methods can effectively reduce metal artifacts, but secondary artifacts are often introduced due to the loss of structural information in the corrected sinograms. Recent works propose to leverage deep neural networks (DNNs) to directly learn the sinogram correction. Park et al. [7] applies U-Net [9] to correct metal-inserted sinogram, and Gjesteby et al. [1] proposes to refine NMAR-corrected sinograms [6] using a convolutional neural network (CNN). Although better sinogram completions are achieved, the results are still subject to secondary artifacts due to the imperfect completion.

The development of DNNs in recent years also enables an *image domain* approach that directly reduces metal artifacts in CT/CBCT images. Specifically, the existing methods [2,11,12] train image-to-image CNNs to transform metal-affected CT images to metal-free CT images. Gjesteby et al. [2] proposes to include the NMAR-corrected CT as the input with a two-stream CNN. Zhang et al. [12] fuses beam hardening corrected and linear interpolated CT images for better correction. All the current image domain approaches use synthesized data to generate the metal-affected and metal-free image pairs for training. However, the synthesized data may not fully simulate the CT imaging under the clinical scenario making the image domain approaches less robust to clinical applications.

In this work, we propose a novel learning-based sinogram domain approach to metal artifact reduction (MAR). Unlike the existing image domain methods, the proposed method does not require synthesized metal artifact during training. Instead, we treat MAR as an image inpainting problem, i.e., we apply random metal traces to mask out artifact-free sinograms, and train a DNN to recover the data within the metal traces. Since metal-affected regions are viewed as missing, factors such as X-ray spectrum and the material of metal implants will not affect the generalizability of the proposed method. Unlike the existing learning-based sinogram domain approaches, our method delivers high-quality sinogram completion with three designs. *First*, we propose a two-stage projection-sinogram[1] completion scheme to achieve more contextually consistent correction results. *Second*, we introduce adversarial learning into the projection-sinogram completion so that more structural and anatomically plausible information can be recovered from the metal regions. *Third*, to make the learning more robust to the various shapes of metallic implants, we introduce a novel mask pyramid network (MPN) to distill the geometry information of different scales and a mask fusion loss to penalize early saturation. Our extensive experiments on both synthetic and clinical datasets demonstrate that the proposed method is indeed effective and perform better than the state-of-the-art MAR approaches.

2   Methodology

An overview of the proposed method is shown in Fig. 1. Our method consists of two major modules: a projection completion module (blue) and a sinogram correction module (green). The projection completion module is an image-to-image

---

[1] We denote the X-ray data that captured at the same view angle as a "projection" and a stack of projections corresponding to the same CT slice as a "sinogram".

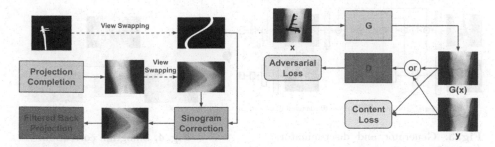

Fig. 1. Method overview.(Color figure online)

Fig. 2. The base framework.

translation model enhanced with a novel mask pyramid network. Given an input projection image and a pre-segmented metal mask, the projection completion module generates anatomically plausible and structurally consistent surrogates within the metal-affected regions. The sinogram correction module predicts a residual map to refine the projection-corrected sinograms. This joint projection-sinogram correction approach enforces inter-projection consistency and makes use of the context information between different viewing angles. Note that we perform projection completion first due to the observation that the projection images contain better structural information that facilitates the learning of an image inpainting model.

Base Framework. Inspired by recent advances in deep generative models [3,8], we formulate the projection and sinogram correction problems under a generative image-to-image translation framework. The structure of the proposed model is illustrated in Fig. 2. It consists of two individual networks: a generator G and a discriminator D. The generator G takes a metal-segmented projection x as the input and generates a metal-free projection $G(x)$. The discriminator D is a patch-based classifier that predicts if the metal-free projection y or $G(x)$, is real or not. Similar to the PatchGAN [3] design, D is constructed as a CNN without fully-connected layers at the end to enable the patch-wise prediction. The detailed structures of G and D are presented in the supplementary material. G and D are trained adversarially with LSGAN [5], i.e.,

$$\min_{D} \mathcal{L}_{\mathrm{GAN}} = \mathbb{E}_y[\|\mathbf{1} - D(y)\|^2] + \mathbb{E}_x[\|D(G(x))\|^2], \tag{1}$$

$$\min_{G} \mathcal{L}_{\mathrm{GAN}} = \mathbb{E}_x[\|\mathbf{1} - D(G(x))\|^2]. \tag{2}$$

In addition, we also expect the generator output $G(x)$ to be close to its metal-free counterpart y. Therefore, we add a content loss $\mathcal{L}_c$ to ensure the pixel-wise consistency between $G(x)$ and y,

$$\min_{G} \mathcal{L}_c = \mathbb{E}_{x,y}[\|G(x) - y\|_1]. \tag{3}$$

Mask Pyramid Network. Metallic implants have various shapes and sizes, such as metallic balls, bars, screws, wires, etc. When X-ray projections are

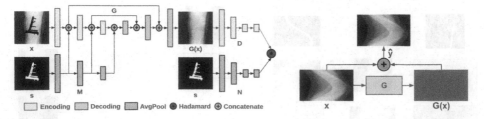

Fig. 3. Generator and discriminator. (Color figure online)

Fig. 4. Sinogram correction.

acquired at different angles, the projected implants would exhibit complicated geometries. Hence, unlike typical image inpainting problems, where the shape of the mask is usually simple and fixed, projection completion is more challenging since the network has to learn how to fuse such diversified mask information of the metallic implants. Directly using metal-masked image as the input requires the metal mask information to be encoded by each layer and passed along to the later layers. For unseen masks, this encoding may not work very well and hence the mask information may be lost. To retain sufficient amount of mask information, we introduce a mask pyramid network (MPN) into the generator to feed the mask information into each layer explicitly.

The architecture of the generator G with this design is illustrated in Fig. 3. The MPN M takes a metal mask s as the input, and each block (in yellow) of M is coupled with an encoding block (in grey) in G. Let l_M^i denote the ith block of M and l_G^i denote the ith block of G. When l_M^i and l_G^i are coupled, the output of l_M^i will be concatenated to the output of l_G^i. In this way, the mask information will then be used by l_G^{i+1}, and a recall of the mask is achieved. Each block l_M^i of M is implemented with an average pooling layer that has the same kernel, stride, and padding size as the convolutional layer in l_G^i. Hence, the metal mask output by l_M^i not only has the same size as the feature maps from l_G^i, but also takes into account the receptive field of the convolution operation in l_G^i.

Mask Fusion Loss. In conventional image-to-image framework, the loss is usually computed on the entire image. On the one hand, this makes the generation less efficient, as a significant portion of the generator's computation will be spent on recovering the already known information. On the other hand, this also introduces early saturation during adversarial training, in which the generator stops improving in the masked regions, since the generator does not have information about the mask. We address this issue with two strategies. First, when computing the loss function, we only consider the content within the metal mask. That is, the content loss is rewritten as

$$\min_{G} \mathcal{L}_c = \mathbb{E}_{x,y}[\|\hat{y} - y\|_1], \tag{4}$$

where $\hat{y} = s \odot G(x) + (1 - s) \odot x$.

Second, we modulate the output score matrix from the discriminator by the metal mask s so that the discriminator can selectively ignore the unmasked regions. As shown in Fig. 3, we implement this design using another MPN N. But this time, we do not feed the intermediate outputs from N to the coupled blocks in D, since the metal mask will, in the end, be applied to the loss. The adversarial part of the mask fusion loss is given as

$$\min_{D} \mathcal{L}_{\text{GAN}} = \mathbb{E}_y[\|N(s) \odot (1 - D(y))\|^2] + \mathbb{E}_x[\|N(s) \odot D(\hat{y})\|^2], \qquad (5)$$

$$\min_{G} \mathcal{L}_{\text{GAN}} = \mathbb{E}_x[\|N(s) \odot (1 - D(\hat{y}))\|^2], \qquad (6)$$

and the total mask fusion loss can be written as

$$\mathcal{L} = \mathcal{L}_{\text{GAN}} + \lambda \mathcal{L}_c, \qquad (7)$$

where λ balances the importance between $\mathcal{L}_{\text{GAN}}$ and $\mathcal{L}_c$.

Sinogram Correction with Residual Map Learning. Although the proposed projection completion framework in previous sections can produce an anatomically plausible result, it only considers the contextual information within a projection. Observing that a stack of consecutive projections form a set of sinograms. We use a simple yet effective model to enforce the inter-projection consistency by having the completion results look like sinograms.

Let x denote a sinogram formed from previous projection completion step. A generator, as shown in Fig. 4, predicts a residual map $G(x)$ which is then added to x to correct the projection completion results. Here, we use the same generator structure as the one introduced in Fig. 3. For the objective function, we apply the same one as used in Eq. 7, except that we have $\hat{y} = s \odot (G(x)+x)+(1-s) \odot x$.

3 Experimental Evaluations

Implementation Details and Baselines. We train the model with the Adam optimization method. For the hyper-parameters, we set learning rate $= 5e^{-4}$, $\beta_1 = 0.5$, $\lambda = 100$, and batch size $= 16$. We compare our projection completion (PC) model and joint projection-sinogram correction (PC+SC) model with the following baseline MAR approaches: (1) LI, sinogram correction by linear interpolation [4]; (2) BHC, beam hardening correction for MAR [10]; (3) NMAR, a state-of-the-art MAR model [6] that produces a prior CT image to correct metal artifacts; and (4) CNNMAR, the state-of-the-art deep learning based method [12] that uses a CNN to output the prior image for MAR.

Datasets and Simulation Details. For the synthesized dataset, we use the images collected from a CBCT scanner that is dedicated for lower extremities. The size of the CBCT projections is 448×512 and the projections contain no metal objects. We randomly apply masks to the projections to obtain masked and unmasked projection pairs. In total, there are 27 CBCT scans, each with

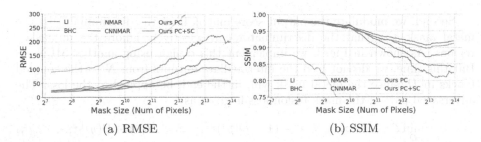

(a) RMSE   (b) SSIM

Fig. 5. Quantitative MAR results of different models with respect to different mask sizes. For RMSE/SSIM, the lower/higher values are better.

600 projections. Projections from 24 of the CBCT scans are used for training, and the rest are held out for testing.

Two types of object masks are collected for the experiments: metal masks and blob masks. For the metal masks, we collect 3D binary metal implant volumes from clinical records and forward project them to obtain 2D metal projection masks. In total, we obtain 18,000 projection masks from 30 binary metal implant volumes. During training, we simulate the metal implants insertion process by randomly placing metal segmentation masks on the metal-free projections. For the blob masks, we adopt the method from [8] by drawing randomly shaped blobs on the image. Results for projection and sinogram completion with the metal and blob masks are provided in the supplementary material.

For a fair comparison, we adopt the same procedures as in [12] to synthesize metal-affected CBCT volumes. We assume a 120 kVp X-ray source with 2×10^7 photons. The distance from the X-ray source to the rotation center is set to 59.5 cm, and 416 projection views are uniformly spaced between 0–360 degrees. The size of the reconstructed volume is $448 \times 448 \times 448$. During simulation, we set the material to iron for all the metal masks. Note that since the metal masks are from clinical records, the geometries and intensities of the metal artifacts are extremely diverse, which makes MAR highly challenging.

For the clinical dataset, we use the vertebrae localization and identification dataset from Spineweb[2]. We first define regions with HU values greater than 2,500 as metal regions. Then, we select images with the largest-connected metal region greater than 400 pixels as metal-affected images and images with the largest HU value smaller than 2,000 as metal-free images. The metal masks for the projections and sinograms are obtained by forward projecting the metal regions in the CT image domain. The training for this dataset is performed on the metal-free images with metal masks obtained from the metal-affected images.

Quantitative Comparisons. We use two metrics: the rooted mean square error (RMSE) and structural similarity index (SSIM) for quantitative evaluations. We conduct a thorough study by evaluating RMSE and SSIM for a wide range of mask sizes. The results are summarized in Fig. 5. We observe that the proposed

---

[2] spineweb.digitalimaginggroup.ca.

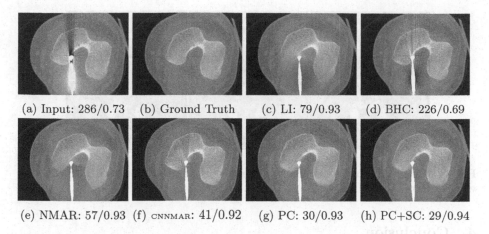

(a) Input: 286/0.73   (b) Ground Truth   (c) LI: 79/0.93   (d) BHC: 226/0.69

(e) NMAR: 57/0.93   (f) CNNMAR: 41/0.92   (g) PC: 30/0.93   (h) PC+SC: 29/0.94

Fig. 6. MAR results (RMSE/SSIM) on images with synthesized metal artifacts. Metallic implants are replaced with constant values (white) after MAR.

method achieves superior performance over the other methods. For example, the RMSE error of the second-best method CNNMAR [12] almost doubles that of the proposed method when the implant size is large. In addition, by further refining in the sinogram domain, improved performance can be achieved especially in terms of the SSIM metric. From Fig. 5, we also perceive that methods which require tissue segmentation (e.g. NMAR and CNNMAR) perform well when the metallic object is smaller than 1000 pixels. However, when the size of the metallic implants becomes larger, these methods deteriorate significantly due to erroneous segmentation. The proposed joint correction approach, which does not rely on tissue segmentation, exhibits less degradation.

Qualitative Comparisons. Figure 6 shows MAR results on synthesized metal-affected images. It is clear that the proposed method successfully restores streaking artifacts caused by metallic implants. Unlike other approaches that generates erroneous surrogates, our method fills in contextually consistent values through generative modeling and joint correction. For the results with clinical data (Fig. 7), we also observe that our method produces qualitatively better results. BHC and NMAR cannot totally reduce the metal artifacts. LI and CNNMAR can recover most of the metal-affected regions. However, they also produce secondary artifacts. We notice a performance degradation for CNNMAR on the clinical data compare to the synthesized data, which demonstrates that image domain approaches relying on synthesizing metal artifact have worse generalizability.

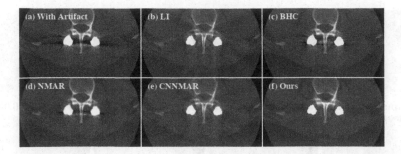

Fig. 7. MAR results on clinical images. Metallic implants are replaced with constant values (white) after MAR.

4 Conclusion

We present a novel MAR approach based on a generative adversarial framework with joint projection-sinogram correction and mask pyramid network. From the experimental evaluations, we show that existing MAR methods does not effectively reduce metal artifact. By contrast, the proposed approach leverages the extra contextual information from sinogram and achieves a superior performance over other MAR methods in both the synthesized and clinical datasets.

Acknowledgement. This work was supported in part by NSF award #1722847, the Morris K. Udall Center of Excellence in Parkinson's Disease Research by NIH, and the corporate sponsor Carestream.

References

1. Gjesteby, L., Yang, Q., Xi, Y., Zhou, Y., Zhang, J., Wang, G.: Deep learning methods to guide ct image reconstruction and reduce metal artifacts. In: SPIE Medical Imaging (2017)
2. Gjesteby, L., et al.: Reducing metal streak artifacts in CT images via deep learning: pilot results. In: The 14th International Meeting on Fully Three-Dimensional Image Reconstruction in Radiology and Nuclear Medicine, pp. 611–614 (2017)
3. Isola, P., Zhu, J.Y., Zhou, T., Efros, A.A.: Image-to-image translation with conditional adversarial networks. In: Proceedings of CVPR, pp. 1125–1134 (2017)
4. Kalender, W.A., Hebel, R., Ebersberger, J.: Reduction of CT artifacts caused by metallic implants. Radiology **164**(2), 576–577 (1987)
5. Mao, X., Li, Q., Xie, H., Lau, R.Y., Wang, Z., Paul Smolley, S.: Least squares generative adversarial networks. In: Proceedings of the IEEE International Conference on Computer Vision, pp. 2794–2802 (2017)
6. Meyer, E., Raupach, R., Lell, M., Schmidt, B., Kachelrieß, M.: Normalized metal artifact reduction in computed tomography. Med. Phys. **37**(10), 5482–5493 (2010)
7. Park, H.S., Chung, Y.E., Lee, S.M., Kim, H.P., Seo, J.K.: Sinogram-consistency learning in CT for metal artifact reduction. arXiv preprint arXiv:1708.00607 (2017)
8. Pathak, D., Krahenbuhl, P., Donahue, J., Darrell, T., Efros, A.A.: Context encoders: feature learning by inpainting. arXiv preprint arXiv:1604.07379 (2016)

9. Ronneberger, O., Fischer, P., Brox, T.: U-Net: convolutional networks for biomedical image segmentation. In: Navab, N., Hornegger, J., Wells, W.M., Frangi, A.F. (eds.) MICCAI 2015. LNCS, vol. 9351, pp. 234–241. Springer, Cham (2015). https://doi.org/10.1007/978-3-319-24574-4_28

10. Verburg, J.M., Seco, J.: CT metal artifact reduction method correcting for beam hardening and missing projections. Phys. Med. Biol. **57**(9), 2803 (2012)

11. Xu, S., Dang, H.: Deep residual learning enabled metal artifact reduction in CT. In: Medical Imaging 2018: Physics of Medical Imaging, vol. 10573, p. 105733O. International Society for Optics and Photonics (2018)

12. Zhang, Y., Yu, H.: Convolutional neural network based metal artifact reduction in x-ray computed tomography. IEEE Trans. Med. Imaging **37**, 1370–1381 (2018)

Multi-class Gradient Harmonized Dice Loss with Application to Knee MR Image Segmentation

Qin Liu[1], Xiongfeng Tang[2], Deming Guo[2], Yanguo Qin[2], Pengfei Jia[1],
Yiqiang Zhan[1], Xiang Zhou[1], and Dijia Wu[1(✉)]

[1] Shanghai United Imaging Intelligence Co., Ltd., Shanghai, China
{qin.liu,dijia.wu}@united-imaging.com
[2] Department of Orthopedics, The Second Hospital of Jilin University,
Changchun, China

Abstract. The Dice loss function is widely used in volumetric medical image segmentation for its robustness against the imbalance between the numbers of foreground and background voxels. However, it is not able to differentiate hard examples from easy ones, which usually comprise the majority of training examples and therefore dominate the loss function. In this work, we propose a novel loss function, termed as *Gradient Harmonized Dice Loss*, to both address the quantity imbalance between classes and focus on hard examples in training, with further generalization to multi-class segmentation. The proposed loss function is employed in a 3D fully convolutional neural network for multiple object segmentation of MRI knee joint images and validated on both public *SKI10* dataset and 637 MRI knee scans collected from local hospitals. The experimental results show that the Gradient Harmonized Dice Loss outperforms the popular loss functions, such as Dice loss and Focal loss, and achieves the state-of-the-art results on the validation data of *SKI10*.

Keywords: Gradient Harmonized Dice Loss · Knee MR image · Segmentation

1 Introduction

Recent years have witnessed the great success of convolutional neural network (CNN)-based methods in various medical image analysis tasks such as object segmentation, highlighting the capabilities of CNNs to solve many challenging problems. However, CNN-based segmentation networks are subject to the two well-known imbalance problems during training, namely the huge difference in quantity between foreground and background examples as well as between easy and hard examples. In order to mitigate the two imbalance problems, strategies such as the weighted cross-entropy function [7], the Dice loss function [6]

Q. Liu and X. Tang—These authors contributed equally to this work.

© Springer Nature Switzerland AG 2019
D. Shen et al. (Eds.): MICCAI 2019, LNCS 11769, pp. 86–94, 2019.
https://doi.org/10.1007/978-3-030-32226-7_10

or the Focal loss function [5], have been proposed. For the inter-class imbalance problem, weighted cross-entropy loss function tries to address it by assigning a weight to each training sample. It requires the pre-computation of pixel-wise weight maps, which are task-specific designed, to force the network to focus on rare examples. Dice loss approaches the inter-class imbalance problem by taking the union region of the ground truth and segmentation result as the guidance of the loss function, see Eq. 1. Thus, examples from a small object would adaptively acquire greater contribution to the loss function than examples from a larger object. In this way, Dice loss is more elegant and efficient than the weighed cross-entropy loss in tacking with the former imbalance problem. However, both Dice loss and cross-entropy loss are not able to address the latter imbalance problem by differentiating hard examples from the easy ones, which usually account for the vast majority of all training examples and therefore dominate the loss function. Focal Loss [5] has been proposed to address it by reshaping the standard cross-entropy loss such that it down-weights the loss assigned to well-classified examples, and thus focuses more on mis-classified examples. Despite Focal loss has achieved state-of-the-art performance in unbalanced segmentation, it adopts two hyper-parameters which need be manually tuned with effort. Moreover, Focal loss is a *static* loss, which means the weight assigned to an example is controlled by the fixed hyper-parameter γ, and therefore is not able to change adaptively according to data distribution in the mini-batch. To tackle with this issue, GHM-C loss [1] embeds gradient harmonization mechanism (GHM) into standard cross-entropy loss. Instead of using a weight factor module controlled by a fixed hyper-parameter, GHM-C loss uses a gradient harmonized weight factor which is calculated every iteration and is more adaptive to current state of model as well as the mini-batch of data.

However, both Focal loss and GHM-C loss are based on the standard cross-entropy loss, which is not as efficient and elegant as the Dice loss behaves in tacking with the former class imbalance problem. Meanwhile, there has been no research on the topic of replacing the standard cross-entropy loss function in GHM-C or Focal loss with the Dice loss function. In this work, we investigate this kind of possibility by proposing a novel loss function, termed as *Gradient Harmonized Dice Loss* (GHDL), to embed GHM in Dice loss and apply it to multiple object segmentation in Knee MR images. To be specific, we first define the gradient norm in the context of Dice loss function and then derive the form of gradient norm density function. Similar to [1], we call gradient norm density as *gradient density* for convenient. Finally, we formulate the form of the GHDL function by embedding the gradient harmonized weight in the Dice loss function.

To evaluate the effectiveness of GHDL, we apply it in an end-to-end fully convolutional neural network with application to knee joint segmentation from MR images. Automatic segmentation of knee cartilage, meniscus and the surrounding bones from MRI is important for the development of biomarkers targeted at different stages of Osteoarthritis (OA) [3], offering opportunities to better understand the pathophysiological processes of OA [4]. However, this is a challenging task due to the severe class imbalance between bones and soft tissues.

Moreover, MRI volumes are often affected by artifacts and distortions due to field inhomogeneity. Experimental results on both public *SKI10* dataset [9] and a dataset of 637 MRI knee scans collected from local hospitals show that without manual hyper-parameter tuning, GHDL outperforms the popular loss functions, such as Dice loss and Focal loss, and contribute to reasonable improvement for segmentation accuracy, achieving state-of-the-art results on the validation data of *SKI10*.

2   Previous Work on Dice Loss

The Dice Similarity Coefficient (DSC) is wildly used as a measurement for pairwise comparison between the predicted probability volume and the ground truth volume. Proposed in [6] as a loss function for binary segmentation, Dice loss can be expressed in terms of vector measures as:

$$DL = \frac{2\boldsymbol{p}^T\boldsymbol{g}}{\|\boldsymbol{p}\|^2 + \|\boldsymbol{g}\|^2} \tag{1}$$

with $\boldsymbol{p}$ the vector of probability volume, and $\boldsymbol{g}$ the vector of ground truth volume. For the i-th voxel of the prediction volume, let $p_i \in [0,1]$ be the probability predicted by the model and $g_i \in \{0,1\}$ be its ground-truth label. This formulation of Dice loss can be differentiated yielding the gradient with respect to the predicted probability of the i-th voxel:

$$\frac{\partial DL}{\partial p_i} = \frac{2}{S}\left(g_i - \frac{2I}{S}p_i\right) \tag{2}$$

where $S = \|\boldsymbol{p}\|^2 + \|\boldsymbol{g}\|^2$, and $I = \boldsymbol{p}^T\boldsymbol{g}$. Specifically, if $\boldsymbol{p}$ is binarized, S can be denoted as the summation of the ground truth region and the predicted region, and I can be denoted as the intersection or overlap of the two regions.

Mean-Class Dice Loss (MDL). The easiest way to extend binary Dice loss to multi-class Dice loss is to consider the mean Dice score:

$$MDL = \frac{1}{L}\sum_{j=1}^{L}\frac{2\boldsymbol{p}_j^T\boldsymbol{g}_j}{\|\boldsymbol{p}_j\|^2 + \|\boldsymbol{g}_j\|^2} \tag{3}$$

where $L \geq 2$ is the number of classes, $\boldsymbol{g}_j$ is the vector of probability volume of class j, and $\boldsymbol{p}_j$ is the vector of ground truth volume of class j. The gradient with respect to the predicted probability of the i-th voxel can be written as:

$$\frac{\partial MDL}{\partial p_i} = \frac{2}{L}\sum_{j=1}^{L}\frac{1}{S_j}\left(g_{ij} - \frac{2I_j}{S_j}p_{ij}\right) \tag{4}$$

Generalized Dice Loss (GDL). The generalized form of multi-class Dice loss is proposed in [8] for highly unbalanced segmentation. It can be written as:

$$GDL = \frac{2\sum_{j=1}^{L} \omega_j \boldsymbol{p}_j^T \boldsymbol{g}_j}{\sum_{j=1}^{L} \omega_j \left(\|\boldsymbol{p}_j\|^2 + \|\boldsymbol{g}_j\|^2\right)} \tag{5}$$

where ω_j is used to weight the contribution of each class.

3 Gradient Harmonized Dice Loss

In this section, we focus on voxel classification in binary segmentation where the classes (foreground/background) of examples are highly imbalanced. Before formulating the formal definition of the GHDL, the concept of gradient norm and gradient density are proposed first. We claim here that although the concept of gradient norm is borrowed from [1], the gradient norm w.r.t the Dice loss is first introduced in this work.

Gradient Norm. Based on the Eq. 2, we define the gradient norm of the i-th voxel w.r.t. the predicted probability as follows:

$$g_i^* = |g_i - \frac{2I}{S}p_i| = \begin{cases} 1 - \frac{2I}{S}p_i & \text{if } g_i = 1 \\ \frac{2I}{S}p_i & \text{if } g_i = 0 \end{cases} \tag{6}$$

with $\frac{2I}{S} \in [0,1]$ being the DSC of the current segmentation. In this definition, we discard the coefficient $\frac{2}{S}$ as shown in Eq. 2 since it is constant to all voxels in the prediction volume. Apparently, $g_i^* \in [0,1]$, and it represents the impact of an example on the global gradient flow.

Gradient Density Function. Given the definition of the gradient norm, the gradient density function is defined in Eq. 7:

$$D(g^*) = \frac{1}{\varepsilon} \sum_{i=1}^{N} \delta_\varepsilon(g_i^* - g^*) \tag{7}$$

where g_i^* is the gradient norm of the i-th example, N is the total number of examples in a training mini-batch, and ε is the size of the bin centered at g_i^*. And

$$\delta_\varepsilon(x) = \begin{cases} 1 & \text{if } |x| \leq \frac{\varepsilon}{2} \\ 0 & \text{otherwise} \end{cases} \tag{8}$$

The gradient density of g^* represents the number of examples lying in the bin centered at g^* and normalized by the bin size.

Gradient Harmonized Dice Loss. We embed the gradient density function in Dice loss function to formulate the definition of GHDL:

$$GHDL = \frac{2\boldsymbol{p}^T \boldsymbol{W} \boldsymbol{g}}{\|\boldsymbol{p}\|^2 + \|\boldsymbol{g}\|^2} = \frac{2\sum_{i=1}^{N} w_i p_i g_i}{\sum_{i=1}^{N}(p_i^2 + g_i^2)} \tag{9}$$

where $W = diag(w_1, w_2, ..., w_n)$, with $w_i = \frac{N}{D(g_i^*)}$. The value of w_i measures the weight of a training example w.r.t. its gradient norm. W can be comprehended as the gradient weight matrix. If training examples are uniformly distributed w.r.t. gradient, then W will be an identity matrix, which means GHDL is identical to Dice loss function. The gradient with respect to the predicted probability of the i-th voxel can be written as:

$$\frac{\partial GHDL}{\partial p_i} = \frac{2w_i}{S}\left(g_i - \frac{2I}{S}p_i\right) \tag{10}$$

with S and I having the same definitions with the variables shown in Eq. 2.

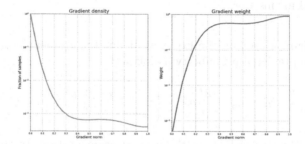

Fig. 1. Left: The gradient distribution from a converged binary segmentation model. Note that the y-axis uses log scale since the number of voxels with different gradient norm can differ by orders of magnitude. Right: The normalized gradient weight of the gradient norm.

Figure 1 (left) shows the gradient density from a converged multi-class segmentation model trained on *SKI10* dataset. We can observe that hard examples, whose gradient norm is usually greater than 0.5, comprise only a small portion of all training examples. Figure 1 (right) shows the normalized gradient weight computed from the same model. With the help of the gradient weight term, the total contribution of hard examples would be significantly improved. Both figures are displayed in log scale.

Although GHDL is formulated for binary segmentation, it can be easily extended to multi-class GHDL. In this work, we simply adopt the mean-class GHDL in a manner similar to Eq. 3 for multi-classification in knee MR images.

4   Experiments and Results

We evaluate the effectiveness of our proposed loss function on both *SKI10* dataset and a private dataset collected from local hospitals (Table 1). Examples of the

typical volumes from both datasets are shown in Fig. 2. Specifically, we employe
V-Net [6] to compare our loss function with other state-of-the-art loss functions,
such as Focal Loss and mean-class Dice loss.

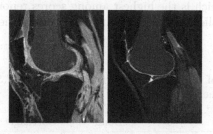

Fig. 2. Two of the MRI knee images with corresponding manual segmentation used in
our experiments, both shown in sagittal plane. Left: image from *SKI10* dataset. Right:
image from our private dataset.

4.1 Datasets

The public *SKI*10 dataset consists of 150 MRI images from the MICCAI SKI10
grand challenge [9], and is divided into 60 training, 40 validation, and 50 test
images. Our own dataset consists of 637 MRI images which were randomly
divided into 500 training and 137 test images. Images from both datasets were
acquired for surgical planning of partial or complete knee replacement, and therefore is representative of the clinical variability and challenges encountered in
clinical settings.

Table 1. Summary of the datasets used for training and validation. All images were
acquired once per patient.

	SKI10 dataset	Private dataset
Number of scans	150	637
Field strength	1.5T (90%), 3T and 1T (10%)	3T (50%), 1.5T (50%)
MRI sequence	T1, T2, GRE, fat suppression	PD fat suppression
Acquisition plane	Sagittal	Sagittal
Image resolution [mm]	$0.39 \times 0.39 \times 1.0$	$0.35 \times 0.35 \times 4.5$
Manual segmentations	Bones, cartilages	Bones, cartilages, meniscus

4.2 Results

Table 2 summarizes the comparison results between GHDL and other state-of-
the-art loss functions on *SKI10* validation dataset. The bone label includes femur

bone (FB) and tibial bone (TB), and the cartilage label includes femoral cartilage (FC) and tibial cartilage (TC). Our proposed loss function achieves the highest score among all the loss functions in terms of the SKI10 metrics [9]. We ensembled the best three models on the validation dataset and achieved a total score of 75.8 ± 8.5, which is the highest among scores reported in previous publications on *SKI10* validation dataset, including the winner of SKI10 challenge [2].

Table 2. Comparison of the state-of-the-art loss functions on *SKI10* validation data, in terms of the SKI10 metrics.

Loss function	Bone	Cartilage	Total score
Cross-entropy	69.0 ± 10.5	65.9 ± 12.1	67.5 ± 12.6
Focal loss	72.5 ± 11.7	70.5 ± 9.3	71.5 ± 7.9
Mean-class Dice loss	73.7 ± 8.7	64.2 ± 13.1	69.0 ± 9.3
Mean-class GHDL	75.9 ± 10.0	72.1 ± 11.0	74.0 ± 8.3
Mean-class GHDL (Ensemble)	$\mathbf{79.3 \pm 9.0}$	$\mathbf{72.3 \pm 12.2}$	$\mathbf{75.8 \pm 8.5}$

Table 3 summarize the comparison results between GHDL and other state-of-the-art loss functions on our own dataset. Our own dataset contains the labels of lateral meniscus (LM) and medial meniscus (MM), which are small tissues lying between the FC and TC as shown in 2 (right).

Table 3. Comparison of the state-of-the-art loss functions on our private dataset, measured in DSC (%).

Loss function	FB	FC	TB	TC	LM	MM
Cross-entropy	94.6 ± 1.3	77.8 ± 4.6	91.8 ± 2.3	70.7 ± 5.3	80.8 ± 6.9	79.5 ± 7.8
Focal loss	94.1 ± 1.4	77.9 ± 4.5	91.8 ± 2.3	70.1 ± 5.4	$\mathbf{82.2 \pm 6.3}$	81.8 ± 7.4
Mean-class Dice loss	94.4 ± 1.3	76.7 ± 4.7	90.8 ± 2.4	69.2 ± 5.8	80.4 ± 7.2	80.5 ± 7.6
Mean-class GHDL	$\mathbf{94.8 \pm 1.4}$	$\mathbf{78.1 \pm 4.7}$	$\mathbf{91.9 \pm 2.3}$	$\mathbf{70.7 \pm 5.3}$	82.0 ± 6.6	$\mathbf{81.8 \pm 7.3}$

To better understand the contribution of GHDL, we investigate the gradient weight maps of different labels from the converged model trained on our own dataset. Each row in Fig. 3 shows the gradient weight map of three representative labels (FB, FC, LM), respectively. To focus on hard examples, we only select those voxels in the gradient weight map with gradient norm higher than 0.5. As shown in Fig. 3 (right column), these hard examples only comprise a very small fraction of all training examples. Much in line with our expectation, we find that the gradient weight map has high response in the edge area where the boundaries are ambiguous, as shown in yellow arrows in Fig. 3.

Our framework was trained and tested in python, using Pytorch 1.0. Computation for the whole segmentation pipeline (end to end) was around 5s on a standard workstation (CPU: Intel Xeon E5-2620 v4, 2.10 GHz; GPU: TITAN Xp with 12G memory). During each training iteration, we augmented dataset through random rotation, random flip along sagittal axis, and histogram matching. For each experiment, we let our model trained for 3000 epochs, and used a momentum of 0.99 and an initial learning rate of 0.0001.

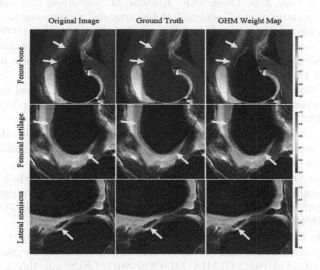

Fig. 3. Illustration of the gradient weight maps from the converged model trained with GHDL on our own dataset. (Color figure online)

5   Conclusion

In this work, we proposed a novel loss function to address the two well-known imbalance problems encountered during the training of multi-class segmentation. To our best knowledge, this is the first work trying to combine Dice loss with adaptive weight regularization mechanism, which has been widely used in state-of-the-art loss functions such as Focal loss and GHM-C loss. We employed our loss function in a 3D fully convolutional neural network for multiple object segmentation of MRI knee joint images and validated on both public *SKI10* dataset and a private dataset. The experimental results showed that the GHDL outperformed the popular loss functions, and achieved the state-of-the-art results on the validation data of *SKI10*.

Acknowledgement. This work was partially supported by the National Key Research and Development Program of China (2018YFC0116400).

References

1. Buyu, L., Liu, Y., Wang, X.: Gradient harmonized single-stage detector. arXiv preprint arXiv: 1811.05181 (2018)
2. Felix, A., Alexander, T., Moritz, E., Zachow, S.: Automated segmentation of knee bone and cartilage combining statistical shape knowledge and convolutional neural networks: data from the osteoarthritis initiative. Med. Image Anal. **52**, 109–118 (2019)
3. Folkesson, J., Dam, E.B., Olsen, O.F., Karsdal, M., Pettersen, P., Christiansen, C.: Automatic quantification of local and global articular cartilage surface curvatures: biomarkers for osteoarthritis? Magn. Reson. Med. **59**, 1340–1346 (2008)
4. Fripp, J., Crozier, S., Warfield, S., Ourselin, S.: Automatic segmentation and quantitative analysis of the articular cartilages from magnetic resonance images of the knee. IEEE Trans. Med. Imaging **29**, 55–64 (2010)
5. Lin, T.Y., Goyal, P., Girshick, R., Kaiming, H., Dollar, P.: Focal loss for dense object detection. In: IEEE International Conference on Computer Vision (ICCV), pp. 2999–3007 (2017)
6. Milletari, F., Navab, N., Ahmadi, S.A.: V-net: fully convolutional neural networks for volumetric medical image segmentation. In: 2016 Fourth International Conference on 3D Vision (3DV), pp. 565–571. IEEE (2016)
7. Ronneberger, O., Fischer, P., Brox, T.: U-Net: convolutional networks for biomedical image segmentation. In: Navab, N., Hornegger, J., Wells, W.M., Frangi, A.F. (eds.) MICCAI 2015. LNCS, vol. 9351, pp. 234–241. Springer, Cham (2015). https://doi.org/10.1007/978-3-319-24574-4_28
8. Sudre, C.H., Li, W., Vercauteren, T., Ourselin, S., Jorge Cardoso, M.: Generalised dice overlap as a deep learning loss function for highly unbalanced segmentations. In: Cardoso, M.J., et al. (eds.) DLMIA/ML-CDS -2017. LNCS, vol. 10553, pp. 240–248. Springer, Cham (2017). https://doi.org/10.1007/978-3-319-67558-9_28
9. Tobias, H., Bryan, J.M., Martin, A.S., Niethammer, M., Simon, K.W.: Generalised dice overlap as a deep learning loss function for highly unbalanced segmentations. In: MICCAI Workshop on Medical Image Analysis for the Clinic, pp. 207–214 (2010)

LSRC: A Long-Short Range Context-Fusing Framework for Automatic 3D Vertebra Localization

Jintai Chen[1,2], Yanjie Wang[1,2], Ruoqian Guo[1,2], Bohan Yu[1,2],
Tingting Chen[1,2], Wenzhe Wang[1,2], Ruiwei Feng[1,2], Danny Z. Chen[3],
and Jian Wu[1,2(✉)]

[1] College of Computer Science and Technology, Zhejiang University,
Hangzhou, China
wujian2000@zju.edu.cn
[2] Real Doctor AI Research Centre, Zhejiang University, Hangzhou, China
[3] Department of Computer Science and Engineering, University of Notre Dame,
Notre Dame, IN 46556, USA

Abstract. Automatic localization and identification of vertebrae in computed tomography (CT) images is a challenging task, due to the specific spine structure, complex pathological conditions, and limited field-of-view in 3D CT images. The local and long-range contextual information is especially useful for solving this problem. To explore both the local and long-range contextual information of vertebrae, in this paper, we propose a new framework called **Long-Short Range Context-fusing framework (LSRC)**, combining a 3D local semantic network and a 2D long-range contextual network. The 3D local semantic network, using 3D CT images, produces 3D heat maps corresponding to the locations of all vertebrae. The 3D heat maps and CT images are respectively projected onto the sagittal plane and coronal plane, and fed to the 2D long-range contextual network, in which a convolutional encoder-decoder module integrates the long-range contextual information of these two views. Two refined heat maps in the sagittal and coronal planes are generated by a globally-refining module, adjusting vertebra locations using the global location information in an attention manner. Experiments on a public dataset of 302 3D spine CT scans with various pathological conditions show that our new framework outperforms state-of-the-art methods.

1 Introduction

Medical imaging techniques have been widely used in clinical practice, including diagnosis, treatment planning, and postoperative assessment. 3D computed tomography (CT) images provide a good view of the spine structure for evaluation of spinal anatomical conditions. However, human vertebrae are highly

---

J. Chen, Y. Wang, R. Guo and B. Yu—These authors contributed equally to this work.

© Springer Nature Switzerland AG 2019
D. Shen et al. (Eds.): MICCAI 2019, LNCS 11769, pp. 95–103, 2019.
https://doi.org/10.1007/978-3-030-32226-7_11

complex anatomy with a specific structure and similar morphological appearance. Besides, the various pathological cases and the restriction of the field-of-view of 3D CT images cause substantial difficulties to accurate localization and identification of vertebrae. Such pathological cases have different conditions, for example, metal implants often cause bright visual imaging artifacts, deformation may result in abnormal curvature of the spine, etc. Thus, it is a challenging task to accurately localize and identify each individual vertebra in 3D CT images.

Recently, deep learning methods have shown a remarkable capability to deal with complicated pattern recognition problems. Recently, many methods [1,3,4,7–10], especially deep learning frameworks, were presented to address the localization and identification of vertebrae. In [1], a joint convolutional neural network (CNN) was utilized after coarse detection by a random forest classifier. In [8], density-based features were extracted and a deep neural network was used for vertebra identification. These two methods outperformed the previous work by a large margin, but their feature extraction was not very effective and may possibly miss some essential features. Later in [10], a 3D deep image-to-image network was used to detect an initial location of each vertebra, and a convolutional long short-term memory (ConvLSTM) model was employed to adjust the locations based on the context of the vertebrae. In [9], the architecture of [10] was modified and a massage passing method was developed to replace ConvL-STM. Since these two frameworks were deployed in end-to-end manner, the 3D deep image-to-image network in the first step limited the receptive field of the frameworks, even if they tried to make use of long-range contextual information via ConvLSTM [10] and the massage passing method [9]. A two-step framework was proposed in [7], utilizing the sagittal and coronal planes of the spine images; this 2D butterfly-shaped network combined information from the sagittal and coronal plane projections and was trained in an energy-based adversarial regime. Comparing with [10], this method had a larger receptive field and emphasized the importance of the vertebra context. However, some spatial information might be missed since it used only the sagittal and coronal planes of 3D CT images.

To effectively extract both the local information and long-range contextual information, in this paper, we propose a new framework for vertebra localization and identification in 3D CT images, called **Long-Short Range Context-fusing framework (LSRC)**. LSRC uses a 3D local semantic network for local information extraction and a 2D long-range contextual network for long-range contextual information extraction. The 3D local semantic network predicts the presence probability of every vertebra in a sequence of 3D heat maps voxel-wise in order. The 2D long-range contextual network, which is used to further extract long-range contextual information, utilizes the 2D sagittal and coronal views of the CT images and heat maps (see Fig. 1) and produces refined 2D heat maps on the sagittal and coronal planes. This 2D long-range contextual network contains a convolutional encoder-decoder module (CEDM) and a globally-refining module (GRM). CEDM extracts long-range contextual information from all the 2D views synchronously, and then GRM optimizes the locations of the vertebrae and produces refined 2D heat maps using the context of the correlative vertebrae in an attention manner. At the end, for every vertebra, a final heat map is predicted via an outer product of a refined 2D sagittal heat map and a refined 2D coronal heat map. The final coordinates of the predicted vertebra centroids are obtained as the maxima in the corresponding heat maps.

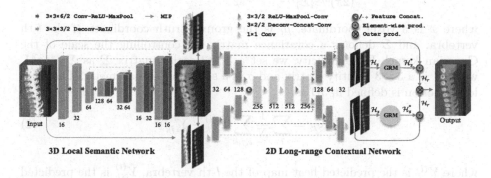

Fig. 1. An overview of our LSRC framework, with the 3D local semantic network and 2D long-range contextual network as two main components. GRM = the globally-refining module. MIP = the maximum intensity projection. The kernel sizes of convolution and stride of max-pooling or deconvolution are denoted as "kernel sizes/stride". The value under each feature map is the number of channels.

We make three main contributions in this work. (**A**) We propose a novel LSRC framework to fuse the long-short range contextual information by combining two 3D and 2D convolutional networks. (**B**) We develop a new globally-refining module to learn the correlations among vertebrae in an attention manner that helps refine the locations of vertebrae. (**C**) Our framework outperforms the previous methods on a public dataset with various pathological conditions.

2   Approach

2.1   3D Local Semantic Network (LSN)

Our local semantic network (denoted by LSN) is a 3D fully convolutional encoder-decoder network. LSN directly operates on the input 3D CT images and produces a sequence of 3D heat maps, each of which corresponds to one vertebra, predicting the presence probability of this vertebra voxel-wise. To keep the local resolution information, feature concatenations bridge every feature map in the encoder part to its corresponding feature map in the decoder part. The details are shown in Fig. 1. $3 \times 3 \times 6$ convolutional kernels in the encoder part are utilized to expand the vertical receptive field in order to cover more context. LSN extracts detailed information of the vertebrae by exploiting the ability of 3D convolutions. As in [10], 3D heat maps are computed in voxel-wise manner under the specification of the mean squared error (MSE) loss function. The ground truth for each vertebra is represented as a 3D Gaussian kernel. For the l-th vertebra ($l = 1, 2, 3, \ldots, C$, with C being the number of vertebrae in a spine), we represent its ground truth as:

$$Y^{(l)} = \frac{1}{(2\pi)^{3/2}|\Sigma|^{1/2}} \exp[-\frac{1}{2}(x - \mu_l)^T \Sigma^{-1}(x - \mu_l)] \tag{1}$$

where x is a voxel coordinate, μ_l is the ground truth coordinate of the l-th vertebra, and Σ denotes a covariance matrix for controlling the scale of the Gaussian kernel. For simplicity, we set a 3×3 scalar matrix Σ as $\Sigma = \sigma^2 I$, where I is a 3×3 identity matrix and σ is a scalar hyper-parameter. The MSE loss function is defined in 3D as:

$$\mathcal{L}_{MSE} = \sum_l \frac{1}{N} \sum_{i,j,k} (\hat{Y}_{ijk}^{(l)} - Y_{ijk}^{(l)})^2 \tag{2}$$

where $\hat{Y}^{(l)}$ is the predicted heat map of the l-th vertebra, $\hat{Y}_{ijk}^{(l)}$ is the predicted presence probability at the coordinate (i, j, k) in $\hat{Y}^{(l)}$, N is the number of voxels in a 3D CT image, and $Y^{(l)}$ is defined as in Eq. (1).

2.2   2D Long-Range Contextual Network (LRCN)

Convolutional Encoder-Decoder Module (CEDM). Inspired by [6,7], our 2D CEDM, with two input branches and two output branches, extracts the long-range contextual information from 3D heat maps and CT images in the sagittal and coronal views, and produces two refined 2D sagittal and coronal heat maps. The detailed architecture of CEDM is shown as the ladder-shaped structure in the middle part of Fig. 1. As discussed in Sect. 2.1, our local semantic network LSN produces a sequence of 3D heat maps. Each 3D heat map and its corresponding CT image are directly projected onto the sagittal and coronal planes by maximum intensity projection (MIP). In CEDM, one input branch takes the heat maps and the corresponding CT images of the sagittal view (after concatenation across channels) as input while the other takes the coronal ones. After fusing features from these two views, CEDM outputs feature maps in two branches: one produces the sagittal "semi-refined" heat maps $\mathcal{H}_s$ and a mask while the other produces the coronal ones. Each output branch produces one mask $\mathcal{M}_{mask}$ and C "semi-refined" heat maps (corresponding to C vertebrae) in 2D. The mask indicates the spine skeleton region. These C heat maps $\mathcal{H}_s$ are further refined by GRM using the global context of vertebrae, and are transformed to $\mathcal{H}_s^*$ (more details of this are given in the next subsection).

Finally, we compute the refined sagittal and coronal heat maps by element-wise product: $\mathcal{H}_r^{(l)} = \mathcal{M}_{mask} \times \mathcal{H}_s^{*(l)}$. Note that the learning of the mask $\mathcal{M}_{mask}$ is easier than that of heat maps; thus, the prediction is of higher confidence, since one can view it as just a localization task without identification. Hence, we can regard this element-wise product operation as a de-noising process. During training, the ground truths of $\mathcal{H}_s$, $\mathcal{H}_s^*$ and $\mathcal{H}_r$ are represented as 2D Gaussian kernels, similar to Eq. (1). The ground truth of mask $\mathcal{M}_{mask}$ is represented as

$$Y_{\mathcal{M}} = \mathcal{X}_A(x) \quad \text{such that} \quad A = \{x' | (x' - \mu)^2 \leqslant \lambda\} \tag{3}$$

where μ is a point on the line segments connecting the ground truth centroids of every two consecutive vertebrae (in each 2D view), x is a voxel in the 2D view, $\mathcal{X}_A(x)$ is an indicator function indicating whether x is in a set A, and the hyper-parameter λ controls the size of the ground truth mask.

CEDM is trained by the specification of the cross-entropy loss and MSE loss $\mathcal{L}_{mse}$ in 2D (similar to Eq. (2)). The cross-entropy loss guides the learning of the mask. $\mathcal{L}_{mse}$ is for the predicted heat maps (including $\mathcal{H}_s$, $\mathcal{H}_s^*$, and $\mathcal{H}_r$).

Globally-Refining Module (GRM). As shown in Figs. 1 and 2, GRM is utilized on every "semi-refined" heat map $\mathcal{H}_s$, generated by the 2D CEDM (as described above). GRM is designed using a novel attention-based method which learns to compute the correlations among vertebrae, in order to refine the pixel-wise predicted presence probabilities of one vertebra by considering those of its correlative vertebrae. When learning the correlations among vertebrae, we exclude other potential influencing factors by down-sampling the C heat maps into one vector of size C. That is, every heat map (corresponding to one vertebra) is down-sampled to a single value by global max-pooling. We compute an attention map of size $C \times C$, obtained by outer product of this vector as initialization and then adjusted by a fully connected layer, as shown in Fig. 2. Next, to produce $\mathcal{H}_s^*$, the "semi-refined" heat map $\mathcal{H}_s$ is enhanced by the attention map and then operated by three 6×3 convolutional layers with ReLU activation. The attention operation is performed as:

$$M_{(i,j)}^{(l)} = \sum_{c=1}^{C} M_{att(l,c)} \times \mathcal{H}_{s(i,j)}^{(c)} \qquad \mathcal{H}_s^* = Conv(M) \tag{4}$$

where M_{att} denotes an attention map and (i,j) is a point of a heat map. Ideally, M_{att} should be trained with the whole training dataset in one "batch" because one single CT often does not contain all vertebrae. However, limited by the GPU memory and computing devices, we need to divide the data into multiple batches of size B each. In the training, we compute the initial M_{att} by $M_{att(C \times C)} = M_{(B \times C)}^T M_{(B \times C)}$, where $M_{(B \times C)}$ is a down-sampled heat map using global max-pooling operation in a batch (stacked by B vectors). In the testing, we use M_{att} averaged by all the learned attention maps obtained in training. GRM is also trained under the guidance of $\mathcal{L}_{mse}$ and the coordinate regression loss $\mathcal{L}_{reg}$, and the ground truth of the heat maps is the 2D Gaussian kernels (which are the same as for the 2D CEDM). The regression loss is defined as:

$$\mathcal{L}_{reg} = \sum_{l=1}^{C} \text{smooth}_{L_1}(y_l - \mu_l) \tag{5}$$

where y_l and μ_l are the predicted coordinates and ground truth coordinates of the l-th vertebra, respectively, and $\text{smooth}_{L_1}(\cdot)$ is the same as in [2]. y_l on the

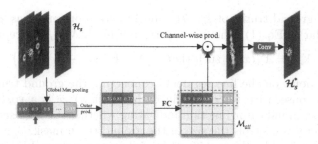

Fig. 2. The architecture of our globally-refining module (GRM). We illustrate the operations with one heat map as an example. FC = a full connected layer. Note that the "channel-wise product" operation is equivalent to the left equation in Eq. (4), and only a single channel of the channel-wise product results is shown for easy viewing.

heat maps is computed by the soft-argmax method [5] which is differentiable, so that it can be updated by back-propagation.

2.3 Training Process

Our training process can be divided into two stages. In the first stage, we randomly crop the CT images as input when training the 3D local semantic network LSN for data augmentation and memory saving. In the second stage, the 2D long-range contextual network LRCN is trained as discussed in Sect. 2.2. The loss function of the whole LSRC network can be presented as:

$$\mathcal{L} = \alpha \mathcal{L}_{MSE} + \beta \mathcal{L}_{mse} + \gamma \mathcal{L}_{ce} + \eta \mathcal{L}_{reg} \tag{6}$$

where $\mathcal{L}_{MSE}$ is the MSE loss operating in 3D as in Eq. (2), and $\mathcal{L}_{mse}$ is the MSE loss operating in 2D used by the 2D LRCN, $\mathcal{L}_{ce}$ denotes the cross entropy for the learning of the mask $\mathcal{M}_{mask}$, and $\mathcal{L}_{reg}$ is defined in Eq. (5). When training the 3D local semantic network, $\beta = \gamma = \eta = 0$. When training the 2D long-range contextual network, $\alpha = 0$. The whole LSRC framework is optimized by back-propagation until convergence. After the two refined heat maps $\mathcal{H}_r$ is obtained (a sagittal heat map and a coronal one, as described in Sect. 2.2), we predict the final heat map with an outer product of them, as $\widetilde{\mathcal{H}}^{(l)} = \mathcal{H}_{r,sag}^{(l)} \times \mathcal{H}_{r,cor}^{(l)}$ for every vertebra. Finally, the final coordinates of the predicted vertebral centroids are obtained as the maxima in the corresponding heat maps.

3   Experiments

As the previous work [7,9,10], we evaluate our LSRC on the dataset provided by [4], which consists of 302 3D CT scans (242 for training and 60 for testing) with various pathological conditions. These pathological cases contain abnormal spinal deformations, bright metal-induced visual imaging artifacts, etc. Moreover, the field-of-view of the CT images is quite limited. To better compare with other results, we set $C = 24$ (ignoring the two sacrums) as in [7] and $C = 26$ as in [1,4,9,10]. We use a routine CT respacing pre-processing to resample the data to 1 mm isotropic resolution and train the LSN and LRCN models with batch-size of 2 and 8, respectively. We conduct experiments following the training process in Sect. 2.3. Additionally, we evaluate every component of LSRC (the 3D local semantic network, 2D encoder-decoder module, and 2D globally-refining module) in ablation study. To show the ability of capturing the global context by the globally-refining module, we compare it with ConvLSTM [10] and the massage passing method [9], using the "local semantic network + encoder-decoder module" as the *baseline*. Every part of LSRC is built as in Sect. 2, with $\sigma = 1$ for Eq. (1). The Adam optimizer is employed with an initial learning rate 1×10^{-3}. $\lambda = 5.0$ in Eq. (3). We set α, β, γ, and η as 1.0 when they are used, as described in Sect. 2.3.

To compare the performance of our LSRC with the previous work, we utilize two metrics as in [4,7,9,10]: the identification rates (Id. rate) and localization distances (d_{mean} and d_{std}, measured in mm). Table 1 shows the performances of the frameworks LSRC-24, Btrfly [7], Btrfly$^-$ [7] (Btrfly without the energy based GAN) using $C = 24$, and the frameworks LSRC-26, DI2IN [10], DI2IN$^+$ [9], DI2IN$^-$ [9] (DI2IN without massage passing), Glocker's [4], and J-CNN [1] using $C = 26$. We do not compare performance on the private dataset in DI2IN$^+$ [9]. We also evaluate the effect of every part of LSRC, shown in Table 2. One can see that our LSRC outperforms previous frameworks (their results came from either the original papers or [7,10]) in terms of all the metrics and the C configurations. To further illustrate the effect of LSRC, we show some qualitative results of LSRC in Fig. 3. As the results of the ablation study in Table 2 show, the three components of LSRC all contribute to the good performance of LSRC. Moreover, comparing Tables 2 and 1, one can see that our combination of the 3D and 2D convolutional networks ("LSN + CEDM", without GRM) remarkably outperforms the 3D networks (DI2IN$^-$) and 2D networks (Btrfly$^-$) alone by 0.10 and 0.05 in Id. rate, and 6.3 mm and 0.2 mm in d_{mean}. On d_{std}, "LSN + CEDM" outperforms DI2IN$^-$ by 28.6 mm, but incurs a slightly larger distance value than Btrfly$^-$.

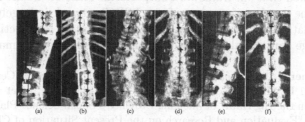

Fig. 3. Some qualitative results of LSRC: (a), (c), and (e) are sagittal views while (b), (d), and (f) are coronal views. The red and blue crosses denote the ground truth locations and the predicted vertebra locations, respectively. (Color figure online)

Table 1. Performance comparison of our LSRC-24, Btrfly [7], Btrfly$^-$ [7], LSRC-26,DI2IN [10], DI2IN$^+$ [9], DI2IN$^-$ [9], J-CNN [1], and the Glocker's [4].

Method	LSRC-24	Btrfly	Btrfly$^-$	LSRC-26	DI2IN	DI2IN$^+$	DI2IN$^-$	J-CNN	Glocker's
Id. rate	**0.88**	0.86	0.81	**0.88**	0.85	0.85	0.76	0.84	0.74
d_{mean} (in mm)	**7.1**	7.4	7.5	**7.4**	8.7	8.6	13.6	8.8	13.2
d_{std} (in mm)	7.7	9.3	**5.4**	8.3	8.5	**7.8**	37.5	13.0	17.8

Table 2. Ablation study of our 3D local semantic network (LSN), convolutional encoder-decoder module (CEDM), and globally-refining module (GRM).

LSN	CEDM	GRM	Id. rate	d_{mean}	d_{std}
✓			0.79	8.7	12.7
✓	✓		0.86	7.3	8.9
✓	✓	✓	0.88	7.1	7.7

Table 3. Comparative experiments for the globally-refining module (GRM), ConvLSTM (CL), and Massage Passing (MP), with "LSN+CEDM" as the *baseline*.

baseline	GRM	CL	MP	Id. rate	d_{mean}	d_{std}
✓	✓			**0.88**	**7.1**	**7.7**
✓		✓		0.87	7.7	8.0
✓			✓	0.87	7.3	**7.7**

The comparison of our globally-refining module, ConvLSTM, and the massage passing method in Table 3 shows that our globally-refining module is better at capturing global context. A reason may be that ConvLSTM is more suitable for learning much longer sequences, and the massage passing method focuses only on every two consecutive vertebrae in each iteration, which may cause errors.

4   Conclusions

In this paper, we proposed a new long-short range contextual-fusing (LSRC) network for automatic 3D vertebra localization and identification. We combined a 3D convolutional network and a 2D convolutional network to extract features. We also developed a novel attention based globally-refining module. Experimental results showed that our framework outperforms state-of-the-art methods. We believe that the good performance of our LSRC network is largely due to our careful combination of 3D convolution and 2D convolution for effectively learning both long-range contextual information and local semantic information.

Acknowledgment. The research of the Real Doctor AI Research Centre was partially supported by the Subject of the Major Commissioned Project "Research on China's Image in the Big Data" of Zhejiang Province's Social Science Planning Advantage Discipline "Evaluation and Research on the Present Situation of China's Image" No. 16YSXK01ZD-2YB, Ministry of Education of China under grant No. 2017PT18, the Zhejiang University Education Foundation under grants No. K18-511120-004, No. K17-511120-017, and No. K17-518051-021, the Major Scientific Project of Zhejiang Lab under grant No. 2018DG0ZX01, the National Natural Science Foundation of China under grant No. 61672453, and the Key Laboratory of Medical Neurobiology of Zhejiang Province. The research of D.Z. Chen was supported in part by NSF Grant CCF-1617735. We like to thank three anonymous reviewers for their helpful suggestions.

References

1. Chen, H., et al.: Automatic localization and identification of vertebrae in spine CT via a joint learning model with deep neural networks. In: Navab, N., Hornegger, J., Wells, W.M., Frangi, A.F. (eds.) MICCAI 2015. LNCS, vol. 9349, pp. 515–522. Springer, Cham (2015). https://doi.org/10.1007/978-3-319-24553-9_63
2. Girshick, R.: Fast R-CNN. In: ICCV, pp. 1440–1448 (2015)
3. Glocker, B., Feulner, J., Criminisi, A., Haynor, D.R., Konukoglu, E.: Automatic localization and identification of vertebrae in arbitrary field-of-view CT scans. In: Ayache, N., Delingette, H., Golland, P., Mori, K. (eds.) MICCAI 2012. LNCS, vol. 7512, pp. 590–598. Springer, Heidelberg (2012). https://doi.org/10.1007/978-3-642-33454-2_73
4. Glocker, B., Zikic, D., Konukoglu, E., Haynor, D.R., Criminisi, A.: Vertebrae localization in pathological spine CT via dense classification from sparse annotations. In: Mori, K., Sakuma, I., Sato, Y., Barillot, C., Navab, N. (eds.) MICCAI 2013. LNCS, vol. 8150, pp. 262–270. Springer, Heidelberg (2013). https://doi.org/10.1007/978-3-642-40763-5_33
5. Luvizon, D., et al.: Human pose regression by combining indirect part detection and contextual information. arXiv preprint arXiv:1710.02322 (2017)
6. Ronneberger, O., Fischer, P., Brox, T.: U-Net: convolutional networks for biomedical image segmentation. In: Navab, N., Hornegger, J., Wells, W.M., Frangi, A.F. (eds.) MICCAI 2015. LNCS, vol. 9351, pp. 234–241. Springer, Cham (2015). https://doi.org/10.1007/978-3-319-24574-4_28
7. Sekuboyina, A., et al.: Btrfly net: vertebrae labelling with energy-based adversarial learning of local spine prior. In: Frangi, A.F., Schnabel, J.A., Davatzikos, C., Alberola-López, C., Fichtinger, G. (eds.) MICCAI 2018. LNCS, vol. 11073, pp. 649–657. Springer, Cham (2018). https://doi.org/10.1007/978-3-030-00937-3_74
8. Suzani, A., Seitel, A., Liu, Y., Fels, S., Rohling, R.N., Abolmaesumi, P.: Fast automatic vertebrae detection and localization in pathological CT scans - a deep learning approach. In: Navab, N., Hornegger, J., Wells, W.M., Frangi, A.F. (eds.) MICCAI 2015. LNCS, vol. 9351, pp. 678–686. Springer, Cham (2015). https://doi.org/10.1007/978-3-319-24574-4_81
9. Yang, D., et al.: Automatic vertebra labeling in large-scale 3D CT using deep image-to-image network with message passing and sparsity regularization. In: Niethammer, M., et al. (eds.) IPMI 2017. LNCS, vol. 10265, pp. 633–644. Springer, Cham (2017). https://doi.org/10.1007/978-3-319-59050-9_50
10. Yang, D., et al.: Deep image-to-image recurrent network with shape basis learning for automatic vertebra labeling in large-scale 3D CT volumes. In: Descoteaux, M., Maier-Hein, L., Franz, A., Jannin, P., Collins, D.L., Duchesne, S. (eds.) MICCAI 2017. LNCS, vol. 10435, pp. 498–506. Springer, Cham (2017). https://doi.org/10.1007/978-3-319-66179-7_57

Contextual Deep Regression Network for Volume Estimation in Orbital CT

Shikha Chaganti[1(⊠)], Cam Bermudez[2], Louise A. Mawn[3],
Thomas Lasko[4], and Bennett A. Landman[5]

[1] Computer Science, Vanderbilt University, Nashville, TN, USA
shikha.chaganti@vanderbillt.edu
[2] Biomedical Engineering, Vanderbilt University, Nashville, TN, USA
[3] Department of Ophthalmology, Vanderbilt University Medical Center,
Nashville, TN, USA
[4] Biomedical Informatics, Vanderbilt University Medical Center,
Nashville, TN, USA
[5] Electrical Engineering, Vanderbilt University, Nashville, TN, USA

Abstract. Diseases of the optic nerve cause structural changes observable through clinical computed tomography (CT) imaging. Previous work has shown that multi-atlas methods can be used to segment and extract volumetric measurements from the optic nerve, which are associated with visual disability and disease. In this work, we trained a weakly supervised convolutional neural network to learn optic nerve volumes directly, without segmentation. Furthermore, we explored the role of contextual electronic medical record (EMR) information, specifically ICD-9 codes, to improve optic nerve volume estimation. We constructed a merged network to combine data from imaging as well as EMR and demonstrated that context improved volume prediction, with a 15% increase in explained-variance (R^2). Finally, we compared disease prediction models using volumes learned from multi-atlas, CNN, and contextual-CNN. We observed that the predicted optic nerve volume from merge-CNN had an AUC of 0.74 for classification of disease, as compared to an AUC of 0.54 using the multi-atlas metric. This is the first work to show that a contextually derived volume biomarker is more accurate than volume estimations through multi-atlas or weakly supervised image CNN. These results highlight the potential for image processing improvements by incorporating non-imaging data.

Keywords: Weak supervision · Optic nerve · CT · Segmentation-free · EMR ·
Volume estimation · Non-imaging data

1 Introduction

Diseases of the optic nerve can have serious consequences such as permanent blindness when not detected and treated within the window of opportunity. These diseases include a wide range of conditions such as glaucoma, thyroid eye disease, optic neuritis, papilledema, idiopathic intracranial hypertension, and orbital infections. A patient with optic neuropathy typically exhibits symptoms of sudden mild to severe vision loss in terms of both visual acuity and visual field defects, due to damage to the optic nerve.

© Springer Nature Switzerland AG 2019
D. Shen et al. (Eds.): MICCAI 2019, LNCS 11769, pp. 104–111, 2019.
https://doi.org/10.1007/978-3-030-32226-7_12

Clinical evaluation of patients with optic nerve diseases is performed by examining their optic nerve structure through modern imaging methods, as well as a thorough examination of their medical history such as past diagnoses. In this work, we present a method to automatically estimate a volumetric measurement of the optic nerve from clinically acquired CT scans, we show that contextual information from a patient's diagnostic history improves this estimate, and we demonstrate that this volumetric estimate is better at disease evaluation than estimates derived in previous studies.

Our hypothesis for this work is based on the notion that a direct volumetric estimate performed by a statistical model is not likely to be made using the typical approach of a human expert. Instead of first segmenting the optic nerve and then calculating the volume of that segment, the model is more likely to find various image features that probabilistically indicate an increase or decrease of the optic nerve volume, and then aggregate the effect of those features to arrive at a volume estimate. We hypothesized that the relevance of these image features to optic nerve volume may be dependent on the presence or absence of certain clinical conditions, so adding that clinical context to the input data may improve the accuracy of the model.

1.1 Role of Medical Imaging

Medical imaging methods, such as computed tomography (CT) and magnetic resonance imaging (MRI), are used to assess the pathology in orbital conditions. The pathophysiology of the optic nerve affected by these conditions is variable, including edema, atrophy, and compression [1]. Volumetric measurements of structural changes in the orbit, computed from medical image processing studies, are associated with visual function, visual acuity and visual field defects [2, 3]. More recently, Chaganti et al. showed that structural measurements obtained from the orbital CT can successfully classify optic nerve disease from healthy controls [4]. Volumetric measurements of the structures in the eye orbit, including the optic nerve, are therefore important biomarkers for objectively establishing eye disease.

1.2 Patient Story: Context from Electronic Medical Record (EMR)

Since many optic nerve conditions are systemic in nature, detection, diagnosis and therapeutic planning of these diseases require careful study of a patient's medical history. In diseases of the optic nerve, searching for system-wide co-morbidities is particularly important. For example, intracranial idiopathic hypertension (optic nerve edema) is associated with several systemic conditions such as Vitamin A deficiency, polycystic ovary syndrome, diabetes, thyroid disease, anemia, stroke, migraine, systemic lupus erythematous, pregnancy, menstrual dysfunction, and side-effects to certain medications [5, 6]. Thyroid eye disease is associated with past hypothyroidism, hyperthyroidism and Grave's disease [7–9]. Interestingly, previous work in image processing of the eye orbit has shown that addition of this contextual information of a subjects' past diagnoses improves image-based prediction of disease [4] and association with visual disability [3].

1.3   Weak Supervision

Previous work in image processing of the optic nerve relied on multi-atlas label fusion to segment structures of importance in the orbit, in order to compute volumetric biomarkers [10]. The preliminary step of segmentation can introduce errors of its own, which can get propagated to metric calculation. Recently, convolutional neural networks have shown success in kidney volume estimation [11] and ventricular volume estimation from 2D views [12]. In these examples, the segmentation step is skipped completely and the networks are trained with image-level labels, i.e., the volumes of the structures of interest. In this paper, we explore the ability of a weakly supervised, fully convolutional network (FCN) to directly learn optic nerve volumes from 3D CT scans of the orbit. The weak labels are obtained from volume estimates of multi-atlas segmentation. We developed a 3D FCN for volume estimation using clinically acquired CT volumes or the orbit. Inspired by previous work in contextual models for image processing of the orbit, we also developed a merged-FCN network that estimates the volume of left and right optic nerves from CT imaging as well as diagnosis data extracted from electronic medical records (EMR). Finally, we compare the performance of the predicted volumes from FCN networks to the multi-atlas volumes to predict disease. The novel contribution of this work is to show that addition of EMR data improves volume prediction and predictive power for disease classification.

2   Methods

2.1   Data

We use data collected under institutional review board at Vanderbilt University Medical Center. The imaging and EMR data of 136 subjects with diseases of the optic nerve: glaucoma, intrinsic optic nerve disease, thyroid eye disease, orbital inflammation and optic nerve edema was obtained. The control group for this study was 534 individuals with hearing loss who were chosen for having similar imaging data available. Clinically acquired CT imaging was collected for each subject, with variable imaging protocols such as CT head, orbital, and maxillofacial. The field of view for each scan included the full view of the orbit, including, optic nerves from the globes to the chiasm. The slice thickness was 1 mm and the in-plane resolution was 1 mm x 1 mm. In addition to imaging, we collected ICD-9 (International Classification of Disease, version 9) codes and demographic data for each subject. The volume regression was performed on all disease and control subjects with five-fold cross validation (Sect. 2.4). The classification task was performed on age-matched disease (n = 104) and control (n = 104) subjects with repeated 10-fold cross validation (Sect. 2.5).

2.2   Multi-atlas Segmentation

Multi-atlas segmentation was used to segment the optic nerve from CT imaging. In this paradigm, a set of 25 example atlases with expertly marked labels for the optic nerve, along with other structures in the orbit, are used to segment the structures in a new target scan. First, the eye orbit is localized in the target image since it can have varying fields of view from a whole head scan to a scan limited to the eye orbit. The example atlases are affinely registered to the target space [13]. The deformation fields from the registration are used to propagate the labels to the target space to form a probability map, and the eye orbit is localized by generating a bounding box around voxels with greater than probability of 0.5. Next, the example atlases are non-rigidly registered to the cropped target space using ANTS SyN registration with cross-correlation metric [14]. The expert labels are propagated to the target space and combined using non-local statistical label fusion [15] to segment the optic nerve. Finally, the volumes of the right and left optic nerve are computed from the segmentation.

2.3   Extraction of EMR Features

For each subject, we extract an EMR feature vector describing their clinical phenotypes from their electronic medical record. A clinical phenotype is described by a phecode, which is based on hierarchical categorization of ICD-9 (International Classification of Disease - 9) codes. A phecode groups a set of related ICD-9 codes together to form a clinically meaningful category [16]. For example, the "optic neuropathy" phecode groups the ICD-9 codes for different types of optic neuritis *(ICD-9 = 377.3, 377.30, 377.31, 377.32, 377.33, 377.34, or 377.39)* or other disorders of the optic nerve *(ICD-9 = 377.4, 377.41, 377.42, 377.43, or 377.49)*. A binary vector, p of length 1865 is formed for each subject, where p_i is 1 is the subject has the ith phecode in their record, and 0 if not. We used an open-source tool to automatically generate these EMR feature vectors, given a list of clinical visits for each subject, including ICD-9 codes recorded at each visit [17].

2.4   Network Architecture

We trained a fully convolutional regression network N_1, to estimate optic nerve volume. The network comprises of five 3D convolutional layers, each followed by max pooling and batch-normalization layers, as shown in the first panel of Fig. 1. At the end of the 5th convolutional layer, the features are flattened and the network is appended with two linear layers with ReLU activation. Finally, a single regression node is used to predict volume. Next, we train a linear regression network N_2, with two hidden layers to estimate volume from clinical phenotypes as seen in the second panel of Fig. 1. Finally, we construct a merged network M, where N_1 and N_2 are merged at the penultimate hidden linear layer, as seen in the third panel of Fig. 1. This is followed by one hidden layer and an output regression node. Network M is initialized with weights of previously trained networks N_1 and N_2 and fine-tuned. All the models are trained in a 5-fold cross-validation paradigm, with weak volume labels provided by the multi-atlas segmentation metrics. The learning rates for all three models were initiated with 1e-5 with a 1% decay each epoch. They were trained using the ADAM optimizer, with a mean squared loss for 1000 epochs.

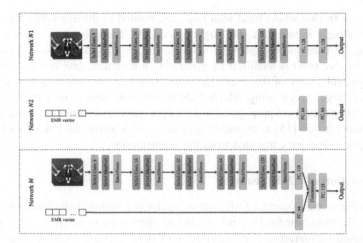

Fig. 1. Network architectures for volume estimation. Top panel: N_1, a regression-CNN to learn the optic nerve volumes from 3D CT images. Middle panel: N_2, a regression network to learn optic nerve volumes from EMR data. Bottom panel: M, a regression network that merges N_1 with N_2 at the penultimate layer, to learn optic nerve volume from both imaging and EMR data.

2.5   Classification

Following the volume estimation procedures described in Sects. 2.2 and 2.4, a logistic regression was trained to use the estimated optic nerve volumes to distinguish subjects belonging to the disease group from the control group. First, age-matching was performed to select a control within 2 years of age at the time of imaging for each disease subject. As a result, we obtain a dataset of 104 case and 104 control subjects. Next, we use 10-fold cross-validation to train a logistic regression model. We model $P(y_i = disease|X = x_i) = \frac{e^{\beta_0 + \beta^T x_i}}{1 + e^{\beta_0 + \beta^T x_i}}$, where $X = [V_l, V_r, sex, age]$. The folds are repeatedly sampled 100 times in order to obtain an estimate of performance for optic nerve volume obtained from each method. Area under the curve (AUC) is computed from the receiver operating curve (ROC) for each volume estimate.

3   Results

We use five-fold cross-validation to train networks N_1, N_2, and M to learn right and left optic nerve volumes. The left and right predicted volumes are denoted by V_{ln1}, V_{ln2}, and V_{lm}, and V_{rn1}, V_{rn2}, and V_{rm} respectively. The results are shown in Fig. 2 and Table 1 in terms of the median absolute loss, R^2, and Pearson's ρ. It can be seen that N_2, the EMR network, has the lowest explanatory power, being close to zero. N_1 learns the optic nerve volumes with a better accuracy with an R^2 of over 0.1 for both optic nerve volumes, and a significant correlation with the multi-atlas volumes of over 0.4. The merged network has the best volume prediction compared to N_1 and N_2, with the lowest median absolute error, and the highest explained variance (R^2 = 0.25, 0.23 for left and right optic nerves respectively) and Pearson correlation ($\rho = 0.52$, 0.49 for left and right optic nerves respectively).

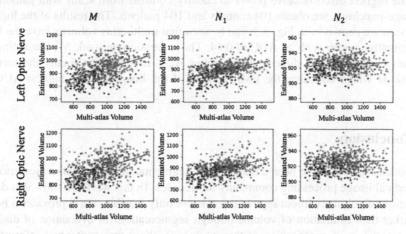

Fig. 2. Results of volume estimation using networks M, N_1, and N_2. The top row shows results for the left optic nerve, and the bottom row shows results for the right optic nerve.

Table 1. Results for volume estimation

	Statistic	Imaging + EMR (V_{l_m})	Imaging ($V_{l_{n1}}$)	EMR ($V_{l_{n2}}$)
Left optic nerve	Median absolute error (mm³)	130.37	134.76	161.62
	R^2	0.25	0.16	0.01
	Pearson's ρ	0.52	0.45	0.11
Right optic nerve	Median absolute error (mm³)	129.96	141.6	159
	R^2	0.23	0.1	0.0
	Pearson's ρ	0.49	0.43	0.12

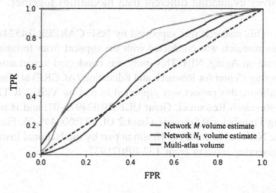

Fig. 3. ROC curves for classification of disease based on volume estimates.

Finally, we compare the predictive power of the volumes learned by N_1, and M to the multi-atlas volumes using a simple logistic regression to test which of the volumes have the highest discriminative power to classify controls from scans with pathology. After age-matching, we obtain 104 controls and 104 patients. The results of the logistic regression are shown in in Fig. 3. It can be seen that multi-atlas volumes have the least discriminative power with an AUC of 0.54. The regression network N_1, that estimates volumes from CT scans directly has a higher AUC of 0.67, and finally the merged network M which considers the EMR context of the image has the highest AUC of 0.74.

4 Conclusion

Multi-atlas methods have been a standard for segmentation and volume prediction in the medical image processing community for decades. In this work we show that direct estimation of volume without segmentation is not only feasible, but it provides a better biomarker than estimation of volume through segmentation for evaluation of disease. However, the main contribution of this work is to show that contextual information from a subject's past diagnostic history improves estimation of volumes of the optic nerve. We proposed a simple architecture to combine imaging data with EMR data. While previous work has shown that contextual information improves computer-aided diagnosis tasks, this is the first work to show that contextual information is helpful in a more traditional image processing task such as volume estimation. The addition of EMR information helps the model to contextualize certain pathology-related image features with their corresponding clinical conditions. In a way, this method helps the network estimate the volumes with an implicit "prior". In addition, it might also be learning implicit changes in other image features that correlate with increase or decrease in volume—features that cannot be measured via segmentation. The contextual network M, showed the highest explained variance in learning the optic nerve volumes and was shown to be the strongest biomarker for disease evaluation, when compared to other estimates (AUC = 0.74), thus proving our hypothesis that clinical context improves accuracy of the model. The methods used in this work are not specific to the optic nerve, and can be generalized to any disease area with a complex presentation that involves evaluating different data modalities together.

Acknowledgement. This research was supported by NSF CAREER 1452485 and NIH grants 5R21EY024036. This research was conducted with the support from Intramural Research Program, National Institute on Aging, NIH. This study was conducted in part using the resources of the Advanced Computing Center for Research and Education (ACCRE) at Vanderbilt University, Nashville, TN. In addition, this project was supported in part by ViSE/VICTR VR3029 and the National Center for Research Resources, Grant UL1 RR024975-01, and is now at the National Center for Advancing Translational Sciences, Grant 2 UL1 TR000445-06. Finally, this work was also supported by the National Institutes of Health in part by the National Institute of Biomedical Imaging and Bioengineering training grant T32-EB021937.

References

1. Becker, M., Masterson, K., Delavelle, J., Viallon, M., Vargas, M.-I., Becker, C.D.: Imaging of the optic nerve. Eur. J. Radiol. **74**(2), 299–313 (2010)
2. Yao, X., et al.: Structural-functional relationships between eye orbital imaging biomarkers and clinical visual assessments. In: SPIE Medical Imaging, p. 101331F (2017)
3. Chaganti, S., Robinson, J.R., Bermudez, C., Lasko, T., Mawn, L.A., Landman, B.A.: EMR-radiological phenotypes in diseases of the optic nerve and their association with visual function. In: Cardoso, M.Jorge, Arbel, T., Carneiro, G., et al. (eds.) DLMIA/ML-CDS -2017. LNCS, vol. 10553, pp. 373–381. Springer, Cham (2017). https://doi.org/10.1007/978-3-319-67558-9_43
4. Chaganti, S., et al.: Electronic medical record context signatures improve diagnostic classification using medical image computing. IEEE J. Biomed. Heal. Informatics **PP**, 1 (2018)
5. Ball, A.K., Clarke, C.E.: Idiopathic intracranial hypertension. Lancet Neurol. **5**(5), 433–442 (2006)
6. Binder, D.K., Horton, J.C., Lawton, M.T., McDermott, M.W.: Idiopathic intracranial hypertension. Neurosurgery **54**(3), 538–552 (2004)
7. Nunery, W.R., Nunery, C.W., Martin, R.T., Truong, T.V., Osborn, D.R.: The risk of diplopia following orbital floor and medial wall decompression in subtypes of ophthalmic Graves' disease. Ophthalmic Plast. Reconstr. Surg. **13**(3), 153–160 (1997)
8. Laurberg, P., Berman, D.C., Bülow Pedersen, I., Andersen, S., Carlé, A.: Double vision is a major manifestation in moderate to severe graves' orbitopathy, but it correlates negatively with inflammatory signs and proptosis. J. Clin. Endocrinol. Metab. **100**(5), 2098–2105 (2015)
9. Ophthalmopathy, G.: Graves' Ophthalmopathy (2010)
10. Harrigan, R.L., et al.: Robust optic nerve segmentation on clinically acquired computed tomography. J. Med. Imaging **1**(3), 34006 (2014)
11. Hussain, M.A., Amir-Khalili, A., Hamarneh, G., Abugharbieh, R.: Segmentation-free kidney localization and volume estimation using aggregated orthogonal decision CNNs. In: Descoteaux, M., Maier-Hein, L., Franz, A., Jannin, P., Collins, D.Louis, Duchesne, S. (eds.) MICCAI 2017. LNCS, vol. 10435, pp. 612–620. Springer, Cham (2017). https://doi.org/10.1007/978-3-319-66179-7_70
12. Luo, G., Dong, S., Wang, K., Zuo, W., Cao, S., Zhang, H.: Multi-views fusion CNN for left ventricular volumes estimation on cardiac MR images. IEEE Trans. Biomed. Eng. **65**(9), 1924–1934 (2018)
13. Heinrich, M.P., Jenkinson, M., Brady, M., Schnabel, J.A.: MRF-based deformable registration and ventilation estimation of lung CT. IEEE Trans. Med. Imaging **32**(7), 1239–1248 (2013)
14. Avants, B.B., Epstein, C.L., Grossman, M., Gee, J.C.: Symmetric diffeomorphic image registration with cross-correlation: evaluating automated labeling of elderly and neurode-generative brain. Med. Image Anal. **12**(1), 26–41 (2008)
15. Asman, A.J., Landman, B.A.: Non-local statistical label fusion for multi-atlas segmentation. Med. Image Anal. **17**(2), 194–208 (2013)
16. Denny, J.C., et al.: PheWAS: demonstrating the feasibility of a phenome-wide scan to discover gene–disease associations. Bioinformatics **26**(9), 1205–1210 (2010)
17. Chaganti, S., Nabar, K., Landman, B.: pyPheWAS (2017). https://github.com/Bennett Landman/pyPheWAS

Multi-scale GANs for Memory-efficient Generation of High Resolution Medical Images

Hristina Uzunova[1(✉)], Jan Ehrhardt[1], Fabian Jacob[2], Alex Frydrychowicz[2], and Heinz Handels[1]

[1] Institute of Medical Informatics, University of Lübeck, Lübeck, Germany
uzunova@imi.uni-luebeck.de
[2] Department for Radiology and Nuclear Medicine,
University Hospital of Schleswig-Holstein, Lübeck, Germany

Abstract. Currently generative adversarial networks (GANs) are rarely applied to medical images of large sizes, especially 3D volumes, due to their large computational demand. We propose a novel multi-scale patch-based GAN approach to generate large high resolution 2D and 3D images. Our key idea is to first learn a low-resolution version of the image and then generate patches of successively growing resolutions conditioned on previous scales. In a domain translation use-case scenario, 3D thorax CTs of size 512^3 and thorax X-rays of size 2048^2 are generated and we show that, due to the constant GPU memory demand of our method, arbitrarily large images of high resolution can be generated. Moreover, compared to common patch-based approaches, our multi-resolution scheme enables better image quality and prevents patch artifacts.

Keywords: Multi-scale GAN · High resolution 3D images

1 Introduction

Generative adversarial networks (GANs) [3] have shown impressive results for photo-realistic image synthesis in the last couple of years [4,6,12]. They also offer numerous applications in medical image analysis, such as generating images for data augmentation, image reconstruction and image synthesis for domain adaptation. Despite the undeniable success and the large variety of applications, GANs still struggle to generate images of high resolution. A reason for that is the fact that generated images are easier to distinguish from real ones at higher resolutions, which hinders the training process [6]. Further reasons are computational demands and memory requirements of current network architectures. To deal with the first issue, Karras et al. [6] recently proposed a progressive

Electronic supplementary material The online version of this chapter (https://doi.org/10.1007/978-3-030-32226-7_13) contains supplementary material, which is available to authorized users.

© Springer Nature Switzerland AG 2019
D. Shen et al. (Eds.): MICCAI 2019, LNCS 11769, pp. 112–120, 2019.
https://doi.org/10.1007/978-3-030-32226-7_13

learning strategy for GANs that starts with low resolution and adds finer details throughout the training. Using this strategy, the authors were able to generate high resolution 2D images of size 1024×1024. However, the training process already requires $\sim$16 GB of GPU RAM, meaning that larger images can only be generated with special and expensive hardware. The problem is further aggravated in 3D imaging typically demanded in clinical routine. An early attempt for the 3D application of GANs is made in [10], where furniture shapes of size 64^3 are generated using a DCGAN architecture. Even though the task of generating only shapes (no texture or intensities) is fairly simple, its computational demands are borderline to most consumer-class GPUs.

The image size limitations make GANs impracticable for many medical image applications, e.g. for thoracic CTs, brain MRIs, or high resolution X-ray images. In [9] the authors claim to be forced to use only half of the image size ($128 \times 128 \times 54$) due to GPU memory limits of the dedicated hardware (NVIDIA DGX system). The largest 3D output size of a GAN found in literature is 128^3 [11], however no memory requirements are mentioned. An usual approach to overcome such computational challenges is slice-/patch-wise generation [5,7]. Unfortunately, those methods suffer from artifacts between patches/slices due to noncontinuous transitions. Dealing with this problem by applying patch overlaps and averaging, leads to blurry results and loss of image detail. The intuition behind patch inconsistencies is that independently generated patches do not have any global intensity information. Thus, [5] proposes to additionally observe a larger area around each patch of the input image to cope with this issue. Even though shown to be well suitable for segmentation and would probably improve patch artifacts in strictly paired image translation (e.g. CT to MR), such an approach cannot be applied to image generation from scratch (or sparsely conditioned), and its effect is limited when the image size drastically exceeds the chosen patch size.

In this work we propose a memory-efficient multi-scale GAN approach for the generation of high-resolution medical images in high quality. Our approach combines a progressive multi-scale learning strategy with a patch-wise approach, where low-resolution image content is learned first, and image patches at higher resolutions are conditioned on the previous scales to preserve global intensity information. We demonstrate the ability to generate realistic large images on thoracic X-rays of size 2048^2 and 3D lung CTs of size 512^3. Further, we show that w.r.t. the growing side length of an isotropic 3D image, the memory requirements for popular GANs grow cubical, while they stay constant for any image size using our approach. Although the presented method is theoretically suitable for from-scratch image generation, in this work, we apply a conditional GAN for unsupervised domain adaptation. This application features topology preserving style transfer, where in contrast to strictly paired image translation, our approach does not assume corresponding images from two domains and enables the possibility to translate arbitrary datasets to a desired domain. We show that image translation from different CT reconstruction kernels, different devices and different acquisition parameters to a particular desired domain is possible,

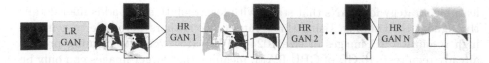

Fig. 1. An overview of our method. Generate the whole image with a low resolution (LR) GAN, then subsequently increase the resolution by generating patches with multiple high resolution (HR) GANs conditioned on the previous scales. Blue: patches of original resolution for the current scale; red: upscaled patches of lower resolution. (Color figure online)

keeping the original 3D image size. The generated images are evaluated with respect to a known ground-truth image emphasizing the quality of generated images.

2 Methods

GANs are generative models that learn to map a random noise vector $\mathbf{z}$ to an output image y using a generator function $G : \mathbf{z} \rightarrow y$ [3]. An extension of regular GANs are the conditional GANs, that learn the mapping from an observed image x additionally, $G : \{x, \mathbf{z}\} \rightarrow y$. To ensure that the generator produces realistically looking images that cannot be distinguished from real ones, an adversarial discriminator D is enclosed in the training process, aiming to perfectly distinguish between real images and generator's fakes.

2.1 Multi-scale Conditional GANs

The idea of multi-scale image generation to obtain high resolutions, is inspired by early works like [2], where, based on a Laplacian pyramid, multiple GANs for increasing resolutions are used, and more recent approaches [12] that achieve photo-realistic image quality by iterative resolution refinement applying successive GANs. However, those methods still assume that at a certain stage the whole full-resolution image is propagated through the network, requiring extremely high GPU capacities especially for 3D images. Here, we propose to overcome this issue by first generating the whole image in a low resolution, then iteratively proceed by generating image patches of constant size but growing resolutions. Since the GANs for each scale are trained separately, a particular maximum size is never exceeded during training, so the GPU demand stays constantly low, facilitating the generation of arbitrarily large images. Further, we enable a consistent and realistic look of the generated images by conditioning each high resolution scale on the previous lower resolution image, thus providing patches with global intensity information and preventing patch artifacts and inconsistencies (see Fig. 1 for a method overview). A further benefit of progressively learning increasing resolutions, is that each GAN has a rather simple task to learn compared to generating the whole high-resolution image from scratch.

This does not only enable a simpler training process, but also ensures sharp results for each scale and thus a consistent high-resolution result.

We also consider conditioning on the object edges to enable topology preserving image domain translation. In the lowest resolution (LR) GAN, the whole low-resolution edge image is used as an input. In the higher-resolution (HR) GANs, two conditions are used: a patch from the image of the previous resolution, upscaled to the size of the current scale; and a patch from the edge image of the current scale. Note, that the patch size of each resolution is constant, however, as the overall image becomes larger after each HR GAN, the relative image fraction per patch decreases, while resolution grows. The objective of this learning process can be described as follows. For multiple conditional images $x_0 \ldots x_n$ with resolutions $0 \ldots n$, output images $y_0 \ldots y_n$, where y_n represents the final output image, are generated using separate generators $G_{0 \ldots n}$ and discriminators $D_{0 \ldots n}$ with the objectives

$$\mathcal{L}_{cGAN}(G_0, D_0) =$$
$$\mathbb{E}_{x_0,y_0}[\log D_0(x_0, y_0)] + \mathbb{E}_{x_0,\mathbf{z}}[\log(1 - D_0(x_0, G_0(x_0, \mathbf{z})))]$$
$$\mathcal{L}_{cGAN}(G_i, D_i) = \mathbb{E}_{x_{p_i},y_{p_i}}[\log D_i(x_{p_i}, y_{p_{i-1}}, y_{p_i})] +$$
$$\mathbb{E}_{x_{p_i},\mathbf{z}}[\log(1 - D_i(x_{p_i}, y_{p_{i-1}}, G_i(x_{p_i}, y_{p_{i-1}}, \mathbf{z})))],$$

where x_{p_i} and y_{p_i} are patches of the conditional image x_i and the generated image y_i respectively, with $i \in [1, n]$.

2.2   Architecture and Training

Different generator's architectures were chosen for G_0 and $G_{1 \ldots n}$, since the tasks of generating whole low resolution images and high resolution patches differ in a variety oCOPDf requirements. The LR GAN uses a U-Net architecture, which is able to filter out many unimportant details and generalize better due to its bottleneck. Its tendency to result in more blurry images is negligible in the context of low-resolution images. For the patch generation by the HR GANs, ResNet blocks are chosen, since they are known to produce sharp results by keeping the input image resolution unchanged. The higher overfitting risk of not having a bottleneck is diminished due to the stronger conditioning (on the previous scales) and the overall large number of patches compared to the number of images used. For the discriminators $D_{0 \ldots n}$ a regular fully-convolutional architecture is chosen. However, the concrete network architectures are interchangeable. Data augmentation is crucial to our method, because cascading approaches are prone to propagate errors up from lower resolutions. To deal with this issue we corrupt a percentage of the low resolution images while training each HR GAN: we apply random noise, Gaussian blurring and vary the image resolution. Also to make the patch generation less dependent on perfect edge extraction, the edge images are perturbed with noise. In our experience those techniques help to overcome overadapting to either of the inputs.

3   Results and Experiments

3.1   Memory Requirements for 3D GANs

GANs are currently rarely applied to 3D images due to computational constrains, therefore in this experiment we investigate the dependence of 3D image side length and memory requirements. Three common GAN architectures are chosen as baselines: DCGAN [10], Pix2Pix [4] and progressive growing GAN (PGGAN) [6], and compared to the two architectures of our method: LR 64 for low resolution images of size 64^3 and HR 32 for high resolution patches of size 32^3. PyTorch [8] is used as implementation framework of choice for all networks. Since Pix2Pix and PGGAN are only implemented for 2D images, a straightforward translation to 3D is obtained (replacing 2D by 3D convolutions, etc.). The RAM demand computation is realized using the summary approach from the keras framework [1]. The assumed lower bound of memory usage here includes one forward and backward pass for the generator and discriminator each, as well as the memory required to store the images, gradients and network's parameters for batch size of one.

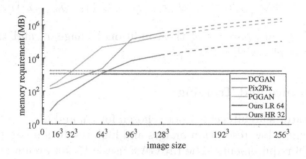

Fig. 2. RAM requirements for 3D GANs. Baselines: DCGAN, Pix2Pix and PGGAN. Dashed lines indicate cubic regression approximation. Our methods: for low resolution images of size 64^3 (LR 64) and high resolution patches of size 32^3 (HR 32), have constant memory requirement regardless the image size. Dotted lines indicate sizes under the assumed minimal size 64^3. Log-scale is used on the y-axis.

The results for different image sizes are shown in Fig. 2. Naturally, all three baseline approaches have an at least cubic memory requirement growth w.r.t. the image side's length. For those approaches calculations for size over 128^3 were not even possible on the used Titan XP 12GB GPU, thus the extrapolated cubic regressed curves are shown. These results underline the infeasibility of straightforward 3D GAN approaches for medical images, as their sizes commonly reach 512^3. In contrast, our method has a constant character and is thus suitable for arbitrary image sizes with predictable memory usage.

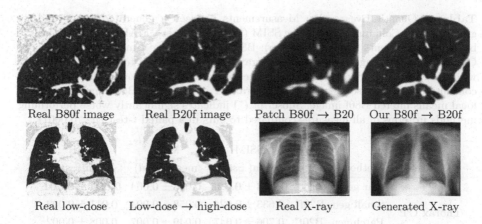

| Real B80f image | Real B20f image | Patch B80f → B20 | Our B80f → B20f |

| Real low-dose | Low-dose → high-dose | Real X-ray | Generated X-ray |

Fig. 3. Exemplary images from the used datasets and results of the experiments. First row: thorax CTs (zoomed) – real B80f image; corresponding B20f; translated B80f to B20f with a standard patch-wise approach; our method. Second row: Real low-dose image; translated low-dose to high-dose; real X-ray; generated X-ray. For larger/further images and brain MRI-based experiments, see supplementary.

3.2 High Resolution Medical Image Generation

Data. Our experiments use the following datasets (see Fig. 3 for examples):

Thorax CT: 3D CT images ($\sim 512^3$) of 56 subjects with varying degree of chronic obstructive pulmonary disease. For each subject the data is reconstructed simultaneously with a soft (B20f) and a sharp (B80f) kernel.

Low-dose thorax CT: Low-dose 4D lung CT images (120kVp, 40mAs) of 12 patients acquired during free breathing, resulting in 166 3D volumes. Image intensities are rescaled with a lung window setting and the images are cropped with a bounding box around the lungs resulting in about 320^3 voxels.

Thorax X-ray: An open access chest X-ray dataset from the Indiana University containing frontal and lateral images usually around the size of 2000^2. In our experiments about 1500 frontal images of size 2048^2 are used.

Experimental Setup. In our experiments the GANs are conditioned on the object's edges and the following scenarios are considered. (1) B80f to B20f CTs domain translation: Since images reconstructed with a sharp B80f kernel are very noisy, a reconstruction with a soft B20f kernel is advantageous for automatic quantitative computations (e.g. emphysema index). Here, the GANs are trained in a 5-fold cross-validation manner on the B20f images from the thorax dataset. In test phase, the edges from the B80f images of the test patients are extracted and translated into the B20f domain using the trained GANs. Note that the B80f reconstructions are not used for training, thus the domain translation is unpaired. (2) Low-dose to high-dose domain translation: In this experiment, we show that translations between different image domains of different devices and protocols are possible with our method, since it does not require paired

Table 1. Quantitative results: Measurements between a generated image and its ground truth. Columns 3–5: average SSIM (higher is better), MAE and MSE (lower is better). Experiments (top and bottom): B80f to B20f image translation on a thorax CT dataset, and image generation on thorax X-Ray. Compared to ground truth (row-wise): For both experiments – our generated images, upscaled low resolution images, conventional patch-wise generation; for thorax CT – the original B80f image and a non-local means filtered B80f image. Subscript (*) indicates significantly worse performing methods in terms of all measures compared to ours in a paired t-test ($p < 0.0001$).

Dataset	Method	SSIM mean($\pm std$)	MAE mean($\pm std$)	MSE mean($\pm std$)
Thorax CT $512 \times 512 \times 512$	Our gen. B20f	**0.773 ± 0.025**	0.033 ± 0.004	**0.004 ± 0.001**
	Small gen. B20f*	0.633 ± 0.024	0.058 ± 0.004	0.011 ± 0.002
	Patch gen. B20f*	0.706 ± 0.047	0.049 ± 0.007	0.008 ± 0.002
	Original B80f*	0.480 ± 0.045	0.065 ± 0.008	0.012 ± 0.003
	Filtered B80f	**0.773 ± 0.048**	**0.031 ± 0.005**	**0.004 ± 0.001**
Thorax X-Ray 2048×2048	Our gen	**0.711 ± 0.067**	**0.104 ± 0.028**	**0.022 ± 0.014**
	Small gen.*	0.673 ± 0.064	0.108 ± 0.027	0.024 ± 0.014
	Patch gen.*	0.520 ± 0.072	0.200 ± 0.024	0.069 ± 0.019

data. Here, the GANs are trained on the high-dose B20f images from the thorax dataset, and in test phase, the edges extracted from the low-dose data are used to enable a translation between the two datasets. (3) Large 2D image generation: To show that our approach is not constricted to 3D images, in this experiment huge X-ray images are generated. The GANs are trained on 90% of the thorax X-ray datasets, whereas the rest of the images is used for testing.

Results. For evaluation of experiment (1) the actual B20f reconstructions of the test B80f images serve as ground truth and for experiment (3) the real X-ray images. Here structural similarity index (SSIM), mean absolute error (MAE) and mean squared error (MSE) between the ground truth and the generated images are used as image quality criterions (Table 1). Our method is compared to other standard methods: generate a smaller image with an LR GAN (64^3 is about our computational limit) and upscale it; develop a straight-forward patch-based approach for the high resolution images (HR GAN without conditioning on previous scales) and apply stitching. The comparison networks were trained in the exact same manner as for our method. In all experiments isotropic sizes of 64 for the LR GAN, and 32 for the HR GANs are used. To avoid padding artifacts on patch borders, only the network's receptive field parts of the generated patches are considered. However, for our method no patch overlaps are needed, whereas for the conventional patch-based method, patch overlaps of 5 pixels are applied. The significantly higher SSIM values and smaller pixel-wise distances for our method show its ability to outperform conventional GAN-based approaches. Visually, the generated images have a consistent appearance, barely any artifacts and high resolution, enabling the visibility of tiny structures within the lungs.

In contrast, when using conventional patch-wise approaches, patch artifacts and inconsistencies are clearly present (Fig. 3).

We further apply a state-of-the-art denoising method, the non-local means filter, to match the B80f and B20f images. In terms of metrics, this approach is comparable to ours, however its computation time is ~100 times longer and it does not apply to any other domain transfer tasks. Also, the filtered images lack important details and have an inconsistent appearance visually.

For the low-dose dataset no ground truth is available, so we evaluate experiment (2) qualitatively and compare the feature space distributions of both domains using the Fréchet inception distance (FID) between: the original low-dose and the original high-dose images (150); the translated and the original high-dose images (131); the translated and the original low-dose images (157). The visual correspondence of the target domain and the translated images is also underlined by the smaller FID value. The large FID between the original low-dose and the translated images indicates that different features are extracted for the same image of various appearances, and thus emphasizes the need for domain translation.

4 Discussion and Conclusion

In this work, we propose a multi-scale GAN-based approach for the generation of arbitrarily large 3D medical images of high resolution and realistic homogeneous appearance. We show that in contrast to existing GANs, that produce the whole image at once, the presented patch-based method, only requires constant GPU memory w.r.t. the image size. Also compared to trivial patch-wise methods, our sophisticated multi-resolution scheme provides higher quality images in terms of image consistency and resolution. Here we show a use-case scenario for medical image domain translation based on conditional GANs, however our method is also suitable for image generation from scratch and it enables various applications and possibilities for medical images.

References

1. Chollet, F., et al.: Keras (2015). https://keras.io. Accessed 15 Sept 2019
2. Denton, E.L., Chintala, S., Szlam, A., Fergus, R.: Deep generative image models using a Laplacian pyramid of adversarial networks. In: Advances in Neural Information Processing Systems, pp. 1486–1494 (2015)
3. Goodfellow, I., et al.: Generative adversarial nets. In: Advances in Neural Information Processing Systems, pp. 2672–2680 (2014)
4. Isola, P., Zhu, J.Y., Zhou, T., Efros, A.A.: Image-to-image translation with conditional adversarial networks. In: IEEE Conference on Computer Vision and Pattern Recognition (CVPR), pp. 5967–5976 (2017)
5. Kamnitsas, K., et al.: Efficient multi-scale 3D CNN with fully connected CRF for accurate brain lesion segmentation (2017)
6. Karras, T., Aila, T., Laine, S., Lehtinen, J.: Progressive growing of GANs for improved quality, stability, and variation. In: International Conference on Learning Representations (2018)

7. Lei, Y., et al.: MRI-based synthetic CT generation using deep convolutional neural network. In: SPIE Medical Imaging, vol. 10949 (2019)
8. Paszke, A., et al.: Automatic differentiation in PyTorch (2017)
9. Shin, H.-C., et al.: Medical image synthesis for data augmentation and anonymization using generative adversarial networks. In: Gooya, A., Goksel, O., Oguz, I., Burgos, N. (eds.) SASHIMI 2018. LNCS, vol. 11037, pp. 1–11. Springer, Cham (2018). https://doi.org/10.1007/978-3-030-00536-8_1
10. Wu, J., Zhang, C., Xue, T., Freeman, W.T., Tenenbaum, J.B.: Learning a probabilistic latent space of object shapes via 3D generative-adversarial modeling. In: Advances in Neural Information Processing Systems, pp. 82–90 (2016)
11. Yu, B., Zhou, L., Wang, L., Fripp, J., Bourgeat, P.: 3D cGAN based cross-modality MR image synthesis for brain tumor segmentation. In: IEEE International Symposium on Biomedical Imaging (ISBI), pp. 626–630 (2018)
12. Zhang, H., et al.: StackGAN++: realistic image synthesis with stacked generative adversarial networks. IEEE Trans. Pattern Anal. Mach. Intell. **47**, 1947–1962 (2018)

Deep Learning Based Metal Artifacts Reduction in Post-operative Cochlear Implant CT Imaging

Zihao Wang[1]([✉]), Clair Vandersteen[2], Thomas Demarcy[3], Dan Gnansia[3], Charles Raffaelli[2], Nicolas Guevara[2], and Hervé Delingette[1]

[1] Université Côte d'Azur, Inria, Epione Team, Nice, France
zihao.wang@inria.fr
[2] Université Côte d'Azur, Nice University Hospital, Nice, France
[3] Oticon Medical, Vallauris, France

Abstract. To assess the quality of insertion of Cochlear Implants (CI) after surgery, it is important to analyze the positions of the electrodes with respect to the cochlea based on post-operative CT imaging. Yet, these images suffer from metal artifacts which often entail a difficulty to make any analysis. In this work, we propose a 3D metal artifact reduction method using convolutional neural networks for post-operative cochlear implant imaging. Our approach is based on a 3D generative adversarial network (MARGANs) to create an image with a reduction of metal artifacts. The generative model is trained on a large number of pre-operative "artifact-free" images on which simulated metal artifacts are created. This simulation involves the segmentation of the scala tympani, the virtual insertion of electrode arrays and the simulation of beam hardening based on the Beer-Lambert law.

Quantitative and qualitative evaluations compared with two classical metallic artifact reduction algorithms show the effectiveness of our method.

Keywords: Generative adversarial networks · Metal artifacts reduction

1 Introduction

The physical imaging process of spiral CT leads to the creation of artifacts in the reconstructed images when dense objects such as metallic parts are fully absorbing the X-rays. Such artifacts are for instance visible in CT post-operative images of the inner ear following the surgical insertion of Cochlea Implants (CI) due to the presence of a metallic electrode array. Figure 1(a) shows the image distortions around the metallic electrodes implanted along the scala tympani,

Electronic supplementary material The online version of this chapter (https://doi.org/10.1007/978-3-030-32226-7_14) contains supplementary material, which is available to authorized users.

© Springer Nature Switzerland AG 2019
D. Shen et al. (Eds.): MICCAI 2019, LNCS 11769, pp. 121–129, 2019.
https://doi.org/10.1007/978-3-030-32226-7_14

one of three ducts constituting the cochlea with the scala vestibuli and scala media (see Fig. 1 Right). Those artifacts make the post-operative assessment of CI implantation very difficult in particular the estimation of the relative positions of the electrodes with respect to scala tympani and the scala vestibuli.

There is a vast body of research efforts for Metal Artifact Reduction (MAR) approaches, for instance based on iterative reconstruction or corrections of the physical effects. Deep learning MAR methods were also recently introduced. Zhang *et al.* [11] introduced CNN as prior for filtered back projections based method. A simulation dataset was built for training the CNN. Huang *et al.* [3] developed CNN (*RL-ARCNN*) directly on the image domain for removing metal artifacts in cervical CT images based on a residual learning method in an end to end manner. A neural network named *DestreakNet* was proposed for streak artifacts reduction [2]. *DestreakNet* is used for quality improvement as post-processing after the application of the state of the art NMAR interpolation-based algorithm. Some details that were lost after the NMAR processing can be recovered by the *DestreakNet* network.

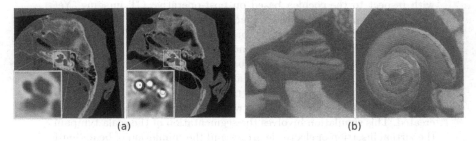

(a)   (b)

Fig. 1. (a) Pre-operative (Left) and post-operative (Right) CT imaging of the inner ear. Cochlear implant creates metallic artifacts. (b) μCT images of the cochlea including the scala tympani (green) and scala vestibuli (orange). (Color figure online)

For CI metal artifacts reduction, conditional generative adversarial networks (cGAN) were proposed by Wang *et al.* [8] to generate artifact-free images. The cGAN operates on each 2D slice and was trained on 76 pairs of registered pre and post-operative images. The registration of those image pairs is very challenging precisely due to those artifacts and the 2D approach does not guarantee spatial consistency of the result from one slice to the next.

In this paper, we propose a 3D generative adversarial network for MAR on cochlear implants. Instead of training the GANs on pairs of pre and postoperative images, our approach relies on the physical simulation of artifacts in CT images from pre-operative CT images. The simulation involves the automatic segmentation of the scala tympani on preoperative CT, the automatic estimation of the positions of the electrode arrays and finally the simulation of beam hardening on fan-beam projections based on the Beer-Lambert law discretized on 5 different energies. This approach was applied on 1090 3D preoperative CT images to create 1090 3D images with simulated artifacts. The 1090 image pairs are then used to train an original 3D generative adversarial network (GANs) named MARGANs for which a generative loss derived from Retinex theory was introduced. This unsupervised approach was successfully tested on 10 post-operative images to generate artifact reduced images and its quantitative performance was favorably compared with two other MAR methods. Unlike [8], our method is unsupervised and does not require any registration of pre and post operative images which is a difficult task. The use of a 3D GAN improves a lot the spatial consistency of the generated images. It is also generic to the type of artifacts without requiring pre and postoperative images which is not available in many surgery procedures.

2   Method

2.1   CI Metal Artifacts Simulation

CI Electrode Array Simulation. The processing pipeline to generate the training set for the MARGANs is displayed in Fig. 2. Given a preoperative cochlea CT image, it is first automatically rigidly registered on a reference cochlea CT image where the modiolus axis is along the Z direction. The segmentation of the cochlea is then performed through a parametric cochlea shape model similarly to the approach proposed by Demarcy et al. [1]. As a result of the segmentation, the scala tympani (ST) is extracted and then a signed distance map of the ST is generated (Step 2). The positions of the simulated electrode array are estimated by thresholding the distance map to create a 3D tubular binary mask near the center of the ST (Step 3). The Hounsfield unit of simulated electrode array was then set to $3071 HU$ (Step 4), which is the maximum observed value on CI metal artifacts.

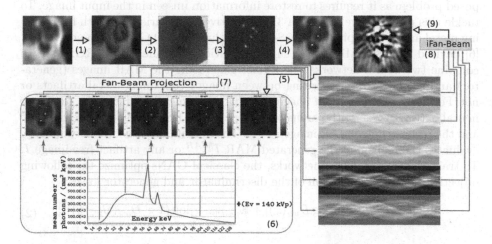

Fig. 2. CI metal artifacts simulation workflow starting from a pre-operative image and ending with the simulated post-operative image after 9 processing steps.

Metal Artifacts Simulation. We rely on the by Beer-Lambert law, relating the number of photons $I(x, y, \delta z)$ for a monoenergetic X-ray source at point (x, y) through a slice δz to the initial photon number I_0 and linear absorption coefficient $\mu(x, y)$: $I(x, y, \delta z) = I_0 e^{-\mu(x,y)\delta z}$. For a polychromatic X-ray beam, the attenuation coefficient depends on the chromatic photon energy $\mu(E_v)$, and the energy spectrum $\phi(E_v)$ must be taken into account. The number of photons received in the entire detector surface is then:

$$I = \int_{E_0}^{E_n} (\phi(E_v)e^{-\iiint \mu(x,y,z,E_v)dxdydz} + S(E_v))dE_v \qquad (1)$$

where E_0 and E_n are the minimum and maximum energies for a fixed tube peak voltage, and where $S(E_v)$ captures X-ray scattering. The energy spectrum $\phi(E_v)$ was downloaded from a CT manufacturer dedicated site[1] for a tungsten anode tube at 140 kVp.

The simulation starts by computing attenuation maps $\mu(x, y, z, E_{v_i})$ (Step 5) for five sample energies shown in Fig. 2(6). This computation is based on the Hounsfield unit formula and the water absorption coefficients as a function of energy [9]. We then perform fan-beam projection (Step 7) of the 5 attenuation maps to produce sinograms-like images representing absorbed energy on CT detectors. Then a weighted sum of the 5 sinograms (Step 8) is computed (including energy spectrum and scatter) as a discretization of Eq. 1. Finally inverse fan beam projection produces the output image with metallic artifacts (Step 9).

2.2 CI CT Image Metal Artifacts Reduction Based on 3D GANs

MARGANs. The issue of removing metal artifact from images is clearly an ill-posed problem as it requires to restore information unseen in the input image. To tackle this problem, we propose a 3D generative adversarial approach for reducing metal artifacts inspired by the Super-Resolution (SR) GANs of Sánchez et al. [6] devised for brain MR images super-resolution. The idea of MARGANs is to combine two neural networks, the former generating the MAR images (generator) and the latter discriminating between images containing metal artifacts or not. Formally, given an input image $I^{metal}(\mathbf{x})$ with metal artifacts, the generator neural networks G_{w_g} with parameters w_g performs the mapping between I^{metal} and the reconstructed MAR image I^{MAR}. The discriminator neural network D_{w_d} evaluates the realism of the generated MAR I^{MAR} or any artifact-free image I. To train the G_{w_g} and D_{w_d} networks, the classical GANs optimize the following objective function as the sum of the discriminator and generator losses:

$$\min_{w_g} \max_{w_d} U = \mathbb{E}_{x \sim I}[\log D_{w_d}(x)] + \mathbb{E}_{y \sim I^{metal}}[\log(1 - D_{w_d}(G_{w_g}(y)))] \qquad (2)$$

Network Architecture. The generator network architecture vastly differs from [6] as it is similar to U-Net with convolution and deconvolution layers, and

---

[1] https://www.oem-xray-components.siemens.com/x-ray-spectra-simulation.

batch normalization layers to improve the training efficiency. Moreover, unlike [6] which is patch-based, the input of the network consist of full 3D images as it easily fits in GPU memory. The number of filters increases from 1 to N_f and then decreases to 1, where N_f is the maximum number of feature maps, which depends on the GPU memory size. The discriminator network follows that of [6] with eight groups of convolution layers and batch normalization layers combined sequentially. Instead of using the original GANs formula, MARGANs is trained by minimizing both the discriminator loss and generator loss.

Discriminator Loss. The discriminator network D_{w_d} loss should consider differently the artifact-free images I from images with metal artifacts I^{metal}. We proposed loss for the discriminator is:

$$L_{discriminator} = \log(|D_{w_d}(I) - 1|) + \log(D_{w_d}(G_{w_g}(I^{metal}))) \tag{3}$$

Generator Loss. We propose a new loss function based on Retinex theory [5] to measure the discrepancy in the reconstruction of the MARGANs. Retinex theory is mostly used to improve images seriously affected by environmental illumination. We propose a novel generator loss based on the Retinex theory consisting in two parts: the content and Retinex penalties. For content penalty, mean square error (MSE), $L_{mse} = \mathbb{E}(I - G_{w_g}(I^{MAR}))$ were used to encourage the generator to generate voxels consistent with the artifact free images. But using only the MSE loss leads to blurred MAR images with a lack of high frequency image details. To avoid this excessive smoothing, we add the Retinex penalty written as follows to get numerically stable evaluations:

$$L_{retinex} = \frac{1}{|I^{metal}|} \sum_{\mathbf{x}} |G_{w_g}(I^{metal}) - e^{\log I^{MAR} - \log I^{MAR} * \mathcal{N}(0,\sigma)}| \tag{4}$$

The Retinex theory assumes that a given image can be expressed by the product of environmental brightness $L(x,y)$ and the object reflectance $R(x,y)$. To get the high frequency information of the object reflectance $R(c,y)$ we use Gaussian function to remove the low frequency part of the image as done in [10] (known as single-Scale Retinex algorithm) for ultrasound image enhancement, $\mathcal{N}(0,\sigma)$ is a Gaussian function of standard deviation σ and $*$ is the convolution operator. This loss enforces salient features in the image that would be attenuated otherwise. Putting it all together with the adversarial term $L_{adv} = \frac{1}{2}|D_{w_d}(G_{w_g}) - 1|^2$ as in [6], the full loss function of the generator is:

$$L_{generator} = \alpha \cdot L_{retinex} + L_{mse} + L_{adv} \tag{5}$$

where α is a parameter controlling the influence of the Retinex loss.

3 Experiments and Evaluation

3.1 Dataset

Simulation Dataset. CT scans of the temporal bones include 493 left and 597 right images collected from 597 patients by a GE LightSpeed CT scanner with a standard protocol (without metal artifact reduction filters) at the Radiology Department of the Nice University Hospital. Imaging voxel size is $0.2 \times 0.2 \times 0.2 \, \text{mm}^3$. All images were registered by a pyramidal blocking-matching algorithm to find the ROI and then cropped as $60 \times 50 \times 50$ volume images.

Evaluation Dataset. The evaluation dataset includes 10 temporal bones images outside the simulation dataset but collected with the same conditions. It additionally includes pre-operative and post-operative pairs of images. Due to resected tissues and artifacts caused by implanted electrodes during surgery, all tested rigid registration algorithms fail to register the pre-operative with post-operative images. Therefore they were manually registered in 3D using landmarks and then both were cropped similarly to the simulation dataset.

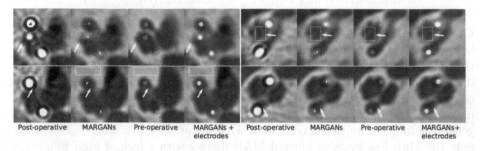

| Post-operative | MARGANs | Pre-operative | MARGANS + electrodes | Post-operative | MARGANS | Pre-operative | MARGANs+ electrodes |

Fig. 3. Results on patients #4 (Left) and #6 (Right) for two middle slices (First and second rows). The 4 columns correspond respectively to: original post-operative images, output of MARGANs, registered pre-operative images with manually positioned electrodes in red and post-operative images with electrodes in yellow. (Color figure online)

3.2   Implementation Details

The proposed GANs were implemented with TensorFlow following Sect. 2. Convolution kernel size is set to $3 \times 3 \times 3$, the number of filters was $N_f = 512$ and the weight of Retinex loss was set as $\alpha = 0.00002$ experimentally. The generator and discriminator were trained by using RMSprop optimizer with learning rate $l_{rg} = 1e-4$ and $l_{rd} = 1e-3$ respectively. The simulation of metal artifacts took about 1 h on a CPU cluster for each of the 1090 images. Training the MARGANs took about 23 h on one NVIDIA 1080Ti GPU.

3.3   Performance on Clinical Data

Performance on Evaluation Dataset. Figure 3 shows the application of the proposed method on two middle slices of two patient images, including registered pre-operative images. The metal artifacts are significantly reduced in the MARGANs generated images without important geometry distortions. Furthermore, some visible internal structures inside the cochlea are restored by the MARGANs as shown with added arrows. The electrodes positions in yellow and red were manually added to allow for the visual assessment of the electrodes with respect to the pre-operative images.

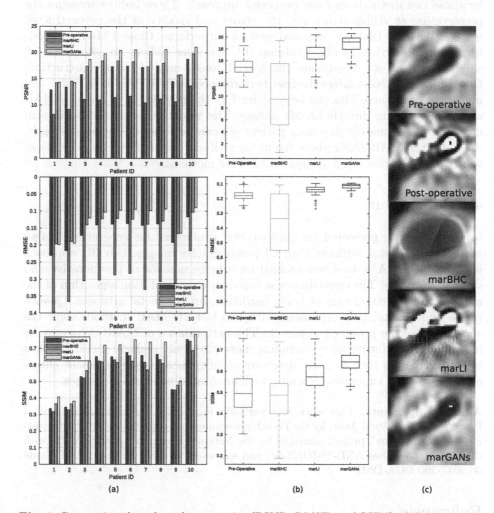

(a)   (b)   (c)

Fig. 4. Comparison based on three metrics (PSNR, RMSE, and SSIM) of the proposed MARGANs methods with two other MAR algorithms: marLI and marBHC. (a) overall performance on 10 clinical post-operative images, (b) the 3D consistency between slices for patient #4, (c) middle slice generated by the different methods.

Performance Comparison. MARGANs is compared with 2 open-source 2D fast metallic artifacts reduction methods: projection linear interpolation replacement [4] (marLI) and beam hardening correction [7] (marBHC). The 10 evaluation dataset images were processed by marLI, marBHC slice by slice. In Fig. 4(a), for each of the 10 images, we compare the Root Mean Square Error (RMSE), Structural Similarity Index (SSIM) and Peak Signal to Noisy Ratio (PSNR) computed between the pre-operative images and the MAR images generated by those two methods and our proposed approach. Those indices measure the preservation of visible structures, the errors and quality of the reconstructed images. We show that our proposed method outperforms those 2 MAR methods for all three metrics. In Fig. 4 column (b), the same indices are shown for all slices of patient #4 to evaluate the spatial consistency of the reconstruction. Clearly MARGANs exhibits the best performances with a lower mean value and much lower variance. This can be explained by the fact that it is the only MAR algorithm working directly on 3D images. The visualization of the 3 different methods on one middle slice from patient #4 can be found in Fig. 4(c). Clearly, the output of MARGANs where the metal artifacts are largely reduced is closer to the pre-operative image compared to other methods.

4   Conclusion

In this paper we presented an unsupervised framework for generating images with reduced metal artifacts from CI postoperative images. Our 3D approach is based on a GANs that was trained on a large number of preoperative and simulated images. The simulation was based on a segmentation algorithm of the cochlea and the simulation of beam hardening for the metal artifacts. Quantitative and qualitative comparisons with two fast 2D MAR methods show the superiority of the proposed approach. The performance of MARGANs may be improved in the future (i) by including more physically realistic metal artifacts in the simulation such as noisy detectors and exponential edge-gradient effects etc. (ii) by using supervised learning with annotated pairs of CT images.

Acknowledgements. This work was partially funded by the regional council of Provence Alpes Côte d'Azur, by the French government through the UCA[JEDI] "Investments in the Future" project managed by the National Research Agency (ANR) with the reference number ANR-15-IDEX-01, and was supported by the grant AAP Santé 06 2017-260 DGA-DSH.

References

1. Demarcy, T., et al.: Automated analysis of human cochlea shape variability from segmented μCT images. Comput. Med. Imaging Graph. **59**, 1–12 (2017)
2. Gjesteby, L., et al.: Deep neural network for CT metal artifact reduction with a perceptual loss function. In: The fifth international conference on Image Formation in X-ray Computed Tomography, Salt Lake city, pp. 439–443, May 2018
3. Huang, X., Wang, J., Tang, F., Zhong, T., Zhang, Y.: Metal artifact reduction on cervical CT images by deep residual learning. BioMed. Eng. OnLine **17**, 175 (2018)
4. Kalender, W.A., Hebel, R., Ebersberger, J.: Reduction of CT artifacts caused by metallic implants. Radiology **164**(2), 576–577 (1987)

5. Land, E.H., McCann, J.J.: Lightness and retinex theory. J. Opt. Soc. Am. **61**(1), 1–11 (1971)
6. Sánchez, I., Vilaplana, V.: Brain MRI super-resolution using 3D generative adversarial networks. In: 1st Conference on Medical Imaging with Deep Learning (MIDL 2018), Amsterdam (2018)
7. Verburg, J.M., Seco, J.: CT metal artifact reduction method correcting for beam hardening and missing projections. Phys. Med. Biol. **57**(9), 2803–2818 (2012)
8. Wang, J., Zhao, Y., Noble, J.H., Dawant, B.M.: Conditional generative adversarial networks for metal artifact reduction in CT images of the ear. In: Frangi, A.F., Schnabel, J.A., Davatzikos, C., Alberola-López, C., Fichtinger, G. (eds.) MICCAI 2018. LNCS, vol. 11070, pp. 3–11. Springer, Cham (2018). https://doi.org/10.1007/978-3-030-00928-1_1
9. Wunderlich, A., Noo, F.: Image covariance and lesion detectability in direct fan-beam X-ray computed tomography. Phys. Med. Biol. **53**(10), 2471–2493 (2008)
10. Zhang, R., Yali, H., Zhen, Z.: A ultrasound liver image enhancement algorithm based on multi-scale Retinex theory. In: 2011 5th International Conference on Bioinformatics and Biomedical Engineering, Wuhan, China, pp. 1–3, May 2011
11. Zhang, Y., Yu, H.: Convolutional neural network based metal artifact reduction in X-ray computed tomography. IEEE Trans. Med. Imaging **37**(6), 1370–1381 (2018)

ImHistNet: Learnable Image Histogram Based DNN with Application to Noninvasive Determination of Carcinoma Grades in CT Scans

Mohammad Arafat Hussain[1(✉)], Ghassan Hamarneh[2], and Rafeef Garbi[1]

[1] BiSICL, University of British Columbia, Vancouver, BC, Canada
{arafat,rafeef}@ece.ubc.ca
[2] Medical Image Analysis Lab, Simon Fraser University, Burnaby, BC, Canada
hamarneh@sfu.ca

Abstract. Renal cell carcinoma (RCC) is the seventh most common cancer worldwide, accounting for an estimated 140,000 global deaths annually. Clear cell RCC (ccRCC) is the major subtype of RCC and its biological aggressiveness affects prognosis and treatment planning. An important ccRCC prognostic predictor is its 'grade' for which the 4-tiered Fuhrman grading system is used. Although the Fuhrman grade can be identified by percutaneous renal biopsy, recent studies suggested that such grades may be non-invasively identified by studying image texture features of the ccRCC from computed tomography (CT) data. Such image feature based identification currently mostly relies on laborious manual processes based on visual inspection of 2D image slices that are time-consuming and subjective. In this paper, we propose a learnable image histogram based deep neural network approach that can perform the Fuhrman low (I/II) and high (III/IV) grade classification for ccRCC in CT scans. Validated on a clinical CT dataset of 159 patients from the TCIA database, our method classified ccRCC low and high grades with 80% accuracy and 85% AUC.

1 Introduction

Renal cell carcinoma (RCC) is the seventh most common cancer accounting for an estimated 140,000 global deaths annually [1]. Clear cell RCC (ccRCC) accounts for approximately 80% of RCC [2] and its biological aggressiveness affects the prognosis and treatment planning [3]. The 'grade' of a ccRCC is one of the important prognostic predictors of 5-year survival where higher grade tumors have an elevated risk of postoperative recurrence [2]. Although the 4-tiered Fuhrman grading system (FGS) [4] is used for ccRCC grading, in current clinical practice, a simplified 2-tiered FGS that reduces variability and improves reproducibility of the tumor grade is preferred by pathologists [1–3]. The 2-tier FGS, which divides grades to low grade (Fuhrman I/II) and high grade (Fuhrman

© Springer Nature Switzerland AG 2019
D. Shen et al. (Eds.): MICCAI 2019, LNCS 11769, pp. 130–138, 2019.
https://doi.org/10.1007/978-3-030-32226-7_15

III/IV), was shown to be as effective as 4-tiered FGS in predicting cancer-specific mortality in a study population of 2,415 ccRCC patients [5].

Clinically, invasive percutaneous renal biopsy is currently used for ccRCC FGS [1]. However, inter-observer reproducibility of grades assigned by pathologists ranges from 31.3% to 97% [1]. Oh et al. [6] tried to assess the correlation between the CT features and Fuhrman grade of ccRCC, where ccRCCs were retrospectively reviewed in consensus by two radiologists. Using logistic regression, they showed a threshold tumor size of 36 mm to predict (AUC: 70%) the high Fuhrman grade. Recently, Sasaguri et al. [7] suggested that RCCs can be characterized and graded based on CT textural features. Ding et al. [1] employed logistic regression on both non-textural features, e.g. pseudocapsule, round mass, as well as textural ones, e.g. histogram, gray-level co-occurrence matrices (GLCM), gray level run length matrix (GLRLM), and reported that textural features better discriminated high from low grade ccRCC. Shu et al. [2] also employed logistic regression on CT textural features, e.g. GLCM, GLRLM, gray level size zone matrix (GLSZM), and achieved an FGS accuracy of 77%. Huhdanpaa et al. [8] used histogram analysis of the peak tumor enhancement, tumor heterogeneity and percent contrast washout in CT, and reported these parameters to be statistically different between low and high grade ccRCC.

Current textural feature identification and quantification nonetheless faces two main challenges: it requires (1) ccRCC segmentation in CT, and (2) manual feature engineering. To our knowledge, there is no automatic ccRCC segmentation method present for CT. On the other hand, manual tumor segmentation relying on human visual inspection for feature identification is laborious, time consuming, and suffers from high intra/inter-observer variability [9].

Avoiding complex manual feature engineering, supervised deep learning using convolutional neural networks (CNN) have exploded in popularity for automatic feature learning, classification, as well as localization and dense labelling. In a classical CNN, the learned features in the first layer typically capture low level features such as edges, the second layer detects motifs by spotting particular arrangements of edges, the third layer assembles motifs into larger combinations representing parts of objects, and subsequent layers detect objects as combinations of these parts [10]. These features of a classical CNN tend to ignore diffuse textural features [11] that are often important for medical imaging applications, e.g. tumor characterization and analysis. In an attempt to learn textural features via CNNs, Andrearczyk et al. [11] proposed deploying a global average pooling over each feature map of the last convolution layer of a conventional CNN to make the model object-shape unaware. However, the pooling still operates on the learned object-edge/motifs that do not capture complex and subtle textural variation in the input image. In a recent study [12], Wang et al. proposed an approach to learn histograms that back-propagates errors to learn optimal bin centers and widths during training. Wang's approach has 2-stages: in stage 1, a conventional CNN learns the appearance feature maps followed by producing a class-likelihood (for classification) or likelihood-map (for segmentation). A learnable histogram is subsequently trained on the stage-1 likelihood estimates, and the resultant features of this histogram are concatenated with the appearance features learned in stage-1. The combined appearance plus histogram features are then used to produce a fine-tuned stage-2 likelihood-map/class-likelihood which resulted in a slightly better (1.9%) prediction accuracy.

Inspired by Wang's approach, which was designed to learn histograms of likelihood-maps (for segmentation) or class-likelihoods (for classification) generated by a conventional CNN, we propose ImHistNet, a deep neural network (DNN) for end to end texture-based image classification. Our proposed work makes the following contributions: (1) we modify the learnable histogram approach by Wang et al. [12] into a learnable image histogram (LIH) layer within a DNN framework capable of learning complex and subtle task-specific textural features from raw images directly, adhering to the classical input-output mapping of a CNN; (2) we remove the requirement for fine pre-segmentation of the ccRCC as the proposed learnable image histogram can stratify tumor and background textures well thus enabling the model to focus specifically on the tumor texture; (3) we demonstrate ImHistNet's capabilities by performing automatic ccRCC grade classification for the 2-tiered FGS on an extended clinical dataset from real patients.

2 Materials and Methods

2.1 Data

We used CT scans of 159 patients from The Cancer Imaging Archive (TCIA) database [13]. These patients were diagnosed with ccRCC, of which 64 were graded Fuhrman low (I/II) and 95 were graded Fuhrman high (III/IV). The images in this database have variations in CT scanner models, contrast administration, field of view, and spatial resolution. The in-plane pixel size ranged from 0.29 to 1.87 mm and the slice thickness ranged from 1.5 to 7.5 mm. We normalized the intensity of all the datasets between [−1000, 3000] Hounsfield Units. We divided the dataset for training/validation/testing as 44/5/15 and 75/5/15 for Fuhrman low and and Fuhrman high, respectively. Note that typical tumor radiomic analysis comprises [14]: (i) 3D imaging, (ii) tumor detection and/or segmentation, (iii) tumor phenotype quantification, and (iv) data integration (i.e. phenotype + genotype + clinical + proteomic) and analysis. Our approach falls under step-iii. The input data to our method are thus 2D image patches of size 64 × 64 pixels, taken from kidney+ccRCC (i.e. both mutually inclusively present) bounding boxes. We do not require any fine pre-segmentation of the ccRCC rather only assume a kidney+ccRCC bounding box, generated in step-ii. For this study, kidney+ccRCC bounding boxes are manually generated. We also do not require any voxel spacing normalization among the datasets. Given data imbalance where samples for Fuhrman low are fewer than for Fuhrman high, we allowed more overlap among adjacent patches for the Fuhrman low dataset. The amount of overlap is calculated to balance the samples from both cohorts.

2.2   Learnable Image Histogram for Classification

Learnable Image Histogram: Our proposed learnable image histogram (LIH) stratifies the pixel values in an image x in different learnable and possibly overlapping intervals (bins of width w_b) with arbitrary learnable means (bin centers β_b). The feature value $h_b(x) : b \in \mathcal{B} \to \mathcal{R}$, corresponding to the pixels in x that fall in the bth bin, is estimated as:

$$h_b(x) = \Phi\{H_b(x)\} = \Phi\{\max(0, 1 - |x - \beta_b| \times \widetilde{w}_b)\}, \tag{1}$$

where $\mathcal{B}$ is the set of all bins, Φ is the global pooling operator, $H_b(x)$ is the piece-wise linear basis function that accumulates positive votes from the pixels in x that fall in the bth bin of interval $[\beta_b - w_b/2, \beta_b + w_b/2]$, and $\widetilde{w}_b$ is the learnable weight related to the width w_b of the bth bin: $\widetilde{w}_b = 2/w_b$. Any pixel may vote for multiple bins with different $H_b(x)$ since there could be an overlap between adjacent bins in our learnable histogram. The final $|\mathcal{B}| \times 1$ feature values from the learned image histogram are obtained using a global pooling Φ over each $H_b(x)$ separately. This pooling can be a 'non-zero elements count' (NZEC), which matches the convention of a traditional histogram, or can be an 'average' or 'max' pooling, depending on the task-specific requirement. Similar to [12], the linear basis function $H_b(x)$ of the LIH is also piece-wise differentiable and can back-propagate (BP) errors to update β_b and $\widetilde{w}_b$ during training. The gradients of β_b and $\widetilde{w}_b$ for a loss $\mathcal{L}$ are estimated as:

$$\frac{\partial \mathcal{L}}{\partial \beta_b} = \begin{cases} \widetilde{w}_b & \text{if } H_b(x) > 0 \text{ and } x - \beta_b > 0, \\ -\widetilde{w}_b & \text{if } H_b(x) > 0 \text{ and } x - \beta_b < 0, \\ 0 & \text{otherwise.} \end{cases} \tag{2}$$

$$\frac{\partial \mathcal{L}}{\partial \widetilde{w}_b} = \begin{cases} |x - \beta_b| & \text{if } H_b(x) > 0, \\ 0 & \text{otherwise.} \end{cases} \tag{3}$$

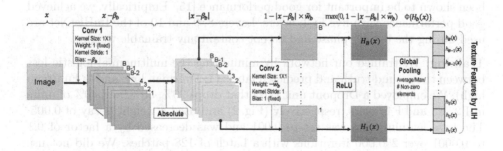

Fig. 1. The architecture of our learnable image histogram using CNN layers.

Design of LIH Using CNN Layers: The proposed LIH is implemented using CNN layers as illustrated in Fig. 1. The input of LIH can be a 2D or vectorized

134   M. A. Hussain et al.

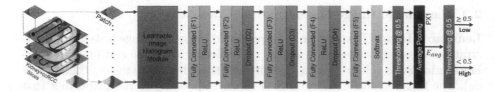

Fig. 2. Multiple instance decisions aggregated ImHistNet for grade classification.

1D image, and the output is a $|\mathcal{B}| \times 1$ histogram feature vector. The operation
$x - \beta_b$ for a bin centered at β_b is equivalent to convolving the input by a 1×1
kernel with fixed weight of 1 (i.e. with no updating by back-propagation [BP])
and a learnable bias term β_b ('Conv 1' in Fig. 1). A total of $B = |\mathcal{B}|$ number of
similar convolution kernels are used for a set of $\mathcal{B}$ bins. Then an absolute value
layer produces $|x - \beta_b|$. This is followed by a set of convolutions ('Conv 2' in
Fig. 1) with a total of B separate (non-shared across channels) learnable 1×1
kernels and a fixed bias of 1 (i.e. no updating by BP) to model the operation of
$1 - |x - \beta_b| \times \widetilde{w}_b$. We use the rectified linear unit (ReLU) to model the $\max(0, \cdot)$
operator in Eq. 1. The final $|\mathcal{B}| \times 1$ feature values $h_b(x)$ are obtained by global
pooling over each feature map $H_b(x)$ separately.

ImHistNet Classifier Architecture: The classification network comprises ten
layers: the LIH layer, five (F1-F5) fully connected layers (FCLs), one softmax
layer, one average pooling (AP) layer, and two thresholding layers (see Fig. 2).
The first seven layers contain trainable weights. The input is a 64×64 pixel
image patch extracted from the kidney+ccRCC slices. During training, randomly shuffled image patches are individually fed to the network. The LIH layer
learns the variables β_b and $\widetilde{w}_b$ to extract representative textural features from
image patches. In implementing the proposed ImHistNet, we chose $B = 128$ and
'average' pooling at $H_b(x)$. We set subsequent FCL (F1-F5) size to 4096×1.
The number of FCLs plays a vital role as the overall depth of the model has
been shown to be important for good performance [15]. Empirically, we achieved
good performance with five FCL layers. Layers 8, 9 and 10 of the ImHistNet are
used during the testing phase and do not contain any trainable weights.

Training: We trained our network by minimizing the multinomial logistic loss
between the ground truth and predicted labels (1: Fuhrman low, and 0: Fuhrman
high). We employed a Dropout unit (Dx) that drops 20%, 30%, and 40% of units
in F2, F3 and F4 layers, respectively (Fig. 2) and used a weight decay of 0.005.
The base learning rate was set to 0.001 and was decreased by a factor of 0.1
to 0.0001 over 250,000 iterations with a batch of 128 patches. We did not use
any batch normalization. Training was performed on a workstation with Intel
4.0 GHz Core-i7 processor, an Nvidia GeForce Titan Xp GPU with 12 GB of
VRAM, and 32 GB of RAM.

ccRCC Grade Classification: After training ImHistNet (layers 1 to 7) by estimating errors at the layer 7 (i.e. Softmax layer), we used the full configuration

Table 1. Automatic ccRCC Fuhrman grade classification performance comparison. NTS: Number of test samples, HE: hand engineered, SVM: support vector machines, xFCV: x-fold cross-validation, LxOCV: leave-x-out cross-validation, '-': Not reported.

Row	Method types	Methods	NTS	Accuracy	AUC
1	Conventional CNNs	Full image+ResNet-50	30	53%	0.4302
2		Full image+AlexNet	30	56%	0.4756
3		Patch+ResNet-50	30	50%	0.6680
4		Patch+AlexNet	30	56%	0.4505
5	HE Features +	Patch+Histogram (128 bins)+SVM	30	56%	0.5046
6	Conventional Machine	Patch+Histogram (256 bins)+SVM	30	63%	0.5140
7	Learning (ConML)	Ding et al. [1]	92	-	0.6700
8		Shu et al. [2] (5FCV on 260 samples)	-	77%	0.8220
9		Fei et al. [16] (L1OCV on 90 samples)	-	70%	-
10		Oh et al. [6]	173	-	0.7000
11	HE Features + Deep	Patch+Histogram (128 bins)+5 FCL	30	50%	0.5664
12	Learning	Patch+Histogram (256 bins)+5 FCL	30	50%	0.6449
13	LIH + ConML	Patch+LIH (128 bins)+AP+SVM	30	60%	0.5885
14	LIH + Different Number	Patch+LIH (128 bins)+NZEC+5 FCL	30	50%	0.5502
15	of FCL/bins + Different	Patch+LIH (128 bins)+AP+4 FCL	30	50%	0.6388
16	Pooling Types	Patch+LIH (128 bins)+AP+6 FCL	30	50%	0.6379
17		Patch+LIH (64 bins)+AP+5 FCL	30	50%	0.6386
18		Patch+LIH (256 bins)+AP+ 5 FCL	30	43%	0.6378
19	Combined LIH &	Patch+LIH (128 bins)+AP+5 FCL	30	53%	0.6501
20	Conventional CNN	Full Image+LIH (128 bins)+AP+ 5 FCL	30	50%	0.4883
21	**Proposed**	ImHistNet [LIH (128 bins)+AP+5 FCL]	30	**80%**	**0.8495**

(from layer 1 to 10) in the testing phase. Although we used patches from only ccRCC-containing kidney slices during training and validation, not all the ccRCC cross-sections contained discriminant features for proper grade identification. Thus our trained network may miss-classify the interrogated image patch. To reduce such misclassification, we adopt a similar multiple instance decision aggregation procedure proposed by Hussain et al. [9]. In this approach, we feed randomly shuffled single image patches as inputs to the model during training. During inference, we feed all candidate image patches of a particular kidney to the trained network and accumulate the patch-wise binary classification labels (0 or 1) at layer 8 (the thresholding layer). We then feed these labels into a $P \times 1$ average pooling layer, where P is the total number of patches of an interrogated kidney. Finally, we feed the estimated average (E_{avg}) from layer 9 to the second thresholding layer (layer 10), where $E_{avg} \geq 0.5$ indicates the Fuhrman low, and Fuhrman high otherwise (see Fig. 2).

3 Results and Discussion

We compared our ccRCC grade classification performance in terms of accuracy (%) and area under the curve (AUC) to a wide range of methods in Table 1. Note that for all our implementations, we trained models with shuffled single image patches, and used multiple instance decision aggregation per kidney during inference. We fixed our patch size to 64×64 pixels across all contrasted methods.

First, we use ResNet-50 and AlexNet (rows 1–4) with transfer learning in order to test the performance of conventional CNNs. Here, we used the full kidney+ccRCC slices as well as patches as inputs. As we mentioned in Sect. 1 that a classical CNN typically fails to capture textural features, it has become evident from the results where such CNNs performed poorly in learning the textural features of ccRCC. Next, in order to evaluate the performance of hand-engineered (HE) features-based conventional machine learning (ConML) approaches, we tested SVM (rows 5–6) employing the conventional image histogram of 128 and 256 bins. We also compared four state-of-the-art methods in rows 7–10. Since we do not have access to their codes and datasets, we conservatively quote authors' best self-reported performances. These methods mostly relied on the ccRCC textural features, and used classical predictive models, e.g. logistic regression. Here, the method by Shu et al. [2] performed the best with 77% classification accuracy. Then, to contrast the performance of a SVM against a DNN, we fed the conventional histogram (128 and 256 bins) features to a DNN of 5 FCL with weight sizes (4096×1)-(4096×1)-(4096×1)-(4096×1)-(2×1) (rows 11–12). We choose this FCL configuration as our ImHistNet contains the same. The better AUC score by the FCL approaches suggest that it better classify tumor grade than that by the SVM (rows 5–6). Next, to evaluate the HE features against LIH features, we used LIH features to train a SVM (row 13). We see that the SVM with LIH features outperformed the SVM with conventional histogram features (row 5). We also varied the number of bins (64/128/256) and FCLs of size 4096×1 (4/5/6), and the pooling types (AP/NZEC) with the LIH layer (rows 14–18). However, the classification performance in terms of AUC by any of these combinations did not exceed ∼65%. After that, in order to evaluate the performance of a DNN, combining a CNN and the ImHistNet, we added a CNN of AlexNet equivalent configuration in parallel to the ImHistNet. The last FCLs of size 4096×1 in both networks were concatenated and the total network was trained end-to-end. We implemented two such approaches using the full kidney+ccRCC images, as well as the patches as inputs (rows 19–20). We observed that the classical CNN affect the performance of the proposed ImHistNet negatively, i.e. results were worse than those by ImHistNet (row 21). In conclusion, our proposed ImHistNet achieved the highest accuracy and AUC performance among all contrasted methods as can be seen in row 21.

4   Conclusions

We proposed a learnable image histogram based DNN framework for end to end image classification. We demonstrated our approach on a cancer grade prediction task providing automatic 2-tiered FGS (Fuhrman low and Fuhrman high) grade classification of ccRCC from CT scans. Our approach learns a histogram directly from the image data and deploys it to extract representative discriminant textural image features. We increased efficacy by using small image patches to increase the number and variability of training samples, as well address class imbalances in the training data via overlap control. We also used multiple instance decision aggregation to further robustify binary classification. Our proposed ImHist-Net outperformed current competing approaches for this task including conventional ML, deep learning, as well as manual human radiology experts. ImHistNet appears well-suited for radiomic studies, where learned textural features using the learnable image histogram may aid in better diagnosis.

Acknowledgement. We thank NVIDIA Corporation for supporting our research through their GPU Grant Program by donating the GeForce Titan Xp.

References

1. Ding, J., et al.: CT-based radiomic model predicts high grade of clear cell renal cell carcinoma. Eur. J. Radiol. **103**, 51–56 (2018)
2. Shu, J., et al.: Clear cell renal cell carcinoma: CT-based radiomics features for the prediction of fuhrman grade. Eur. J. Radiol. **109**, 8–12 (2018)
3. Ishigami, K., Leite, L.V., Pakalniskis, M.G., Lee, D.K., Holanda, D.G., Kuehn, D.M.: Tumor grade of clear cell renal cell carcinoma assessed by contrast-enhanced computed tomography. SpringerPlus **3**(1), 694 (2014)
4. Fuhrman, S.A., Lasky, L.C., Limas, C.: Prognostic significance of morphologic parameters in renal cell carcinoma. Am. J. Surg. Pathol. **6**(7), 655–663 (1982)
5. Becker, A., et al.: Critical analysis of a simplified fuhrman grading scheme for prediction of cancer specific mortality in patients with clear cell renal cell carcinoma-impact on prognosis. Eur. J. Surg. Oncol. (EJSO) **42**(3), 419–425 (2016)
6. Oh, S., et al.: Correlation of ct imaging features and tumor size with fuhrman grade of clear cell renal cell carcinoma. Acta Radiologica **58**(3), 376–384 (2017)
7. Sasaguri, K., Takahashi, N.: CT and MR imaging for solid renal mass characterization. Eur. J. Radiol. **99**, 40–54 (2018)
8. Huhdanpaa, H., et al.: Ct prediction of the fuhrman grade of clear cell renal cell carcinoma (RCC): towards the development of computer-assisted diagnostic method. Abdom. Imaging **40**(8), 3168–3174 (2015)
9. Hussain, M.A., Hamarneh, G., Garbi, R.: Noninvasive determination of gene mutations in clear cell renal cell carcinoma using multiple instance decisions aggregated CNN. In: Frangi, A.F., Schnabel, J.A., Davatzikos, C., Alberola-López, C., Fichtinger, G. (eds.) MICCAI 2018. LNCS, vol. 11071, pp. 657–665. Springer, Cham (2018). https://doi.org/10.1007/978-3-030-00934-2_73
10. LeCun, Y., Bengio, Y., Hinton, G.: Deep learning. Nature **521**(7553), 436 (2015)
11. Andrearczyk, V., Whelan, P.F.: Using filter banks in convolutional neural networks for texture classification. Pattern Recognit. Lett. **84**, 63–69 (2016)
12. Wang, Z., Li, H., Ouyang, W., Wang, X.: Learnable histogram: statistical context features for deep neural networks. In: Leibe, B., Matas, J., Sebe, N., Welling, M. (eds.) ECCV 2016. LNCS, vol. 9905, pp. 246–262. Springer, Cham (2016). https://doi.org/10.1007/978-3-319-46448-0_15
13. Clark, K., et al.: The cancer imaging archive (TCIA): maintaining and operating a public information repository. J. Digit. Imaging **26**(6), 1045–1057 (2013)
14. Aerts, H.J.: The potential of radiomic-based phenotyping in precision medicine: a review. JAMA Oncol. **2**(12), 1636–1642 (2016)

15. Zeiler, M.D., Fergus, R.: Visualizing and understanding convolutional networks. In: Fleet, D., Pajdla, T., Schiele, B., Tuytelaars, T. (eds.) ECCV 2014. LNCS, vol. 8689, pp. 818–833. Springer, Cham (2014). https://doi.org/10.1007/978-3-319-10590-1_53
16. Meng, F., Li, X., Zhou, G., Wang, Y.: Fuhrman grade classification of clear-cell renal cell carcinoma using computed tomography image analysis. J. Med. Imaging Health Inform. **7**(7), 1671–1676 (2017)

DPA-DenseBiasNet: Semi-supervised 3D Fine Renal Artery Segmentation with Dense Biased Network and Deep Priori Anatomy

Yuting He[1], Guanyu Yang[1,4(✉)], Yang Chen[1,4], Youyong Kong[1,4],
Jiasong Wu[1,4], Lijun Tang[3], Xiaomei Zhu[3], Jean-Louis Dillenseger[2,4],
Pengfei Shao[5], Shaobo Zhang[5], Huazhong Shu[1,4], Jean-Louis Coatrieux[2],
and Shuo Li[6]

[1] LIST, Key Laboratory of Computer Network and Information Integration
(Southeast University), Ministry of Education, Nanjing, China
yang.list@seu.edu.cn
[2] Univ Rennes, Inserm, LTSI - UMR1099, 35000 Rennes, France
[3] Department of Radiology, The First Affiliated Hospital
of Nanjing Medical University, Nanjing, China
[4] Centre de Recherche en Information Biomédicale Sino-Français (CRIBs),
Strasbourg, France
[5] Department of Urology, The First Affiliated Hospital
of Nanjing Medical University, Nanjing, China
[6] Department of Medical Biophysics, University of Western Ontario,
London, ON, Canada

Abstract. 3D fine renal artery segmentation on abdominal CTA image targets on the segmentation of the complete renal artery tree which will help clinicians locate the interlobar artery's corresponding blood feeding region easily. However, it is still a challenging task that no one has reported success due to the large intra-scale changes, large inter-anatomy variation, thin structures, small volume ratio and limitation of labeled data. Hence, in this paper, we propose a novel semi-supervised learning framework named DPA-DenseBiasNet for 3D fine renal artery segmentation. The dense biased connection method is presented for multi-receptive field feature maps merging and implicit deep supervision [5] which enable the network to adapt to large intra-scale changes and improve its training process. The dense biased network (DenseBiasNet) is designed based on this method. We develop deep priori anatomy (DPA) for semi-supervised learning of thin structures. Differ from other semi-supervised methods, it embeds priori anatomical features to segmentation network which avoids inaccurate results sensitive to thin structures as optimizing targets, so that the network achieves generalization of different anatomies with the help of unlabeled data. Only 26 labeled and 118 unlabeled images were used to train our framework and it achieves satisfactory results on the testing dataset. The mean centerline voxel distance is 1.976 which

© Springer Nature Switzerland AG 2019
D. Shen et al. (Eds.): MICCAI 2019, LNCS 11769, pp. 139–147, 2019.
https://doi.org/10.1007/978-3-030-32226-7_16

reduced by 3.094 compared to 3D U-Net. The results illustrate that our framework has great prospects in the diagnosis and treatment of kidney disease.

1   Introduction

3D fine renal artery segmentation on abdominal CTA image targets on achieving 3D renal artery tree that reaches the end of interlobar arteries. If successful, clinicians will locate the blood feeding region corresponding to each interlobar artery easily which is important for the diagnosis and pre-operative planning of kidney disease [7,11,12]. For example, it will show the tumor-feeding artery branches for segmental renal arteries clamping before laparoscopic partial nephrectomy [11,12]. With the increasing probability of kidney disease [1], 3D fine renal artery segmentation will play an important role in its diagnosis and treatment.

However, no one has reported success in 3D fine renal artery segmentation because it is a challenging task [10]: (1) Large intra-scale changes. The thickest renal artery of a patient can up to 7.4 mm, which can be more than 5 times of the thinnest artery as is shown in Fig. 1(a). This makes the network have to sensitive to different scale features, which increases the difficulty in feature extraction. (2) Large inter-anatomy variation. 11 different renal artery structures were found just from 461 patients [10]. The number of ostia, branch and accessory renal artery are variable between patients as Fig. 1(b) shows. This makes it difficult for a small dataset to cover all variation and causes the network to overfit easily. (3) Thin structure. The thinnest artery is less than 1.5 mm which is much smaller than other organs in the same region so that the network is prone to lose these structures. (4) Small volume ratio. Renal arteries just account for 0.27% of the kidney region which will cause serious class imbalance problem, so the network is difficult to train. (5) Limitation of labeled data. It is difficult to learn the feature representation of different renal artery anatomies on a small data set, which limits the network's generalization ability. Therefore, how to overcome these challenges and to achieve 3D fine renal artery segmentation is an urgent problem.

There is no success to achieve 3D fine renal artery segmentation automatically, although some rough segmentation methods [6,13] that only segmented up to segmental arteries have been proposed. Li et al. [6] only segmented the main and the thick segmental renal arteries using 400 images. Taha et al. [13] used 99 cases to achieve the main arteries out of the renal. These methods cannot be applied to our task directly for two reasons: (1) The rough results. Main and segmental arteries usually correspond to multi blood feeding regions so that these rough results cannot be used to locate the specific blood feeding region of each vessel. (2) Large labeled dataset requirements. These methods used supervised learning which relies on a large labeled dataset and made it difficult to achieve satisfactory results when the 3D fine renal artery labeled dataset is small.

Semi-supervised learning gives us a tool to solve the limitation of labeled data because it uses unlabeled data to improve the model's performance [15].

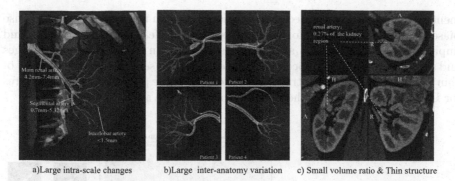

a)Large intra-scale changes   b)Large inter-anatomy variation   c) Small volume ratio & Thin structure

Fig. 1. The challenges of 3D fine renal artery segmentation. (a) The thickest artery of a patient is up to 7.4 mm which can be more than 5 times of the thinnest artery. (b) The number of ostia, branch and accessory renal artery are variable between patients. (c) Renal arteries account for 0.27% of the kidney region and are much thinner than other organs.

Nie et al. [9] designed an attention-based network trained by 35 labeled and 20 unlabeled data to achieve the segmentation on a pelvic dataset. Bia et al. [2] applied CRF to a full convolutional network, and achieved the cardiac MR image segmentation with 240 unlabeled and 80 labeled images. **However**, these methods cannot be used for our tasks directly because they use unlabeled data to get inaccurate labels which lose thin structures easily so that the model is optimized in wrong targets and its performance is weak in our task.

We propose a novel semi-supervised framework (DPA-DenseBiasNet) for 3D fine renal artery segmentation in this paper. Our work has the following contributions: (1) To the best of our knowledge, this work is the first achievement in 3D fine renal artery segmentation. (2) It presents a dense biased connection method which merges multi-receptive field feature maps to adapt to large intra-scale changes. Further, each layer has direct access to the gradients from the loss function, leading to deep supervision [5], to simplify the training process. Dense biased network (DenseBiasNet) is designed based on this method. (3) Deep priori anatomy (DPA) is proposed for semi-supervised learning of thin structures. It embeds priori anatomical features from the encoder trained by unlabeled data to the DenseBiasNet to avoid inaccurate results sensitive to thin structures as optimizing target like other semi-supervised methods. Therefore, DenseBiasNet trained by a small labeled dataset has a higher generalization of different anatomies and keeps the segmentation ability of thin structures. The experimental results show that our framework has enormous potential for clinical application.

2   Methodology

As is illustrated in Fig. 2, DPA-DenseBiasNet adopts a dense biased network (DenseBiasNet) and deep priori anatomy (DPA) for 3D fine renal artery segmentation. DenseBiasNet (Sect. 2.1) is a segmentation network which uses dense biased connection method for multi-receptive field feature maps merging and implicit deep supervision to achieve the segmentation with large scale changes and simplify the training process. DPA (Sect. 2.2) is a semi-supervised method of thin structures which uses a trained encoder to provide priori anatomical features for DenseBiasNet to guide the adaptation of variable anatomical structures.

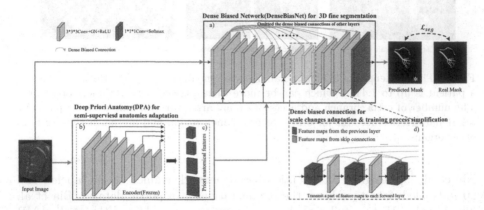

Fig. 2. The framework of DPA-DenseBiasNet: (a) and (d) are DenseBiasNet and dense biased connection method which introduced in Sect. 2.1. (b) is the encoder network from denoising autoencoder trained by numerous unlabeled data and (c) is the priori anatomical features from the encoder. (b) and (c) constitutes DPA which introduced in Sect. 2.2.

2.1   Dense Biased Network (DenseBiasNet) for Fine Segmentation

DenseBiasNet is a 3D fine renal artery segmentation network which based on dense biased connection method. It connects a part of feature maps in each layer to every other forward layer to build dense connectivity pattern. These feature maps are optimized by richer gradients and play a more important role in the network. Hence, we call the method dense biased connection.

Advantages of Dense Biased Connection: (1) It allows the network to adapt to large intra-scale changes via merging multi-receptive field feature maps which have different sensitivities to different scale vessels in each convolutional layer. (2) It simplifies the training process because the gradients from the loss function optimize each layer along the dense biased connection directly.

Dense Biased Connection: As is illustrated in Fig. 2(d), each layer gets a part of feature maps from all preceding layers as additional inputs and transmits a part of its output feature maps to all forward layers. If the sizes of feature maps do not match, maxpooling or upsample method will be used. We denoted the output of the lth layer as F_l. The lth layer receives a part of feature maps of previous layers, $F_0, \ldots, F_{l-2}$, and all the feature maps of F_{l-1} as input: $F_l = H_l(F_{l-1} \circ F_{l-2}[0 : k_{l-2}] \circ \ldots \circ F_0[0 : k_0])$. Where $H_l(\cdot)$ can be a composite function of operations such as group normalization (GN), rectified linear units(ReLU), pooling, upsampling, or convolution (Conv). The symbol '$\circ$' refers to the concatenation of the feature maps. $\{k_0, \ldots, k_{l-2}\}$ is the number of the feature maps the l_{th} layer can receive from $\{0, \ldots, l - 2\}$ layers. In our experiments, we set $\{k_0, \ldots, k_{l-2}\} = 1$.

Structure and Loss Function of DenseBiasNet: Figure 2(a) illustrates DenseBiasNet's structure. It comprises of 14 3D convolution layers which followed a GN and a ReLU, 3 maxpooling layers, 3 3D deconvolution layers used to change scales and a $1 \times 1 \times 1$ convolution layer followed a softmax as the output layer to reduce the number of channels to classes. The dense biased connection is used throughout the network to adapts to different scale arteries.

The network is trained by minimizing the loss function consisting of dice coefficient loss and cross-entropy loss. The dice coefficient loss $\mathcal{L}_{dice}$ helps to establish a balance between artery and background from a global perspective, and the cross-entropy loss $\mathcal{L}_{ce}$ is used for correct classification of each voxel at a local perspective:

$$\mathcal{L}_{seg} = \lambda(1 - \underbrace{\frac{1}{C}\sum_c^C \frac{2\sum_n^N y_{n,c}\hat{y}_{n,c}}{\sum_n^N y_{n,c}^2 + \sum_n^N \hat{y}_{n,c}^2}}_{\mathcal{L}_{dice}}) - \underbrace{\frac{1}{N}\sum_c^C \sum_n^N y_{n,c}\log\hat{y}_{n,c}}_{\mathcal{L}_{ce}} \quad (1)$$

where C is the number of channels output from the network, and N is the size of each channel. $\hat{y}_{n,c}$ is the predicted result and $y_{n,c}$ indicates the label. λ is used to balance these loss functions. In our experiments, we set $\lambda = 0.1$.

2.2 Deep Priori Anatomy (DPA) Based Semi-supervised Learning

DPA is a novel semi-supervised method that avoids inaccurate optimizing targets which sensitive to thin structures during training. It first trains an autoencoder [14] with numerous unlabeled data, and then uses the encoder part to extract input image's priori anatomical features of different semantic levels in different depth in order to guide the anatomical adaptation of the segmentation network which trained with a small labeled dataset as shown in Fig. 2(b)(c).

Advantages of DPA: (1) Deep priori anatomical feature representation learned from unlabeled data which adapts to more anatomical structures than manual priori features. (2) It focuses on both local and global anatomical information because different semantic levels features are extracted from different depths. (3) It improves the network's generalization ability utilizing these priori features. (4) It is suitable for thin structures compared with other semi-supervised methods [2,9] because embedding priori knowledge will not introduce inaccurate labels that are easy to lose thin structures.

DPA for Semi-supervised Anatomical Adaptation: Figure 2 shows the process of extracting and embedding deep prior anatomical features into the DenseBiasNet. Prior to this, a convolutional denoising autoencoder was trained with numerous unlabeled data, and then its encoder part was frozen and used to extract anatomical features (Fig. 2(b)). The image x is putted into the encoder to obtain priori anatomical features at different depths $\{F_{f1}, F_{f2}, F_{f3}, F_{f4}\} = f(x; \theta_f)$. These feature maps (Fig. 2(c)) together with input image x are putted into the DenseBiasNet's different convolution layers to predict fine renal artery segmentation $\hat{y} = d(x, F_{f1}, F_{f2}, F_{f3}, F_{f4}; \theta_d)$. The learning process is minimizing the loss function $\mathcal{L}_{seg}(y, \hat{y})$ to optimize the DenseBiasNet. y is the renal artery mask, $f(\cdot)$ is the encoder operation and $d(\cdot)$ is the DenseBiasNet operation.

3   Experiments and Results

Setting: Abdominal contrast-enhanced CT images of 170 patients who underwent LPN surgery were included in this study. The pixel size of these CT images is between $0.59\,\mathrm{mm}^2$ to $0.74\,\mathrm{mm}^2$. The slice thickness and the spacing in z-direction were fixed at $0.75\,\mathrm{mm}$ and $0.5\,\mathrm{mm}$ respectively. 52 of these images have renal artery mask, half of them were used as the training sets and the other half as the test set. The remaining 118 unlabeled images are used to train the denoising autoencoder. On the training set, we mirrored each image on three axes to expand the training data to 104 images. The kidney region of interest which size was $152 \times 152 \times Z$ was extracted firstly. The denoising autoencoder and DenseBiasNet are all trained with Adam where the batch size was 1, the learning rate was 1×10^{-4} and the decay rate was 1×10^{-5}. They all trained 200 epochs on their corresponding data sets.

   To demonstrate the advantage of our framework, we compared our method with 2 supervised methods (3D U-Net and VNet) and 2 semi-supervised methods (SemiFCN and ASDNet). We adopt the following evaluation metrics to evaluate our proposed method: mean dice coefficient (Dice), mean centerline distance (MCD) and mean surface distance (MSD).

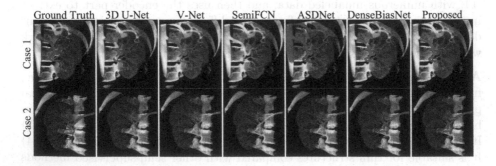

Fig. 3. The visual superiority of our framework (DPA-DenseBiasNet).

Table 1. The advantages of our method (DPA-DenseBiasNet) on each metrics.

Network	Dice	MCD	MSD
V-Net [8]	0.787 (0.113)	2.872 (2.196)	2.213 (2.155)
3D U-Net [4]	0.750 (0.162)	5.070 (4.949)	4.385 (4.208)
(semi)SemiFCN [3]	0.388 (0.259)	8.772 (10.085)	7.921 (10.593)
(semi)ASDNet [9]	0.555 (0.191)	8.557 (5.124)	7.484 (5.132)
DenseBiasNet	0.851 (0.110)	2.478 (2.090)	1.920 (2.354)
(semi)Proposed	**0.861 (0.095)**	**1.976 (1.394)**	**1.472 (1.738)**

Visual Superiority: Figure 3 shows the visual superiority of our framework. Case 1 is a left kidney region whose artery has many singular anatomical structures which difficult to segment. Case 2 is a right kidney region whose artery has great scale changes at the branches. Compared with ground truth, DPA-DenseBiasNet achieves fine segmentation in these cases thanks to the dense biased connection which merges multi-receptive field feature maps and DPA which ensures the segmentation quality of thin structures and generalization of different anatomies. Without the help of DPA, DenseBiasNet loses some parts in case1. SemiFCN cannot realize our task, because CRF removes thin renal arteries so that the inaccurate optimize target weakens the network's performance. ASDNet has serious mis-segmentations due to the more serious class imbalance caused by the confidence map and the instability caused by adversarial learning.

Evaluation Metrics Advantages: The advantages of our DPA-DenseBiasNet on each metric are demonstrated in Table 1. DPA-DenseBiasNet achieves the best segmentation results compared with other methods. The dice coefficient, mean centerline distance and mean surface distance are 0.861, 1.976 and 1.472, and their corresponding standard deviations are 0.095, 1.394 and 1.738. Ablation experiments in the last two rows validate the importance of DPA which improves the segmentation accuracy obviously.

Training Process Improvement: Figure 4 illustrates the improvement of the training process due to dense biased connection. We compared DenseBiasNet, 3D

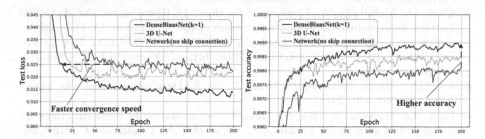

Fig. 4. The improvement of the training process by the dense biased connection. DenseBiasNet has faster convergence speed and higher accuracy than the other two networks.

U-Net (3 layers have skip connections) and the network without skip connections. DenseBiasNet has faster convergence speed and higher test accuracy because the gradients from the loss function optimize each convolution layer directly.

4   Conclusion

This paper proposed a novel semi-supervised framework which achieved 3D fine renal artery segmentation. The proposed framework used dense biased connection method to enable DenseBiasNet to adapt to large intra-scale changes and simplify its training process. Further, our developed semi-supervised method of thin structures, DAP, embedded priori anatomical features from an encoder network to DenseBiasNet to improve its generalization of different anatomies. The performance of our framework was compared with other methods. The results showed that our framework had great prospects in the diagnosis and treatment of kidney disease.

Acknowledgements. This research was supported by the National Key Research and Development Program of China (2017YFC0107903), National Natural Science Foundation under grants (31571001, 61828101), the Short-Term Recruitment Program of Foreign Experts (WQ20163200398), Key Research and Development Project of Jiangsu Province (BE2018749) and Southeast University-Nanjing Medical University Cooperative Research Project (2242019K3DN08).

References

1. Cancer stat facts: Kidney and renal pelvis cancer. https://seer.cancer.gov/statfacts/html/kidrp.html. Accessed 12 Feb 2019
2. Bai, W., et al.: Semi-supervised learning for network-based cardiac MR image segmentation. In: Descoteaux, M., Maier-Hein, L., Franz, A., Jannin, P., Collins, D.L., Duchesne, S. (eds.) MICCAI 2017. LNCS, vol. 10434, pp. 253–260. Springer, Cham (2017). https://doi.org/10.1007/978-3-319-66185-8_29
3. Baur, C., Albarqouni, S., Navab, N.: Semi-supervised deep learning for fully convolutional networks. In: Descoteaux, M., Maier-Hein, L., Franz, A., Jannin, P., Collins, D.L., Duchesne, S. (eds.) MICCAI 2017. LNCS, vol. 10435, pp. 311–319. Springer, Cham (2017). https://doi.org/10.1007/978-3-319-66179-7_36
4. Çiçek, Ö., Abdulkadir, A., Lienkamp, S.S., Brox, T., Ronneberger, O.: 3D U-Net: learning dense volumetric segmentation from sparse annotation. In: Ourselin, S., Joskowicz, L., Sabuncu, M.R., Unal, G., Wells, W. (eds.) MICCAI 2016. LNCS, vol. 9901, pp. 424–432. Springer, Cham (2016). https://doi.org/10.1007/978-3-319-46723-8_49
5. Lee, C.Y., Xie, S., Gallagher, P., Zhang, Z., Tu, Z.: Deeply-supervised nets. Eprint Arxiv, pp. 562–570 (2014)
6. Li, J., Lo, P., Taha, A., Wu, H., Zhao, T.: Segmentation of renal structures for image-guided surgery. In: Frangi, A.F., Schnabel, J.A., Davatzikos, C., Alberola-López, C., Fichtinger, G. (eds.) MICCAI 2018. LNCS, vol. 11073, pp. 454–462. Springer, Cham (2018). https://doi.org/10.1007/978-3-030-00937-3_52

7. Ljungberg, B., et al.: Eau guidelines on renal cell carcinoma: 2014 update. Eur. Urol. **67**(5), 913–924 (2015)
8. Milletari, F., Navab, N., Ahmadi, S.A.: V-net: fully convolutional neural networks for volumetric medical image segmentation. In: 2016 Fourth International Conference on 3D Vision (3DV), pp. 565–571. IEEE (2016)
9. Nie, D., Gao, Y., Wang, L., Shen, D.: ASDNet: attention based semi-supervised deep networks for medical image segmentation. In: Frangi, A.F., Schnabel, J.A., Davatzikos, C., Alberola-López, C., Fichtinger, G. (eds.) MICCAI 2018. LNCS, vol. 11073, pp. 370–378. Springer, Cham (2018). https://doi.org/10.1007/978-3-030-00937-3_43
10. Petru, B., Elena, Ş., Dan, I., Klara, B., Radu, B., Constantin, D.: Morphological assessments on the arteries of the superior renal segment. Surg. radiol. Anat. **34**(2), 137–144 (2012)
11. Shao, P., et al.: Laparoscopic partial nephrectomy with segmental renal artery clamping: technique and clinical outcomes. Eur. Urol. **59**(5), 849–855 (2011)
12. Shao, P., et al.: Precise segmental renal artery clamping under the guidance of dual-source computed tomography angiography during laparoscopic partial nephrectomy. Eur. Urol. **62**(6), 1001–1008 (2012)
13. Taha, A., Lo, P., Li, J., Zhao, T.: Kid-net: convolution networks for kidney vessels segmentation from CT-volumes. arXiv preprint arXiv:1806.06769 (2018)
14. Vincent, P., Larochelle, H., Bengio, Y., Manzagol, P.A.: Extracting and composing robust features with denoising autoencoders. In: Proceedings of the 25th International Conference on Machine Learning, pp. 1096–1103. ACM (2008)
15. Zhu, X.J.: Semi-supervised learning literature survey, Technical report. University of Wisconsin-Madison Department of Computer Sciences (2005)

Semi-supervised Segmentation of Liver Using Adversarial Learning with Deep Atlas Prior

Han Zheng[1,3], Lanfen Lin[1(✉)], Hongjie Hu[2(✉)], Qiaowei Zhang[2],
Qingqing Chen[2], Yutaro Iwamoto[3], Xianhua Han[3],
Yen-Wei Chen[1,3,4(✉)], Ruofeng Tong[1], and Jian Wu[1]

[1] College of Computer Science and Technology, Zhejiang University,
Hangzhou, China
llf@zju.edu.cn
[2] Department of Radiology, Sir Run Run Shaw Hospital, Hangzhou, China
hongjiehu@zju.edu.cn
[3] College of Information Science and Engineering, Ritsumeikan University,
Kusatsu, Japan
chen@is.ritsumei.ac.jp
[4] Zhejiang Lab, Hangzhou, China

Abstract. Medical image segmentation is one of the most important steps in computer-aided intervention and diagnosis. Although deep learning-based segmentation methods have achieved great success in computer vision domain, there are still several challenges in medical image domain. In comparison with natural images, medical image databases are usually small because the annotation is extremely time-consuming and requires expert knowledge. Thus, effective use of unannotated data is essential for medical image segmentation. On the other hand, medical images have many anatomical priors in comparison to non-medical images such as the shape and position of organs. Incorporating the anatomical prior knowledge in deep learning is a vital issue for accurate medical image segmentation. To address these two problems, in this paper we proposed a semi-supervised adversarial learning model with Deep Atlas Prior (DAP) to improve the accuracy of liver segmentation in CT images. We trained the semi-supervised adversarial learning model using both annotated and unannotated images. The DAP, which is based on the probability atlas of organ (liver) and contains prior information such as the shape and position, is combined with the conventional focal loss to aid segmentation. We call the combined loss as Bayesian loss and the conventional focal loss that utilizes the predicted probabilities of training data in the previous learning epoch as a likelihood loss. Experiments on ISBI LiTS 2017 challenge dataset showed that the performance of the semi-supervised network was significantly improved by incorporating with DAP.

Keywords: Liver segmentation · Semi-supervised · Deep Atlas Prior · Adversarial learning

© Springer Nature Switzerland AG 2019
D. Shen et al. (Eds.): MICCAI 2019, LNCS 11769, pp. 148–156, 2019.
https://doi.org/10.1007/978-3-030-32226-7_17

1   Introduction

The liver is one of the vital organs of the human body. Liver segmentation from abdominal computed tomography (CT) images is a crucial step in computer-aided intervention and diagnosis [1]. Thus, different techniques have been developed for automatic liver segmentation. Although deep learning-based image semantic segmentation techniques [2–4] have been achieved state-of-the-art performance, the models need to be trained with a large amount of annotated data to prevent over-fitting and improve the generalization ability. Therefore, applying deep learning to medical image segmentation still faces some challenges due to the limitation of annotated data.

In comparison with natural images, medical image datasets are usually small because the annotation is extremely time-consuming and requires expert knowledge. Semi-supervised learning which can make effective use of unannotated data seems particularly important for medical image segmentation. Many of the current semi-supervised deep learning frameworks are based on Generative Adversarial Network (GAN). Most of them have focused on non-medical images. For example, Hung [5] proposed a semi-supervised semantic segmentation based on adversarial network with a discriminator, which can distinguish between the predicted probability maps and the ground truth. Souly [6] also proposed a semi-supervised segmentation network based on GAN, utilizing the generator network to provide extra training samples while the discriminator assigns a label to samples. For medical image segmentation, there are few studies based on semi-supervised technology [7, 8]. Nie [8] introduced a semi-supervised learning strategy according to [5] with an attention based mechanism inspired by the focal loss [12] to segment pelvic images. In addition, these studies have not taken into account the prior information of medical images.

Medical images have many anatomical priors in comparison to non-medical images such as shape and position of organs. Incorporating the anatomical prior knowledge in deep learning is a vital issue for accurate medical image segmentation. Probabilistic atlas is the statistical information about the spatial distribution of organs in medical images, which is widely applicable in the field of medical image research. In the study of traditional machine learning of medical images, Dong [9] used an iterative probabilistic atlas in template matching framework for liver and spleen segmentation. Tong [10] generated a probabilistic atlas by using dictionary learning and sparse coding techniques for multi-organ segmentation and then they obtained the final segmentation results after post-processing based on a graph-cuts method. Recent studies have combined deep learning methods with probabilistic atlas. Vakalopoulou [11] presented AtlasNet, which used multiple forward transformers mapping all training images to common subspace to generate a new atlas. Our work also mapped all the images to a subspace by registration, but furthermore, we extracted the probabilistic atlas as a prior knowledge to assist in network training.

It is a challenging task to incorporate the probabilistic atlas into the deep learning. In this paper, we proposed a prior loss based on probability atlas for medical image segmentation, which is called as deep atlas prior (DAP). We address the imbalance of the positive and negative samples, by proposing an asymmetric DAP loss to relatively increase the weights of small positive samples relatively. The conventional losses, such as focal loss [12] use the predicted probabilities of the training samples in the previous learning epoch without any prior information, known as likelihood losses. The proposed prior loss and the conventional likelihood losses are equivalent to the prior and the likelihood in a Bayesian framework respectively. Finally, we propose a Bayesian loss that combines the prior and likelihood losses.

The main contributions of this paper are summarized as follows.

(1) We propose a novel semi-supervised liver segmentation approach based on adversarial learning framework, which can incorporate prior knowledge with deep learning to improve the segmentation accuracy.
(2) We extract the liver probabilistic atlas and define a kind of prior loss, i.e., DAP loss. We further propose a Bayesian loss by combining the DAP loss with the focal loss according to the principle of Bayesian model which consists of a likelihood and a prior.
(3) Experiments on ISBI LiTS 2017 challenge dataset proved that the performance of the semi-supervised network was significantly improved by incorporating with DAP.

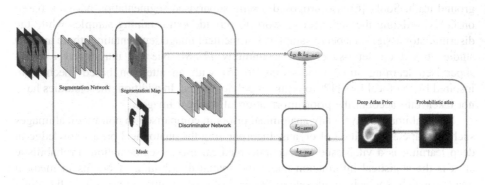

Fig. 1. Overview of the proposed semi-supervised adversarial learning segmentation network with Deep Atlas Prior.

2   Method

Figure 1 shows an overview of the proposed framework, which is made up of two main parts: adversarial learning network and Deep Atlas Prior. The former is the backbone of segmentation model including a Segmentation Network and a Discriminator Network. The latter is transformed from the probabilistic atlas to assist the model learning.

2.1   Adversarial Learning

Adversarial learning comes from the generative adversarial network (GAN) proposed by Goodfellow [13]. GAN was initially used for image generation. In this paper we adapted GAN for image segmentation by replacing the generator in GAN with a semantic segmentation network. Therefore, the model consists of two networks, namely, the Segmentation Network (SN) and the Discriminator Network (DN).

As the name suggests, the primary goal of the SN is to segment the input images and generate a segmentation map with the probability of each class. To capture space context along z-axis, the input image X has three channels, including the segmented, upper and lower slices. The DN receives the ground truths with label 1 and the segmentation maps from the SN with label 0. In the learning phase, the DN attempts to distinguish between the feature maps and the ground truths, as the SN is also trying to deceive the DN, that is, to make the segmentation maps closer to the ground truths.

To take advantage of the unannotated images, we utilized the DN's ability to distinguish between the segmentation maps and the ground truths to choose a reliable mask for unannotated samples, as same as the strategy in [5]. We treated the output of the DN as a confidence map and set a threshold to select the pixels with higher confidence map value to backpropagation.

2.2   Deep Atlas Prior (DAP)

Probabilistic Atlas

The organ probabilistic atlas can serve as a prior probability image of the organ. We used the manually segmented liver masks in the training data to build a probability atlas for the liver. In the initial step, we register the liver mask in different CT cases to the location of the reference volume, which is selected from the training volumes with the largest scan range. The registration was performed by using extracted bones [9]. Probabilistic atlas is obtained by averaging the manually segmented liver masks after registration of all annotated volumes. The value of each point represents the prior statistical probability that the liver appears at this space location.

Deep Atlas Prior

Inspired by the focal loss [12], we proposed a DAP loss. The author of focal loss observed that there are many easy to classify samples with small losses when training the neural network, which dominates the final loss because such samples are large in number. Focal loss decreases the weight of the easy to classify samples to make the network focus on the difficult to classify samples.

Focal loss, which focused on hard samples, by the previous learning epoch is referred to as the likelihood loss. We predefine the hard samples by the anatomical prior (probabilistic atlas) of the liver data, which can be called as the prior loss. Each value in the liver probabilistic atlas represents the probability that the liver will appear at that point; we assume that the atlas values of the hard samples are close to 0.5, meaning the prior probability of liver and non-liver are close. To decrease the weight of easy samples, we choose a Gaussian function to convert the probabilistic atlas to the weight of our DAP loss:

$$W_{DAP} = exp\left(-\frac{(PA - 0.5)^2}{2\sigma^2}\right) \tag{1}$$

where PA is the probabilistic atlas and σ is a hyper-parameter to control the minimal weight. The value of PA is between 0 and 1, meaning the liver has never appeared in the point if the value of probabilistic atlas in this point is 0; if the value is 1, it means that the liver appeared in this point in all training volumes. Points with value 0 or 1 are easy samples with minimal weight and points with value is close to 0.5 are hard samples with maximal weight because it is difficult to determine if they are liver or non-liver. By the Gaussian function, we decrease the weight of the easy samples and increase the weight of the hard samples with middle values relatively.

To address the imbalance of the positive and negative samples, we further proposed an asymmetrical Gaussian function to improve the weight of positive samples:

$$W_{a-DAP} = \begin{cases} exp\left(-\frac{(PA-0.5)^2}{2\sigma_1^2}\right) & 0 \le PA \le 0.5 \\ exp\left(-\frac{(PA-0.5)^2}{2\sigma_2^2}\right) & 0.5 < PA \le 1 \end{cases} \tag{2}$$

where σ_1 and σ_2 are the hyper-parameters to control the minimal value of negative (non-liver) and positive (liver) samples. We set $\sigma_1 < \sigma_2$ to ensure the weight of positive samples are upper than negative samples. By the experimental results in Table 1, we set $\sigma_1 = 0.5$ and $\sigma_2 = 1$ to optimize the DAP.

2.3   Loss Functions

There are four losses in our model: L_D, L_{S-adv}, L_{S-seg} and L_{S-semi}.

L_D is the binary cross entropy loss of the DN, which is used to discriminate the ground truths and the segmentation maps:

$$L_D = -\sum_{h,w} (1 - y_n)log\left(1 - D(D_{in})\right) + y_nlog\left(D(D_{in})\right) \tag{3}$$

where h and w are the height and weight of the input images. D is the DN and D_{in} is the input of DN, which can be the segmentation maps or the ground truths after one-hot coded, and $D(D_{in})$ is the output of the DN with the input of D_{in}. If $y_n = 0$, the D_{in} is the segmentation maps, otherwise, the D_{in} is the ground truths. The calculation of L_D requires the ground truths, so that the unannotated volumes are not included.

The other losses are proposed for training the SN. L_{S-adv} is the adversarial loss to deceive the DN:

$$L_{S-adv} = -\sum_{h,w} log\left(D(S(X_n))\right) \tag{4}$$

where X_n is the input volumes and D, S are the DN, SN, respectively.

L_{S-seg} is the segmentation loss of the annotated volumes, which can be conventional losses, such as the cross entropy loss, dice loss and focal loss. In this paper, we proposed a variance of the cross entropy loss by our DAP:

$$L_{DAP} = -\sum_{h,w} W_{a-DAP}((1 - \alpha)(1 - y_n)log\left(1 - S(X_n)\right) + \alpha y_nlog\left(S(X_n)\right)) \tag{5}$$

where α (set to 0.8) is a hyper-parameter for balancing the positive and negative samples, y_n is the ground truths and $S(X_n)$ is the segmentation maps outputted by the SN. The detail of W_{a-DAP} is shown in Eq. (2). Our DAP loss included the anatomical prior knowledge of the liver, called the prior loss. The conventional losses employ the predicted probabilities of the training samples in the previous learning epoch without any prior anatomic information, called as the likelihood losses. Therefore, we incorporated our DAP loss (prior loss) and the focal loss (likelihood loss) into a Bayesian loss. The Bayesian loss is the final L_{S-seg} in our model.

$$L_{S-seg} = L_{DAP} + \delta L_{focal} \tag{6}$$

where δ was set to 2 in our experiments.

L_{S-semi} is the segmentation loss of the unannotated volumes. Without the ground truths, we trust some segmentation results of the segmentation maps according the output of the DN and use them to calculate the loss:

$$L_{S-semi} = -\sum_{h,w} W_{a-DAP} D(S(X_n)) I(D(S(X_n)) > T_{semi}) f_{bce} \tag{7}$$

$$\text{where } f_{bce} = (1 - \alpha)(1 - y_n) \log(1 - S(X_n)) + \alpha y_n log(S(X_n)) \tag{8}$$

where $D(S(X_n))$ is the output of the DN of the unannotated samples, which is the confidence score of the segmentation results from the SN, which also is a likelihood information in some context. The f_{bce} means the binary cross entropy, where the y_n is the segmentation results from the SN because the unannotated volumes are without ground truth. If $D(S(X_n))$ upper to a threshold T_{semi} (set to 0.3), we trust the related segmentation results and use an indicator function to select them. We then multiply the f_{bce} with the W_{a-DAP} and the $D(S(X_n))$.

The final loss of the SN is the combination of L_{S-adv}, L_{S-semi} and L_{S-seg}:

$$L_S = L_{S-seg} + \lambda_{semi} L_{S-semi} + \lambda_{adv} L_{S-adv} \tag{9}$$

where the λ_{semi} was set to 0.01 and λ_{adv} was set to 0.05.

3   Experiments and Results

3.1   Dataset

The dataset for liver segmentation was from the ISBI LiTS 2017 Challenge, which consists of 131 volumes with 103 training volumes and 28 testing volumes. All the volumes are 3D and with different sizes. In the semi-supervised training process, we built our atlas only with the annotated training volumes, not including the unannotated training volumes or testing volumes.

3.2   Experiments

We chose the DeepLab (Resnet101) as the SN. The DN is a convolutional neural network with four convolutional layers and an up-sample layer, and the activation function is the Leaky ReLU. We chose the SGD optimizer with weight decay of 5e−4. The batch size was set to five. The Dice per case score is chosen as the evaluate metric. We first trained the model with the annotated images and then re-trained the model by unannotated images and annotated images alternately. In every step of the re-train phase, the model was used to segment a batch of unannotated images and the selected unannotated pixels by Eqs. (7) and (8), where the segmentation results were used as their ground truth, were used to re-train the model. After that, we re-trained the model by a batch of annotated images.

Table 1. Comparison of symmetrical and asymmetrical DAP. The results in the diagonal are with symmetrical DAP losses ($\sigma_1 = \sigma_2$), and the other are with asymmetrical losses ($\sigma_1 < \sigma_2$).

$\sigma_1 \backslash \sigma_2$	0.25	0.50	1.00	2.00
0.25	91.80%	92.41%	91.84%	91.96%
0.50	–	93.37%	**93.90%**	93.52%
1.00	–	–	93.47%	93.85%
2.00	–	–	–	93.76%

Table 2. Effects of unannotated data and DAP. The last row is the proposed method.

Annotated data	Unannotated data	DAP	Annotation: 30%	Annotation: 70%
✓			91.30%	92.12%
✓		✓	93.03%	94.38%
✓	✓		92.16%	93.97%
✓	✓	✓	**94.21%**	**94.76%**

Table 3. Comparison of the proposed method with state-of-the-art semi-supervised methods.

Annotated: unannotated	0.1: 0.9	0.3: 0.7	0.5: 0.5	0.7: 0.3	1.0: 0.0
Hung et al. [5]	90.52%	92.16%	93.60%	93.97%	92.28%
Nie et al. [8]	90.79%	92.82%	94.13%	94.03%	93.24%
Proposed method	**93.12%**	**94.21%**	**94.78%**	**94.76%**	**95.23%**

Symmetrical vs. Asymmetrical DAP

We adjusted the σ_1 and σ_2 in Eq. (2) to compare different DAP; Table 1 shows the results. We did not perform the experiments in lower left corner of the table ($\sigma_1 > \sigma_2$) because we wanted to focus on the positive samples, which means the weight of negative samples will not be higher than positive samples and σ_1 will not be higher than σ_2. The results in the diagonal are with symmetrical DAP losses ($\sigma_1 = \sigma_2$) while other results were with asymmetrical DAP losses ($\sigma_1 < \sigma_2$). From the experimental results, we found that the asymmetrical DAP performed better than the symmetrical DAP did. For all subsequent experiments, we set $\sigma_1 = 0.5$ and $\sigma_2 = 1$, which achieved the best results.

Effects of Unannotated Data and DAP
We introduced a semi-supervised segmentation based on adversarial learning to include the unannotated data and DAP. Table 2 shows the results of experiments conducted using a different volume of annotated data. The results in the first and second rows were only with the annotated data, and the first row was a result without DAP. The results in the last two rows were with both annotated and unannotated data. DAP was used for the last row (the proposed method). We found that the segmentation accuracy can be improved by adding DAP and the accuracy can be further improved by including the unannotated data (semi-supervised segmentation).

Comparison With State-of-the-Art Semi-supervised Methods
Table 3 shows the results of comparing our proposed losses with state-of-the-art semi-supervised methods (without anatomic priors) [5, 8] with different rate of unannotated data. The results in rightmost column are supervised with 100% annotated data in the dataset. From the results, we found that our proposed loss performed better than state-of-the-art semi-supervised methods in all cases, which proved that the anatomic prior knowledge is meaningful in liver segmentation.

4 Conclusion

In this paper, we proposed a semi-supervised adversarial learning model with DAP to segment liver in CT images. The semi-supervised model includes unannotated data in the training dataset to minimize the need for annotation of medical images. DAP is a statistical anatomical prior knowledge of medical images. The focal loss which utilizing the predicted probabilities of the training samples in the previous learning epoch as a likelihood loss and our DAP as a prior loss. We also proposed a Bayesian loss based on the Bayesian model, which consists of a prior and a likelihood. The experimental results showed that the proposed method is useful in semi-supervised liver segmentation.

Acknowledgements. This work was supported in part by Major Scientific Research Project of Zhejiang Lab under the Grant No. 2018DG0ZX01, in part by the Key Science and Technology Innovation Support Program of Hangzhou under the Grant No. 20172011A038, and in part by the Grant-in Aid for Scientific Research from the Japanese Ministry for Education, Science, Culture and Sports (MEXT) under the Grant No. 18H03267 and No. 17H00754.

References

1. Lu, F., Wu, F., Hu, P., Peng, Z., Kong, D.: Automatic 3D liver location and segmentation via convolutional neural network and graph cut. Int. J. Comput. Assist. Radiol. Surg. **12**(2), 171–182 (2017)
2. Long, J., Shelhamer, E., Darrell, T.: Fully convolutional networks for semantic segmentation. In: Proceedings of the IEEE Conference on Computer Vision and Pattern Recognition, pp. 3431–3440 (2015)

3. Ronneberger, O., Fischer, P., Brox, T.: U-Net: convolutional networks for biomedical image segmentation. In: Navab, N., Hornegger, J., Wells, W.M., Frangi, A.F. (eds.) MICCAI 2015. LNCS, vol. 9351, pp. 234–241. Springer, Cham (2015). https://doi.org/10.1007/978-3-319-24574-4_28

4. Chen, L.C., Papandreou, G., Kokkinos, I., Murphy, K., Yuille, A.L.: DeepLab: semantic image segmentation with deep convolutional nets, atrous convolution, and fully connected CRFs. IEEE Trans. Pattern Anal. Mach. Intell. **40**, 834–848 (2018)

5. Hung, W.C., Tsai, Y.H., Liou, Y.T., Lin, Y.Y., Yang, M.H.: Adversarial learning for semi-supervised semantic segmentation. arXiv preprint arXiv:1802.07934 (2018)

6. Souly, N., Spampinato, C., Shah, M.: Semi-supervised semantic segmentation using generative adversarial network. In: Proceedings of the IEEE International Conference on Computer Vision, pp. 5688–5696 (2017)

7. Liu, X., et al.: Semi-supervised automatic segmentation of layer and fluid region in retinal optical coherence tomography images using adversarial learning. IEEE Access **7**, 3046–3061 (2019)

8. Nie, D., Gao, Y., Wang, L., Shen, D.: ASDNet: attention based semi-supervised deep networks for medical image segmentation. In: Frangi, A.F., Schnabel, J.A., Davatzikos, C., Alberola-López, C., Fichtinger, G. (eds.) MICCAI 2018. LNCS, vol. 11073, pp. 370–378. Springer, Cham (2018). https://doi.org/10.1007/978-3-030-00937-3_43

9. Dong, C., et al.: Segmentation of liver and spleen based on computational anatomy models. Comput. Biol. Med. **67**, 146–160 (2015)

10. Tong, T., et al.: Discriminative dictionary learning for abdominal multi-organ segmentation. Med. Image Anal. **23**(1), 92–104 (2015)

11. Vakalopoulou, M., et al.: AtlasNet: multi-atlas non-linear deep networks for medical image segmentation. In: Frangi, A.F., Schnabel, J.A., Davatzikos, C., Alberola-López, C., Fichtinger, G. (eds.) MICCAI 2018. LNCS, vol. 11073, pp. 658–666. Springer, Cham (2018). https://doi.org/10.1007/978-3-030-00937-3_75

12. Lin, T.Y., Goyal, P., Girshick, R., He, K., Dollár, P.: Focal loss for dense object detection. In: Proceedings of the IEEE International Conference on Computer Vision, pp. 2980–2988 (2017)

13. Goodfellow, I., et al.: Generative adversarial nets. In: Advances in Neural Information Processing Systems, pp. 2672–2680 (2014)

Pairwise Semantic Segmentation via Conjugate Fully Convolutional Network

Renzhen Wang[1,2], Shilei Cao[2(✉)], Kai Ma[2], Deyu Meng[1], and Yefeng Zheng[2]

[1] School of Mathematics and Statistics, Xi'an Jiaotong University, Xi'an, China
[2] Youtu Lab, Tencent, Shenzhen, China
eliasslcao@tencent.com

Abstract. Semantic segmentation has been popularly addressed using fully convolutional networks (FCNs) with impressive results if the training set is diverse and large enough. However, FCNs often fail to achieve satisfactory results due to a limited number of manually labelled samples in medical imaging. In this paper, we propose a conjugate fully convolutional network (CFCN) to address this challenging problem. CFCN is a novel framework where pairwise samples are input and synergistically segmented in the network for capturing a rich context representation. To avoid overfitting introduced by appearance and shape changes in a small number of training samples, a fusion module is designed to provide proxy supervision for the network training process. Quantitative evaluation shows that the proposed method has a significant performance improvement on pathological liver segmentation.

Keywords: Semantic segmentation · Pairwise segmentation · Conjugate fully convolutional network · Proxy supervision

1 Introduction

Semantic segmentation, a computer vision task, aims at predicting semantic labels for each pixel of an image. Benefiting from the recent development of deep learning, it has achieved great success in natural image segmentation [4,8]. While the 2D/3D medical image segmentation can leverage similar technologies (e.g., U-Net [13] and V-Net [9]) to achieve a sound result, there are a few challenges that deserve broad attention. Firstly, semantic segmentation is a task to assign a consistent semantic label to a category of objects, rather than to each single pixel. Actually, all the objects, not only the ones to be segmented, in medical images/volumes usually lie in a low-dimensional manifold and modeling the intrinsic relations of them is of great significance for segmentation. For example, in liver segmentation, the relative positions of the surrounding organs are very important for locating the liver and helpful to the liver segmentation. Secondly, individual differences such as smoothness and pixel intensity of target objects in different images need a large number of training samples to be discriminative. With limited training samples, how to trade-off between exactly modeling the

© Springer Nature Switzerland AG 2019
D. Shen et al. (Eds.): MICCAI 2019, LNCS 11769, pp. 157–165, 2019.
https://doi.org/10.1007/978-3-030-32226-7_18

manifold of target objects and robustly representing the individual difference is a bottleneck to a fully convolutional network (FCN) and its variants, e.g., U-Net [13] and V-Net [9].

There are some remarkable works for modeling the manifold or prior knowledge of the target objects. One group leveraged the intrinsic relations among the same category of pixels to improve the performance of FCNs. For example, a dense conditional random field (CRF) was attached to the FCN as a post-processing step to preserve the boundary of the object in [3]. Similarly, Ke et al. [6] proposed an adaptive affinity field to encode spatial structural information and geometric regularities through the label relations in the training process. Another group of methods improved the segmentation performance of FCNs by explicitly or implicitly modeling high-order prior knowledge in-between different objects in medical images/volumes, such as shape, topological structure, etc. Chen et al. [2] took gland objects and contours as auxiliary information under a multi-task learning framework to boost the gland segmentation from histology images. In [12], a non-linear shape model was pre-learned by convolutional autoencoders (CAE) to model the shape manifold space and then incorporated in an FCN. Ravishankar et al. [11] proposed a novel framework based on deep learning to jointly learn the foreground, background and shape to improve segmentation accuracy. In [1], a topology-aware loss was proposed to train the FCN for coding geometric and topological priors of containment and detachment on histology gland segmentation.

Considering semantic segmentation is a structured prediction task, a target object lying in different images/volumes should have consistent labels. This implies that objects in different slices of volumes or different patches of images usually have intrinsic relations among context, shape and location. To model these intrinsic relations, we propose a conjugate fully convolutional network (CFCN) to pairwisely segment the medical objects. Generally speaking, our CFCN has two conjugate sub-networks, each for segmenting one single sample of a paired input. To capture the intrinsic relations of pairwise input and encode the manifold of target objects, the two sub-networks share the same weights in the encoder backbone, which implies that the low-level features captured by CFCN should be sufficient to represent the target object and robust for distinguishing backgrounds. In the remaining layers, the two conjugate sub-networks have independent weights, which enables CFCN to learn discriminative features for representing each of the two inputs. As medical image segmentation is a location-aware task where the relative position of the anatomical structure is very important for locating the target object, we design a fusion sub-network to provide proxy supervision for modeling intra-class inconsistency and prior shape knowledge. Different from the mini-batch training manner of FCNs, in the CFCN, features of the pairwise input interact and guide each other in the fusion module, which offers a new data augmentation method that one sample could be paired with (multi-shot by) different samples.

We demonstrate the efficiency of our approach on the typical problem of pathological liver segmentation. Compared with the traditional FCNs, the main

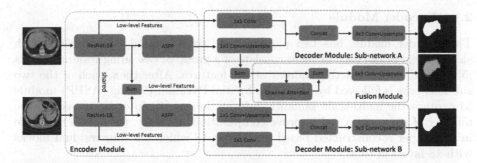

Fig. 1. The overview of the proposed conjugate fully convolutional network. The architecture consists of three parts: encoder module, decoder module, and fusion module. The network takes two different inputs and outputs the corresponding probability maps for the segmentation throughout two sub-networks of the decoder module. Besides, an additional output of the fusion module is employed to fit the proxy supervision.

contributions of this paper are three-fold: Firstly, a new conjugate network framework is proposed to pairwisely mine the semantic information of samples and implicitly model the correlation between the two input samples. Secondly, a novel fusion module is designed to provide proxy supervision for eliminating intra-class inconsistency and modeling shape prior of target objects to improve segmentation accuracy. Thirdly, pairwise input can augment the magnitude of training samples and provide a new solution for medical image segmentation with limited training samples.

2   Method

In this section, we present the details of the proposed pairwise segmentation network CFCN. The CFCN model consists of three parts: an encoder module, a decoder module and a fusion module. The encoder module takes a pair of samples as inputs and jointly captures their representations. The decoder module consists of two conjugate sub-networks which take the low-level and high-level features from the encoder module as their input and learn the discriminative features for segmenting each input under the supervision of their own groundtruth maps. The fusion module uses the summation of low-level features from the encoder module, and the summation of high-level features from the decoder module, as its input to capture the location-aware representation under the proxy supervision. Our CFCN for medical image segmentation is illustrated in Fig. 1.

Before detailed description, we summarize the notations used in this paper. The training data is composed of an image sequence $\mathbf{X} = \{\mathbf{x}^1, \mathbf{x}^2, \cdots, \mathbf{x}^N\}$ from 3D medical volumes and a corresponding mask sequence $\mathbf{Y} = \{\mathbf{y}^1, \mathbf{y}^2, \cdots, \mathbf{y}^N\}$, with $\mathbf{x}^i \in \mathbb{R}^{h \times w}$ and $\mathbf{y}^i \in \{0,1\}^{h \times w}, i = 1, 2, \cdots, N$, where h, w denote the height and width of the medical image, respectively.

2.1   Encoder Module

The encoder module has two parallel fully convolutional sub-networks with shared weights and each of them consists of a group of cascading residual blocks [5] for gradually extracting more abstract features. After then, each of the two sub-networks is followed by an Atrous Spatial Pyramid Pooling (ASPP) module to capture the multi-scale semantic information as [4]. In order to reduce the number of parameters and improve computation efficiency, the encoder module in this paper is constructed based on ResNet-18 which has four residual blocks with 18 layers in total.

Different from the traditional medical image segmentation networks, our encoder module takes pairwise samples as inputs and try to make the siamese sub-networks guide each other during the training process. As aforementioned, the medical image/volume globally lies in a low-dimensional manifold and pairwise input usually has intrinsic relations in context, shape, location, etc. Using this strategy, the encoder module can learn rich semantic information representing the target object while robustly distinguishing it from the background. In the fusion module we further exploit the intrinsic relations of paired inputs. The outputs of each sub-networks are high-level and low-level features from ASPP and the first residual blocks of ResNet-18, respectively, which serve as the inputs of the decoder module and the fusion module.

2.2   Decoder Module

The decoder module consists of two conjugate convolutional sub-networks (Sub-network A and Sub-network B) for segmenting each sample of the paired inputs. Each decoder sub-network uses the same architecture as [4], where the high-level features from the encoder's ASPP module are filtered by a convolutional layer and up-sampled to the same size of the low-level features, and then concatenated with the low-level features from ResNet-18. The resulting feature maps are fed into a convolutional layer with 3×3 convolutions and bilinearly up-sampled to the same size as the mask maps. Note that, if removed one of the two conjugate sub-networks, the other one attached with the encoder module can be separately regarded as DeepLabv3+ [4] with a ResNet-18 backbone, which is a state-of-the-art architecture in semantic segmentation. Please refer to [4] for more details.

2.3   Fusion Module

The fusion module is designed by considering the following motivations: the first one is intra-class inconsistency where the target objects in different images/volumes share the same semantic label but different appearances. For example, in liver segmentation, individual anatomy difference and imaging device difference can both result in intra-class inconsistency as shown in Fig. 2(a). Especially with limited training data, the network is sensitive to intra-class inconsistency and prone to overfitting. The second motivation is shape learning in an end-to-end manner. As shown in Fig. 2(b), if the two inputs are sampled from

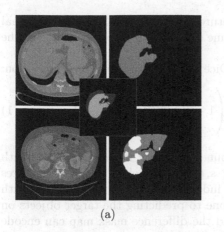 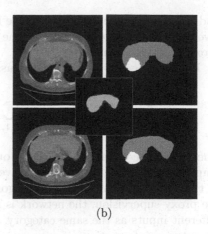

        (a)   (b)

Fig. 2. Two typical challenges faced in the medical image segmentation. (a) Intra-class inconsistency: a pair of slices are from two different volumes, where the livers differ greatly in appearance. And the local contexts are very different on the below pathological liver. Synergistically predicting the intersection and difference of the two masks can eliminate intra-class inconsistency, as shown in the central subgraph. (b) Shape modeling in an end-to-end manner. To address this, a pair of slices are sampled from one volume with a small interval along the axial direction, and the difference of the two masks can encode the shape prior of the liver, as the central subgraph shows. Note that the lesions are masked for better visualization. (Color figure online)

the same volume with a small interval along the axial direction, then the difference of the mask (where region masked in red denotes only one of the two inputs' pixels belonging to the target objects) can encode the shape prior of the target object. To this end, we design a fusion module to learn location-aware features through a proxy supervision in the training process. Suppose $\mathbf{x}^i$ and $\mathbf{x}^j$ are a pair of inputs, $\mathbf{y}^i$ and $\mathbf{y}^j$ are their corresponding groundtruth maps, then the proposed proxy is simply implemented by $\mathbf{y}^{ij} = \mathbf{y}^i + \mathbf{y}^j$, where the mask $\mathbf{y}^{ij} \in \{0,1,2\}^{h \times w}$ and 0, 1, 2 imply the two inputs' pixels, at the index, are both belonging to the background, one for the target object and both belonging to the target object, respectively. In other words, we can implement the proxy supervision by an additional 3-category segmentation task, where the labels constitute three maps, including the intersection of background, the difference and intersection of the target object (corresponding to the label 0, 1, 2), respectively.

As aforementioned, the proxy supervision is abstract prior knowledge which requires the fusion module to exploit semantic information of the low-level and high-level features of the paired inputs. To this end, we element-wisely add the low-level and high-level features, and take the overall features as the input of the fusion module. Furthermore, inspired by [14], we adopt a channel attention block to refine the low-level features. With this design, the fusion module can adaptively learn global context information with a negligible computation cost. In pursuit of further fusion, we sum the features from the channel attention block and the high-level features. Then, the features are fed into a 3×3 convolutional layer and bilinearly up-sampled to the same size as output corresponding to the proxy supervision maps.

In this paper, we employ multi-class Dice loss to learn the proxy supervision:

$$\mathcal{L}_{proxy}\left(\mathbf{y}^{ij},\mathbf{p}^{ij}\right) = \frac{1}{3} \sum_{\ell \in \{0,1,2\}} \left(1 - \frac{2\sum_{s,t} \mathbf{y}_{st}^{ij\ell} \mathbf{p}_{st}^{ij\ell}}{\sum_{s,t} \left(\mathbf{y}_{st}^{ij\ell} + \mathbf{p}_{st}^{ij\ell} \right)} \right), \quad (1)$$

where $\mathbf{p}^{ij}$ and $\mathbf{y}^{ij}$ are the CFCN's output probability maps and groundtruth maps corresponding to $\mathbf{x}^{ij}$, respectively; s, t are the height and width indices of the two maps; and ℓ is the category index of the proxy supervision. With the proxy supervision, the network is prone to predicting the target objects on different inputs as the same category, and the difference mask map can encode the contour information.

The overall loss of the proposed CFCN model can then be presented:

$$\mathcal{L}(\mathbf{y}^i, \mathbf{p}^i, \mathbf{y}^j, \mathbf{p}^j, \mathbf{y}^{ij}, \mathbf{p}^{ij}; \mathbf{\Theta}) = \left(\mathcal{L}_1(\mathbf{y}^i, \mathbf{p}^i) + \mathcal{L}_2(\mathbf{y}^j, \mathbf{p}^j)\right) + \lambda \mathcal{L}_{proxy}(\mathbf{y}^{ij}, \mathbf{p}^{ij}), \quad (2)$$

where $\mathbf{y}^i$ and $\mathbf{y}^j$ are the mask maps of $\mathbf{x}^i$ and $\mathbf{x}^j$; $\mathbf{p}^i$ and $\mathbf{p}^j$ are their corresponding predicted probability maps output by the Sub-network A and Sub-network B of the decoder module, respectively; $\mathcal{L}_1$ and $\mathcal{L}_2$ refer to the pixel-level segmentation losses for $\mathbf{x}^i$ and $\mathbf{x}^j$, respectively. In this paper, the Dice loss is adopted for $\mathcal{L}_1$ and $\mathcal{L}_2$. Note that λ is a user-preset weight used to balance the contribution of the paired inputs' loss and the proxy loss.

3   Experiments and Discussions

We then substantiate the robustness and generalization capability of our proposed framework on the 2D segmentation of abnormal liver. Since the presence of any pathology or abnormality may seriously distort the scanned texture, accurate pathological liver segmentation remains a challenge to deep FCNs, especially with small or moderate amount of training data.

Dataset: We evaluate our method on the public benchmark dataset of the Liver Tumor Segmentation Challenge Dataset[1] (LiTS), which consists of 201 contrast-enhanced abdominal CT volumes acquired from multiple clinical sites. Since the challenge organizers only provide a subset of 131 volumes with manually labelled liver masks, we perform all our experiments on this subset.

Implementation: All experiments are implemented with the PyTorch framework [10]. We use the Adam Optimizer [7] with batch size of 20, weight decay of $5e^{-4}$, and learning rate of $1e^{-4}$ in training. As for λ, we empirically set it as 0.2. For each of paired inputs, we adopt a 2.5D input with five adjacent slices.

We use a fixed proportion 20% (26 volumes) of the 131 volumes as the test set and the remaining volumes as the training set. In order to verify that our

---

[1] https://competitions.codalab.org/competitions/17094.

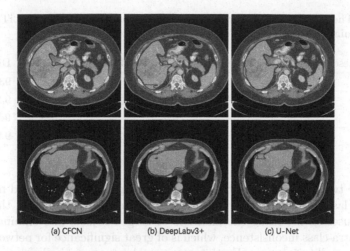

(a) CFCN   (b) DeepLabv3+   (c) U-Net

Fig. 3. Examplar segmentation results (lined in red) of CFCN, DeepLabv3+ [4] and U-Net [13] on the LiTS dataset. Here blue lines manifest the groundtruth. (Color figure online)

Table 1. Comparison of segmentation performance (Average Dice, %) between our approach and U-Net [13], DeepLabv3+ [4] on the LiTS dataset with 80%, 5% and 1% proportions of training samples (training radio), and the test set is always set as a fixed proportion of 20%.

Training ratio	U-Net	DeepLabv3+	CFCN
80%	95.88	95.93	96.43
5%	92.15	92.59	94.45
1%	80.19	81.13	85.26

model can achieve a reasonable segmentation accuracy with a limited number of training samples, additional experiments are designed with 5% and 1% of the training subset (corresponding to 7 volumes and 1 volume, respectively), and the training samples are augmented by the aforementioned multi-shot ways, i.e. paired inputs are sampled from two random volumes with each slice paired twice, and sampled from one volume at intervals of 5, 9, and 13 slices. We use the average Dice score of all volumes to evaluate the performance of the proposed method, and compare the results with U-Net [13] and DeepLabv3+ [4] with a ResNet-18 backbone due to their sound performance and close relation with our CFCN model, as mentioned in Sect. 2.2.

The results are listed in Table 1. As shown, our CFCN achieves a Dice score of 96.43% with 80% training data, which outperforms U-Net [13] and DeepLabv3+ [4] with Dice scores of 95.88% and 95.93%, respectively. Especially, with 5% training data, the performance of CFCN is 94.45%, outperforming 1.8% compared with the two state-of-the-art networks. As shown in Fig. 3, CFCN is supe-

Table 2. The performance (Average Dice, %) of ablation study on the LiTS dataset with 5% training samples, and the test set remains fixed as Table 1.

Siamese DeepLabv3+	Heterogeneous inputs	Homogeneous inputs	Dice
✓			93.10
✓	✓		93.69
✓		✓	94.11
✓	✓	✓	94.45

rior to the two comparison methods in delineating the boundary and maintaining intra-class consistency of the liver segmentation. Unsurprisingly, the CFCN model focuses on modeling the manifold of target objects and eliminating the effect of intra-class inconsistence, which is of great significance for network training with a small training set. Furthermore, we also try to train deep models with a extremely limited training set of one volume, and the performance of CFCN is 85.26%, outperforming 4.1% compared with U-Net [13] and DeepLabv3+ [4].

To investigate the effect of each component of our CFCN model, we perform an ablation study on the training set with 5% volumes. We respectively study the ablation for the fusion module, pairwise input from different volumes as Fig. 2(a) shows, and pairwise input from the same volume as Fig. 2(b) shows. For simplicity, we call the three ablation schemes as Siamese DeepLabv3+, heterogeneous inputs and homogeneous inputs, respectively. Note that the latter two are with the fusion module. As Table 2 shows, these schemes can gradually and effectively improve the segmentation performance with a limited training set.

4   Conclusion

In this paper, we proposed the CFCN model to pairwisely segment pathological livers on CT, which employs location correlation to eliminate intra-class inconsistence and shape priors to model the manifold of target objects in an end-to-end training manner. The experimental result demonstrates that CFCN can significantly improve segmentation accuracy with a limited number of training data. The model can be naturally extended to other medical segmentation applications and we will further exploit relevant prior knowledge to incorporate into deep learning models.

Acknowledgments. This work was supported by the China NSFC (11690011, 61661166011, 61721002, 81830053, U1811461) and the Key Area Research and Development Program of Guangdong Province, China (2018B010111001).

References

1. BenTaieb, A., Hamarneh, G.: Topology aware fully convolutional networks for histology gland segmentation. In: Ourselin, S., Joskowicz, L., Sabuncu, M.R., Unal, G., Wells, W. (eds.) MICCAI 2016. LNCS, vol. 9901, pp. 460–468. Springer, Cham (2016). https://doi.org/10.1007/978-3-319-46723-8_53
2. Chen, H., Qi, X., Yu, L., Heng, P.A.: DCAN: deep contour-aware networks for accurate gland segmentation. In: CVPR, pp. 2487–2496 (2016)
3. Chen, L.C., Papandreou, G., Kokkinos, I., et al.: DeepLab: semantic image segmentation with deep convolutional nets, atrous convolution, and fully connected CRFs. IEEE TPAMI **40**(4), 834–848 (2018)
4. Chen, L.-C., Zhu, Y., Papandreou, G., Schroff, F., Adam, H.: Encoder-decoder with atrous separable convolution for semantic image segmentation. In: Ferrari, V., Hebert, M., Sminchisescu, C., Weiss, Y. (eds.) ECCV 2018. LNCS, vol. 11211, pp. 833–851. Springer, Cham (2018). https://doi.org/10.1007/978-3-030-01234-2_49
5. He, K., Zhang, X., Ren, S., Sun, J.: Deep residual learning for image recognition. In: CVPR, pp. 770–778 (2016)
6. Ke, T.-W., Hwang, J.-J., Liu, Z., Yu, S.X.: Adaptive affinity fields for semantic segmentation. In: Ferrari, V., Hebert, M., Sminchisescu, C., Weiss, Y. (eds.) ECCV 2018. LNCS, vol. 11205, pp. 605–621. Springer, Cham (2018). https://doi.org/10.1007/978-3-030-01246-5_36
7. Kingma, D.P., Ba, J.: Adam: a method for stochastic optimization. arXiv preprint arXiv:1412.6980 (2014)
8. Long, J., Shelhamer, E., Darrell, T.: Fully convolutional networks for semantic segmentation. In: CVPR, pp. 3431–3440 (2015)
9. Milletari, F., Navab, N., Ahmadi, S.A.: V-Net: fully convolutional neural networks for volumetric medical image segmentation. In: Fourth International Conference on 3D Vision, pp. 565–571 (2016)
10. Paszke, A., Gross, S., Chintala, S., et al.: Automatic differentiation in PyTorch. In: NIPS Workshop Autodiff, pp. 1–4 (2017)
11. Ravishankar, H., Thiruvenkadam, S., Venkataramani, R., Vaidya, V.: Joint deep learning of foreground, background and shape for robust contextual segmentation. In: Niethammer, M., et al. (eds.) IPMI 2017. LNCS, vol. 10265, pp. 622–632. Springer, Cham (2017). https://doi.org/10.1007/978-3-319-59050-9_49
12. Ravishankar, H., Venkataramani, R., Thiruvenkadam, S., Sudhakar, P., Vaidya, V.: Learning and incorporating shape models for semantic segmentation. In: Descoteaux, M., Maier-Hein, L., Franz, A., Jannin, P., Collins, D.L., Duchesne, S. (eds.) MICCAI 2017. LNCS, vol. 10433, pp. 203–211. Springer, Cham (2017). https://doi.org/10.1007/978-3-319-66182-7_24
13. Ronneberger, O., Fischer, P., Brox, T.: U-Net: convolutional networks for biomedical image segmentation. In: Navab, N., Hornegger, J., Wells, W.M., Frangi, A.F. (eds.) MICCAI 2015. LNCS, vol. 9351, pp. 234–241. Springer, Cham (2015). https://doi.org/10.1007/978-3-319-24574-4_28
14. Yu, C., Wang, J., Peng, C., et al.: Learning a discriminative feature network for semantic segmentation. In: CVPR, pp. 1857–1866 (2018)

Unsupervised Deformable Image Registration Using Cycle-Consistent CNN

Boah Kim[1] , Jieun Kim[2], June-Goo Lee[2], Dong Hwan Kim[2], Seong Ho Park[2], and Jong Chul Ye[1]($\boxtimes$)

[1] Korea Advanced Institute of Science and Technology, Daejeon, South Korea
{boahkim,jong.ye}@kaist.ac.kr
[2] Asan Medical Center, University of Ulsan College of Medicine, Seoul, South Korea

Abstract. Medical image registration is one of the key processing steps for biomedical image analysis such as cancer diagnosis. Recently, deep learning based supervised and unsupervised image registration methods have been extensively studied due to its excellent performance in spite of ultra-fast computational time compared to the classical approaches. In this paper, we present a novel unsupervised medical image registration method that trains deep neural network for deformable registration of 3D volumes using a cycle-consistency. Thanks to the cycle consistency, the proposed deep neural networks can take diverse pair of image data with severe deformation for accurate registration. Experimental results using multiphase liver CT images demonstrate that our method provides very precise 3D image registration within a few seconds, resulting in more accurate cancer size estimation.

Keywords: Deep learning · Medical image registration · Unsupervised learning · Cycle consistency

1 Introduction

Radiologists often diagnose the progress of disease by comparing medical images at different temporal phases. In case of diagnosis of liver tumor such as hepatocellular carcinoma (HCC), the contrast of normal liver tissue and tumor region in contrast enhanced CT (CECT) distinctly varies before and after the infection of contrast agent. This provides radiologists an important clue to diagnose cancers and plan surgery or radiation therapy [7]. However, liver images taken at different phases are usually different in their shape due to disease progress, breathing, patient motion, etc, so image registration is important to improve accuracy of dynamic studies.

Classical image registration methods [4,10] are usually implemented in a variational framework that solves an energy minimization problem over the space of deformations. Since the diffeomorphic image registration ensures the preservation of topology and one-to-one mapping between the source and target images, the algorithmic extensions to large deformation such as LDDMM [3] and

© Springer Nature Switzerland AG 2019
D. Shen et al. (Eds.): MICCAI 2019, LNCS 11769, pp. 166–174, 2019.
https://doi.org/10.1007/978-3-030-32226-7_19

SyN [1] have been applied to various image registration studies. However, these approaches usually require substantial time and extensive computation.

To address this issue, recent image registration techniques are often based on deep neural networks that instantaneously generate deformation fields. In supervised learning approaches [11], the ground-truths of deformation fields are required for training neural networks, which are typically generated by the traditional registration method. However, the performance of these existing supervised methods depends on the quality of the ground-truth registration fields, or they do not explicitly enforce the consistency criterion to uniquely describe the correspondences between two images.

In order to overcome the aforementioned limitations and provide topology-preserving guarantee, many unsupervised learning methods have been developed in these days. Balakrishnan et al. [2] propose 3D medical image registration algorithm using a spatial transform network. Zhang [12] presents a CNN framework that enforces an inverse-consistent constraint for the deformation fields. However, for the registration of large deformable volumes such as livers, the existing unsupervised learning methods often result in inaccurate registration due to the potential for the degeneracy of the mapping. Although Dalca et al. [5] tried to address this problem by incorporating a diffeomorphic integration layer, we found that its application of the liver registration is still limited.

In this paper, we present a novel unsupervised registration method using convolutional neural networks (CNN) with cycle-consistency [13]. We show that the cyclic constraint can be adopted for the image registration case naturally, and this cycle consistency improves topology preservation in generating fewer folding problems. Also, our network is trained with diverse source and target images in multiphase CECT acquisition so that a single neural network of our method provides deformable registration between every pairs once the network is trained. Experimental results demonstrate that the proposed method performs accurate 3D image registration for any pair of images within a few seconds in the challenging problem of 3D liver registration in multiphase CECT.

2   Proposed Method

The overall framework of our method is illustrated in Fig. 1. For the input images, A and B, in different phases, we define two registration networks as G_{AB} : $(A, B) \rightarrow \phi_{AB}$ and $G_{BA} : (B, A) \rightarrow \phi_{BA}$, where ϕ_{AB} (resp. ϕ_{BA}) denotes the 3-D deformation field from A to B (resp. B to A). We use a 3D spatial transformation layer T in the networks to warp the moving image by the estimated deformation field, so that the registration networks are trained to minimize the dissimilarity between the deformed moving source image and fixed target image. Accordingly, once a pair of images are given to the registration networks, the moving images are deformed into the fixed images.

To guarantee the topology preservation between the deformed and fixed images, we here adopt the cycle consistency constraint between the original moving image and its re-deformed image. That is, the deformed volumes are

168   B. Kim et al.

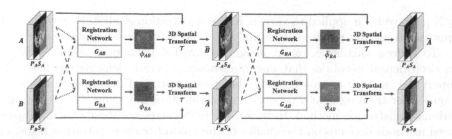

Fig. 1. The overall framework of the proposed method for image registration. The input images in different phases are denoted as A and B, and their phase and shape are denoted as P and S, respectively. The short-dashed line indicates the floating image and the long-dashed line denotes the fixed image.

given as the inputs to the networks again by switching their order to impose the cycle consistency. This constraint ensures that the shape of deformed images successively returns to the original shape.

2.1   Loss Function

We train the networks by solving the following loss function:

$$\mathcal{L} = \mathcal{L}_{regist}^{AB} + \mathcal{L}_{regist}^{BA} + \alpha \mathcal{L}_{cycle} + \beta \mathcal{L}_{identity}, \tag{1}$$

where $\mathcal{L}_{regist}$, $\mathcal{L}_{cycle}$, and $\mathcal{L}_{identity}$ are registration loss, cycle loss, and identity loss, respectively (see Fig. 2), and α and β are hyper-parameters. Based on this loss function, our method is trained in an unsupervised manner without ground-truth deformation fields.

Registration Loss. The registration loss function is based on the energy function of classical variational image registration. For example, the energy function for the registration of floating image A to the target volume B is composed of two terms:

$$\mathcal{L}_{regist}^{AB} = \mathcal{L}_{sim}\left(\mathcal{T}(A,\phi), B\right) + \mathcal{L}_{reg}(\phi), \tag{2}$$

where A is the moving image, and B is the fixed image. $\mathcal{L}_{sim}$ computes image dissimilarity between the deformed image by the estimated deformation field ϕ and the fixed image, and $\mathcal{L}_{reg}$ evaluates the smoothness of the deformation field. Here, $\mathcal{T}$ denotes the 3D spatial transformation function. In particular, we employ the cross-correlation as the similarity function to deal with the contrast change during CECT exam, and the L2-loss for regularization function. Accordingly, our registration loss function can be written as:

$$\mathcal{L}_{regist}^{AB} = -(\mathcal{T}(A,\phi_{AB}) \otimes B) + \lambda \|\phi_{AB}\|_2, \tag{3}$$

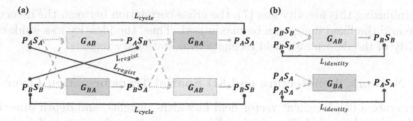

Fig. 2. The diagram of loss function structure in our proposed method. The short- and long-dashed lines are for floating image and fixed image, respectively.

where $\otimes$ denotes the cross-correlation defined by

$$x \otimes y = \frac{|\langle x - \bar{x}, y - \bar{y} \rangle|^2}{\|x - \bar{x}\|\|y - \bar{y}\|},$$ (4)

where $\bar{x}$ and $\bar{y}$ denote the mean value of x and y, respectively.

Cycle Loss. The cycle consistency condition is implemented by minimizing the loss function as shown in Fig. 2(a). Since an image A is first deformed to an image $\hat{B}$, which is then deformed again by the other network to generate image $\tilde{A}$, the cyclic consistency imposes $A \simeq \tilde{A}$. Similarly, an image B should be successively deformed by the two networks to generate image $\tilde{B}$. Then, the cyclic consistency is to impose that $B \simeq \tilde{B}$.

As shown in Fig. 2(a), since the network in our registration receives both the moving image and the fixed image, the implementation of the cycle consistency loss should be given by as the vector-form of the cycle consistency condition:

$$\begin{bmatrix} A \\ B \end{bmatrix} \simeq \begin{bmatrix} \mathcal{T}(\hat{B}, \hat{\phi}_{BA}) \\ \mathcal{T}(\hat{A}, \hat{\phi}_{AB}) \end{bmatrix} = \begin{bmatrix} \mathcal{T}\left(\mathcal{T}(A, \phi_{AB}), \hat{\phi}_{BA}\right) \\ \mathcal{T}\left(\mathcal{T}(B, \phi_{BA}), \hat{\phi}_{AB}\right) \end{bmatrix}$$ (5)

where $(\hat{B}, \hat{A}) := (\mathcal{T}(A, \phi_{AB}), \mathcal{T}(B, \phi_{BA}))$. Thus, the cycle loss is computed by:

$$\mathcal{L}_{cycle} = \left\| \begin{bmatrix} \mathcal{T}(\hat{B}, \hat{\phi}_{BA}) \\ \mathcal{T}(\hat{A}, \hat{\phi}_{AB}) \end{bmatrix} - \begin{bmatrix} A \\ B \end{bmatrix} \right\|_1,$$ (6)

where $\| \cdot \|_1$ denotes the l_1-norm.

Identity Loss. Another important consideration for the design of loss function is that the network should not change the stationary regions of the body, i.e. the stationary regions should be the fixed points of the network. As shown in Fig. 2(b), this constraint can be implemented by imposing that the input image should not be changed when the identical images are used as the floating and reference volumes. More specifically, we use the following identity loss:

$$\mathcal{L}_{identity} = -(\mathcal{T}(A, G_{AB}(A, A)) \otimes A) - (\mathcal{T}(B, G_{BA}(B, B)) \otimes B).$$ (7)

By minimizing this identity loss (7), the cross-correlation between the deformed image and the fixed image can be maximized. Thus, the identity loss guides the stability of the deformable field estimation in stationary regions.

2.2 Network Architecture and 3D Spatial Transformation Layer

To generate a displacement vector field in width-, height-, and depth direction, we adopt VoxelMorph-1 [2] as our baseline network. Note that our model without both the cycle and identity loss is equivalent to VoxelMorph-1. This 3D network consists of encoder, decoder and their skip connections similar to U-Net [9].

The 3D spatial transformation layer [6] is to deform the moving volume with the deformation field ϕ. We use the spatial transformation function $\mathcal{T}$ with trilinear interpolation for warping the image A by ϕ, which can be written as:

$$\mathcal{T}(A, \phi) = \sum_{y \in \mathcal{N}(x + \phi(x))} A(y) \prod_{d \in \{i,j,k\}} (1 - |x_d + \phi(x_d) - y_d|), \qquad (8)$$

where x indicates the voxel index, $\mathcal{N}(x + \phi(x))$ denotes the 8-voxel cubic neighborhood around $x + \phi(x)$, and d is three directions in 3D image space.

3 Experiments

To verify the performance of our method, we conducted liver registration from multiphase CT images. The dataset was collected from liver cancer (HCC) patients at Asan Medical Center, Seoul, South Korea. Each scans has pathologically proven hepatic nodules and four-phase liver CT (unenhanced, arterial, portal, and 180-s delayed phases). The slice thickness was 5 mm. We did not perform pre-processing such as affine transformation except for matching the number of slices for the moving and fixed images. Here, we extracted slices only including liver by a pre-trained liver segmentation network and performed zero-padding to the above and below volumes based on the center of mass of liver.

We used 555 scans for training and 50 scans for testing. For the network training, we stacked two volumes with different phases as the input. We normalized the input intensity with the maximum value of each volume. Also, we randomly down-sampled the training data from $512 \times 512 \times depth$ to $128 \times 128 \times depth$ to fit in the GPU memory, while we evaluated the test data with original size of $512 \times 512 \times depth$, where $depth$ is different for each pair of input. For data augmentation, we adopted random horizontal/vertical flipping and rotation with 90° for each pair of training volume. Our proposed method was implemented with pyTorch library. We applied Adam with momentum optimization algorithm to train the models with a learning rate of 0.0001, and set the batch size 1. The model was trained for 50 epochs using a NVIDIA GeForce GTX 1080 Ti GPU.

3.1 Registration Results

We evaluated the registration performance using the target registration error (TRE) based on the 20 anatomical points in the liver and adjacent organs at the portal phases, which are marked by radiologists. Also, we measured the tumor size that verifies the registration performance in the view point of tumor diagnosis. We compared our method to Elastix [8] that is known to have its state-of-the-art performance among the classical approaches. We also compared with VoxelMorph-1 [2]. Additionally, we performed ablation studies by excluding the cycle loss or identity loss. Apart from the loss, different ablated networks were subjected to the same training procedure for fair comparison.

Figure 3 shows the registration performance. We visualize the TRE values of the deformed arterial and delayed images with respect to each test data, and also show the average TRE values of all subjects with respect to the deformed arterial and delayed images into the fixed portal image. We can observe that the proposed method achieves significant improvement compared to VoxelMorph-1, while the error of the proposed method is slightly higher than Elastix. Also, in Table 1, we can confirm that the tumor size of deformed images from our proposed method is the most accurate for the case of delay to portal registration, and comparable in arterial to portal registration.

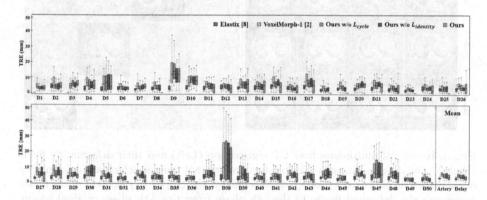

Fig. 3. Results of the target registration errors (TRE) of all 20 anatomical points in the deformed arterial and delayed images of 50 test data. Mean graph represents the mean TRE of the points for all subjects. D# in the x-axis indicates the patient number.

Table 1. Tumor size differences, TRE values (mm) between the deformed arterial/delayed images and the fixed portal image, and their average time (min) to be deformed on test set.

Method	Arterial → Portal				Delayed → Portal			
	Tumor size		TRE	Time	Tumor size		TRE	Time
	Major	Minor			Major	Minor		
Elastix [8]	0.98	**0.61**	**3.26**	19.64	0.91	0.58	**2.96**	19.64
VoxelMorph [2]	**0.79**	1.64	6.67	0.18	0.61	0.87	5.35	0.20
Ours	0.89	1.16	4.91	0.22	**0.59**	**0.43**	3.76	0.20

Table 2. Percentage of voxels with a non-positive Jacobian determinant and normalized mean square error (NMSE) on test set.

Method	Arterial → Portal		Delayed → Portal	
	% of $\det(J_\phi) \leq 0$	NMSE	% of $\det(J_\phi) \leq 0$	NMSE
VoxelMorph [2]	0.0327	0.0278	0.0311	0.0213
Ours w/o $\mathcal{L}_{cycle}$	0.0270	0.0279	0.0284	0.0214
Ours w/o $\mathcal{L}_{identity}$	0.0218	0.0279	0.0205	0.0208
Ours	**0.0175**	**0.0277**	**0.0181**	**0.0199**

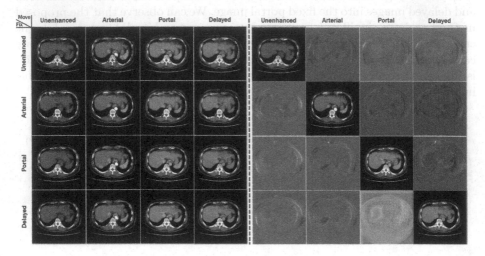

Fig. 4. Results of multiphase liver CT registration (Left) and their deformation fields (Right). The diagonal images with red-box are original images, which are deformed to other phases as indicated by each row. Specifically, the $(i, j), i \neq j$ element of the figure represents the deformed image to the i-th phase from the j-th phase original image. (Color figure online)

To demonstrate the effect of the cycle consistency, we also computed the percentage of voxels with a non-positive Jacobian determinant on the deformation fields and the normalized mean square error (NMSE) between the original moving image and re-deformed image. As shown in Table 2, we confirm that the proposed method is less prone to folding problem and improves topological preservation for liver registration.

Figure 4 illustrates an example of registration results that deforms the multiphase 3D images with the four distinct phases. Moreover, we calculated the time required for the proposed method to deform one image into the fixed image (see Table 1). Specifically, the conventional Elastix takes approximately 19.6 min for the image registration, while the proposed method takes only 10 s.

4   Conclusion

We presented an unsupervised image registration method using a cycle consistent convolutional neural network. Using two registration networks, our proposed method is trained to satisfy the cycle consistency that imposes inverse consistency between a pair of images. However, once the networks are trained, a single network can provide accurate 3D image registration with any pair of new data, so the computational complexity is same as VoxelMorph-1. Our liver registration results demonstrated that the proposed method works well for any image pairs with different contrast.

Acknowledgements. This work was supported by the Industrial Strategic technology development program (10072064, Development of Novel Artificial Intelligence Technologies To Assist Imaging Diagnosis of Pulmonary, Hepatic, and Cardiac Diseases and Their Integration into Commercial Clinical PACS Platforms) funded by the Ministry of Trade Industry and Energy (MI, Korea).

References

1. Avants, B.B., Epstein, C.L., Grossman, M., Gee, J.C.: Symmetric diffeomorphic image registration with cross-correlation: evaluating automated labeling of elderly and neurodegenerative brain. Med. Image Anal. **12**(1), 26–41 (2008)
2. Balakrishnan, G., Zhao, A., Sabuncu, M.R., Guttag, J., Dalca, A.V.: An unsupervised learning model for deformable medical image registration. In: Proceedings of the IEEE Conference on Computer Vision and Pattern Recognition, pp. 9252–9260 (2018)
3. Beg, M.F., Miller, M.I., Trouvé, A., Younes, L.: Computing large deformation metric mappings via geodesic flows of diffeomorphisms. Int. J. Comput. Vis. **61**(2), 139–157 (2005)
4. Christensen, G.E., Johnson, H.J.: Consistent image registration. IEEE Trans. Med. Imaging **20**(7), 568–582 (2001)
5. Dalca, A.V., Balakrishnan, G., Guttag, J., Sabuncu, M.R.: Unsupervised learning for fast probabilistic diffeomorphic registration. In: Frangi, A.F., Schnabel, J.A., Davatzikos, C., Alberola-López, C., Fichtinger, G. (eds.) MICCAI 2018. LNCS, vol. 11070, pp. 729–738. Springer, Cham (2018). https://doi.org/10.1007/978-3-030-00928-1_82
6. Jaderberg, M., Simonyan, K., Zisserman, A., et al.: Spatial transformer networks. In: Advances in Neural Information Processing Systems, pp. 2017–2025 (2015)
7. Kim, K.W., Lee, J.M., Choi, B.I.: Assessment of the treatment response of HCC. Abdom. Imaging **36**(3), 300–314 (2011)
8. Klein, S., Staring, M., Murphy, K., Viergever, M.A., Pluim, J.P.: Elastix: a toolbox for intensity-based medical image registration. IEEE Trans. Med. Imaging **29**(1), 196–205 (2010)
9. Ronneberger, O., Fischer, P., Brox, T.: U-Net: convolutional networks for biomedical image segmentation. In: Navab, N., Hornegger, J., Wells, W.M., Frangi, A.F. (eds.) MICCAI 2015. LNCS, vol. 9351, pp. 234–241. Springer, Cham (2015). https://doi.org/10.1007/978-3-319-24574-4_28
10. Thirion, J.P.: Image matching as a diffusion process: an analogy with Maxwell's demons. Med. Image Anal. **2**(3), 243–260 (1998)

11. Yang, X., Kwitt, R., Styner, M., Niethammer, M.: Quicksilver: fast predictive image registration-a deep learning approach. NeuroImage **158**, 378–396 (2017)
12. Zhang, J.: Inverse-consistent deep networks for unsupervised deformable image registration. arXiv preprint arXiv:1809.03443 (2018)
13. Zhu, J.Y., Park, T., Isola, P., Efros, A.A.: Unpaired image-to-image translation using cycle-consistent adversarial networks. In: Proceedings of the IEEE International Conference on Computer Vision, pp. 2223–2232 (2017)

Volumetric Attention for 3D Medical Image Segmentation and Detection

Xudong Wang[1,2(✉)], Shizhong Han[1], Yunqiang Chen[1], Dashan Gao[1],
and Nuno Vasconcelos[2]

[1] 12 Sigma Technologies, San Diego, USA
{Shan,yunqiang,dgao}@12sigma.ai
[2] Department of Electrical and Computer Engineering, University of California,
San Diego, USA
{xuw080,nuno}@ucsd.edu

Abstract. A volumetric attention (VA) module for 3D medical image segmentation and detection is proposed. VA attention is inspired by recent advances in video processing, enables 2.5D networks to leverage context information along the z direction, and allows the use of pre-trained 2D detection models when training data is limited, as is often the case for medical applications. Its integration in the Mask R-CNN is shown to enable state-of-the-art performance on the Liver Tumor Segmentation (LiTS) Challenge, outperforming the previous challenge winner by 3.9 points and achieving top performance on the LiTS leader board at the time of paper submission. Detection experiments on the DeepLesion dataset also show that the addition of VA to existing object detectors enables a 69.1 sensitivity at 0.5 false positive per image, outperforming the best published results by 6.6 points.

Keywords: Volumetric Attention · 3D images · LiTS · DeepLesion

1 Introduction

A natural solution to 3D medical image segmentation and detection problems is to rely on 3D convolutional networks, such as the 3D U-Net of [5] or the extended 2D U-Net of [15]. However, current GPU memory limitations prevent the processing of 3D volumes with high resolution. This is problematic, because the use of low-resolution volumes leads to low precision or miss-detection of small lesions and tumors and blur in lesion mask predictions, especially on boundaries. Hence, there is a need to trade-off the spatial resolution of each 2D slice for the number of slices processed. This implies a trade-off between the precision with which segmentation or detection can be performed and the amount of contextual information, in the z direction, that can be leveraged. A popular solution is to

---

X. Wang—This work was fully conducted during the internship in 12 Sigma Technologies, USA.

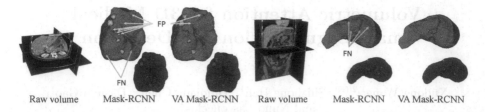

Raw volume   Mask-RCNN   VA Mask-RCNN   Raw volume   Mask-RCNN   VA Mask-RCNN

Fig. 1. Comparison of 3D segmentations by the Mask-RCNN and the proposed VA Mask-RCNN on the LiTS `val` set. Red denotes segmented liver, green segmented lesions. 3D ground truth is shown on the bottom right, with liver in dark red and lesions in dark green. Left: while the Mask-RCNN misses two lesions (false negative, FN) and has six false positive (FP) instances, the VA Mask-RCNN detects all lesions with only two FPs. Right: VA Mask RCNN detects 5 very small lesions, 4 of which are missed by the Mask-RCNN. These examples illustrate how the VA module *both* enhances small lesion prediction and enables the network to avoid false positives. (best viewed in color) (Color figure online)

a use a 2D network to segment or detect the structures of interest in 2D or 2.5D slices and then concatenate the results to build a 3D segmentation mask or bounding box.

Christ et al. proposed a 2D U-Net for liver and tumor segmentation, followed by a conditional random field for segmentation refinement [4]. Li et al. proposed a hybrid Dense 2D/3D UNet of three-stages [13]. They found that a pre-trained 2D model can significantly boost performance of their network. Han proposed a 2.5D (adjacent slices) residual U-Net for liver lesion segmentation [9]. These approaches are limited by the lack of contextual information. Since even human experts need to inspect multiple slices to reach confident assessments of confusing lesions, this is likely to upper bound their performance. To address this problem, Yan et al. [18] proposed a 3D context enhanced region-based CNN. However, their method is based on a region proposal network (RPN) and cannot be implemented as a single-stage detector, such as SSD and YOLO, or a segmentation network, such as U-Net, without an RPN component. Furthermore, because only the feature map derived from a central image is processed by the RPN to generate proposals, the proposal generation process has no access to 3D context. Given that missed proposals can not be recovered, this places an upper bound on detection performance.

In this work, we propose to address these limitations with ideas inspired by recent video processing work, where a similar problem is posed by the need to trade off the modeling of long-range dependencies between video frames and the spatial resolution of each frame. The proposed approach is inspired by [17], which added a non-local network to a 3D convolutional network (C3D/I3D) for video classification, using a spacetime dependency/attention mechanism. We generalize this method into a flexible and computationally efficient Volumetric Attention (VA) module, which sequentially infers 3D enhanced attention maps along two separate dimensions, channel and spatial. The attention maps produced by this module are multiplied by the input feature map to enable adaptive feature

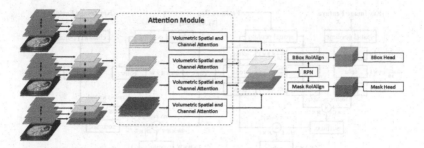

Fig. 2. Architecture of the Volumetric Attention (VA) Mask-RCNN. Three continuous 2.5D images, each composed of 3 adjacent slices, are shown as example.

refinement, using a 2D network. Similar to [12], global spatial pooling and global channel pooling are used to reduce computational cost.

The VA module has several interesting properties. First, it enables the processing of high spatial resolution images, while leveraging contextual information over multiple slices of the 3D CT volume. Second, it can be combined with any CNN architecture, including one-stage and two-stage detectors and segmentation networks. Third, it is computationally efficient, due to extensive use of spatial and channel pooling. Fourth, because the VA module can operate on image sub-regions, it can also benefit RPN networks. Fifth, since VA can be used with 2D networks, it can leverage pre-trained 2D CNN weights for transfer learning. The proposed VA attention module is implemented within the Mask-RCNN, leading to an architecture denoted the VA Mask-RCNN. As illustrated in Fig. 1, this not only reduces segmentation false positives, but also enables the retrieval of very small lesions that are missed by the Mask-RCNN model. The VA Mask-RCNN is shown to obtain state-of-the-art performance, 74.1 dice per case, on the LiTS liver tumor segmentation challenge **test** set, significantly outperforming (3.9 points) the winner of last year's challenge. It is the top method on the challenge leaderboard at the time of submission of this paper. To assess the generalization ability of the VA Mask-RCNN to 3D CT volumes, we have also performed experiments on the DeepLesion dataset. The VA Faster-RCNN achieved a sensitivity of 69.1 at 0.5 false positives (FPs)/image, outperforming the best published results by 6.6 points.

2   Volumetric Attention

The overall architecture of the VA Mask R-CNN is shown in Fig. 2. The VA attention module operates on the Mask R-CNN feature pyramids extracted from a *target* 2.5D image, where detection takes place, and neighboring *contextual* 2.5D images. The 2.5D images are each composed of 3 adjacent slices. The attention module has three components: bag of long-range features, volumetric channel attention, and volumetric spatial attention. Unlike the self-attentive feature map of [17], VA uses long-range features from neighboring slices, which are combined with the feature map of the target slice to generate spatial and channel attention

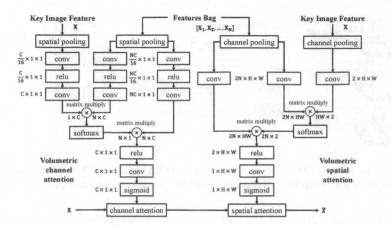

Fig. 3. Volumetric spatial and channel attention module. N is the bag size, C, H, W the feature map channel size, height and width, respectively. Spatial and channel pooling are used to reduce computation.

responses. A detailed scheme of the attention module is given in Fig. 3. We next discuss the three components combined with Mask-RCNN in detail.

2.1 Bag of Long-Range Features

To account for dependencies along the z direction of the 3D CT volume, the VA Mask R-CNN complements the target 2.5D image, with neighboring images, both above and below the target image. These are denoted as contextual images. The features extracted from these images are concatenated for each level of the spatial pyramid, according to

$$\mathbf{X}_{long}^i = [\mathbf{X}_1, \mathbf{X}_2, ..., \mathbf{X}_N] \in \mathbb{R}^{N \times C^i \times H^i \times W^i}, \tag{1}$$

where i is the pyramid level, $C^i \times H^i \times W^i$ its dimensions (chanel, height, and width, respectively), $\mathbf{X}_{long}^i$ the corresponding bag of long-range features, and N the number of contextual images. The features $\mathbf{X}_k$ are sorted by the order of the corresponding images along the z direction of the 3D volume.

2.2 Volumetric Channel Attention

This attention mechanism is inspired by that of [12,17]. The bag of features $\mathbf{X}_{long} \in \mathbb{R}^{N \times C \times H \times W}$ and corresponding target image feature map $\mathbf{X}_{tgt} \in \mathbb{R}^{C \times H \times W}$ are each subject to a global average pooling operator $\mathbf{F}_{avg}^c$. Following [12], computation is reduced by replacing the linear embedding layer of the original non-local blocks of [17] by two 1×1 convolutional layers with reduction ratio of 16. This is implemented as $\mathbf{F}_{emb}^c(\mathbf{X}) = W_2 \delta(W_1 \mathbf{F}_{avg}^c(\mathbf{X}))$, where $W_1 \in \mathbb{R}^{\frac{C}{16} \times C}$, $W_2 \in \mathbb{R}^{C \times \frac{C}{16}}$ and δ is the RELU function. The slices attention signal is finally computed with a softmax

$$\mathbf{S}_{att}^c = \text{softmax}(\mathbf{F}_{emb}^c(\mathbf{X}_{tgt}) \cdot \mathbf{F}_{emb}^c(\mathbf{X}_{long})) \in \mathbb{R}^{1 \times N} \qquad (2)$$

along dimension N, where $\mathbf{F}_{emb}^c(\mathbf{X}_{tgt}) \in \mathbb{R}^{1 \times C}$, $\mathbf{F}_{emb}^c(\mathbf{X}_{long}) \in \mathbb{R}^{C \times N}$ and $\cdot$ refers to matrix multiplication. The slice attention signal $\mathbf{S}_{att}^c$ is then applied to $\mathbf{F}_{emb}^c(\mathbf{X}_{long}) \in \mathbb{R}^{N \times C}$ according to $\mathbf{S}_{att}^c \cdot \mathbf{F}_{emb}^c(\mathbf{X}_{long})$ and this is followed by a relu layer, a 1×1 conv layer and a sigmoid layer, to learn a nonlinear interaction $\mathbf{S}_c \in \mathbb{R}^{C \times 1 \times 1}$ between channels. Then channel-wise multiplication is applied on $\mathbf{X}_{tgt} \in \mathbb{R}^{C \times H \times W}$.

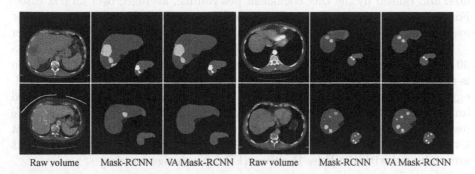

Raw volume   Mask-RCNN   VA Mask-RCNN   Raw volume   Mask-RCNN   VA Mask-RCNN

Fig. 4. 2D visualization of segmentations by Mask-RCNN and VA Mask R-CNN on LiTS **val** set. Segmented liver is shown in red and lesions in green. Zoomed out ground truth masks are shown on bottom right, with liver in gray and lesions in white. The VA Mask-RCNN produces smoother segmentation boundaries and lower FP and miss rates. In the top left, the gallbladder area is easily confused with the lesion area. VA Mask-RCNN leverages contextual slices to remove this FP. (Best viewed in color and zoom in for details) (Color figure online)

2.3   Volumetric Spatial Attention

The volumetric spatial attention module uses max and average pooling to shrink feature maps along the channel dimension, concatenating them into two channel feature maps $\mathbf{F}_{pool}^s(\mathbf{X}) = [\mathbf{F}_{max}^s(\mathbf{X}), \mathbf{F}_{avg}^s(\mathbf{X})] \in \mathbb{R}^{2 \times H \times W}$. An embedding function is then implemented as $\mathbf{F}_{emb}^s(\mathbf{X}) = W\mathbf{F}_{pool}^s(\mathbf{X})$, where W is a learned convolutional weight layer. The slice attention signal is finally computed with a softmax

$$\mathbf{S}_{att}^s = \text{softmax}(\mathbf{F}_{emb}^s(\mathbf{X}_{tgt}) \cdot \mathbf{F}_{emb}^s(\mathbf{X}_{long})) \in \mathbb{R}^{1 \times N} \qquad (3)$$

along dimension N. A spatial attention map $S_s \in \mathbb{R}^{1 \times H \times W}$ is then generated with an architecture similar to that of Sect. 2.2 and element-wise multiplied with $\mathbf{X}_{tgt}$.

3   Experiments

The volumetric attention was evaluated on two public datasets, Liver Tumor Segmentation (LiTS) [1] and DeepLesion [19]. All experiments used a PyTorch implementation [2] of the Mask-RCNN and Faster R-CNN. Unless otherwise noted, all hyperparameters are as in [14] for the Faster-RCNN and [10] for the Mask-RCNN.

3.1 Datasets and Evaluation

LiTS is a dataset of liver lesions, including 131 training and 70 test CT scans, acquired in six different clinical sites. Lesion segmentation performance is evaluated and ranked by the Dice coefficient per volume, averaged over all test cases. For additional insight on the quality of the segmentation, we also break down the average Dice/lesion per lesion size: the coefficients measured for small (diameter $< 15\,mm$), medium (diameter between [$15\,mm$, $30\,mm$] and large (diameter $> 30\,mm$) legions are denoted as $Dice_s$, $Dice_m$ and $Dice_l$ respectively. DeepLesion is a dataset with a larger variety of lesions, including 33,688 bookmarked radiology images from 10,825 studies of 4,477 unique patients. For each bookmarked image, a bounding box is generated to indicate the location of each lesion. We use the official split (70% training, 15% validation and 15% test) at the patient level, for training and testing. For consistency with prior art, detection results are evaluated with the False Positives (FPs) per Image metric.

3.2 LiTS Experiments

Pre-processing: For 3D liver/lesion detection and segmentation, we stack three adjacent axial slices into a 3-channel image and apply the Mask-RCNN to detect and segment the liver/lesion for the center slice. 3D segmentation results are then obtained by stacking the masks generated for all slices. The Mask-RCNN is trained to detect both liver and lesions, to enable the removal of false lesions outside the liver by simply computing the logical AND of the predicted liver and lesion masks. Since the focus of this task is on the liver and lesions, the CT scan's Hounsfield unit (HU) is clamped between $[-200, 300]$ and normalized to a floating point between $[0, 1]$. Each slice is scaled to 1024×1024 pixels and the slice-thickness resampled to $1.5\,mm$.

Benchmark Results: To evaluate performance on LiTS, the feature bag size of (1) was set to 9, the weights of the feature extractor and RPN copied from detectors pretrained on the MS-COCO and DeepLesion datasets, and the smallest image scale set to 1024. Table 1 presents a copy of the LiTS leaderboard, at the

Table 1. Comparison with LiTS challenge leaderboard, as of July 1st, 2019

Team	Model	Dice per case
3D U-Net (Ours) [5]	3D U-Net	55.0
Chlebus [3]	2D U-Net	65.0
Vorontsov et al. [16]	2D + 3D FCN	65.0
Yuan [20]	Deconv-Conv Net	65.7
Han [9]	2D U-Net	67.0
LeHealth	-	70.2
Mask-RCNN (Ours) [10]	Mask-RCNN	70.3
Li et al. [13]	H-DenseUNet	72.2
Volumetric Attention	VA Mask-RCNN	**74.1**

time of submission of this paper. All algorithms are evaluated on the LiTS test set. The VA Mask R-CNN achieves state-of-the-art performance, with 74.10 dice per case. This outperforms the previous LiTS challenge winner by 3.9 points and the best published results by 1.9 points.

Ablation Study and Evaluation: To better understand the proposed architecture, the LiTS dataset was split, using 75% of the train data to create a training set and the remaining 25% as a val set for a local ablation study. Table 2 summarizes the resulting dice per volume, averaged over all cases, and dice per cases, averaged over small, medium and large lesions. All these are control experiments, all hyper-parameters and settings remaining the same as in the benchmark experiments, unless otherwise noted.

Benefits of VA Attention: Three conclusions can be drawn from Table 2a. First, the 2D approaches outperform the 3D U-Net, even before addition of the VA attention module. This shows that 2D networks are at least competitive for 3D mask segmentation. Since the Mask-RCNN achieved the best performance on these experiments, we use it as base model in the remainder of the paper. It should, however, be pointed out that VA could equally be combined with the 2D U-Net. Second, the addition of the VA module further increases performance, increasing the Dice coefficient per case by 4.1 points. Third, this gain is especially large for small lesions. Note how the lack of contextual information along the z direction severely compromises the small lesion performance of the mask R-CNN. Figure 4 illustrates how VA attention enables the Mask R-CNN to reject confusing FP lesions and produce smoother segment boundaries.

Table 2. Evaluation on LiTS val set, in terms of dice per volume, averaged over all cases, and dice per lesions, averaged over small, medium and large lesions.

	Dice	Dice_s	Dice_m	Dice_l
3D U-Net	35.3	17.0	39.2	61.3
2D U-Net	48.8	39.7	58.2	68.3
Mask-RCNN	56.7	44.3	70.6	78.4
Ours	**60.8**	**52.2**	**71.4**	**78.7**

(a) Dice comparison.

Pre-training dataset				Dice per case	Dice	Dice_s	Dice_l
+ImageNet	✓	✓	✓				
+MS-COCO		✓	✓				
+DeepLesion			✓				
				Dice per case	60.8	61.9	**63.3**

(b) Pre-training dataset.

Scale	Dice	Dice_s	Dice_m	Dice_l
512	50.2	35.8	65.1	77.9
800	61.1	52.1	71.6	79.3
1024	**63.3**	54.3	**73.7**	80.3
1333	**63.5**	**54.8**	73.5	**80.4**

(c) Influence of image scales.

	Dice	Dice_s	Dice_m	Dice_l
Baseline	56.7	44.3	70.6	78.4
+channel att	61.5	52.2	72.7	78.7
+spatial att	**63.3**	**54.3**	**73.7**	**80.3**

(d) Influence of VA modules.

	Dice	Dice_s	Dice_m	Dice_l
Baseline	56.7	44.3	70.6	78.4
RPN	**63.3**	**54.3**	**73.7**	**80.3**
RCNN	61.3	51.7	71.8	79.9

(e) Influence of VA location.

# Slices	Dice	Dice_s	Dice_m	Dice_l
9(3 × 3)	61.7	52.2	71.6	79.5
21(3 × 7)	62.5	52.6	72.2	79.8
27(3 × 9)	**63.3**	**54.3**	**73.7**	80.3
33(3 × 11)	63.1	53.6	73.4	**80.6**

(f) Influence of number of slices.

Influence of Pre-training: [11] claims that ImageNet pre-training does not improve accuracy of networks trained with as few as 10k COCO images. As shown in Table 2b, this does not hold for medical imaging where, due to the difficulties of collecting and labeling datasets, few datasets have 10k examples. Furthermore, while MS-COCO has ∼5 objects/image, this number is much smaller for medical image datasets. For LiTS the number is smaller than 1, especially when the 3D volume is split into 2D slices and these are considered different examples. Table 2b shows that, in this case, ImageNet pre-training still has an important role in combating overfitting. Adding MS-COCO to the pre-training dataset further improves performance by 1.1 points. This is mostly because the COCO tasks encourage the network to more accurately localize objects. Finally, due to the non-trivial domain shift between MS-COCO and LiTS, further pre-training on DeepLesion improves performance by an additional 1.4 points.

Image Scales: Table 2c shows that larger image scales lead to better performance, especially for small lesions. However, performance saturates at a scale of 1333 pixels. This is only marginally better than a scale of 1024 but requires substantially more memory. For this reason, a scale of 1024 is adopted in the remainder of the paper.

Spatial vs. Channel Attention: To compare the relative importance of the two attention mechanisms, the two modules were incrementally added to the 2D Mask-RCNN, with the results of Table 2d. These experiments use 9 slices. The addition of channel attention enhances performance by more than 4 points, and the subsequent addition of spatial attention increases performance by another 1.8 points. In summary, both attention mechanisms are important.

Location of Attention Module: The VA module can be added as shown in Fig. 2, i.e. to the last stage of feature extraction, before the RPN, or after the bounding box ROI align and mask ROI align steps, i.e. before the RCNN. Table 2e shows that attention is more effective if introduced before the RPN. While this improves performance by 6.6 Dice points per case, the gain is only 4.6 points when attention is introduced after the RCNN. This shows that 3D context is important for high quality proposal generation. Since only RPN detected ROIs are used to crop feature maps, addition of attention after the RPN only improves the ability to reject FPs. In this case, attention cannot improve the retrieval of lesions that are otherwise missed.

Feature Bags Size: Table 2f compares the network performance as the feature bag size. While dice per case increases with feature bag size, the small and medium lesion performance starts to worsen beyond a bag size of 9. We note that for applications sensitive to inference time, smaller bag size may be preferable.

3.3 Extension Experiments on DeepLesion

To test the effectiveness of volumetric attention for the processing of 3D CT volume datasets, we performed some extension experiments on DeepLesion. This dataset enables the use of part of the 3D CT volume as context for 2D bounding box prediction on target slices. Since DeepLesion does not provide mask groundtruth, the VA module was implemented on Faster-RCNN-FPN and Deformable Faster-RCNN-FPN detectors, with ResNet50 backbones. As usual for DeepLesion, performance is evaluated with FPs per image. AP_{50} is also presented in Table 4. All experiments in this section are based on training with the

Table 3. Sensitivity (%) at 0.5, 1 and 2 FPs per image on the DeepLesion **test** set.

Model	Backbone	0.5	1	2
Faster-RCNN [8]	VGG-16	56.9	67.3	75.6
R-FCN [6]	VGG-16	55.7	67.3	75.4
Improved R-FCN [6]	VGG-16	56.5	67.7	76.9
Data-level fusion, 11 slices	VGG-16	58.5	70.0	77.9
3-DCE, 9 Slices [18]	VGG-16	59.3	70.7	79.1
3-DCE, 27 Slices [18]	VGG-16	62.5	73.4	80.7
Faster-RCNN+VA, 9 Slices	ResNet50	**67.6**	**75.6**	**82.5**
Deformable Faster-RCNN+VA	ResNet50	**69.1**	**77.9**	**83.8**

Table 4. Sensitivity (%) at 1 FPs/ image and AP_{50} on the DeepLesion **test** set.

Model	Backbone	1 FPs	AP_{50}
Faster-RCNN [8]	ResNet152	77.4	64.9
Faster-RCNN [8]	ResNet101	75.1	61.8
Faster-RCNN [8]	ResNet50	73.4	60.0
Deformable Faster-RCNN [7]	ResNet50	76.3	62.4
Faster-RCNN+VA	ResNet50	75.6	63.0
Deformable Faster-RCNN+VCA	ResNet50	76.8	63.8
Deformable Faster-RCNN+VSA	ResNet50	76.9	64.1
Deformable Faster-RCNN+VA	ResNet50	**77.9**	**65.0**

DeepLesion **train** and **val** sets, and testing on **test** set. Each 2.5D image is formed by concatenating 3 contiguous slices and scaled to 512×512 pixels as in [19], the Faster-RCNN-FPN backbone is pretrained on ImageNet. Feature bag size is fixed to be 3, i.e. 9 slices.

Tables 3 and 4, compare the proposed networks to several methods from the literature. The proposed networks achieve state of the art results, increasing sensitivity by 6.6 points at 0.5 FPs/image, 4.4 points at 1 Fp/image and 3.1 at 2 FPs/image. Table 4, shows that the proposed network with the ResNet50 backbone is comparable with the heavier Faster-RCNN with ResNet101 backbone. Independently adding Volumetric Channel Attention (VCA) and Volumetric Spatial Attention (VSA) to Deformable Faster-RCNN with ResNet50 can get 1.4 and 1.6 points performance increase separately, integrating VSA and VCA got 2.6 points performance improvement, this result is even slightly higher than much heavier Faster-RCNN with ResNet152 backbone.

4 Conclusion

In this paper, we proposed a volumetric attention module that enables 2.5D methods to leverage contextual information along the z direction and the use of pretrained 2D detection models when training data is limited, as is often the case for medical applications. VA can be combined with any CNN architecture, including one-stage and two-stage detectors and segmentation networks. It was shown that 2.5D networks with VA achieve state of the art results for *both* lesion segmentation and detection.

References

1. Bilic, P., et al.: The liver tumor segmentation benchmark (LITS). arXiv:1901.04056 (2019)
2. Chen, K., et al.: MMDetection (2018). https://github.com/open-mmlab/mmdetection
3. Chlebus, G., et al.: Neural network-based automatic liver tumor segmentation with random forest-based candidate filtering. arXiv:1706.00842 (2017)
4. Christ, P.F., et al.: Automatic liver and lesion segmentation in CT using cascaded fully convolutional neural networks and 3D conditional random fields. In: Ourselin, S., Joskowicz, L., Sabuncu, M.R., Unal, G., Wells, W. (eds.) MICCAI 2016. LNCS, vol. 9901, pp. 415–423. Springer, Cham (2016). https://doi.org/10.1007/978-3-319-46723-8_48
5. Çiçek, Ö., Abdulkadir, A., Lienkamp, S.S., Brox, T., Ronneberger, O.: 3D U-Net: learning dense volumetric segmentation from sparse annotation. In: Ourselin, S., Joskowicz, L., Sabuncu, M.R., Unal, G., Wells, W. (eds.) MICCAI 2016. LNCS, vol. 9901, pp. 424–432. Springer, Cham (2016). https://doi.org/10.1007/978-3-319-46723-8_49
6. Dai, J., et al.: R-FCN: object detection via region-based fully convolutional networks. In: NIPS (2016)
7. Dai, J., et al.: Deformable convolutional networks. In: ICCV (2017)
8. Girshick, R., et al.: Fast R-CNN. In: ICCV (2015)
9. Han, X.: Automatic liver lesion segmentation using a deep convolutional neural network method. arXiv:1704.07239 (2017)
10. He, K., et al.: Mask R-CNN. In: ICCV (2017)
11. He, K., et al.: Rethinking imagenet pre-training. arXiv:1811.08883 (2018)
12. Hu, J., et al.: Squeeze-and-excitation networks. In: CVPR (2018)
13. Li, X., et al.: H-DenseUNet: hybrid densely connected UNet for liver and tumor segmentation from CT volumes. IEEE Trans. Med. Imaging 37(12), 2663–2674 (2018)
14. Lin, T.Y., et al.: Feature pyramid networks for object detection. In: CVPR (2017)
15. Ronneberger, O., Fischer, P., Brox, T.: U-Net: convolutional networks for biomedical image segmentation. In: Navab, N., Hornegger, J., Wells, W.M., Frangi, A.F. (eds.) MICCAI 2015. LNCS, vol. 9351, pp. 234–241. Springer, Cham (2015). https://doi.org/10.1007/978-3-319-24574-4_28
16. Vorontsov, E., et al.: Liver lesion segmentation informed by joint liver segmentation. In: ISBI (2018)
17. Wang, X., et al.: Non-local neural networks. In: CVPR (2018)
18. Yan, K., Bagheri, M., Summers, R.M.: 3D context enhanced region-based convolutional neural network for end-to-end lesion detection. In: Frangi, A.F., Schnabel, J.A., Davatzikos, C., Alberola-López, C., Fichtinger, G. (eds.) MICCAI 2018. LNCS, vol. 11070, pp. 511–519. Springer, Cham (2018). https://doi.org/10.1007/978-3-030-00928-1_58
19. Yan, K., et al.: DeepLesion: automated mining of large-scale lesion annotations and universal lesion detection with deep learning. J. Med. Imaging 5(3), 036501 (2018)
20. Yuan, Y.: Hierarchical convolutional-deconvolutional neural networks for automatic liver and tumor segmentation. arXiv:1710.04540 (2017)

Improving Deep Lesion Detection Using 3D Contextual and Spatial Attention

Qingyi Tao[1,2(✉)], Zongyuan Ge[1,3], Jianfei Cai[2], Jianxiong Yin[1], and Simon See[1]

[1] NVIDIA AI Technology Center, Santa Clara, USA
[2] Nanyang Technological University, Singapore, Singapore
qtao002@e.ntu.edu.sg
[3] Monash University, Melbourne, Australia

Abstract. Lesion detection from computed tomography (CT) scans is challenging compared to natural object detection because of two major reasons: small lesion size and small inter-class variation. Firstly, the lesions usually only occupy a small region in the CT image. The feature of such small region may not be able to provide sufficient information due to its limited spatial feature resolution. Secondly, in CT scans, the lesions are often indistinguishable from the background since the lesion and non-lesion areas may have very similar appearances. To tackle both problems, we need to enrich the feature representation and improve the feature discriminativeness. Therefore, we introduce a dual-attention mechanism to the 3D contextual lesion detection framework, including the cross-slice contextual attention to selectively aggregate the information from different slices through a soft re-sampling process. Moreover, we propose intra-slice spatial attention to focus the feature learning in the most prominent regions. Our method can be easily trained end-to-end without adding heavy overhead on the base detection network. We use DeepLesion dataset and train a universal lesion detector to detect all kinds of lesions such as liver tumors, lung nodules, and so on. The results show that our model can significantly boost the results of the baseline lesion detector (with 3D contextual information) but using much fewer slices.

1 Introduction

As one of the essential computer-aided detection/diagnosis (CADe/CADx) technologies, lesion detection has been studied by the medical imaging community for automatic disease screening and examination. With the great success of deep convolutional neural network (CNN) adoption in object detection in natural images [1,2], many researchers utilized CNN based algorithms for detecting diseases in different modalities of medical images such as lesion detection in color retinal images [3], disease detection in X-ray [4], etc.

Electronic supplementary material The online version of this chapter (https://doi.org/10.1007/978-3-030-32226-7_21) contains supplementary material, which is available to authorized users.

© Springer Nature Switzerland AG 2019
D. Shen et al. (Eds.): MICCAI 2019, LNCS 11769, pp. 185–193, 2019.
https://doi.org/10.1007/978-3-030-32226-7_21

Despite the progress, lesion detection in computed tomography (CT) images is challenging due to the difficulty of learning discriminative feature representation. The primary reasons accounting for such difficulty include: (1) the lesion size can be extremely small compared to natural objects in a general object detection task, and this degrades the richness in the existing feature representation; (2) the inter-class variance is small, i.e., lesions and non-lesions often have very similar appearances.

To enrich the lesion features, lesion detection methods in CT images often take advantage of the intrinsic 3D context information. The works in [5,6] exploit 3D CNNs to encode richer spatial and context information for more discriminative features. However, 3D CNN requires more computational resources and at the same time, it requires more efforts to annotate 3D bounding boxes. This motivates [7] to use $(2+1)$D information which aggregates 2D features from multiple consecutive CT slices. Particularly, in 3DCE [7], a set of consecutive slices are fed into a 2D detection network to generate feature maps separately, which are then aggregated along the channel dimension for the final detection task. Nevertheless, with the increasing number of neighbouring slices, the information extracted from some of the slices may be irrelevant whereas some of the slices may have higher importance for the correct prediction.

To solve this problem, we propose an attentive feature aggregation mechanism through a 3D contextual attention module to adaptively select important and relevant slices to be focused on. Moreover, to further improve the feature discrimintiveness for small regions in each CT slice, we introduce a similar spatial attention network as used in [8,9] to mine the discriminative regions and concentrate the learning on these regions in each feature map. The self-attentive feature maps could enhance the differentiation between lesion and non-lesion proposals.

2   Methods

Figure 1 gives an overview of the proposed lesion detection framework. In particular, we adopt an improved version of R-FCN [2] as the backbone object detection network which contains a region proposal network (RPN) to generate region proposals, followed by a position-sensitive pooling layer and two fully connected layers. The final classification branch distinguishes between lesion and non-lesion classes and the regression branch refines the bounding box coordinates for more accurate localization. To incorporate 3D context, we group $3M$ slices into M 3-channel images which include the key slice and $(3M-1)$ neighbouring slices before and after the key slice. Similar to [7], instead of performing data-level fusion, we adopt feature integration by forwarding M grouped images to the shared convolutional layers and then concatenating the features right before the position-sensitive ROI (PSROI) pooling layer. Finally, the lesion area is predicted with the aggregated features from all $3M$ slices. The loss functions including the lesion classification loss and the bounding-box regression loss in both RPN and the improved R-FCN are optimized jointly.

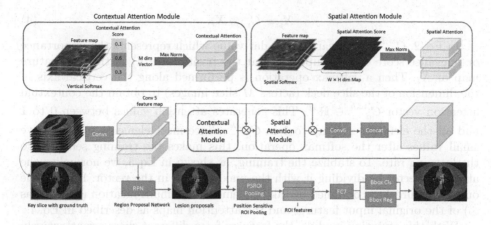

Fig. 1. Overview of network architecture: using 3DCE [7] as the base framework, we introduce two attention modules: (a) contextual attention module to re-weight the feature importance across all input slices; (b) spatial attention module to amplify the learning of the most prominent regions within each feature map.

The unique part of our framework lies in the introduced two attention modules: contextual attention module and spatial attention module, which are able to extract more important and discriminative features. In the following subsections, we describe our dual-attention mechanism including the contextual attention module to reweight the importance of contextual information, and the spatial attention module to focus on discriminative regions.

2.1 3D Contextual Attention Module

The 3D contextual attention module aims to selectively aggregate features from M input images by attending to the relevant context information among all neighbouring slices. We denote the input feature map ($relu\_5\_3$ for vgg 16) of input image i as $X_i \in \mathbb{R}^{(D \times W \times H)}$ ($i = [1, 2, ..M]$), where D is the number of feature channels, H and W is the height and width of the feature map. The contextual attention module contains a convolutional layer denoted as ϕ_C in Eq. 1. The contextual attention is calculated through a softmax function followed by a normalization operation.

$$C_i = \phi_C(X_i) \tag{1}$$

$$C_{i,d}^{'w,h} = \frac{exp(C_{i,d}^{w,h})}{\sum_{i=1}^{M} exp(C_{i,d}^{w,h})} \tag{2}$$

$$C_{i,d}^{''w,h} = \frac{C_{i,d}^{'w,h}}{\max_i |C_{i,d}^{'w,h}|} \tag{3}$$

$$X_i^{'} = C_i^{''} \otimes X_i. \tag{4}$$

In Eq. 2, $C_{i,d}^{w,h}$ is the learnable scalar value which represents the importance or relevance score of each input slice at the position (w, h) in the dth feature map of X_i. Then a softmax operation is performed along the vertical axis in the dimension of the slice deck (across M slice images) to obtain the contextual attention vector $C_d^{'w,h} \in \mathbb{R}^M$. This generates attention values between 0 to 1 and all the elements sum up to 1 in $C_d^{'w,h}$. Since most elements tend to have small values after the softmax operation, this makes the training sensitive to the learning rate. To stablize the training, as shown in Eq. 3, we normalize the attention vector by dividing it with the max element in the vector. Finally, the output feature $X_i^{'}$ is obtained by taking element-wise multiplication (denoted as $\otimes$) of the original input features and the attention maps as described in Eq. 4.

With this attention module, the features from different slices are attentively aggregated with a learnable cross-slice attention vector to amplify the relevant contextual features and suppress irrelevant ones.

2.2 Spatial Attention Module

Spatial attention module is designed to optimize the feature learning for prominent regions by applying intra-slice attention on each feature plane. Similar to the contextual attention module, it contains a convolution layer (ϕ_S) followed by a softmax function and a max normalization operation. As shown in Fig. 1, the spatial attention module takes refined features $X_i^{'}$ of all input images and generates spatial attention weight matrix for each feature map. The process can be mathematically written as:

$$S_i = \phi_S(X_i^{'}) \tag{5}$$

$$S_{i,d}^{'w,h} = \frac{exp(S_{i,d}^{w,h})}{\sum_{w=1}^{W} \sum_{h=1}^{H} exp(S_{i,d}^{w,h})} \tag{6}$$

$$S_{i,d}^{''w,h} = \frac{S_{i,d}^{'w,h}}{\max_{w,h} |S_{i,d}^{'w,h}|} \tag{7}$$

$$X_i^{''} = S_i^{''} \otimes X_i^{'}. \tag{8}$$

The spatial attention module generates attentive feature maps by amplifying prominent regions within each feature plane in order to improve the richness in features for small lesions and increase the feature discrepancy between lesion and non-lesion regions.

3   Experiments

Dataset: To validate the effectiveness of our approach, we use DeepLesion [10] dataset that provides 32,120 axial CT slices with 2D bounding box annotations of lesion regions. The CT images are pre-processed in the same way as that in 3DCE [7]. We use the official split of samples which includes ~22k samples for training, ~5k for validation and another ~5k for testing. Following the practice in [7], 35 noisy lesion annotations mentioned in the dataset are removed for training and testing.

Table 1. Sensitivity (%) at different false false positives (FPs) per image on the test set of the official data split of DeepLesion. Note that the results of 3DCE are obtained from our experiments which are higher than the reported results in the original paper.

Sensitivity @	0.5	1	2	4	8	16
Improved R-FCN, 3 Slices [7]	56.5	67.7	76.9	82.8	87.0	89.8
3DCE, 9 Slices [7]	61.7	71.9	79.2	84.3	87.8	89.7
3DCE, 15 Slices [7]	63.0	73.1	80.2	85.2	87.8	89.7
3DCE, 21 Slices [7]	63.2	73.4	80.9	85.6	88.4	90.2
3DCE_CS_Att, 9 Slices (Ours)	67.8	76.3	82.9	86.6	89.3	90.7
3DCE_CS_Att, 15 Slices (Ours)	70.8	78.6	83.9	87.5	89.9	**91.4**
3DCE_CS_Att, 21 Slices (Ours)	**71.4**	**78.5**	**84.0**	**87.6**	**90.2**	**91.4**

Table 2. Sensitivity (%) at 4 FPs per image on the test set of DeepLesion using the baseline model (3DCE) and the proposed model (3DCE_CS_Att), both using 15 slices.

	Lesion type								Lesion diameter			Slice interval	
	LU	ME	LV	ST	PV	AB	KD	BN	<10	10–30	>30	<2.5	>2.5
3DCE	90.9	88.1	90.4	73.5	82.1	81.3	82.1	**75.0**	80.9	87.8	82.9	85.8	85.1
3DCE_CS_Att	**92.0**	**88.5**	**91.4**	**80.3**	**85.0**	**84.4**	**84.3**	**75.0**	**82.3**	**90.0**	**85.0**	**87.6**	**87.6**

Network and Training: We initialize the network using pre-trained ImageNet vgg-16 model. In the proposed attention modules, we use a softmax with temperature of 3 for spatial attention and 2 for contextual attention. During the training, each mini-batch has 2 samples and each sample has M three-channel images. Stochastic gradient decent (SGD) with momentum of 0.9 and decay of $5e-5$ is used as the optimizer. We train 6 epochs using the base learning rate of 0.001, which is then reduced it by a factor of 10 after the 4th and 5th epochs.

Evaluation Metrics: Following the standard practice, we use intersection-over-union (IoU) > 0.5 as the measure for overlap to evaluate the prediction results. We study sensitivities at [0.5, 1, 2, 4, 8, 16] to evaluate the performance by different model variants.

190   Q. Tao et al.

3.1 Results Using Contextual and Spatial Attention

Firstly, we evaluate the effectiveness of our overall model, using the framework described in Sect. 2. We compare our method with the baseline methods as shown in Table 1. The improved R-FCN uses only 3 input slices fused at data-level. 3DCE improves the performance by adding more neighbouring slices and enabling the feature-level aggregation. Our method improves on 3DCE by introducing the contextual and spatial attention modules for attentive feature aggregation. We reproduce the results of 3DCE with different numbers of slices and achieve slightly higher results than those reported in their paper. Then we evaluate our model using the same numbers of slices as used in 3DCE. The results show that our method constantly boosts the accuracy at various FPs per image by around 7–8% in sensitivity at 0.5 and 2% in sensitivity at 4. More surprisingly, it is observed that our model using only 9 slices can greatly outperform the original 3DCE using 21 slices by a large margin while using much less computing resources in terms of GPU memory and computation time.

We further analyze the detection accuracy on different lesions types and image properties by splitting the test set according to three criteria: (1) Lesion type; (2) Lesion diameter (in mm) and (3) Slice interval (in mm) of the CT scans. The results for each split are shown in Table 2. There are eight types of lesions, including lung (LU), mediastinum (ME), liver (LV), soft tissue (ST), pelvis (PV), abdomen (AB), kidney (KD), and bone (BN) [10]. It is found that our method surpasses 3DCE in almost all lesion types. Especially for soft tissue lesion, our model achieves a large increase of 6.8% when compared with the baseline. In term of lesion diameter, the proposed method is slightly more effective on lesions that are larger than 10 mm. This is probably because the lesions smaller than 10 mm are less than 20 pixels in the CT image and have very low resolution at the attention maps (not greater than 2 × 2 patches). Therefore, the attentive feature enhancement on very small lesions could be less effective than on lesions with slightly larger size. Lastly, our method can achieve a constant improvement for CT scans with different slice intervals since our model attentively aggregates the relevant information from different slices with a cross-slice normalization.

3.2 Ablation Study

Table 3. Sensitivity (%) at various FPs per image on the test set of the official data split of DeepLesion using different attention components with 15 slices.

C_Att	S_Att	0.5	1	2	4	8	16
		63.0	73.1	80.2	85.2	87.8	89.7
✓		64.0	74.0	81.4	86.0	88.6	90.5
	✓	69.0	77.4	83.1	86.7	89.1	90.8
✓	✓	**70.8**	**78.6**	**83.9**	**87.5**	**89.9**	**91.4**

In this section, we investigate the effectiveness of each proposed component. We study the sensitivity at different FPs per image by comparing the baseline 3DCE model with the following variants: (1) adding contextual attention (C_Att); (2) adding spatial attention (S_Att); and (3) adding both contextual and spatial attention. As shown in Table 3, applying contextual attention alone brings a slight and constant improvement to the baseline method, whereas the spatial attention module alone performs very well and boosts the sensitivity at 0.5 from 63% to 69% with 6% performance gain. While adding both C_Att and S_Att modules, we achieve a higher sensitivity of 70.8% at 0.5 and further improve the sole S_Att model by 1.8%.

It is observed that at fewer FPs per image (0.5, 1), the performance gain is mainly from spatial attention, indicating that the spatial attention is essential to improve the prediction confidence for positive boxes. On the other hand, at higher FPs contextual attention gets more and more important for the performance gain.

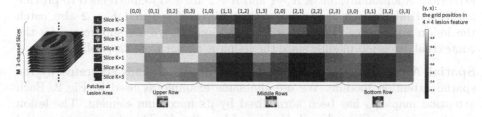

Fig. 2. Visualization of cross-slice contextual attention vectors based on our model with 7 three-channel images ($M = 7$). We visualize the slice patches corresponding to the lesion area in the key slice K as well as its previous and subsequent slices. The lesion region corresponds to 4×4 grids in Conv 5 feature. Therefore, we obtain 16 attention vectors for each feature grid from the contextual attention module. The vectors are visualized as a heatmap where each column (with a (y, x) coordinate in sub feature map of lesion patch) shows a normalized cross-slice attention vector.

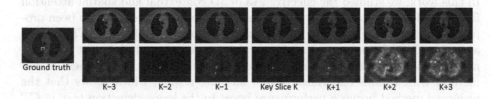

Fig. 3. Visualization of spatial attention map based on our model with 7 three-channel images. We can obtain 7 attention maps that are self-normalized to re-weight the feature importance within each feature map.

3.3   Qualitative Results and Visualization

In this section, to better understand how spatial and contextual attentions work for discriminative region mining, we illustrate some intermediate results of cross-slice contextual attention for soft-sampling and the intra-slice spatial attention for feature re-weighting. Some examples of detection results are shown in supplementary materials.

Contextual Attention: We visualize the contextual attention vectors at the lesion area in Fig. 2. There are $3 \times M$ input slices that are grouped in M 3-channel images. For simplicity, we denote each 3-channel image as a "Slice" in the figure. Each column of the heatmap shows a weight vector $v = C_d^{''y,x} \in \mathbb{R}^M$ to determine the importance of each slice ($K - 3$ to $K + 3$) at position (y, x) of the lesion feature map. Note that each vector has been normalized by its maximum element. It shows that at the upper part of the lesion area, all the slices almost have the same importance since there are no prominent features in this area. Near the center of the lesion area, the key slice is given the largest attention. Additionally, Slices $K - 1$ and $K - 2$ are also well-attended to provide additional information of the lesion since Slices $K - 1$ and $K - 2$ also catch the lesion appearance. Slices $K + 1$, $K + 2$ and $K + 3$ are suppressed by the contextual attention module since the lesion is absent from these slices.

Spatial Attention: In Fig. 3, we show the attention maps generated by the spatial attention module. We use the same example as used in Fig. 2. Each attention map $S_{i,d}^{''}$ has been normalized by its maximum element. The lesion clearly appears in Slices $K - 2$, $K - 1$ and key slice K. Therefore, in the spatial attention map, we can see a clear pulse at the lesion area. Since the lesion disappears from Slices $K + 1$, $K + 2$ and $K + 3$, the attention maps become plainer by which most feature grids are treated equally.

4   Conclusion

In this work, we studied the effectiveness of 3D contextual and spatial attention for lesion detection task in CT scans. The 3D contextual attention has been proposed to attentively aggregate the information from multiple slices. The spatial attention could help to concentrate the feature learning at the most discriminative regions within each feature map. We validated the effectiveness of our method with various experimental and analytic results, which shows that the proposed method brings a performance boost in the lesion detection task in CT scans.

References

1. Ren, S., He, K., Girshick, R., Sun, J.: Faster R-CNN: towards real-time object detection with region proposal networks. In: NIPS, pp. 91–99 (2015)
2. Dai, J., Li, Y., He, K., Sun, J.: R-FCN: object detection via region-based fully convolutional networks. In: NIPS, pp. 379–387 (2016)

3. Lam, C., Caroline, Y., Huang, L., Rubin, D.: Retinal lesion detection with deep learning using image patches. Investig. Ophthalmol. Vis. Sci. **59**(1), 590–596 (2018)
4. Li, Z., et al.: Thoracic disease identification and localization with limited supervision. In: IEEE CVPR, pp. 8290–8299 (2018)
5. Liao, F., Liang, M., Li, Z., Hu, X., Song, S.: Evaluate the malignancy of pulmonary nodules using the 3-D deep leaky noisy-or network. IEEE Trans. Neural Netw. Learn. Syst. (2019)
6. Dou, Q., Chen, H., Lequan, Y., Qin, J., Heng, P.-A.: Multilevel contextual 3-D CNNs for false positive reduction in pulmonary nodule detection. IEEE Trans. Biomed. Eng. **64**(7), 1558–1567 (2017)
7. Yan, K., Bagheri, M., Summers, R.M.: 3D context enhanced region-based convolutional neural network for end-to-end lesion detection. In: Frangi, A.F., Schnabel, J.A., Davatzikos, C., Alberola-López, C., Fichtinger, G. (eds.) MICCAI 2018. LNCS, vol. 11070, pp. 511–519. Springer, Cham (2018). https://doi.org/10.1007/978-3-030-00928-1_58
8. Wang, F., et al.: Residual attention network for image classification. In: IEEE CVPR, pp. 3156–3164 (2017)
9. Woo, S., Park, J., Lee, J.-Y., Kweon, I.S.: CBAM: convolutional block attention module. In: Ferrari, V., Hebert, M., Sminchisescu, C., Weiss, Y. (eds.) ECCV 2018. LNCS, vol. 11211, pp. 3–19. Springer, Cham (2018). https://doi.org/10.1007/978-3-030-01234-2_1
10. Yan, K., et al.: Deep lesion graphs in the wild: relationship learning and organization of significant radiology image findings in a diverse large-scale lesion database. In: IEEE CVPR, pp. 9261–9270 (2018)

MULAN: Multitask Universal Lesion Analysis Network for Joint Lesion Detection, Tagging, and Segmentation

Ke Yan[1]([✉]), Youbao Tang[1], Yifan Peng[2], Veit Sandfort[1],
Mohammadhadi Bagheri[1], Zhiyong Lu[2], and Ronald M. Summers[1]

[1] Imaging Biomarkers and Computer-Aided Diagnosis Laboratory, Clinical Center,
National Institutes of Health, Bethesda, MD 20892, USA
yankethu@gmail.com, {youbao.tang,mohammad.bagheri,rms}@nih.gov,
veit.sandfort@googlemail.com
[2] National Center for Biotechnology Information, National Library of Medicine,
National Institutes of Health, Bethesda, MD 20892, USA
{yifan.peng,zhiyong.lu}@nih.gov

Abstract. When reading medical images such as a computed tomography (CT) scan, radiologists generally search across the image to find lesions, characterize and measure them, and then describe them in the radiological report. To automate this process, we propose a multitask universal lesion analysis network (MULAN) for joint detection, tagging, and segmentation of lesions in a variety of body parts, which greatly extends existing work of single-task lesion analysis on specific body parts. MULAN is based on an improved Mask R-CNN framework with three head branches and a 3D feature fusion strategy. It achieves the state-of-the-art accuracy in the detection and tagging tasks on the DeepLesion dataset, which contains 32K lesions in the whole body. We also analyze the relationship between the three tasks and show that tag predictions can improve detection accuracy via a score refinement layer.

1 Introduction

Detection, classification, and measurement of clinically important findings (lesions) in medical images are primary tasks for radiologists [8]. Generally, they search across the image to find lesions, and then characterize their locations, types, and related attributes to describe them in radiological reports. They may also need to measure the lesions, e.g., according to the RECIST guideline [2], for quantitative assessment and tracking. To reduce radiologists' burden and improve accuracy, there have been many efforts in the computer-aided diagnosis area to automate this process. For example, detection, attribute estimation,

Electronic supplementary material The online version of this chapter (https://doi.org/10.1007/978-3-030-32226-7_22) contains supplementary material, which is available to authorized users.

D. Shen et al. (Eds.): MICCAI 2019, LNCS 11769, pp. 194–202, 2019.
https://doi.org/10.1007/978-3-030-32226-7_22

and malignancy prediction of lung nodules have been extensively studied [5,11]. Other works include detection and malignancy prediction of breast lesions [7] and classification of three types of liver lesions [1]. Variants of Faster R-CNN [5,7] have been used for detection, whereas patch-based dictionaries [1] or networks [5,11] have been studied for classification and segmentation.

Most existing work on lesion analysis focused on certain body parts (lung, liver, etc.). In practice, a radiologist often needs to analyze various lesions in multiple organs. Our goal is to build such a universal lesion analysis algorithm to mimic radiologists, which to the best of our knowledge is the first work on this problem. To this end, we attempt to integrate the three tasks in one framework. Compared to solving each task separately, the joint framework will be not only more efficient to use, but also more accurate, since different tasks may be correlated and help each other [10,11].

We present the multitask universal lesion analysis network (MULAN) which can detect lesions in CT images, predict multiple tags for each lesion, and segment it as well. This end-to-end framework is based on an improved Mask R-CNN [3] with three branches: detection, tagging, and segmentation. The tagging (multilabel classification) branch learns from tags mined from radiological reports. We extracted 185 fine-grained and comprehensive tags describing the body part, type, and attributes of the lesions. The relation between the three tasks is analyzed by experiments in this paper. Intuitively, lesion detection can benefit from tagging, because the probability of a region being a lesion is associated with its attribute tags. We propose a score refinement layer in MULAN to explicitly fuse the detection and tagging results and improve the accuracy of both. A 3D feature fusion strategy is developed to leverage the 3D context information to improve detection accuracy.

MULAN is evaluated on the DeepLesion [14] dataset, a large-scale and diverse dataset containing measurements and 2D bounding-boxes of over 32K lesions from a variety of body parts on computed tomography (CT) images. It has been adopted to learn models for universal lesion detection [10,12], measurement [9], and classification [13]. On DeepLesion, MULAN achieves the state-of-the-art accuracy in detection and tagging and performs comparable in segmentation. It outperforms the previous best detection result by 10%.

2 Method

The flowchart of the multitask universal lesion analysis network (MULAN) is displayed in Fig. 1(a). Similar to Mask R-CNN [3], MULAN has a backbone network to extract a feature map from the input image, which is then used in the region proposal network (RPN) to predict lesion proposals. Then, an ROIAlign layer [3] crops a small feature map for each proposal, which is used by three head branches to predict the lesion score, tags, and mask of the proposal.

2.1 Backbone with 3D Feature Fusion

A good backbone network is able to encode useful information of the input image into the feature map. In this study, we adopt the DenseNet-121 [4] in

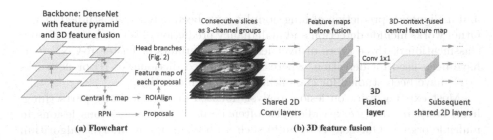

Fig. 1. Flowchart of MULAN and the 3D feature fusion strategy.

the backbone with the last dense block and transition layer removed, as we found removing them slightly improved accuracy and speed. Next, we employ the feature pyramid strategy [6] to add fine-level details into the feature map. This strategy also increases the size of the final feature map, which will benefit the detection and segmentation of small lesions. Different from the original feature pyramid network [6] which attaches head branches to each level of the pyramid, we attach the head branches only to the finest level [5,11].

3D context information is very important when differentiating lesions from non-lesions [12]. 3D CNNs have been used for lung nodule detection [5]. However, they are memory-consuming, thus smaller networks need to be used. Universal lesion detection is much more difficult than lung nodule detection, so networks with more channels and layers are potentially desirable. Yan et al. [12] proposed 3D context enhanced region-based CNN (3DCE) and achieved better detection accuracy than a 3D CNN in the DeepLesion dataset. They first group consecutive axial slices in a CT volume into 3-channel images. The upper and lower images provide 3D context for the central image. A feature map is then extracted for each image with a shared 2D CNN. Lastly, they fuse the feature maps of all images with a convolutional (Conv) layer to produce the 3D-context-enhanced feature map for the central image and predict 2D boxes for the lesions on it.

The drawback of 3DCE is that the 3D context information is fused only in the last Conv layer, which limits the network's ability to learn more complex 3D features. As shown in Fig. 1(b), we improve 3DCE to relieve this issue. The basic idea is to fuse features of multiple slices in earlier Conv layers. Similar to 3DCE, feature maps (FMs) are fused with a Conv layer (i.e., the 3D fusion layer). Then, the fused central FM is used to replace the original central FM, while the upper and lower FMs are kept unchanged. All FMs are then fed to subsequent Conv layers. Because the new central FM contains 3D context information, sophisticated 3D features can be learned in subsequent layers with nonlinearity. This 3D fusion layer can be inserted between any two layers of the original 2D CNN. In MULAN, one 3D fusion layer is inserted after dense block 2 and another one after the last layer of the feature pyramid. We found fusing 3D context in the beginning of the CNN (before dense block 2) is not good possibly because the CNN has not yet learned good semantic 2D features by then. At the end of the network, only the central feature map is used as the FM of the central image.

2.2 Head Branches and Score Refinement Layer

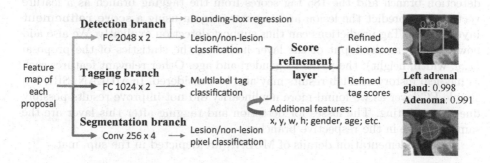

Fig. 2. Illustration of the head branches and the score refinement layer of MULAN.

The structure and function of the three head branches are shown in Fig. 2. The **detection branch** consists of two 2048D fully connected layers (FC) and predicts the lesion score of each proposal, i.e., the probability of the proposal being a lesion. It also conducts bounding-box regression to refine the box [3].

The **tagging branch** predicts the body part, type, and attributes (intensity, shape, etc.) of the lesion proposal. It applies the same label mining strategy as that in LesaNet [13]. We first construct the lesion ontology based on the RadLex lexicon. To mine training labels, we tokenize the sentences in the radiological reports of DeepLesion, and then match and filter the tags in the sentences using a text mining module. 185 tags with more than 30 occurrences in DeepLesion are kept. A weighted binary cross-entropy loss is applied on each tag. The hierarchical and mutually exclusive relations between the tags were leveraged in a label expansion strategy and a relational hard example mining loss to improve accuracy [13]. The score propagation layer and the triplet loss in [13] are not used. Due to space constraints, we refer readers to the supplementary material (sup. mat.) and [13] for more implementation details in this branch.

For the **segmentation branch**, we follow the method in [10] and generate pseudo-masks of lesions for training. The DeepLesion dataset does not contain lesions' ground-truth masks. Instead, each lesion has a RECIST measurement [2], namely a long axis and a short axis annotated by radiologists. They are utilized to generate four quadrants as the estimation of the real mask [10], since most lesions have ellipse-like shapes. We use the Dice loss [11] as it works well in balancing foreground and background pixels. The predicted mask can be easily used to compute the contour and then the RECIST measurement of the lesion, see Fig. 2 for an example.

Intuitively, detection (lesion/non-lesion classification) is closely related to tagging. One way to exploit their synergy is to combine them in one branch to make them share FC features. However, this strategy led to inferior accuracy for both tasks in our experiments probably because detecting a variety of lesions is a hard problem and requires rich features with high nonlinearity, thus a dedicated branch is necessary. In this study, we propose to combine them at the decision level. Specifically, for each lesion proposal, we join its lesion score from the detection branch and the 185 tag scores from the tagging branch as a feature vector, then predict the lesion and tag scores again using a **score refinement layer** (SRL). Tag predictions can thus support detection explicitly. We also add new features as the input of the layer including the statistics of the proposal $(x, y$, width, height), the patient's gender, and age. Other relevant features such as medical history and lab results may also be considered. In MULAN, SRL is a simple FC layer as we found more nonlinearity did not improve results possibly due to overfitting. The losses for detection and tagging after this layer are the same as those in the respective branches.

More implementation details of MULAN are depicted in the sup. mat.

3 Experiments and Discussion

Implementation: MULAN was implemented in PyTorch based on the maskrcnn-benchmark[1] project. The DenseNet backbone was initialized with an ImageNet pretrained model. The score refinement layer was initialized with an identity matrix so that the scores before and after it were the same when training started. Other layers were randomly initialized. Each mini-batch had 8 samples, where each sample consisted of three 3-channel images for 3D fusion (Fig. 1). We used SGD to train MULAN for 8 epochs and set the base learning rate to 0.004, then reduced it by a factor of 10 after the 4th and 6th epochs. It takes MULAN 30 ms to predict a sample during inference on a Tesla V100 GPU.

Data: The DeepLesion dataset [14] contains 32,735 lesions and was divided into training (70%), validation (15%), and test (15%) sets at the patient level. When training, we did data augmentation for each image in three ways: random resizing with a ratio of 0.8–1.2; random translation of −8–8 pixels in x and y axes; and 3D augmentation. A lesion in DeepLesion was annotated in one axial slice, but the actual lesion also exists in approximately the same position in several neighboring slices depending on its diameter and the slice interval. Therefore, we can do 3D augmentation by randomly shifting the slice index within half of the lesion's short diameter. Each of these three augmentation methods improved detection accuracy by 0.2–0.4%. Some examples of DeepLesion are presented in Sect. 1 of the sup. mat.

Metrics: For detection, we compute the sensitivities at 0.5, 1, 2, and 4 false positives (FPs) per image [12] and average them, which is similar to the evaluation metric of the LUNA dataset [5]. For tagging, we use the 500 manually tagged lesions in [13] for evaluation. The area under the ROC curve (AUC) and F1 score are computed for each tag and then averaged. Since there are no ground-truth (GT) masks in DeepLesion except for RECIST measurements [9], we use the average distance from the endpoints of the GT measurement to the predicted contour as a surrogate criterion (see sup. mat. Sect. 2). The second criterion is

---

[1] https://github.com/facebookresearch/maskrcnn-benchmark.

the average error of length of the estimated RECIST diameters, which are very useful values for radiologists and clinicians [2].

Qualitative and quantitative results are presented in Fig. 3 and Table 1, respectively. Note that in Table 1, tagging and segmentation accuracy were calculated by predicting tags and masks based on GT bounding-boxes, so that they were under the same setting as previous studies [9,13] and independent of the detection accuracy. We will discuss the results of each task below.

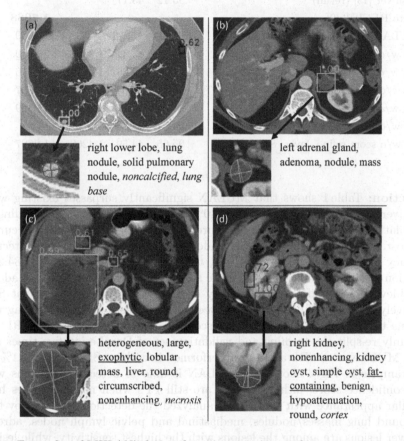

Fig. 3. Examples of MULAN's lesion detection, tagging, and segmentation results on the test set of DeepLesion. For detection, boxes in green and red are predicted TPs and FPs, respectively. The number above each box is the lesion score (confidence). For tagging, tags in black, red (underlined), and blue (italic) are predicted TPs, FPs, and FNs, respectively. They are ranked by their scores. For segmentation, the green lines are ground-truth RECIST measurements; the orange contours and lines show predicted masks and RECIST measurements, respectively. More visual examples are provided in sup. mat. Sect. 3. (TP: true positive; FP: false positive; FN: false negative) (Color figure online)

Table 1. Accuracy comparison and ablation studies on the test set of DeepLesion. Bold results are the best ones. Underlined results in the ablation studies are the worst ones, indicating the ablated strategy is the most important for the criterion.

	Detection (%)	Tagging (%)		Segmentation (mm)	
	Avg. sensitivity	AUC	F1	Distance	Diam. err
ULDor [10]	69.22	–	–	–	–
3DCE [12]	75.55	–	–	–	–
LesaNet [13] (rerun)	–	95.12	43.17	–	–
Auto RECIST [9]	–	–	–	–	**1.7088**
MULAN	**86.12**	**96.01**	**45.53**	1.4138	1.9660
(a) w/o feature pyramid	79.73	95.51	43.44	<u>1.6634</u>	<u>2.3780</u>
(b) w/o 3D fusion	<u>79.57</u>	95.88	44.28	1.4120	1.9756
(c) w/o detection branch	–	<u>95.16</u>	<u>40.03</u>	**1.2445**	1.7837
(d) w/o tagging branch	84.79	–	–	1.4230	1.9589
(e) w/o mask branch	85.21	95.87	43.76	–	–
(f) w/o score refine. layer	84.24	95.65	44.59	1.4260	1.9687

Detection: Table 1 shows that MULAN significantly surpasses existing work on universal lesion detection by over 10% in average sensitivity. According to the ablation study, 3D fusion and feature pyramid improve detection accuracy the most. If the tagging branch is not added (ablation study (d)), the detection accuracy is 84.79%; When it is added, the accuracy slightly drops to 84.24% (ablation study (f)). However, when the score refinement layer (SRL) is added, we achieve the best detection accuracy of 86.12%. We hypothesize that SRL effectively exploits the correlation between the two tasks and uses the tag predictions to refine the lesion detection score. To verify the impact of SRL, we randomly re-split the training and validation set of DeepLesion five times and found MULAN with SRL always outperformed it without SRL by 0.7–1.1%.

Examples in Fig. 3 show that MULAN is able to detect true lesions with high confidence score, although there are still FPs when normal tissues have a similar appearance with lesions. We analyzed the detection accuracy by tags and found lung masses/nodules, mediastinal and pelvic lymph nodes, adrenal and liver lesions are among the lesions with the highest sensitivity, while lesions in pancreas, bone, thyroid, and extremity are relatively hard to detect. These conclusions can guide us to collect more training samples with the difficult tags in the future.

Tagging: MULAN outperforms LesaNet [13], a multilabel CNN designed for universal lesion tagging. According to ablation study (c), adding the detection branch improves tagging accuracy. This is probably because detection is hard and requires comprehensive features to be learned in the backbone of MULAN, which are also useful for tagging. Figure 3 shows that MULAN is able to predict the body part, type, and attributes of lesions with high accuracy.

Segmentation: Our predicted RECIST diameters have an average error of 1.97 mm compared with the GT diameters. From Fig. 3, we can find that MULAN performs relatively well on lesions with clear borders, but struggles on those with indistinct or irregular borders, e.g., the liver mass in Fig. 3(c). Ablation studies show that feature pyramid is the most crucial strategy. Another interesting finding is that removing the detection branch (ablation study (c)) markedly improves segmentation accuracy. The detection task impairs segmentation, which could be a major reason why the multitask MULAN cannot beat Auto RECIST [9], a framework dedicated to lesion measurement. It implies that better segmentation results may be achieved using a single-task CNN.

More detailed results are shown in supplementary material.

4 Conclusion and Future Work

In this paper, we proposed MULAN, the first multitask universal lesion analysis network which can simultaneously detect, tag, and segment lesions in a variety of body parts. The training data of MULAN can be mined from radiologists' routine annotations and reports with minimum manual effort [14]. An effective 3D feature fusion strategy was developed. We also analyzed the interaction between the three tasks and discovered that: (1) Tag predictions could improve detection accuracy via a score refinement layer; (2) The detection task improved tagging accuracy but impaired segmentation performance.

Universal lesion analysis is a challenging task partially because of the large variance of appearances of the normal and abnormal tissues. Therefore, the 22 K training lesions in DeepLesion are still not sufficient for MULAN to learn, which is a main reason for its FPs and FNs. In the future, more training data need to be mined. We also plan to apply or finetune MULAN on other applications of specific lesions. We hope MULAN can be a useful tool for researchers focusing on different types of lesions.

Acknowledgments. This research was supported by the Intramural Research Programs of the National Institutes of Health (NIH) Clinical Center and National Library of Medicine (NLM). It was also supported by NLM of NIH under award number K99LM013001. We thank NVIDIA for GPU card donations.

References

1. Diamant, I., et al.: Improved patch-based automated liver lesion classification by separate analysis of the interior and boundary regions. IEEE J. Biomed. Health Inform. **20**(6), 1585–1594 (2016)
2. Eisenhauer, E.A., et al.: New response evaluation criteria in solid tumours: revised RECIST guideline (version 1.1). Eur. J. Cancer **45**(2), 228–247 (2009)
3. He, K., Gkioxari, G., Dollar, P., Girshick, R.: Mask R-CNN. In: ICCV, pp. 2980–2988 (2017)
4. Huang, G., Liu, Z., Weinberger, K.Q., van der Maaten, L.: Densely connected convolutional networks. In: CVPR (2017)

5. Liao, F., Liang, M., Li, Z., Hu, X., Song, S.: Evaluate the malignancy of pulmonary nodules using the 3D deep leaky noisy-or network. IEEE Trans. Neural Netw. Learn. Syst. (2019)
6. Lin, T.Y., Dollár, P., Girshick, R., He, K., Hariharan, B., Belongie, S.: Feature pyramid networks for object detection. In: CVPR (2017)
7. Ribli, D., Horváth, A., Unger, Z., Pollner, P., Csabai, I.: Detecting and classifying lesions in mammograms with deep learning. Sci. Rep. 8(1), 4165 (2018)
8. Sahiner, B., et al.: Deep learning in medical imaging and radiation therapy. Med. Phys. 46(1), e1–e36 (2019)
9. Tang, Y., Harrison, A.P., Bagheri, M., Xiao, J., Summers, R.M.: Semi-automatic RECIST labeling on CT scans with cascaded convolutional neural networks. In: Frangi, A.F., Schnabel, J.A., Davatzikos, C., Alberola-López, C., Fichtinger, G. (eds.) MICCAI 2018. LNCS, vol. 11073, pp. 405–413. Springer, Cham (2018). https://doi.org/10.1007/978-3-030-00937-3_47. http://arxiv.org/abs/1806.09507
10. Tang, Y., Yan, K., Tang, Y.X., Liu, J., Xiao, J., Summers, R.M.: ULDor: a universal lesion detector for CT scans with pseudo masks and hard negative example mining. In: ISBI (2019)
11. Wu, B., Zhou, Z., Wang, J., Wang, Y.: Joint learning for pulmonary nodule segmentation, attributes and malignancy prediction. In: ISBI, pp. 1109–1113 (2018)
12. Yan, K., Bagheri, M., Summers, R.M.: 3D context enhanced region-based convolutional neural network for end-to-end lesion detection. In: Frangi, A.F., Schnabel, J.A., Davatzikos, C., Alberola-López, C., Fichtinger, G. (eds.) MICCAI 2018. LNCS, vol. 11070, pp. 511–519. Springer, Cham (2018). https://doi.org/10.1007/978-3-030-00928-1_58
13. Yan, K., Peng, Y., Sandfort, V., Bagheri, M., Lu, Z., Summers, R.M.: Holistic and comprehensive annotation of clinically significant findings on diverse CT images: learning from radiology reports and label ontology. In: CVPR (2019)
14. Yan, K., Wang, X., Lu, L., Summers, R.M.: DeepLesion: automated mining of large-scale lesion annotations and universal lesion detection with deep learning. J. Med. Imaging 5(3) (2018). https://doi.org/10.1117/1.JMI.5.3.036501

Artifact Disentanglement Network for Unsupervised Metal Artifact Reduction

Haofu Liao[1](✉), Wei-An Lin[2], Jianbo Yuan[1], S. Kevin Zhou[3,4], and Jiebo Luo[1]

[1] Department of Computer Science, University of Rochester, Rochester, NY, USA
haofu.liao@rochester.edu
[2] Department of ECE, University of Maryland, College Park, MD, USA
[3] Institute of Computing Technology, Chinese Academy of Sciences, Beijing, China
[4] Peng Cheng Laboratory, Shenzhen, China

Abstract. Current deep neural network based approaches to computed tomography (CT) metal artifact reduction (MAR) are supervised methods which rely heavily on synthesized data for training. However, as synthesized data may not perfectly simulate the underlying physical mechanisms of CT imaging, the supervised methods often generalize poorly to clinical applications. To address this problem, we propose, to the best of our knowledge, the first unsupervised learning approach to MAR. Specifically, we introduce a novel artifact disentanglement network that enables different forms of generations and regularizations between the artifact-affected and artifact-free image domains to support unsupervised learning. Extensive experiments show that our method significantly outperforms the existing unsupervised models for image-to-image translation problems, and achieves comparable performance to existing supervised models on a synthesized dataset. When applied to clinical datasets, our method achieves considerable improvements over the supervised models. The source code of this paper is publicly available at https://github.com/liaohaofu/adn.

1 Introduction

Metal artifact is one of the commonly encountered artifacts in computed tomography (CT) images. It is introduced by the metallic implants during the imaging and reconstruction process. The formation of metal artifact involves several mechanisms such as beam hardening, scatter, noise, and the non-linear partial volume effect [1], which make it very challenging to be modeled and removed by traditional methods. Therefore, recent approaches [2,4,9,11] to metal artifact reduction (MAR) propose to use deep neural networks (DNNs) to inherently address the modeling of metal artifacts, and their experimental results show promising MAR performances.

All the existing DNN-based approaches are supervised methods requiring pairs of anatomically identical CT images, one with and the other without metal artifacts, for training. As it is clinically impractical to obtain such pairs of images,

© Springer Nature Switzerland AG 2019
D. Shen et al. (Eds.): MICCAI 2019, LNCS 11769, pp. 203–211, 2019.
https://doi.org/10.1007/978-3-030-32226-7_23

most of the supervised methods rely on synthesized images to train their models. However, due to the complexity of metal artifacts and the variations of CT devices, the synthesized images may not fully simulate the real clinical scenarios, and the performances of these supervised methods may degrade in clinical applications.

In this work, we aim to address the challenging yet more practical unsupervised setting where *no paired CT images are available for training*. To this end, we propose a novel artifact disentanglement network to separate the metal artifacts from clinical CT images in a latent space. The disentanglement enables manipulations between the artifact-affected and artifact-free image domains so that different forms of adversarial- and self-regularizations can be achieved to support unsupervised learning. *To the best of our knowledge, this is the first unsupervised learning approach to MAR.* Extensive experiments show that our method achieves comparable performance to the existing supervised methods on a synthesized dataset. When applied to clinical datasets, all the supervised methods demonstrate certain degrees of degradation, whereas our method outperforms the supervised methods with significantly better clinical MAR results.

2   Related Work

Unsupervised Image-to-Image Translation. Image artifact reduction can be regarded as a form of image-to-image translation. One of the earliest unsupervised works in this category is CycleGAN [12] where a cycle-consistency design is proposed for unsupervised learning. Later works [5,6] improve CycleGAN for diverse and multimodal image generation. However, these unsupervised methods target at image synthesis and do not have suitable components for artifact reduction. Another recent work that is specialized for artifact reduction is deep image prior (DIP) [8], which, however, only works for less structured artifacts such as noise and compression artifacts.

Deep Metal Artifact Reduction. A number of studies have recently been proposed to address MAR with DNNs. RL-ARCNN [4] introduces residual learning to a deep convolutional neural network (CNN) and achieves better MAR performance than ordinary CNN. DesteakNet [2] proposes a two-streams approach that can take a pair of preprocessed CT images as the input to jointly reduce metal artifact. CNNMAR [11] uses CNN to generate prior images in the CT image domain to help the correction in the sinogram domain. Both DesteakNet and CNNMAR show significant improvements over the existing non-DNN based methods on synthesized datasets. cGANMAR [9] leverages generative adversarial networks (GANs) [3] to further improve DNN-based MAR performance.

3   Methodology

Let $\mathcal{I}$ be the domain of all artifact-free CT images and $\mathcal{I}^a$ be the domain of all artifact-affected CT images, the proposed artifact disentanglement network

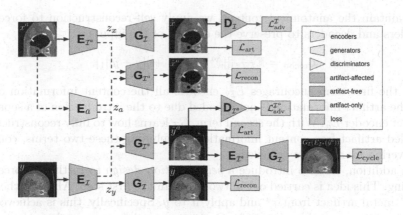

Fig. 1. Overview of the artifact disentanglement network.

(ADN) aims to learn a mapping from $\mathcal{I}^a$ to $\mathcal{I}$ without paired data. As illustrated in Fig. 1, ADN contains a set of artifact-free image encoder, generator and discriminator $\{E_\mathcal{I}, G_\mathcal{I}, D_\mathcal{I}\}$, a set of artifact-affected image encoder, generator and discriminator $\{E_{\mathcal{I}^a}, G_{\mathcal{I}^a}, D_{\mathcal{I}^a}\}$ and an artifact-only encoder E_a. The architectures of these building components are inspired from the state-of-the-art studies for image-to-image translation [5,13].

Components. Given two unpaired images $x^a \in \mathcal{I}^a$ and $y \in \mathcal{I}$, the encoders $E_{\mathcal{I}^a}$ and $E_\mathcal{I}$ map the artifact-free content information from x^a and y to a common content space $\mathcal{C}$, respectively. E_a maps the artifact-only information from x^a to an artifact space $\mathcal{A}$,

$$z_x = E_{\mathcal{I}^a}(x^a), z_y = E_\mathcal{I}(y), z_a = E_a(x^a), \quad \{z_x, z_y\} \subset \mathcal{C}, z_a \in \mathcal{A}. \quad (1)$$

The generator $G_{\mathcal{I}^a}$ takes an artifact-free code, z_x or z_y, and an artifact-only code z_a as the input and outputs an artifact-affected image. $G_\mathcal{I}$ takes an artifact-free code, z_x or z_y, as the input and outputs an artifact-free image,

$$\hat{x} = G_\mathcal{I}(z_x), \quad \hat{x}^a = G_{\mathcal{I}^a}(z_x, z_a),$$
$$\hat{y} = G_\mathcal{I}(z_y), \quad \hat{y}^a = G_{\mathcal{I}^a}(z_y, z_a). \quad (2)$$

During testing, only $E_{\mathcal{I}^a}$ and $G_\mathcal{I}$ are required to obtain an artifact-corrected output, i.e., $\hat{x} = G_\mathcal{I}(E_{\mathcal{I}^a}(x^a))$. The discriminators $D_{\mathcal{I}^a}/D_\mathcal{I}$ decides whether an input is sampled from $\mathcal{I}^a/\mathcal{I}$ or generated by $G_{\mathcal{I}^a}/G_\mathcal{I}$.

Loss Functions. A good MAR model should (i) reduce the artifacts as much as possible and (ii) keep the anatomical content of the input CT images. To remove the artifacts, we train $D_\mathcal{I}$ and $G_\mathcal{I}$ adversarially to encourage the output $\hat{x}$ to appear similar to an artifact-free image,

$$\mathcal{L}_{adv}^\mathcal{I} = \mathbb{E}_\mathcal{I}[\log D_\mathcal{I}(y)] + \mathbb{E}_{\mathcal{I}^a}[1 - \log D_\mathcal{I}(\hat{x})] \quad (3)$$

To maintain the anatomical content, we apply self-reconstruction to force the encoders and decoders to preserve the content of the inputs,

$$\mathcal{L}_{\text{recon}} = \mathbb{E}_{\mathcal{I},\mathcal{I}^a}[|| \hat{x}^a - x^a||_1 + ||\hat{y} - y||_1]. \tag{4}$$

Here, the first term encourages $E_{\mathcal{I}^a}$ encodes all the content information of x^a and the artifact information is not encoded due to the introduction of a separate artifact encoder E_a. With the second term, $G_{\mathcal{I}}$ learns how to fully reconstruct the encoded artifact-free content information. Combining these two terms, content persevering for $\hat{x}$ can be achieved.

In addition, we also introduce a *self-reduction design* to further enforce the learning. This idea is carried out in two steps. In the first step, ADN synthesizes "real" metal artifact from x^a and apply it to y. Specifically, this is achieved by decoding from z_y and z_a, i.e., $\hat{y}^a = G_{\mathcal{I}^a}(z_y, z_a)$, and we use another adversarial loss to guarantee $\hat{y}^a$ looking "real",

$$\mathcal{L}_{\text{adv}}^{\mathcal{I}^a} = \mathbb{E}_{\mathcal{I}^a}[\log D_{\mathcal{I}^a}(x^a)] + \mathbb{E}_{\mathcal{I},\mathcal{I}^a}[1 - \log D_{\mathcal{I}^a}(\hat{y}^a)] \tag{5}$$

In the second step, ADN reduces artifacts from the synthesized data to recover back to y. This is regularized by a cycle-consistent loss

$$\mathcal{L}_{\text{cycle}} = \mathbb{E}_{\mathcal{I},\mathcal{I}^a}[||G_{\mathcal{I}}(E_{\mathcal{I}^a}(\hat{y}^a)) - y||_1]. \tag{6}$$

Finally, due to the use of the same metal artifact, the difference map between x^a and $\hat{x}$ and that between $\hat{y}^a$ and y should be close. Thus, we employ an *artifact-consistent* loss to constrain the artifact difference,

$$\mathcal{L}_{\text{art}} = \mathbb{E}_{\mathcal{I},\mathcal{I}^a}[||(x^a - \hat{x}) - (\hat{y}^a - y)||_1]. \tag{7}$$

The full objective function is given by

$$\mathcal{L} = \lambda_{\text{adv}}^{\mathcal{I}} \mathcal{L}_{\text{adv}}^{\mathcal{I}} + \lambda_{\text{adv}}^{\mathcal{I}^a} \mathcal{L}_{\text{adv}}^{\mathcal{I}^a} + \lambda_{\text{recon}} \mathcal{L}_{\text{recon}} + \lambda_{\text{cycle}} \mathcal{L}_{\text{cycle}} + \lambda_{\text{art}} \mathcal{L}_{\text{art}}, \tag{8}$$

where the λ's are hyper-parameters that control the importance of each term.

4   Experiments

Datasets. We evaluate the proposed method on one synthesized dataset and two clinical datasets. We refer to them as SYN, CL1 and CL2, respectively. For SYN, we randomly select 4,118 artifact-free CT images from DeepLesion [10] and follow the method from CNNMAR [11] to synthesize metal artifacts. We use 3,918 of the synthesized pairs for training and the rest 200 pairs for testing.

For CL1, we choose the vertebrae localization and identification dataset from Spineweb[1]. We split the CT images from this dataset into two groups, one with artifacts and the other without artifacts. First, we identify regions with HU

---

[1] spineweb.digitalimaginggroup.ca.

Table 1. Quantitative evaluation on the SYN dataset.

	Supervised			Unsupervised				
	CNNMAR[11]	UNet [7]	cGANMAR [9]	Ours	CycleGAN [13]	DIP [8]	MUNIT [5]	DRIT [6]
PSNR	32.5	**34.8**	**34.1**	<u>33.6</u>	30.8	26.4	14.9	25.6
SSIM	91.4	**93.1**	**93.4**	<u>92.4</u>	72.9	75.9	7.5	79.7

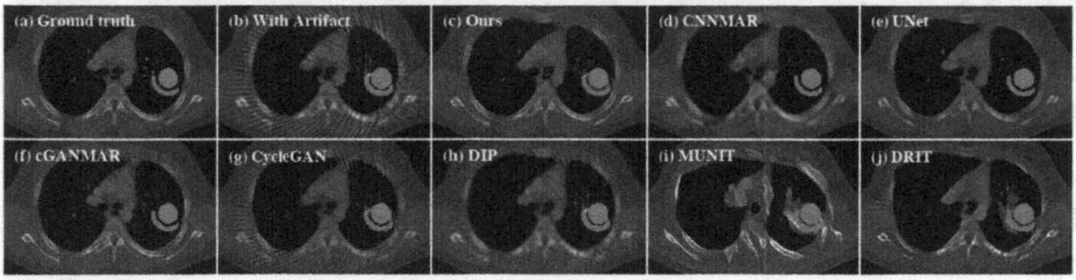

Fig. 2. Qualitative evaluation on the SYN dataset. For better visualization, we obtain the metal region through thresholding and color it with red. (Color figure online)

values greater than 2,500 as the metal regions. Then, CT images whose largest-connected metal regions have more than 400 pixels are selected as artifact-affected images. CT images with the largest HU values less than 2,000 are selected as artifact-free images. After this selection, the artifact-affected group contains 6,270 images and the artifact-free group contains 21,190 images. We withhold 200 images from the artifact-affected group for testing.

For CL2, we investigate the performance of the proposed method under a more challenging *cross-modality* setting. Specifically, the artifact-affected images of CL2 are from a cone-beam CT (CBCT) dataset collected during spinal interventions. Images from this dataset are very noisy and the majority of them contain metallic implants. There are in total 2,560 CBCT images from this dataset, among which 200 images are withheld for testing. For the artifact-free images, we reuse the CT images collected from CL1.

Baselines. We compare the proposed method with seven state-of-the-art methods that are closely related to our problem. Three of the compared methods are supervised: CNNMAR [11], UNet [7] and cGANMAR [9]. CNNMAR and cGANMAR are two recent approaches that are dedicated to MAR. UNet is a general DNN framework that shows effectiveness in many image-to-image problems. The other four compared methods are unsupervised: CycleGAN [12], DIP [8], MUNIT [5] and DRIT [6]. These methods are currently state-of-the-art approaches to unsupervised image-to-image translation problems. All the compared methods except UNet are trained with their officially released code. For UNet, a publicly available implementation[2] is used.

---

[2] github.com/milesial/Pytorch-UNet.

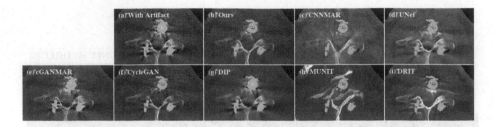

Fig. 3. Qualitative evaluation on the CL1 dataset. For better visualization, we obtain the metal region through thresholding and color it with red. (Color figure online)

Training and Testing. We implement our method under the PyTorch deep learning framework[3] and use the Adam optimizer with 1×10^{-4} learning rate to minimize the objective function. For the hyper-parameters, we use $\lambda^{\mathcal{I}}_{adv} = \lambda^{\mathcal{I}^a}_{adv} = 1.0$, $\lambda_{recon} = \lambda_{cycle} = \lambda_{art} = 20.0$ for SYN and CL1, and use $\lambda^{\mathcal{I}}_{adv} = \lambda^{\mathcal{I}^a}_{adv} = 1.0$, $\lambda_{recon} = \lambda_{cycle} = \lambda_{art} = 5.0$ for CL2.

To simulate the unsupervised setting for SYN, we evenly divide the 3,918 synthesized training pairs into two groups. For one group, only artifact-affected images are used and their corresponding artifact-free images are withheld. For the other group, only artifact-free images are used and their corresponding artifact-affected images are withheld. During training of the unsupervised methods, we randomly select one image from each of the two groups as the input. For the supervised methods, all the 3,918 synthesized training pairs are used.

To train the supervised methods with CL1, we first synthesize metal artifacts using the images from the artifact-free group of CL1. Then, we train the supervised methods with the synthesized pairs. During testing, the trained models are applied to the testing set containing only clinical metal artifact images. To train the unsupervised methods, we randomly select one image from the artifact-affected group and the other from the artifact-free group as the input.

For CL2, synthesizing metal artifacts is not possible due to the unavailability of artifact-free CBCT images. Therefore, for the supervised methods we directly use the models trained for CL1. The supervised methods are trained on synthesized CT images (from CL1) and tested on clinical CBCT images (from CL2). For the unsupervised models, each time we randomly select one artifact-affected CBCT image and one artifact-free CT image as the input for training.

Performance on Synthesized Data. SYN contains paired data, allowing for both quantitative and qualitative evaluations. Following the convention in the literature, we use peak signal-to-noise ratio (PSNR) and structural similarity index (SSIM) as the metrics. For both metrics, the higher the better. Table 1 and Fig. 2 show the quantitative and qualitative evaluation results, respectively.

We observe that the proposed method performs significantly better than the other unsupervised methods. MUNIT focuses more on diverse and realistic outputs (Fig. 2i) with less constraint on structural similarity. CycleGAN and

---

[3] pytorch.org.

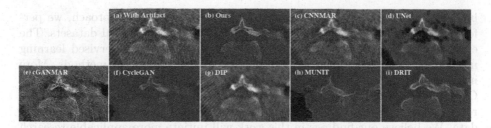

Fig. 4. Qualitative evaluation on the CL2 dataset.

DRIT perform better as both the two models also require the artifact-corrected outputs to be able to transform back to the original artifact-affected images. Although this helps preserve content information, it also encourages the models to keep the artifacts. Therefore, as shown in Fig. 2g and j, the artifacts cannot be greatly reduced. DIP does not reduce much metal artifact in the input image (Fig. 2h) as it is not designed to handle the more structured metal artifact.

We also find that the performance of our method is on a par with the supervised methods. The performance of UNet is close to that of cGANMAR which at its backend uses an UNet-like architecture. However, owing to the use of GAN, it produces sharper outputs (Fig. 2e) than UNet (Fig. 2f). As for PSNR and SSIM, both methods only slightly outperform our method and, surprisingly, our method performs better than CNNMAR.

Performance on Clinical Data. Next, we investigate the performance of the proposed method on clinical data. Since there are no ground truths available for the clinical images, only qualitative comparisons are performed. The qualitative evaluation results of CL1 are shown in Fig. 3. Here, all the supervised methods are trained with paired images that are synthesized from the artifact-free group of CL1. We can see that UNet and cGANMAR generalize poorly when applied to clinical images (Fig. 3d and e). CNNMAR is more robust as it corrects the artifacts in the sinogram domain. However, such a sinogram domain correction also introduces secondary artifacts (Fig. 3c). For the more challenging cross-modality artifact reduction task with CL2 (Fig. 4), all the supervised methods fail. This is not totally unexpected as the supervised methods are trained using only CT images because of the lack of artifact-free CBCT images. Similar to the cases with SYN, the other unsupervised methods also show inferior performances when evaluated on both the CL1 and CL2 datasets. By contrast, our method consistently delivers high-quality artifact reduced results on clinical images.

5 Conclusion

We presented a novel unsupervised learning approach to MAR. Through the development of an artifact disentanglement network, we showed how to leverage different forms of regularizations to eliminate the requirement of paired images for training. To understand the effectiveness of this approach, we performed extensive evaluations on one synthesized and two clinical datasets. The evaluation results demonstrated the feasibility of using unsupervised learning method to achieve comparable performance to the supervised methods. More importantly, the results also showed that directly learning MAR from clinical CT images under an unsupervised setting was a more feasible and robust approach than transferring the knowledge learned from synthesized data to clinical data. We believe our findings in this work will initiate more applicable research for medical image artifact reduction even under an unsupervised setting.

Acknowledgement. This work was supported in part by NSF award #1722847 and the Morris K. Udall Center of Excellence in Parkinson's Disease Research by NIH.

References

1. Gjesteby, L., et al.: Metal artifact reduction in CT: where are we after four decades? IEEE Access **4**, 5826–5849 (2016)
2. Gjesteby, L., et al.: Deep neural network for CT metal artifact reduction with a perceptual loss function. In: Proceedings of the Fifth International Conference on Image Formation in X-Ray Computed Tomography (2018)
3. Goodfellow, I., et al.: Generative adversarial nets. In: Advances in Neural Information Processing Systems (2014)
4. Huang, X., Wang, J., Tang, F., Zhong, T., Zhang, Y.: Metal artifact reduction on cervical CT images by deep residual learning. Biomed. Eng. Online **17**(1), 175 (2018)
5. Huang, X., Liu, M.-Y., Belongie, S., Kautz, J.: Multimodal unsupervised image-to-image translation. In: Ferrari, V., Hebert, M., Sminchisescu, C., Weiss, Y. (eds.) ECCV 2018. LNCS, vol. 11207, pp. 179–196. Springer, Cham (2018). https://doi.org/10.1007/978-3-030-01219-9_11
6. Lee, H.-Y., Tseng, H.-Y., Huang, J.-B., Singh, M., Yang, M.-H.: Diverse image-to-image translation via disentangled representations. In: Ferrari, V., Hebert, M., Sminchisescu, C., Weiss, Y. (eds.) ECCV 2018. LNCS, vol. 11205, pp. 36–52. Springer, Cham (2018). https://doi.org/10.1007/978-3-030-01246-5_3
7. Ronneberger, O., Fischer, P., Brox, T.: U-Net: convolutional networks for biomedical image segmentation. In: Navab, N., Hornegger, J., Wells, W.M., Frangi, A.F. (eds.) MICCAI 2015. LNCS, vol. 9351, pp. 234–241. Springer, Cham (2015). https://doi.org/10.1007/978-3-319-24574-4_28
8. Ulyanov, D., Vedaldi, A., Lempitsky, V.S.: Deep image prior. In: The IEEE Conference on Computer Vision and Pattern Recognition (CVPR), June 2018
9. Wang, J., Zhao, Y., Noble, J.H., Dawant, B.M.: Conditional generative adversarial networks for metal artifact reduction in CT images of the ear. In: Frangi, A.F., Schnabel, J.A., Davatzikos, C., Alberola-López, C., Fichtinger, G. (eds.) MICCAI 2018. LNCS, vol. 11070, pp. 3–11. Springer, Cham (2018). https://doi.org/10.1007/978-3-030-00928-1_1
10. Yan, K., Wang, X., Lu, L., Summers, R.M.: DeepLesion: automated mining of large-scale lesion annotations and universal lesion detection with deep learning. J. Med. Imaging (2018)
11. Zhang, Y., Yu, H.: Convolutional neural network based metal artifact reduction in X-ray computed tomography. IEEE Trans. Med. Imaging **37**(6), 1370–1381 (2018)

12. Zhu, J.Y., Park, T., Isola, P., Efros, A.A.: Unpaired image-to-image translation using cycle-consistent adversarial networks. In: The IEEE Conference on Computer Vision and Pattern Recognition (CVPR) (2017)
13. Zhu, J., Park, T., Isola, P., Efros, A.A.: Unpaired image-to-image translation using cycle-consistent adversarial networks. CoRR abs/1703.10593 (2017)

AirwayNet: A Voxel-Connectivity Aware Approach for Accurate Airway Segmentation Using Convolutional Neural Networks

Yulei Qin[1,2], Mingjian Chen[1,2], Hao Zheng[1,2], Yun Gu[1,2], Mali Shen[4],
Jie Yang[1,2(✉)], Xiaolin Huang[1,2], Yue-Min Zhu[3], and Guang-Zhong Yang[2,4]

[1] Institute of Image Processing and Pattern Recognition,
Shanghai Jiao Tong University, Shanghai, China
`jieyang@sjtu.edu.cn`
[2] Institute of Medical Robotics, Shanghai Jiao Tong University, Shanghai, China
[3] CREATIS (CNRS UMR 5220, INSERM U1206), INSA Lyon, Lyon, France
[4] Hamlyn Centre for Robotic Surgery, Imperial College London, London, UK

Abstract. Airway segmentation on CT scans is critical for pulmonary disease diagnosis and endobronchial navigation. Manual extraction of airway requires strenuous efforts due to the complicated structure and various appearance of airway. For automatic airway extraction, convolutional neural networks (CNNs) based methods have recently become the state-of-the-art approach. However, there still remains a challenge for CNNs to perceive the tree-like pattern and comprehend the connectivity of airway. To address this, we propose a voxel-connectivity aware approach named AirwayNet for accurate airway segmentation. By connectivity modeling, conventional binary segmentation task is transformed into 26 tasks of connectivity prediction. Thus, our AirwayNet learns both airway structure and relationship between neighboring voxels. To take advantage of context knowledge, lung distance map and voxel coordinates are fed into AirwayNet as additional semantic information. Compared to existing approaches, AirwayNet achieved superior performance, demonstrating the effectiveness of the network's awareness of voxel connectivity.

1 Introduction

Pulmonary diseases, including chronic obstructive pulmonary diseases (COPD) and lung cancer, pose high risks to human health. The standard computed tomography (CT) helps radiologists detect pathological changes. For tracheal and bronchial surgery, airway tree modeling on CT scans is often considered a prerequisite. Meticulous efforts are required to manually segment airway due to its tree-like structure and variety in size, shape, and intensity.

This research is partially supported by National Natural Science Foundation of China (No. 61572315, 61603248), IMR2018QY01, 973 Plan of China (No. 2015CB856004), and Committee of Science and Technology, Shanghai, China (No. 17JC1403000).

© Springer Nature Switzerland AG 2019
D. Shen et al. (Eds.): MICCAI 2019, LNCS 11769, pp. 212–220, 2019.
https://doi.org/10.1007/978-3-030-32226-7_24

Several methods have been proposed for airway segmentation on CT images. Van Rikxoort et al. [10] proposed a region growing method with adaptive thresholding. Xu et al. [11] combined two tubular structure enhancement techniques within the fuzzy connectedness segmentation framework. Lo et al. [6] designed a learning-based approach that models airway appearance and utilized vessel orientation similarity. In the EXACT'09 challenge, fifteen airway extraction algorithms were summarized by Lo et al. [7]. Most algorithms adopted region growing with additional constraints such as tube likeness. Although successfully segmenting bronchi of large size, these conventional methods performed worse on peripheral bronchi.

Recently, convolutional neural networks (CNNs) were increasingly used in segmentation tasks [2,9]. For airway extraction, CNNs-based methods [1,3,4,8,12] were developed and proved superior to previous methods in [7]. Charbonnier et al. [1] and Yun et al. [12] respectively used two-dimensional (2-D) and 2.5-D CNNs on already coarsely segmented bronchi to reduce false positives and increase detected tree length. Meng et al. [8] embedded CNNs-based segmentation into the airway volume of interest (VOI) tracking framework. Jin et al. [3] employed graph-based refinement on the probability output of CNNs. Juarez et al. [4] designed an end-to-end CNN model with simple pre- and post-processing. Despite their satisfactory performance, these methods did not specifically take airway connectivity into consideration, leaving room for improvement.

In this paper, we propose AirwayNet, a CNNs-based approach for accurate airway segmentation. Considering that the tree-like structure of airway is rather complex and the prediction of airway candidates is prone to discontinuity, we put emphasis on the connectivity of airway voxels. Unlike previous methods, we do not directly train the network to classify foreground and background voxels. Instead, binary segmentation task is transformed into 26 tasks of predicting whether a voxel is connected to its neighbors. Since airway voxels are stretching from the main bronchus towards bronchiole end as a whole connected region, we consider it a good solution to enable the model being aware of voxel connectivity. Previous work on salient segmentation [5] demonstrated that connectivity modeling spontaneously encodes the relation between two pixels. Therefore, we design a voxel connectivity-aware approach to better comprehend the inherent structure of airway. Our main contributions can be summarized as follows: (1) The voxel connectivity of airway is modeled using conventional binary ground-truth labels to better serve the airway segmentation task. The proposed AirwayNet automatically learns relationship between adjacent voxels and discriminates airway from the background. For each voxel, the network predicts not only its probability of being airway but also its connectivity to neighbors. (2) To effectively utilize wide-range context knowledge, voxels' coordinates and their distance to lung borders are leveraged by the model as additional semantic information. (3) Trained using 20 cases and evaluated on 10 additional cases, AirwayNet achieved the highest Dice coefficient and true positive rate of 90.2%, 84.7%, respectively, compared to state-of-the-art methods.

2   Method

In this section, we first introduce how to model voxel connectivity and transform the segmentation problem into connectivity prediction problem. Then, details about CT pre-processing and the 3-D CNNs-based connectivity prediction are provided. Finally, we discuss the generation process of airway candidates. The flowchart of the proposed AirwayNet is depicted in Fig. 1.

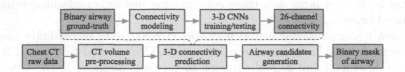

Fig. 1. Flowchart of the proposed AirwayNet.

2.1   Connectivity Modeling Using Binary Ground-Truth Labels

In a three-dimensional (3-D) CT, 26-connectivity describes well the relation between one voxel and its 26 neighbors (see Fig. 2). Given a voxel $P = (x, y, z)$ and its neighbor $Q = (u, v, w)$, the distance between P and Q is restricted by $d(P, Q) = max(\|(x - u)\|, \|(y - v)\|, \|(z - w)\|) \leq 1$, which means that Q is located within a $3 \times 3 \times 3$ cube centered at P. We index neighbors Q from 1 to 26 and denote each voxel pair $(P, Q_i), i \in \{1, 2, ..., 26\}$ as a connectivity orientation. Each orientation is encoded using a 1-channel binary label. If both P and Q_i are airway voxels, then the pair (P, Q_i) is connected and the corresponding position "P" on the i-th label is marked as 1. Otherwise, we mark 0 on the i-th label to represent disconnected pair (P, Q_i). By sliding such a $3 \times 3 \times 3$ window over each voxel, we obtain 26 binary labels and concatenate them into a 26-channel connectivity label. Zero padding is performed on CT volume borders to keep the size of generated labels unchanged. Such connectivity label encodes both ground-truth position and 26-connectivity relation between airway voxels. Note that all operations are performed on conventional binary labels of airway ground-truth. We do not require extra manual annotation for connectivity labels.

After modeling the 3-D connectivity, the original airway ground-truth label is reformed, and the conventional segmentation task is then transformed into 26 connectivity prediction tasks. The objective here is to classify and merge connected airway voxels along each connectivity orientation. An advantage of decomposing one task into 26 different tasks is that multi-task learning strategy helps the network learn more generalized features. These 26 tasks are correlated in depicting voxel connectivity, so that our AirwayNet can extract essential and robust features. Furthermore, the connectivity label emphasizes airway's structure attribute. The network trained using such label is encouraged to grasp the tree-like pattern of bronchial airway.

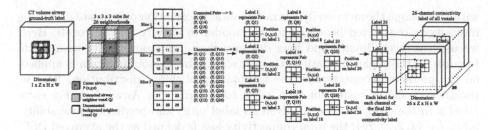

Fig. 2. Illustration of 26-connectivity modeling. The binary ground-truth of airway (Dim: $1 \times Z \times H \times W$) is transformed into a connectivity label (Dim: $26 \times Z \times H \times W$).

2.2 CT Volume Pre-processing

One challenge in airway segmentation is that the foreground voxels only occupy a small proportion of all CT voxels. To avoid feature learning from irrelevant parts (e.g., ribs and skin), we restrict the valid airway candidate region inside the lung area. To extract lung mask, each CT slice is first filtered with a Gaussian filter ($\sigma = 1$) and binarized with a threshold (-600 Hounsfield unit). The connected component analysis is applied to remove unconfident candidates and the largest two components are chosen as left and right lungs, respectively. To avoid under-segmentation, we replace the lung area by its convex hull on each slice if the convex hull has 50% more area. We also perform Euclidean distance transform on the lung mask to calculate the distance map. Each voxel on the distance map records its minimum distance to the lung border. We add such map into the network because the airway's relative position to lung border is considered anatomically meaningful. To prepare for network training, CT voxel intensity is clipped by a window $[-1000, 600]$ (HU) and normalized to $[0, 255]$. Due to the limit of GPU memory, the bounding box of lungs is further cropped into smaller cubes using a sliding window technique. The cropped size is $32 \times 224 \times 224$ and the sliding stride is $[8, 56, 56]$. Such cubes include abundant context knowledge for our model to distinguish between the airway and the background.

2.3 Connectivity Prediction Based on 3-D CNNs

Given a cropped CT cube, the objective is to use 3-D CNNs to predict voxel connectivity of the cube. The proposed AirwayNet (see Fig. 3) is based on the U-Net [2] backbone. Our full 3-D architecture captures more spatial information than the 2-D or 2.5-D CNNs used in [1,12] and is more suitable for learning the bronchial continuity and branching patterns. The AirwayNet consists of a contracting path and an expansive path with four resolution scales. At each resolution scale, the contracting path has two convolution layers (Conv) with batch normalization (BN) and rectified linear unit (ReLU), followed by a max-pooling layer. In the expansive path, finer features from lower resolution scale are linearly upsampled first and then concatenated with coarse features from skip connection to preserve details of thin bronchi. Since airway voxels are distributed within the large thoracic cavity, extra semantic information other than grayscale intensity is considered beneficial for the model to classify airway voxels. Here we use voxel coordinates and lung distance map, and concatenate them with features on the expansive path at the last scale. The sigmoid function is applied on the predicted connectivity cube to obtain probability distribution. We use the Dice similarity coefficient (DSC) loss to optimize our AirwayNet. For each voxel x in the cropped cube X, given its label $y_i(x)$ and prediction probability $p_i(x), i \in \{1, 2, ..., 26\}$, the total connectivity loss is defined as the averaged DSC loss over all channels:

$$\mathcal{L} = 1 - \frac{1}{26} \sum_{i=1}^{26} \frac{2 \sum_{x \in X} p_i(x) y_i(x)}{\sum_{x \in X} (p_i(x) + y_i(x)) + \epsilon}, \tag{1}$$

where ϵ is used to avoid division by zero.

2.4   Airway Candidates Generation

The final step is to generate airway candidates based on the predicted connectivity cube. First, a threshold $t = 0.5$ is used to binarize prediction results. Here we consider that pairwise voxels should agree with each other in connectivity. For example, if voxel P is connected to its neighbor Q_{14} (see Fig. 2), then voxel P on the 14-th connectivity channel is marked as 1. Meanwhile, on the 13-th channel, voxel Q_{14} is marked as 1 because P is also at the position "Q_{13}" of the $3 \times 3 \times 3$ neighborhood of Q_{14}. The connectivity between P and Q_{14} is coded in both the 13-th and the 14-th channels. Therefore, we only keep voxels that comply with such pairwise agreement. Then, channel-wise summation is performed on the connectivity cube and those non-zero voxels are marked as airway candidates. The segmentation results are multiplied with the lung field mask to filter out false positives. Finally, we follow [3] to apply fuzzy connectedness segmentation on the generated candidates to consolidate the bronchial distal ends.

3   Experiments and Results

The experiment dataset contains 30 chest CT scans. All CT axial slices have the same size of 512×512, with a pixel spacing ranging from 0.5 to 0.781 mm.

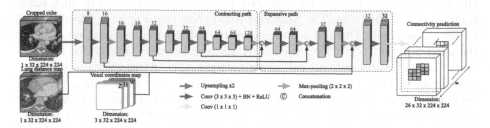

Fig. 3. The architecture of the 3-D CNNs used in the proposed AirwayNet. The number of channels is denoted above each feature map.

Table 1. Comparison of airway segmentation results (%) on 10 chest CT scans.

Case	AirwayNet				Jin et al. [3]				Juarez et al. [4]			
	DSC	TPR	FPR	PPV	DSC	TPR	FPR	PPV	DSC	TPR	FPR	PPV
1	92.4	86.5	0.003	99.2	90.4	84.4	0.010	97.2	91.0	83.8	0.002	99.5
2	87.5	78.5	0.003	98.8	73.8	60.8	0.011	94.0	76.9	62.6	0.000	99.8
3	91.1	85.3	0.004	97.7	88.9	83.1	0.008	95.6	91.1	84.6	0.002	98.8
4	82.9	73.1	0.009	95.7	79.6	66.5	0.002	99.1	70.8	55.6	0.004	97.4
5	90.8	86.2	0.015	95.9	90.6	85.3	0.012	96.6	89.3	81.4	0.003	99.1
6	91.5	89.2	0.025	94.0	84.5	88.3	0.091	81.0	92.3	87.9	0.012	97.1
7	90.6	87.6	0.025	93.7	88.2	85.3	0.034	91.2	90.3	85.1	0.014	96.2
8	91.7	88.9	0.017	94.7	86.4	88.1	0.054	84.8	90.2	86.5	0.018	94.2
9	93.1	88.8	0.009	97.8	90.5	84.3	0.009	97.7	85.9	75.9	0.004	98.9
10	90.4	83.2	0.003	98.9	88.2	79.3	0.002	99.4	88.3	79.4	0.001	99.5
Mean	**90.2**	**84.7**	0.011	96.6	86.1	80.5	0.023	93.7	86.6	78.3	**0.006**	**98.1**
Std.	**2.8**	**4.9**	0.008	1.9	5.2	8.9	0.027	5.9	6.7	10.3	**0.006**	**1.7**

The slice thickness varies from 0.5 to 1.0 mm. These scans were acquired using different scanners, protocols, dose level, and reconstruction kernels. The dataset contains cases from both healthy volunteers and patients with severe pulmonary diseases (e.g., emphysema and pneumonia). The ground-truth labels of airway were annotated and screened by well-trained experts for verification. We randomly chose 20 CT scans for training and fine-tuning hyper-parameters. Our approach was evaluated on the remaining 10 scans.

During training, cropped cubes were augmented on-the-fly via random horizontal flipping, with a probability of 0.5. We densely sampled cubes near airway region and discarded cubes near lung border randomly. This results in around 5000 training samples for each epoch. The Adam optimizer ($\beta_1 = 0.5, \beta_2 = 0.999$) was used and the learning rate was set to 10^{-4}. The training converged after 15 epochs. Our AirwayNet was implemented in Keras with 4 NVIDIA Titan Xp GPUs. During testing, the stride of the sliding window was [16, 128, 128] and the prediction results were averaged on overlapping margins. Four evaluation metrics were used: (a) Dice coefficient (DSC), (b) True positive rate (TPR), (c) False positive rate (FPR), and (d) Positive predictive value (PPV).

We compared our AirwayNet with two state-of-the-art approaches, Jin's method [3] and Juarez's method [4]. They both employ 3-D CNNs with a sliding window technique for airway extraction. In Table 1, it is observed that our method achieved the highest DSC and TPR of 90.2%, 84.7%, respectively, with the comparable FPR of 0.011% and PPV of 96.6%. The smallest standard deviation of DSC and TPR was achieved by AirwayNet, confirming its robustness. With lower DSC, TPR, and FPR but higher PPV, Juarez et al. [4] segmented more conservatively than AirwayNet and the proposed method slightly tended to

218   Y. Qin et al.

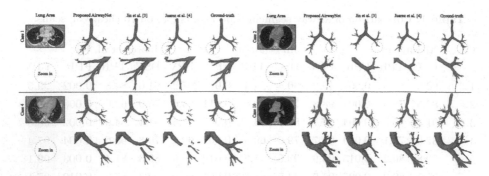

Fig. 4. Comparison of airway segmentation results. Local bronchial branches are highlighted with **circles** and zoomed in to better see performance difference.

classify background voxels as airway. But our TPR is 6.4% higher than theirs on average, meaning that more airway voxels were detected by AirwayNet. In addition, qualitative results of the proposed AirwayNet are shown in Fig. 4, together with its comparison with [3,4]. Owing to connectivity modeling, our method enriched details of segmented peripheral bronchi. In contrast, more holes and cracks appear on the predicted bronchial airway of other methods.

We also conducted ablation study (see Table 2) to validate whether each component of the proposed method is useful. Compared to AirwayNet without Conn and D&C, the slightly higher FPR and lower PPV of AirwayNet may be due to the introduction of connectivity modeling and semantic information, making the model more sensitive and perceptive to airway than background. Meanwhile, the improvement in DSC and TPR proves that it is worthwhile to enable the model being aware of connectivity and semantic knowledge. These two components do contribute to the performance improvement.

According to Table 1 and Fig. 4, our AirwayNet clearly improves the connectivity and shape reconstruction of airway but is not yet 100% perfect, mainly due to the fact that the used training samples did not reflect all the situations including weak intensity contrast between airway lumen and wall, blurring from low quality imaging, and pathological changes of pulmonary diseases.

Table 2. Results (%) of ablation study of AirwayNet (mean ± standard deviation). The Conn and D&C represent connectivity modeling and distance map & coordinates, respectively. Note that without Conn, the task of AirwayNet becomes a common segmentation task and the network is directly trained to output binary masks of airway.

Methods	DSC	TPR	FPR	PPV
AirwayNet w/o Conn	87.1 ± 6.4	79.3 ± 9.6	**0.007 ± 0.008**	**97.6 ± 2.5**
AirwayNet w/o D&C	88.4 ± 5.4	81.6 ± 8.7	0.009 ± 0.009	97.1 ± 2.1
AirwayNet	**90.2 ± 2.8**	**84.7 ± 4.9**	0.011 ± 0.008	96.6 ± 1.9

4 Conclusion

This paper proposed a CNNs-based approach, AirwayNet, for airway segmentation on CT scans. It explicitly learns voxel connectivity to perceive airway's inherent structure. By connectivity modeling, conventional segmentation task is transformed into 26 tasks of connectivity prediction, with each task classifying airway voxels along a certain connectivity orientation. The lung distance map and voxel coordinates are introduced as additional semantic information to better utilize context knowledge. Experimental results corroborated the two main strengths of AirwayNet: (1) the model's attention paid on the connectivity of airway structure and (2) the extra knowledge about voxels' position and their distance to lung borders. Consequently, the performance improvement is achieved on peripheral airway segmentation. In the future, the proposed method could further be improved by working on (1) the adoption of generative adversarial networks to produce various training samples to improve robustness on unhealthy patients' scans and (2) the exploration of specific enhancement mechanisms for thin bronchus details in low quality CT scans to improve performance.

References

1. Charbonnier, J.P., et al.: Improving airway segmentation in computed tomography using leak detection with convolutional networks. MedIA **36**, 52–60 (2017)
2. Çiçek, Ö., Abdulkadir, A., Lienkamp, S.S., Brox, T., Ronneberger, O.: 3D U-Net: learning dense volumetric segmentation from sparse annotation. In: Ourselin, S., Joskowicz, L., Sabuncu, M.R., Unal, G., Wells, W. (eds.) MICCAI 2016. LNCS, vol. 9901, pp. 424–432. Springer, Cham (2016). https://doi.org/10.1007/978-3-319-46723-8_49
3. Jin, D., Xu, Z., Harrison, A.P., George, K., Mollura, D.J.: 3D convolutional neural networks with graph refinement for airway segmentation using incomplete data labels. In: Wang, Q., Shi, Y., Suk, H.-I., Suzuki, K. (eds.) MLMI 2017. LNCS, vol. 10541, pp. 141–149. Springer, Cham (2017). https://doi.org/10.1007/978-3-319-67389-9_17
4. Juarez, A.G.-U., Tiddens, H.A.W.M., de Bruijne, M.: Automatic airway segmentation in chest CT using convolutional neural networks. In: Stoyanov, D., et al. (eds.) RAMBO/BIA/TIA-2018. LNCS, vol. 11040, pp. 238–250. Springer, Cham (2018). https://doi.org/10.1007/978-3-030-00946-5_24
5. Kampffmeyer, M., Dong, N., Liang, X., Zhang, Y., Xing, E.P.: ConnNet: a long-range relation-aware pixel-connectivity network for salient segmentation. IEEE TIP **28**(5), 2518–2529 (2019)
6. Lo, P., Sporring, J., Ashraf, H., Pedersen, J.J., de Bruijne, M.: Vessel-guided airway tree segmentation: a voxel classification approach. MedIA **14**(4), 527–538 (2010)
7. Lo, P., et al.: Extraction of airways from CT (EXACT'09). IEEE TMI **31**(11), 2093–2107 (2012)
8. Meng, Q., Roth, H.R., Kitasaka, T., Oda, M., Ueno, J., Mori, K.: Tracking and segmentation of the airways in chest CT using a fully convolutional network. In: Descoteaux, M., Maier-Hein, L., Franz, A., Jannin, P., Collins, D.L., Duchesne, S. (eds.) MICCAI 2017. LNCS, vol. 10434, pp. 198–207. Springer, Cham (2017). https://doi.org/10.1007/978-3-319-66185-8_23

9. Ronneberger, O., Fischer, P., Brox, T.: U-Net: convolutional networks for biomedical image segmentation. In: Navab, N., Hornegger, J., Wells, W.M., Frangi, A.F. (eds.) MICCAI 2015. LNCS, vol. 9351, pp. 234–241. Springer, Cham (2015). https://doi.org/10.1007/978-3-319-24574-4_28

10. Van Rikxoort, E.M., Baggerman, W., van Ginneken, B.: Automatic segmentation of the airway tree from thoracic CT scans using a multi-threshold approach. In: Proceedings of Second International Workshop on Pulmonary Image Analysis, pp. 341–349 (2009)

11. Xu, Z., Bagci, U., Foster, B., Mansoor, A., Udupa, J.K., Mollura, D.J.: A hybrid method for airway segmentation and automated measurement of bronchial wall thickness on CT. MedIA **24**(1), 1–17 (2015)

12. Yun, J., et al.: Improvement of fully automated airway segmentation on volumetric computed tomographic images using a 2.5 dimensional convolutional neural net. MedIA **51**, 13–20 (2019)

Integrating Cross-modality Hallucinated MRI with CT to Aid Mediastinal Lung Tumor Segmentation

Jiang Jue[1], Hu Jason[1], Tyagi Neelam[1], Rimner Andreas[2], Berry L. Sean[1], Deasy O. Joseph[1], and Veeraraghavan Harini[1(✉)]

[1] Medical Physics, Memorial Sloan Kettering Cancer Center, New York, USA
veerarah@mskcc.org
[2] Radiation Oncology, Memorial Sloan Kettering Cancer Center, New York, USA

Abstract. Lung tumors, especially those located close to or surrounded by soft tissues like the mediastinum, are difficult to segment due to the low soft tissue contrast on computed tomography images. Magnetic resonance images contain superior soft-tissue contrast information that can be leveraged if both modalities were available for training. Therefore, we developed a cross-modality educed learning approach where MR information that is educed from CT is used to hallucinate MRI and improve CT segmentation. Our approach, called cross-modality educed deep learning segmentation (CMEDL) combines CT and pseudo MR produced from CT by aligning their features to obtain segmentation on CT. Features computed in the last two layers of parallelly trained CT and MR segmentation networks are aligned. We implemented this approach on U-net and dense fully convolutional networks (dense-FCN). Our networks were trained on unrelated cohorts from open-source the Cancer Imaging Archive CT images (N = 377), an internal archive T2-weighted MR (N = 81), and evaluated using separate validation (N = 304) and testing (N = 333) CT-delineated tumors. Our approach using both networks were significantly more accurate (U-net $P < 0.001$; denseFCN $P < 0.001$) than CT-only networks and achieved an accuracy (Dice similarity coefficient) of 0.71 ± 0.15 (U-net), 0.74 ± 0.12 (denseFCN) on validation and 0.72 ± 0.14 (U-net), 0.73 ± 0.12 (denseFCN) on the testing sets. Our novel approach demonstrated that educing cross-modality information through learned priors enhances CT segmentation performance.

Keywords: Hallucinating MRI from CT for segmentation · Lung tumors · Adversarial cross-domain deep learning

1 Introduction

Precision medical treatments including image-guided radiotherapy require accurate target tumor segmentation [1]. Computed tomography (CT), the standard-

© Springer Nature Switzerland AG 2019
D. Shen et al. (Eds.): MICCAI 2019, LNCS 11769, pp. 221–229, 2019.
https://doi.org/10.1007/978-3-030-32226-7_25

of-care imaging modality lacks sufficient soft-tissue contrast, which makes visualizing tumor boundaries difficult, especially for those that are adjacent to soft-tissue structures. With the advent of new MRI simulator technologies, radiation oncologists can delineate target structures on MRI acquired in simulation position, which then have to be transferred using image registration to the planning CTs acquired at a different time in treatment position for radiation therapy planning [2]. Image registration itself is prone to errors and thus accurate segmentation on CT itself is more desirable for improving accuracy of clinical radiation treatment margins. More importantly, driven by the lack of simultaneously acquired CT and MR scans, current methods are restricted to CT alone. Therefore, we developed a novel approach, called cross-modality educed deep learning (CMEDL), that uses unpaired cross-domain adaptation between unrelated CT and MR datasets to hallucinate MR-like images or pseudo MR (pMR) from CT scans. The pMR image is combined with CT image to regularize training of a CT segmentation network. This is accomplished by aligning the features of the CT with the pMR features during training (Fig. 1).

Ours is not a method for data augmentation using cross-domain adaptation [3–5]. Our work is also unlike methods that seek to reduce the datashift differences between same imaging modalities [6–8]. Instead, our goal in this work is to maximize the segmentation performance in a single less informative imaging modality, namely, CT using learned information modeling the latent tissue relationships with a more informative modality, namely MRI. The key insight here is that the features dismissed as uninterpretable on CT can provide inference information when learning proceeds from a more informative modality such as MRI.

Our approach is most similar in its goal to compute shared representations for improving segmentations as in the work by [9], where several shared representations between CT and MRI were constructed using fully convolutional networks. Our approach, that is based on GANs for cross-modality learning, shares some similarities to [10] that also used a GAN as a backbone framework, and implemented dual networks for performing segmentations on both CT and MRI. However, our approach substantially differs from prior works in its use of the cross-modality tissue relations as priors to improve inference on the less informative source (or CT) domain. Though applied to segmenting lung tumors, this method is generally applicable to other structures and imaging modalities.

Our contributions in this work are as follows: (i) first, we developed a novel approach to generate segmentation on CT by leveraging more informative MRI through cross-modality priors. (ii) second, we implemented this approach on two different segmentation networks to study feasibility of segmenting lung tumors located in the mediastinum, an area where there is diminished contrast between tumor and the surrounding soft-tissue. (iii) third, we evaluated our approach on a large dataset of 637 tumors.

2   Methods

We use a supervised cross-modality and CT segmentation approach with a reasonably large number of expert segmented CT scans (X_{CT}, y_{CT}) and a few MR scans with expert segmentation $(\{X_{MR}, y_{MR}\}$, where, $N_{X_{MR}} \ll N_{X_{CT}})$. The cross-modality educed deep learning (CMEDL) segmentation consists of two sub-networks that are optimized alternatively. The first sub-network (Fig. 1A) generates a pMR image given a CT image. The second sub-network (Fig. 1B), trains its CT segmentation network constrained using features from another network trained using pMRI. The alternative optimization enables the approach to regularize both the segmentation and pMR generation, such that the pMR is specifically tuned to increase segmentation accuracy. In other words, pMR acts as an informative regularizer for CT segmentation, while the gradients of segmentation errors serve to constrain the generated pMR images.

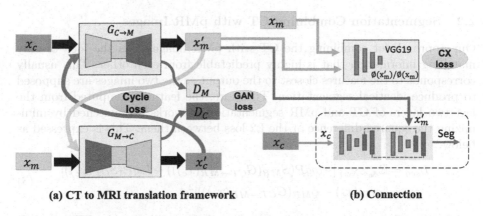

(a) CT to MRI translation framework   (b) Connection

Fig. 1. Overview of the comparison of different combinations. x_c is the CT image; x_m is the MRI image; $G_{C \to M}$ and $G_{M \to C}$ are the CT and MRI transfer networks; x'_m is the translated MRI image from x_c; x'_c is the translated MRI image from x_m.

2.1   Cross-domain Adaptation for Hallucinating Pseudo MR Images

A pair of conditional GANs [11] are trained with unpaired CT and T2-weighted (T2w) MR images arising from different sets of patients. The first GAN transforms CT into a pseudo MR (pMR) image $(G_{C \to M})$ while the second, transforms a MR image into its corresponding pseudo CT (pCT) $(G_{M \to C})$ image. The GANs are optimized using the standard adversarial loss $(L_{adv} = L^{CT}_{adv} + L^{MR}_{adv})$ and cycle consistency losses $(L_{cycl} = L^{CT}_{cycl} + L^{MR}_{cycl})$. In addition, we employed a contextual loss that was introduced for real-world images [12] in order to handle learning from image sets lacking spatial correspondence. The contextual loss facilitates such transformations by treating images as collection of features and computing a global similarity between all pairs of features between the two images

($\{g_{j \in N}, m_{i \in M}\}$) used in computing domain adaptation. The contextual similarity is expressed as:

$$CX(g, m) = \frac{1}{N} \sum_j \max_i CX(g_j, m_i), \qquad (1)$$

where, N corresponds to the number of features. The contextual similarity is computed by normalizing the inverse of cosine distances between the features in the two images as described in [12]. The contextual loss is computed as:

$$L_{cx} = -log(CX(f(G(X_{CT})), f(X_{MR})). \qquad (2)$$

The total loss for the cross-modality adaptation is then expressed as the summation of all the aforementioned losses. The pMR generated from this step is passed as an additional input for training the CT segmentation network.

2.2   Segmentation Combining CT with pMR Images

Our approach for combining the CT with pMR images uses the idea of only matching information that is highly predictable from each other. This usually corresponds to the features closest to the output as the two images are supposed to produce identical segmentation. Therefore, the features computed from the last two layers of CT and pMR segmentation networks are matched by minimizing the squared difference or the L2 loss between them. This is expressed as below.

$$L_{seg} = \mathbb{E}_{x_c \sim X_{CT}}[-logP(S_{MR}(G_{CT \to MR}(x_c))) - logP(S_{CT}(x_c))] \\ + \|\phi_{CT}(x_c) - \phi_{MR}(G_{CT \to MR}(x_c))\|_F^2, \qquad (3)$$

where S_{CT}, S_{MR} are the segmentation networks trained using the CT and pMR images, ϕ_{CT}, ϕ_{MR} are the features computed from these networks, and $G_{CT \to MR}$ is the cross-modality network used to compute the pMR image, and F stands for Frobenius norm.

The total loss computed from the cross-modality adaptation and the segmentation networks is expressed as:

$$\text{Loss} = L_{adv} + \lambda_{cyc}L_{cyc} + \lambda_{cx}L_{CX} + \lambda_{seg}L_{seg}, \qquad (4)$$

where λ_{cyc}, λ_{cx} and λ_{seg} are the weighting coefficients for each loss. During training, we alternatively update the cross-domain adaptation network and the segmentation network with the following gradients, $-\Delta_{\theta_G}(L_{adv} + \lambda_{cyc}L_{cyc} + \lambda_c L_c + \lambda_{cx}L_{cx})$, $-\Delta_{\theta_D}(L_{adv})$ and $-\Delta_{\theta_{seg}}L_{seg}$. More concretely, the segmentation network is fixed when updating the cross-modality translation and vice versa in each iteration.

2.3   Segmentation Architecture

We implemented the U-net [13] and dense fully convolutional networks (dense-FCN) [14] to evaluate the feasibility of combining hallucinated MR for improving CT segmentation accuracy. These networks are briefly described below.

1. **U-net** was modified using batch normalization after each convolution filter in order to standardize the features computed at the different layers.
2. **Fully Convolutional DenseNets** (Dense-FCN) that is based on [14], uses dense feature maps computed using a sequence of dense feature blocks and concatenated with feature maps from previous computations through residual connections. Specifically, a dense feature block is produced by iterative summation of previous feature maps within that block. As features computed from all image resolutions starting from the image resolution to the lowest resolution are iteratively concatenated, features at all levels are utilized. This in turn facilitates an implicit dense supervision to stabilize training.

2.4   Implementation and Training

All networks were implemented using the Pytorch [15] library and trained end to end on Tesla V100 with 16 GB memory and a batch size of 2. The ADAM algorithm [16] with an initial learning rate of 1e-4 was used during training. The segmentation networks were trained with a learning rate of 2e-4. We set $\lambda_{adv} = 10$, $\lambda_{cx} = 1$, $\lambda_{cyc} = 1$ and $\lambda_{seg} = 5$. For the contextual loss, we use the convolution filters after the Con7, Conv8 and Conv9 due to memory limitations.

3   Datasets and Evaluation

We used patients obtained from three different cohorts consisting of (a) the Cancer Imaging Archive (TCIA) [17] with non-small cell lung cancers (NSCLC) [18] consisting of 377 patients (training), (b) 81 longitudinal T2-weighted MR scans (scanned on Philips 3T Ingenia) from 21 patients treated with radiation therapy, and (training) (c) 637 contrast-enhanced tumors treated with immunotherapy at our institution for validation (N = 304) and testing (N = 333) such that different sets of patients were used for validation and testing. Early stopping was used during the training to prevent overfitting and the best model selected using validation set was used for testing. Identical CT datasets were used in both CT only and CMEDL approach for equitable comparisons. Expert segmentations were available on all scans.

The segmentation accuracies were evaluated using Dice similarity coefficient (DSC) and Hausdorff distance at 95th percentile (HD95) as recommended in [19]. In addition, we computed the detection rate for the tumors where tumors with at least 50% DSC overlap with expert segmentations were considered as detected.

4   Results

4.1   Tumor Detection Rate

Our method achieved the most accurate detection using both U-net and Dense-FCN methods for validation and test sets. In comparison the CT-only method resulted in much lower detection rates for both networks (Table 1).

Table 1. Detection and segmentation accuracy using the two networks.

Method	Validation			Test		
	Detection rate	DSC	HD95 mm	Detection rate	DSC	HD95 mm
U-net CT	80%	0.67 ± 0.18	7.44 ± 7.18	79%	0.68 ± 0.17	9.35 ± 7.08
DenseFCN CT	77%	0.70 ± 0.15	7.25 ± 6.71	75%	0.68 ± 0.16	9.34 ± 9.68
U-net CMEDL	85%	0.71 ± 0.15	6.57 ± 7.15	85%	0.72 ± 0.14	8.22 ± 6.89
DenseFCN CMEDL	84%	0.74 ± 0.12	5.89 ± 5.87	84%	0.73 ± 0.12	7.19 ± 8.55

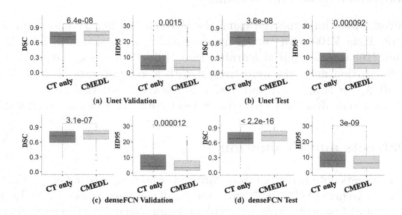

Fig. 2. Box plots comparing CT-only and CMEDL-based networks.

4.2   Segmentation Accuracies

The CMEDL approach resulted in more accurate segmentations than CT-only segmentations (see Table 1). In addition, both of the U-net and denseFCN networks trained using CMEDL approach were significantly more accurate than CT only segmentations when evaluated with both DSC ($P < 0.001$) and HD95 ($P < 0.001$) metrics. Figure 2 shows the box plots for the validation and test sets using the two metrics and the two networks. P-values computed using paired Wilcoxon two-sided tests are also shown.

4.3   Visual Comparisons

Figure 3 shows visual segmentation results produced by the different networks for representative cases when trained using CT-only and with the CMEDL approach. As seen, in both networks, the CMEDL method closely follows the expert-segmentation that is missed using CT-only networks. Figure 4 shows the feature map activations produced using U-net CT only and with Unet CMEDL. As seen, the feature activations are minimal when using CT-only but shows a clear preferential boundary activation when incorporating the MR information. Figure 4(b) also shows a pseudo MR produced from a CT (Fig. 4(a)).

5   Discussion

We developed a novel approach for segmenting lung tumors located in areas with low soft-tissue contrast by leveraging learned prior information from more informative MR modality. These cross-modality priors are learned from unrelated patients and are used to hallucinate MRI to inform CT segmentation. Through extensive experiments on two different network architectures, we showed that leveraging a more informative modality (MRI) to inform inference in a less informative modality (CT), improves segmentation. Our work is limited by lack of sufficiently large MR datasets to potentially improve the accuracy of cross-domain adaptation models. Nevertheless, this is the first approach to our knowledge that used the cross-modality information in a novel way to generate CT segmentation.

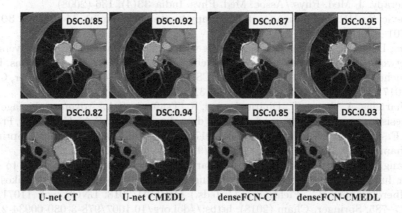

Fig. 3. Representative segmentations produced using CT-only and CMEDL-based segmentations for U-net and DenseFCN networks. The Dice similarity coefficient (DSC) is also shown for each method. Red corresponds to algorithm, green to expert and yellow to overlap between algorithm and expert. (Color figure online)

228   J. Jue et al.

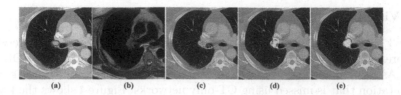

Fig. 4. Feature map activations from the 21 channel of last layer of Unet. (a) the original CT (b) the translated pMRI (c) activation from CT only (d) activation from pMRI (e) activation from CMEDL

6 Conclusions

We introduced a novel approach for segmenting on CT datasets that can leverage more informative MR modality through cross-modality learning. Our approach implemented on two different segmentation architectures shows improved performance over CT-only methods.

Acknowledgements. This work was supported by the MSK Cancer Center support grant/core grant P30 CA008748, and NCI R01 CA198121-03.

References

1. Njeh, C.: Tumor delineation: the weakest link in the search for accuracy in radiotherapy. J. Med. Phys./Assoc. Med. Phys. India **33**(4), 136 (2008)
2. Devic, S.: MRI simulation for radiotherapy treatment planning. Med. Phys. **39**(11), 6701–6711 (2012)
3. Nie, D., et al.: Medical image synthesis with context-aware generative adversarial networks. In: Descoteaux, M., Maier-Hein, L., Franz, A., Jannin, P., Collins, D.L., Duchesne, S. (eds.) MICCAI 2017. LNCS, vol. 10435, pp. 417–425. Springer, Cham (2017). https://doi.org/10.1007/978-3-319-66179-7_48
4. Chartsias, A., Joyce, T., Dharmakumar, R., Tsaftaris, S.A.: Adversarial image synthesis for unpaired multi-modal cardiac data. In: Tsaftaris, S.A., Gooya, A., Frangi, A.F., Prince, J.L. (eds.) SASHIMI 2017. LNCS, vol. 10557, pp. 3–13. Springer, Cham (2017). https://doi.org/10.1007/978-3-319-68127-6_1
5. Jiang, J., et al.: Tumor-aware, adversarial domain adaptation from CT to MRI for lung cancer segmentation. In: Frangi, A.F., Schnabel, J.A., Davatzikos, C., Alberola-López, C., Fichtinger, G. (eds.) MICCAI 2018. LNCS, vol. 11071, pp. 777–785. Springer, Cham (2018). https://doi.org/10.1007/978-3-030-00934-2_86
6. Zhu, J.Y., Park, T., Isola, P., Efros, A.: Unpaired image-to-image translation using cycle-consistent adversarial networks. In: International Conference Computer Vision (ICCV), pp. 2223–2232 (2017)
7. Long, M., Zhu, H., Wang, J., Jordan, M.I.: Deep transfer learning with joint adaptation networks. In: Proceedings of the 34th International Conference on Machine Learning, vol. 70, pp. 2208–2217. JMLR. org (2017)
8. Kamnitsas, K., et al.: Efficient multi-scale 3D CNN with fully connected CRF for accurate brain lesion segmentation. Med. Image Anal. **36**, 61–78 (2017)

9. Vanya, V.V., et al.: Multi-modal learning from unpaired images: application to multi-organ segmentation in CT and MRI. In: 2018 IEEE Winter Conference on Applications of Computer Vision, WACV 2018, Lake Tahoe, NV, USA, 12–15 March 2018, pp. 547–556 (2018)
10. Cai, J., Zhang, Z., Cui, L., Zheng, Y., Yang, L.: Towards cross-modal organ translation and segmentation: a cycle-and shape-consistent generative adversarial network. Med. Image Anal. **52**, 174–184 (2019)
11. Goodfellow, I., et al.: Generative adversarial nets. In: Advances in Neural Information Processing Systems (NIPS), pp. 2672–2680 (2014)
12. Mechrez, R., Talmi, I., Zelnik-Manor, L.: The contextual loss for image transformation with non-aligned data. In: Ferrari, V., Hebert, M., Sminchisescu, C., Weiss, Y. (eds.) Computer Vision – ECCV 2018. LNCS, vol. 11218, pp. 800–815. Springer, Cham (2018). https://doi.org/10.1007/978-3-030-01264-9_47
13. Ronneberger, O., Fischer, P., Brox, T.: U-net: convolutional networks for biomedical image segmentation. In: Navab, N., Hornegger, J., Wells, W.M., Frangi, A.F. (eds.) MICCAI 2015. LNCS, vol. 9351, pp. 234–241. Springer, Cham (2015). https://doi.org/10.1007/978-3-319-24574-4_28
14. Jégou, S., Drozdzal, M., Vazquez, D., Romero, A., Bengio, Y.: The one hundred dred layers tiramisu: fully convolutional densenets for semantic segmentation. In: 2017 IEEE Conference on Computer Vision and Pattern Recognition Workshops (CVPRW), pp. 1175–1183. IEEE (2017)
15. Paszke, A., et al.: Automatic differentiation in pytorch (2017)
16. Kingma, D.P., Ba, J.: Adam: a method for stochastic optimization. In: Proceedings of the 3rd International Conference on Learning Representations (ICLR) (2014)
17. Clark, K., et al.: The cancer imaging archive (TCIA): maintaining and operating a public information repository. J. Digit. Imaging **26**(6), 1045–1057 (2013)
18. Aerts, H.J., et al.: Decoding tumour phenotype by noninvasive imaging using a quantitative radiomics approach. Nat. Commun. **5**, 4006 (2014)
19. Menze, B.H., et al.: The multimodal brain tumor image segmentation benchmark (BRATS). IEEE Trans. Med. Imaging **34**(10), 1993 (2015)

Bronchus Segmentation and Classification by Neural Networks and Linear Programming

Tianyi Zhao[1,2], Zhaozheng Yin[1(✉)], Jiao Wang[2], Dashan Gao[2],
Yunqiang Chen[2], and Yunxiang Mao[2]

[1] Missouri University of Science and Technology, Rolla, MO, USA
yinz@mst.edu
[2] 12 Sigma Technologies, San Diego, CA, USA

Abstract. Airway segmentation is a critical problem for lung disease analysis. However, building a complete airway tree is still a challenging problem because of the complex tree structure, and tracing the deep bronchi is not trivial in CT images because there are numerous small airways with various directions. In this paper, we develop two-stage 2D+3D neural networks and a linear programming based tracking algorithm for airway segmentation. Furthermore, we propose a bronchus classification algorithm based on the segmentation results. Our algorithm is evaluated on a dataset collected from 4 resources. We achieved the dice coefficient of 0.94 and F1 score of 0.86 by a centerline based evaluation metric, compared to the ground-truth manually labeled by our radiologists.

Keywords: Airway segmentation · 2D+3D neural network · Linear programming · Tracking · Bronchus classification

1 Introduction

Airway segmentation is to segment the airway tree volume from the lung CT images. The airway tree can provide valuable information (e.g., the length and thickness of airways, the bronchus wall thickness [9], bronchus categories [10], etc.) for airway disease diagnosis (e.g. Chronic Obstructive Pulmonary Disease (COPD)). Morphological and machine learning [6,9] algorithms have been developed to solve the airway segmentation problem. Recently, the airway segmentation also draws a lot of attentions in the deep learning community, e.g., 3D Unet [1,2,4,7], Convolutional Neural Networks (CNN) with leakage detection [8], and 2.5D CNN [5].

However, the complex tree structure of lung airways makes the airway segmentation and bronchus classification problem challenging. There are three main challenges to be solved: (1) Horizontal airways. Since in CT the resolution on z-axis is not as high as x/y-axis, the horizontal airway sometimes is not tube-like, as shown in Fig. 1(a). Horizontal airways frequently appear in the middle lobe

D. Shen et al. (Eds.): MICCAI 2019, LNCS 11769, pp. 230–239, 2019.
https://doi.org/10.1007/978-3-030-32226-7_26

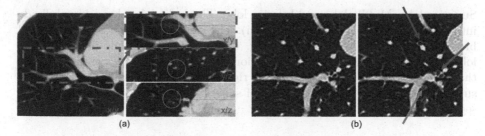

(a)   (b)

Fig. 1. Two airway segmentation challenges: (a) horizontal airway (indicated by yellow circle regions) at the y/z and x/z plane does not show a tube-like transection; (b) thin airways from different segmental bronchi (indicated by different arrows). (Color figure online)

and the anterior portion in the superior lobe, as shown in Fig. 2; (2) Thin airways. The thickness of airways gradually decreases from the trachea to the tips of airway tree, which leads to many thin airways, as shown in Fig. 1(b). Segmenting the large amount of thin airways is critical to obtain the complete airway tree. (3) Various bronchi. Although each bronchus has some common characteristics (direction, sequence order) summarized by radiologists, the practical bronchi from different patients exhibit various appearances and shapes (e.g., Fig. 9).

The above challenges motivate us to propose a new framework for airway segmentation and bronchus classification with three contributions: (1) a 2D+3D Neural Network (NN) is proposed to segment both vertical tube-like airways and horizontal airways; (2) a 2-stage NN with a tracking algorithm is proposed to segment and link small airway branches. The first-stage NN focuses on the trachea and main bronchus. The second-stage NN focuses on the lobar and segmental bronchus. A linear-programming based object tracking algorithm is deployed to connect the segmented airways from the two stages; and (3) a linear programming based bronchus classification algorithm is proposed to classify bronchus segments based on their characteristics in the airway tree structure.

2   Preliminaries

2.1   Airway Structure

Figure 2 shows the airway structure of a human. Each person has left lung and right lung. The trachea enters each lung and then separates into left main bronchus and right main bronchus. The right main bronchus divides into 3 lobar bronchi (secondary bronchi):

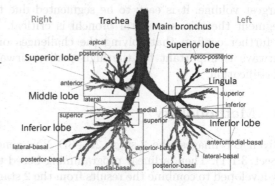

Fig. 2. Airway structure.

Superior lobe, Middle lobe and Inferior lobe. Then, the lobar bronchi subdivide into segmental bronchi (tertiary bronchi). The right lung contains 10 segmental bronchi in total. Unlike the right lung, the left main bronchus divides into 2 lobar bronchi (Superior lobe and Inferior lobe). The left lung contains a part that is similar to the middle lobe in the right lung, but it is inside the left lung's superior lobe, which is called Lingula of superior lobe. The left lung contains 8 segmental bronchi.

Table 1. Mean and distribution of the bronchus direction.

Bronchi	apical	posterior	anterior	lateral	medial	superior	anterior-basal	...
Direction (x,y,z)	(-0.83, 0.02, 0.56)	(-0.92, -0.01, 0.37)	(-0.92, 0.37, 0.11)	(-0.91, 0.33, -0.24)	(-0.81, 0.47, -0.36)	(-0.51, 0.09, -0.86)	(-0.55, 0.22, -0.81)	...
Distribution								...

Table 2. The volume and transection area of bronchi at different levels.

Bronchi	Trachea	Main bronchus	Lobar bronchus	Segmental bronchus
Volume	$14.53 \, cm^3$	$4.70 \, cm^3$	$3.11 \, cm^3$	$6.14 \, cm^3$
Area	$2.61 \, cm^2$	$0.93 \, cm^2$	$0.25 \, cm^2$	$0.09 \, cm^2$

2.2 Statistics on Horizontal Airways and Thin Airways

The average direction and the distribution of the angle between each bronchus and the xy-plane in the right lung are shown in Table 1. The posterior, anterior, lateral and medial bronchi are more horizontal than others. The total volume (amount) and the transection area (thickness) of bronchi at different levels are summarized in Table 2. We observe that segmental bronchus is very thin, but its quantity is the second largest in the lung. Though the large trachea has the largest volume, it is easy to be segmented due to its large size. Thus, how to segment the thin segmental bronchi is critical. The statistics in Tables 1 and 2 further confirm that solving the challenges on horizontal airways and thin airways is important for the high-quality airway segmentation and bronchus classification.

3 Methodology

Given CT images, the 2-stage 2D+3D NNs generate the airway segmentation (Sect. 3.1.1). Then, a linear programming based tracking algorithm (Sect. 3.1.2) is developed to combine the results from the 2 stages. The bronchus classification algorithm is introduced in Sect. 3.2, based on the airway segmentation result.

3.1 Airway Segmentation

3.1.1 2-Stage 2D+3D Neural Networks

In CT images, the resolution on z axis is not as high as x/y axis. 3D networks can segment tube-like vertical airways but it may not work well on the horizontal bronchus due to its large appearance difference compared to the vertical airways. Thus, we propose a 2D network on the xy-plane to better detect horizontal airways and a 3D network focusing on other airways.

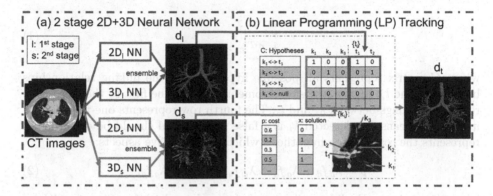

Fig. 3. Airway segmentation framework.

Our 3D NN structure is similar to the 3D Unet structure [1]. It contains 15 fully convolutional layers. The first 9 layers downsize the feature map and the following layers upsize the feature map following the deconvlotional layer with skip connection. Our 2D NN structure is a simple fully convolutional network [3], which contains 11 layers. The filter size is fixed as 3 for each layer. The number of kernels in each layer is: 64, 64, 128, 128, 256, 256, 128, 128, 64, 64, and 2.

Since the thickness from the trachea to the segmental bronchus decreases dramatically, one network may not segment the complete airway structure well. We propose a 2-stage design to handle the large-scale change: the first-stage 2D+3D network ($2D_l + 3D_l$) is trained by the whole airway data; the second-stage 2D+3D network ($2D_s + 3D_s$) is trained by the segmental bronchus data.

As shown in Fig. 3(a), $2D_l$ NN and $3D_l$ NN are ensembled by the average operation, resulting in a 'big picture' of the airway (d_l), and $2D_s$ NN and $3D_s$ NN are ensembled by the maximum operation, yielding the fine details of the airway structure (d_s). d_l and d_s are connected by the following Linear Programming based tracking algorithm.

3.1.2 Linear Programming Based Tracking

After ensembling the segmentation results from the 2-stage 2D+3D Networks and applying the thresholding (threshold h) and 3D connected component analysis, there are some false positive segmentation and some segmented airways may be broken from the airway tree. Thus, we propose a linear programming based tracking (LP-Tracking) to filter out false positives and connect the broken components to the airway tree.

Firstly, the overlapped segmentation between d_l and d_s is removed from d_s: $d'_s = d_s \setminus d_l$. In one CT slice (xy-plane), a list of 2D connected components are included in d'_s: $\{k_i\} \in d'_s$. In the previous and current slice, a list of 2D connected components are included in d_l: $\{t_i\} \in d_l$. Then, the linear programming based tracking is to find the best linking relationship between $\{k_i\}$ and $\{t_i\}$ by solving the following optimization problem:

$$\min_x p^T x$$
$$s.t.\ C^T x \geq 1 \tag{1}$$

where C matrix represents all possible hypotheses of the linking relationships between k_i and t_i. Figure 3(b) shows some examples. The first to the third rows represent linkings between k_i and t_i. The fourth row represents one-to-null linking, which means the detected k_i is a false positive and should be discarded. p represents the cost of each hypothesis which considers five aspects:

$$p = \lambda_d f_d + \lambda_a f_a + \lambda_w f_w + \lambda_r f_r + \lambda_g f_g. \tag{2}$$

where (1) f_d is the Euclidean distance between k_i and t_i, $f_d = ||centroid(k_i) - centroid(t_i)||$, as shown in Fig. 4; (2) f_a measures the area change from k_i to t_i, $f_a = max(area(k_i)/area(t_i), area(t_i)/area(k_i))$; (3) f_w is the length of the minor axis of the fitting ellipse that has the same normalized second central moments as k_i; (4) f_r = the aspect ratio of the ellipse. When the airway transection is long and thin, it probably is a missed airway; and (5) f_g is the angle between two directions: the first direction is from the centroid of t_i to the centroid of k_i, and the second direction is from the centroid of the trachea to the centroid of t_i. The five costs are normalized by dividing their maximum values. If in a hypothesis, k_i is a false-positive, p is set as a constant value 0.5. Solution x is the best linking relationship corresponding to the lowest cost. If $x_i = 1$, the ith

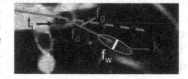

Fig. 4. f_d, f_w, and f_g costs.

hypothesis is chosen, i.e., the connection represented by the hypothesis is established. Otherwise, the connection hypothesis is discarded. The constraint in the optimization in Eq. 1 enforces the 2D connected component k_i or t_i to appear at least once.

3.2   Bronchus Classification

Based on the above segmentation, we develop a bronchus classification algorithm to classify bronchi into one of the 5 lobes and 18 segmental bronchi as shown in Fig. 2. The classification algorithm consists of 6 steps:

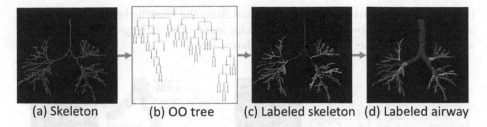

(a) Skeleton   (b) OO tree   (c) Labeled skeleton   (d) Labeled airway

Fig. 5. Bronchus classification flow.

(1) A skeleton is extracted from the segmented result, as shown in Fig. 5(a). The $3 \times 3 \times 3$ neighborhood of each pixel is examined and the exterior pixels are removed iteratively, until the data do not change.

(2) An object-oriented (OO) tree is generated from the skeleton based on the width-first search from the root (the start of the trachea), as shown in Fig. 5(b). From the root of the skeleton to the leaf, if a voxel has only one neighbor, it is considered as an end (root or leaf) voxel. If a voxel has two neighbors, it is considered as an edge voxel. If a voxel has more than two neighbors, it is considered as a vertex voxel (a division point). The edge or vertex object in the tree contains the corresponding voxels as attributes. Two vertexes are connected by an edge (edge objects are attributes of the vertex class).

(3) After the tree is constructed, some short **edges are removed**. Firstly if two vertexes are connected by a short edge, these two vertexes and the edge will be combined as one vertex. Secondly, if an end has a low depth in the tree, and the edge between this end and the vertex is short (<7). This end and the edge is discarded. Note that a leaf end usually has a depth more than 10.

(4) The lobar bronchi are classified based on the anatomy of the airway structure in Fig. 2, i.e., the superior lobar bronchi are first divided from the main bronchi, then the middle and inferior lobes.

(5) The segmental bronchi in each lobe are classified by a linear programming algorithm. After the lobar bronchi are labeled, we get the vertex of the root of the lobar bronchus. The descendants of the lobar root are collected as the segmental bronchi candidates $\{a_i\}$. The defined segmental bronchi in a lobe is noted as $\{b_i\}$, i.e., the 18 segmental bronchi in Fig. 2. The linear programming hypotheses are defined as shown in Fig. 6. p is calculated by the difference between the angle of the candidate (a_i in Fig. 6) and the average angle of the segmental bronchi (Table 1). Unlike the LP-tracking algorithm, the bronchus classification algorithm does not consider the false positive. All candidates should be assigned to the corresponding segmental bronchi. For the n-to-1 linking (e.g., the 3rd row in Fig. 6), p adds an additional term: the angle between two candidates. Different from Eq. 1, the constraint here is $C^T x = 1$, which enforces that the component k_i or t_i can not appear in two conflict hypotheses. Finally, a skeleton is constructed based on the tree with bronchus labels, as shown in Fig. 5(c).

(6) **The labeled airway tree** is rendered from the classified skeleton, as shown in Fig. 5(d). The label of each voxel in the segmented airway (from Sect. 3.1) is assigned by the label of the nearest skeleton voxel.

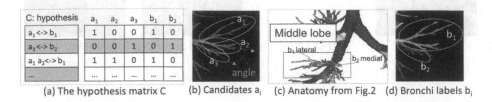

C: hypothesis	a_1	a_2	a_3	b_1	b_2
$a_1 \leftrightarrow b_1$	1	0	0	1	0
$a_3 \leftrightarrow b_2$	0	0	1	0	1
$a_1 a_2 \leftrightarrow b_1$	1	1	0	1	0
...	...	...	...	...	...

(a) The hypothesis matrix C   (b) Candidates a_i (c) Anatomy from Fig.2   (d) Bronchi labels b_i

Fig. 6. Linear programming for bronchus classification.

4   Experiments

4.1   Dataset

We validate our approach on a dataset collected from 4 resources: The Lung Image Database Consortium (LIDC) [11] (9 sets of CT images), The Lung Tissue Research Consortium (LTRC) [12] (20 sets of CT images), The National Lung Screening Trial (NLST) [13] (15 sets of CT images), and one from our collaborative hospital (PH, 30 sets of CT images). In total, 72 sets of CT images are collected and annotated by our radiologists. 40 sets are used for training. 10 sets are used for validation. The rest 22 sets are used for testing.

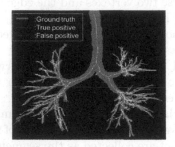

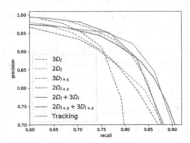

Fig. 7. Centerline based evaluation.   **Fig. 8.** Precision and recall curves.

4.2   Training Details

Feeding the whole 3D lung volume into a 3D segmentation network is too memory consuming. We crop volume of interests (VOIs) with $80 \times 80 \times 72$ pixels. The stride size is 48. During training, a VOI with any positive pixel inside is fed to the input to the 3D NN. A VOI without any positive pixel has a probability of 20% to be fed into the network. If one VOI is not discarded, 5 VOIs are randomly selected around the VOI. For the 2D NN, the input is a Region-of-Interest (ROI) with the size of 256×256 at the center of the slice. Both 2D and 3D NNs are trained by cross-entropy loss and stochastic gradient descent (SGD). The learning rate decreases from $1e-4$ to $1e-6$.

4.3   Evaluation

Table 3. Comparing different segmentation methods by the centerline based evaluation.

Method	Precision	Recall	F1-score
$3D_l$ [2]	0.911	0.751	0.824
$2D_l$ [3]	0.950	0.691	0.800
$3D_{l+s}$	0.820	0.848	0.833
$2D_{l+s}$	0.862	0.784	0.821
$2D_l + 3D_l$	**0.950**	0.768	0.849
$2D_{l+s} + 3D_{l+s}$	0.719	**0.900**	0.800
Tracking	0.931	0.810	**0.866**

We achieved the dice coefficient of 0.94 by comparing our segmentation with the ground truth. However, since the trachea is the main proportion of the airway volume and the trachea is not the main challenging part, the pixel-wise dice coefficient might not be the most suitable evaluation metric for this study. Thus, we proposed a centerline based evaluation metric, as shown in Fig. 7. To calculate the recall, the centerline of the ground truth is extracted, and the recall is the percentage that the centerline is detected in the predicted result. To calculate the precision, the centerline of the segmentation result is extracted, and the precision is the percentage that the detected centerline is true regarding to the ground truth. Quantitative comparisons are summarized in Table 3. Seven methods are compared: (1) $3D_l$ uses only one 3D Unet to generate the segmentation result; (2) $2D_l$ uses only one 2D FCN to generate the segmentation result; (3) $3D_{l+s}$ or (4) $2D_{l+s}$ ensemble **3D** or **2D** models from 2 stages, respectively; (5) $2D_l + 3D_l$ ensembles $2D_l$ and $3D_l$ model from the first stage; (6) $2D_{l+s} + 3D_{l+s}$ ensembles all four models; Finally, (7) **Tracking** combines the result from $2D_l + 3D_l$ and $2D_s + 3D_s$ by our LP-tracking algorithm. As we can see, the $2D_l + 3D_l$ method gets the best precision. When ensembling all 4 models, the precision decreases but the recall increases, which leads to the F1-score decreases. This is because of too many false-positives. Our LP-tracking algorithm combines the segmentation results from 4 models, filters out false-positives, and obtains the best F1-score. The precision and recall curve is shown in Fig. 8. The threshold h in Sect. 3.1.2 is selected from 0.1 to 0.6. We can see that the tracking result has a good balance on the precision and recall.

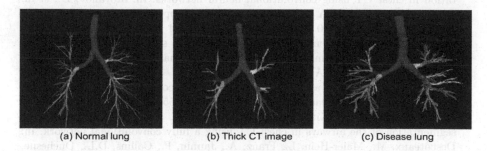

(a) Normal lung   (b) Thick CT image   (c) Disease lung

Fig. 9. Bronchus classification examples.

Our segment-wise segmental bronchus classification accuracy is 85%. Some examples are shown in Fig. 9. Figure 9(a) is from a healthy lung. Figure 9(b)

shows the result when the resolution on z-axis is low, causing the difficulties in airway segmentation and bronchus classification. Figure 9(c) is from a patient with lung diseases.

5   Conclusion

In this paper, we present 2-stage 2D+3D networks and linear programming based algorithms to attack the challenges in airway segmentation and bronchus classification, such as horizontal and thin airways, and bronchi with various appearances and shapes. The effectiveness of our method is evaluated on a dataset collected from four resources, showing competitive performance.

Acknowledgements. Tianyi Zhao and Zhaozheng Yin were partially supported by National Science Foundation (NSF) CAREER award IIS-1351049.

References

1. Ronneberger, O., Fischer, P., Brox, T.: U-net: convolutional networks for biomedical image segmentation. In: Navab, N., Hornegger, J., Wells, W.M., Frangi, A.F. (eds.) MICCAI 2015. LNCS, vol. 9351, pp. 234–241. Springer, Cham (2015). https://doi.org/10.1007/978-3-319-24574-4_28
2. Jin, D., Xu, Z., Harrison, A.P., George, K., Mollura, D.J.: 3D convolutional neural networks with graph refinement for airway segmentation using incomplete data labels. In: Wang, Q., Shi, Y., Suk, H.-I., Suzuki, K. (eds.) MLMI 2017. LNCS, vol. 10541, pp. 141–149. Springer, Cham (2017). https://doi.org/10.1007/978-3-319-67389-9_17
3. Zhao, T., Yin, Z.: Pyramid-based fully convolutional networks for cell segmentation. In: Frangi, A.F., Schnabel, J.A., Davatzikos, C., Alberola-López, C., Fichtinger, G. (eds.) MICCAI 2018. LNCS, vol. 11073, pp. 677–685. Springer, Cham (2018). https://doi.org/10.1007/978-3-030-00937-3_77
4. Juarez, A.G.-U., Tiddens, H.A.W.M., de Bruijne, M.: Automatic airway segmentation in chest CT using convolutional neural networks. In: Stoyanov, D., et al. (eds.) RAMBO/BIA/TIA -2018. LNCS, vol. 11040, pp. 238–250. Springer, Cham (2018). https://doi.org/10.1007/978-3-030-00946-5_24
5. Yun, J., et al.: Improvement of fully automated airway segmentation on volumetric computed tomographic images using a 2.5 dimensional convolutional neural net. Med. Image Anal. (MedIA) **51**, 13–20 (2019)
6. Bian, Z., et al.: Small airway segmentation in thoracic computed tomography scans: a machine learning approach. Phys. Med. Biol. **63**, 155024 (2018)
7. Meng, Q., Roth, H.R., Kitasaka, T., Oda, M., Ueno, J., Mori, K.: Tracking and segmentation of the airways in chest CT using a fully convolutional network. In: Descoteaux, M., Maier-Hein, L., Franz, A., Jannin, P., Collins, D.L., Duchesne, S. (eds.) MICCAI 2017. LNCS, vol. 10434, pp. 198–207. Springer, Cham (2017). https://doi.org/10.1007/978-3-319-66185-8_23
8. Charbonnier, J.-P., et al.: Improving airway segmentation in computed tomography using leak detection with convolutional networks. Med. Image Anal. (MedIA) **36**, 52–60 (2017)

9. Xu, Z., et al.: A hybrid method for airway segmentation and automated measurement of bronchial wall thickness on CT. Med. Image Anal. (MedIA) **24**, 1–17 (2015)
10. Mori, K., et al.: Automated anatomical labeling of the bronchial branch and its application to the virtual bronchoscopy system. IEEE-TMI **19**(2), 103–114 (2000)
11. Bidaut, L., et al.: The lung image database consortium (LIDC) and image database resource initiative (IDRI): a completed reference database of lung nodules on CT scans. Med. Phys. **38**, 915–931 (2011)
12. Bartholmai, B., et al.: The Lung Tissue Research Consortium: an extensive open database containing histological, clinical, and radiological data to study chronic lung disease. In: MICCAI Open Science Workshop (2006)
13. Clark, K., et al.: The Cancer Imaging Archive (TCIA): maintaining and operating a public information repository. J. Digit. Imaging **26**(6), 1045–1057 (2013)

Unsupervised Segmentation of Micro-CT Images of Lung Cancer Specimen Using Deep Generative Models

Takayasu Moriya[1], Hirohisa Oda[1], Midori Mitarai[1], Shota Nakamura[2], Holger R. Roth[1], Masahiro Oda[1], and Kensaku Mori[1,3,4(✉)]

[1] Graduate School of Informatics, Nagoya University, Nagoya, Japan
kensaku@is.nagoya-u.ac.jp
[2] Nagoya University Graduate School of Medicine, Nagoya, Japan
[3] Information Technology Center, Nagoya University, Nagoya, Japan
[4] Research Center for Medical Bigdata, National Institute of Informatics, Tokyo, Japan

Abstract. This paper presents a novel unsupervised segmentation method for the three-dimensional microstructure of lung cancer specimens in micro-computed tomography (micro-CT) images. Micro-CT scanning can nondestructively capture detailed histopathological components of resected lung cancer specimens. However, it is difficult to manually annotate cancer components on micro-CT images. Moreover, since most of the recent segmentation methods using deep neural networks have relied on supervised learning, it is also difficult to cope with unlabeled micro-CT images. In this paper, we propose an unsupervised segmentation method using a deep generative model. Our method consists of two phases. In the first phase, we train our model by iterating two steps: (1) inferring pairs of continuous and categorical latent variables of image patches randomly extracted from an unlabeled image and (2) reconstructing image patches from the inferred pairs of latent variables. In the second phase, our trained model estimates te probabilities of belonging to each category and assigns labels to patches from an entire image in order to obtain the segmented image. We apply our method to seven micro-CT images of resected lung cancer specimens. The original sizes of the micro-CT images were $1024 \times 1024 \times (544-2185)$ voxels, and their resolutions were $25-30\,\mu\text{m}$/voxel. Our aim was to automatically divide each image into three regions: invasive carcinoma, noninvasive carcinoma, and normal tissue. From quantitative evaluation, mean normalized mutual information scores of our results are 0.437. From qualitative evaluation, our segmentation results prove helpful for observing the anatomical extent of cancer components. Moreover, we visualize the degree of certainty of segmentation results by using values of categorical latent variables.

© Springer Nature Switzerland AG 2019
D. Shen et al. (Eds.): MICCAI 2019, LNCS 11769, pp. 240–248, 2019.
https://doi.org/10.1007/978-3-030-32226-7_27

1 Introduction

Recent research on deep generative models, such as variational auto-encoders (VAEs) [1] and generative adversarial networks (GANs) [2], have accelerated studies of unsupervised representation learning using neural networks. Meanwhile, however, most of the segmentation methods using neural networks still rely on supervised learning using manually labeled data. In this study, we present a deep generative model that can be used as a segmentation method by setting the number of categories in a dataset.

The proposed deep generative model has two major advantages. The first is that we can learn representations by considering the number of categories. In previous unsupervised segmentation methods using deep neural networks, the number of clusters had to be set to a value larger than the number of actual categories in a dataset [3,4]. Therefore, learned features are not necessarily suitable for segmenting into the desired number of categories. Our deep generative models overcome this problem. The second advantage is that we can assign labels to images without the use of external clustering algorithms such as k-means [5]. Previous unsupervised segmentation methods have adopted different methods for the feature learning and for the segmentation respectively (e.g. [3]). In that case, the features learned by unsupervised methods are not necessarily suitable for a clustering algorithm used in segmentation. Using our deep generative models, we eliminate the need to choose an appropriate clustering algorithm.

In this work, we evaluate our method on the micro-computed tomography (micro-CT) images of lung cancer specimens. Micro-CT scanning of resected lung specimens can nondestructively capture detailed structures of lung cancer specimens. If the observation of cancer components in 3D became possible with micro-CT images, histopathological diagnosis using micro-CT images could be used to support the current histopathological diagnosis based on microscopic images [6]. However, due to the difficulty of manually annotating cancer components on micro-CT images, it is not easy to acquire a sufficiently large dataset for training supervised segmentation methods using deep neural networks. Therefore, micro-CT images of lung cancer specimens are suitable for applying our proposed unsupervised segmentation method.

2 Methods

2.1 Overview

The underlying idea of our method is that deep generative models that allow the inference of the posterior category probabilities are applicable to image segmentation. Our method consists of a training phase and a segmentation phase. In the training phase, our method iterates two steps: (1) inferring of pairs of continuous and categorical latent variables of image patches randomly extracted from unlabeled 3D images and (2) reconstructing image patches from the inferred pairs of latent variables. In the segmentation phase, our trained network assigns labels to patches from a target image.

2.2   Deep Generative Model with Categorical Latent Variables

The proposed deep generative model learns feature representation for reconstructing an input image with categorical latent variables representing posterior category probabilities. Our deep generative model consists of three networks: (1) the encoder, (2) the generator, and (3) the code discriminator. The training process of our deep generative model is illustrated in Fig. 1.

The encoder estimates both continuous latent variables $z \in \mathbb{R}^d$ and categorical variables $y \in \mathbb{R}^k$ from observed input x. In the training phase, categorical variables are intended to play the role of controlling which categories of images the generator creates, while in the segmentation phase they become the posterior probabilities for determining segmentation labels. Note that the number of dimensions of the categorical variables is the same as the desired number of categories k. The generator reconstructs images based on both continuous latent variables z and categorical latent variables y of corresponding inputs.

The code discriminator distinguishes between the estimated latent variables and a certain prior distribution. It is used to impose latent variables on a more tractable distribution than the true distribution. In our method, a tractable prior of a continuous latent variable z is noise from the Gaussian distribution, and a prior of a categorical latent variable y is a one-hot vector from the uniform distribution. Unlike the previous code discriminators used in [7] and [8], our code discriminator copes with both continuous and categorical latent variables. To distinguish our code discriminator from the previous one, we call the new one a *unified code discriminator*. The architecture of the unified code discriminator is based on a projection discriminator [9], which distinguishes between real and generated images given both the image and the corresponding label. In the unified code discriminator, we take inner product between the embedded categorical latent variables and the intermediate features of continuous latent variables. There are two reason why we simultaneously cope with both latent variables in one network. One reason is that we can reduce parameters of our model. The other reason is to learn feature space where features belonging to different categories can be transformed smoothly and continuously each other. An explicit constraint of both latent variables is difficult, we adopt adversarial training.

2.3   Objective Function

Let $q_\eta(y, z|x)$, $G_\theta(y, z)$ and $C_\omega(y, z)$ denote the encoder, generator and unified code discriminator, respectively. Note that $q_\eta(y, z|x)$ is represented as an approximation of the true posterior $p(y, z|x)$. Moreover, let the distribution of the observed data be $p(x)$. The training of our the deep generative model is carried out to optimize the parameters of the encoder η, the generator θ, and the unified code discriminator ω. An objective function $\mathcal{L}$ of our deep generative model is defined as

$$\mathcal{L}(\theta, \eta, \omega) = \mathbb{E}_{p(x)} \left[\mathbb{E}_{q_\eta(y,z|x)} \left[\lambda \|x - G_\theta(y, z)\|_1 \right] \right.$$
$$\left. + D(q_\eta(y, z) \| p(y, z)) \right],$$

(1)

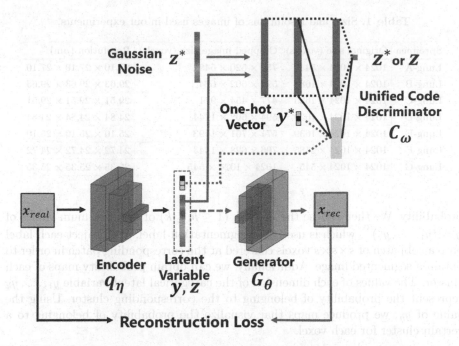

Fig. 1. Illustration of our deep generative model. We first input a real image x_{real} into the encoder q_η and obtain a categorical latent variable y and a continuous latent variable z. Next, the generator G_θ reconstructs an image x_{rec} from a pair of the latent variables. The unified code discriminator C_ω distinguishes between the pair of y^* and z^* and the pair of y and z. We update the parameters of networks using the unified code discriminator loss and L_1-norm reconstruction loss between x_{real} and x_{rec}.

where D is a divergence between $q_\eta(y, z|x)$ and $p(y, z)$, and λ is a hyperparameter for adjusting the L_1-norm reconstruction loss. While the VAE is not theoretically suitable for handing two type of latent variables, our objective function is similar to that of the Wasserstein auto-encoder (WAE) [10], that is, to minimize the optimal transport cost between the distributions of real images and generated images. Our deep generative model can be viewed as an extension of WAE designed to cope with categorical latent variables. In order to optimize the objective function, we alternately update θ, η and ω. As a training dataset, we extract N patches of $w \times w \times w$ voxels from the unlabeled target image to which we apply segmentation.

2.4 Segmentation

After training the deep generative models, we conduct labeling to obtain a segmentation result using a trained encoder. We first extract a certain number of patches of $w \times w \times w$ voxels from the target image separated by s voxels each and input them into the trained encoder. Given each patch, the trained encoder produces categorical latent variable y, which represents the posterior category

244   T. Moriya et al.

Table 1. Sizes and resolutions of images used in our experiments.

Specimen	Original size (voxels)	Cropped image size (voxels)	Resolution (μm)
Lung-A	1024 × 1024 × 544	756 × 520 × 545	27.10 × 27.10 × 27.10
Lung-B	1024 × 1024 × 1083	594 × 602 × 624	29.63 × 29.63 × 29.63
Lung-C	1024 × 1024 × 1625	477 × 454 × 971	29.51 × 29.51 × 29.51
Lung-D	1024 × 1024 × 1639	594 × 602 × 1244	24.84 × 24.84 × 24.84
Lung-E	1024 × 1024 × 1639	571 × 761 × 1193	25.10 × 25.10 × 25.10
Lung-F	1024 × 1024 × 2185	706 × 628 × 1243	24.72 × 24.72 × 24.72
Lung-G	1024 × 1024 × 545	1024 × 1024 × 545	25.35 × 25.35 × 25.35

probability. We then choose the index h ($1 \leq h \leq k$) of the maximum values of $\mathbf{y} = (y_1, \ldots, y_k)^{\mathrm{T}}$, which is used as a segmentation label. We project each label onto a subpatch of $s \times s \times s$ voxels centered at the corresponding patch in order to obtain a segmented image. Additionally, we can obtain probability maps of each cluster. The values of each dimension of the categorical latent variable $y_1, \ldots, y_k$ represent the probability of belonging to the corresponding cluster. Using the value of y_h, we produce maps that visualize the probability of belonging to a certain cluster for each voxel.

3   Experiments

3.1   Datasets

We used seven specimens of resected lung cancer tissue scanned with a micro-CT scanner (inspeXio SMX-90CT Plus, Shimadzu Corporation, Kyoto, Japan) to evaluate our proposed method. The lung cancer specimens from different patients were scanned with similar isotropic resolutions in the range of 25–30 μm. Each micro-CT volume consists of 544, 1083 and 1625 slices of 1024 × 1024 pixels. In order to eliminate background regions, which are not relevant to our task, and to reduce computational cost, we used cropped images. Detailed information for each image is shown in Table 1. We attempted to divide the images into three histopathological regions: (a) invasive carcinoma, (b) noninvasive carcinoma, and (c) normal tissue.

3.2   Parameter Settings

For training the deep generative model, we used 10,000 randomly extracted patches setting N to 10,000 and w to 32. We set the dimension of continuous and categorical latent variables d and k to 10 and 3, respectively. After the training, we extracted 32 × 32 × 32-voxel patches from unlabeled micro-CT images, setting a stride s to 5. We input them into the trained encoder and then assigned labels based on the values of categorical latent variables to obtain a segmented image. We also obtained probability maps directly using the values of categorical latent variables.

Table 2. Comparison of mean NMIs.

	Multi-Otsu	k-means	Deep generative model (proposed)
Lung-A	0.258	0.243	**0.457**
Lung-B	0.392	0.357	**0.436**
Lung-C	0.307	0.281	**0.424**
Lung-D	0.224	0.199	**0.423**
Lung-E	0.215	0.169	**0.377**
Lung-F	0.260	0.199	**0.459**
Lung-G	0.363	0.336	**0.484**

3.3 Evaluations

For quantitative evaluation, we used normalized mutual information (NMI). The range of NMI is 0 to 1, where a larger NMI value means better segmentation results. We measured mean NMI of several manually annotated slices. We used five annotated slices for Lung-A, six for Lung-B, seven for Lung-C and Lung-D, one for Lung-E, and 10 for Lung-F and Lung-G. We compared the proposed method with k-means segmentation and the multithreshold Otsu method. Table 2 shows comparisons of NMIs. Our proposed methods accomplished higher NMIs for all specimens.

Figure 2 shows the segmentation results and probability maps of Lung-F. In the segmentation results, the colors red, green, and blue are assigned to invasive carcinoma, noninvasive carcinoma, and normal tissue, respectively, after obtaining segmentation results whose colors were initially assigned at random. In the probability maps, voxel values represent probability, and their range is 0 to 1. Here, the red parts represent higher probability and the dark blue parts represent lower probability. The segmentation results show that our method effectively divided images into the three histopathological regions. Moreover, the probability map of each histopathological region shows high probabilities in that region.

We also visually evaluated the segmentation results by 3D volume rendering. Figure 3 shows the volume rendering of Lung-F and the results of labeling the segmentation results of the proposed methods. We only overlaid labels of invasive carcinoma and noninvasive carcinoma to emphasize cancer regions. In the volume rendering, we can observe the anatomical extent of lung cancer. Concretely, regions labeled as invasive carcinoma are seen as solid components, while regions labeled as noninvasive carcinoma are seen as thick walls of alveoli.

4   Discussion

The segmentation results show that our method succeeded in learning suitable features for separating histopathological regions. Furthermore, they suggest that features learned by our models are suitable not only for image reconstruction

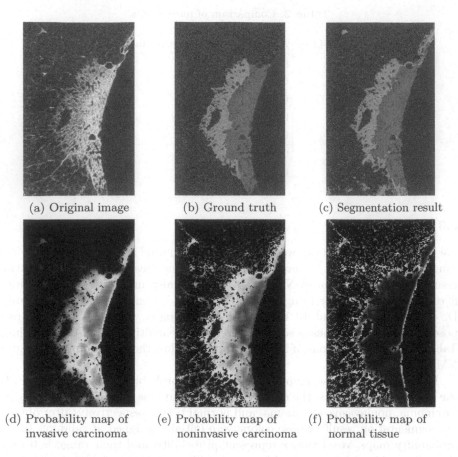

(a) Original image   (b) Ground truth   (c) Segmentation result

(d) Probability map of   (e) Probability map of   (f) Probability map of
invasive carcinoma   noninvasive carcinoma   normal tissue

Fig. 2. Segmentation results and probability maps of Lung-F. In (b) and (c), red, green and blue regions correspond to regions of invasive carcinoma, non-invasive carcinoma, and normal tissue, respectively. In (c), colors indicate the same cluster, but assigned at random. In (d), (e), and (f), red parts represent higher probability and blue parts represent lower probability. (Color figure online)

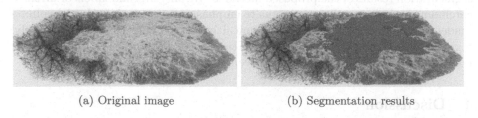

(a) Original image   (b) Segmentation results

Fig. 3. Volume rendering of segmentation results of Lung-F. In (b), red and green regions correspond to the region of invasive carcinoma and non-invasive carcinoma, respectively. For visibility, we omitted labels of normal tissue. (Color figure online)

but also for unsupervised segmentation. The probability maps, moreover, show that the result of our representation learning is close to the human sense of visual recognition. While the highest values of the probability maps of invasive carcinoma and normal tissue exceeded 0.9, those of noninvasive carcinoma were about 0.8. Generally, distinguishing noninvasive carcinoma from other regions on micro-CT images is more difficult for humans, even medical experts, than distinguishing invasive carcinoma from normal tissue. In our probability maps of each histopathological region, furthermore, the closer to the boundary of the region, the lower the probability becomes. These results suggest that regions with high probability mostly coincide with regions that are easy for humans to identify. Interestingly, our deep generative model mimics the human ability of visual recognition on micro-CT images without comparing image patches using an external clustering algorithm or using annotated labels.

5   Conclusion

We proposed a deep generative model specifically designed for unsupervised segmentation. Our method produced promising segmentation results for micro-CT images of lung cancer specimens. Moreover, the probability maps of the three histopathological regions functioned in a highly similar way to the capabilities of the human sense of visual recognition.

Acknowledgements. Parts of this work was supported by MEXT/JSPS KAKENHI (26108006, 17H00867, 17K20099, 26560255, 15H01116, 15K19933), the JSPS Bilateral Joint Research Project, AMED (19lk1010036h0001) and the Hori Sciences and Arts Foundation.

References

1. Kingma, D.P., Welling, M.: Auto-encoding variational bayes (2014)
2. Goodfellow, I., et al.: Generative adversarial nets. In: Advances in Neural Information Processing Systems, pp. 2672–2680 (2014)
3. Moriya, T., et al.: Unsupervised segmentation of 3D medical images based on clustering and deep representation learning. In: Medical Imaging 2018: Biomedical Applications in Molecular, Structural, and Functional Imaging, vol. 10578, p. 1057820. International Society for Optics and Photonics (2018)
4. Bulten, W., Litjens, G.: Unsupervised prostate cancer detection on H&E using convolutional adversarial autoencoders. In: Medical Imaging with Deep Learning (2018)
5. MacQueen, J., et al.: Some methods for classification and analysis of multivariate observations. In: Proceedings of the Fifth Berkeley Symposium on Mathematical Statistics and Probability, Oakland, CA, USA, vol. 1, pp. 281–297 (1967)
6. Nakamura, S., et al.: Micro-computed tomography of the lung: imaging of alveolar duct and alveolus in human lung. In: D55. Lab Methodology and Bioengineering: Just Do It, pp. A7411–A7411. American Thoracic Society (2016)
7. Makhzani, A., Shlens, J., Jaitly, N., Goodfellow, I.: Adversarial autoencoders. In: International Conference on Learning Representations (2016)

8. Rosca, M., Lakshminarayanan, B., Warde-Farley, D., Mohamed, S.: Variational approaches for auto-encoding generative adversarial networks. CoRR abs/1706.04987 (2017)
9. Miyato, T., Koyama, M.: cGANs with projection discriminator. In: International Conference on Learning Representations (2018)
10. Tolstikhin, I., Bousquet, O., Gelly, S., Schoelkopf, B.: Wasserstein auto-encoders. In: International Conference on Learning Representations (2018)

Normal Appearance Autoencoder for Lung Cancer Detection and Segmentation

Mehdi Astaraki[1,2(✉)], Iuliana Toma-Dasu[2], Örjan Smedby[1],
and Chunliang Wang[1]

[1] Department of Biomedical Engineering and Health Systems,
KTH Royal Institute of Technology, Hälsovägen 11C, 14157 Huddinge, Sweden
{mehast, chunwan}@kth.se

[2] Department of Oncology-Pathology, Karolinska Institutet,
Karolinska Universitetssjukhuset, Solna, 17176 Stockholm, Sweden

Abstract. One of the major differences between medical doctor training and machine learning is that doctors are trained to recognize normal/healthy anatomy first. Knowing the healthy appearance of anatomy structures helps doctors to make better judgement when some abnormality shows up in an image. In this study, we propose a normal appearance autoencoder (NAA), that removes abnormalities from a diseased image. This autoencoder is semi-automatically trained using another partial convolutional in-paint network that is trained using healthy subjects only. The output of the autoencoder is then fed to a segmentation net in addition to the original input image, i.e. the latter gets both the diseased image and a simulated healthy image where the lesion is artificially removed. By getting access to knowledge of how the abnormal region is supposed to look, we hypothesized that the segmentation network could perform better than just being shown the original slice. We tested the proposed network on the LIDC-IDRI dataset for lung cancer detection and segmentation. The preliminary results show the NAA approach improved segmentation accuracy substantially in comparison with the conventional U-Net architecture.

Keywords: Lung nodule segmentation · Anomaly detection · Convolutional variational autoencoder

1 Introduction

Lung cancer is the most frequently diagnosed cancer in the world which accounts for 12.9% of all cancers and 19.4% of cancer-related deaths. Approximately 70% of all lung cancers are diagnosed at advanced stages which resulted in a 5-year survival rate of 10–16%. However, the 5-year survival rate increases by 70% if lung cancer is diagnosed at early stages. Automatic detection of lung cancer and delineation of lung nodules/masses have been the focus of many research efforts of building Computer Aided Diagnosis (CAD) systems to help doctors to detect lung cancer early and classify them. Conventional CAD systems utilize rule-based algorithms including intensity-based approach, statistical modelling, and energy minimization schemes for nodule detection. Although many powerful rule-based methods have been proposed,

© Springer Nature Switzerland AG 2019
D. Shen et al. (Eds.): MICCAI 2019, LNCS 11769, pp. 249–256, 2019.
https://doi.org/10.1007/978-3-030-32226-7_28

accurately detection of non-trivial cases such as juxta-pleural or sub-solid nodules with cavities remains as challenging. Benefiting from hierarchical feature learning, Convolutional Neural Networks (CNN) shown promising results in lung nodule detection [1]. Accurately detecting/segmenting the pulmonary nodules have been achieved by supervised deep learning approaches that classify image patches or pixel centered in a receptive field to be lung nodule or not [2]. The majority of these methods rely on a large number of training samples to exhaustively cover all possible distributions of the image features of both classes. Therefore, the performance of CNN methods depends heavily on the quantity and quality of the training data. On the other hand, there are always theoretic risks of some rare disease appearances missing or under-represented in the training data, which could lead to detection failure [3]. One example is the ground-glass nodules that are known to be challenging even for CNNs. In contrast, radiologists are trained with a limited number of image samples and perform more robustly against different appearances of abnormalities [4]. One of the major differences between medical doctor training and machine learning is that doctors are trained to recognize normal/healthy anatomy first. Knowing the healthy appearance of anatomy structures helps doctors to make better judgement when some abnormality shows up in an image. In the field of deep learning, this idea has been recognized as "anomaly detection" and mostly implemented with autoencoders due to their ability in compressed representation [3, 5].

In this paper, we propose a normal appearance autoencoder (NAA), that removes abnormalities from a diseased image. This autoencoder is semi-automatically trained using another partial convolutional in-painting network. The output of the autoencoder is then fed to a segmentation net in addition to the original input image, i.e. the latter gets both the diseased image and a simulated healthy image where the lesion is artificially removed. By getting access to knowledge of how the abnormal region is supposed to look, we hypothesized that the segmentation network could perform better than just being shown the original slice. We tested the proposed network on the LIDC-IDRI dataset for lung cancer detection and segmentation. We demonstrate that the proposed approach outperformed the conventional ones and is comparable to state-of-the-art patch-based schemes.

2   Methods

The proposed method consists of three major steps. First, we train a partial convolutional network to in-paint the tumor/nodule region with healthy appearance. This is a semi-automatic step where manual annotation of the tumor region is required. In a second step, we used the trained inpainting network to generate training samples to train a NAA to automatically remove lung nodule/mass from the input images. Finally, the differences between the output of NAA and the original image are input to a U-Net like segmentation network, in addition to the original input image, for lung nodule segmentation. A schematic summary of the three steps is shown in Fig. 1. The individual steps are explained in detail in the following sections.

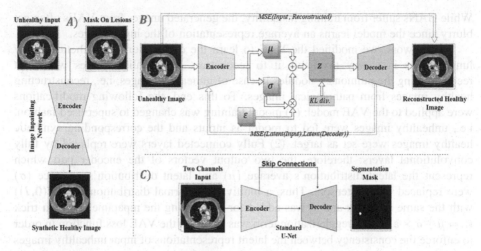

Fig. 1. Schematic illustration of the pipeline: (A) Partial-convolutional network for inpainting the nodules, (B) Semi-supervised fully convolutional variational autoencoder for reconstructing the unhealthy images without the nodules, (C) Two-channels U-Net for nodule segmentation.

2.1 Healthy Image Synthesis with Partial Convolutional Network

Removing a tumor from a lung image can be seen as an image inpainting problem, i.e., we consider the nodule location in the lung image as a hole and use the characteristics of rest of the lung region to produce semantically meaningful patterns in order to smoothly fill the hole. Partial convolutional network is a new inpainting technique that was recently introduced by NVIDIA, which is able to robustly handle holes with different sizes and arbitrary shapes at random locations [6]. In our study, the network is trained with chest CT images from healthy subjects with randomly generated corruption holes. In the testing phase, we used the segmentation masks of the nodules which were already provided by radiologist experts to identify the nodule locations which were, then, filled with healthy-appearing lung tissue by the trained network. Because the need of human annotation, this method is not suited for fully automatic lung cancer detection and segmentation tasks. However, this network provides training image pairs in which the lung nodules are artificially removed. Later we use the outputs of the inpainting network (mixed with other healthy training samples) to train an autoencoder to perform the same operation on diseased images, but automatically. All the results from this step were manually inspected and refined, if necessary. Therefore, for each of the unhealthy images, a synthetic healthy image is paired which is exactly similar to the main image except the nodule location that is replaced by healthy tissues.

2.2 Normal Appearance Autoencoder

We hypothesized that a lung image with nodules would be mapped into a highly similar representative latent space as the same image without the nodules. In deep learning field, Generative Adversarial Networks (GAN) and Variational Autoencoder (VAE) are two main approaches to estimate the complicated distributions of high-dimensional data.

While GANs suffer from training instability, the generated images from VAEs often get blurry since the model learns an average representation of the input images.

In this work, we modified the VAE to learn the distribution of synthetic-healthy lung images in a way to enable it to reconstruct high-quality images while not reconstructing the pulmonary nodules in case of unhealthy images, i.e., reconstructing healthy images from pathological images. To this end, the following modifications were applied to the VAE model: (1) model training was changed to supervised fashion, i.e., unhealthy images were fed to model as inputs and the corresponding synthetic healthy images were set as target. (2) Fully connected layers were replaced by fully convolutional layers; therefore, the two output vectors of the encoder part which represent the latent distribution's average (μ) and latent distribution's variance (σ) were replaced by two tensors. Thus, a multivariate normal distribution ($\varepsilon = N(0, I)$) with the same size of μ and σ, was added for performing the reparameterization trick ($z = \mu + \sigma \times \varepsilon$). (3) A regularization term was added to the VAE loss function in order to enforce the consistency between the latent representations of input unhealthy images and reconstructed healthy images [4]. (4) A weighting map was applied to the reconstruction loss in order to assign lower weight in the loss minimization process for the regions outside the lungs. Accordingly, we optimize our proposed framework with a multi-loss function which is not only beneficial for more accurate results but also minimizes the risk of overfitting:

$$
\begin{aligned}
L_{VAE} &= W.L_{rec} + L_{prior} + \alpha L_{reg} \\
&= W.MSE(x, \hat{x}) + D_{KL}\{z, N(0, I)\} \\
&\quad + \alpha.MSE\{z(x), z(\hat{x})\}
\end{aligned}
\tag{1}
$$

In the first term, MSE (mean square error) indicates the reconstruction loss between the input image and the reconstructed image. W represents a weighting map which contains values equals to one for the regions inside the lungs and declining values followed by a one-sided Gaussian pattern for the regions outside the lungs. In the second term, D_{KL} refers to Kullback-Leibler divergence between the distribution of the latent representation and a multivariate normal distribution. The third term represents the regularization term which minimizes the differences between the latent of the input and latent of the reconstructed images. The training samples used to train the NAA is a mixture of healthy image pairs (same image used on both ends) and the lung-nodule/synthetic-healthy image pairs.

2.3   Nodule Segmentation

Most of the anomaly detection-based models have been focused on detecting/segmenting the lesions by finding the differences between the input and reconstructed images of the VAEs following by post-processing steps. Such approaches have yielded encouraging results in brain lesion segmentation in magnetic resonance images [3, 4, 7]. However, in lung CT images the intensity similarity between the nodules and surrounding tissues will result in a large number of false positives after thresholding the differences between the input images and the reconstructed ones. Furthermore, the size of the nodules is too small to be retained after the post-processing steps. This issue also yields the presence of a remarkable number of false negatives. Hence, instead of performing the mentioned steps, we utilized the differences between the input and reconstructed images (ΔI) of the proposed VAE as a priori knowledge for the segmentation network to guide the attention of the model toward the candidates [8]. To this end, a two-channels input including original unhealthy images, and image differences (ΔI) were fed into the standard U-Net segmentation model. Since the nodules are highlighted in the second channel (ΔI), they catch more concentrations from hierarchical feature learning process and, thus, help the model to better identify the small nodules.

3 Experiments and Results

The Lung Image Database Consortium and Image Database Resource Initiative (LIDC–IDRI) has provided 1018 chest CT scans of diagnosed lung cancer patients. In this dataset, the acquisition parameters varied significantly. For example, slice thickness ranged from 0.6 mm to 5 mm and spatial resolution ranged from 0.5 mm to 1 mm. Regarding the very small size of the nodules, there is a high risk of losing critical information while isotropically resampling the 3D images. On the other hand, 2D image slices are not affected by slice thickness. Accordingly, we used 2D image slices in the axial view; however, in order to compensate for the lack of volumetric information we extracted three consecutive image slices around the nodule centers from each case. In total, we extracted 1175 image slices corresponding to the nodule centers, 1175 image slices prior to the centers and 1175 posterior images. Image intensities were converted to Hounsfield units and then normalized in the range of 0 to 1.

The inpainting model was identical to the one proposed in the original paper [6]. It was only modified to match the input image size of 512×512. The encoder part of the VAE includes 6 convolutional layers followed by a sampling layer to prepare the decoder inputs. The decoder part contains 6 transpose convolutional layers. The model was fed by a 3-channel input (prior, center and posterior slices) and therefore 3 images were reconstructed at the end. The reconstructed center image slices from the test-sets were then saved and their differences from the original inputs were calculated (ΔI) and set as the second channel for the segmentation network. The standard U-Net architecture was slightly modified to be matched with the input size of $512 \times 512 \times 2$, where the first channel is the original unhealthy images and the second channel is the corresponding image differences (ΔI). Both VAE and U-Net models were trained with Adam optimizer, and a batch size of 8. In order to perform a fair comparison, another experiment was performed by only feeding the original input images to the same segmentation network. The segmentation results were evaluated with 3 metrics including Dice coefficient, sensitivity, and Positive Predictive Value (PPV), and compared against the state of the art methods on the same dataset (see Table 1). Finally, it should be noticed that all the steps, including inpainting, nodule removal, and nodule segmentation were performed in a patient-wise 5-fold cross validation fashion. Figure 2 illustrates step by step examples of the pipeline.

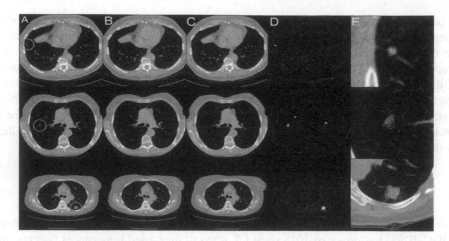

Fig. 2. Step by step examples of the results. Column A: represents the original input images containing nodules. Column B: shows the results of synthetic healthy images from inpainting model. Column C: represents the high-quality reconstructed images without the nodules from the VAE model. Column D: shows the differences between the input images and reconstructed images. Column E: segmentations resulted from two-channels U-Net model; the images are magnified around the nodules to better visualize the agreement between the manual (green) and algorithm (red) contours. (Color figure online)

Table 1. Segmentation accuracy over the test-sets. * denotes the results reported at [9] and ** refers to the reference [10]. For each case, the highest value is marked in bold.

Method	Criteria (Mean ± SD)		
	Dice	Sensitivity	Positive predictive value
A priori-based U-Net	**85.86 ± 1.24**	83.17 ± 2.67	**90.32 ± 2.38**
Single-channel U-Net	66.69 ± 2.85	59.22 ± 12.72	78.30 ± 10.78
Level Set*	60.63 ± 17.39	64.38 ± 22.75	71.03 ± 24.35
2-D Patch Branch*	80.47 ± 11.23	91.36 ± 14.40	74.64 ± 13.16
CF-CNN*	82.15 ± 10.76	**92.75 ± 12.83**	75.84 ± 13.14
TLBO**	82.73 ± 5.41	87.29 ± 9.52	86.03 ± 18.84

4 Discussion and Conclusion

The main contributions of the proposed method include: proposing a NAA to automatically replace lung nodules/masses with healthy appearing tissue, incorporation the output of NAA into a segmentation network for robust tumor segmentation, and proposing a NAA training scheme using semi-automated inpainting network. As the evaluation results show, adding the NAA a priori-knowledge to the segmentation network is beneficial and significantly improves the segmentation accuracy. It is worth noting that most previous studies have suggested patch base lung nodule segmentation methods are superior to the fully convolutional networks (such as U-net) [9, 10]. To the best of our knowledge, it is the first time to demonstrate a fully convolutional setup can deliver comparable results, if not better, to the patch-based solutions.

One of the underlying reasons for using unsupervised anomaly detection methods is the availability of healthy datasets in order to learn the distribution of healthy anatomical structures. However, in the case of lung images, the appearance of small nodules is very similar to healthy structures which confuse the learned latent representation and the model performance would significantly decrease. To address this issue, we trained the VAE model in a semi-supervised fashion by synthetically producing paired images. In our experiments, the unsupervised VAE worked only as a denoising autoencoder and was not able to remove even mid-size nodules. However, having changed the method to semi-supervised learning, the model was enforced to learn the healthy anatomical parts and successfully remove the nodules from reconstructed images.

Another advantage of the proposed pipeline is the high-quality reconstructed images of the VAE. In conventional VAEs, substantial spatial information will not be preserved due to the presence of fully-connected layers and therefore the reconstructed images will be too blurry to be useful for anomaly detection. In other words, many healthy tissues and vessels will be removed, and the reconstructed image will miss the valuable information. Even remarkably increasing the number of neurons in fully-connected layers or employing more sophisticated tricks such as matrix-variate normal distributions [11] was not helpful to improve the image quality in our experiments. On the other hand, we showed that using fully-convolutional layers in the latent space instead of fully-connected layers is not only helpful to preserve spatial information but also is quite beneficial to reconstruct high-quality images without the nodules and noise.

Although the complexity of the nodule characteristics makes it impossible to directly achieve accurate segmentation results from the output of the VAE, adding the difference images (ΔI) as a priori-information to the second channels of the U-Net inputs seems to be helpful to improve segmentation accuracy. Surprisingly, the presence of the a priori-information has increased the segmentation accuracy up to 19% in terms of Dice coefficient compared to one-channel U-Net. The overall segmentation accuracy of the proposed pipeline was compared against the results reported by the state of the art studies [9, 10], although they used different subsets of the same dataset. The superiority of the proposed method can be seen when the a priori-based U-Net outperformed the complicated patch-based methods in terms of Dice and PPV.

In conclusion, we have proposed an a priori-based image segmentation pipeline based on the ability of deep autoencoders to detect anomalies. The preliminary results are promising, and further developments will include adding adversarial learning to the proposed pipeline.

Acknowledgment. This study was supported by the Swedish Childhood Cancer Foundation (grant no. MT2016-0016) and the Swedish innovation agency Vinnova (grant no. 2017-01247).

256   M. Astaraki et al.

References

1. Zhang, J., Xia, Y., Cui, H., Zhang, Y.: Pulmonary nodule detection in medical images: a survey. Biomed. Signal Process. Control **43**, 138–147 (2018). https://doi.org/10.1016/j.bspc.2018.01.011
2. Setio, A.A.A., et al.: Pulmonary nodule detection in CT images: false positive reduction using multi-view convolutional networks. IEEE Trans. Med. Imaging **35**, 1160–1169 (2016). https://doi.org/10.1109/TMI.2016.2536809
3. Baur, C., Wiestler, B., Albarqouni, S., Navab, N.: Deep autoencoding models for unsupervised anomaly segmentation in brain MR images. In: Crimi, A., Bakas, S., Kuijf, H., Keyvan, F., Reyes, M., van Walsum, T. (eds.) BrainLes 2018. LNCS, vol. 11383, pp. 161–169. Springer, Cham (2019). https://doi.org/10.1007/978-3-030-11723-8_16
4. Chen, X., Konukoglu, E.: Unsupervised detection of lesions in brain MRI using constrained adversarial auto-encoders (2018)
5. Schlegl, T., Seeböck, P., Waldstein, S.M., Schmidt-Erfurth, U., Langs, G.: Unsupervised anomaly detection with generative adversarial networks to guide marker discovery. In: Niethammer, M., et al. (eds.) IPMI 2017. LNCS, vol. 10265, pp. 146–157. Springer, Cham (2017). https://doi.org/10.1007/978-3-319-59050-9_12
6. Liu, G., Reda, F.A., Shih, K.J., Wang, T.-C., Tao, A., Catanzaro, B.: Image inpainting for irregular holes using partial convolutions (2018)
7. Alex, V., Mohammed Safwan, K.P., Chennamsetty, S.S., Krishnamurthi, G.: Generative adversarial networks for brain lesion detection. Presented at the 24 February (2017)
8. Wang, C., Smedby, Ö.: Automatic whole heart segmentation using deep learning and shape context. In: Pop, M., et al. (eds.) STACOM 2017. LNCS, vol. 10663, pp. 242–249. Springer, Cham (2018). https://doi.org/10.1007/978-3-319-75541-0_26
9. Wang, S., et al.: Central focused convolutional neural networks: developing a data-driven model for lung nodule segmentation. Med. Image Anal. **40**, 172–183 (2017). https://doi.org/10.1016/j.media.2017.06.014
10. Shakibapour, E., Cunha, A., Aresta, G., Mendonça, A.M., Campilho, A.: An unsupervised metaheuristic search approach for segmentation and volume measurement of pulmonary nodules in lung CT scans. Expert Syst. Appl. **119**, 415–428 (2019). https://doi.org/10.1016/j.eswa.2018.11.010
11. Wang, Z., Yuan, H., Ji, S.: Spatial variational auto-encoding via matrix-variate normal distributions (2017)

mlVIRNET: Multilevel Variational Image Registration Network

Alessa Hering[1,2]([✉]), Bram van Ginneken[2], and Stefan Heldmann[1]

[1] Fraunhofer MEVIS, Lübeck, Germany
alessa.hering@mevis.fraunhofer.de
[2] Diagnostic Image Analyse Group, Radboudumc, Nijmegen, The Netherlands

Abstract. We present a novel multilevel approach for deep learning based image registration. Recently published deep learning based registration methods have shown promising results for a wide range of tasks. However, these algorithms are still limited to relatively small deformations. Our method addresses this shortcoming by introducing a multilevel framework, which computes deformation fields on different scales, similar to conventional methods. Thereby, a coarse-level alignment is obtained first, which is subsequently improved on finer levels. We demonstrate our method on the complex task of inhale-to-exhale lung registration. We show that the use of a deep learning multilevel approach leads to significantly better registration results.

Keywords: Image registration · Multilevel · Deep learning · Thoracic CT

1 Introduction

Image registration is the process of aligning two or more images to achieve point-wise spatial correspondence. This is a fundamental step for many medical image analysis tasks and has been an active field of research for decades. Since recently, deep learning based approaches have been successfully employed for image registration [2,4,6,7,13,16]. They have shown promising results in a wide range of application. However, capturing large motion and deformation with deep learning based registration is still an open challenge. In common iterative image registration approaches, this is typically addressed with a multilevel coarse-to-fine registration strategy [1,11,15]. Starting on a coarse grid with smoothed and down-sampled versions of the input images a deformation field is computed which is subsequently prolonged on the next finer level as a initial guess. Hereby, a coarse level alignment is obtained first that typically captures the large motion components and which is later improved on finer levels for the alignment of more local details. Most of the recently presented deep learning based approaches also make use of a multilevel strategy as they are based on the U-Net architecture [2,6,7,13]. Thereby, the first half of the "U" is used to generate features on different scales starting at the highest resolution and reducing the resolution

© Springer Nature Switzerland AG 2019
D. Shen et al. (Eds.): MICCAI 2019, LNCS 11769, pp. 257–265, 2019.
https://doi.org/10.1007/978-3-030-32226-7_29

through pooling operations. In this procedure, however, only feature maps on different levels are calculated but neither different image resolutions are used nor deformation fields are computed. Only a few approaches implement a multi-resolution or hierarchical strategy in the sense of multilevel strategies associated with conventional methods. In [8] the authors proposed an architecture which is divided into a global and a local network, which are optimized together. In [4] a multilevel strategy is incorporated into the training of a U-net. Here, a CNN is grown and trained progressively level-by-level. In [16] a patch based approach is presented, where multiple CNNs (ConvNets) are combined additive into a larger architecture for performing coarse-to-fine image registration of patches. The results from the patches are then combined into a deformation field warping the whole image. In this work, we address this challenge and present a multilevel strategy for deep learning based image registration to advance state-of-the-art approaches. The contribution of this paper includes:

- We present deep learning based multilevel registration that is able to compensate and handle large deformations by computing deformation fields on different scales and functionally compose them.
- Our method is a theoretically sound and a direct transference of coarse-to-fine registration from conventional, iterative registration schemes to the deep learning based methods.
- We do not rely on patches. We take the whole image information into account and always consider the full field of view on all levels.
- A robust and fast registration method for the complex task of inhale-to-exhale registration validated on a large dataset of 270 thoracic CT scan pairs of the multi-center COPDGene study and on the publicly available DIR-LAB dataset [3].

2 Method

Our deep learning based framework for deformable image registration consists of two main building blocks. The first one is the specific design of the convolutional neural network and the loss function. In general, several architectures together with different distance measures, regularizer and penalty terms can be used. However, we focus on a U-Net based architecture, combined with a loss function that has shown good results for the task of pulmonary registration [14]. The second main building block is the embedding into a multilevel approach from coarse to fine. In the following, we give a brief outline of the variational setup, then we describe our particular architecture and loss function and, finally, we present its embedding into a multilevel approach.

Variational Registration Approach

Following [10], let $\mathcal{F}, \mathcal{M} : \mathbb{R}^3 \to \mathbb{R}$ denote the fixed image and moving image, respectively, and let $\Omega \subset \mathbb{R}^3$ be a domain modeling the field of view of $\mathcal{F}$. We aim to compute a deformation $y : \Omega \to \mathbb{R}^3$ that aligns the fixed image $\mathcal{F}$ and the moving image $\mathcal{M}$ on the field of view Ω such that $\mathcal{F}(x)$ and $\mathcal{M}(y(x))$ are similar for $x \in \Omega$. The deformation is defined as a mimimizer of a suitable cost function that typically takes the form

$$\mathcal{J}(\mathcal{F}, \mathcal{M}, y) = \mathcal{D}(\mathcal{F}, \mathcal{M}(y)) + \alpha\mathcal{R}(y) \tag{1}$$

with so-called distance measure $\mathcal{D}$ that quantifies the similarity of fixed image $\mathcal{F}$ and deformed moving image $\mathcal{M}(y)$ and so-called a regularizer $\mathcal{R}$ that forces smoothness of the deformation typically by penalizing of spatial derivatives. Typical examples for the distance measure are, e.g., the squared L_2 norm of the difference image (SSD), cross correlation (CC) or mutual information (MI). In our experiments, we follow the approach of [14] using the edge based normalized gradient fields distance measure (NGF) and second order curvature regularization.

Deep Learning Based Image Registration

In contrast to conventional registration [10], we do not employ iterative optimization during inference of new unseen images but use a convolutional neural network (CNN) that takes images $\mathcal{F}$ and $\mathcal{M}$ as input and yields the deformation y as output. Thus, in the context of CNNs we can consider y as a function of a trainable CNN model parameter vector $\theta \in \mathbb{R}^P$ and input images $\mathcal{F}$, $\mathcal{M}$, i.e. $y(x) \equiv y(\theta; \mathcal{F}, \mathcal{M}, x)$. In an unsupervised learning approach, we set up a loss function $\mathcal{L}$ that depends on $\mathcal{F}$, $\mathcal{M}$ and y, and then θ is learned by training, i.e., minimizing the expected value of $\mathcal{L}$ among a set of representative input images w.r.t. θ. A natural choice would $\mathcal{L} = \mathcal{J}$. However, in our particular application, we have additional information available during training and we perform a weakly supervised approach. To this end, we define our loss function as suggested in [7]

$$\mathcal{L}(\mathcal{F}, \mathcal{M}, b_{\mathcal{F}}, b_{\mathcal{M}}, y) = \mathcal{J}(\mathcal{F}, \mathcal{M}, y) + \frac{\beta}{2}\|b_{\mathcal{F}} - b_{\mathcal{M}}(y)\|_{L_2}^2 \tag{2}$$

with binary segmentation masks $b_{\mathcal{F}}$ and $b_{\mathcal{M}}(y)$ of the fixed and warped moving image, respectively. Note that these segmentations are only used to evaluate the loss function for training and their are not used as network input.

Single Level Architecture

Our CNN $y \equiv y(\theta, \mathcal{M}, \mathcal{F})$ is based on a U-Net which takes the concatenated 3D moving and fixed image as input and predicts a 3D dense displacement field. The network consists of three resolution levels starting with 16 filters in the first layer, which are doubled after each downsampling step. We apply 3D convolutions in both encoder and decoder stage with a kernel size of 3 followed by a batch normalization and a ReLU layer. For downsampling the feature maps during the encoder path, an $2 \times 2 \times 2$ average pooling operation with a stride of 2 is used. Transposed convolutions upsample and halve the feature maps in the decoder path. At the final layer, a $1 \times 1 \times 1$ convolution is used to map each 16 component feature vector to a three dimensional displacement vector.

Multilevel Deep Learning Based Registration

Multilevel continuation and scale space techniques have been proven very efficient in conventional variational registration approaches to avoid local minima, to reduce topological changes or foldings and to speed up runtimes [1,9,11,15]. However, beside carrying over these properties, our major motivation here is, to overcome the limitation of deep learning based registration to small and local deformations.

We follow the ideas of standard multilevel registration and compute coarse grid solutions that are prolongated and refined on the subsequent finer level. To this end, first we create image pyramids $\mathcal{F}_\ell, \mathcal{M}_\ell$ for $\ell = 1, \ldots, L$ with coarsest level L. We start on finest level $\ell = 1$ and subsequently halve image size and resolution from level to level. Registration starts on coarsest level L and we compute deformation y_L from images $\mathcal{F}_L$ and $\mathcal{M}_L$ as network input. On all finer levels $\ell < L$, we incorporate the deformations from all preceding coarse levels as initial guess. Therefore, we combine them by functional composition and warp the moving image at current level. Let X_ℓ denote the cell-centered image grid on level ℓ, we compute the warped moving $\mathcal{M}_\ell(Y_\ell)$ with

$$Y_\ell := y_{\ell+1} \circ y_{\ell+2} \circ \ldots \circ y_L(X_\ell)$$

and use it together with fixed image $\mathcal{F}_\ell$ as network input, yielding the deformation field y_ℓ on the current level. The final output deformation y is then given by composition of the whole sequence of coarse-to-fine solutions, i.e., $y = y_1 \circ y_2 \circ \ldots \circ y_L$. To evaluate deformations and images at non-grid grid points, we use trilinear interpolation. Our scheme is summarized in Algorithm 1.

In our experiments we use in particular a three level scheme ($L = 3$). And we create image pyramid with three reduced resolution images generated from the original 3D images by applying a low-pass filter with a stride of two, four and eight. During training, the three networks are learned progressively. First, the network on the coarsest level is trained for a fixed amount of epochs. Afterwards, the parameters of the middle network are learned while the coarsest network stays fixed and is only used to produce the initial deformation field. The same procedure is repeated on the finest level. The same architecture is used on all levels. The convolution parameters on the coarsest level are initialized with Xavier uniform [5]. Whereas, all other networks are using the learned parameters of the previous network as initialization. Note that the receptive field in voxel is the same for all used networks, however, due to the decreased resolution on the coarse levels, the receptive field in mm is much higher.

3 Experiments and Results

We demonstrate our deep learning based registration method by registration of inhale-to-exhale lung CT scans. We use data from 500 patients for training and a disjoint set of 50 patients for validation from the COPDGene study, a large multi-center clinical trial with over 10,000 subjects with chronic obstructive

Algorithm 1: Multilevel Deep Learning Registration

IN   : Fixed image $\mathcal{F}$, moving image $\mathcal{M}$, image grid X
OUT: Corse-to-fine deformations $y_L, ..., y_1$, transformed grid $Y = y_1 \circ ... \circ y_L(X)$

1   Create image pyramid $\mathcal{F}_\ell, \mathcal{M}_\ell$ for $\ell = 1, 2, ..., L$ with finest level $\ell = 1$ and L coarsest.
2   On coarsest level Compute deformation $y_L = \text{CNN}(\mathcal{F}_L, \mathcal{M}_L)$
3   **for** $\ell = L - 1, L - 2, ..., 1$ **do**
4   Compute transformed grid $Y_\ell = y_{\ell+1} \circ ... \circ y_L(X_\ell)$
5   Compute deformation $y_\ell = \text{CNN}(\mathcal{F}_\ell, \mathcal{M}_\ell(Y_\ell))$
6   **end**

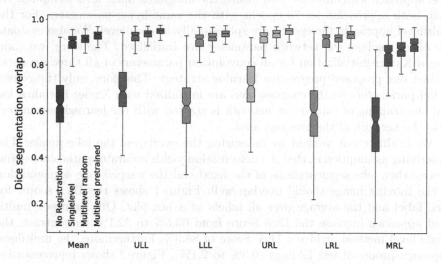

Fig. 1. Comparison of Dice overlaps for all test images and each anatomical label (average of all labels ■, upper left lobe (ULL) ■, lower left lobe (LLL) ■, upper right lobe (URL) ■, lower right lobe (LRL) ■, middle right lobe (MRL) (LRL) ■). For each one the distributions of Dice coefficients after an before registration, after single level dl registration, multilevel dl registration without pretrained CNNs and after multilevel registration with pretrained CNNs. (Color figure online)

pulmonary disease (COPD) [12]. The dataset was acquired across 21 imaging centers using a variety of scanner makes and models. Each patient had received two breath hold 3D CT scans, one on full inspiration (200 mAs) and one at the end of normal expiration (50 mAs). For all scans segmentations of the lobes are available, which were computed automatically and manually corrected and verified by trained human analysts. The original images have sizes in the range of $512 \times 512 \times \{430, ..., 901\}$ voxels. Due to memory and time limitations, we create low-resolution images by resampling to a fixed size of $160 \times 160 \times 160$ voxels. The low-resolution images are then used during training for the computation of the deformation field and for evaluating of the loss function. Note that, our method is generally not limited to any fixed input size. Although we use images with 160^3 voxels, the computed deformation field are defined on full field-of-view and can be evaluated on grids with arbitrary resolution by using trilinear interpolation. Consequently, we use original full-resolution images for the evaluation of our method.

Multilevel vs. Single Level

First, we evaluate our multilevel approach on a disjoint subset of 270 patients from the COPDGene study. We compare our proposed method against a single level approach with only one U-Net using the images on finest level as inputs. We train both approaches for 75 epochs with the same hyper-parameters. For the multilevel approach, the epochs are split equally at each level. We also evaluate the effect on how the network parameter are initialized. Therefore, we compare a Xavier initialization for all convolution parameters of all three networks against our proposed progressive learning strategy. Therefore, only the convolution parameters on the coarsest level are initialized with Xavier initialization and the training of subsequent network is started with the learned parameters form the network of the previous level.

We evaluate our method by measuring the overlap of the lobe masks. The underlying assumption is, that if a deformation yields accurate spatial correspondences, then lobe segmentations of the fixed and the warped lobe segmentation of the moving image should overlap well. Figure 1 shows the Dice scores for each label and the average over all labels as a box-plot. Our proposed multilevel approach increase the Dice Score from 63.5% to 92.1%. In contrast, the single level method archive a Dice Score of 88.3%. Furthermore, the multilevel approach produced less foldings (0.3% to 2.1%). Figure 2 shows representative qualitative results for of two scan pairs before registration and after our single level and multilevel registration. In both cases the respiratory motion was successfully recovered. Although the single level registration produces reasonable Dice scores, it does not well align the inner structures. This is also reflected by the landmark errors in the following section. Comparing the results of the pretrained initialization to the random initialization, an improvement of about 2% in terms of the Dice Score could be reached.

Comparison with State-of-the-Art

Additionally, we evaluate our method and compare it to others on the public available DIR-LAB dataset [3]. It is a collection of ten inspiration-expiration cases with 300 expert-annotated landmarks in the lung. The landmarks are used for evaluating our deformable registration method. The mean (and standard deviation) for all ten scans for the deep learning based multi-resolution approaches of Eppenhof [4] and de Vos (DLIR) [16], the single VIRNET and our proposed method are listed in Table 1. The overall average landmark error is 2.19 mm with a standard deviation of 1.62 mm. In contrast to the other methods, our mlVIRNET is more robust against outliers and can better handle large initial landmark distances without training on this specific dataset.

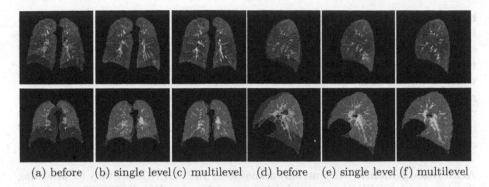

(a) before   (b) single level (c) multilevel   (d) before   (e) single level (f) multilevel

Fig. 2. Visualization of two inspiration-expiration registration results: (a)–(c) show coronal views before and after single and multilevel registration, (d) and (f) sagittal views, respectively. The color overlays show the inhale scan in orange and the exhale in blue; due to addition of RGB values, aligned structures appear gray or white. In both cases the respiratory motion was successfully recovered. However, the single level registration does not well align the inner structures. (Color figure online)

Table 1. Mean (standard deviation) of the registration error in mm determined on DIR-Lab 4D-CT data. From left to right: initial landmark error, the multi-resolution approaches of [4] and [16] and the single level VIRNET and the proposed multilevel VIRNET.

Scan	Initial	Eppenhof [4]	DLIR [16]	Single VIRNET	mlVIRNET
Case 1	3.89(2.78)	2.18(1.05)	1.27(1.16)	1.73(0.83)	1.33(0.73)
Case 2	4.34(3.90)	2.06(0.96)	1.20(1.12)	2.38(1.11)	1.33(0.69)
Case 3	6.94(4.05)	2.11(1.04)	1.48(1.26)	3.01(1.86)	1.48(0.94)
Case 4	9.83(4.85)	3.13(1.60)	2.09(1.93)	4.28(2.37)	1.85(1.37)
Case 5	7.48(5.50)	2.92(1.70)	1.95(2.10)	3.17(2.2)	1.84(1.39)
Case 6	10.89(6.96)	4.20(2.00)	5.16(7.09)	4.85(3.04)	3.57(2.15)
Case 7	11.03(7.42)	4.12(2.97)	3.05(3.01)	3.67(1.82)	2.61(1.63)
Case 8	14.99(9.00)	9.43(6.28)	6.48(5.37)	5.75(3.93)	2.62(1.52)
Case 9	7.92(3.97)	3.82(1.69)	2.10(1.66)	4.90(2.25)	2.70(1.46)
Case 10	7.30(6.34)	2.87(1.96)	2.09(2.24)	3.49(2.21)	2.63(1.93)
Total	8.46(6.58)	3.68(3.32)	2.64(4.32)	3.72(2.45)	2.19(1.62)

4   Discussion and Conclusion

We presented an end-to-end multilevel framework for deep learning based image registration which is able to compensate and handle large deformations by computing deformation fields on different scales. Our method takes the whole image information into account and predicts a dense 3D deformation field. We validated our framework on the challenging task of large motion inhale-to-exhale registration using large image data of the multi-center COPDGene study. We have shown that our proposed method archives better results than the comparable single level variant. In particular with regard to the alignment of inner lung structures and the presence of foldings. Only less than 0.3% voxel positions of the images showed a folding. Additionally, we demonstrated that using the network parameter of the previous level as initialization, yields to better registration results. Moreover, we demonstrated the transferability of our approach to new datasets by evaluating our learned method on the publicly available DIRLAB dataset and showing a lower landmark error than other deep learning based registration methods.

Acknowledgements. We gratefully acknowledge the COPDGene Study for providing the data used. COPDGene is funded by Award Number U01 HL089897 and Award Number U01 HL089856 from the National Heart, Lung, and Blood Institute. The COPDGene project is also supported by the COPD Foundation through contributions made to an Industry Advisory Board comprised of AstraZeneca, Boehringer Ingelheim, GlaxoSmithKline, Novartis, Pfizer, Siemens and Sunovion.

References

1. Bajcsy, R., Kovačič, S.: Multiresolution elastic matching. Comput. Vis. Graph. Image Process. **46**(1), 1–21 (1989)
2. Balakrishnan, G., Zhao, A., Sabuncu, M.R., Guttag, J., Dalca, A.V.: VoxelMorph: a learning framework for deformable medical image registration. IEEE TMI (2019)
3. Castillo, R., et al.: A reference dataset for deformable image registration spatial accuracy evaluation using the copdgene study archive. Phys. Med. Biol. **58**(9), 2861 (2013)
4. Eppenhof, K.A., Lafarge, M.W., Pluim, J.P.: Progressively growing convolutional networks for end-to-end deformable image registration. In: Medical Imaging 2019: Image Processing, vol. 10949, p. 109491C. International Society for Optics and Photonics (2019)
5. Glorot, X., Bengio, Y.: Understanding the difficulty of training deep feedforward neural networks. In: Proceedings of the Thirteenth International Conference on Artificial Intelligence and Statistics, pp. 249–256 (2010)
6. Hering, A., Heldmann, S.: Unsupervised learning for large motion thoracic CT follow-up registration. In: SPIE Medical Imaging: Image Processing, vol. 10949, p. 109491B (2019)
7. Hering, A., Kuckertz, S., Heldmann, S., Heinrich, M.P.: Enhancing label-driven deep deformable image registration with local distance metrics for state-of-the-art cardiac motion tracking. In: Handels, H., Deserno, T., Maier, A., Maier-Hein, K., Palm, C., Tolxdorff, T. (eds.) Bildverarbeitung für die Medizin 2019. I, pp. 309–314. Springer, Wiesbaden (2019). https://doi.org/10.1007/978-3-658-25326-4_69
8. Hu, Y., et al.: Label-driven weakly-supervised learning for multimodal deformable image registration. In: Proceedings of ISBI 2018, pp. 1070–1074. IEEE (2018)
9. Kabus, S., Lorenz, C.: Fast elastic image registration. Med. Image Anal. Clinic: A Grand Challenge, 81–89 (2010)
10. Modersitzki, J.: FAIR: Flexible Algorithms for Image Registration. SIAM (2009)
11. Modersitzki, J., Haber, E.: COFIR: coarse and fine image registration, chap. 14. In: Computational Science & Engineering: Real-Time PDE-Constrained Optimization, pp. 277–288. SIAM (2007)

12. Regan, E.A., et al.: Genetic epidemiology of COPD (COPDGene) study design. COPD: J. Chronic Obstructive Pulm. Dis. **7**(1), 32–43 (2011)
13. Rohé, M.-M., Datar, M., Heimann, T., Sermesant, M., Pennec, X.: SVF-Net: learning deformable image registration using shape matching. In: Descoteaux, M., Maier-Hein, L., Franz, A., Jannin, P., Collins, D.L., Duchesne, S. (eds.) MICCAI 2017. LNCS, vol. 10433, pp. 266–274. Springer, Cham (2017). https://doi.org/10.1007/978-3-319-66182-7_31
14. Rühaak, J., et al.: Estimation of large motion in lung CT by integrating regularized keypoint correspondences into dense deformable registration. IEEE TMI **36**(8), 1746–1757 (2017)
15. Schnabel, J.A., et al.: A generic framework for non-rigid registration based on non-uniform multi-level free-form deformations. In: Niessen, W.J., Viergever, M.A. (eds.) MICCAI 2001. LNCS, vol. 2208, pp. 573–581. Springer, Heidelberg (2001). https://doi.org/10.1007/3-540-45468-3_69
16. de Vos, B.D., Berendsen, F.F., Viergever, M.A., Sokooti, H., Staring, M., Išgum, I.: A deep learning framework for unsupervised affine and deformable image registration. Med. Image Anal. **52**, 128–143 (2019)

NoduleNet: Decoupled False Positive Reduction for Pulmonary Nodule Detection and Segmentation

Hao Tang[1,2], Chupeng Zhang[2], and Xiaohui Xie[1(✉)]

[1] Department of Computer Science,
Univeresity of California Irvine, Irvine, USA
{htang6,xhx}@uci.edu
[2] Deep Voxel Inc., Costa Mesa, USA
chupengz@deep-voxel.com

Abstract. Pulmonary nodule detection, false positive reduction and segmentation represent three of the most common tasks in the computer aided analysis of chest CT images. Methods have been proposed for each task with deep learning based methods heavily favored recently. However training deep learning models to solve each task separately may be sub-optimal - resource intensive and without the benefit of feature sharing. Here, we propose a new end-to-end 3D deep convolutional neural net (DCNN), called NoduleNet, to solve nodule detection, false positive reduction and nodule segmentation jointly in a multi-task fashion. To avoid friction between different tasks and encourage feature diversification, we incorporate two major design tricks: (1) decoupled feature maps for nodule detection and false positive reduction, and (2) a segmentation refinement subnet for increasing the precision of nodule segmentation. Extensive experiments on the large-scale LIDC dataset demonstrate that the multi-task training is highly beneficial, improving the nodule detection accuracy by 10.27%, compared to the baseline model trained to only solve the nodule detection task. We also carry out systematic ablation studies to highlight contributions from each of the added components. Code is available at https://github.com/uci-cbcl/NoduleNet.

Keywords: Pulmonary nodule detection and segmentation · Deep convolutional neural network

1 Introduction

Lung cancer has the highest incidence and mortality rates worldwide [3]. Early diagnosis and treatment of pulmonary nodules can increase the survival rate of patients. Computed tomography (CT) has been widely used and proved effective for detecting pulmonary nodules. However, manually identifying nodules in CT scans is often time-consuming and tedious, because a radiologist needs to read the CT scans slice by slice, and a chest CT may contain over 200 slices. Accurate

© Springer Nature Switzerland AG 2019
D. Shen et al. (Eds.): MICCAI 2019, LNCS 11769, pp. 266–274, 2019.
https://doi.org/10.1007/978-3-030-32226-7_30

and precise nodule segmentation can provide more in-depth assessment of the shape, size and change rate of the nodule. When nodule is identified, a follow up scan in 3–12 months is usually required to assess its growth rate [7]. The growth of the lung tumor may be an indicator for malignancy, and an accurate nodule segmentation can be used for measuring the growth rate of the nodule.

In recent years, deep convolutional neural network has emerged as a leading method for automatically detecting and segmenting pulmonary nodules and have achieved great success. State-of-the-art frameworks for nodule detection often utilize the 3D region proposal network (RPN) [12] for nodule screening [10,14,15,19], followed by a 3D classifier for false positive reduction [5,16]. Although single stage detector has also been proposed in [8], their hit criteria was different from what was more commonly adopted [14]. Moreover, the refinement provided by the extra classifiers may correct some errors made by the detectors. In terms of nodule segmentation, U-Net [13] and V-Net [11] like structure is predominantly used [1,17,18]. In practice, a computer aided diagnosis (CAD) system for pulmonary nodule detection and segmentation often consists of several independent subsystems, optimized separately.

There are some limitations on handling each task completely independent. First, it is time-consuming and resource intensive to train several deep convolutional neural networks. Although each component is designed for different purposes, they share the common procedure of extracting feature representations that characterize pulmonary nodules. Second, the performance of the whole system may not be optimal, because separately training several systems prevents communication between each other and learning intrinsic feature representations. Intuitively, the segmentation mask of the nodule should provide a strong guide for the neural network to learn discriminative features, which may in turn improve the performance of nodule detection.

Although multi-task learning (MTL) and feature sharing offer an attractive solution to combine different tasks, a naive implementation may cause other problems [4]. First, because of the mismatched goals of localization and classification, it may be sub-optimal if these two tasks are performed using the same feature map. Second, a large receptive field may integrate irrelevant information from other parts of the image, which may negatively affect and confuse the classification of nodules, especially small ones. [4] decoupled localization and classification to address the problem in natural imaging. However, completely separating the two tasks without sharing any feature extraction backbone, still prevents cross-talk between two networks and may not be the most efficient. Therefore, a decoupled false positive reduction, that pools features from early scales of the feature extraction backbone, is proposed to address this problem, which allows learning both task-independent and task-dependant features.

Here, we propose a new end-to-end framework, called NoduleNet, for solving pulmonary nodule candidate screening, false positive reduction and segmentation jointly. NoduleNet consists of three parts: nodule candidate screening, false positive reduction and segmentation refinement (Fig. 1). These three components share the same underlying feature extraction backbone and the whole network is trained in an end-to-end manner.

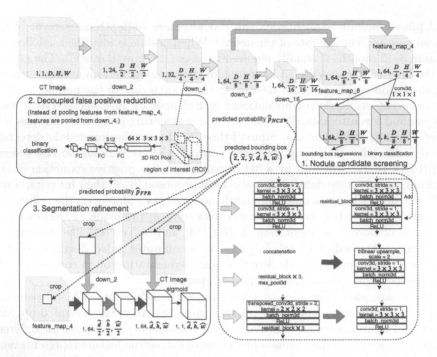

Fig. 1. Overview of NoduleNet. NoduleNet is an end-to-end framework for pulmonary nodule detection and segmentation, consisting of three sequential stages: nodule candidate screening, false positive reduction and segmentation refinement. k is the number of anchors. FC is short for fully connected layer.

Our main contributions are summarized as follows:

- We propose a unified model to integrate nodule detection, false positive reduction and nodule segmentation within a single framework, trained end-to-end in a multi-task fashion.
- We demonstrate the effectiveness of the model, improving nodule detection accuracy by 10.27% compared to the baseline model trained only for nodule detection, and achieving a state-of-the-art nodule segmentation accuracy of 83.10% on Dice-Sørensen coefficient (DSC).
- We carry out systematic ablation studies to verify the contributions of several design tricks underlying NoduleNet, including decoupled features maps, segmentation refinement subnet, and multi-task training.

2   NoduleNet

Nodule Candidate Screening (NCS). To generate nodule candidates, a $3 \times 3 \times 3$ 3D convolutional layer is applied to the feature map (feature_map_4 in Fig. 1), followed by two parallel $1 \times 1 \times 1$ convolutional layers to generate classification probability and six regression terms associated with each anchor at each voxel on the feature map. An anchor is a 3D box, which requires six parameters to specify: central z-, y-, x- coordinates, depth, height and width. We chose cube of size 5, 10, 20, 30 and 50 as the 5 anchors in this work. Then, we minimize the same multi-task loss function as [12].

Decoupled False Positive Reduction (DFPR). Unlike [12] that performs classification using features pooled from the same feature map as RPN (feature_map_4). Learning using coupled feature map may lead to sub-optimal solutions of the two tasks. Instead, we use 3D region of interest (ROI) pooling layer to pool features from early feature map that has a small receptive field (down_4). This not only ensures the false positive reduction network has a small receptive field and can learn feature representations that are substantially different from nodule candidate screening network, but also allows sharing of a few feature extraction blocks. The false positive reduction network minimizes the same multi-task in loss function as the NCS.

Segmentation Refinement (SR). As shown in Fig. 1, segmentation is performed at the same scale of the original input CT image, by progressively upsampling the cropped high-level feature map (feature_map_4) and concatenating them with low-level semantically strong features.

This approach is fundamentally different from the mask branch proposed in [6]. In [6], the authors perform segmentation by only using downsampled feature map and then resize the predicted mask back to the original image scale, which may lose precision due to bounding box regression errors and loss of more fine-grained local features.

Another advantage is that, only the regions have nodules are upsampled to the original image scale, which only accounts for a small area of the whole input image. This saves a large amount of GPU memory, making whole volume input feasible during training and testing, as compared to upsampling the whole feature map to original input scale in [11].

The segmentation refinement network minimizes the soft dice loss of the predicted mask sets $\{m\}$ and the ground truth mask sets $\{g\}$ of the input image.

3   Results

Data and Experiment Configurations. We used LIDC-LDRI [2] for evaluating the performance of NoduleNet. LIDC-LDRI is a large-scale public dataset for studying lung cancers, which contains 1018 sets of CT scans collected from multiple sites with various slice thickness. Nodules with diameter equal or greater than 3 mm in this dataset have contour outlined by up to four radiologists. We included only those CT scans met the selection criteria of LUNA16 [14] in this work. If the two segmentation masks provided by two radiologists have an intersection over union (IoU) larger than 0.4, we consider the two masks are referring to the same nodule. We consider nodules annotated by at least 3 out of 4 radiologists the ground truth, resulting in a total number of 586 CT scans with 1131 nodules. Note that the number of CT scans and nodules included in this work may be different from previous work [1,17,18], due to different inclusion criteria.

A six-fold cross validation was performed to demonstrate the performance of NoduleNet. All models in the experiment were trained using stochastic gradient descent (SGD) with initial learning rate 0.01, momentum 0.9 and $l2$ penalty 0.0001, for 200 epochs. The learning rate was scheduled to decrease to 0.001 after 100 epochs and to 0.0001 after another 60 epochs.

Free-Response Receiver Operating Characteristic (FROC) [9] analysis was adopted for evaluating the performance of nodule detection. We used the same hit criterium and competition performance metric (CPM) as in the LUNA16 [14]. Intersection over union (IoU) and Sørensen-Dice coefficient (DSC) were used for evaluating the performance of nodule segmentation.

Nodule Detection Performance. In order to fully verify and understand our aforementioned assumptions, we conducted extensive experiments using different network architectures and design choices. We use N_1 to represent network that only has NCS branch, N_2 for network has both NCS and FPR branches, and N_3 for network has all NCS, FPR and SR branches. F_c represents the FPR branch is built on the same feature map as NCS, and F_d means the FPR branch is built on the decoupled feature map mentioned in previous section. R means the training data is extraly augmented with xy - plane rotation. **NCS** means the predicted probability comes from NCS branch, **FPR** means the predicted probability comes from FPR branch, and **FU** means the predicted probability is fused from NCS and FPR. Note that N_1 is the widely used 3D RPN for nodule detection [10,15,16,19], which was served as a strong baseline for evaluating the performance of each added component. The results are summarized in Table 1.

As seen from Table 1, the sensitivity at 8 false positives per patient rate has a consistent improvement of 1.0% to 1.5% by adding the segmentation refinement network (N_3), which demonstrates the effectiveness of using the extra nodule segmentation information.

The average sensitivity of the NoduleNet using decoupled false positive reduction (F_d) has around 3% to 4% improvement over the NoduleNet using coupled false positive (F_c). Moreover, by adding rotation in data augmentation (R), the performance of **FPR** branch is further improved by around 2.5% while the performance of **NCS** branch remains almost the same. This verifies our assumption that classification should learn invariant features, while localization may learn co-variant features. Those findings demonstrate the importance of decoupling modules that are essentially learning different tasks.

By fusing the predicted probability from NCS and FPR, the performance was consistently improved by 0.7%–1.0%, demonstrating that combining predictions from branches that perceive different level of context information is important.

By adding false positive reduction and segmentation refinement network, the performance of the baseline detector (**NCS**) is correspondingly improved, showing the effectiveness of multi-task learning and feature sharing.

All together, NoduleNet outperforms a strong baseline single stage detector by 10.27%. Note that performance reported in LUNA16 may not be directly comparable to this work, because of different nodule selection criteria, and training and testing data splits. Also, this work focuses on the joint learning of nodule detection and segmentation, whereas the LUNA16 focuses only on nodule detection.

Table 1. CPM of different methods on the LIDC dataset based on six-fold cross validation. Shown are nodule detection sensitivities (unit: %) with each column denoting the threshold false positive rate per CT scan (FPs/scan). The last column denotes the average sensitivities across the seven pre-defined FPs/scan thresholds.

Method	0.125	0.25	0.5	1.0	2.0	4.0	8.0	Avg.
N_1 (NCS) [10, 15, 16, 19]	52.17	62.51	71.09	80.46	87.27	91.07	94.43	77.00
$N_2 + F_c$ (NCS)	53.85	62.07	71.09	79.22	86.74	90.98	93.28	76.75
$N_2 + F_c$ (FPR) [16]	55.79	66.93	75.77	82.40	88.68	91.78	93.10	79.21
$N_3 + F_c$ (NCS)	53.67	63.84	74.62	83.20	88.51	92.04	94.96	78.69
$N_3 + F_c$ (FPR)	57.38	65.96	77.19	84.97	89.92	93.28	95.40	80.59
$N_2 + F_d$ (NCS)	56.15	66.93	74.54	82.23	88.59	92.22	95.05	79.39
$N_2 + F_d$ (FPR)	61.98	71.26	78.78	85.41	89.30	92.22	95.31	82.04
$N_3 + F_d$ (NCS)	61.45	70.20	78.16	84.62	90.27	93.63	96.20	82.08
$N_3 + F_d$ (FPR)	68.08	73.56	81.70	85.94	90.80	93.90	96.55	84.36
$N_3 + F_d$ (FU)	68.70	75.60	82.23	87.36	92.04	94.96	96.46	85.34
$N_3 + F_d + R$ (NCS)	62.78	70.65	78.43	84.44	89.74	93.10	95.49	82.09
$N_3 + F_d + R$ (FPR)	69.23	77.01	84.70	89.48	93.37	95.23	**96.55**	86.51
$N_3 + F_d + R$ (FU)	**70.82**	**78.34**	**85.68**	**90.01**	**94.25**	**95.49**	96.29	**87.27**

Nodule Segmentation Performance. In Table 2, we compared the segmentation performance of NoduleNet to other deep learning based methods trained and tested on LIDC dataset [1, 17, 18]. NoduleNet outperformed previous state-of-the-art deep learning based method by 0.95% on DSC, without the need to train a separate and dedicated 3D DCNN for nodule segmentation. We randomly selected several nodules for visualizing the segmentation quality (Fig. 2).

Table 2. IoU (%) and DSC (%) performance of nodule segmentation between different methods. "# Consensus" means each method includes nodules that are annotated by at least "# Consensus" experts.

Approach	# Nodules		# Consensus	IoU (%)	DSC (%)
	Train	Test			
Wu et al. [18]	1404	1404	3	N\A	73.89 ± 3.87
Aresta et al. [1]	1593	1593	3	55.00 ± 14.00	N\A
Wang et al. [17]	350	493	4	71.16 ± 12.22	82.15 ± 10.76
NoduleNet	1131	1131	3	69.98 ± 10.80	81.80 ± 8.65
NoduleNet	1131	712	4	**71.85 ± 10.48**	**83.10 ± 8.85**

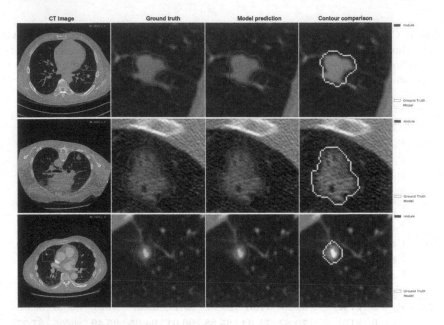

Fig. 2. Examples of nodule segmentation generated by NoduleNet.

4   Conclusion

In this work, we propose a new end-to-end 3D DCNN, named NoduleNet, for solving pulmonary nodule detection, false positive reduction and segmentation jointly. We performed systematic analysis to verify the assumptions and intuitions behind the design of each component in the architecture. Cross validation results on LIDC dataset demonstrate that our model achieves a final CPM score of 87.27% on nodule detection and DSC score of 83.10% on nodule segmentation, representing current state-of-the-arts on this dataset. The techniques introduced here are general, and can be readily transferred to other models.

References

1. Aresta, G., et al.: iW-Net: an automatic and minimalistic interactive lung nodule segmentation deep network. arXiv preprint arXiv:1811.12789 (2018)
2. Armato, S.G., et al.: The lung image database consortium (LIDC) and image database resource initiative (IDRI): a completed reference database of lung nodules on CT scans. Med. Phys. **38**(2), 915–931 (2011)
3. Bray, F., Ferlay, J., Soerjomataram, I., Siegel, R.L., Torre, L.A., Jemal, A.: Global cancer statistics 2018: GLOBOCAN estimates of incidence and mortality worldwide for 36 cancers in 185 countries. CA: Cancer J. Clin. **68**(6), 394–424 (2018)
4. Cheng, B., Wei, Y., Shi, H., Feris, R., Xiong, J., Huang, T.: Revisiting RCNN: on awakening the classification power of faster RCNN. In: Ferrari, V., Hebert, M., Sminchisescu, C., Weiss, Y. (eds.) ECCV 2018. LNCS, vol. 11219, pp. 473–490. Springer, Cham (2018). https://doi.org/10.1007/978-3-030-01267-0_28
5. Ding, J., Li, A., Hu, Z., Wang, L.: Accurate pulmonary nodule detection in computed tomography images using deep convolutional neural networks. In: Descoteaux, M., Maier-Hein, L., Franz, A., Jannin, P., Collins, D.L., Duchesne, S. (eds.) MICCAI 2017. LNCS, vol. 10435, pp. 559–567. Springer, Cham (2017). https://doi.org/10.1007/978-3-319-66179-7_64
6. He, K., Gkioxari, G., Dollár, P., Girshick, R.: Mask R-CNN. In: Proceedings of the IEEE International Conference on Computer Vision, pp. 2961–2969 (2017)
7. Kalpathy-Cramer, J., et al.: A comparison of lung nodule segmentation algorithms: methods and results from a multi-institutional study. J. Digit. Imaging **29**(4), 476–487 (2016)
8. Khosravan, N., Bagci, U.: *S4ND*: single-shot single-scale lung nodule detection. In: Frangi, A.F., Schnabel, J.A., Davatzikos, C., Alberola-López, C., Fichtinger, G. (eds.) MICCAI 2018. LNCS, vol. 11071, pp. 794–802. Springer, Cham (2018). https://doi.org/10.1007/978-3-030-00934-2_88
9. Kundel, H., Berbaum, K., Dorfman, D., Gur, D., Metz, C., Swensson, R.: Receiver operating characteristic analysis in medical imaging. ICRU Rep. **79**(8), 1 (2008)
10. Liao, F., Liang, M., Li, Z., Hu, X., Song, S.: Evaluate the malignancy of pulmonary nodules using the 3-D deep leaky noisy-or network. IEEE Trans. Neural Networks Learn. Syst. (2019)
11. Milletari, F., Navab, N., Ahmadi, S.A.: V-net: fully convolutional neural networks for volumetric medical image segmentation. In: 2016 Fourth International Conference on 3D Vision (3DV), pp. 565–571. IEEE (2016)
12. Ren, S., He, K., Girshick, R., Sun, J.: Faster R-CNN: towards real-time object detection with region proposal networks. In: Advances in Neural Information Processing Systems, pp. 91–99 (2015)
13. Ronneberger, O., Fischer, P., Brox, T.: U-net: convolutional networks for biomedical image segmentation. In: Navab, N., Hornegger, J., Wells, W.M., Frangi, A.F. (eds.) MICCAI 2015. LNCS, vol. 9351, pp. 234–241. Springer, Cham (2015). https://doi.org/10.1007/978-3-319-24574-4_28
14. Setio, A.A.A., et al.: Validation, comparison, and combination of algorithms for automatic detection of pulmonary nodules in computed tomography images: the luna16 challenge. Med. Image Anal. **42**, 1–13 (2017)
15. Tang, H., Kim, D.R., Xie, X.: Automated pulmonary nodule detection using 3D deep convolutional neural networks. In: 2018 IEEE 15th International Symposium on Biomedical Imaging (ISBI 2018), pp. 523–526. IEEE (2018)

16. Tang, H., Liu, X., Xie, X.: An end-to-end framework for integrated pulmonary nodule detection and false positive reduction. In: 2019 IEEE 16th International Symposium on Biomedical Imaging (ISBI 2019). IEEE (2019)
17. Wang, S., et al.: Central focused convolutional neural networks: developing a data-driven model for lung nodule segmentation. Med. Image Anal. **40**, 172–183 (2017)
18. Wu, B., Zhou, Z., Wang, J., Wang, Y.: Joint learning for pulmonary nodule segmentation, attributes and malignancy prediction. In: 2018 IEEE 15th International Symposium on Biomedical Imaging (ISBI 2018), pp. 1109–1113. IEEE (2018)
19. Zhu, W., Liu, C., Fan, W., Xie, X.: DeepLung: 3D deep convolutional nets for automated pulmonary nodule detection and classification. arXiv preprint arXiv:1709.05538 (2017)

Encoding CT Anatomy Knowledge for Unpaired Chest X-ray Image Decomposition

Zeju Li[1], Han Li[2], Hu Han[3,4](✉), Gonglei Shi[5], Jiannan Wang[6], and S. Kevin Zhou[3,4](✉)

[1] Biomedical Image Analysis Group, Imperial College London, London, UK
zeju.li18@imperial.ac.ukk
[2] University of Chinese Academy of Sciences, Beijing, China
[3] Medical Imaging, Robotics, Analytic Computing Laboratory/Engineering
(MIRACLE), Key Laboratory of Intelligent Information Processing of Chinese
Academy of Sciences (CAS), Institute of Computing Technology, CAS, Beijing, China
{hanhu,zhoushaohua}@ict.ac.cn
[4] Peng Cheng Laboratory, Shenzhen, China
[5] Department of Computer Science and Technology,
Southest University, Nanjing, China
[6] College of Electronic Information and Optical Engineering,
Nankai University, Tianjin, China

Abstract. Although chest X-ray (CXR) offers a 2D projection with overlapped anatomies, it is widely used for clinical diagnosis. There is clinical evidence supporting that decomposing an X-ray image into different components (e.g., bone, lung and soft tissue) improves diagnostic value. We hereby propose a decomposition generative adversarial network (DecGAN) to anatomically decompose a CXR image but **with unpaired data**. We leverage the anatomy knowledge embedded in CT, which features a 3D volume with clearly visible anatomies. Our key idea is to embed CT priori decomposition knowledge into the latent space of unpaired CXR autoencoder. Specifically, we train DecGAN with a decomposition loss, adversarial losses, cycle-consistency losses and a mask loss to guarantee that the decomposed results of the latent space preserve realistic body structures. Extensive experiments demonstrate that DecGAN provides superior unsupervised CXR bone suppression results and the feasibility of modulating CXR components by latent space disentanglement. Furthermore, we illustrate the diagnostic value of DecGAN and demonstrate that it outperforms the state-of-the-art approaches in terms of predicting 11 out of 14 common lung diseases.

1 Introduction

Chest X-ray (CXR) and computed tomography (CT) are two closely related medical imaging modalities given that a 3D CT is reconstructed from a set of

This work was done when Z. Li, G. Shi and J. Wang were interns at MIRACLE.

X-ray projections. However, CXR is only a 2D projection image which contains overlapped anatomies and ambiguous structure details. A possible connection between CXR and CT is via a digitally reconstructed radiograph (DRR), which is a virtual CXR-like projection image calculated from a CT volume based on ray-tracing and rigid transform. The decomposition of DRR is readily accessible.

In terms of economy and health, it could be of great importance to improve the diagnostic value of CXR. There is clinical evidence supporting that decomposing an X-ray image into different components (e.g. bone, lung and soft tissue) improves diagnostic value [5]. This paper aims to propose a method to decompose a CXR into different components such as bone, lung and other soft-tissue structures, thereby boosting the CXR diagnosis accuracy of lung diseases. Existing approaches to X-ray image decomposition are supervised, requiring paired original and decomposed images in training. For example, the paired dual energy (DE) imaging is always needed for supervised bone suppression and serves as the learning targets of neural networks [8,10]. DE radiography provides bone-free CXR by capturing two radiographs at two energy levels. However, these methods are limited because only few hospitals could provide DE images, and the obtained learning models might do not work well on other CXR datasets. We attempt to offer a solution *without DE images*. As shown in Fig. 1, the main idea of our proposed method, called a decomposition generative adversarial network (DecGAN), is to integrate the decomposition knowledge from the CT domain into the latent space of CXR autoencoder. The DRR decomposition is generated by projecting separate CT anatomic components obtained in a 3D CT volume.

DecGAN is developed upon the theory of domain adaptation based on generative adversarial network (GAN) [11]. For medical imaging, it is more crucial to resolve the domain adaptation problem because medical data is always limited [9]. However, currently all these domain adaptation methods for medical imaging are designed for the tasks of image segmentation or classification but not for image decomposition, which is more difficult for domain adaptation because it is required to preserve a lot of detail information. To the best of our knowledge, DecGAN is *the first approach* to tackle the problem of cross-domain medical image decomposition under an unpaired setting.

In this paper, we overcome three main challenges in cross-domain image decomposition: (1) creating a corresponding latent space, (2) building a powerful and robust decoder, and (3) preserving anatomical reliability. We demonstrate that our method outperforms other state-of-the-art methods on the task of unsupervised CXR bone suppression and allows modulating CXR components, which is of great clinical value. Our preliminary study shows that DecGAN can enhance the diagnostic potential of CXR and benefit the diagnosis of lung diseases.

2   Method

DecGAN is designed upon the backbone of CylceGAN with latent space disentanglement, as shown in Fig. 2. Given a CXR X as input, we want to build a function F to produce the modulated reconstruction X_m, in which different chest

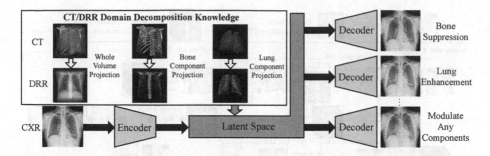

Fig. 1. We aim to decompose a chest X-ray (CXR) into multiple components by utilizing priori decomposition knowledge provided by computed tomography (CT) domain.

components can be modulated by changing the corresponding factors $[\alpha_b, \alpha_l, \alpha_o]$:

$$X_m = F(X, \alpha_b, \alpha_l, \alpha_o) = G_X(G_{Dec}(G_D(X, \alpha_b, \alpha_l, \alpha_o))), \qquad (1)$$

In order to tackle the problem of CXR decomposition, we mainly make three contributions: (1) An additional latent space decomposition discriminator D_{Dec} is designed to encourage the embedding of priori CT decomposition knowledge and the separation of different components in the generated DRR. (2) The DRR decomposition network G_{Dec} is embedded into the backbone of CycleGAN to provide the decoder enough knowledge to tackle the decomposition information in the latent space. (3) A soft bone mask $\mathcal{M}$, generated using the bone components in the latent space, serves as additional constraints to make the components separated and realistic in the reconstruction results.

2.1 DRR Decomposition Network G$_{Dec}$

The decomposition network is designed based on the architecture of U-net [6]. The components of a 3D CT volume are projected using the same parameters and concatenated into channels to serve as the ground truths of DRR decomposition:

$$I_{Dec} = [I_{bone}, I_{lung}, I_{other}], \qquad (2)$$

where I_{bone}, I_{lung} and I_{other} are the components of DRR for bone, lung and other soft-tissue, respectively.

Based on the input DRR image D and its separated components I_{Dec}, the decomposition network can be trained in a supervised way by using the decomposition loss:

$$\mathcal{L}_{Dec}(G_{Dec}) = \mathbb{E}_{D \sim p_{data}(D)}[\|G_{Dec}(D) - I_{Dec}\|_2^2]. \qquad (3)$$

2.2 Generative Models G$_D$ and G$_X$

The generative models are trained in an unsupervised way based on unpaired CXR and DRR. The DRR generation network G_D is trained to generate realistic

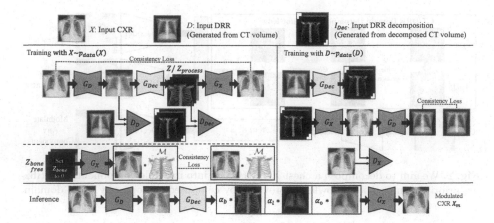

Fig. 2. The illustration of the proposed method. **Training phase:** Decomposition network G_{Dec} and decomposition discriminator network D_{Dec} are embedded into the backbone of CycleGAN which is designed to connect the domains of CXR and digitally reconstructed radiograph (DRR). A mask loss is provided to guarantee the corresponding relationship of non-bone components between the latent space and the reconstructed images. **Inference phase:** The components of reconstructed CXR can be modulated by changing the weight of probability maps in the latent space.

DRR based on input CXR, while the CXR generation network G_X is trained to reconstruct a realistic CXR based on the input DRR components.

Training with CXR. Taking the CXR X as input, the probability maps of decomposed components can be obtained using G_D and G_{Dec}:

$$Z = G_{Dec}(G_D(X)) = [Z_{bone}, Z_{lung}, Z_{other}], \tag{4}$$

where Z_{bone}, Z_{lung} and Z_{other} refer to the probability maps of bone, lung and other soft-tissue structures, respectively, which also correspond to (2). Thereafter, these maps are encoded into $Z_{process}$ to ensure the information is complete in the latent space:

$$Z_{process} = [Z_{bone}, Z_{lung}, G_D(X) - Z_{bone} - Z_{lung}]. \tag{5}$$

Once different CXR components are encoded separately into $Z_{process}$, it is possible to highlight or suppress specific CXR components by modulating the weights of different components in $Z_{process}$.

Another decomposition discriminator D_{Dec} is added in DecGAN to help separate different CXR components in the latent space. Thus, the generation loss is given as:

$$\mathcal{L}_{GXD}(G_D, D_D, D_{Dec}) = \mathbb{E}_{X \sim p_{data}(X)}[log(1 - D_D(G_D(X)))$$
$$+ log(1 - D_{Dec}(Z_{process}))] + \mathbb{E}_{D \sim p_{data}(D)}[log(D_D(D)) + log(D_{Dec}(I_{Dec}))]. \tag{6}$$

The discriminators are designed to reduce the gap between DRR and the generated CXR as well as the gap between DRR decomposition and CXR decomposition in the latent space.

At last, the cycle-consistency loss is applied to constrain the reconstruction results:

$$\mathcal{L}_{cycX}(G_D, G_X) = \mathbb{E}_{X \sim p_{data}(X)}[\|G_X(Z_{process}) - X\|_1]. \tag{7}$$

Training with DRR. The training cycle of DRR is conventional except that the cycle of DRR starts from its decompositions instead of the original images. The generation loss and cycle-consistency loss are defined as:

$$\mathcal{L}_{GDX}(G_X, D_X) = \mathbb{E}_{X \sim p_{data}(X)}[log(D_X(X)))$$
$$+\mathbb{E}_{D \sim p_{data}(D)}[log(1 - D_X(G_X(I_{Dec})))], \tag{8}$$

$$\mathcal{L}_{cycD}(G_D, G_X) = \mathbb{E}_{D \sim p_{data}(D)}[\|G_D(G_X(I_{Dec})) - D\|_1]. \tag{9}$$

Mask Loss. In early experiments of DecGAN, we find that the reconstruction results lack fidelity when changing the probability maps $Z_{process}$. It is because there is little priori knowledge for G_X to generate results with changed $Z_{process}$. To resolve this issue, we propose to put more constraints on the generative model for the CXR decomposition. Bone component is suitable for this task because it only appears in certain regions of CXR, and it is distinguishable from other components. In addition, it is always of no use for lung disease diagnosis. Therefore, we decide to optimize the generative model by putting less 'emphasis' on bone structures.

Different from the complete probability maps $Z_{process}$ in (5), we first eliminate the bone components in the latent space:

$$Z_{bonefree} = [0, Z_{lung}, G_D(X) - Z_{bone} - Z_{lung}]. \tag{10}$$

A soft mask $\mathcal{M}$ is then generated based on the existing bone probability map over 95% confidence. As the images are normalized to [0,1], the soft mask is defined as:

$$\mathcal{M} = 1 - (Z_{bone} - t)/(1 - t) * \delta[Z_{bone}], \tag{11}$$

where t is a threshold (we set $t = 0.95$) and the binary function $\delta[Z_{bone}]$ is defined as:

$$\delta[Z_{bone}] = \begin{cases} 0 & Z_{bone} < t; \\ 1 & Z_{bone} \geq t. \end{cases} \tag{12}$$

Based on the mask $\mathcal{M}$ in (11), the reconstruction results without bone components or the bone suppression results can be restricted by the input CXRs. The mask loss drives the non-bone regions of the reconstruction results become more similar to the original images:

$$\mathcal{L}_{mask}(G_X) = \mathbb{E}_{X \sim p_{data}(X)}[\|G_X(Z_{bonefree}) * \mathcal{M} - X * \mathcal{M}\|_1]. \tag{13}$$

Table 1. The quantitative results of unsupervised CXR bone suppression.

Method	CXR	Blind signal separation [2]	No Adaptation [6]	CycleGAN [11]	DecGAN	DecGAN (no D_{Dec}, no $\mathcal{L}_{mask}$)
$r_l(10^4)$	3.82	2.75	1.41	1.50	**0.854**	1.03
PSNRs	–	28.2	26.7	27.1	**29.6**	27.5

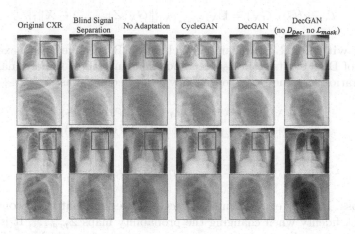

Fig. 3. Qualitative results of CXR bone suppression. We build several constraints in DecGAN to not only decompose different components separately but also produce realistic results. DecGAN can not only suppress bone to the greatest extent but also preserve the most realistic results of non-bone regions.

2.3   Inference and Modulation

In the inference phase, as the CXR components can be separated in the latent space and we have built the generative model to decode this information, we can modulate the CXR components to highlight specific component (e.g., lung) by changing the weights of probability maps, $[\alpha_b, \alpha_l, \alpha_o]$ and generating the modulated CXR reconstruction like:

$$X_m = G_X([\alpha_b * Z_{bone}, \alpha_l * Z_{lung}, \alpha_o * (G_D(X) - Z_{bone} - Z_{lung})]). \qquad (14)$$

3   Experiments

3.1   Datasets

We collect 246 CT volumes from LIDC-IDRI [1]. The bone regions in 3D CT volumes are labeled manually. The lung regions in CT volumes are labeled based on intensity and dilatation. We generate DRRs using those 246 CT volumes with augmentation based on rotation and rescaling. We collect 662 and 112,120 CXRs from Shenzhen Hospital X-ray Set [4] and ChestX-ray14 [7], respectively. We randomly select 99 cases from Shenzhen Hospital X-ray Set as test data and use the official split of ChestX-ray14 in our experiments.

3.2   CXR Bone Suppression

We first assess the quality of CXR decomposition through the task of unsupervised bone suppression. We evaluate the results based on CXR from the Shenzhen Hospital X-ray Set because its superior image quality makes it easier for manual bone annotation. Like the previous studies [2], we calculate the *line response* r_l to provide the quantitative evaluation of bone elimination, which is defined as the squared errors between the two eigenvalues of the Hessian matrix to reflect the elimination of high frequency bone borders. The lower is the metric, the less visible are the bone components in the CXRs. We also calculate *peak signal to noise ratio* (PSNR) of the non-bone regions based on manual annotations to gauge how well the non-bone regions are preserved. The quantitative and qualitative results are summarized in Table 1 and Fig. 3, respectively. DecGAN clearly outperforms the traditional solution which is based on blind signal suppression. Without domain adaptation, deep learning based methods would fail when the test CXR looks different from DRR: the bone suppression always lacks precision and the non-bone components are suppressed too. Similar failures happen to CycleGAN as the decoder has little knowledge of modified probability maps, the non-bone regions of the reconstruction results tend to be disturbed and collapse. Integrating G_{Dec} can make the generative model generate more reasonable bone suppression results, as shown in the results of 'DecGAN (no D_{Dec}, no $\mathcal{L}_{mask}$)'. However, the probability maps of different components are not separated clearly and the non-bone components sometimes look different from the original CXR. Therefore, the D_{Dec} component is added to encourage the components to separate in the latent space and an additional mask loss based on bone regions is further designed for DecGAN to guarantee the components of the lung and other soft-tissue structures can remain unchanged through the generative model.

3.3   Modulating CXR Components and Application to Diagnosis

CXR components can be modulated by changing the weights of $Z_{process}$, according to (14). The results of modulating components are shown in Fig. 4. The weights α_b and α_l are changed with the other weights always remaining the same. It is quite noticeable that the components of bone and lung are accordingly suppressed or enhanced while other components unchanged. This modulation feature has the potential of largely increasing the diagnosis value of CXR especially when the disease exists in a single component but overlaps with others.

In order to directly demonstrate the effectiveness of DecGAN for lung diseases diagnosis, the decomposition results are fed into the lung disease prediction system based on DenseNet-121. The lung enhancement results are generated with weights $[\alpha_b, \alpha_l, \alpha_o]$ being $[1, 2, 1]$. The lung enhancement results are concatenated with the original CXRs and stacked as the inputs of pretrained DenseNet-121 [3] model. The quantitative prediction results are summarized in Table 2, along with others' results which are also evaluated based on the official splits. Our method achieves the state-of-the-art results on 11 out of 14 common

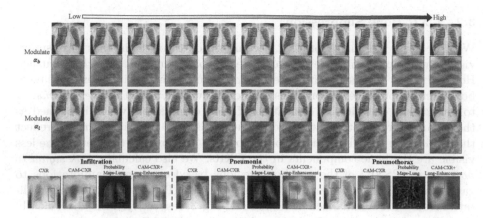

Fig. 4. (top half) Illustration of CXR modulation. DecGAN can modulate specific components with others unchanged. (bottom half) Examples of the unsupervised detection of lung diseases. The lung enhancement results can help better recognize and detect both the lung opacities, which are related to infiltration or pneumonia, and the lung collapse, which is caused by pneumothorax.

Table 2. The area under curve (AUC) of predicting 14 lung diseases from the ChestX-ray14 dataset. DecGAN can boost the prediction performance of the majority of lung diseases based on the prediction model of DenseNet-121.

Method	Atelectasis	Cardiomegaly	Effusion	Infiltration	Mass	Nodule	Pneumonia
Wang et al. [7]	0.700	0.810	0.759	0.661	0.693	0.669	0.658
DenseNet-121 [3]	0.777	0.879	0.825	0.696	**0.836**	0.773	0.730
Ours	**0.781**	**0.881**	0.827	**0.703**	0.835	**0.778**	**0.737**

Method	Pneumothorax	Consolidation	Edema	Emphysema	Fibrosis	Hernia	Pleura Thicken
Wang et al. [7]	0.799	0.703	0.805	0.833	0.786	0.872	0.684
DenseNet-121 [3]	0.842	0.761	0.847	**0.920**	0.823	**0.938**	0.779
Ours	**0.843**	**0.762**	**0.851**	0.917	**0.837**	0.929	**0.783**

lung diseases. While this performance boost is achieved *under an unpaired training setting*, we believe that this boost will be more conspicuous with supervised training data. The class activation mapping (CAM) results are shown in Fig. 4. The lung enhancement results by DecGAN are especially helpful in highlighting the lung abnormalities such as opacities in infiltration. In addition, the abnormal regions always show heterogeneity in the probability map of lung. For example, some disease patterns such as lung collapse in pneumothorax are more obvious in the probability map.

4   Conclusion

In this paper, we propose to learn a DecGAN *under an unpaired setting*, which decomposes a CXR image into different components based on priori CT anatomy knowledge. We demonstrate the effectiveness of DecGAN in the tasks of unsupervised bone suppression and lung diseases diagnosis, achieving the state-of-the-art performances. We believe DecGAN can enhance the diagnostic potential of CXR.

Acknowledgements. H. Han's work is supported in part by the Natural Science Foundation of China (grants 61732004 and 61672496), External Cooperation Program of Chinese Academy of Sciences (CAS) (grant GJHZ1843), and Youth Innovation Promotion Association CAS (grant 2018135). We thank Cheng Ouyang for helpful comments.

References

1. Armato III, S.G., McLennan, G., et al.: The lung image database consortium (LIDC) and image database resource initiative (IDRI): a completed reference database of lung nodules on CT scans. Med. Phys. **38**(2), 915–931 (2011)
2. Hogeweg, L., Sanchez, C.I., van Ginneken, B.: Suppression of translucent elongated structures: applications in chest radiography. IEEE Trans. Med. Imaging **32**(11), 2099–2113 (2013)
3. Huang, G., Liu, Z., Van Der Maaten, L., Weinberger, K.Q.: Densely connected convolutional networks. In: IEEE CVPR, pp. 4700–4708 (2017)
4. Jaeger, S., Candemir, S., et al.: Two public chest X-ray datasets for computer-aided screening of pulmonary diseases. Quant. Imaging Med. Surg. **4**(6), 475–477 (2014)
5. Laskey, M.A.: Dual-energy X-ray absorptiometry and body composition. Nutrition **12**(1), 45–51 (1996)
6. Ronneberger, O., Fischer, P., Brox, T.: U-net: convolutional networks for biomedical image segmentation. In: Navab, N., Hornegger, J., Wells, W.M., Frangi, A.F. (eds.) MICCAI 2015. LNCS, vol. 9351, pp. 234–241. Springer, Cham (2015). https://doi.org/10.1007/978-3-319-24574-4_28
7. Wang, X., Peng, Y., et al.: ChestX-ray8: hospital-scale chest X-ray database and benchmarks on weakly-supervised classification and localization of common thorax diseases. In: IEEE CVPR, pp. 3462–3471 (2017)
8. Yang, W., et al.: Cascade of multi-scale convolutional neural networks for bone suppression of chest radiographs in gradient domain. Med. Image Anal. **35**, 421–433 (2017)
9. Zhang, Y., Miao, S., Mansi, T., Liao, R.: Task driven generative modeling for unsupervised domain adaptation: application to X-ray image segmentation. In: Frangi, A.F., Schnabel, J.A., Davatzikos, C., Alberola-López, C., Fichtinger, G. (eds.) MICCAI 2018. LNCS, vol. 11071, pp. 599–607. Springer, Cham (2018). https://doi.org/10.1007/978-3-030-00934-2_67
10. Zhou, B., Lin, X., Eck, B., Hou, J., Wilson, D.: Generation of virtual dual energy images from standard single-shot radiographs using multi-scale and conditional adversarial network. In: Jawahar, C.V., Li, H., Mori, G., Schindler, K. (eds.) ACCV 2018. LNCS, vol. 11361, pp. 298–313. Springer, Cham (2019). https://doi.org/10.1007/978-3-030-20887-5_19
11. Zhu, J.Y., Park, T., Isola, P., Efros, A.A.: Unpaired image-to-image translation using cycle-consistent adversarial networks. In: IEEE ICCV, pp. 2242–2251 (2017)

Targeting Precision with Data Augmented Samples in Deep Learning

Pietro Nardelli$^{(\boxtimes)}$ ⓘ and Raúl San José Estépar ⓘ

Applied Chest Imaging Laboratory, Brigham and Women's Hospital,
Harvard Medical School, Boston, MA, USA
{pnardelli,rsanjose}@bwh.harvard.edu

Abstract. In the last five years, deep learning (DL) has become the state-of-the-art tool for solving various tasks in medical image analysis. Among the different methods that have been proposed to improve the performance of Convolutional Neural Networks (CNNs), one typical approach is the augmentation of the training data set through various transformations of the input image. Data augmentation is typically used in cases where a small amount of data is available, such as the majority of medical imaging problems, to present a more substantial amount of data to the network and improve the overall accuracy. However, the ability of the network to improve the accuracy of the results when a slightly modified version of the same input is presented is often overestimated. This overestimation is the result of the strong correlation between data samples when they are considered independently in the training phase. In this paper, we emphasize the importance of optimizing for accuracy as well as precision among multiple replicates of the same training data in the context of data augmentation. To this end, we propose a new approach that leverages the augmented data to help the network focus on the precision through a specifically-designed loss function, with the ultimate goal to improve both the overall performance and the network's precision at the same time. We present two different applications of DL (regression and segmentation) to demonstrate the strength of the proposed strategy. We think that this work will pave the way to a explicit use of data augmentation within the loss function that helps the network to be invariant to small variations of the same input samples, a characteristic that is always required to every application in the medical imaging field.

Keywords: Deep learning · Data augmentation · Accuracy · Precision

This work has been partially funded by the National Institutes of Health NHLBI awards R01HL116931, R01HL116473, and R21HL14042. We gratefully acknowledge the support of NVIDIA Corporation with the donation of the GPU used for this research.

D. Shen et al. (Eds.): MICCAI 2019, LNCS 11769, pp. 284–292, 2019.
https://doi.org/10.1007/978-3-030-32226-7_32

1   Introduction

Thanks to their demonstrated great performance and potential, deep learning (DL) techniques are quickly becoming the main tools for medical imaging analysis. In recent years, several new architectures and DL applications have been proposed in the literature trying to solve various problems [5,9]. However, depending on the complexity of the task that a DL model has to perform, the number of parameters that need to be tuned to reduce the loss might be very high.

Therefore, in order to get good performance, a proportionally high amount of examples should be shown to the network, as a model's performance typically increases as the quality, diversity, and the amount of training data increases. However, especially in medical imaging tasks, collecting enough data is often highly complicated and one of the biggest problems developers have to face when creating a new DL tool is over-fitting to the training dataset, which happens when the network is robust with the shown examples, but it is not able to generalize well the output if initial conditions are even slightly modified.

The most typical approach used to overcome this issue is the augmentation of the training data-set by means of various synthetic transformations of the input image, a method that is particularly helpful when only a small amount of data is available, and that may help increase the level of invariance of the network to known transformation of the input image space.

In recent years, much effort has been spent trying to improve and automatize augmentation techniques in order to get the network to learn varying conditions and improve the overall accuracy and robustness [2]. Recently, adversarial neural networks (GANs) have been proposed [4], and one possible application domain for these techniques is data augmentation [1,3].

However, in addition to accuracy and robustness an important metric that should also be taken into account, especially when trying to solve medical imaging issues, is precision. Precision is a metric that indicates that the network is able to output the same values when replicas of the same input, although slightly modified, are presented. In the majority of proposed works though, this aspect is underestimated, and the overall performance is the only metric considered during the training phase of the network.

In this paper, we present a novel approach to augmented samples that takes into account both accuracy and precision during the training phase. We propose to use a specifically-designed loss function that can be modified according to the problem into consideration and combines both metrics to improve the network ability to learn image characteristics regardless of varying conditions properly.

To demonstrate the strength of the proposed strategy, two applications of DL with and without the presented approach are shown. First, a regression problem where 25 modified replicas of the same input are used to measure airway lumen radius on CT images accurately is presented. Then, a segmentation of the lung region is shown to demonstrate the improvement achieved both in accuracy and precision when 20 synthetically modified versions of each input example are used.

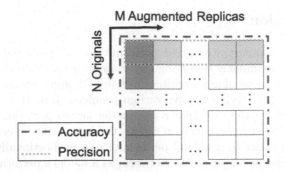

Fig. 1. Scheme of accuracy-precision loss. Accuracy is computed over all N × M images (red square), while precision is calculated over the M image replicas (purple square). (Color figure online)

2   Material and Methods

In order to properly target precision for DL techniques, we propose the development of a customized loss function that can be designed around the problem of interest to take into account augmented data and simultaneously improve the overall accuracy as well as the network's precision. The basic idea is that when a synthetically modified version of the same input is presented to the network, the exact same output should be expected. In this section, we first introduce the general loss, and we then present two different versions of it as we adapt it to two separate problems.

2.1   Accuracy-Precision Loss

In this paper, we propose the usage of a new loss for DL algorithms that consists of two terms; a term that represents the loss of the accuracy over all images, $\mathcal{L}_\mu$, and a second term that takes into account the precision over the synthetically augmented replicas of the original inputs, $\mathcal{L}_\sigma$.

If we represent all input and augmented images in a N × M matrix where the first column contains the N original inputs and all other columns contain M augmented replicas (one column for each augmentation) then, the precision loss, $\mathcal{L}_\sigma$, is computed over each row N of the matrix, while the accuracy loss, $\mathcal{L}_\mu$, is given over all N × M inputs, as shown in Fig. 1. More formally, the accuracy-precision loss, $\mathcal{L}_{AP}$, is given by the following expression:

$$\mathcal{L}_{AP}(\boldsymbol{y}, \widehat{\boldsymbol{y}}) = \omega \cdot \mathcal{L}_\mu(\boldsymbol{y}, \widehat{\boldsymbol{y}}) + \lambda \cdot \mathcal{L}_\sigma(\boldsymbol{y}, \widehat{\boldsymbol{y}}) \tag{1}$$

where $\boldsymbol{y}$ is the true value of the input, $\widehat{\boldsymbol{y}}$ is the predicted value, and ω, λ define how the two terms of the loss are weighted. From this it follows that:

$$\mathcal{L}_{AP}(\boldsymbol{y}, \widehat{\boldsymbol{y}}) = \omega \cdot \frac{1}{N \times M} \sum_{i=0, j=0}^{N,M} \mathcal{L}_\mu(y_{i,j}, \widehat{y}_{i,j}) + \lambda \cdot \frac{1}{N} \sum_{i=0}^{N} \left(\frac{1}{M} \sum_{j=0}^{M} \mathcal{L}_\sigma(y_{i,j}, \widehat{y}_{i,j}) \right) \tag{2}$$

Depending on the specific task that the deep learning model has to perform, $\mathcal{L}_\mu$ and $\mathcal{L}_\sigma$ can be specifically designed according to Eq. 2. In the following two sections we show two examples of accuracy-precision loss as it might adapted to regression and segmentation tasks.

2.2 Accuracy-Precision Loss for Regression

In this section, we present an accuracy-precision loss applied to a regression task to measure the lumen nominal radius of small airways from chest CT images. For this problem, we developed a model-generator that creates 2D synthetic patches of 32×32 pixels (with a resolution of 0.5 mm) on the reformatted axial plane that resemble patches around real airways.

Thanks to this generative model, training examples are not an issue, as they can be generated at will with known lumen size. The regressor consists of a 9-layer 2D network with seven convolutional and two fully-connected layers, as proposed in [6], and is trained on 2,500,000 synthetic patches, generated as 100,000 individual images for which 25 augmented replicas are created by maintaining the same lumen and wall thickness and varying point spread function (PSF), rotation, flipping, and translation, and adding a various number of additional vessels around the airway.

While trying to reduce the relative error (RE) over all images (accuracy), we want the regressor to also learn that the same measurement for airway lumen radius should be provided across all replicas regardless of possible confounding factors inside the patch. Therefore, the accuracy loss is given by the RE:

$$\mathcal{L}_\mu(\boldsymbol{y}, \widehat{\boldsymbol{y}}) = \frac{1}{N \times M} \cdot \sum_{i=0, j=0}^{N,M} \frac{|y_{i,j} - \widehat{y}_{i,j}|}{y_{i,j}} \tag{3}$$

where $\boldsymbol{y}$ indicates the ground-truth measure of a synthetic patch provided by the generative model, $\widehat{\boldsymbol{y}}$ the measure predicted by the regressor, N is the total number of individual patches (N = 100,000), and M is the number of replicas (M = 25). Conversely, for the precision loss we want to minimize the error across the M replicas by:

$$\mathcal{L}_\sigma(\boldsymbol{y}, \widehat{\boldsymbol{y}}) = \frac{1}{N} \cdot \sum_{i=0}^{N} \left(\frac{1}{M} \cdot \sum_{j=0}^{M} \left(y_{i,j} - \widehat{y}_{i,j} \right)^2 - \left(\frac{1}{M} \cdot \sum_{j=0}^{M} (y_{i,j} - \widehat{y}_{i,j}) \right)^2 \right) \tag{4}$$

Moreover, in this specific case we want to give more importance to precision with respect to accuracy. Therefore, we set $\omega = 1$ and $\lambda = 2$ and the final accuracy-precision loss for the presented regression problem is given by:

$$\mathcal{L}(\boldsymbol{y}, \widehat{\boldsymbol{y}}) = \frac{1}{N \times M} \cdot \sum_{i=0, j=0}^{N,M} \frac{|y_{i,j} - \widehat{y}_{i,j}|}{y_{i,j}} +$$

$$2.0 \cdot \frac{1}{N} \cdot \sum_{i=0}^{N} \left(\frac{1}{M} \cdot \sum_{j=0}^{M} \left(y_{i,j} - \widehat{y}_{i,j} \right)^2 - \left(\frac{1}{M} \cdot \sum_{j=0}^{M} (y_{i,j} - \widehat{y}_{i,j}) \right)^2 \right) \tag{5}$$

2.3 Accuracy-Precision Loss for Segmentation

The same concept can also be applied to a segmentation task. In this paper, we use a 2D intra-parenchymal lung segmentation from CT images to show a different application domain for the proposed technique. Since our final goal is to show the ability of our method to improve results compared to traditional approaches, and not to obtain an optimal segmentation, we used a modified version of U-Net [7] as segmenter.

In this case, as ground-truth we used axial lung labels obtained with the method described in [8] and visually evaluated for correctness. We randomly extracted 2,100 2D axial CT slices and corresponding label maps from 300 cases from high-resolution chest CT scans of the COPDGene study phase 2.

For memory reasons, we resampled images to a size of 256×256 pixels. To create the augmented data, we generated 10 replicas for each original image by introducing random noise, rotation, flipping, translation, and skew, and shear transformations. As a main metric for the segmentation, we used the dice coefficient score to compare the label produced by our segmenter to the ground-truth. However, while we want the dice coefficient as high as possible over all images, we also want an as small as possible standard deviation of the error across the 10 image replicas. To this end, we used an accuracy loss given by:

$$\mathcal{L}_\mu(y, \widehat{y}) = 1.0 - 2.0 \cdot \frac{|y \cap \widehat{y}|}{|y| + |\widehat{y}|} \tag{6}$$

where y indicates the ground-truth label, $\widehat{y}$ the label provided by the network, $N = 2,100$ is the total number of individual images, and $M = 10$ is the number of synthetically augmented replicas. In this case, the precision loss is computed as the standard deviation of the dice coefficient loss over the $M = 10$ replicas:

$$\mathcal{L}_\sigma(y, \widehat{y}) = \frac{1}{N} \cdot \sum_{i=0}^{N} \sqrt{\mathrm{VAR}_M\left(1.0 - 2.0 \cdot \frac{|y \cap \widehat{y}|}{|y| + |\widehat{y}|}\right)} \tag{7}$$

where VAR_M indicates the variance across the M replicas. As in the regression case, we set $\omega = 1$ and $\lambda = 3.0$ to obtain the global accuracy-precision loss as:

$$\mathcal{L}(y, \widehat{y}) = 1.0 - 2.0 \cdot \frac{|y \cap \widehat{y}|}{|y| + |\widehat{y}|} + 3.0 \cdot \frac{1}{N} \cdot \sum_{i=0}^{N} \sqrt{\mathrm{VAR}_M\left(1.0 - 2.0 \cdot \frac{|y \cap \widehat{y}|}{|y| + |\widehat{y}|}\right)} \tag{8}$$

3 Experimental Setup

To evaluate the proposed approach, we compared the results obtained for the regression and the segmentation tasks with the presented accuracy-precision loss and its accuracy-only version.

For airway lumen measurement, we first used 200,000 randomly generated synthetic patches to evaluate the overall mean RE. Then, we created a dataset by varying the level of noise in the range $\sigma_n \in [0, 40]$ HU (smoothing level fixed at

1.3 mm) and generating 100 synthetic replicas for each noise value, and a second dataset fixing the level of noise at 25 HU and changing the applied smoothness in the range $\sigma_s \in [0.4, 0.9]$ mm to generate 100 synthetic replicas per degree of smoothing.

To create the two datasets, we fixed the wall thickness at 1.5 mm and used three airway lumen values (small: 0.5 mm; medium: 2.5 mm; large: 4.5 mm) randomly varying all other parameters of the geometric model. For these two datasets, we computed the mean RE (in %) across the 100 patches for each level of noise and smoothness, to demonstrate that the proposed loss function helps improve not only the accuracy but also the precision of network when initial conditions change. For the accuracy-only method, we used a simple mean RE loss.

On the other hand, to demonstrate the improved ability to segment the lung region of a U-net that uses the proposed loss function, we used the 55 cases from the Lobe and Lung Analysis 2011 (LOLA11) challenge that were first segmented with the method presented in [8], and were then visually inspected and manually refined. We used the Dice coefficient score for the comparison. The same process was finally repeated using the same neural network architecture, but only with a Dice coefficient loss.

4 Results

The mean RE when using the proposed accuracy-precision loss to measure the airway lumen was 2.06%, while when a mean RE loss is used the mean RE is 3.01%. Results obtained when fixing three values of airway lumen (0.5, 2.5, and 4.5 mm) and varying the level of noise and smoothing for the two methods are presented in Fig. 2. As shown, the RE obtained with both methods and for both measurements is stable across the different levels of noise and smoothness.

However, while with the proposed loss a very high accuracy is obtained (RE close to 0 for large and medium structures, RE around -10 for small airways), using a traditional loss function a bigger RE is obtained for all structures. Also, the standard deviation is much smaller when a precision-accuracy loss function is used. This effect is visible when varying both the noise (first row in Fig. 2) and the smoothness (second row in Fig. 2).

For the segmentation analysis, the mean Dice score -in comparison with the method proposed in [8]- when using the loss function presented in Eq. 8 was 97.6% $\pm$ 0.027, while a traditional loss is used, a mean Dice score of 95.8% $\pm$ 0.029 was obtained.

Dice coefficient results stratified by lung volume (low and high volume defined as being below or above the median lung volume of the LOLA datasets) and by lung size (right vs. left) are presented in Fig. 4. As shown, while the Dice scores are consistent for both lungs and by level of volume lung for both methods independently, the proposed loss has a consistent higher Dice score ($p < 0.001$) with a lower variance implying a more robust result.

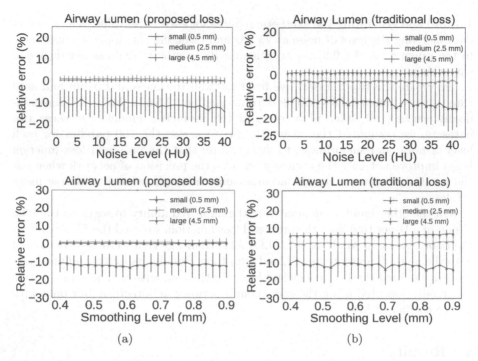

Fig. 2. Results obtained for airway lumen regression when varying the level of noise (first row) and smoothing (second row). In both cases, the RE (reported in %) obtained with proposed loss (a) is lower than that obtained when precision is not taken into account (b). Also, a precision-accuracy loss function greatly reduces the standard deviation for the RE.

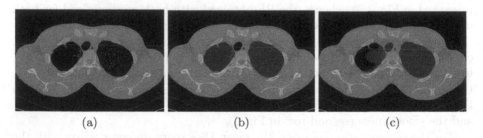

Fig. 3. Example of lung segmentation for case 23 from the LOLA11 dataset. A slice from the original CT (a), and the same slice overlaid with the segmentation obtained using (b) the proposed loss function and (c) a Dice loss function are presented.

From an accurate analysis of segmentation of single cases, it was clear that with a traditional loss the segmentation has a higher tendency to leak inside the trachea, whereas the proposed loss function seems to help the network segment the lung region in a more accurate and precise way (see Fig. 3).

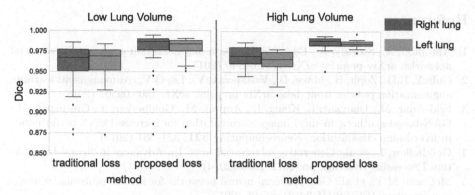

Fig. 4. Dice coefficient results obtained with the traditional and the proposed method when considering right and left lung independently and separating the cases by lung volume.

5 Discussion and Conclusion

In this paper, we presented a novel approach to data augmentation for deep learning tasks that instead of focusing only on the overall performance of the network may help increase both accuracy and precision of a neural network.

The modified data is used not only to increase the amount of data presented to the network but also to reduce the variance of the output when similar inputs are presented. To this end, we introduce a new generalized loss function that leverages the information provided by the augmented data and can be adapted to the specific problem of interest. Results from the application of the loss function to regression and segmentation tasks showed that while the presented technique helps improve the overall accuracy, the precision of the DL model is also increased.

For the lung segmentation task, we want to point out that the final goal was not to obtain an optimal segmentation, but to demonstrate that if the proposed function is utilized, results improve compared to the usage of a traditional loss. For future work, we will validate the proposed loss function by showing that the best performing deep neural network reported for LOLA11 trained with the proposed loss function improves the final segmentation. Also, a classification task will also be considered for further testing.

The main limitation of the proposed loss function is given by the fact that when big image data is required the batch size will necessarily get smaller, significantly reducing the number of replicas that can be shown to the network.

In conclusion, we believe that the proposed approach to data augmentation will pave the way to a new way of using the synthetically modified data and will help to improve the performance of DL techniques in a field where a significant amount of data is not available at no cost.

References

1. Antoniou, A., Storkey, A., Edwards, H.: Data augmentation generative adversarial networks. arXiv preprint arXiv:1711.04340 (2017)
2. Cubuk, E.D., Zoph, B., Mane, D., Vasudevan, V., Le, Q.V.: Autoaugment: learning augmentation policies from data. arXiv preprint arXiv:1805.09501 (2018)
3. Frid-Adar, M., Diamant, I., Klang, E., Amitai, M., Goldberger, J., Greenspan, H.: GAN-based synthetic medical image augmentation for increased CNN performance in liver lesion classification. Neurocomputing **321**, 321–331 (2018)
4. Goodfellow, I., et al.: Generative adversarial nets. In: Advances in Neural Information Processing Systems, pp. 2672–2680 (2014)
5. McCann, M.T., et al.: Convolutional neural networks for inverse problems in imaging: a review. IEEE SPM **34**(6), 85–95 (2017)
6. Nardelli, P., et al.: Accurate measurement of airway morphology on chest CT images. In: Stoyanov, D., et al. (eds.) RAMBO/BIA/TIA -2018. LNCS, vol. 11040, pp. 335–347. Springer, Cham (2018). https://doi.org/10.1007/978-3-030-00946-5_34
7. Ronneberger, O., Fischer, P., Brox, T.: U-net: convolutional networks for biomedical image segmentation. In: Navab, N., Hornegger, J., Wells, W.M., Frangi, A.F. (eds.) MICCAI 2015. LNCS, vol. 9351, pp. 234–241. Springer, Cham (2015). https://doi.org/10.1007/978-3-319-24574-4_28
8. Ross, J.C., et al.: Lung extraction, lobe segmentation and hierarchical region assessment for quantitative analysis on high resolution computed tomography images. In: Yang, G.-Z., Hawkes, D., Rueckert, D., Noble, A., Taylor, C. (eds.) MICCAI 2009. LNCS, vol. 5762, pp. 690–698. Springer, Heidelberg (2009). https://doi.org/10.1007/978-3-642-04271-3_84
9. Suzuki, K.: Overview of deep learning in medical imaging. Radiol. Phys. Technol. **10**(3), 257–273 (2017)

Pulmonary Vessel Segmentation Based on Orthogonal Fused U-Net++ of Chest CT Images

Hejie Cui[1,2], Xinglong Liu[1], and Ning Huang[1]([⊠])

[1] SenseTime Research, Beijing, China
huangning@sensetime.com
[2] Emory University, Atlanta, GA, USA

Abstract. Pulmonary vessel segmentation is important for clinical diagnosis of pulmonary diseases, while is also challenging due to the complicated structure. In this work, we present an effective framework and refinement process of pulmonary vessel segmentation from chest computed tomographic (CT) images. The key to our approach is a 2.5D segmentation network applied from three orthogonal axes, which presents a robust and fully automated pulmonary vessel segmentation result with lower network complexity and memory usage compared to 3D networks. The slice radius is introduced to convolve the adjacent information of the center slice and the multi-planar fusion optimizes the presentation of intra and inter slice features. Besides, the tree-like structure of pulmonary vessel is extracted in the post-processing process, which is used for segmentation refining and pruning. In the evaluation experiments, three fusion methods are tested and the most promising one is compared with the state-of-the-art 2D and 3D structures on 300 cases of lung images randomly selected from LIDC dataset. Our method outperforms other network structures by a large margin and achieves by far the highest average DICE score of 0.9272 and a precision of 0.9310, as per our knowledge from the pulmonary vessel segmentation models available in literature.

Keywords: Pulmonary vessel segmentation · U-Net++ · 2.5D CNN

1 Introduction

Pulmonary vessel segmentation is a topic of high interest in the field of medical image analysis: accurate vascular analysis has extremely important research and application value for treatment planning and clinical effect evaluation. Pulmonary vessel segmentation is a basis for common pulmonary vascular diseases diagnosis such as lobectomy and pulmonary embolism [2].

However, the lung of the human body is the exchange place for metabolically produced gases, which is rich in trachea and vascular tissues, so its structure is relatively complicated. At the same time, due to factors such as noise and

© Springer Nature Switzerland AG 2019
D. Shen et al. (Eds.): MICCAI 2019, LNCS 11769, pp. 293–300, 2019.
https://doi.org/10.1007/978-3-030-32226-7_33

volume effect, CT images might suffer from poor contrast and blurred boundaries. Moreover, the pulmonary venous arteries and veins are intertwined and accompanied, which further increases the difficulty of segmentation [4].

A number of earlier vessel segmentation methods like tracking algorithms [9], seed point based [3], edge-based or region-based deformable model [11] have been applied and tested in different anatomical regions or imaging modalities, such as retina images. These methods, however, depend on hand-crafted features, thus having limited feature representation abilities. Besides, few supervised methods have been applied on pulmonary vessel segmentation. This is due to the inaccessibility of complex, fully-annotated dataset, which has become an important factor limiting the development of deep learning algorithms in this task [6]. Besides, relevant vessel segmentation studies have proposed the use of synthetic data for 2D or 3D neural network training [7], but considering the complexity of real blood vessel distribution and the influence of pathological tissue variability, hardly can synthetic data truly and comprehensively reflect the pattern of vascular tree.

Fully connected neural networks (FCNs) have achieved general success on segmentation tasks. In order to find an effective segmentation method for pulmonary vessel segmentation task, we do early-stage experiments on both 2D FCNs and 3D FCNs architecture with volumetric input. Result shows that 2D FCNs ignore the context information along the stacked axis, which contains important connection information for the upper and lower levels of the vascular tree; while 3D FCNs suffer from high computational cost and GPU memory consumption, which impedes the performance for large scale dataset [13].

To better solve the problems mentioned above, we have proposed a fused 2.5D U-Net++ applied from three orthogonal axes. We use volumetric ground truth generated by unsupervised methods and then manually corrected by professional radiologists as the input of 2D convolutional network for each direction. The voxel prediction results of adjacent slices are employed for the prediction of the center slice, and segmentation volume of each axis is gained by stacking the segmentation maps of the center slices. This 2.5D convolution process is applied from three axes, where 3D contexts are effectively extracted and jointly optimized for an accurate pulmonary vessel tree segmentation. The evaluation of our proposed network achieves a reliably better result compared with several state-of-the-art segmentation networks. Besides, we also propose a post-processing process where the tree-like skeleton is generated for the refining of the segmentation result. Our contributions mainly lie in:

- We propose a 2.5D convolution network, which employs the 2D convolutional network on a stack of adjacent slices and fuses the features extracted from three orthogonal axes.
- A whole automated segmentation framework is given and we introduce a post-processing where the segmentation result is refined by the graph information of pulmonary vessel tree.
- Our method gives a very competitive performance and ranks 1st till now on DICE Similarity Coefficient and Precision compared with the results reported by other state-of-the-art methods.

2 Methods

We combine the idea of 2.5D network [13] and orthogonal fusion of multi-planar network to obtain a new architecture: an orthogonal fused 2.5D U-Net++. Figure 1 shows the pipeline of our proposed method for pulmonary vessel segmentation.

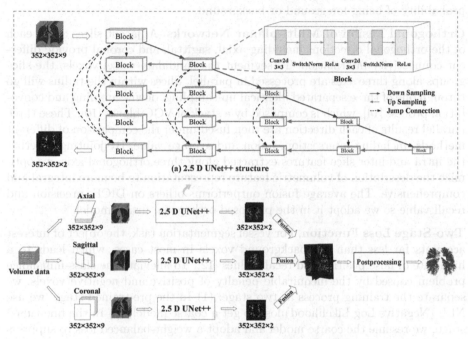

Fig. 1. Overall architecture of the proposed pulmonary vessel segmentation framework. Each volume data is sampled as adjacent slice groups along three orthogonal axes and then fed to a 2.5D U-Net++ network; The features extracted by the three parallel 2.5D networks are fused to optimize the volumetric representation; In the post processing, a structure graph is extracted to refine the segmentation result. (a) The structure of 2.5D U-Net++, whose output is the two-channel probability map of the center slice. (b) The whole framework, including the orthogonal fusion of multi-planar networks and the post-processing for segmentation refinement.

2.5D Network Based on U-Net++. In the clinical practice, the experienced radiologists usually observe and judge the full structure of pulmonary vessel based on several successive slices along a specific axis. Therefore, a conventional 2D based network will easily ignore the context information while extracting the intra slice features, thus restricting the segmentation accuracy [5].

In order to include the adjacency information between slices while doing the vessel segmentation, we design a 2.5D network which digests multiple channels cropped from the original CT images. Slice radius is introduced, where slices within the radius will be convolved during the feature map extraction process. The input channel is 9, and the ground-truth of the middle slice will be provided. The upper and lower 4 pieces of the middle slice are used to generate the feature maps. Since the information within radius range will be convolved, the inter slice information is preserved as much as possible to help the segmentation of middle slices. The output channel of the 2.5D network is 2, indicating the voxel-wise probability of being foreground or background.

Orthogonal Fusion of Multi-planar Networks. Adjacent slices along each of the orthogonal directions including axial, sagittal, and coronal provide different connectivity information. To segment the candidate vessel voxels, the slice groups along three axes are processed in parallel. Slices within the radius will go through one of three separated identical up-sampling, down-sampling and convolution process [14], which is composed by a stack of VGG blocks [10]. These three parallel results of each direction are then fused under the comparison of different methods, including intersection, union and average value. By jointing together the intra and inter slice features extracted along three orthogonal axis, we optimize the description of volumetric feature representation to be more integral and comprehensive. The average fusion outperforms others on DICE, precision and recall value so we adopt it in the proposed orthogonal fusion model.

Two-Stage Loss Function. For vessel segmentation task, the object of interest accounts far less than the background voxels in most cases, which leads to a high rate of false positive and recall values [12]. To alleviate the class-imbalance problem caused by the inequitable penalty of positive and negative voxels, we separate the training process as two stage: (1) In the pre-trained stage, we use NLL (Negative Log Likelihood) loss to get a coarse model; (2) In the fine-tuned stage, we resume the coarse model and adopt a weight-balanced loss to suppress the over-segmentation and high false-positive rate: the calculated voxel-wised losses of both positive and negative positions are sorted, and the negative sorted list is much longer than the positive one considering the small occupancy of interest regions. We cut the negative list to make it the same length as the positive list. The top part of negative list is taken for loss function in order to balance the weight between the proportion of two kinds of voxels. The weighted loss function employed is described as below:

$$L = L_{Y_+(W)} + L_{Y_-(W)} \tag{1}$$

$$L_{Y_+(W)} = -\sum_{i \in Y_+}^{N} log P(y_i = 1 | X; W) \tag{2}$$

$$L_{Y_-(W)} = -\sum_{j \in \widetilde{Y}_-}^{N} log P(y_j = 0 | X; W) \tag{3}$$

where $\widetilde{Y}_-$ represents the top N loss value selected from the sorted list of negative samples and N is the number of elements in positive list.

Vessel Structure Generation. In the post-processing stage, vessel structure is used to refine the segmentation result. We generate the morphology representation of tree-like graph from the skeleton of segmentation result. The graph includes nodes and edges, and the connected components can be calculated. This tree-like graph of pulmonary vessel can express plenty of potential useful information at very fine scales. In the post-processing, connected components with less than 10 nodes are trimmed on the graph, then the refined graph is filled edge by edge to get a refined segmentation result. The input of the post-processing is segmentation result of the end-to-end segmentation network and the output is refined vessel tree segmentation composed by the main connected components with more than 10 nodes [8].

In addition to pruning the segmentation result, the topological structure represented by edges and nodes also indicates meaningful information for clinical practice, such as the location of junction points, the number of individual branches, and the connection relationship between bifurcations and end-points. We will continue to explore its application in future work.

3   Experiments

Dataset and Pre-processing. We randomly select a subset of 300 cases of chest CTs from publicly available LIDC [1] dataset and split them into 270 cases for training and 30 cases for validating. 10% of the selected dataset is utilized as testing set. To ensure the data variability, both challenging and visible vessels are included to cover a comprehensive situation. The ground truth mask for training is first generated using unsupervised method and then refined and validated by expert radiologists.

Pre-processing includes two parts: resolution regularization and Hounsfield Unit (HU) Value normalization. The original resolution varies from $0.6 \times 0.6 \times 1.25 \, mm^3$ to $0.9 \times 0.9 \times 2.5 \, mm^3$. For resolution regularization, we resample the data to $1 \, mm^3$ resolution cube. For intensity normalization, we adopt a lung window of $[-1200, 600]$ HU. The HU value of all data is cropped and adjusted to the range of lung window and then normalized to $[0, 1]$.

Implementation Details. The training of our model is performed on a workstation with a CPU of Intel(R) Core(R) i7-7700 @ 3.6 GHz and a NVIDIA GTX 1080 Ti GPU with 11 GB of memory. In the training process of the fused 2.5D network, we use the SGD optimizer with a momentum of 0.99 and a weight decay of 1e-8. The initial learning rate is 0.001 and we apply a stepped learning rate scheduler with the initial value multiplied by a specific gamma value every several epochs. The loss function is divided into two stages: in the pre-trained stage, we use NLL-loss; and in the fine-tuned stage, we propose the weight-balanced loss to alleviate the disproportionate rate between the foreground and background.

Table 1. Comparison of six fusion methods.

Methods	Min dice	Max dice	Avg. dice	Precision/Recall
Axial	0.8618	0.9584	0.9162	0.9250/0.9144
Sagittal	0.8444	0.9575	0.9114	0.9232/0.9080
Coronal	0.7474	0.9547	0.8964	0.9024/0.9020
Union	0.8252	0.9580	0.9118	0.8714/0.9634
Intersection	0.7946	0.9555	0.9096	0.9518/0.8772
Average	**0.8779**	**0.9627**	**0.9262**	**0.9310/0.9272**

Results and Discussion. The evaluation experiments include two parts.

First, we compare the single axis model with three fusion methods, including intersection, union and average value, to find the best one in keeping information of three axes. The pulmonary vessel segmentation result of each fusion method is presented in Table 1. Grid search in the range of $(0.05, 0.5)$ is used to find the best threshold value of the prediction result map for each fusion method. We record the minimal, maximum, average dice value and precision/recall ratio under the best threshold of each method. Results show that the average fusion method achieves the highest performance in all statistical indicators.

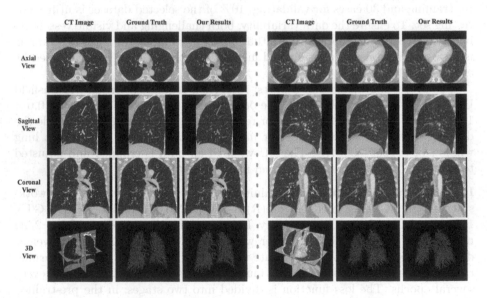

Fig. 2. The visual comparison between the ground truth and result of the proposed 2.5D Average Orthogonal Fused U-Net++.

Second, we further compare the average fused 2.5D network structure with several state-of-the-art network structures, including 2D U-Net++, 3D U-Net++ as well as several 3D FCNs. The quantitive results of U-Net++ based model are shown in Table 2 for comparison on a single-model basis. The promising 2.5D network significantly outperforms 2D and 3D FCNs models, which validates the advantage of our proposed structure.

Table 2. Comparison of three state-of-art structures.

Structures	Min dice	Max dice	Avg. dice	Precision/Recall
2D U-net++	0.5201	0.7376	0.6628	0.6629/0.6767
3D U-Net++	0.4385	0.8038	0.7286	0.7425/0.7436
2.5D U-Net++	**0.8779**	**0.9627**	**0.9262**	**0.9310/0.9272**

Figure 2 shows the qualitative results of our methods compared with the ground truth. Results of more cases are displayed in Fig. 3 to prove the robustness of model on different quality CT images.

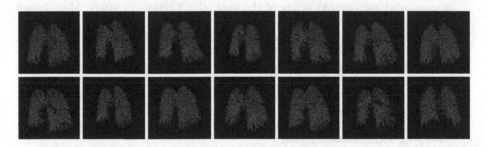

Fig. 3. Qualitative results of average fusion 2.5D U-Net++ on more CT images. Note that the position and shape of lung are varied from case to case, and the vessel segmentation results remain high performance on different quality CT images.

4 Conclusion

Pulmonary Vessel Segmentation is one of the most challenging tasks in medical image analysis. The segmentation must overcome the complexity of the pulmonary structure as well as the limited resolution of CT images. In this paper, we propose a novel framework for automated pulmonary vessel segmentation based on a fused 2.5D convolution network structure. Slice radius is introduced to convolve adjacent information and the multi-planar fusion optimizes the presentation of intra and inter slice features. Besides, a post-processing is designed to refine the segmentation results using main components information of the pulmonary vessel tree. Our method excels others by a large margin on pulmonary vessel segmentation task and achieves very competitive results on DICE and Precision value.

Acknowledgments. This work is partially funded by Beijing Posdoctoral Research Foundation.

References

1. Armato, S.G., et al.: The lung image database consortium (LIDC) and image database resource initiative (IDRI): a completed reference database of lung nodules on CT scans. Med. Phys. **38**(2), 915–931 (2011)
2. El-Baz, A., Suri, J.S.: Lung Imaging and Computer Aided Diagnosis. CRC Press, Boca Raton (2011)
3. Kaftan, J.N., Kiraly, A.P., Bakai, A., Das, M., Novak, C.L., Aach, T.: Fuzzy pulmonary vessel segmentation in contrast enhanced CT data. In: Medical Imaging 2008: Image Processing, vol. 6914, p. 69141Q. International Society for Optics and Photonics (2008)
4. Lesage, D., Angelini, E.D., Bloch, I., Funka-Lea, G.: A review of 3D vessel lumen segmentation techniques: models, features and extraction schemes. Med. Image Anal. **13**(6), 819–845 (2009)
5. Li, X., Chen, H., Qi, X., Dou, Q., Fu, C.W., Heng, P.A.: H-DenseUNet: hybrid densely connected UNet for liver and tumor segmentation from CT volumes. IEEE Trans. Med. Imaging **37**(12), 2663–2674 (2018)
6. Rudyanto, R.D., et al.: Comparing algorithms for automated vessel segmentation in computed tomography scans of the lung: the VESSEL12 study. Med. Image Anal. **18**(7), 1217–1232 (2014)
7. Schneider, M., Reichold, J., Weber, B., Székely, G., Hirsch, S.: Tissue metabolism driven arterial tree generation. Med. Image Anal. **16**(7), 1397–1414 (2012)
8. Shang, Y., et al.: Vascular active contour for vessel tree segmentation. IEEE Trans. Biomed. Eng. **58**(4), 1023–1032 (2011)
9. Shikata, H., Hoffman, E.A., Sonka, M.: Automated segmentation of pulmonary vascular tree from 3D CT images. In: Medical Imaging 2004: Physiology, Function, and Structure from Medical Images, vol. 5369, pp. 107–117. International Society for Optics and Photonics (2004)
10. Simonyan, K., Zisserman, A.: Very deep convolutional networks for large-scale image recognition. arXiv preprint arXiv:1409.1556 (2014)
11. Staal, J., Abràmoff, M.D., Niemeijer, M., Viergever, M.A., Van Ginneken, B.: Ridge-based vessel segmentation in color images of the retina. IEEE Trans. Med. Imaging **23**(4), 501–509 (2004)
12. Tetteh, et al.: DeepVesselNet: vessel segmentation, centerline prediction, and bifurcation detection in 3-D angiographic volumes. arXiv preprint arXiv:1803.09340 (2018)
13. Yun, J., et al.: Improvement of fully automated airway segmentation on volumetric computed tomographic images using a 2.5 dimensional convolutional neural net. Med. Image Anal. **51**, 13–20 (2019)
14. Zhou, Z., Rahman Siddiquee, M.M., Tajbakhsh, N., Liang, J.: UNet++: a nested U-Net architecture for medical image segmentation. In: Stoyanov, D., et al. (eds.) DLMIA/ML-CDS -2018. LNCS, vol. 11045, pp. 3–11. Springer, Cham (2018). https://doi.org/10.1007/978-3-030-00889-5_1

Attentive CT Lesion Detection Using Deep Pyramid Inference with Multi-scale Booster

Qingbin Shao[1,2], Lijun Gong[1(✉)], Kai Ma[1], Hualuo Liu[2], and Yefeng Zheng[1]

[1] Tencent Youtu Lab, Shenzhen, China
lijungong@tencent.com
[2] Jilin University, Changchun, China

Abstract. Accurate lesion detection in computer tomography (CT) slices benefits pathologic organ analysis in the medical diagnosis process. More recently, it has been tackled as an object detection problem using the Convolutional Neural Networks (CNNs). Despite the achievements from off-the-shelf CNN models, the current detection accuracy is limited by the inability of CNNs on lesions at vastly different scales. In this paper, we propose a Multi-Scale Booster (MSB) with channel and spatial attention integrated into the backbone Feature Pyramid Network (FPN). In each pyramid level, the proposed MSB captures fine-grained scale variations by using Hierarchically Dilated Convolutions (HDC). Meanwhile, the proposed channel and spatial attention modules increase the network's capability of selecting relevant features response for lesion detection. Extensive experiments on the DeepLesion benchmark dataset demonstrate that the proposed method performs superiorly against state-of-the-art approaches.

Keywords: Deep lesion detection · Attentive multi-scale inference

1 Introduction

Automatically detecting lesions in CT slices is important to computer-aided detections/diagnosis (CADe/CADx). The identification and analysis of lesions in the clinic practice benefit the diagnosis of diseases at the early stage. The recent progress of the CADx mainly focuses on the visual recognition. By using the Convolutional Neural Networks (CNNs), the automatic detection of lesions has reduced the workload of the manual examinations. These lesion detection approaches arise from the object detection frameworks such as Faster R-CNN [8] and Feature Pyramid Network (FPN) [7], which typically employ a two-stage process. First, they draw a set of bounding box samples indicating the potential

---

Q. Shao and L. Gong contribute equally and share the first authorship. This work was done when Q. Shao was an intern in Tencent Youtu Lab. The source code and results are available at https://github.com/shaoqb/multi_scale_booster.

© Springer Nature Switzerland AG 2019
D. Shen et al. (Eds.): MICCAI 2019, LNCS 11769, pp. 301–309, 2019.
https://doi.org/10.1007/978-3-030-32226-7_34

region-of-interest (ROI) on the feature maps of CT slices. Then, each sample is classified as either lesion or background by a binary classifier. The two-stage CNN based detection frameworks have been trained in an end-to-end fashion and achieved the state-of-the-art performance.

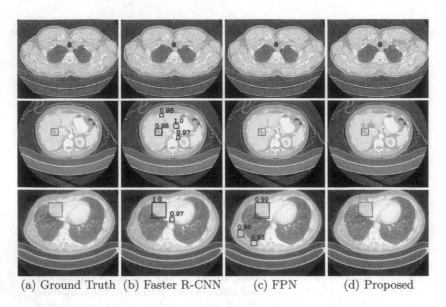

(a) Ground Truth (b) Faster R-CNN   (c) FPN   (d) Proposed

Fig. 1. Lesion detection results. The red bounding boxes represent ground truth annotations. The black, blue and green bounding boxes are the predicted results by Faster R-CNN [8], FPN [7] and the proposed method, respectively. (Color figure online)

To further improve the detection accuracy of CT data where blur and artifacts rarely exist [9,11,12], several methods [2,3,6,13] have been proposed to leverage the 3D spatial information. Ding et al. [2] proposed a 3D-CNN classifier to refine the detection results of the pulmonary cancer from the 2D-CNN framework. Furthermore, Dou et al. [3] explored a 3D-CNN for false positive reduction in pulmonary nodules detections. On the other side, Liao et al. [6] extended the region proposal network (RPN) [8] to 3D-RPN to generate 3D proposals. Although spatial representations extracted from 3D space improve the network performance on certain tasks, these methods suffer from tremendous memory and computational consumption. To tackle the computation efficiency problem, Yan et al. [13] proposed a 3D context enhanced region-based CNN (3DCE) to produce 3D context from feature maps of 2D input images. It achieved similar performance to 3D-CNN while consuming the same speed of the traditional 2D-CNN, which deserves further improvement with more advanced networks.

In real-world scenarios, body lesions usually have arbitrary size. For instance, in the DeepLesion [14] dataset, the lesion size ranges from 0.21 mm to 342.5 mm. Since most of the established CNNs are not robust to handle such spatial scale

variations, they have unpredictable behavior in the varying cases. As shown in
Fig. 1, both Faster R-CNN and FPN fail to detect tiny lesions in the first row,
while they produce small false positive lesions around the actual large lesion
locations in the second and third rows.

In this paper, we propose a fine-grained lesion detection approach with a
novel multi-scale attention mechanism. We use 2D FPN as the backbone to construct the feature pyramid in a relatively coarse scale. Within each level of the
feature pyramid, we propose to use a Multi-Scale Booster (MSB) to facilitate
lesion detection across fine-grained scales. Given the feature maps from one pyramid level, MSB first performs Hierarchically Dilated Convolution (HDC) that
consists of several dilated convolution operations with different dilation rates
[15]. The feature responses from HDC contain fine-grained information that is
complementary to the original feature pyramid, which is achieved by extensive
feature extraction in 2D space. The over-sampled feature responses are then
concatenated and further exploited by channel-wise and spatial-wise attention.
The channel attention module in MSB explores different lesion responses from
the subchannels of the concatenated feature maps. The spatial attention module
in MSB locates lesion response within each attentive channel. The channel-wise
and spatial-wise attention modules enable the network to focus on particular
lesion responses offered by the fine-grained features, while annealing the irrelevant and interference information. Thorough experiments demonstrate that MSB
improves the deep pyramid prediction results and performs favorably against
state-of-the-art approaches on the DeepLesion benchmarks.

2   Proposed Method

Figure 2 shows an overview of the pipeline. Our method uses a pre-trained FPN
network to extract features from the input image at different pyramid levels. The
extracted features are further processed by channel and spatial attention modules
to capture fine-grained information to handle large spatial scale variations. The
output of the MSB modules is used to make the final prediction at each pyramid
feature map respectively.

2.1   Revisiting FPN

The FPN [7] consists of three components for object detection: the bottom-up
pathway, top-down pathway and skip connections in between. The bottom-up
pathway computes feature maps at several different scales with a down-sampling
factor of 2. We use C_i^D to denote the feature maps at the i-th down-sampled
pyramid. The C_i^D has strides of 2^{i+1} pixels with respect to the input image. In
the top-down pathway, the feature maps from the coarse levels are upsampled
gradually to the finer resolutions with an up-sampling factor of 2. We denote
the upsampled feature maps at the i-th upsampled pyramid as C_i^U. The skip
connections merge the downsampled and upsampled feature maps together at
each pyramid level and the fused feature maps can be written as:

$$P_i = C_i^D \oplus C_i^U \tag{1}$$

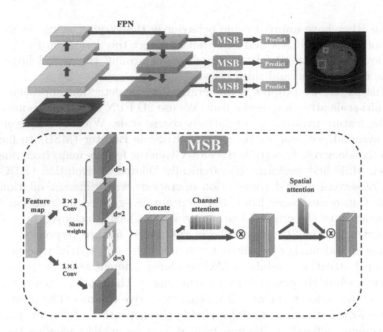

Fig. 2. Frameworks of the proposed approach. The detailed architecture of the Multi-Scale Booster (MSB) module is shown in the second row.

where $\oplus$ is the element-wise addition operation. After generating the feature maps P_i, the potential objects are then detected at each feature pyramid level.

2.2 Hierarchically Dilated Convolution

The dilated convolution is commonly used to expand the reception fields without loss of the original resolution. In ASPP [1], dilated convolution provided precise scale estimations for pixel-level semantic segmentation. Given the input feature map C_i^D, the dilated convolution can be written as:

$$y(x) = \sum_k C_i^D(x + r \cdot k) \cdot W(x) \tag{2}$$

where x is the location of the current pixel under processing; k is the supporting pixels in the convolution process; W is the filter weight; and r is the dilation rate. The dilation rate corresponds to the stride that we use to sample input feature map C_i^D. We denote the dilated convolution in a general form as $\mathcal{D}_r(C_i^D)$ where $\mathcal{D}_r$ is the dilated convolution operator with dilation rate r.

The HDC performs multiple dilated convolutions with different dilation rates. In our method, we use three dilated convolutions (i.e., d_1, d_2, and d_3) and keep the filter weight W fixed. The HDC output of the input feature map C_i^D can be formulated in the following:

$$\mathcal{H}(C_i^D) = \{\mathcal{D}_{r_1}(C_i^D); \mathcal{D}_{r_2}(C_i^D); \mathcal{D}_{r_3}(C_i^D); \mathcal{M}(C_i^D)\} \tag{3}$$

where $\mathcal{H}$ is the concatenation of the dilated convolution results $\mathcal{D}(C_i^D)$ and dimension mapping results $\mathcal{M}(C_i^D)$. We denote the concatenated results as H_i^D. The dimension mapping operation $\mathcal{M}$ is a 1×1 convolution on the input feature maps to ensure the channel consistency with respect to the dilated convolution results, while maintaining the original feature information from the FPN. We use different dilation rates to capture the lesion responses from each pyramid feature map respectively. These fine-grained feature responses of HDC contain multiple scales of reception fields within each feature pyramid level C_i^D. In order to only capture the scale variation responses on the pyramid feature maps, we share weights among HDC to overcome other interferences such as rotation and deformation.

2.3 Channel Attention

We refine the HDC result using a squeeze-and-excitation network as shown in Fig. 2 following [5]. The HDC result H_i^D captures the feature responses of the potential lesions from the multi-scale perspective. For a particular lesion with a certain dimension, high feature response may reside in one of the dilated convolution scales. Therefore it is intuitive to attend the network to the subchannels of H_i^D. We propose a channel attention module as shown in Fig. 2. It first squeezes H_i^D by a global pooling operation and then activates the reduced feature maps by a 1×1 convolution layer. The channel attention can be written as:

$$\mathcal{F}_{ch}(H_i^D) = \mathcal{P}_{avg}(H_i^D) * W_{1 \times 1} \tag{4}$$

where $\mathcal{P}_{avg}$ and $W_{1 \times 1}$ represent the global pooling and the convolution operation, respectively. The channel attention output $\mathcal{F}_{ch}(H_i^D)$ is a one dimensional vector re-weighting C_i^D. The network is learned to pay more attention to the subchannels of H_i^D where the precise scale response of the lesion region resides. The reweighted feature maps from channel attention can be written as:

$$H_i^{Dch} = \mathcal{F}_{ch}(H_i^D) \otimes H_i^D \tag{5}$$

where $\otimes$ is the element-wise multiplication operation.

2.4 Spatial Attention

The channel attention ensures the network to focus on H_i^{Dch}, where the response of the scale estimation from HDC resides. To increase the network's attention to the lesion response within H_i^{Dch}, we propose a spatial attention module that reduces the distraction outside of the ROIs. The proposed spatial attention module first squeezes H_i^{Dch} by using a max pooling operation along channel axis to generate the spatial feature map $\mathcal{F}_{sp}(H_i^{Dch})$, which encodes where to emphasize. The spatial attention activation process can be written as:

$$\mathcal{F}_{sp}(H_i^{Dch}) = \mathcal{P}_{max}(H_i^{Dch}) \tag{6}$$

306   Q. Shao et al.

Table 1. An ablation study with various configurations of the proposed modules. Lesion detection sensitivity is reported at different false positive (FP) rates on the DeepLesion [14] test set.

Method	Backbone	FPs per image				
		0.5	1	2	4	8
FPN	ResNet-50	0.621	0.728	0.807	0.864	0.890
FPN+HDC (weights sharing)	ResNet-50	0.622	0.734	0.818	0.873	0.910
FPN+HDC+CH (weights sharing)	ResNet-50	0.645	0.746	0.820	0.880	0.911
FPN+HDC+SP (weights sharing)	ResNet-50	0.629	0.743	0.821	0.881	0.914
FPN+MSB	ResNet-50	0.637	0.748	0.819	0.871	0.917
FPN+MSB (weights sharing)	ResNet-50	**0.670**	**0.768**	**0.837**	**0.890**	**0.920**

where $\mathcal{P}_{max}$ is the max pooling. The spatial attention $\mathcal{F}_{sp}(H_i^{Dch})$ is a one-channel feature map with size $H \times W$ used to filer out the irrelevant information of H_i^{Dch}. As a result, the network will attentively focus around the lesion region. The refined output feature map can be formulated as:

$$\hat{P}_i = \mathcal{F}_{sp}(H_i^{Dch}) \otimes H_i^{Dch} \tag{7}$$

where $\otimes$ is the same as that in Eq. 1. The output feature map $\hat{P}_i$ is then used for lesion detection.

3   Experiments

We evaluate the proposed method on the large-scale benchmark dataset DeepLesion [14]. It includes 32,735 lesions from 32,120 CT slices, which are captured from 4,427 patients. The lesion areas cover liver, lung nodules, bone, kidney, and other organs. We follow the dataset configuration to split into the training, validation and test sets. In the training process, we use ResNet50 [4] as the feature extraction backbone. The initial weights from conv1 to conv5 are from the ImageNet pretrained model [10] and the remaining weights are randomly initialized. We resize the CT slices to 512×512 pixels and concatenate three consecutive CT slides as the input to predict lesions of the central slice. The five anchor scales and three anchor ratios are set as $(8, 16, 32, 64, 128)$, $\{1:2, 1:1, 2:1\}$ respectively at each level while training RPN. The learning rate is set as 0.01 and the learning process is around 10 epochs.

3.1   Ablation Study

The proposed network consists of four major components. They are FPN, HDC, CH (channel attention), and SP (spatial attention). To evaluate the effectiveness of each module and weights sharing, we ablatively study on the DeepLesion dataset. The evaluation metric is the average sensitivity values at different false positives rates of the whole test set. The evaluation configuration is shown in Table 1. The comparisons among different configurations demonstrate that the proposed MSB achieves highest sensitivity under different false positives rates.

Table 2. Comparison of the proposed method (FPN + MSB) with state-of-the-art methods on the DeepLesion [14] test set. Lesion detection sensitivity values are reported at different false positive (FP) rates.

Method	Backbone	Number of slices	FPs per image				
			0.5	1	2	4	8
3DCE [13]	VGG-16	3	0.569	0.673	0.756	0.816	0.858
	VGG-16	9	0.593	0.707	0.791	0.843	0.878
	VGG-16	27	0.625	0.737	0.807	0.857	0.891
Faster R-CNN [8]	ResNet-50	3	0.560	0.677	0.763	0.832	0.867
FPN [7]	ResNet-50	3	0.621	0.728	0.807	0.864	0.890
FPN+MSB (weights sharing)	ResNet-50	3	**0.670**	**0.768**	**0.837**	**0.890**	**0.920**

Table 3. Sensitivity values at four false positives per image on five test subsets categorized by different lesion size.

Method	Backbone	Number of slices	Lesion diameters (mm)				
			<10	10–30	30 60	60 100	>100
3DCE [13]	VGG-16	27	0.78	0.86	0.84		
Faster R-CNN [8]	ResNet-50	3	0.77	0.86	0.81	0.88	0.72
FPN [7]	ResNet-50	3	0.83	0.88	0.82	0.91	0.77
FPN+HDC (weights sharing)	ResNet-50	3	0.85	0.89	**0.88**	**0.93**	0.79
FPN+MSB (weights sharing)	ResNet-50	3	**0.86**	**0.91**	0.86	**0.93**	**0.86**

3.2   Comparisons with State-of-the-Art

We compare the proposed method with state-of-the-art approaches including 3DCE [13], Faster R-CNN [8] and FPN [7]. Yan et al. [13] sent multiple slices into the 2D detection network (i.e., Faster R-CNN [8]) to generate feature maps separately, and then aggregated them to incorporate 3D context information for final prediction. We note that the results of 3DCE [13] are the only available results reported on this dataset. We perform the evaluation from two perspectives. The first one is to compute the sensitivity values at different false positives rates as illustrated in Sect. 3.1. It reflects the averaged performance of each method for test set. The other one is to compute the sensitivity values generated based on different sizes of lesions. It reflects how effective each method is to detect lesions at different scales.

Table 2 shows the evaluation results. It demonstrates that the proposed method performs superiorly against existing methods. We note that there are different numbers of CT slices used as input for 3DCE to produce different sensitivity values. The result shows that sensitivity value increases when more CT slices are taken as input. As these CT slices are captured on the same organ of the patient, using more slices will provide sufficient information to the network to detect. Nevertheless, we show that the proposed method achieves higher sensitivity values when using only three slices as input.

To evaluate how the proposed method performs when detecting different size of lesions, we divide the test set into five categories. Each category consists of lesions in a fixed range of size and the range does not overlap with each other. Table 3 shows the evaluation results. The proposed method shows better performance to detect lesions in different sizes. Meanwhile, the sensitivity values of the proposed method exceed those of existing methods more when the size of the testing lesions becomes extremely large or small (i.e., the diameters of the lesions are above 100 mm or below 10 mm). It indicates that the proposed method is more effective to detect extreme scales of the input lesions.

4   Conclusion

We proposed a multi-scale booster (MSB) to detect lesion in large scale variations. We use FPN to decompose the feature map response into several coarse-grained pyramid levels. Within each level, we increase the network awareness of the scale variations by using HDC. The HDC offers fine-grained scale estimations to effectively capture the scale responses. To effectively select meaningful responses, we proposed a cascaded attention module consists of channel and spatial attentions. Evaluations on the DeepLesion benchmark indicated the effectiveness of the proposed method to detect lesions at vastly different scales.

Acknowledgments. This work was founded by the Key Area Research and Development Program of Guangdong Province, China (No. 2018B010111001).

References

1. Chen, L.C., Papandreou, G., Kokkinos, I., Murphy, K., Yuille, A.L.: DeepLab: semantic image segmentation with deep convolutional nets, atrous convolution, and fully connected CRFs. IEEE Trans. Pattern Anal. Mach. Intell. **40**, 834–848 (2017)
2. Ding, J., Li, A., Hu, Z., Wang, L.: Accurate pulmonary nodule detection in computed tomography images using deep convolutional neural networks. In: Descoteaux, M., Maier-Hein, L., Franz, A., Jannin, P., Collins, D.L., Duchesne, S. (eds.) MICCAI 2017. LNCS, vol. 10435, pp. 559–567. Springer, Cham (2017). https://doi.org/10.1007/978-3-319-66179-7_64
3. Dou, Q., Chen, H., Yu, L., Qin, J., Heng, P.A.: Multilevel contextual 3-D CNNs for false positive reduction in pulmonary nodule detection. IEEE Trans. Biomed. Eng. **64**, 1558–1567 (2017)
4. He, K., Zhang, X., Ren, S., Sun, J.: Deep residual learning for image recognition. In: IEEE Conference on Computer Vision and Pattern Recognition (2016)
5. Hu, J., Shen, L., Sun, G.: Squeeze-and-excitation networks. In: IEEE Conference on Computer Vision and Pattern Recognition (2018)
6. Liao, F., Liang, M., Li, Z., Hu, X., Song, S.: Evaluate the malignancy of pulmonary nodules using the 3D deep leaky noisy-or network. IEEE Trans. Neural Netw. Learn. Syst. **PP** (2017). https://doi.org/10.1109/TNNLS.2019.2892409
7. Lin, T.Y., Dollár, P., Girshick, R., He, K., Hariharan, B., Belongie, S.: Feature pyramid networks for object detection. In: International Conference on Computer Vision (2017)
8. Ren, S., He, K., Girshick, R., Sun, J.: Faster R-CNN: towards real-time object detection with region proposal networks. In: Neural Information Processing Systems (2015)
9. Roy, A.G., Navab, N., Wachinger, C.: Concurrent spatial and channel 'squeeze & excitation' in fully convolutional networks. In: Frangi, A., Schnabel, J., Davatzikos, C., Alberola-López, C., Fichtinger, G. (eds.) MICCAI 2018. LNCS, vol. 11070, pp. 421–429. Springer, Cham (2018). https://doi.org/10.1007/978-3-030-00928-1_48
10. Russakovsky, O., et al.: ImageNet large scale visual recognition challenge. Int. J. Comput. Vis. **115**, 211–252 (2015)
11. Song, Y., Zhang, J., Bao, L., Yang, Q.: Fast preprocessing for robust face sketch synthesis. In: International Joint Conference on Artificial Intelligence (2017)
12. Song, Y., et al.: Joint face hallucination and deblurring via structure generation and detail enhancement. Int. J. Comput. Vis. **127**, 785–800 (2018)
13. Yan, K., Bagheri, M., Summers, R.M.: 3D context enhanced region-based convolutional neural network for end-to-end lesion detection. In: Frangi, A.F., Schnabel, J.A., Davatzikos, C., Alberola-López, C., Fichtinger, G. (eds.) MICCAI 2018. LNCS, vol. 11070, pp. 511–519. Springer, Cham (2018). https://doi.org/10.1007/978-3-030-00928-1_58
14. Yan, K., Wang, X., Lu, L., Summers, R.M.: DeepLesion: automated deep mining, categorization and detection of significant radiology image findings using large-scale clinical lesion annotations. arXiv:1710.01766 (2017)
15. Yu, F., Koltun, V.: Multi-scale context aggregation by dilated convolutions. arXiv:1511.07122 (2015)

Deep Variational Networks
with Exponential Weighting
for Learning Computed Tomography

Valery Vishnevskiy[(✉)], Richard Rau, and Orcun Goksel

Computer-assisted Applications in Medicine, ETH Zurich, Zürich, Switzerland
valeryv@vision.ee.ethz.ch

Abstract. Tomographic image reconstruction is relevant for many medical imaging modalities including X-ray, ultrasound (US) computed tomography (CT) and photoacoustics, for which the access to full angular range tomographic projections might be not available in clinical practice due to physical or time constraints. Reconstruction from incomplete data in low signal-to-noise ratio regime is a challenging and ill-posed inverse problem that usually leads to unsatisfactory image quality. While informative image priors may be learned using generic deep neural network architectures, the artefacts caused by an ill-conditioned design matrix often have global spatial support and cannot be efficiently filtered out by means of convolutions. In this paper we propose to learn an inverse mapping in an end-to-end fashion via unrolling optimization iterations of a prototypical reconstruction algorithm. We herein introduce a network architecture that performs filtering jointly in both sinogram and spatial domains. To efficiently train such deep network we propose a novel regularization approach based on deep exponential weighting. Experiments on US and X-ray CT data show that our proposed method is qualitatively and quantitatively superior to conventional non-linear reconstruction methods as well as state-of-the-art deep networks for image reconstruction. Fast inference time of the proposed algorithm allows for sophisticated reconstructions in real-time critical settings, demonstrated with US SoS imaging of an *ex vivo* bovine phantom.

1 Introduction

Tomographic image reconstruction with sparse or limited angular (LA) data arises in a number of applications including image guided interventions [17], photoacoustics [8], and US speed-of-sound (SoS) imaging [3,13,14]. Such underdetermined problems usually require suitable problem-specific regularization for meaningful reconstructions, e.g. free from streaking artefacts. Setting regularization parameters manually can be cumbersome and often generalizes poorly. Using learning-based methods as in [22] can greatly improve reconstruction accuracy and account for non-Gaussian noise models. Unfortunately the method in [22] is based on patch-based clustering leading to very slow reconstruction. Straightforward application of computationally efficient convolutional network directly

© Springer Nature Switzerland AG 2019
D. Shen et al. (Eds.): MICCAI 2019, LNCS 11769, pp. 310–318, 2019.
https://doi.org/10.1007/978-3-030-32226-7_35

to measurements might be tempting, but is unjustified, because sinogram values have global spatial dependence on image intensities. In practice, such generic networks are not likely to generalize well for LA-CT problems [10]. Many deep-learning inspired methods employ artificial neural networks to learn filtering or weighting [16,21] of the input sinograms prior to the backprojection step, after which the result might be postprocessed by another network [5]. Unfortunately such sinogram preprocessing requires problem-specific weighting schemes, which would constrain applicable acquisition geometries. Variational Networks (VN) learn convolutional filters in *spatial* domain by employing adjoint imaging operator [1]. For compressed sensing in MRI, a landmark VN architecture was introduced by Hammernik et al. [4], which in practice relies on unitarity of Fourier transform. This was later addressed in [19] with sophisticated unrolled iterations of a momentum-based gradient descent, which largely improved USCT reconstructions and allowed for the *detection* of coarse blob-looking inclusions.

In order to allow for accurate image reconstruction with ill-conditioned spatial encoding operators, in this paper we extend VN architecture by introducing sinogram filters that are learned as preconditioners, inspired by filtered backprojection. We also propose an efficient network regularization scheme that promotes a stable training, inspired by Landweber iterations [7] and deep supervision [9].

2   Methods

Tomographic reconstruction problem involves estimating image intensities x from set of measurements (sinogram) b_i (e.g., time-of-flight or ray attenuation) that are modelled, e.g., as line integrals $b_i = \int_{\text{ray}_i} x(\mathbf{r})ds$. Given a set of measurements $\mathbf{b} \in \mathbb{R}^M$, algebraic reconstruction methods solve for discretized spatial encoding equations in a maximum-a-posteriori (MAP) sense, i.e.:

$$\hat{\mathbf{x}}(\mathbf{b}; \lambda, p) = \underset{\mathbf{x}}{\text{argmin}} \, \|\mathbf{L}\mathbf{x} - \mathbf{b}\|_p^p + \lambda \mathcal{R}(\mathbf{x}), \tag{1}$$

where $\mathbf{x} \in \mathbb{R}^{n_1 n_2}$ is $n_1 \times n_2$ image and $\mathbf{L} \in \mathbb{R}^{M \times n_1 n_2}$ is a sparse, ray-discretization matrix that depends on the acquisition geometry. The norm p determines data inconsistency penalty, e.g. $p = 2$ assumes Gaussian acquisition noise while $p = 1$ assumes Laplace noise, the latter of which is often considered to be more robust. Non-negative weight λ controls the influence of regularizer. Similarly to [6], we herein consider total variation $\mathcal{R}_{\text{TV}}(\mathbf{x}) = \|\nabla\mathbf{x}\|_1$ and total generalized variation $\mathcal{R}_{\text{TGV}}(\mathbf{x}) = \min_{\mathbf{u}} \|\nabla\mathbf{x} - \mathbf{u}\|_1 + 2\|\mathcal{E}\mathbf{u}\|_1$ regularizers. Here ∇ denotes first-order forward finite derivative matrix and $\mathcal{E}$ is the symmetrized vector field derivative operator. Both TV and TGV regularizers yield convex optimization problems for $p = \{1, 2\}$, which we hereafter refer as LpTV and LpTGV.

A Variational Network can be seen as a sequence of K unrolled iterations of a numerical optimization scheme, inspired by a prototypical objective as in (1). For additional learning capacity, these iterations are further relaxed, e.g. by adding variable filters and activations that can be tuned during training. As illustrated

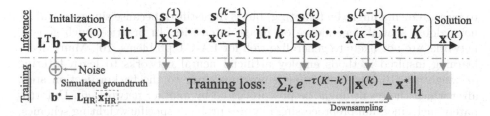

Fig. 1. Structure of variational network and its training strategy.

in Fig. 1, we initialize VN inference by $\mathbf{L}^{\mathsf{T}}\mathbf{b}$. Then, at each network layer (iteration) k, a *gradient* term $\mathbf{g}^{(k)}$ is accumulated via running average governed by momentum coefficient $\alpha^{(k)}$ and used to update current image estimate $\mathbf{x}^{(k)}$ as follows:

$$
\mathbf{g}^{(k)} \leftarrow \left(\mathbf{P}^{(k)}\mathbf{L}\mathbf{Q}^{(k)}\right)^{\mathsf{T}} \mathbf{W}_d^{(k)} \varphi_d^{(k)} \left\{ \mathbf{W}_d^{(k)} \left(\mathbf{P}^{(k)}\mathbf{L}\mathbf{Q}^{(k)}\mathbf{x}^{(k-1)} - \mathbf{b}\right)\right\} +
$$
$$
\left(\mathbf{D}^{(k)}\right)^{\mathsf{T}} \mathbf{W}_r^{(k)} \varphi_r^{(k)} \left\{ \mathbf{W}_r^{(k)}\mathbf{D}^{(k)}\mathbf{x}^{(k-1)}\right\}, \tag{2}
$$
$$
\mathbf{s}^{(k)} \leftarrow \alpha^{(k)}\mathbf{s}^{(k-1)} + \mathbf{g}^{(k)}, \qquad \mathbf{x}^{(k)} \leftarrow \mathbf{x}^{(k-1)} - \mathbf{s}^{(k)}.
$$

We define the gradient term $\mathbf{g}^{(k)}$ with the following tunable operations that all allow backpropagation of gradients: (i) multiplication with diagonal *preconditioner* $\mathbf{W}_d^{(k)}$ and spatial regularization *weighting* $\mathbf{W}_r^{(k)}$; (ii) convolution with left ($\mathbf{P}^{(k)}$) and right ($\mathbf{Q}^{(k)}$) preconditioners, and several (herein, $n_f = 50$) regularization filters $\mathbf{D}^{(k)}$; (iii) nonlinear data ($\varphi_d^{(k)}$) and regularization ($\varphi_r^{(k)}$) activation functions that are parametrized via linear interpolation on a regular grid, herein, of size $n_g = 35$; i.e. $\varphi\{t\} = (1 - t + \lfloor t \rfloor)\phi_{\lfloor t \rfloor} + (t - \lfloor t \rfloor)\phi_{\lfloor t \rfloor + 1}$. To avoid bilinear ambiguities, every $n_k \times n_k$ (herein, $n_k = 7$) convolution $\mathbf{D}, \mathbf{Q}, \mathbf{P}$ with kernel $\mathbf{d}$ is reparametrized to be zero-centered unit-norm, i.e. $\mathbf{d} = n_k(\mathbf{d}' - \mathrm{mean}(\mathbf{d}'))/\mathrm{std}(\mathbf{d}')$, while diagonal terms are also ensured to be nonnegative and bounded via sigmoid: $\mathbf{W} = \mathrm{diag}(\sigma(w_i))$. Stochastic minimization of the *exponentially weighted* ℓ_1 reconstruction loss is then conducted to tune parameter set $\Theta = \{\mathbf{P}^{(k)}, \mathbf{Q}^{(k)}, \mathbf{D}^{(k)}, \mathbf{W}_r^{(k)}, \mathbf{W}_f^{(k)}, \phi_r^{(k)}, \phi_d^{(k)}, \alpha^{(k)}\}$:

$$
\min_{\Theta} \ \mathbb{E}_{\{\mathbf{b}, \mathbf{x}^*\} \in \mathcal{T}} \sum_{k=1}^{K} e^{-\tau(K-k)} \|\mathbf{x}^{(k)}(\mathbf{b}; \Theta) - \mathbf{x}^*\|_1, \tag{3}
$$

on the training set $\mathcal{T}$. Here $\tau \geq 0$ controls the regularization of the network: at $\tau = 0$, the reconstruction on all layers is weighted equally, therefore all network parameters have low variance of gradients, which allows for stable training. For $\tau \to +\infty$, only the last network output $\mathbf{x}^{(K)}$ is used for training, which allows the network to be tuned accurately for the final objective. We accordingly increase τ during the training procedure, in order to gradually relax the constraints on the network. Intuitively, such regularization encourages VN to provide reconstruction as early as possible, which is inspired by *early stopping*—a common image reconstruction strategy used to prevent degenerate solutions and which is equivalent to Tikhonov regularization in certain cases [7].

Training. We employ a $K = 10$ layer VN and perform $5 \cdot 10^4$ iterations of Adam algorithm (learning rate 10^{-3}, $\beta_1 = 0.85$, $\beta_1 = 0.98$, batch size of 10) for training, during which we continually adjust $\tau = j \cdot 10^{-3}$ with j being the iteration number. To avoid overfitting to the discretization scheme employed in the simulation, we use higher resolution images x_{HR} to compute line integrals defined by L_{HR} while training for these to be reconstructed in the desired resolution defined by the discretization of L. The network was implemented using Tensorflow framework, where multiplication with the design matrix L was carried out as a generic sparse matrix-vector multiplication. For comparison with iterative reconstruction, we employ ADMM algorithm [2] to solve (1) by approximating the regularized inversion of L with 5 iterations of LSQR solver [11]. For each experimental scenario, an optimal value of λ was tuned on a single test image.

3   Experiments and Results

X-Ray CT Dataset. We used 3DIRCADb dataset [18] that consists of 3080 axial CT scans from 22 patients with inplane resolution varying from 0.56^2 to 0.961^2 mm^2 and slice thickness of 1.6 to 4 mm. The forward simulation was conducted on original 512×512 images, which then were downsampled to 256×256 grid, yielding the ground truth (GT). We simulated parallel beam acquisition geometry for limiter-angle (LA) and sparse-view (SV) scenarios. In the LA scenario we simulated angular ranges of $120°$, $90°$ and $60°$, where projections were acquired in $1°$ increments. For the SV scenario we simulated $180°$ range with 60, 30, and 15 uniformly-acquired projections. To simulate realistic acquisition noise, we employ a Poisson+Gaussian model [22], i.e.

$$b = \log \left| \text{Poisson}(I_0 \exp(-b^\star)) + \text{Gauss}(0, \sigma_E) \right|, \qquad (4)$$

with $I_0 = 2 \cdot 10^4$ and $\sigma_E = 8 \cdot \text{Unif}(0, 1)$ to model variable SNR. We used 20 patient scans for training and two for testing.

US Speed-of-Sound Tomography. We follow [19] to model reflector-based USCT reconstruction problem [13,15] with a 128-element transducer and a square imaging field-of-view. Synthetic inclusion masks were generated at 256×256 resolution as levelsets of random, spatially-smooth functions. The inclusion SoS values were then randomly sampled from $[1350, 1650]$ m/s. Acquisition noise was modelled as Gaussian with $\sigma_N = 2 \cdot 10^{-8}$ and the reconstruction was conducted on a coarser 64×64 grid to avoid overfitting to the discretization. The training set contains 15000 random synthetic inclusions, while the test set includes 13 geometric primitives consisting of oval and polygonal inclusions.

Evaluation. For quantitative comparison of reconstruction and ground truth, we calculated structural similarity index measurement (SSIM) [20], Root Mean

Table 1. Mean reconstruction RMSE computed on corresponding training sets with standard deviations indicated in parentheses. Errors in Hounsfield units [H] for X-ray CT and speed-of-sound [m/s] for USCT. Methods proposed herein are highlighted.

Dataset	L2TV	L1TV	L2TGV	VN0 [4]	VN1 [19]	PC-VN	expPC-VN
	RMSE	RMSE	RMSE	RMSE	RMSE	RMSE	RMSE
LA-CT 90° [H]	216 (9)	238 (16)	205 (6)	210 (9)	128 (15)	119 (19)	**103 (8)**
SV-CT #30 [H]	93 (5)	91 (4)	98 (6)	97 (4)	87 (8)	88 (9)	**65 (5)**
SoS USCT [m/s]	1.48 (0.44)	1.62 (0.48)	1.89 (0.35)	1.80 (0.33)	1.35 (0.43)	1.19 (0.41)	**1.00 (0.35)**

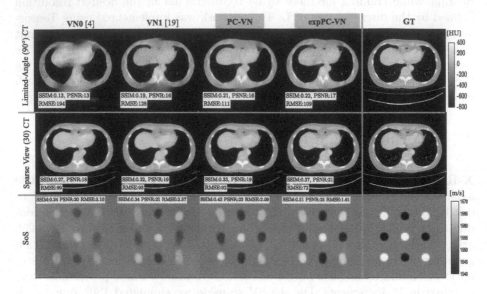

Fig. 2. Performance comparison of VN architectures on X-ray CT and SoS simulations. Proposed architectures are highlighted in green. (Color figure online)

Square Error (RMSE), and peak signal-to-noise ratio (PSNR) as follows:

$$\text{RMSE}(\mathbf{x}, \mathbf{y}) = \sqrt{\frac{\|\mathbf{x} - \mathbf{y}\|_2^2}{N}}, \qquad \text{PSNR}(\mathbf{x}, \mathbf{y}) = 10 \log_{10} \frac{R^2 N}{\|\mathbf{x} - \mathbf{y}\|_2^2}, \qquad (5)$$

where R is the dynamic range of the ground truth image. The corresponding values are reported in Hounsfield units (HU) and m/s, respectively, for X-ray CT and USCT SoS experiments. We denote the architectures employed in [4] and [19] as VN0 and VN1, respectively. As seen in Fig. 2 the proposed preconditioned network (PC-VN) with sinogram convolutions improves reconstruction accuracy and quality for all X-ray CT acquisition scenarios and USCT as suggested by RMSE and SSIM values. As reported in Table 1, training the proposed network using exponentially weighted loss (expPC-VN) defined in Eq. (3) further improves reconstruction quality and reduces the variance of error, which can be explained by the introduced regularization effect. Figure 3 shows that expPC-VN outperforms iterative methods both in terms of accuracy and image

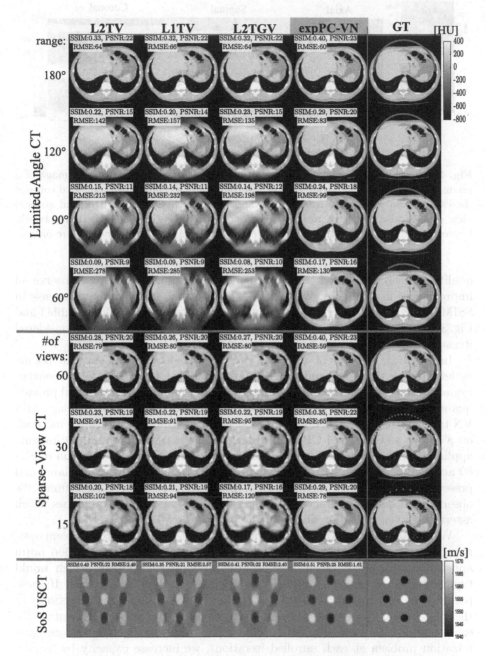

Fig. 3. Reconstruction results for X-ray CT and USCT acquisitions. For sparse view and limited angle experiments, acquired angular positions of projections are depicted in the GT column.

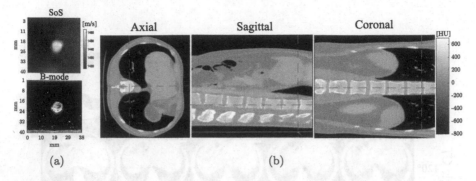

Fig. 4. (a) expPC-VN SoS reconstruction and the corresponding B-mode image of a phantom with an *ex vivo* bovine sample inserted inside a gelatin phantom. Red contour shows inclusion segmented from the B-mode image. (b) Axial, sagittal and coronal view of slice-wise reconstruction of the proposed expPC-VN reconstruction network. Corresponding slice positions are indicated with red dashed line. (Color figure online)

quality. Namely, compared to nonlinear reconstruction methods, we observe an improvement in RMSE by 49% in the CT-LA-60° scenario, and an increase in SSIM by 38% in the CT-SV-15 experiment. Quantitative results from Table 1 and Fig. 3 show that our proposed reconstruction method outperforms all considered iterative and deep learning-based approaches.

In Fig. 4(a), we present a USCT SoS reconstruction from *ex vivo* bovine skeletal muscle tissue embedded in a gelatin phantom. Compared to the conventional B-Mode image, we could accurately identify inclusion location and provide quantitative estimates of local tissue SoS. Reconstruction of a single image with VN takes 0.03 s on NVIDIA Titan Xp GPU and 1–4 min with iterative methods on a 6-core 3.7 GHz Intel CPU. In order to demonstrate potential 3D imaging applications of our method, we also conducted X-ray CT reconstruction of SV-60 acquisition scenario with test images rotated by 90° in the axial plane, and present in Fig. 4(b) cross-sectional views from the reconstructed 3D volume. We observe high spatial coherence and contrast in coronal and sagittal planes which asserts high generalization ability of the proposed expPC-VN method.

We herein learn the parameters required for an effective inverse problem optimization, such as regularization choice, weight, data and regularization norm approximations, optimization step lengths, and preconditioners, which would typically need to be set empirically, which may thus be suboptimal. If these parameters were linked between K iteration layers, a single cost function can then be solved. Nevertheless, by allowing to learn parameters separately for each unfolded iteration step (thus solving potentially a slightly different optimization problem at each unrolled iteration), we increase capacity by leaving further flexibility to the network to arrive at desired reconstruction. By fixing the imaging operator $\mathbf{L}$, hence the physical problem, and accordingly learning only the somewhat ad-hoc parameters required for a stable optimization and noise modeling, we show that learning from fully synthetic data can be generalized to actual imaging data. Bridging the gap between deep learning and classical numerical algorithms will allow for leveraging the decades-long understanding and know-how from the latter, as we show here with preconditioner learning and early stopping.

4 Conclusions

In this paper we have presented a novel network architecture for preconditioned reconstruction and a regularization scheme for its efficient training via exponential weighting. The proposed network has been shown to outperform conventional algebraic and learning-based reconstruction methods in terms of accuracy and image quality for various challenging X-ray CT and SoS USCT scenarios. Such effectiveness and versatility of our approach may suggest its potential for solving other image reconstruction problems such as ultrasound attenuation [12] and reflector-free SoS [14] and those in tomosynthesis [17], photoacoustics [8], MRI, and PET imaging, as well as other intriguing optimization and inverse problems such as denoising and super-resolution and even outside the imaging and image analysis fields.

Funding. It was provided by the Swiss National Science Foundation (SNSF).

References

1. Adler, J., Öktem, O.: Learned primal-dual reconstruction. IEEE Trans. Med. Imaging **37**(6), 1322–1332 (2018)
2. Boyd, S., Parikh, N., Chu, E., Peleato, B., Eckstein, J.: Distributed optimization and statistical learning via the alternating direction method of multipliers. Found. Trends ML **3**(1), 1–122 (2011)
3. Cheng, A., et al.: Deep learning image reconstruction method for limited-angle ultrasound tomography in prostate cancer. In: Proceedings of SPIE Medical Imaging, p. 1095516 (2019)
4. Hammernik, K., et al.: Learning a variational network for reconstruction of accelerated MRI data. MRM **79**(6), 3055–3071 (2018)
5. Hammernik, K., Würfl, T., Pock, T., Maier, A.: A deep learning architecture for limited-angle computed tomography reconstruction. Bildverarbeitung für die Medizin 2017. INFORMAT, pp. 92–97. Springer, Heidelberg (2017). https://doi.org/10.1007/978-3-662-54345-0_25
6. Knoll, F., Bredies, K., Pock, T., Stollberger, R.: Second order total generalized variation (TGV) for MRI. MRM **65**(2), 480–491 (2011)
7. Landweber, L.: An iteration formula for Fredholm integral equations of the first kind. Am. J. Math. **73**(3), 615–624 (1951)
8. Lin, H., Azuma, T., Unlu, M.B., Takagi, S.: Evaluation of adjoint methods in photoacoustic tomography with under-sampled sensors. In: Frangi, A.F., Schnabel, J.A., Davatzikos, C., Alberola-López, C., Fichtinger, G. (eds.) MICCAI 2018. LNCS, vol. 11070, pp. 73–81. Springer, Cham (2018). https://doi.org/10.1007/978-3-030-00928-1_9

318   V. Vishnevskiy et al.

9. Liu, Y., Lew, M.S.: Learning relaxed deep supervision for better edge detection. In: CVPR, pp. 231–240 (2016)
10. Maier, A., Syben, C., Lasser, T., Riess, C.: A gentle introduction to deep learning in medical image processing. Zeitschrift für Medizinische Physik **29**, 86–101 (2019)
11. Paige, C.C., Saunders, M.A.: LSQR: an algorithm for sparse linear equations and sparse least squares. ACM TOMS **8**(1), 43–71 (1982)
12. Rau, R., Unal, O., Schweizer, D., Vishnevskiy, V., Goksel, O.: Attenuation imaging with pulse-echo ultrasound based on an acoustic reflector. In: MICCAI (2016, accepted). arXiv:1906.11615
13. Sanabria, S.J., Goksel, O.: Hand-held sound-speed imaging based on ultrasound reflector delineation. In: Ourselin, S., Joskowicz, L., Sabuncu, M.R., Unal, G., Wells, W. (eds.) MICCAI 2016. LNCS, vol. 9900, pp. 568–576. Springer, Cham (2016). https://doi.org/10.1007/978-3-319-46720-7_66
14. Sanabria, S.J., Ozkan, E., Rominger, M., Goksel, O.: Spatial domain reconstruction for imaging speed-of-sound with pulse-echo ultrasound: simulation and in vivo study. Phys. Med. Biol. **63**(21), 215015 (2018)
15. Sanabria, S., Rominger, M., Goksel, O.: Speed-of-sound imaging based on reflector delineation. IEEE Trans. Biomed. Eng. **66**(7), 1949–1962 (2019)
16. Schwab, J., Antholzer, S., Haltmeier, M.: Learned backprojection for sparse and limited view photoacoustic tomography. In: Proceedings of SPIE Photons Plus Ultrasound: Imaging and Sensing, p. 1087837 (2019)
17. Siewerdsen, J., et al.: Multimode C-arm fluoroscopy, tomosynthesis, and cone-beam CT for image-guided interventions: from proof of principle to patient protocols. In: Proceedings of SPIE Medical Imaging, p. 65101A (2007)
18. Soler, L., et al.: 3D image reconstruction for comparison of algorithm database: a patient specific anatomical and medical image database. Technical report. IRCAD, Strasbourg, France (2010)
19. Vishnevskiy, V., Sanabria, S.J., Goksel, O.: Image reconstruction via variational network for real-time hand-held sound-speed imaging. In: Knoll, F., Maier, A., Rueckert, D. (eds.) MLMIR 2018. LNCS, vol. 11074, pp. 120–128. Springer, Cham (2018). https://doi.org/10.1007/978-3-030-00129-2_14
20. Wang, Z., Bovik, A.C., Sheikh, H.R., Simoncelli, E.P., et al.: Image quality assessment: from error visibility to structural similarity. IEEE Trans. Image Process. **13**(4), 600–612 (2004)
21. Würfl, T., et al.: Deep learning computed tomography: learning projection-domain weights from image domain in limited angle problems. IEEE Trans. Med. Imaging **37**(6), 1454–1463 (2018)
22. Zheng, X., Ravishankar, S., Long, Y., Fessler, J.A.: PWLS-ULTRA: an efficient clustering and learning-based approach for low-dose 3D CT image reconstruction. IEEE Trans. Med. Imaging **37**(6), 1498–1510 (2018)

R²-Net: Recurrent and Recursive Network for Sparse-View CT Artifacts Removal

Tiancheng Shen[1], Xia Li[2], Zhisheng Zhong[2], Jianlong Wu[2,3], and Zhouchen Lin[2(✉)]

[1] Center for Data Science, Peking University, Beijing 100871, China
tianchengShen@pku.edu.cn
[2] Key Laboratory of Machine Perception (MOE), School of EECS, Peking University, Beijing 100871, China
{ethanlee,zzs1994,jlwu1992,zlin}@pku.edu.cn
[3] School of Computer Science and Technology, Shandong University, Tsingtao 266000, China

Abstract. We propose a novel neural network architecture to reduce streak artifacts generated in sparse-view 2D Computed Tomography image reconstruction. This architecture decomposes the streak artifacts removal into multiple stages through the recurrent mechanism, which can fully utilize information in previous stages and guide the learning of later stages. In each recurrent stage, the key components of the architecture operate recursively. The recursive mechanism is helpful to save parameters and enlarge the receptive field efficiently with exponentially increased dilation of convolution. To verify its effectiveness, we conduct experiments on the AAPM's CT dataset through 5-fold cross-validation. Our proposed method outperforms the state-of-the-art methods both quantitatively and qualitatively.

Keywords: Computed Tomography · Sparse-view reconstruction · Convolutional recurrent neural network

1 Introduction

In the past twenty years, the radiation risk issue of CT receives much attention and the demand for radiation dose reduction becomes more intense. One way to reduce radiation dose and shorten acquisition time is the sparse-view CT reconstruction, which is achieved by reducing the number of radiation angles,

T. Shen and X. Li—Equal contribution.

Electronic supplementary material The online version of this chapter (https:// doi.org/10.1007/978-3-030-32226-7_36) contains supplementary material, which is available to authorized users.

© Springer Nature Switzerland AG 2019
D. Shen et al. (Eds.): MICCAI 2019, LNCS 11769, pp. 319–327, 2019.
https://doi.org/10.1007/978-3-030-32226-7_36

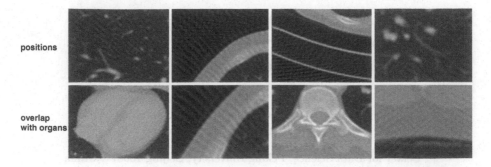

positions

overlap
with organs

Fig. 1. Streak artifacts in different positions or overlapped with different organs have different characteristics.

i.e., views. However, this process introduces some streak artifacts, thus reduces the image quality and causes it confusing for doctors to diagnose.

Great efforts have been devoted to improving sparse-view CT reconstruction's quality. Existing approaches to address the streak artifacts can be mainly divided into two categories: (1) Classical methods: ASD-POCS [5] and PICCS [6] are based on the compressed sensing theory; AwTV [7] and TVS-POCS [8] are total variation based methods; ASDL [9] and AS-LNLM [10] develop from dictionary learning, and so on. (2) Deep learning methods: almost all state-of-the-art (SOTA) deep learning methods are based on U-Net [11] framework, such as Tight Frame U-Net (TF U-Net) [3], cascade of U-Nets [12], etc. In terms of PSNR and SSIM, deep learning methods outperform traditional ones.

In most mainstream deep learning algorithms, there always exist two weaknesses. (1) It is supposed that a sparse-view CT image I_s can be decomposed into a dense-view CT image I_d and a streak artifacts image A as follows:

$$I_s = I_d + A. \tag{1}$$

However, if we observe the sparse-view CT images more carefully, we will find that the streak artifacts in different positions or overlapped with different organs have different characteristics, which is shown in Fig. 1. So it is more proper to decompose the original sparse-view CT image into a dense-view CT image and several different mixture modes of streak artifacts, which can be formulated as:

$$I_s = I_d + \sum_{i=1}^{n} \alpha_i A_i, \tag{2}$$

where A_i represents a certain mixture mode of streak artifacts' image, and α_i denotes the intensity of this certain kind of streak artifacts mixture mode. (2) In order to enlarge the receptive field size, U-Net adopts the "contracting path" and "expansive path" [11]. This feature's downsampling design saves the computation, however, introduces many more parameters. Most SOTA deep learning methods are based on U-Net, so they also suffer from this weakness.

In order to address the above two issues, we propose an architecture, named R^2-Net. On the one hand, we decompose the streak artifacts removal into multiple stages and adopt the **recurrent** mechanism. The visualization results about different mixture modes of streak artifacts in various stages and the progressive learning process are shown in Fig. 4. Moreover, we incorporate the SE block [1] to explicitly learn the α_i in Eq. (2). On the other hand, our proposed network also has a large receptive field without contracting and expanding. This scheme is achieved by the **recursive** mechanism and exponentially increased dilation of convolution. Because of the two mechanisms, we call our model **R^2-Net**.

Main contributions of this paper are listed as follows:

1. We propose a novel network with the recurrent mechanism to remove streak artifacts in sparse-view CT images stage by stage. Besides, SE blocks [1] are used to assign different alpha-values to various mixture modes of streak artifacts in one recurrent stage.
2. In order to achieve capability comparable to U-Net-like networks, recursive mechanism and exponentially increased dilation are utilized in our proposed model. Our network requires fewer parameters than U-Net-like networks.
3. To the best of our knowledge, this is the first paper to introduce recurrent and recursive mechanisms into the artifacts removal of sparse-view CT. Experiments show that R^2-Net outperforms several SOTA methods on the American Association of Physicists in Medicine (AAPM) CT dataset [13].

2 Method

2.1 Overview

Our proposed R^2-Net consists of several components, including an encoder network **E** to transform a 2D CT image to feature maps, a recursive transformer **T** in the feature space and a decoder network **D** to estimate the streak artifacts.

For the overall framework, it contains several **recurrent** stages, and each recurrent stage has several **recursive** stages. In one recurrent stage, firstly, a sparse-view CT image I_s is used as input of the encoder network **E**. Then the recursive transformer **T** extracts feature maps recursively.

Later on, the decoder **D** aggregates refined feature maps from different recursive stages of **T** and estimates the streak artifacts. In the next recurrent stage, the output and feature maps of the previous recurrent stage are used as input and hidden states to predict the streak artifacts more precisely.

In the following, we first describe the architecture of the base model, i.e., the model in one recurrent stage. Then we describe the recurrent mechanism.

2.2 Base Model

The base model, i.e., the model in one recurrent stage, of our proposed method is illustrated in Fig. 2. It is a forward network that transforms I_s to an ideally artifacts-free image $\widehat{I_d}$ that looks like the dense-view CT image I_d.

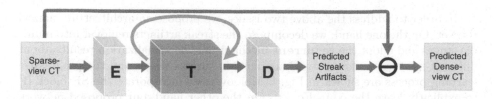

Fig. 2. The architecture of our proposed method in one recurrent stage.

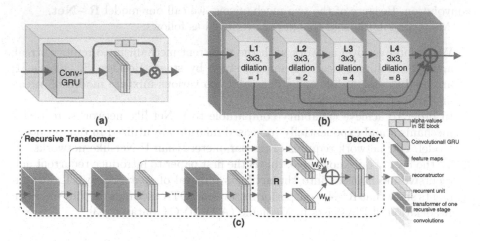

Fig. 3. (a) Basic unit. (b) The recursive transformer in one recursive stage, i.e., a ConvGRU group with exponentially increasing dilations and the sum of all layers' output. (c) Unrolling recursive transformer, reconstructor, the weighted sum of feature maps and final convolutions, i.e., $\mathbf{T}$ and $\mathbf{D}$ in Fig. 2. The number of the recursive stages is M in the figure.

Basic Unit. In our proposed model, we choose Convolutional GRU (ConvGRU) as the basic component, which is shown in Fig. 3(a). ConvGRU includes two convolutional kernels: one on the input tensor and the other on the hidden state tensor. The input tensor comes from the previous layer. The hidden state tensor comes from the same layer in the previous recurrent stage, which is 'zeroes' for the first stage. This design intends to adapt to our recurrent mechanism.

Besides, we regard each channel of ConvGRU's output as the embedding of one mixture mode of streak artifacts. So we extend ConvGRU with the SE block [1] to explicitly compute the alpha-value (α_i) for every channel. Through multiplying alpha-values, feature maps are reweighted to better fit the distribution of streak artifacts with different characteristics.

Encoder E. The encoder is comprised of a basic unit and designed to transform a sparse-view CT image to feature maps.

Recursive Transformer T. This module is recursively used in the base model and can be unrolled as Fig. 3(c). $\mathbf{T}$'s convolution parameters are shared. Through this recursive mechanism, we can enlarge the receptive field without introducing more convolution parameters. In detail, if the recursive number is M and the original receptive field size is S^2, the final receptive field size will be $(MS)^2$.

As for the inner structure of $\mathbf{T}$, due to that larger receptive field is very helpful to acquire more contextual information, dilation scheme is adopted in our recursive transformer. As shown in Fig. 3(b), for layers L1 to L4, the dilation increases from $1(2^{1-1})$ to $8(2^{4-1})$ exponentially, which leads to the exponential growth in receptive field size of every element in high-level feature maps. In each recursive stage, the outputs of each basic unit are added up to create new feature maps as the input of the next recursive stage. This design allows the low-level contextual information to be used directly together with the high-level contextual information, which is helpful to the next recursive stage.

Decoder D. While the recursive module is simple and powerful, we find training a deeply-recursive module is difficult due to the gradients vanishing and exploding. To solve the above issue, we feed outputs of all recursive stages to the reconstructor $\mathbf{R}$, and compute their weighted sum, as shown in Fig. 3(c). Through this design, those feature maps are simultaneously supervised during training.

In detail, $\mathbf{D}$ is comprised of $\mathbf{R}$ and two convolutions. $\mathbf{R}$ is built on a basic unit, whose weights are shared for feature maps from each recursive stage. All outputs of $\mathbf{R}$, as shown in Fig. 3(c), are summed by optimal weights which are automatically learned during training. The next part of $\mathbf{D}$ consists of a 3×3 convolution and a 1×1 convolution, which transforms feature maps to streak artifacts. Finally, the predicted steak artifacts are subtracted from the sparse-view CT image to create the prediction of the dense-view CT image.

2.3 Recurrent Model

As it is not easy to remove all streak artifacts in one stage, we incorporate the recurrent mechanism to remove streak artifacts in multiple stages. ConvGRU containing memory mechanism is selected to fully investigate the recurrent connections between different recurrent stages. The recurrent model is shown in Fig. 4. What's more, the feature map size is not changed in R²-Net's process.

In each recurrent stage, our proposed model predicts the whole residual, i.e., streak artifacts. Our scheme can be formulated as:

$$I_s^1 = I_{ori}, \; H^0 = Zeroes, \tag{3}$$

$$\widehat{Res^i} = F_i(I_s^i, H^{i-1}), \; 1 \le i \le N, \tag{4}$$

$$I_s^{i+1} = \widehat{I_d^i} = I_{ori} - \widehat{Res^i}, \tag{5}$$

where I_{ori} indicates the original sparse-view CT image, I_s^i represents the input of the i-th recurrent stage, N is the number of recurrent stages, F_i indicates the computing process of the i-th recurrent stage, H^{i-1} represents the hidden states, i.e., the feature maps of the $i-1$-th stage, $\widehat{Res^i}$ indicates the output of the i-th recurrent stage, and $\widehat{I_d^i}$ is the predicted dense-view CT image as well as intermediate artifacts-free image after the i-th recurrent stage.

The overall loss function is defined as the sum of all recurrent stages' loss, which is formulated as:

$$L(\Theta) = \sum_{i=1}^{N} \left\| \widehat{Res^i} - Res \right\|_F^2 , \tag{6}$$

where Res is the residual between the original sparse-view CT image and dense-view CT image, and Θ represents the network's parameters.

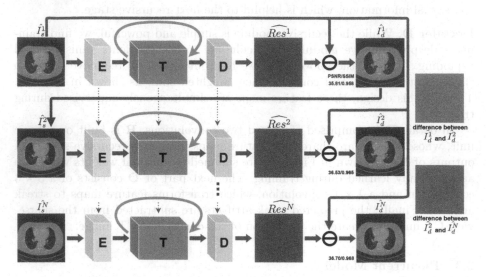

Fig. 4. The unrolling architecture of our proposed method. The two images on the far right show the differences of streak artifacts learned between different stages, which demonstrates that the recurrent mechanism can refine the outputs progressively. **Best viewed on the screen.**

3 Experiments

3.1 Dataset

We evaluate our proposed neural network architecture on the normal-dose part of the AAPM [13] dataset, which consists of 2,378 normal dose CT images from 10 patients and is the most commonly used benchmark dataset in the field. The 3D volumes contain from 128 to 343 slices per patient.

3.2   Experimental Setup

The performance is reported on 5-fold cross-validation. In each cross-validation loop, among the 10 patients, 8 patients' data are used for training and the other 2 patients' data are used for testing.

For the training set, we use the 2D FBP reconstruction images from 30, 60, 120, 180, and 240 projection views as input. The signals of 30, 60, 120, 180, and 240 projection views are generated through simulated downsampling in the transform domain, as the well-known Radon Transform algorithm. And the residual images, i.e., streak artifacts, are used as the label. The residual images are the difference between the dense view (720 views) reconstructions and the sparse view reconstructions. On account of fully utilizing the receptive field, we use the original 512×512 images without cropping as input. What's more, in order to avoid the influence of outliers, we normalize the dataset according to the upper and lower 25 points of all pixels' values.

All architectures are trained by Adam algorithm. As for learning rate, we choose the best decrease range and scheduler for each method, such as 10^{-3} to 10^{-5} for R²-Net, 5×10^{-4} to 10^{-5} for DD-Net [2] and 10^{-3} to 10^{-6} for TF U-Net [3]. The decrease range and scheduler are chosen based on experiments of that method. For evaluation metrics, we adopt SSIM and PSNR.

Table 1. Quantitative comparison (SSIM/PSNR(dB)) between R²-Net and other SOTA methods on the AAPM CT dataset.

SSIM/PSNR	30 views	60 views	120 views	180 views	240 views
FBP [4]	0.459/19.83	0.661/25.54	0.904/33.56	0.976/39.88	0.992/44.83
TF U-Net [3]	0.948/33.87	0.957/36.42	0.979/40.31	0.992/44.16	0.997/48.66
DD-Net [2]	0.945/33.74	0.963/37.13	0.983/40.54	0.993/43.66	0.995/47.11
R²-Net	0.951/34.31	0.971/38.07	0.991/43.97	0.996/47.19	0.998/49.68

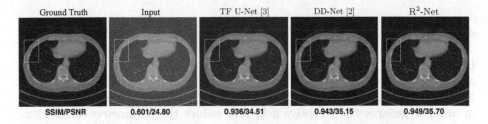

Fig. 5. Qualitative results of R²-Net and other SOTA methods on 60 views. **Best viewed at the screen.** More visualization results are in supplementary material.

3.3 Experimental Results

Comparison Between R²-Net and Other SOTA Models. In Table 1, we present the average SSIM and PSNR values of FBP, other SOTA methods and R²-Net. All methods are significantly better than FBP. Our R²-Net achieves much better results than other two SOTA methods. Qualitative results of 60 view are shown in Fig. 5. More visualization results of different views are presented in supplementary material.

As for the parameters cost, we calculate the number of parameters used in the three methods, which is illustrated in Table 2. R²-Net costs only 4.94% parameters of DD-Net and 0.05% parameters of TF U-Net. Small parameter number makes it easy to deploy and store.

What's more, we present the GPU memory cost of the inference stage in supplementary material.

Ablation Study About Recurrent and Recursive Mechanisms. In this part, we conduct experiments to compare the effect of different settings of recurrent and recursive numbers. This study may help us to understand how important roles are these two mechanisms playing in the architecture. In Table 3, we report the ablation study's results. In the table, M indicates the number of recursive stages, N indicates the number of recurrent stages. It's obvious that both recurrent and recursive mechanisms are beneficial to the performance. In detail, the recurrent mechanism contributes more than the recursive mechanism.

Table 2. Parameters cost comparison among TF U-Net, DD-Net and R²-Net.

	Number of params (K)
TF U-Net [3]	40,837
DD-Net [2]	423
R²-Net	21

Table 3. Quantitative measures comparison among different numbers of recursive(M) and recurrent(N) stages of R²-Net of 120 views.

(M, N)	(1, 1)	(3, 1)	(1, 3)	(3, 3)
SSIM	0.9885	0.9889	0.9908	0.9912
PSNR	42.66	43.03	43.71	43.97

4 Conclusion

In this work, we propose a novel neural network architecture based on recurrent and recursive mechanisms. We incorporate the recurrent mechanism and SE block to progressively suppress streak artifacts stage by stage. What's more, in order to enlarge the receptive field and reduce the parameters number, we introduce the exponentially increased dilation and recursive mechanism into our architecture. Benefited from these two mechanisms, R²-Net outperforms SOTA methods of streak artifacts removal.

Acknowledgment. We thank Dr. Cynthia McCollough (the Mayo Clinic, USA) for providing CT data of Low Dose CT Grand Challenge for research purpose.

Zhouchen Lin is supported by National Basic Research Program of China (973 Program) (grant no. 2015CB352502), National Natural Science Foundation (NSF) of China (grant nos. 61625301 and 61731018), and Microsoft Research Asia.

References

1. Hu, J., Shen, L., Sun, G.: Squeeze-and-excitation networks. In: IEEE conference on Computer Vision and Pattern Recognition, pp. 7132–7141 (2018)
2. Zhang, Z., Liang, X., Dong, X., et al.: A sparse-view CT reconstruction method based on combination of DenseNet and deconvolution. IEEE Trans. Med. Imaging **37**(6), 1407–1417 (2018)
3. Han, Y., Ye, J.C.: Framing U-Net via deep convolutional framelets: application to sparse-view CT. IEEE Trans. Med. Imaging **37**(6), 1418–1429 (2018)
4. Kak, A.C., Slaney, M., Wang, G.: Principles of computerized tomographic imaging. Med. Phys. **29**(1), 107 (2002)
5. Sidky, E.Y., Pan, X.: Image reconstruction in circular cone-beam computed tomography by constrained, total-variation minimization. Phys. Med. Biol. **53**(17), 4777 (2008)
6. Chen, G.H., Tang, J., Leng, S.: Prior image constrained compressed sensing (PICCS): a method to accurately reconstruct dynamic CT images from highly undersampled projection data sets. Med. Phys. **35**(2), 660–663 (2008)
7. Liu, Y., Ma, J., Fan, Y., et al.: Adaptive-weighted total variation minimization for sparse data toward low-dose x-ray computed tomography image reconstruction. Phys. Med. Biol. **57**(23), 7923 (2012)
8. Liu, Y., Liang, Z., Ma, J., et al.: Total variation-stokes strategy for sparse-view X-ray CT image reconstruction. IEEE Trans. Med. Imaging **33**(3), 749–763 (2014)
9. Chen, Y., Shi, L., Feng, Q., et al.: Artifact suppressed dictionary learning for low-dose CT image processing. IEEE Trans. Med. Imaging **33**(12), 2271–2292 (2014)
10. Chen, Y., Yang, Z., Hu, Y., et al.: Thoracic low-dose CT image processing using an artifact suppressed large-scale nonlocal means. Phys. Med. Biol. **57**(9), 2667 (2012)
11. Ronneberger, O., Fischer, P., Brox, T.: U-Net: convolutional networks for biomedical image segmentation. In: Navab, N., Hornegger, J., Wells, W.M., Frangi, A.F. (eds.) MICCAI 2015. LNCS, vol. 9351, pp. 234–241. Springer, Cham (2015). https://doi.org/10.1007/978-3-319-24574-4_28
12. Kofler, A., Haltmeier, M., Kolbitsch, C., Kachelrieß, M., Dewey, M.: A U-Nets cascade for sparse view computed tomography. In: Knoll, F., Maier, A., Rueckert, D. (eds.) MLMIR 2018. LNCS, vol. 11074, pp. 91–99. Springer, Cham (2018). https://doi.org/10.1007/978-3-030-00129-2_11
13. AAPM Low Dose CT Grand Challenge Homepage. https://www.aapm.org/grandchallenge/lowdosect/. Accessed 3 July 2019

Stereo-Correlation and Noise-Distribution Aware ResVoxGAN for Dense Slices Reconstruction and Noise Reduction in Thick Low-Dose CT

Rongjun Ge[1,2,3,5,6], Guanyu Yang[1,2,3], Chenchu Xu[5,6], Yang Chen[1,2,3,4(✉)], Limin Luo[1,2,3], and Shuo Li[5,6(✉)]

[1] Laboratory of Image Science and Technology, School of Computer Science and Engineering, Southeast University, Nanjing, China
chenyang.list@seu.edu.cn
[2] Centre de Recherche en Information Biomedicale Sino-Francais (LIA CRIBs), Rennes, France
[3] Key Laboratory of Computer Network and Information Integration, Southeast University, Ministry of Education, Nanjing, China
[4] School of Cyber Science and Engineering, Southeast University, Nanjing, China
[5] Department of Medical Imaging and Medical Biophysics, Western University, London, ON, Canada
sli287@uwo.ca
[6] Digital Imaging Group of London, London, ON, Canada

Abstract. The low-dose computed tomography (CT) scan with thick slice thickness (3 mm) dramatically improves the imaging efficiency and reduces the radiation risk in clinical. However, the low-dose CT acquisition inherently compromises the signal-to-noise ratio, and the sparse sampled thick slices poorly reproduce the coronal/sagittal anatomy. We propose a Residual Voxel Generative Adversarial Nets (ResVoxGAN), the first powerful work to densely reconstruct slices into the thin thickness (1 mm), and simultaneously denoise the CT image into the more readable pattern, directly from the widely accessible thick low-dose CT. The framework is achieved in a voxel-wise conditional GAN constituted by the following: (1) a generator is composed of consecutive 3D multi-scale residual blocks that richly extracts multi-scale stereo feature for fine-granted and latent spatial structure mining from the noisy volume, and a followed Subpixel Convnet further interpretively reconstructs dense slices from the features for high-resolution and denoising volume; (2) a stereo-correlation constraint elegantly penalizes gradient deviation in voxel adjacent region (i.e., 3D 26-neighborhoods) to guide structural detail, together with a image-expression constraint on perceptual feature representations transformed from a pretrained deep convolution autoencoder to keep scene content; and (3) a pair of coupled discriminators advantageously fuse the prior-knowledge from the thick low-dose CT with the generated image and residual noise via self-learning to drive the generation towards into both realistic anatomic structure distribution and valid noise-reduction distribution. The experiment validated on

© Springer Nature Switzerland AG 2019
D. Shen et al. (Eds.): MICCAI 2019, LNCS 11769, pp. 328–338, 2019.
https://doi.org/10.1007/978-3-030-32226-7_37

Mayo dataset shows that the ResVoxGAN successfully reconstruct the low-dose CT of 3 mm thickness into 1 mm, and meanwhile keeps the with peak signal to noise ratio of 40.80 for noise reduction, and structural similarity index of 0.918 for dense slices reconstruction. These advantages reveal our method a great potential in clinical CT imaging.

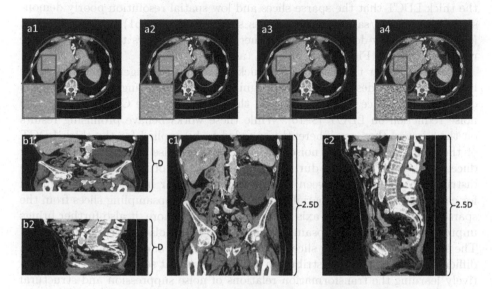

Fig. 1. (1) Thick CT has more clear imaging quality, obviously supported by the red box enlarged region in (a1) thick NDCT vs. (a2) thin NDCT, (a3) thick LDCT vs. (a4) thin LDCT; (2) Thick CT has poor coronal/sagittal anatomy demonstration with sparse slices and low spatial resolution as (b1) coronal thick NDCT vs. (c1) coronal thin NDCT, (b2) sagittal thick NDCT vs. (c2) sagittal thin NDCT; (3) LDCT inherently compromises the signal-to-noise ratio as (a1) vs. (a3), (a2) vs. (a4) (Color figure online)

1   Introduction

The low-dose computed tomography (CT) imaging with thick slice thickness (thick LDCT) is of great clinical significance to dramatically improve the imaging efficiency and reduce the radiation risk for patients. (1) CT technology is one of the most widely used imaging modality in medical diagnosis [1], image-guided surgery [2], and radiation therapy [3], due to its noninvasive procedures, high-contrast resolution and multiplanar reformatted imaging. (2) CT scan of thick slice thickness (i.e., thick CT. It is normally accompanied with bigger interval, but for concise text, we often mention about slice thickness in this paper, that actually indicates about both thickness and interval) is widely set in clinical imaging. It is characterized with the advantages of higher dose efficiency, more reduced storage (e.g., a thick CT of $512 \times 512 \times 343$ only needs $172\,\mathrm{MB}$ storage space, while the corresponding thin CT needs $431\,\mathrm{MB}$), faster iterative reconstruction speed and more clear imaging quality (as shown in Fig. 1, (a1) vs. (a2), (a3) vs. (a4)) [4,5], than the thin one. (3) Low-dose acquired CT image (i.e., LDCT) directly decrease the x-ray radiation flux mainly from lower operating current, voltage or exposure time, to reduces the risk of inducing genetic, cancerous, and disease conditions [6,7]. But there sill exist several problems impede the thick LDCT that the sparse slices and low spatial resolution poorly demonstrate the coronal/sagittal anatomy (as shown in Fig. 1, (b1) vs. (c1), (b2) vs. (c2)), and the low-dose acquisition inherently compromises the signal-to-noise ratio (as shown in Fig. 1, (a1) vs. (a3), (a2) vs. (a4)).

However, so far the solution for thick LDCT is still urgent, and has never been investigated despite its clinical significance. The existing works only focus on either dense slice reconstruction on thick standard dose CT (SDCT) [5], or noise reduction on LDCT [8–10]. While these works behave promising results on their issues, they are inherently impeded to be applied for the thick LDCT of the sparse volume with noise, due to: (1) The noise in thick LDCT introduces the serious inference during the reconstruction of upsampling. The huge distribution difference between noisy images and clear images cause confusion for capturing valid latent spatial structure of densely upsampling slices from the sparse input along the long axis of the body. What's more, it also further brings unpredicted noise on the upsampled slice because of noise covering content. (2) The sparse mapping among slices with thick thickness and thin thickness makes difficulty to extract their distribution difference, so that seriously hampers effectively learning the transformation relations of noise suppression and structural preservation between noisy CT image and clear one, while the strict dense bijection is need in the normal denoising [8–10]. (3) The lack of the unified scheme that reciprocally fuses the dense slices reconstruction and the noise reduction on thick LDCT for elegantly promoting a expressive ultimate-object aware learning to avoid frequently information loss between each other in the handcraftedly phased scheme.

In this study, we propose the first reliable solution, Residual Voxel Generative Adversarial Nets (ResVoxGAN) for widely accessible thick LDCT, to densely reconstruct thick slices ($3\,\mathrm{mm}$) with big interval ($2\,\mathrm{mm}$) into the thin thickness ($1\,\mathrm{mm}$) with small interval ($0.8\,\mathrm{mm}$), and simultaneously denoise the CT image into the more readable pattern. It is achieved with a voxel-wise conditional GAN architecture, as: (1) A novel generator (Sect. 2.1) is proposed by utilizing the consecutive 3D multi-scale residual blocks to richly extract the multi-scale stereo feature for fine-granted and latent spatial structure mining from the noisy volume, and a Subpixel Convnet further interpretively extracts and reconstructs the dense slices from the features of fine-granted latent spatial structure embedded for high-resolution and denoising. Then, (2) a creative stereo-correlation constraint (Sect. 2.2) is proposed by elegantly penalizing the gradient deviation in the voxel adjacent region (i.e., 3D 26-neighborhoods) for guiding the structural detail, together with a image-expression constraint on the perceptual feature representations that are transformed from the pretrained deep convolution autoencoder for maintaining the scene content. And (3) a pair of coupled discriminators (Sect. 2.3) is newly proposed by advantageously fusing the prior-knowledge from the inputting thick LDCT with both the generated image and the residual noise via self-learning for comprehensively driving the generation towards into both realistic anatomic structure distribution and valid noise-reduction distribution. At the end, the thick LDCT is reconstructed with the excellent coronal/sagittal anatomy demonstration and image quality, so that clinically promotes the high imaging efficiency and the low radiation risk for patient.

2 Methodology

As shown in Fig. 2, the proposed ResVoxGAN is performed on the voxel in the thick LDCT volume to acquire and exploit substantial 3D spatial context information. It thus enables the expressive volumetric representations with inter-slice correlation embedded, which breaks the limitation in the 2D cross-section. Specifically, it is implemented with three cooperative elements: (1) a generator (denoted as G, detailed in Sect. 2.1) consists of 3D multi-scale residual blocks and Subpixel Convnet, that maps the thick LDCT into reconstructing dense slices and reducing noise; (2) a stereo-correlation constraint (denoted as $\mathcal{L}_{SteCor}$, detailed in Sect. 2.2) together with a image-expression constraint (denoted as $\mathcal{L}_{ImgExp}$) maintain the structural detail and scene content for the generated images; and (3) a pair of coupled discriminators (denoted as D_{Img} & D_{Res}, detailed in Sect. 2.3) play the adversary against the generator to drive it capture realistic anatomic structure distribution and valid noise-reduction distribution, with the adversarial loss $\mathcal{L}_{Adv}(G, D_{Img}, D_{Res})$.

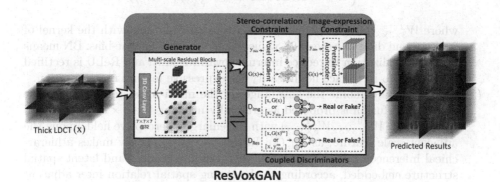

Fig. 2. ResVoxGAN promotes dense slice reconstruction and noise reduction for thick LDCT, via (1) MSVGenerator of consecutive 3D multi-scale residual blocks and Subpixel Convnet for fine-granted stereo feature extraction and latent spatial structure reconstruction; (2) Stereo-correlation & Image-expression Constraints for structural detail and scene content; and (3) Coupled discriminators for realistic anatomic structure distribution and valid noise-reduction distribution.

Summarily, given the thick LDCT, thin NDCT and thick NDCT as x, y_{thin} and y_{thick}, the object of ResVoxGAN is formulated as:

$$\min_{\substack{G}} \max_{\substack{D_{Img} \\ D_{Res}}} \mathcal{L}_{ResVoxGAN} = \mathcal{L}_{Adv}(G, D_{Img}, D_{Res}) + \alpha \mathcal{L}_{SteCor}(G) + \beta \mathcal{L}_{ImgExp}(G)$$

$$(1)$$

2.1   Generator

The generator (denoted as MSVGenerator) in Fig. 3(a) utilizes the multi-scale residual blocks and Subpixel Convnet to generate the candidate results of dense slices reconstruction and noise reduction, directly from the thick LDCT.

Multi-scale Residual Block. As shown in Fig. 3(b), the multi-scale residual block innovatively deploys collateral 3D atrous convolutions, the hierarchical fusion and the residual connection, to mine the fine-granted and latent spatial structure in the sparse and noisy volume.

(1) The atrous convolution is an efficient operation that flexibly enlarges the effective receptive field with the adjustable dilation rate and simplified kernel parameters. To handle our issue of the noise reduction and slices reconstruction in the thick LDCT, the triple collateral 3D atrous convolutions with various dilation rate are used to make an essential stereo feature extraction, as Eq. (2). Being beneficial from them, the different-range stereo context is acquired to capture the multi-scale anatomic structure information and learn the inherent correlation inter slices.

$$\begin{cases} H^{s0} = ReLU(BN(I * W^{2^0}_{3\times3\times3} + b^{s0})) \\ H^{s1} = ReLU(BN(I * W^{2^1}_{3\times3\times3} + b^{s1})) \\ H^{s2} = ReLU(BN(I * W^{2^2}_{3\times3\times3} + b^{s2})) \end{cases} \tag{2}$$

where $W^{2^i}_{3\times3\times3}$ $(i = 0, 1, 2)$ is the 3D atrous convolutions with the kernel of $3 \times 3 \times 3$ and dilation rate of 2^i, while b^{s0}, b^{s1} and b^{s2} are the bias. BN means batch normalization to reduce internal covariate shift, and ReLU is rectified linear unit to introduce nonlinearity for expressive feature representation.

(2) To effectively combine the advantages of the multi-scale stereo feature, the hierarchical fusion is proposed as gradually utilizing the $3 \times 3 \times 3$ standard convolution ($W^{f0}_{3\times3\times3}$, $W^{f1}_{3\times3\times3}$) with the enlarged perceptive field among the adjacent scale feature, as Eq. (3). In this way, it explicitly makes a hierarchical inference on the CT volume, with the fine-granted and latent spatial structure embedded, according to the strong spatial relation inter adjacent scale.

$$H^f = ReLU(BN([ReLU(BN([H^0, H^1] * W^{f0}_{3\times3\times3} + b^{f0})), H^2] * W^{f1}_{3\times3} + b^{f1}))$$

$$(3)$$

where $[\cdot]$ denotes concatenation for grouping the adjacent scale features.

(3) Aims to greatly reduce the computational complexity and efficiently improve the information transmission during the feature extraction, the residual connection is used between the inputs and the outputs of the multi-scale residual block, as:

$$O = ReLU(BN(H^f * W^o_{1 \times 1 \times 1} + b^o) + I) \tag{4}$$

where $W^o_{1 \times 1 \times 1}$ with the kernel of $1 \times 1 \times 1$ is used to reduce the feature channels for decreasing the computational cost and matching with the input feature I.

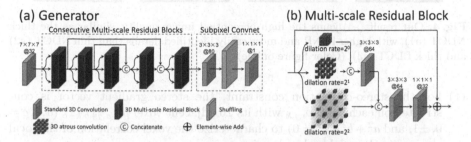

(a) Generator

(b) Multi-scale Residual Block

Fig. 3. (1) (a) MSVGenerator is composed multi-scale residual blocks and Subpixel Convnet for the candidate results of dense slices reconstruction and noise reduction; (b) Multi-scale residual block is constructed by collateral 3D atrous convolutions, hierarchical fusion and residual connection, for fine-granted and latent spatial structure in sparse and noisy volume.

Subpixel Convnet. To interpretively reconstruct the dense slices from the features for high-resolution and denoising volume recovery, we further develop the Subpixel Convnet [12] onto the long-axis direction from the plane. The Subpixel Convnet firstly releases the embedded fine-granted and latent spatial structure information among the slices of the stereo feature with size of $M \times N \times D \times C$ by mapping it into the domain of dimension $M \times N \times D \times (C \cdot S)$ with a learnable $3 \times 3 \times 3$ convolution, where S is the scaling factor for matching the slices reconstruction. Then, a shuffling operation is performed along the long axis to arrange into $M \times N \times (S \cdot D) \times C$. Finally, a convolution of $1 \times 1 \times 1$ integrates all feature channel to map into the desired domain of $M \times N \times (S \cdot D)$ for generating the expected results.

2.2   Stereo-Correlation Constraint and Image-Expression Constraint

The stereo-correlation constraint and image-expression constraint are creatively added into the optimization function Eq. (1) of ResVoxGAN, to naturally guide the structural detail and scene content in the generated image and improve the generalization of the framework. Specifically, the stereo-correlation constraint is proposed to measures the similarity of the inter-voxel changes, namely stereo gradient, between the generated image and the corresponding thin NDCT. Analogously, the image-expression constraint is performed on the high-level feature representations space that encodes the perceptual and semantic information [13].

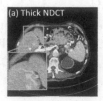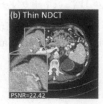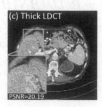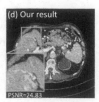

Fig. 4. Our result (a4) gains the high perceptual image quality, similar as the thick NDCT (a1), with higher PSNR and more easily identified details than thin NDCT (a2) and thick LDCT (a3). (Color figure online)

(1) For the stereo-correlation constraint, the stereo gradient vector is constructed on each voxel $p_{i,j,k}$ with its 26 adjacent voxel $p_{i+a,j+b,k+c}$ ($a, b, c = 0, \pm 1$, and $a^2 + b^2 + c^2 \neq 0$) to characterize the voxel correlation of the local changes in the neighborhood region, as:

$$g_{i,j,k} = [p_{i,j,k} - p_{i+a,j+b,k+c}], \quad for \ a, b, c = 0, \pm 1, \ and \ a^2 + b^2 + c^2 \neq 0 \quad (5)$$

Then this penalty item on gradient deviation is implemented as Eq. (6), to guide the structural detail. In Eq. (6), $g_{i,j,k}$ and $\hat{g}_{i,j,k}$ are from the thin NDCT label $y_{thin} \in \mathbb{R}^{M_p \times N_p \times D_p}$ and generated results $G(x) \in \mathbb{R}^{M_p \times N_p \times D_p}$, respectively, and $\|\cdot\|_2$ is L2 norm.

$$\mathcal{L}_{SteCor}(G) = \frac{1}{M_p N_p D_p} \sum_{i,j,k} \|g_{i,j,k} - \hat{g}_{i,j,k}\|_2^2, \quad (6)$$

(2) For the image-expression constraint, the high-level feature representations is transformed by the pretrained 3D deep convolutional autoencoder (DCAE). DCAE, as an alternative loss network, does not need any labeled data, and unsupervisedly encodes the input into the expressive feature that allows a perfect reconstruction of the input with its simple symmetric decoder [14], while the widely recognized pretrained 3D vgg network, unlike the typical 2D version, is lacked so far due to the lack of labeled 3D data. Such remarkable reconstruction from the DCAE feature and the large perceptive field of its each element obviously indicate the intrinsic expression for the global content of the scene. This extracted feature ($\in \mathbb{R}^{M_f \times N_f \times D_f \times C_f}$) from the encoder in DCAE is used for the image-expression constraint, as:

$$\mathcal{L}_{ImgExp}(G) = \frac{1}{M_f N_f D_f C_f} \|DCAE(y_{thin}) - DCAE(G(x))\|_2^2 \quad (7)$$

2.3 Coupled Discriminators

The coupled discriminators innovatively consists of two adversarial nets (D_{Img} & D_{Res}) with different function to assess the generated results weather fits the anatomic structure distribution in the dense slices CT volume and the valid noise-reduction distribution in the high-quality noise-free CT. With the rich experience granted from the determination on real or fake, the coupled discriminators drives the generator to refine and improve the ability of learning dense slices reconstruction and denoising that toward to cheat the discriminators, by using the adversarial loss:

$$\mathcal{L}_{Adv}(G, D_{Img}, D_{Res}) = \mathcal{L}_{Adv-Img}(G, D_{Img}) + \mathcal{L}_{Adv-Res}(G, D_{Res}) \quad (8)$$

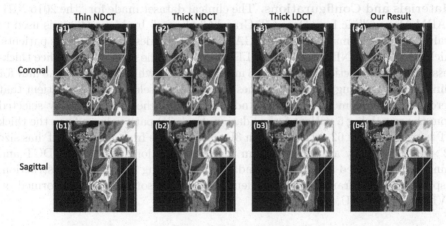

Fig. 5. Our result (a4) & (b4) achieves powerful coronal and sagittal anatomy demonstration, similar as the thin NDCT (a1) & (b1), with the pathological information along the long-axis more easily acquired than thick NDCT (a2) & (b2) and thick LDCT (a3) & (b3).

(1) For the anatomic structure distribution, the discriminator D_{Img} takes the thin NDCT y_{thin} with dense slices that has great coronal/sagittal anatomy demonstration [16,17] as the real data, together with the prior-knowledge from the original input x as reference for self learning more reasonable determination as the conditional GAN [15] does. And the adversarial loss $\mathcal{L}_{Adv-Img}(G, D_{Img})$ promoted by D_{Img} adopts Wasserstein distance [11] for better optimization, as:

$$\mathcal{L}_{Adv-Img}(G, D_{Img}) = -\mathbb{E}_{y_{thin}}[D_{Img}(x, y_{thin})] + \mathbb{E}_x[D_{Img}(x, G(x))] \quad (9)$$

(2) For the valid noise-reduction distribution, the discriminator D_{Res} takes the residual noise y_{thick}^{res} from the thick NDCT y_{thick} between the original input

x as the real data. As the comparison of Fig. 1 (a1) and (a2), the thick NDCT y_{thick} behaves the higher-quality readable pattern [16,18] that has the great signal-to-noise ratio and enables the pathological information to be clear and easy extracted, than the thin NDCT. Therefore, the residual noise y_{thick}^{res} is further used to characterize the real noise distribution, so that drives the generator to learn the valid noise-reduction distribution for candidate results. The $\mathcal{L}_{Adv-Res}(G, D_{Res})$ of D_{Res} is defined in Eq. (10), where $G(x)^{res}$ is the estimated residual noise of the generated result $G(x)$.

$$\mathcal{L}_{Adv-Res}(G, D_{Res}) = -\mathbb{E}_{y_{thick}}[D_{Res}(x, y_{thick}^{res})] + \mathbb{E}_x[D_{Res}(x, G(x)^{res})] \quad (10)$$

3 Experiments

Materials and Configurations. The clinical dataset made for "the 2016 NIH-AAPM-Mayo Clinic Low Dose CT Grand Challenge" by Mayo Clinic is used to evaluate the performance of ResVoxGAN, which includes 10 anonymous patients' thick NDCT, thin NDCT and thick LDCT images. The thick CT has slice thickness and reconstruction interval of 3 mm and 2 mm, while 1 mm and 0.8 mm for thin CT. For training, 8128 3D patches are randomly selected from 5 patient that were randomly from the dataset. And 4096 3D patches are randomly selected from the remaining 5 patient for validating. Each 3D path volume from the thick CT has size of $62 \times 62 \times 12$, and each 3D path volume from the thin CT has size $62 \times 62 \times 30$. They are selected from the same position. The thick NDCT and thin NDCT are used as the gold standard for denoising and slice reconstruction, respectively. The framework is implemented by Tensorflow, and performed on NVIDIA P100 GPU.

3.1 Results and Analysis

As shown in Table 1, the proposed ResVoxGAN achieves effective performance, with peak signal to noise ratio (PSNR) of 40.80 for noise reduction, and structural similarity index (SSIM) of 0.918 for dense slices reconstruction.

Table 1. The quantitative analysis of the proposed method under different configurations. ("MSV-WGAN" denotes using MSVGenerator in 3D-cWGAN, "+Constraint" means adding Stereo-correlation & Image-expression Constraints)

Method	3D-cWGAN	MSV-WGAN	MSV-WGAN+Constraint	**ResVoxGAN**
PSNR	35.42 ± 1.74	36.51 ± 1.61	39.13 ± 1.55	**40.80 ± 1.43**
SSIM	0.885 ± 0.045	0.892 ± 0.031	0.907 ± 0.029	**0.918 ± 0.025**

Visual Analysis. (1) Visually, the instance in Fig. 4 directly illustrates that the result from ResVoxGAN simultaneously gets excellently denoising with higher PSNR as can be seen in the enlarged ROI from the green box, and structure preserving with details more easily identified as the vessel indicated by the yellow arrow, than the thin NDCT and thick LDCT. Obviously our result behaves the high perceptual image quality as the thick NDCT does. (2) Furthermore, as shown in Fig. 5, our ResVoxGAN also promotes the powerful coronal and sagittal anatomy demonstration, as the vessel gets the clear recovering and the osteoarthritis has the unambiguous boundary, compared to the thick NDCT and LDCT (stretched along the long-axis for the comparison). So that, the result of ResVoxGAN effectively enables the easy acquisition of the pathological information along the long-axis, as the thin NDCT does. It can be said that, thanks to the cooperation of thick CT and thin CT, our framework combines the both advantages both of them.

Quantitative Analysis. As shown in Table 1, the performance gets robust improvement by (1) adopting MSVGenerator instead of the normal single-scale voxel generator, (2) adding Stereo-correlation & Image-expression Constraints and (3) introducing Coupled Discriminators on the base model of the 3D conditional WGAN (3D-cWGAN), evaluated by the quantitative analysis of PSNR and SSIM. Since no existing works for thick LDCT slices densely reconstruction and noise reduction, we do not conduct extra comparisons.

4   Conclusion

In this paper, we propose ResVoxGAN, the first powerful work for widely accessible thick LDCT, to densely reconstruct thick slices (3 mm) with big interval (2 mm) into the thin thickness (1 mm) with small interval (0.8 mm), and simultaneously denoise the CT image into the more readable pattern. The net creatively consists of (1) 3D multi-scale residual blocks and Subpixel Convnet for fine-granted stereo feature extraction and latent spatial structure reconstruction; (2) stereo-correlation & image-expression constraint for guiding structural detail and scene content; and (3) Coupled discriminators for driving generator capturing realistic anatomic structure distribution and valid noise-reduction distribution. Extensive experiments with promising results on the excellent coronal/sagittal anatomy demonstration and image quality have revealed the high imaging efficiency and the low radiation risk of ResVoxGAN for patient.

Acknowlegements. This study was supported by the Postgraduate Research & Practice Innovation Program of Jiangsu Province (No. KYCX17_0104), the China Scholarship Council (No. 201706090248), the State's Key Project of Research and Development Plan (No. 2017YFA0104302, No. 2017YFC0109202 and No. 2017YFC0107900), the National Natural Science Foundation (No. 81530060 and No. 61871117).

References

1. Coxson, H.O., Rogers, R.M., Whittall, K.P., D'yachkova, Y., Par, P.D., Sciurba, F.C.: A quantification of the lung surface area in emphysema using computed tomography. Am. J. Respir. Crit. Care Med. **159**(3), 851–856 (1999)
2. Rodrigues, J.C., Pierre, A.F., Hanneman, K., Cabanero, M., Kavanagh, J., et al.: CT-guided microcoil pulmonary nodule localization prior to video-assisted thoracoscopic surgery: diagnostic utility and recurrence-free survival. Radiology **291**, 214–222 (2019). 181674
3. Huynh, E., et al.: CT-based radiomic analysis of stereotactic body radiation therapy patients with lung cancer. Radiother. Oncol. **120**(2), 258–266 (2016)
4. Kanal, K.M., Stewart, B.K., Kolokythas, O., Shuman, W.P.: Impact of operator-selected image noise index and reconstruction slice thickness on patient radiation dose in 64-MDCT. Am. J. Roentgenol. **189**(1), 219–225 (2007)
5. Bae, W., Lee, S., Park, G., Park, H., Jung, K.H.: Residual CNN-based image super-resolution for CT slice thickness reduction using paired CT scans: preliminary validation study. In: Medical Imaging with Deep Learning (2018)
6. National Lung Screening Trial Research Team: Reduced lung-cancer mortality with low-dose computed tomographic screening. N. Engl. J. Med. **365**(5), 395–409 (2011)
7. Wen, N., et al.: Dose delivered from Varian's CBCT to patients receiving IMRT for prostate cancer. Phys. Med. Biol. **52**(8), 2267 (2007)
8. Liu, J., et al.: Discriminative feature representation to improve projection data inconsistency for low dose CT imaging. IEEE TMI **36**(12), 2499–2509 (2017)
9. Chen, H., et al.: Low-dose CT with a residual encoder-decoder convolutional neural network. IEEE TMI **36**(12), 2524–2535 (2017)
10. Yang, Q., et al.: Low-dose CT image denoising using a generative adversarial network with Wasserstein distance and perceptual loss. IEEE TMI **37**(6), 1348–1357 (2018)
11. Gulrajani, I., Ahmed, F., Arjovsky, M., Dumoulin, V., Courville, A.C.: Improved training of Wasserstein GANs. In: NIPS, pp. 5767–5777 (2017)
12. Shi, W., et al.: Real-time single image and video super-resolution using an efficient sub-pixel convolutional neural network. In: CVPR, pp. 1874–1883 (2016)
13. Johnson, J., Alahi, A., Fei-Fei, L.: Perceptual losses for real-time style transfer and super-resolution. In: Leibe, B., Matas, J., Sebe, N., Welling, M. (eds.) ECCV 2016. LNCS, vol. 9906, pp. 694–711. Springer, Cham (2016). https://doi.org/10.1007/978-3-319-46475-6_43
14. Hinton, G.E., Salakhutdinov, R.R.: Reducing the dimensionality of data with neural networks. Science **313**(5786), 504–507 (2006)
15. Isola, P., Zhu, J.Y., Zhou, T., Efros, A.A.: Image-to-image translation with conditional adversarial networks. In: CVPR, pp. 1125–1134 (2017)
16. Goldman, L.W.: Principles of CT: multislice CT. J. Nuclear Med. Technol. **36**(2), 57–68 (2008)
17. Ford, J.M., Decker, S.J.: Computed tomography slice thickness and its effects on three-dimensional reconstruction of anatomical structures. J. Forensic Radiol. Imaging **4**, 43–46 (2016)
18. Chadwick, J.W., Lam, E.W.: The effects of slice thickness and interslice interval on reconstructed cone beam computed tomographic images. Oral Surg. Oral Med. Oral Pathol. Oral Radiol. Endodontol. **110**(4), e37–e42 (2010)

Harnessing 2D Networks and 3D Features for Automated Pancreas Segmentation from Volumetric CT Images

Huai Chen[1], Xiuying Wang[2], Yijie Huang[1], Xiyi Wu[1], Yizhou Yu[3], and Lisheng Wang[1]([✉])

[1] Institute of Image Processing and Pattern Recognition, Department of Automation, Shanghai Jiao Tong University, Shanghai 200240, People's Republic of China
`lswang@sjtu.edu.cn`
[2] School of Computer Science, The University of Sydney, Sydney, Australia
[3] Deepwise AI Lab, Beijing, People's Republic of China

Abstract. Segmenting pancreas from abdominal CT scans is an important prerequisite for pancreatic cancer diagnosis and precise treatment planning. However, automated pancreas segmentation faces challenges posed by shape and size variances, low contrast with regard to adjacent tissues and in particular negligibly small proportion to the whole abdominal volume. Current coarse-to-fine frameworks, either using triplanar schemes or stacking 2D pre-segmentation as prior to 3D networks, have limitation on effectively capturing 3D information. While iterative updates on region of interest (ROI) in refinement stage alleviate accumulated errors caused by coarse segmentation, extra computational burden is introduced. In this paper, we harness 2D networks and 3D features to improve segmentation accuracy and efficiency. Firstly, in the 3D coarse segmentation network, a new bias-dice loss function is defined to increase ROI recall rates to improve efficiency by avoiding iterative ROI refinements. Secondly, for a full utilization of 3D information, dimension adaptation module (DAM) is introduced to bridge 2D networks and 3D information. Finally, a fusion decision module and parallel training strategy are proposed to fuse multi-source feature cues extracted from three sub-networks to make final predictions. The proposed method is evaluated in NIH dataset and outperforms the state-of-the-art methods in comparison, with mean Dice-Sørensen coefficient (DSC) of 85.22%, and with averagely 0.4 min for each instance.

Keywords: Pancreas segmentation · Bias-dice · Dimension adaptation module · Fusion decision module

1 Introduction

Pancreatic cancer, the main cause of several distinct neoplasms in the gland, is the seventh most common cause of cancer death [8]. Accurate pancreas segmentation is vital to effective detection of pancreatic cancer and more accurate

© Springer Nature Switzerland AG 2019
D. Shen et al. (Eds.): MICCAI 2019, LNCS 11769, pp. 339–347, 2019.
https://doi.org/10.1007/978-3-030-32226-7_38

treatment planning [3]. Nevertheless, since pancreas have complex anatomical structures, high diversity of shapes and negligibly small ratio with regard to abdominal volume, automated segmentation of pancreas from volumetric CT images remains a challenging task.

More recently, research efforts have been devoted to automated pancreas segmentation with convolutional neural networks [3,6,9–12]. The coarse-to-fine segmentation frameworks [10–12] assembling networks for coarse ROIs segmentation first and then further refinements, have been proposed to tackle the challenges introduced by the small ratio of pancreas in contrast to the whole abdominal CT volume. However, since the coarse segmentation network may not be able to produce a complete ROI initialization for the refining network, the coarse ROIs are often fed into refining network and updated according to current refining results in several iterators [10,11]. While these iterative ROI refinements further improve the segmentation accuracy, the computational cost would be remarkably increased.

Due to its memory and computational efficiency, 2D pre-trained networks are often utilized to improve performance of pancreas segmentation [3,6]. However, the lack of capturing the third dimensional information limits the segmentation performance of 2D networks. Consequently, tri-planar schemes [6,10,11] have been proposed to capture features along three orthogonal planes. However, features captured in such way cannot fully utilize 3D contents. Method in [9] tries to stack tri-planar predictions and forward them into a 3D network for further capturing of 3D features. However, the cascade of 2D and 3D networks is time-consuming and the independent training of 2D and 3D networks cannot be effectively harnessed for information propagation.

In this paper, we propose an improved coarse-to-fine framework to better utilize 3D information for segmenting small tissue/organ with high computational efficiency. To avoid additional computational cost introduced by iterative ROI refinements, we present bias-dice to 3D coarse segmentation network to raise the recall rate. In the refinement network, we utilize all pre-trained 3D encoder of coarse segmentation network and pre-trained 2D networks, specializing in capturing intra-slice features, to enhance predicted results. The dimension adaptation module (DAM) is proposed to capture interdependencies of adjacent slices. The fusion decision module and parallel training strategy are proposed to effectively fuse aforementioned multi-source features. We evaluate our method in the dataset of NIH [5] and obtain state-of-the-art results.

2   Methods

As illustrated in Fig. 1, our framework is composed of 3D lightweight coarse segmentation network and multi-source refinement architecture. In coarse segmentation, bias-dice loss for the 3D U-Net is designed for optimal ROI extraction. In the refinement stage, the dimension adaptation module (DAM) is introduced to mine 3D information from pre-trained 2D networks. Multi-source 3D features are deconvoluted by 3D decoders for fusion decision module to make predictions.

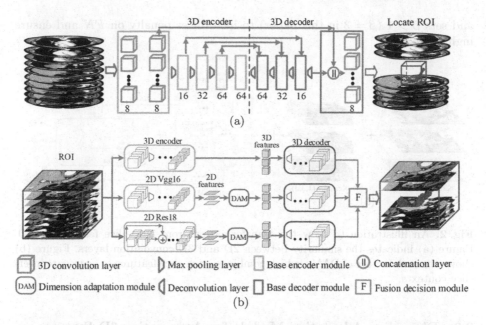

Fig. 1. An illustration of our framework. (a) 3D coarse segmentation network trained with bias-dice loss proposes ROIs with high recall rates. (b) Refinement network that uses DAMs to transform intra-features of pre-trained networks into 3D and the fusion decision module to combine multi-source features to make accurate predictions.

2.1 3D Coarse Segmentation Network

A lightweight 3D U-Net [2], containing a 3D encoder to capture deep content features and a 3D decoder to make end-to-end classifications, is utilized for coarse segmentation. The output from decoder is fed into a decision module, composing of a 3D convolution layer and a sigmoid layer for generating probability map. From this probability map, ROI is defined as the bounding box containing the biggest connective region as the output of this coarse segmentation stage.

To reduce subsequent computational cost due to iterative updates on ROI definitions in the current coarse-to-fine methods [10,11], we define a new bias-dice loss function to increase recall rates and thereby to alleviate incomplete ROI definitions. The bias-dice loss function is defined as below:

$$Loss_{bias\_dice} = 1 - \frac{2(\sum_{i=1}^{N} p_i g_i + \epsilon)}{\sum_{i=1}^{N} p_i(1 - g_i) + 2\sum_{i=1}^{N} g_i p_i + \beta \times \sum_{i=1}^{N} g_i(1 - p_i) + \epsilon} \quad (1)$$

Where p_i denotes predicted probability map and g_i is the ground truth, ϵ is smoothness term to avoid the risk of division by 0. Actually, the item of $\sum_{i=1}^{N} p_i(1 - g_i)$, $\sum_{i=1}^{N} g_i p_i$ and $\sum_{i=1}^{N} g_i(1 - p_i)$ are respectively soft items of TP, FP and FN. Compared to original dice loss, which sets $\beta = 1$ in the soft FN item of $\sum_{i=1}^{N} g_i(1 - p_i)$, the bias-dice loss emphasizes importance of recall and sets $\beta > 1$ ($\beta = 3$ in this paper) to introduces penalty on FN and ensure high recall rates.

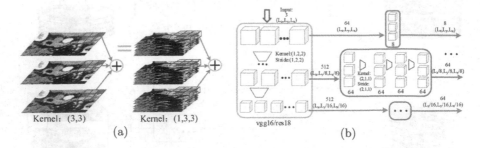

Fig. 2. An illustration to show the transformation from intra-slice features to 3D. Figure (a) indicates the similarity between 2D and 3D convolution layers. Figure (b) shows the architecture of DAMs, which combines intra-slice features to aggregate inter-slice contexts.

2.2 Dimension Adaptation Module for Aggregating 3D Features

2D networks can be effectively initialized by pre-trained models to capture powerful intra-slice features from volumetric CT images. However, only using 2D networks to segment pancreas neglects important information along z-axis, which therefore limits the segmentation performance. In order to utilize pre-trained 2D networks to extract intra-slice features without missing of inter-slice features, we firstly transform 2D pre-trained networks into 3D for direct prediction of volumetric images and propose DAMs to aggregate contexts along z-axis.

Transforming 2D Layers into 3D Layers: As shown in the Fig. 2(a), a 2D convolution layer with kernel of (h, w) can be equivalently expressed as a 3D convolution layer with kernel of $(1, h, w)$. Similarly, the 2D pooling operations can be transformed into the corresponding 3D pooling layers. So we can replace 2D convolution and 2D max-pooling layers with 3D layers to transform 2D pre-trained networks, such as Vgg16 and Res18, into 3D versions to directly obtain intra-slice features of a volumetric image.

Dimension Adaptation Module to Capture 3D Features: Aforementioned intra-slice features can be fed into DAMs to capture inter-slice features. The architecture of DAM is shown in Fig. 2(b), in which, the first 3D convolution layer compresses channel number of intra-slice features by eight times to relieve memory cost. And the following convolution layers with kernel of $(3, 3, 3)$ and max-pooling layers, which only compress features along z-axis to broaden receptive field, are utilized to mine relationship of adjacent 2D sectional slices.

2.3   Parallel Training Strategy and Inferencing

Parallel Training Strategy. In the refinement stage, to effectively capture 3D features, 3D encoder of coarse segmentation network, Vgg16 accompanied with DAMs and Res18 accompanied with DAMs, are simultaneously adopted. To effectively utilize them and unify multi-source cues, we propose a parallel training strategy. As shown in Fig. 3, we respectively set three decoders and add three extra decision modules supplement supervisions of the conventional fusion decision module for the multi-source features. The updated loss is defined as below:

$$loss_{total} = \sum_{i=1}^{N} Loss_i + Loss_{fused} \qquad (2)$$

Where $Loss_i$ denotes the additional supervision of the i-th decision module and $Loss_{fused}$ is the loss of fusion decision module. N is the number of sub-networks and is 3 in refining network. All of these losses are dice loss.

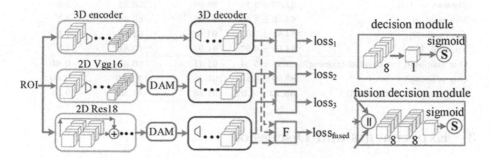

Fig. 3. An illustration of parallel training.

From Whole Volumes to ROIs. To effectively utilize all data, we first respectively train three sub-networks on the whole data, and then we integrate pre-trained models into a unified one. Then, we further train the total network on the data of ROIs by parallel training strategy.

For the training of networks on whole volumes, we forward $64 \times 192 \times 192$ volume images into networks at batch size of 2 each time. For the training of networks based on pre-trained 2D networks, we first freeze encoders and warm up decoders and DAMs with Adam with $lr = 0.001$. Then, we fine-tune encoders with $lr = 0.0001$. We divide 8 instances as validation data, so early stopping can be conducted to stop training if validation loss does not improve in 10 epochs. The max epoch is 200 and networks are updated 60 times each epoch.

For the training on the data of ROIs, we put a whole volumetric ROI into networks every time. We first spend 5 epochs to warm up fusion decision module. Then the lr is set as 0.0001 for Vgg16 and Res18, while other parts with the $lr = 0.001$. If the validation loss does not decrease in 10 epochs, we will set $lr = 0.0001$ for all networks, meanwhile, early stopping strategy is conducted to stop training after 10 epochs without improvement.

Inferencing. The region of abdomen is firstly segmented from the whole volumetric CT image using OTSU [4] to shrink the searching region. Then, the volumetric image of abdomen is fed into the coarse segmentation network to obtain initial results, which will be further binarized by a threshold value of 0.1. The biggest connective region of binary result will be set as ROI, and the margins of ROI region will be extended by 8, 32, 32 on z, y, x axis to provide sufficient spatial contexts. Finally, the extended ROI will be entered into the refinement segmentation network to get fine results. The predicted results will be binarized by 0.5 and the biggest connective region will be the final segmentation result.

Table 1. Comparison of segmentation results and inference times of different methods.

Method	Mean DSC (%)	Max DSC (%)	Min DSC (%)	Time (m)
Roth et al. [5]	71.42 ± 10.11	86.29	23.99	6–8
Roth et al. [6]	78.01 ± 8.20	88.65	34.11	2–3
Roth et al. [7]	81.27 ± 6.27	88.96	50.69	2–3
Cai et al. [1]	82.4 ± 6.7	90.10	60.00	N/A
Zhou et al. [11]	82.50 ± 6.14	89.98	56.33	0.9
Zhu et al. [12]	84.59 ± 4.86	91.45	69.62	4.1
Xia et al. [9]	84.63 ± 5.07	**91.57**	61.58	1.4
Yu et al. [10]	84.50 ± 4.97	91.02	62.81	1.3
Our proposed (no parallel training)	83.99 ± 5.34	91.41	66.62	**0.40**
Our proposed	85.09 ± 4.13	91.26	**71.42**	**0.40**
Our proposed (integrated)	**85.22 ± 4.07**	91.36	71.40	0.44

3   Experiments and Discussion

3.1   Dataset and Evaluation Metrics

Experiments are conducted on the NIH pancreas segmentation dataset [5], which contains 82 abdominal CT volumes. The size of each CT scan is $512 \times 512 \times D$, where D ranges from 181 to 466. We perform 4-fold cross-validation. Every CT is evaluated by computing the DSC: $DSC = \frac{2|P \times G|}{|P|+|G|}$, where P is the binary results of predictions and G is the ground truth.

3.2   Results

We compare our proposed method with extensive state-of-the-art methods. The DSC values and inference times of different methods are shown in Table 1. In addition to presenting the results of single fusion decision module, we also show the results of integrating all four decision modules using average operation.

According to results shown in Table 1, our proposed method has the better mean DSC, where the mean DSC is 85.09% for fusion decision module and is 85.22% for integrated one. And the worst instance can still have a DSC of 71.42%, which shows the good robustness of the proposed method. What's more, the method proposed is much more time-effective with only about 0.4 min to realize the segmentation of one single instance.

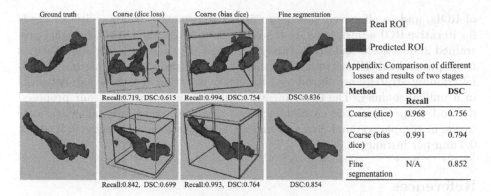

Fig. 4. Comparison of coarse segmentation methods with different loss functions and refinement segmentation. The left figure shows two instances of different methods. And the right one is a table shows the average ROI recall and mean DSC.

3.3 Discussion

The Contribution of Bias-Dice: As shown in Fig. 4, coarse segmentation method based on bias-dice loss has a better performance in the average ROI recall with 99.1% and mean DSC with 79.4% than based on original dice loss. The bias-dice makes network pay more attention on recall rate, therefore, the results have less FNs, which reduces the missing of meaningful pancreas regions.

The Contribution of Parallel Training: Both results of methods with and without parallel training are shown in Table 1. Compared to method without parallel training with mean DSC of 83.99% and minimum DSC of 66.62%, method with parallel training can be much more stable and effective with mean DSC of 85.09% and minimum DSC of 71.42%. The utilization of parallel training can effectively alleviate over-fitting caused by massive parameters and improve the performance of unified network.

The Optimal "Speed-Accuracy Tradeoff": Our method provides an optimal "speed-accuracy tradeoff" with both improved accuracy and reduced inference time in comparison to the state-of-the-art methods with best accuracy and fastest speed. Compared with the method with highest mean DSC, our method remarkably accelerates inference from 1.4 min to 0.44 min. In comparison with the fastest method, our method increases mean DSC from 82.5% to 85.2% and further reduces inference time from 0.9 min to 0.44 min.

4 Conclusion

In this paper, we improve the coarse-to-fine framework for faster and more accurate pancreas segmentation. In the coarse segmentation stage, our proposed bias-dice loss function adds a penalty in the soft FN item to achieve high recall rates of ROIs, and to effectively alleviate missing informative regions without needs for iterative ROI adjustments. In the refinement stage, the DAMs, bridging pre-trained 2D networks and 3D features, is presented to capture inter-slice features from pre-trained 2D networks. Further, a fusion decision module and parallel training strategy are introduced to effectively train the three sub-networks in a unified manner. The experimental results demonstrate that our proposed method outperforms the current methods based on convolutional neural networks in comparison and achieved highest computational efficiency with about 0.4 min per instance.

References

1. Cai, J., Lu, L., Zhang, Z., Xing, F., Yang, L., Yin, Q.: Pancreas segmentation in MRI using graph-based decision fusion on convolutional neural networks. In: Ourselin, S., Joskowicz, L., Sabuncu, M.R., Unal, G., Wells, W. (eds.) MICCAI 2016. LNCS, vol. 9901, pp. 442–450. Springer, Cham (2016). https://doi.org/10.1007/978-3-319-46723-8_51
2. Falk, T., et al.: U-Net: deep learning for cell counting, detection, and morphometry. Nat. Methods 16(1), 67 (2019)
3. Farag, A., Lu, L., Turkbey, E., Liu, J., Summers, R.M.: A bottom-up approach for automatic pancreas segmentation in abdominal CT scans. In: Yoshida, H., Näppi, J., Saini, S. (eds.) ABD-MICCAI 2014. LNCS, vol. 8676, pp. 103–113. Springer, Cham (2014). https://doi.org/10.1007/978-3-319-13692-9_10
4. Otsu, N.: A threshold selection method from gray-level histograms. IEEE Trans. Syst. Man Cybern. 9(1), 62–66 (1979)
5. Roth, H.R., et al.: DeepOrgan: multi-level deep convolutional networks for automated pancreas segmentation. In: Navab, N., Hornegger, J., Wells, W.M., Frangi, A.F. (eds.) MICCAI 2015. LNCS, vol. 9349, pp. 556–564. Springer, Cham (2015). https://doi.org/10.1007/978-3-319-24553-9_68
6. Roth, H.R., Lu, L., Farag, A., Sohn, A., Summers, R.M.: Spatial aggregation of holistically-nested networks for automated pancreas segmentation. In: Ourselin, S., Joskowicz, L., Sabuncu, M.R., Unal, G., Wells, W. (eds.) MICCAI 2016. LNCS, vol. 9901, pp. 451–459. Springer, Cham (2016). https://doi.org/10.1007/978-3-319-46723-8_52
7. Roth, H.R., et al.: Spatial aggregation of holistically-nested convolutional neural networks for automated pancreas localization and segmentation. Med. Image Anal. 45, 94–107 (2018)
8. Stewart, B., Wild, C.P., et al.: World cancer report 2014 (2014)
9. Xia, Y., Xie, L., Liu, F., Zhu, Z., Fishman, E.K., Yuille, A.L.: Bridging the gap between 2D and 3D organ segmentation with volumetric fusion net. In: Frangi, A.F., Schnabel, J.A., Davatzikos, C., Alberola-López, C., Fichtinger, G. (eds.) MICCAI 2018. LNCS, vol. 11073, pp. 445–453. Springer, Cham (2018). https://doi.org/10.1007/978-3-030-00937-3_51
10. Yu, Q., Xie, L., Wang, Y., Zhou, Y., Fishman, E.K., Yuille, A.L.: Recurrent saliency transformation network: incorporating multi-stage visual cues for small organ segmentation. In: Proceedings of the IEEE Conference on Computer Vision and Pattern Recognition, pp. 8280–8289 (2018)

11. Zhou, Y., Xie, L., Shen, W., Wang, Y., Fishman, E.K., Yuille, A.L.: A fixed-point model for pancreas segmentation in abdominal CT scans. In: Descoteaux, M., Maier-Hein, L., Franz, A., Jannin, P., Collins, D.L., Duchesne, S. (eds.) MICCAI 2017. LNCS, vol. 10433, pp. 693–701. Springer, Cham (2017). https://doi.org/10.1007/978-3-319-66182-7_79

12. Zhu, Z., Xia, Y., Shen, W., Fishman, E., Yuille, A.: A 3D coarse-to-fine framework for volumetric medical image segmentation. In: 2018 International Conference on 3D Vision (3DV), pp. 682–690. IEEE (2018)

Tubular Structure Segmentation Using Spatial Fully Connected Network with Radial Distance Loss for 3D Medical Images

Chenglong Wang[1]([✉]), Yuichiro Hayashi[2], Masahiro Oda[2], Hayato Itoh[2], Takayuki Kitasaka[3], Alejandro F. Frangi[4], and Kensaku Mori[2,5,6]

[1] Graduate School of Information Science, Nagoya University, Nagoya, Japan
cwang@mori.m.is.nagoya-u.ac.jp
[2] Graduate School of Informatics, Nagoya University, Nagoya, Japan
[3] Aichi Institute of Technology, Toyota, Japan
[4] School of Computing and School of Medicine, University of Leeds, Leeds, UK
[5] Information Technology Center, Nagoya University, Nagoya, Japan
[6] Research Center for Medical Bigdata, National Institute of Informatics, Tokyo, Japan

Abstract. This paper presents a new spatial fully connected tubular network for 3D tubular-structure segmentation. Automatic and complete segmentation of intricate tubular structures remains an unsolved challenge in the medical image analysis. Airways and vasculature pose high demands on medical image analysis as they are elongated fine structures with calibers ranging from several tens of voxels to voxel-level resolution, branching in deeply multi-scale fashion, and with complex topological and spatial relationships. Most machine/deep learning approaches are based on intensity features and ignore spatial consistency across the network that are otherwise distinct in tubular structures. In this work, we introduce 3D slice-by-slice convolutional layers in a U-Net architecture to capture the spatial information of elongated structures. Furthermore, we present a novel loss function, coined *radial distance loss*, specifically designed for tubular structures. The commonly used methods of cross-entropy loss and generalized Dice loss are sensitive to volumetric variation. However, in tiny tubular structure segmentation, topological errors are as important as volumetric errors. The proposed radial distance loss places higher weight to the centerline, and this weight decreases along the radial direction. Radial distance loss can help networks focus more attention on tiny structures than on thicker tubular structures. We perform experiments on bronchus segmentation on 3D CT images. The experimental results show that compared to the baseline U-Net, our proposed network achieved improvement about 24% and 30% in Dice index and centerline over ratio.

Keywords: Tubular structure segmentation · Spatial FCN · Radial distance loss · Blood vessel · Bronchus

© Springer Nature Switzerland AG 2019
D. Shen et al. (Eds.): MICCAI 2019, LNCS 11769, pp. 348–356, 2019.
https://doi.org/10.1007/978-3-030-32226-7_39

1   Introduction

The extraction and quantification of bronchi and blood vessels remains a fundamental problem with relevance to many computer aided diagnosis (CAD) systems. Automatic and complete segmentation of intricate tubular structures remains a major challenge in medical image-processing field. Airways and vasculature pose high demands on image analysis as they are elongated fine structures with calibers ranging from several tens of voxels to voxel-level resolution, branching in deeply multi-scale fashion, and with complex topological and spatial relationships. Over the past few years, deep learning methods have become the dominant approach in many data analysis fields and have achieved remarkable advances in the medical image analysis [1]. Recently, airways and vasculature image analysis have also been approached using deep convolutional neural networks (ConvNets) instead of the traditional filter banks and machine learning methods.

Many studies have been made using 2D/2.5D image patches to train their networks [2,3]. Similarly, Yun et al. [2] used 2D patches on three anatomical planes to train three ConvNets as classifiers to classify whether a voxel belongs to the bronchus. To explore the inherent relationship between such orthogonal 2D patches, Tetteh et al. [3] presented 2D orthogonal cross-hair filters to make use of 3D context information but with a reduced computational burden. The above approaches made use of local contexts to address the tubular-structure segmentation. Although, they achieved good performance, the problem remains of taking full advantages of large-range information in the field of view (FOV), which can provide global queues unavailable from small local patches. Meng et al. [4] attempted to use an original 3D U-Net combined with a traditional bronchus tracking method to improve bronchus segmentation accuracy. Huang et al. [5] presented a liver-vessel segmentation method using a 3D U-Net with variant Dice loss function. Both works used a large 3D sub-volume size of around $100 \times 100 \times 100$ voxels.

Compared to 2D local patch-based methods, 3D FCNs for tubular-structure segmentation has some limitations that need to be addressed. Foremost is the severe imbalance in the sizes of the large background area when compared to the small foreground (tubular structure). Second, it's unclear whether FCNs can learn useful features from the abundant contexts of 3D data that while capturing coarse-scale long-range interrelationships are also accurate to detect tubular details and topological correctness at finer scales. The motivation of this work is to improve the accuracy of tubular-structure segmentation in respect to these two concerns.

The main contributions of this work can be summarized as follows. **(1)** We introduce 3D recurrent convolutional layer in FCN architecture for tubular-structure segmentation. **(2)** We propose a novel radial distance loss for 3D tubular-structure segmentation that helps the networks to recover tiny tubular structures. **(3)** Both 3D recurrent convolution layer and radial distance loss are generic and flexible, so they can be easily incorporated in other state-of-the-art networks and used in other applications.

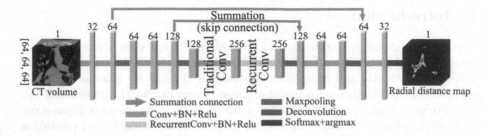

Fig. 1. Overview architecture

2   Method

Our main contribution is twofold from the viewpoint of tackling both network architecture and its loss function. The motivation of this work is to design a new end-to-end FCN for 3D-tubular structure segmentation. Compared with traditional layer-by-layer convolutional layers, the proposed slice-by-slice convolutional layer permits messages to efficiently pass slices. Our proposed loss function places more weight on the centerline of a tubular structure than on the outer border which can help the network pay more attention to tiny structures. A simple illustration of our architecture is shown in Fig. 1.

2.1   3D Spatial FCN

Spatial-CNN was first proposed to address the traffic lane detection problem [6]. The main contribution of spatial-CNN is the introduction of a slice-by-slice convolutional layer. Different from the traditional layer-by-layer CNN, slice-by-slice convolutions perform like recurrent neural networks. The in-layer recurrent convolutions provide more efficient message-passing between neurons in the same layer. This can help networks reinforce structures with strong spatial constraints [6].

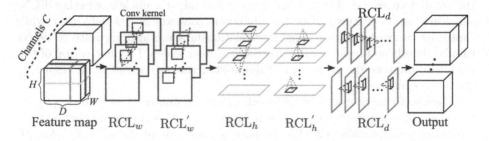

Fig. 2. RCL architecture: feature map represents the output of the last convolutional layer with a shape of $N \times C \times W \times H \times D$. Slice-by-slice recurrent convolutions are performed in each RCL.

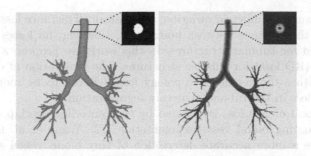

Fig. 3. Volume rendering of binary ground truth and corresponding radial distance map. Radial distance map shown on the right is rendered with pseudo color mapping 0 to blue, and 1 to red. (Color figure online)

In this work, we incorporated Recurrent Convolutional Layers (RCLs) in a 3D FCN architecture for 3D medical imaging applications. Detailed structure of RCLs is illustrated in Fig. 2. Convolutions are performed in both forward and backward directions along the width, height, and depth dimensions. As shown in Fig. 2, RCL_w, RCL_h, and RCL_d denote RCLs with convolutions in front-to-back direction along the three dimensions. RCL'_w, RCL'_h, and RCL'_d denote RCLs with convolutions in the reverse direction. Forward computation of RCL_w can be defined as

$$\mathbfcal{Z}_{c,i,j,k} = \begin{cases} \mathbfcal{X}_{c,i,j,k}, & \text{if } i = 0 \\ \mathbfcal{X}_{c,i,j,k} + f(\mathbfcal{Z}_{c,i-1,j,k} * K), & \text{if } 0 < i < W, \end{cases} \tag{1}$$

where $\mathbfcal{X}$ denote an input 4D feature tensor of size $C \times W \times H \times D$, and $\mathbfcal{Z}$ denotes the output of RCL_w. Let c, i, j, k denote the index of channel, width, height and depth dimensions. K is a 3D convolution kernel of size $w \times w \times w$. $f(\cdot)$ denotes a nonlinear activation function. RELU is used in this work. Similarly, forwarding for RCL_h and RCL_d can be easily derived based on Eq. 1.

In this work, we chose U-Net architecture [7,8] with three multi-scale levels as our backbone FCN. As shown in Fig. 1, we placed the RCLs directly after the deepest feature map, i.e. the compressed low-dimensional representation. In previous spatial-CNN [6], the authors placed the RCLs after the output of CNN, under the assumption that the top hidden layer with rich semantic information is an ideal place to apply RCLs. However, in our FCN architecture, applying RCLs to the deepest representation provides better performance than using top hidden layer.

2.2   Radial Distance Loss

The use of Dice loss for medical segmentation tasks was first proposed by Milletari et al. [9]. They showed that Dice loss outperformed other losses, especially in severe data-imbalance situations [9]. More recently, Hausdorff distance loss and contour loss were proposed for localization and segmentation tasks [10,11].

Dice loss measures volumetric variation, and Hausdorff distance loss and contour loss measure the distance between boundaries. However, no losses were specifically designed for tubular structures. In this work, we propose a novel radial distance loss (RD loss) for tubular structures. The motivation of our proposed loss is to capture the geometric topology loss believed to be more important than volume loss in the tubular-structure segmentation.

The proposal of RD loss is inspired by the centerline overlap (CO) metric used for evaluating blood vessel segmentation [12]. Wang et al. used the CO metric to give a more accurate description of tiny blood vessel segmentation than conventional Dice similarity coefficient (DSC). To take advantage of the CO metric while keeping a volumetric measurement, our proposed RD loss is defined as

$$L = -\frac{1}{2}\sum_{k=0}^{1} \mathcal{W}_k \left(\frac{2\sum_i^N p_{i,k}d_{i,k}}{\sum_i^N p_{i,k}^2 + \sum_i^N d_{i,k}^2} \right),$$ (2)

where $p_i \in \mathbf{P}$ and $d_i \in \mathbf{D}$ denote the i-th voxel predicted binary result and the radial distance map. Voxel index $i \in [1, N]$. $k \in [0, 1]$ denote class. Class weights $\mathcal{W}$ is defined as reciprocal volume ratio of each class. Notice that Eq. 2 is similar to traditional Dice loss [9] except that we use radial distance map $\mathbf{D}$ instead of binary ground truth $\mathbf{G}$. $\mathbf{D}$ is defined as:

$$\mathbf{D} = -\frac{1}{\max(\mathbf{F})}\mathbf{F} + 1,$$ (3)

where $\mathbf{F} = \{f_i, i \in N\}$ denotes a distance map created by a Euclidean distance transformation from the centerline of ground truth. $\mathbf{F}$ is defined as:

$$f_i = \begin{cases} \min\{d(f_i, s_j); s_j = 1\}, & \text{if } s_j = 0, \\ 0, & \text{if } s_j = 1 \text{ or } g_i = 0. \end{cases}$$ (4)

Here, $s_j \in \mathbf{S}$ denotes the j-th voxel of centerline data $\mathbf{S}$ extracted from $\mathbf{G}$. Finally, we obtained radial distance map $\mathbf{D}$ by normalizing $\mathbf{F}$ from 0 to 1 using a simple monomial form. An example of a radial distance map is shown in Fig. 3. RD loss can be weighted combination of centerline loss and Dice loss.

3 Experiments and Results

To evaluate our proposed method, we performed bronchus segmentation experiments on 3D clinical CT scans acquired with a standard dose. The sizes of CT slices were 512×512 pixels with a resolution of 0.63–0.97 mm. The number of CT slices ranged from 238 to 851 with varying thickness of 0.63–1.00 mm. Monte Carlo cross-validation (MCCV) was conducted three times. All 38 CT images were randomly divided into training and validation subsets containing 35 and 3 cases. The model with the best validation accuracy is tested on three unseen datasets acquired in a different hospital than those used for training.

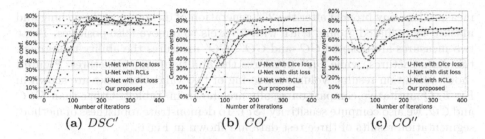

(a) *DSC′*   (b) *CO′*   (c) *CO″*

Fig. 4. Validation results. Dot markers represent actual validation scores. For a clearer visualization, we plot smoothed results in dashed line using Gaussian filter.

Since we chose U-Net as our backbone FCN, we performed comparison experiments using U-Net with Dice loss as a baseline. U-Net with only RCL structures and U-Net with only radial distance loss were also validated to prove the effectiveness of each proposal. We also compared our proposed method with two other methods, one is a variant U-Net architecture, V-Net [9] (Dice loss and RD loss), and the other is 3D voxelwise residual networks, VoxResNet [13].

Table 1. Quantitative comparison results. All measurement was shown with mean ± standard values.

Method	Dataset	DSC' (%)	DSC''(%)	Se (%)	CO' (%)	CO'' (%)
(1) In-house dataset						
Yun et al. [2]	Train: 59 Test:8	89.9 ± 8.9	–	–	–	–
Meng et al. [4]	Train: 30 Test:20	86.6	–	79.6	–	–
(2) Our bronchus dataset						
VoxResNet (Dice loss) [13]	MCCV Test:3	79.6 ± 3.7	90.0 ± 3.4	72.3 ± 5.0	39.2 ± 2.7	31.0 ± 2.1
V-Net (Dice loss) [9]		65.4 ± 9.9	91.0 ± 2.0	69.0 ± 2.0	28.3 ± 3.9	19.8 ± 1.1
V-Net (RD loss)		83.3 ± 2.0	88.4 ± 0.7	76.3 ± 4.6	53.8 ± 1.0	66.6 ± 4.9
U-Net (Dice loss) [8]		64.0 ± 19.5	92.4 ± 1.6	82.9 ± 5.7	47.2 ± 18.1	54.3 ± 9.0
Our proposed		88.7 ± 1.2	94.5 ± 0.8	86.5 ± 1.0	76.6 ± 6.0	80.6 ± 5.6

In training phase, for each epoch, 4 sub-volumes with a size of $64 \times 64 \times 64$ voxels were randomly cropped from each CT image for all 35 training cases. No data augmentation was performed in our experiments. Random cropping was performed in this work. The initial learning rate was set to 0.01, and it decayed by 0.2 every 150 epochs. The optimization was realized via stochastic gradient descent (SGD).

DSC and CO were used for quantitative validation. To validate the general segmentation ability of each method, DSC' was measured on the segmentation results with no post-processing, and DSC'' was only measured on thick branches (before 2nd generation of dichotomous branching). We computed CO scores on the results with two post-processing strategies. One is measured on the largest connected component extracted from the segmentation results. The other one is measured on tiny bronchi after the 2nd generation of dichotomous branching and masked by a dilated ground truth with 5 voxels to remove false positives. These two measures are denoted CO' and CO''. CO' measures the ability to segment tubular structures, while CO'' measures the ability of tiny structures. Figure 4 shows validation results. Volume rendering of two validation cases are shown in Fig. 5. Quantitative comparison results are shown in Table 1. Other than DSC and CO, we also compute sensitivity (Se). To demonstrate robustness of method, segmentation results of three test data are shown in Fig. 6.

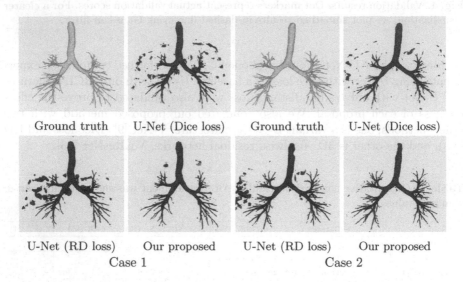

Ground truth   U-Net (Dice loss)   Ground truth   U-Net (Dice loss)

U-Net (RD loss)   Our proposed   U-Net (RD loss)   Our proposed
Case 1   Case 2

Fig. 5. Volume rendering of segmentation results of two validation cases. No post-processing was performed. Trained models at 300th iteration were used for prediction.

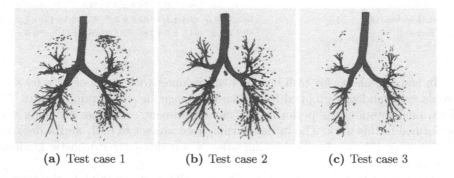

(a) Test case 1   (b) Test case 2   (c) Test case 3

Fig. 6. Segmentation results of three test data. For a clearer visualization, we removed outliers under volume size of 10 voxels.

4   Discussion and Conclusions

In this work, we proposed 3D recurrent convolutional layer and radial distance loss, and demonstrated the implementation of these proposals in a widely used U-Net architecture. As experimental results showed, our proposed approaches achieved significant improvement over our baseline architecture, and obtained competitive results with state-of-the-art methods. Our proposed extensions, viz. 3D RCL and radial distance loss, are generic and flexible component that they can be easily incorporated in other deep learning architectures. We demonstrated an application on V-Net architecture using our RD loss, remarkable improvement was obtained comparing with the one use Dice loss.

Figures 5 and 6 show thick bronchi are under-segmented. This is a side effect of radial distance loss, since we decreased the weight of the most peripheral voxels. The normalization strategy in Eq. 3 can be improved to use more complex functions beyond a simple monomial. However, from Table 1, DSC'' shows our segmentation accuracy of thick branches is still better than baseline U-Net. Segmentation results of three unseen datasets acquired in different hospital illustrated the robustness of our method. Visually, good segmentation accuracy was achieved.

In conclusion, we choose the challenging bronchus segmentation task to prove the effectiveness of our proposed method regarding general tubular structure segmentation. Experimental results showed that our proposed approaches are proven to be effective in bronchus segmentation task. However, we only evaluate the segmentation performance on bronchus segmentation. Our approaches should theoretically work on blood vessel segmentation problem. Application on blood vessel segmentation will be one of our future works. Additionally, more state-of-the-art networks incorporated with our approaches need to be investigated.

Acknowledgement. Parts of this research was supported by MEXT/JSPS KAK-ENHI (26108006, 26560255, 17H00867, 17K20099), and the JSPS Bilateral Collaboration Grant and AMED (191k1010036h0001).

References

1. Litjens, G., et al.: A survey on deep learning in medical image analysis. Med. IA **42**, 60–88 (2017)
2. Yun, J., et al.: Improvement of fully automated airway segmentation on volumetric computed tomographic images using a 2.5 dimensional convolutional neural net. Med. IA **51**, 13–20 (2019)
3. Tetteh, G., et al.: DeepVesselNet: Vessel segmentation, centerline prediction, and bifurcation detection in 3-D angiographic volumes. arXiv preprint arXiv:1803.09340 (2018)
4. Meng, Q., Roth, H.R., Kitasaka, T., Oda, M., Ueno, J., Mori, K.: Tracking and segmentation of the airways in chest CT using a fully convolutional network. In: Descoteaux, M., Maier-Hein, L., Franz, A., Jannin, P., Collins, D.L., Duchesne, S. (eds.) MICCAI 2017. LNCS, vol. 10434, pp. 198–207. Springer, Cham (2017). https://doi.org/10.1007/978-3-319-66185-8_23

5. Huang, Q., Sun, J., Ding, H., Wang, X., Wang, G.: Robust liver vessel extraction using 3D U-Net with variant dice loss function. Comput. Biol. Med. **101**, 153–162 (2018)
6. Pan, X., Shi, J., Luo, P., Wang, X., Tang, X.: Spatial as deep: spatial CNN for traffic scene understanding. In: AAAI, pp. 7276–7283 (2018)
7. Çiçek, Ö., Abdulkadir, A., Lienkamp, S.S., Brox, T., Ronneberger, O.: 3D U-net: learning dense volumetric segmentation from sparse annotation. In: Ourselin, S., Joskowicz, L., Sabuncu, M.R., Unal, G., Wells, W. (eds.) MICCAI 2016. LNCS, vol. 9901, pp. 424–432. Springer, Cham (2016). https://doi.org/10.1007/978-3-319-46723-8_49
8. Roth, H., et al.: Towards dense volumetric pancreas segmentation in CT using 3D fully convolutional networks. In: SPIE MI 2018, vol. 10574, p. 105740B (2018)
9. Milletari, F., Navab, N., Ahmadi, S.A.: V-Net: fully convolutional neural networks for volumetric medical image segmentation. In: 2016 Fourth International Conference on 3D Vision (3DV), pp. 565–571 (2016)
10. Ribera, J., Güera, D., Chen, Y., Delp, E.: Weighted Hausdorff distance: A loss function for object localization. arXiv preprint arXiv:1806.07564 (2018)
11. Jia, S., et al.: Automatically segmenting the left atrium from cardiac images using successive 3D U-nets and a contour loss. In: Pop, M., et al. (eds.) STACOM 2018. LNCS, vol. 11395, pp. 221–229. Springer, Cham (2019). https://doi.org/10.1007/978-3-030-12029-0_24
12. Wang, C., et al.: Tensor-based graph-cut in riemannian metric space and its application to renal artery segmentation. In: Ourselin, S., Joskowicz, L., Sabuncu, M.R., Unal, G., Wells, W. (eds.) MICCAI 2016. LNCS, vol. 9902, pp. 353–361. Springer, Cham (2016). https://doi.org/10.1007/978-3-319-46726-9_41
13. Chen, H., Dou, Q., Yu, L., Qin, J., Heng, P.A.: Voxresnet: deep voxelwise residual networks for brain segmentation from 3D MR images. NeuroImage **170**, 446–455 (2018)

Bronchial Cartilage Assessment with Model-Based GAN Regressor

Pietro Nardelli[✉] [iD], George R. Washko, and Raúl San José Estépar [iD]

Applied Chest Imaging Laboratory, Brigham and Women's Hospital,
Harvard Medical School, Boston, MA, USA
{pnardelli,rsanjose}@bwh.harvard.edu

Abstract. In the last two decades, several methods for airway segmentation from chest CT images have been proposed. The following natural step is the development of a tool to accurately assess the morphology of the bronchial system in all its aspects to help physicians better diagnosis and prognosis complex pulmonary diseases such as COPD, chronic bronchitis and bronchiectasis. Traditional methods for the assessment of airway morphology usually focus on lumen and wall thickness and are often limited due to resolution and artifacts of the CT image. Airway wall cartilage is an important characteristic related to airway integrity that has shown to be deteriorated during the airway disease process. In this paper, we propose the development of a Model-Based GAN Regressor (MBGR) that, thanks to a model-based GAN generator, generate synthetic airway samples with the morphological components necessary to resemble the appearance of real airways on CT at will and that simultaneously measures lumen, wall thickness, and amount of cartilage on pulmonary CT images. The method is evaluated by first computing the relative error on generated images to show that simulating the cartilage helps improve the morphological quantification of the airway structure. We then propose a cartilage index that summarizes the degree of cartilage of bronchial trees structures and perform an indirect validation with subjects with COPD. As shown by the results, the proposed approach paves the way for the use of CNNs to precisely and accurately measure small lung airways morphology, with the final goal to improve the diagnosis and prognosis of pulmonary diseases.

Keywords: COPD · Bronchial tree analysis · Airway cartilage · Deep learning

1 Introduction

In the last two decades, several methods have been proposed to help physicians accurately locate small pulmonary bronchi on chest CT images, that otherwise requires a tedious and time-consuming analysis of the data.

This work has been partially funded by the National Institutes of Health NHLBI awards R01HL116931, R01HL116473, and R21HL14042. We gratefully acknowledge the support of NVIDIA Corporation with the donation of the GPU used for this research.

D. Shen et al. (Eds.): MICCAI 2019, LNCS 11769, pp. 357–365, 2019.
https://doi.org/10.1007/978-3-030-32226-7_40

Once the structures are identified, an equally important step is represented by a quantitative measurement and morphological analysis of the bronchial tree, as this is the part that is commonly affected by inflammatory and infectious lung diseases. As an example, the smaller conducting airways are the structures most affected in patients with chronic obstructive pulmonary disease (COPD) [4], while emphysema has been related to a diminished presence of cartilage in the airway walls [15]. For this reason, a method that provides accurate and precise information about the airway cartilage amount may greatly improve the diagnosis and prognosis of lung diseases.

To the best of our knowledge, while methods have attempted to characterize only wall thickness and lumen size on CT images [10,12], information about the cartilage amount is not provided. One of the reasons why prior work has not been proposed to quantify airway wall cartilage is the complexities to define a ground truth. Histological studies are limited, and it is extremely complex to have imaging data with a well-characterized histological correlate for each airway point. That being said, the histological model of an airway is well understood and can be easily parameterized. On the other hand, the imaging reconstruction process can also be modeled to some extent.

Deep learning [6] is quickly becoming the de-facto approach for solving various tasks in the medical imaging field. One of the advantages of deep learning approaches is the ability to learn from a given domain that can be synthetically generated. In our context, where properly labeled airway morphology data is highly complicated to obtain as a tedious and prone to error analysis of CT images is required, this learning paradigm from a synthetic model is appealing.

In this paper, we propose the development of a Model-Based GAN Regressor (MBGR) that automatically generates 2D patches of synthetic airways resembling real small bronchi (radius $< 6.0\,\mathrm{mm}$) on CT images with known morphometric characteristics of cartilage, wall thickness, and lumen size. Due to the generative nature of our approach, infinite training samples with varying imaging characteristics are available to train a regressor that can estimate those morphometric quantities.

To validate the method, we first compute the relative error (RE) obtained on synthetic patches and we demonstrate that generating a more accurate airway model that takes into account the cartilage improves the estimation of the airway morphology (wall thickness and lumen) with respect to a model without cartilage. Then, we perform an indirect validation that shows that in the cartilage assessment in a population of 547 smoking subjects with and without COPD, our measurements relates to disease severity in a consistent manner with prior histological studies [15].

2   Materials and Methods

Figure 1 shows the flow diagram of the proposed MBGR that automatically generates synthetic CT airways, refines them to resemble real bronchi and simultaneously predicts cartilage amount, wall thickness, and lumen size. Although less

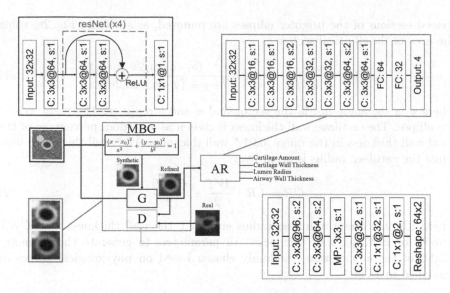

Fig. 1. Workflow of the model-based GAN regressor. MBG (green square) indicates the model-based generator that creates the synthetic airways (black box), G (purple box) is the image-to-image generator, D (yellow box) is the discriminator, and AR (blue box) represents the airway regressor that provides the 4 airway morphology measurements. In the big squares the schemes of the three neural networks used in this paper are presented. C indicates a 2D convolutional layer, FC a fully connected, MP stands for max pooling, and s indicates the layer's strides. (Color figure online)

clinically relevant, for completeness and to help the network better learn airway characteristics, the size of the cartilage wall thickness is also measured.

The model-based generator, MBG, is characterized by an airway geometric model that creates 2D images of 32×32 pixels on the reformatted axial plane, a reasonable simulation as in in-vivo CT images this plane can be extracted along the axis given by the first eigenvector of the Hessian matrix. The geometric model consists of two bright ellipses (inner and outer walls) and a central dark area (lumen) with tangent vessels represented by bright ellipses randomly rotated around the airway.

To simulate the presence of cartilage, two ellipses are created at the center of the airway walls with higher intensity and varying wall thickness. As reported in [15], the percentage of cartilage varies depending both on lumen size (based on Weibel dichotomous morphometry [16]) and amount of emphysema. Therefore, for each airway a random percentage of cartilage is selected between minimum and maximum values of each bronchial order and level of emphysema, in accordance to Table 1 in [15]. Based on the selected cartilage percentage, equally-spaced sections of the brighter ellipses are removed, as shown in Fig. 2a, using the area of the elliptical sector:

$$F(\theta) = \frac{ab}{2}\left[\theta - \arctan\left(\frac{(b-a)\sin 2\theta}{b+a+(b-a)\cos(2\theta)}\right)\right] \tag{1}$$

where θ is the angle inside the sector and a and b represent the main axis of the ellipse. The cartilage wall thickness is chosen as a random percentage of the total wall thickness in the range [0.01 * wall thickness, 0.6 * wall thickness] mm, while the cartilage radius is given by:

$$CR = LR + \frac{WT}{2} - \frac{CWT}{2} \tag{2}$$

where LR indicates the lumen radius size, WT the wall thickness, and CWT stands for cartilage wall thickness. All parameters to generate the geometry model of the airway were randomly chosen based on physiological values as described in Table 1.

Table 1. Parameter ranges used for the creation of the airway model. All values were uniformly distributed within the specified ranges. LR stands for lumen radius, WT for airway wall thickness, and CWT indicates the cartilage wall thickness.

Parameter	Range
LR	[0.5, 6.0] mm
WT	[0.1 * LR + 0.2, 0.3 * LR + 1.5] mm
CWT	[0.01 * WT, 0.6 * WT] mm
Number of vessels	[0, 2]
Vessel radius	[LR, LR + 0.8] mm
Skewness of reconstruction	[−40, 40] degrees
Airway Lumen Intensity	[−1100, −1050] HU
Airway Wall Intensity	[−500, −100] HU
Cartilage Intensity	[−250, 50] HU
Vessel Intensity	[−50, 50] HU

To mimic the structure of the parenchyma, first a Gaussian smoothing (with a standard deviation of 5) was applied to Gaussian distributed noise, to create some broadly correlated noise, which made a texture of multiple structures. Then, the correlated noise was altered to have a mean intensity of −900 HU and a standard deviation of 150. All values were empirically chosen. A super-resolution of 0.05 mm/pixel in a sampling grid of 640 × 640 pixels that is then down-sampled to a resolution of 0.5 mm/pixel is used to create the initial patches (Fig. 2b). Next, a PSF is simulated under the assumption that the PSF can be approximated by means of a spatially locally invariant Gaussian function [13].

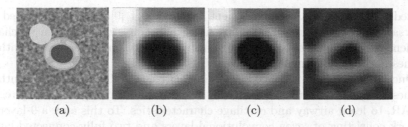

(a)   (b)   (c)   (d)

Fig. 2. An example of generated synthetic airway patch with cartilage mimicking (lumen radius = 3.5 mm, wall thickness = 2.55 mm, cartilage amount = 38%). The geometry model (a) is generated at a super resolution of 0.05 mm/pixel in a sampling grid of 640 × 640 pixels. A point spread function (PSF) is then simulated to obtain the final resolution of 0.5 mm/pixel, the patch is cropped to a 32 × 32 pixels grid (b), and the GAN makes it more realistic (c). An example of airway from a CT is shown in (d).

The standard deviation of the Gaussian filter was randomly chosen in an empirically determined range of 0.4 to 0.9 mm to simulate the differences in the PSF across CT scanners and manufacturers, and a spatially correlated Gaussian noise was added to the image based on Gaussian distributed random noise smoothed with a Gaussian filter (standard deviation of 2), with the empirically determined mean of zero and random standard deviation in a range [0, 40]. As a last step, the image is cropped to a 32 × 32 pixels grid, a size chosen to include enough neighborhood information for big structures, without losing specificity for small and thin features.

The generated patch is then passed to an neural generator that is meant to improve the realism of the synthetic airway while preserving its main characteristics by comparing it to unlabeled real airways extracted from clinical CTs. To this end, a generative adversarial network (GAN) approach is leveraged to add realism.

A pixel-to-pixel fully convolutional neural network with ResNet blocks is used as generator, G (purple box in Fig. 1), which is trained with an adversarial loss with self-regularization (originally introduced in [14]) to preserve the patch global structure. By minimizing the generator's loss function, G tries to "fool" a discriminator network, D (yellow box in Fig. 1), into classifying the refined airways as real. This is modeled as a minimax game, where the weights of G and D (optimized through a binary cross-entropy loss) are updated alternately.

Following the approach presented in [14], the receptive field of D is also limited to local regions, so that multiple local adversarial losses per image are considered. Also, to improve the stability of the network, a mini-batch of refined images (randomly selected from a buffer of refined images generated on previous iterations) are included into the training batch. An example of the refining step result is shown in Fig. 2c.

To train this model-based GAN, we extracted 273,600 real airways patches of 32 × 32 pixels and a resolution of 0.5 mm on the reformatted axial plane of 30 clinical CTs, using the multi-resolution particles method described in [5], initialized with the feature enhancement technique of [9]. We then trained the adversarial network for 10,000 steps using a batch size of 512, a stochastic gradient descent update and learning rate of 0.001, until real and synthetic patches become indistinguishable by D.

Once G is trained, 2,500,000 training and 1,000,000 validation synthetic patches are generated and automatically refined while training the airway regressor, AR, to learn airway and cartilage characteristics. To this end, a 9-layer 2D network consisting of seven convolutional layers and two fully-connected layers, (see the blue box in Fig. 1) is used. An Adam update ($\beta_1 = 0.9$, $\beta_2 = 0.999$, $\epsilon = 1e^{-08}$, decay $= 0.0$), a learning rate of 0.001, and a customized loss function that combines accuracy and precision, as presented in [8], were used to train AR for 100 epochs with a batch size of 1,000:

$$\mathcal{L}(\boldsymbol{y}, \widehat{\boldsymbol{y}}) = \frac{1}{N \times M} \cdot \sum_{i=0, j=0}^{N,M} \frac{|y_{i,j} - \widehat{y}_{i,j}|}{y_{i,j}} +$$

$$2.0 \cdot \frac{1}{N} \cdot \sum_{i=0}^{N} \left(\frac{1}{M} \cdot \sum_{j=0}^{M} \left(y_{i,j} - \widehat{y}_{i,j} \right)^2 - \left(\frac{1}{M} \cdot \sum_{j=0}^{M} (y_{i,j} - \widehat{y}_{i,j}) \right)^2 \right) \quad (3)$$

where N is the total number of images, M is the number of augmented replicas for each original patch, and y and $\widehat{y}$ indicate the true and the predicted values, respectively. In this work, M = 25 has been used.

Finally, in order to help the network focus more on geometry than intensity values, during training we applied a data augmentation that in addition to randomly inverting intensity values inside the patches it also randomly shifts and flips the images.

All networks were trained on a NVIDIA Titan X GPU machine, using the deep learning framework Keras [2] on top of TensorFlow [1].

2.1 Experimental Setup

To evaluate the proposed approach, we used both synthetic and in-vivo experiments. To demonstrate that having a more accurate airway geometric model helps the neural network better measure the structures of interest, we first generated a dataset of 200,000 synthetic patches and we compared the mean relative error (RE) obtained with the proposed MBGR and with the same network trained with a model without the cartilage.

For validation on clinical cases, since a reliable ground-truth cannot be obtained in an accurate way, we performed an indirect validation that leverages a physiological evaluation and demonstrates the clinical relevance of the proposed technique.

We analyzed the associations between the amount of cartilage in bronchi of various orders and the presence of COPD in 547 smoking subjects with and without COPD. To this end, we propose a cartilage index defined by the regression coefficient in a random sample consensus (RANSAC) regression [3] between the

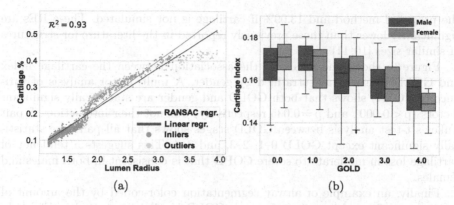

(a)   (b)

Fig. 3. (a) Example of RANSAC regression in comparison to linear regression. The cartilage percentage is plotted against the lumen radius in the range [1.19, 3,95]. (b) Results for the indirect validation on 390 smoking subjects with and without COPD.

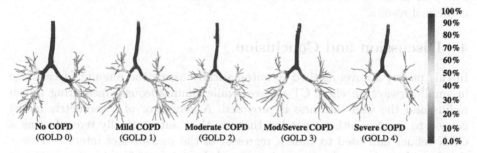

Fig. 4. Example of airway segmentation color-coded by the percentage of cartilage for 5 subjects based on the COPD level. (Color figure online)

airway lumen and cartilage percentage across airway points with a lumen radius $l_r \in [1.19, 3.95]$ mm, similar to what was proposed for the Pi10 calculation [7]. Subjects whose regression fitting was poor ($R^2 < 0.8$) were excluded from the analysis. The total number of subjects after exclusion was 390. An example of regression for one case is shown in Fig. 3a.

3 Results

The mean absolute RE obtained with MBGR for wall thickness, airway lumen, and cartilage percentage across the 200,000 generated patches was 6.19%, 1.73%, and 11.75%, respectively. If the geometric model is generated excluding the cartilage simulation (cartilage percentage set to 0%), the RE was 7.25% for wall thickness and 2.95 for lumen. When considering airways with a wall thickness of 1.0 mm, a mean absolute RE of 6.47% is obtained with the proposed MBGR and 7.93% with the same version without cartilage, whereas when the wall thickness is at the image resolution (0.5 mm) the mean absolute RE was at 12.90% for the proposed method and 13.09% if cartilage is not simulated. These REs are significantly lower than those previously reported in the literature for structures of similar sizes [10,11].

Figure 3b shows the results of the association between the cartilage index and GOLD disease stage stratified by gender. A multi-factor analysis of variance (ANOVA) shows that both GOLD and gender are statistically significant factors ($p < 0.0001$ and $p = 0.035$ respectively) but not their interaction. A pair Tukey's t-test analysis between GOLD stages shows that all pairs are statistically significant except GOLD 0–1, 2–3, and 3–4. This suggests a tendency of cartilage loss in moderate to severe COPD that is consistent in both males and females.

Finally, an example of airway segmentation color-coded by the amount of cartilage for five subjects (one for each GOLD level) is presented in Fig. 4. In this example, it is possible to notice a bigger amount of cartilage (around 50%) in peripheral airways of subjects with no or little COPD (GOLD 0 and 1) while this percentage decreases in subjects with more disease as suggested by our numerical results.

4 Discussion and Conclusion

In this paper, a novel method to automatically assess the amount of cartilage in small airways on chest CT images, while simultaneously measuring lumen radius and the wall thickness is proposed. A generator of a geometric model is used to create synthetic patches that are then automatically refined using a GAN refiner and used to train a regressor of the measures of interest. This is the first time that an automated approach is proposed for the assessment of in-vivo airway cartilage. Our results show that the cartilage area percentage had a small relative error. The indirect validation with subjects with and without COPD showed consistent results with results previously reported in histological studies. These findings indicate that the method here proposed may potentially be used to help physicians toward early diagnosis and prognosis of lung disorders.

Results from the validation on synthetic patches showed a lower absolute relative error for bronchial lumen and wall thickness when the cartilage is included in the geometric model, indicating that creating a more accurate geometric model helps the network better regress the structures of interest.

For future work, we are planning on improving in-vivo validation by comparing the MGBR regression of the three structures to manual measurement, improve the generation of the synthetic model by reducing the level of approximation of the PSF and additive noise, and define a method to properly validate the refining process of the synthetic patches, which is currently done only by visual inspection.

References

1. Abadi, M., Agarwal, A., Barham, P., et al.: Tensorflow: Large-scale machine learning on heterogeneous distributed systems. arXiv preprint arXiv:1603.04467 (2016)

2. Chollet, F., et al.: Keras (2015). https://keras.io
3. Fischler, M.A., Bolles, R.C.: Random sample consensus: a paradigm for model fitting with applications to image analysis and automated cartography. Commun. ACM **24**(6), 381–395 (1981)
4. Hogg, J.C., McDonough, J.E., Suzuki, M.: Small airway obstruction in COPD: new insights based on micro-CT imaging and MRI imaging. CHEST **143**(5), 1436–1443 (2013)
5. Kindlmann, G.L., San José Estépar, R., Smith, S.M., Westin, C.F.: Sampling and visualizing creases with scale-space particles. IEEE TVCG **15**(6), 1415–1424 (2009)
6. LeCun, Y., Bengio, Y., Hinton, G.: Deep learning. Nature **521**(7553), 436 (2015)
7. Nakano, Y., Wong, J.C., de Jong, P.A., et al.: The prediction of small airway dimensions using computed tomography. AJRCCM **171**(2), 142–146 (2005)
8. Nardelli, P., et al.: Accurate measurement of airway morphology on chest CT images. In: Stoyanov, D., et al. (eds.) RAMBO/BIA/TIA -2018. LNCS, vol. 11040, pp. 335–347. Springer, Cham (2018). https://doi.org/10.1007/978-3-030-00946-5_34
9. Nardelli, P., Ross, J.C., Estépar, R.S.J.: CT image enhancement for feature detection and localization. In: Descoteaux, M., Maier-Hein, L., Franz, A., Jannin, P., Collins, D.L., Duchesne, S. (eds.) MICCAI 2017. LNCS, vol. 10434, pp. 224–232. Springer, Cham (2017). https://doi.org/10.1007/978-3-319-66185-8_26
10. Reinhardt, J.M., D'Souza, N., Hoffman, E.A.: Accurate measurement of intrathoracic airways. IEEE TMI **16**(6), 820–827 (1997)
11. Estépar, R.S.J., Washko, G.G., Silverman, E.K., Reilly, J.J., Kikinis, R., Westin, C.-F.: Accurate airway wall estimation using phase congruency. In: Larsen, R., Nielsen, M., Sporring, J. (eds.) MICCAI 2006. LNCS, vol. 4191, pp. 125–134. Springer, Heidelberg (2006). https://doi.org/10.1007/11866763_16
12. Schwab, R.J., Gefter, W.B., Pack, A.I., Hoffman, E.A.: Dynamic imaging of the upper airway during respiration in normal subjects. J. Appl. Physiol. **74**(4), 1504–1514 (1993)
13. Schwarzband, G., Kiryati, N.: The point spread function of spiral CT. Phys. Med. Biol. **50**(22), 5307 (2005)
14. Shrivastava, A., Pfister, T., Tuzel, O., Susskind, J., Wang, W., Webb, R.: Learning from simulated and unsupervised images through adversarial training. In: IEEE CVPR, vol. 3, p. 6 (2017)
15. Thurlbeck, W., Pun, R., Toth, J., Frazer, R.: Bronchial cartilage in chronic obstructive lung disease. Am. Rev. Respir. Dis. **109**(1), 73–80 (1974)
16. Weibel, E.R., Cournand, A.F., Richards, D.W.: Morphometry of the Human Lung, vol. 1. Springer, Heidelberg (1963). https://doi.org/10.1007/978-3-642-87553-3

Adversarial Optimization for Joint Registration and Segmentation in Prostate CT Radiotherapy

Mohamed S. Elmahdy[1]([⊠]), Jelmer M. Wolterink[2], Hessam Sokooti[1], Ivana Išgum[2], and Marius Staring[1,3]

[1] Division of Image Processing, Department of Radiology,
Leiden University Medical Center, 2300 RC Leiden, The Netherlands
m.s.e.elmahdy@lumc.nl
[2] Image Sciences Institute, University Medical Center Utrecht,
Utrecht, The Netherlands
[3] Department of Radiation Oncology,
Leiden University Medical Center, 2300 RC Leiden, The Netherlands

Abstract. Joint image registration and segmentation has long been an active area of research in medical imaging. Here, we reformulate this problem in a deep learning setting using adversarial learning. We consider the case in which fixed and moving images as well as their segmentations are available for training, while segmentations are not available during testing; a common scenario in radiotherapy. The proposed framework consists of a 3D end-to-end generator network that estimates the deformation vector field (DVF) between fixed and moving images in an unsupervised fashion and applies this DVF to the moving image and its segmentation. A discriminator network is trained to evaluate how well the moving image and segmentation align with the fixed image and segmentation. The proposed network was trained and evaluated on follow-up prostate CT scans for image-guided radiotherapy, where the planning CT contours are propagated to the daily CT images using the estimated DVF. A quantitative comparison with conventional registration using elastix showed that the proposed method improved performance and substantially reduced computation time, thus enabling real-time contour propagation necessary for online-adaptive radiotherapy.

Keywords: Deformable image registration · Adversarial training · Image segmentation · Contour propagation · Radiotherapy

1 Introduction

Joint image registration and segmentation (JRS) has long been an active area of research in medical imaging. Image registration and segmentation are closely

Electronic supplementary material The online version of this chapter (https://doi.org/10.1007/978-3-030-32226-7_41) contains supplementary material, which is available to authorized users.

related and complimentary in applications such as contour propagation, disease monitoring, and data fusion from different modalities. Image registration could be enhanced and improved using an accurate segmentation, and vice versa registration algorithms could be used to improve image segmentation.

An important application in which coupling of image registration and segmentation is crucial, is online adaptive image-guided radiotherapy. In this application, clinically approved contours are propagated from an initial *planning* CT scan to *daily* inter-fraction CT scans of the same patient. Image registration can be used to correct for anatomical variations in shape and position of the underlying organs, as well as to compensate for any misalignment in patient setup. Ideally, contours should be propagated quickly to allow immediate computation of a new dose distribution. With these propagated contours, margins can be smaller and treatment-related complications may be reduced. Thus, it is important that the daily contours are of high quality, are consistent with the planning contours, and are generated in near real-time.

In the last decade, researchers have been working on fusing image registration and segmentation. Lu *et al.* [1] proposed a Bayesian framework for modelling segmentation and registration such that these could alternatingly constrain each other. Yezzi *et al.* [2] proposed using active contours to register and segment images. Unal *et al.* [3], generalizing on [2], proposed to use partial differential equations without any shape prior. Most of these methods require long computation times and complex parameter tuning. Recently, the widespread adoption of deep learning techniques has led to remarkable achievements in the field of medical imaging [4]. Among these techniques are generative adversarial networks (GANs), which are defined by joint optimization of a generator and discriminator network [5]. GANs have boosted the performance of traditional networks for image segmentation [6] as well as registration [7]. Recently, Mahapatra *et al.* [8] proposed a GAN for joint registration and segmentation of 2D chest X-ray images. However, this method requires reference deformation vector fields (DVFs) for training. In practice, these are often unavailable and it may be more practical to perform unsupervised registration [9], i.e. training without reference DVFs.

In this paper, we introduce a fast unsupervised 3D GAN to jointly perform deformable image registration and segmentation. A generator network estimates the DVF between two images, while a discriminator network is trained simultaneously to evaluate the quality of the registration and the segmentation and propagate the feedback to the generator network. We consider the use-case in which fixed and moving images as well as their segmentations are available for training, which is a common scenario in radiation therapy. However, no segmentations are required for DVF estimation during testing. This paper has the following contributions. First, we propose an end-to-end 3D network architecture, which is trained in an adversarial manner for joint image registration and segmentation. Second, we propose a strategy to generate well-aligned pairs to train the discriminator network with. Third, we leverage PatchGAN as a local quality measure of image alignment. Fourth, the proposed network is much faster and more accurate than conventional registration methods.

We quantitatively evaluate the proposed method on a prostate CT database, which shows that the method compares favorably to elastix software [10].

2   Methods

Image registration is the transformation of a moving image I_m to the coordinate system of a fixed image I_f. In this paper, we assume that all image pairs are affinely registered beforehand, and we focus on local non-linear deformations.

In conventional contour propagation algorithms, registration and segmentation are disjoint. First, the DVF Φ is estimated using image registration, and then Φ is used to warp the contours S_m to the fixed coordinate space. Afterwards, during system evaluation, a similarity measure such as the Dice similarity coefficient (DSC) can be used to measure the quality of the propagated contours w.r.t. ground truth contours, but this information is not fed back to the registration algorithm. We call this an *open loop* system. In contrast, this paper proposes an end-to-end *closed loop* system to improve image registration based on feedback on the registration as well as the segmentation quality.

2.1   Adversarial Training

We propose to train a GAN containing two CNNs: a generator network that predicts the DVF Φ given I_f and I_m, and a discriminator network that assesses the alignment of $I_f(\boldsymbol{x})$ and $I_m(\Phi(\boldsymbol{x}))$ as well as the overlap between $S_f(\boldsymbol{x})$ and $S_m(\Phi(\boldsymbol{x}))$. Hence, we assume that S_f and S_m are both available, but during training only. The GAN is trained using a Wasserstein objective [11], which has empirically been shown to improve training stability and convergence compared to the GAN objective in [5]. Equations (1) and (2) list the generator loss L_G^{GAN} and the discriminator loss L_D^{GAN} of WGAN:

$$L_G^{GAN} = -E\left[D(I_f(\boldsymbol{x}), I_m(\Phi(\boldsymbol{x})), S_m(\Phi(\boldsymbol{x})))\right], \tag{1}$$

$$L_D^{GAN} = E\left[D(I_f(\boldsymbol{x}), I_m(\Phi(\boldsymbol{x})), S_m(\Phi(\boldsymbol{x})))\right] - \left[D(I_f, \Theta(I_f), S_f)\right], \tag{2}$$

where G and D denote the generator and discriminator networks with trainable parameters and Φ is the DVF provided by G. In a GAN, the discriminator is trained to distinguish between *real* and *fake* samples. In this case, fake samples are the triple $(I_f, I_m(\Phi), S_m(\Phi))$, while real samples should be well-aligned images. As we perform unsupervised registration, and assume no knowledge about the ideal alignment of two images, we synthesize such image based on the fixed image and its segmentation alone: $(I_f, \Theta(I_f), S_f)$. Hence, Θ in Eq. (2) is a random combination of disturbance functions, as follows. First, to mimic imaging noise, Gaussian noise and Gaussian smoothing are added with zero mean and a standard deviation of 0.04. Second, to mimic contrast variations, we apply gamma correction with a random gamma factor in the range $[-0.4, 0.4]$. Third,

we mimic interpolation errors by applying a random deformation of less than
0.5 mm and resample the images using that deformation using linear interpolation.

In addition to these image-based quality measures, we include the segmentation of the deformed moving image as input to the discriminator in order to
enforce DVFs that are consistent with the moving segmentation. We test two
designs. The first design concatenates the segmentation as a third input channel
in the discriminator, next to the fixed and moving image channels. The second
design multiplies the fixed and moving image channel with the corresponding
segmentation, so that the network learns to focus on the target structures and
organs-at-risk instead of on the bowels and other less relevant soft tissue. These
designs are named JRS-GAN^a and JRS-GAN^b, respectively.

We found that training the network using WGAN loss only, resulted in slow
convergence and suboptimal registrations. Thus, a similarity loss L_{sim}, based on
image similarity and segmentation overlap, was added to the generator:

$$L_{sim} = (1 - \mathrm{DSC}(S_m(\varPhi(x)), S_f(x))) + (1 - \mathrm{NCC}(I_m(\varPhi(x)), I_f(x))), \qquad (3)$$

where DSC is the Dice similarity coefficient and NCC is normalized cross-
correlation. Adding the DSC to L_{sim} ensures that the registration improves
the segmentation and vice versa. Furthermore, to ensure smooth and continuous DVFs, the bending energy penalty of the DVF, L_{smooth}, was added as a
regularization term to the overall generator loss, which was defined as:

$$L_G = L_{sim} + \lambda_1 L_{smooth} + \lambda_2 L_G^{GAN}, \qquad (4)$$

where λ_1 and λ_2 are weights for the DVF smoothness and the generator loss.

During training of the network, for every iteration of the generator we used
100 iterations of the discriminator, for the first 25 iterations. After that we used
the ratio 1:5. In each iteration, weights of the discriminator were clipped to the
range $[-0.01, 0.01]$ [11].

2.2 Network Architectures

Generator Network. To estimate the parametric mapping function $\varPhi$ between
the fixed and moving images we use a 3D network similar to the U-net [12].
Figure 1 shows the network design in more detail. The input to the network is
the concatenation of I_f and I_m. The network encodes the image pairs through a
set of $3 \times 3 \times 3$ convolution layers followed by LeakyReLU and batch normalization layers. Strided convolutions are used in the contractive path and upsampling
layers are used in the expanding path. The output size of the network is smaller
than the input size in order to consider a larger field of view. A resampling network adopted from NiftyNet [13] is used to warp the images using the estimated
DVF during training time so that the network can be trained end-to-end.

Discriminator Network. The discriminator is responsible for assessing
whether the image pairs are well-aligned or not, as well as assessing whether

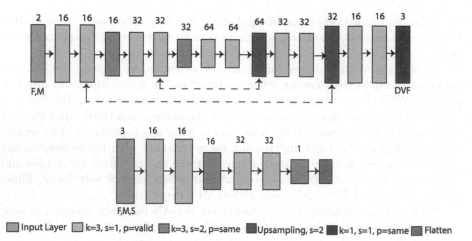

Fig. 1. The proposed generator (top) and discriminator (bottom) networks, where k, s, and p represent the kernel size, stride size, and padding option, respectively. The numbers above the different layers represent the feature maps.

the segmentations overlap. Figure 1 shows the network design, which is similar to the contracting path of the generator. The discriminator network was trained using PatchGAN [16]. Hence, instead of representing the quality of the whole patch with a single number, the network could quantify the sub-patch quality locally.

3   Experiments and Results

3.1   Dataset, Evaluation Criteria and Implementation Details

This study includes eighteen patients who underwent intensity-modulated radiation therapy for prostate cancer in 2007 at Haukeland university hospital [14]. Each patient had a planning CT as well as 7 to 10 inter-fraction repeat CT scans. The prostate, lymph nodes, seminal vesicles, as well as the rectum and bladder were annotated. Each scan has 90 to 180 slices with a slice thickness of around 2 to 3 mm. All the slices were of size 512×512 with an in-plane resolution of around 0.9 mm. All the volumes were affinely registered using elastix. The volumes were resampled to isotropic voxel size of $1 \times 1 \times 1$ mm. All volumes intensities were scaled to $[-1, 1]$. We split the dataset into 111 image pairs (from 12 patients) for training and validation and 50 image pairs (6 patients) for testing.

The quality of registration is quantified geometrically in 3D by comparing the manual delineations of the daily CT with the automatically propagated contours. We use the mean surface distance (MSD), and the 95% Hausdorff distance (HD). A Wilcoxon signed rank test at $p = 0.05$ is used to compare results.

The networks were implemented using TensorFlow (version 1.13) [15] with the RMSProp optimizer using a learning rate of 10^{-5}. The networks were trained and tested on an NVIDIA Tesla V100 GPU with 16 GB of memory. From each image pair, 1000 patches of size $96 \times 96 \times 96$ voxels were sampled within the torso mask. To improve stability, the network was trained to warp the fixed patch to the moving patch and vice versa at the same training iteration. The magnitude of the three loss terms in Eq. (3) was scaled by setting $\lambda_1 = 1$ and $\lambda_2 = 0.01$.

Table 1. MSD (mm) values for different experiments, where † and ‡ represent a significant difference compared to **elastix**-MI and Reg-CNN, respectively.

Evaluation	Prostate	Seminal vesicles	Lymph nodes	Rectum	Bladder
	$\mu \pm \sigma$	$\mu \pm \sigma$	$\mu \pm \sigma$	$\mu \pm \sigma$	$\mu \pm \sigma$
elastix-NCC	1.81 ± 0.7	2.80 ± 1.6	1.19 ± 0.4	3.79 ± 1.2	5.31 ± 2.6
elastix-MI	1.73 ± 0.7	2.70 ± 1.6	1.18 ± 0.4	3.68 ± 1.2	5.26 ± 2.6
Reg-CNN	$1.44 \pm 0.5^\dagger$	$2.09 \pm 1.7^\dagger$	1.22 ± 0.3	$2.59 \pm 1.3^\dagger$	$4.18 \pm 2.6^\dagger$
JRS-CNN	$1.18 \pm 0.4^{\dagger\ddagger}$	$1.91 \pm 1.6^{\dagger\ddagger}$	$1.02 \pm 0.3^{\dagger\ddagger}$	$2.32 \pm 1.3^{\dagger\ddagger}$	$2.37 \pm 2.0^{\dagger\ddagger}$
Reg-GAN	$1.40 \pm 0.5^\dagger$	$2.14 \pm 1.7^\dagger$	$1.06 \pm 0.3^{\dagger\ddagger}$	$2.72 \pm 1.3^\dagger$	$4.31 \pm 2.8^\dagger$
JRS-GAN^a	$\mathbf{1.13 \pm 0.4^{\dagger\ddagger}}$	$\mathbf{1.81 \pm 1.6^{\dagger\ddagger}}$	$\mathbf{1.00 \pm 0.3^{\dagger\ddagger}}$	$\mathbf{2.21 \pm 1.3^{\dagger\ddagger}}$	$\mathbf{2.29 \pm 2.0^{\dagger\ddagger}}$
JRS-GAN^b	$1.17 \pm 0.4^{\dagger\ddagger}$	$1.90 \pm 1.5^{\dagger\ddagger}$	$1.01 \pm 0.3^{\dagger\ddagger}$	$2.34 \pm 1.3^{\dagger\ddagger}$	$2.41 \pm 2.1^{\dagger\ddagger}$

Table 2. %95HD (mm) values for different experiments, where † and ‡ represent a significant difference compared to **elastix**-MI and Reg-CNN, respectively.

Evaluation	Prostate	Seminal vesicles	Lymph nodes	Rectum	Bladder
	$\mu \pm \sigma$	$\mu \pm \sigma$	$\mu \pm \sigma$	$\mu \pm \sigma$	$\mu \pm \sigma$
elastix-NCC	4.2 ± 1.8	6.1 ± 3.3	$\mathbf{2.8 \pm 1.0^\ddagger}$	11.0 ± 5.2	$15.4 \pm 8.4^\ddagger$
elastix-MI	4.0 ± 1.7	6.0 ± 3.7	$2.8 \pm 1.0^\ddagger$	10.9 ± 5.2	$15.3 \pm 8.3^\ddagger$
Reg-CNN	5.3 ± 2.5	6.2 ± 3.5	4.4 ± 1.4	11.0 ± 6.5	16.6 ± 9.3
JRS-CNN	$3.6 \pm 1.5^{\dagger\ddagger}$	$5.4 \pm 3.4^{\dagger\ddagger}$	$3.1 \pm 0.9^\ddagger$	$10.3 \pm 6.7^{\dagger\ddagger}$	$11.6 \pm 10.5^{\dagger\ddagger}$
Reg-GAN	$4.3 \pm 2.1^\ddagger$	6.0 ± 3.6	$3.4 \pm 1.0^\ddagger$	11.1 ± 6.4	$16.2 \pm 9.6^\ddagger$
JRS-GAN^a	$\mathbf{3.4 \pm 1.4^{\dagger\ddagger}}$	$\mathbf{5.3 \pm 3.3^{\dagger\ddagger}}$	$3.1 \pm 0.9^\ddagger$	$\mathbf{10.0 \pm 6.7^{\dagger\ddagger}}$	$\mathbf{11.0 \pm 10.3^{|\ddagger}}$
JRS-GAN^b	$3.5 \pm 1.4^{\dagger\ddagger}$	$5.6 \pm 3.7^\ddagger$	$3.0 \pm 1.0^\ddagger$	$10.5 \pm 6.8^{\dagger\ddagger}$	$11.4 \pm 10.6^{\dagger\ddagger}$

3.2 Experiments and Results

Tables 1 and 2 provide quantitative results comparing the following methods. First, we include conventional iterative methods using **elastix** software [10] with NCC (**elastix**-NCC) and MI (**elastix**-MI) similarity measures, using the settings from [17]. Second, we evaluate two unsupervised deep learning-based methods without adversarial feedback: One uses the generator trained with the NCC loss (Reg-CNN), similar to [9]; the other uses the generator with both the NCC and DSC loss (JRS-CNN). Third, we evaluate several versions of our GAN-based approach. To study the effect of adversarial training without added segmentations, we perform an experiment named Reg-GAN. Finally, we evaluate the proposed JRS-GAN^a and JRS-GAN^b methods. See supplemental document for Dice Similarity Coefficient (DSC).

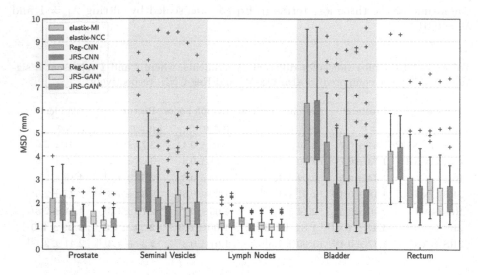

Fig. 2. Boxplots for the evaluated methods in terms of MSD (mm).

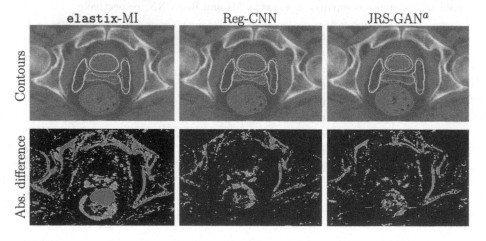

Fig. 3. An example result for three of the methods. Top row shows the fixed image with propagated contours (solid line is manual; dotted is automatic result). The red, yellow, cyan, violet, and green contours represent the bladder, lymph nodes, prostate, rectum, and seminal vesicles, respectively. Bottom row shows heatmaps of absolute difference images between fixed and deformed moving image. (Color figure online)

The MSD values in Table 1 show that for all organs, the GAN-based methods significantly improved over `elastix`. This is further shown in Fig. 2. The results indicate a significant improvement when performing joint registration and segmentation instead of disjoint registration. Furthermore, the boxplot indicates that performance for JRS-GAN^a and JRS-GAN^b was very similar. Similarly, the 95% HD values in Table 2 show improvements in contour accuracy when the GAN-based method is used. Especially the organs-at-risk showed large improvements. The standard deviations of the Jacobian determinant of the estimated DVFs were 0.08 ± 0.01 and 0.17 ± 0.04 for `elastix`-MI and JRS-GAN^a, respectively. The average runtime for the proposed pipeline is 0.6 s on the GPU for a volume of size 256^3 voxels, while the average runtime of `elastix` at 100 iterations is 13 s per volume on an Intel Xeon E51620 CPU using 4 cores. Figure 3 illustrates the segmentation and registration for an example case (see supplemental document for more examples).

4   Discussion and Conclusion

In this study, we investigated the performance of an end-to-end joint registration and segmentation network for adaptive image-guided radiotherapy. Unlike conventional registration methods, our network encodes and learns the most relevant features for joint image registration and segmentation, and exploits the combined knowledge on unseen images without segmentations.

We demonstrate that including the segmentation during training boosts the system's performance by a margin. Furthermore, adversarial feedback had a small benefit on performance, when comparing Reg-CNN with Reg-GAN. Results indicate a noticeable benefit of including segmentation masks as input to the discriminator during training. How exactly segmentation masks were embedded during training was less relevant, with only small differences observed for the seminal vesicles. This could be due to the small size and irregular nature of the seminal vesicles. A key advantage of the proposed deep learning-based contour propagation method is its runtime on new and unseen data, i.e. 0.6 s.

This work has shown that adversarial feedback can help improve registration, i.e. that a discriminator can learn a measure of image alignment. This is a promising aspect that could be further explored in future work. This will include improved GAN objectives, such as the use of gradient penalty regularization.

To conclude, we have proposed a 3D adversarial network for joint image registration and segmentation with a focus on prostate CT radiotherapy. The proposed method demonstrated the effectiveness of training the registration and segmentation jointly. Moreover, it showed a substantial reduction in the computation time making it a strong candidate for online adaptive image-guided radiotherapy of prostate cancer. Since the proposed method did not only improve accuracy for the target areas, but substantially so for the organs-at-risk, this may aid reducing treatment-induced complications.

Acknowledgements. This study was financially supported by Varian Medical Systems and ZonMw, the Netherlands Organization for Health Research and Development, grant number 104003012. The dataset with contours were collected at Haukeland University Hospital, Bergen, Norway and were provided to us by responsible oncologist Svein Inge Helle and physicist Liv Bolstad Hysing; they are gratefully acknowledged.

References

1. Lu, C., et al.: An integrated approach to segmentation and nonrigid registration for application in image-guided pelvic radiotherapy. Med. Image Anal. 15(5), 772–785 (2011)
2. Yezzi, A., et al.: A variational framework for integrating segmentation and registration through active contours. Med. Image Anal. 7(2), 171–185 (2003)
3. Unal, G., Slabaugh, G.: Coupled PDEs for non-rigid registration and segmentation. In: IEEE CVPR (2005)
4. Litjens, G., et al.: A survey on deep learning in medical image analysis. Med. Image Anal. 42, 60–88 (2017)
5. Goodfellow, I., et al.: Generative adversarial nets. In: Advances in Neural Information Processing Systems, vol. 27, pp. 2672–2680 (2014)
6. Kazeminia, S., et al.: GANs for Medical Image Analysis. arXiv:1809.06222v2 (2018)
7. Haskins, G., et al.: Deep Learning in Medical Image Registration: A Survey. arXiv:1903.02026v1 (2019)
8. Mahapatra, D., Ge, Z., Sedai, S., Chakravorty, R.: Joint registration and segmentation of Xray images using generative adversarial networks. In: Shi, Y., Suk, H.-I., Liu, M. (eds.) MLMI 2018. LNCS, vol. 11046, pp. 73–80. Springer, Cham (2018). https://doi.org/10.1007/978-3-030-00919-9_9
9. de Vos, B.D., et al.: A deep learning framework for unsupervised affine and deformable image registration. In: Medical Image Analysis, pp. 204–212. Springer, Heidelberg (2019)
10. Klein, S., et al.: Elastix: a toolbox for intensity-based medical image registration. IEEE Trans. Med. Imaging. 29(1), 196–205 (2010)
11. Arjovsky, M., et al.: Wasserstein GAN. arXiv:1701.07875v3 (2017)
12. Ronneberger, O., Fischer, P., Brox, T.: U-net: convolutional networks for biomedical image segmentation. In: Navab, N., Hornegger, J., Wells, W.M., Frangi, A.F. (eds.) MICCAI 2015. LNCS, vol. 9351, pp. 234–241. Springer, Cham (2015). https://doi.org/10.1007/978-3-319-24574-4_28
13. Gibson, E., et al.: NiftyNet: a deep-learning platform for medical imaging. Comput. Methods Programs Biomed. 158, 113–122 (2018)
14. Muren, L.P., et al.: Intensity-modulated radiotherapy of pelvic lymph nodes in locally advanced prostate cancer: planning procedures and early experiences. Int. J. Radiat. Oncol. Biol. Phys. 71, 4, 1034–1041 (2008)
15. Matin, et al.: TensorFlow: Large-Scale Machine Learning on Heterogeneous Distributed Systems. arXiv:1603.04467 (2017)
16. Isola, et al.: Image-to-Image Translation with Conditional Adversarial Networks. arXiv:1611.07004v3 (2016)
17. Qiao, Y.: Fast optimization methods for image registration in adaptive radiation therapy. Ph.D. thesis, Chapter 5, Leiden University Medical Center (2017). http://elastix.isi.uu.nl/marius/downloads/2017_t_Qiao.pdf

Probabilistic Point Cloud Reconstructions for Vertebral Shape Analysis

Anjany Sekuboyina[1,2(✉)], Markus Rempfler[3], Alexander Valentinitsch[2],
Maximilian Loeffler[2], Jan S. Kirschke[2], and Bjoern H. Menze[1]

[1] Department of Informatics, Technical University of Munich, Munich, Germany
[2] Department of Neuroradiology, Klinikum rechts der Isar, Munich, Germany
anjany.sekuboyina@tum.de
[3] Friedrich Miescher Institute for Biomedical Research, Basel, Switzerland

Abstract. We propose an auto-encoding network architecture for point clouds (PC) capable of extracting shape signatures without supervision. Building on this, we (i) design a loss function capable of modelling data variance on PCs which are unstructured, and (ii) regularise the latent space as in a variational auto-encoder, both of which increase the auto-encoders' descriptive capacity while making them probabilistic. Evaluating the reconstruction quality of our architectures, we employ them for detecting vertebral fractures without any supervision. By learning to efficiently reconstruct only healthy vertebrae, fractures are detected as anomalous reconstructions. Evaluating on a dataset containing ~1500 vertebrae, we achieve area-under-ROC curve of >75%, without using intensity-based features.

1 Introduction

One of the consequences of the numerous algorithms proposed for segmenting organs, tissues, the spine etc. involves analysing their anatomical shapes, eventually contributing towards population studies [1], disease characterisation [2], survival analysis [3], etc. Employing convolutional neural networks (CNN) for this task involves processing voxelised data due to its Euclidean nature. Such voluminous representation, however, is inefficient, especially when the masks are binary and the *shape information* corresponds to its surface profile. Alternatively, surface meshes (a collection of vertices, edges, and faces) or active contours could be used. Since the data is no longer Euclidean, a conventional CNN is unusable. Graph convolutional networks (GCN) [4] were thus developed by redefining the notion of 'neighbourhood' and 'convolution' for meshes and graphs. However,

---

J. S. Kirschke and B. H. Menze—Joint supervising authors.

Electronic supplementary material The online version of this chapter (https://doi.org/10.1007/978-3-030-32226-7_42) contains supplementary material, which is available to authorized users.

© Springer Nature Switzerland AG 2019
D. Shen et al. (Eds.): MICCAI 2019, LNCS 11769, pp. 375–383, 2019.
https://doi.org/10.1007/978-3-030-32226-7_42

if the number of nodes is high, GCNs (esp. spectral) become bulky. Moreover, each mesh is treated as a domain, making mesh registration a requisite.

An alternative surface representation is a set of 3D points in space, referred to as the **point clouds** (PC). A PC represents the surface just with a set of N vertices, thus avoiding both the cubic-complexity of voxel-based representations and the $N \times N$ dimensional, sparse, adjacency matrix of meshes. However, despite their representational effectiveness, PCs are permutation invariant and do not describe data on a structured grid, preventing the usage of standard convolution. To this end, we work with an architecture capable of processing PCs (*point-net*, [5]), and design a network capable of reconstructing PCs thereby extracting shape signatures in an unsupervised manner.

Uncertainty and Latent Space Modelling. Unlike supervised learning on PCs [6], we set out to obtain shape signatures from PCs without supervision, building towards a relatively less explored topic of *auto-encoding* point clouds. This involves mapping the PC to a latent vector and reconstructing it back. Since the PCs are unordered, PC-specific reconstruction losses replace traditional ones [7,8]. Extending auto-encoders (AE) based on such a loss, we propose to improve its representational capacity by regularising the latent space to make it compact and by modelling the variance that exists in a PC population. We claim that this results in learning improved shape signatures, validating the claim by employing the extracted features for unsupervised vertebral fracture detection.

Vertebral Fracture Detection. There exists an inherent shape variation in vertebral shapes within the spine of a single patient (e.g. cervical–thoracic–lumbar) along with a natural variation in a vertebra's shape in a population (e.g. L1 across patients, cf. Fig. 1). Additionally, osteoporotic fractures start without significant shape change and progress into a vertebral collapse. Hence, fracture detection in vertebrae is non-trivial. Added to this, limited availability of fractured vertebrae makes the learning of supervised classifiers non-trivial. In literature, several classification systems exist mainly based on vertebral height measurement [9] or

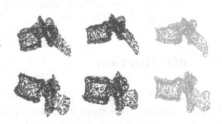

Fig. 1. Variation among vertebral shapes: compare the higher variation between healthy (blue) vertebrae of different classes (T3, top and L1, bottom) w.r.t the relatively lower variation within-class between fractured (red) and healthy vertebrae. (Color figure online)

analysing sub-regions of the spine in sagittal slices [10]. However, an explicit shape-based approach seems absent. Evaluating the representational ability of the proposed AE architectures, we seek to analyse vertebral shapes and eventually detect vertebral fractures using the extracted latent shape features.

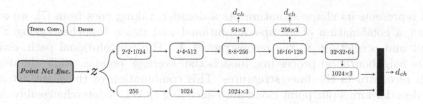

Fig. 2. Point cloud auto-encoder (*pAE*): architectural details of decoding path constructing a point cloud from a latent vector. Top arm is convolutional while bottom arm is fully-connected. Transposed convolution ($- \cdot - \cdot$ channels) have a stride of 2. Since encoder is an adapted *point-net* [5], we detail its architecture in the supplement.

Our Contribution. Summarising the contributions of this work: (1) We build on existing point-net-based architectures to propose a point-cloud auto encoder (*pAE*). (2) Reinforcing this architecture, we incorporate latent space modelling and a more challenging uncertainty quantification. (3) We present a comprehensive analysis of the reconstruction capabilities of our *pAEs* by investigating their utility in detecting vertebral fractures. We work with an in-house, clinical dataset ($\sim$1500 vertebrae) achieving an area-under-curve (AUC) of >75% in detecting fractures, even without employing texture or intensity-based features.

2   Methodology

We present this section in two stages: First, we introduce the notation used in this work and describe a point-net-based architecture capable of efficiently auto-encoding point clouds. Second, we build on this architecture to model the natural variance in vertebrae while regularising the latent space.

2.1   Auto-Encoding Point Clouds

Given accurate voxel-wise segmentation of a vertebra, a *point cloud* (PC) can be extracted as a set of N points denoted by $X = \{p_i\}_{i=0}^{N}$, where p_i represents a point by its 3D coordinate (x_i, y_i, z_i). Additionally, p_i could also represent other point specific features such as normal, radius of curvature etc. So, each vertebra is represented by a PC of dimension $N \times m$ (in this work, $N = 2048$ vertices and $m = 3$ coordinates, with the vertices randomly subsampled from a higher resolution mesh). Recall the lack of a regular coordinate space associated with the PC and that any permutation of these N points represents the same PC. Thus, a unique variant of deep networks is incorporated for processing PCs.

Architecture. An AE consists of an encoder mapping the PC to the latent vector and a decoder reconstructing the PC back from this latent vector, i.e $X \mapsto z \mapsto X$. As the encoder, we employ a variant of the point-net architecture [5]. The latent vector, z, respects the permutation invariance of the PC and represents its shape signature. As a decoder, taking cues from [7], we construct a combination of an up-convolutional and dense branches taking z as input and predicting $\hat{X}$, the reconstructed X. The convolutional path, owing to its neighbourhood processing, models the 'average' regions, while the dense path reconstructs the finer structures. This combination of the point-net and the decoder forms our point cloud auto-encoding (pAE, or interchangeably AE) architecture as illustrated in Fig. 2.

Loss. Reconstructing point clouds requires comparing the predicted PC with the actual PC to back-propagate the loss during training. However, owing to the unordered nature of PCs, usual regression losses cannot be employed. Two prominent candidates for such a task are the Chamfer distance and the Earth Mover (EM) distance [7]. We observed that minimising EM distance ignores the natural variation in shapes (e.g. the processes of the vertebrae) and reconstructs only a mean representation (e.g. the vertebral body), as validated in [7]. Since we intend to model the natural variance in the data, using EM distance is undesirable in our case. We thus employ the Chamfer distance computed as:

$$d_{ch}(X, \hat{X}) = \mathcal{L}_{ae} = \sum_{p \in X} \min_{\hat{p} \in \hat{X}} ||p - \hat{p}||_2^2 + \sum_{\hat{p} \in \hat{X}} \min_{p \in X} ||p - \hat{p}||_2^2. \quad (1)$$

In essence, d_{ch} is the distance between a point in X and its nearest neighbour in $\hat{X}$ and vice versa.

2.2   Probabilistic Reconstruction

From a generative modelling perspective, an AE can be seen to predict the parameters of Gaussian distribution imposed on X, i.e. $p_\Theta(X) = \mathcal{N}(X|\hat{X}, \hat{\Sigma})$, parameterised by the weights of the AE denoted by Θ. Determining the distribution parameters, viz. optimising for the AE weights, now involves maximising the log-likelihood of X, resulting in:

$$\Theta^* = \arg \max_\Theta \log p_\Theta(X) = \arg \min_\Theta \frac{1}{2}(X - \hat{X})^T \hat{\Sigma}^{-1}(X - \hat{X}) + \frac{1}{2}\log|\hat{\Sigma}|. \quad (2)$$

This perspective towards auto-encoding enables us to extend the pAE to encompass the data variance ($\hat{\Sigma}$) while modelling the latent space, as described in following sections. It is important to note that the difference $X - \hat{X}$ is not well defined for point clouds, requiring us to opt for alternatives.

Assuming $\Sigma = \mathbb{I}$, implying an independence among the elements of X and an element-wise unit variance, results in the familiar mean squared error (MSE), $\mathcal{L} = ||X - \hat{X}||^2$. Based on the parallels between MSE and the Chamfer distance (Eq. 1), we design σ-AE and σ-VAE, as illustrated in Fig. 3.

σ-AE. The assumption of unit covariance, as in AE, is inherently restrictive. However, modelling an unconstrained covariance matrix is infeasible due to quadratic complexity. A practical compromise is the independence assumption. Thus, representing covariance as, $\Sigma = diag\{\hat{\sigma}_{p_1}^2, \ldots, \hat{\sigma}_{p_i}^2, \ldots, \hat{\sigma}_{p_N}^2\}$, where

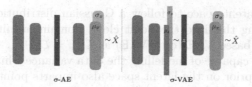

Fig. 3. Probabilistic reconstruction architectures: $\sim$ indicates a sampling operation. Since a point's variance has a smaller scale compared to its mean, the variance is predicted using a softplus activation (added with $\epsilon = 10^{-6}$ for stabilising divisions) and uses a layer parallel to the one predicting the mean.

$\hat{\sigma}_{p_i}^2$ denotes the variance corresponding to p_i, Eq. (2) morphs to a loss function as:

$$\mathcal{L} = \sum_{\hat{p} \in \hat{X}} \sigma_{\hat{p}}^{-2} ||p_i - \hat{p}_i||^2 + \log \sigma_{\hat{p}}^2 \qquad (3)$$

This optimisation models the aleoteric uncertainty [11]. Equation 3 is an attenuated MSE, where a high variance associated to a point down-weighs its contribution to the loss. However, due to the lack of a reference grid in the point cloud space, the notion of uncertainty being associated to a data point (eg. pixel, spatial location etc.) is absent. We propose to associate the notion of variance to every point, $\hat{p}_i$. This results in the variance-modelling Chamfer distance:

$$\mathcal{L}_{\sigma ae} = \sum_{p \in X} \min_{\hat{p} \in \hat{X}} \sigma_{\hat{p}}^{-2} ||p - \hat{p}||_2^2 + \sum_{\hat{p} \in \hat{X}} \sigma_{\hat{p}}^{-2} \min_{p \in X} ||p - \hat{p}||_2^2 + \log \sigma_{\hat{p}}^2 \qquad (4)$$

Observe the slight abuse of notation in Eq. 4, wherein the variance at a predicted point, $\sigma_{\hat{p}}$, actually represents the variance of the coordinate elements of p, i.e $\{\sigma_{\hat{x}}, \sigma_{\hat{y}}, \sigma_{\hat{z}}\}$. Current notation is chosen to avoid clutter.

Variational and σ-Variational AE. An alternative approach for modelling $p(X)$ involves modelling its dependency over a latent variable z, which is distributed according to a known prior $p(z)$. A variational auto-encoder (VAE) operates on these principles and involves maximising a lower bound on the log-evidence (referred to as ELBO) of the data described as below:

$$\log p(X) \geq \mathbb{E}_{z \sim q_\phi(z|X)} \left[\log p_\theta(X|z) \right] - \text{KL}\left[q_\phi(z|X) \,||\, p_\theta(z) \right], \qquad (5)$$

where $q_\phi(z|x)$ is the approximate posterior of z learnt by the encoder and parameterised by ϕ. $p_\theta(X|z)$ is the data likelihood modelled by the decoder and parameterised by θ. $p_\theta(z)$ is the prior on z.

Maximising ELBO is equivalent to maximising the log-likelihood of X while minimising the Kullback-Leibler divergence between the approximate and true prior. Representing the combination as $\mathcal{L}_{rec} + \beta \mathcal{L}_{KL}$, where $\mathcal{L}_{rec}$ is the reconstruction loss seen is earlier sections. β is a scaling factor weighing the contribution of the two losses appropriately. Standard practice assigns Gaussian distributions for $q_\phi(z|x) \sim \mathcal{N}(z|\boldsymbol{\mu}_z, \boldsymbol{\sigma}_z)$ and $p(z) \sim \mathcal{N}(z|\mathbf{0}, \mathbf{1})$ (cf. Fig. 3). Thus,

$\mathcal{L}_{KL}$ models the latent space to follow a Gaussian distribution inline with the prior. Incorporating this into the point cloud domain, results in an objective function for a PC-based VAE (or σ-VAE) as $\mathcal{L}_{vae} = \mathcal{L}_{ae/\sigma ae} + \beta \mathcal{L}_{KL}$. Thus, σ-VAE acts as a AE capable of modelling the data variance while regularising the latent space. The prior on the latent space also imparts point cloud generation capabilities to σ-VAE.

2.3 Detecting Fractures as Anomalies

Examining the descriptive ability of our pAE architectures in auto-encoding PCs, we utilise them for detecting vertebral fractures. Assuming the AE is trained only on 'normal' patterns, a fracture can be detected as an 'anomaly' based on its 'position' in latent space. We inspect two measures for this purpose:

1. Reconstruction error or Chamfer distance: AEs trained on healthy samples fail to accurately reconstruct anomalous ones, resulting in a high d_{ch}.
2. Reconstruction probability or likelihood [12]: Expected likelihood $\mathbb{E}\left[p_\Theta(X)\right]$ of an input can be computed for σ – architectures (cf. Eq. 2). For any input PC, X_{in}, it is computed by $\mathcal{N}(X_{in}|\mu_\Theta, \Sigma_\Theta)$ with the predicted mean and variances. We expect fractured vertebrae to be less *likely* than healthy ones.

Intuitively, relying on the reconstruction error or likelihood for detecting anomalies requires the learnt 'healthy' latent space to be representative. Both σ-AE and the VAE work towards this objective. In σ-AE, predictive variance down-weighs the loss due to highly uncertain points in the PC. This suppresses the interference due to natural variation in the vertebral PCs. On the other hand, VAE acts directly on the latent space by modelling the encoding uncertainty ($X \mapsto z$). The σ-VAE encompasses both these features.

Inference. A given vertebral PC is reconstructed and the reconstruction error and (or) likelihood are computed. This vertebra is said to be fractured if the reconstruction error is greater than a threshold, T_{rec}, or its likelihood is lesser than a threshold, T_l. T_{rec} and T_l and determined on the validation set.

3 Experiments and Discussion

We present this section in two parts: first, we explore the auto-encoding, variance modelling, and generative capabilities of our AE networks. Second, we deploy these architecture to detect vertebral fractures without supervision.

Data preparation: We evaluate our architecture on an in-house dataset with accurate voxel-level segmentations converted into PCs. The dataset consists of 1525 healthy and 155 fractured vertebrae, denoted as $(1525H + 155F)$ vertebrae. Since we intend to learn the distribution of healthy vertebrae, we do not use any fractured vertebrae during training. The validation and test sets consists of $(50H + 55F)$ and $(100H + 100F)$ vertebrae, respectively. For the supervised baselines, the train set needs to contain fractured vertebrae. Thus, validation and test sets were altered to contain $(50H + 55F)$ and $(55H + 55F)$ vertebrae. *Training*: The architecture of the encoder and the decoder is similar across all architectures (cf. Fig. 3) except for the layers predicting variance. PCs are augmented online by perturbing the points with Gaussian noise and random rotations ($\pm15°$). Finally, the PCs are median-centred to origin and normalised to have the same surface area. The networks are trained until convergence using an Adam optimiser with an initial learning rate of 5×10^{-4}. Specific to the VAE, we use KL-annealing by increasing β from 0 to 0.1.

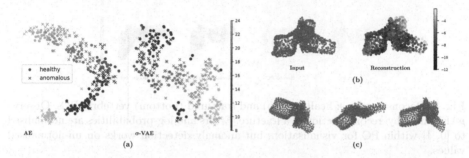

Fig. 4. Characteristics of σ-VAE: (a) Comparison of TSNE embeddings of simple pAE with σ-VAE. Observe transition in clusters being inline with vertebral indices. Note that embedding becomes compact for a VAE. (b) A PC and its reconstruction coloured with $\log(\sigma^2)$ of every point. Observe high variance in vertebral processes. (c) Example generations from decoder with $z \sim \mathcal{N}(0, 1)$. (Color figure online)

Qualitative Evaluation of AE Architectures. We investigate if meaningful shape features can be learnt without supervision. Validating this, in Fig. 4a, we plot a TSNE embedding of the test set latent vectors learnt by a naive pAE and σ-VAE trained only on healthy vertebrae. Observe the clusters formed based on the vertebral index and the transition between the indices. This corresponds to the natural variation of vertebral shapes in a human spine. Indicating the fractured vertebrae in the embedding, we highlight their degree of similarity with the healthy counterparts. Also, observe that embedding is more regularised representing a Gaussian in case of σ-VAE, indicating the continuity of the learnt latent space. Figure 4b shows the predictive variance modelled by the σ-VAE. Posterior elements of a vertebrae are the most varying among population. Observe this being captured by the variance in the vertebral process regions. Lastly, illustrating σ-VAE's generative capabilities, Fig. 4c shows vertebral PC samples generated by sampling the latent vector, $z \sim \mathcal{N}(0, 1)$.

Vertebral Fracture Detection. Evaluating the reconstruction quality of our pAE architectures, we employ them to detect fractures as anomalies. As baselines, we choose two supervised approaches: (1) point-net (PN), the encoding part in our pAE architectures, cast as a binary classifier and (2) the same point-net trained with median frequency balancing the classes (ref. as PN_{bal}) to accentuate the loss from minority fractured class. We report their performance in Table 1, over 3-fold cross-validation while retaining the ratio of healthy to fractured vertebrae in the data splits. Frequency balancing improves the F1 score significantly, albeit not at the level of the proposed anomaly detection schemes.

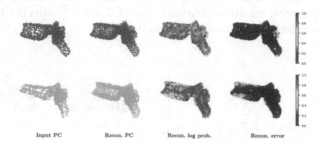

Input PC   Recon. PC   Recon. log prob.   Recon. error

Fig. 5. Reconstructions: healthy (top) and fractured (bottom) vertebral PCs. Observe pAE's 'healthy' reconstruction of a fracture. Errors and log-probabilities are normalised to [0, 1] within PC for visualisation, but anomaly detection works on un-normalised values.

Table 1. Performance comparison of unsupervised and supervised fracture detection approaches. Measures: Precision (P), Recall (R), F1-score, and area-under-ROC curve (AUC) computed by varying thresholds on recon. error and recon. log-probabilities. Since supervised models have no threshold selection, AUC is not reported.

Measures	PN	PN_{bal}	recon. error				recon. log-likelihood	
			AE	VAE	σ-AE	σ-VAE	σ-AE	σ-VAE
P	100 ± 0.0	68.6 ± 3.4	57.6 ± 4.1	61.1 ± 1.9	67.1 ± 6.5	$\mathbf{68.4 \pm 3.3}$	62.3 ± 4.3	61.6 ± 1.4
R	13.9 ± 3.1	57.6 ± 7.5	$\mathbf{85.0 \pm 9.8}$	79.0 ± 3.6	74.3 ± 4.0	71.7 ± 4.1	72.7 ± 6.1	$\mathbf{79.7 \pm 2.5}$
$F1$	24.7 ± 4.7	62.5 ± 5.8	68.0 ± 0.9	68.5 ± 1.7	67.5 ± 5.1	$\mathbf{69.6 \pm 1.2}$	66.7 ± 1.3	$\mathbf{69.5 \pm 0.6}$
AUC	n.a	n.a	70.8 ± 2.2	74.8 ± 3.0	$\mathbf{75.9 \pm 2.0}$	75.9 ± 1.5	70.2 ± 2.2	$\mathbf{73.8 \pm 2.0}$

Reconstruction for fracture detection: When detecting fractures based on reconstruction error (d_{ch}), we observe that a naive pAE already out-performs the supervised classifiers (cf. Table 1). On top of this, we see that latent space modelling and variance modelling individually offer an improvement in F1-scores while increasing the AUC, indicating a stable detection of fractures. The performance of both σ-AE and σ-VAE is similar indicating the role of loss attenuation. However, the advantage of explicitly regularising the latent space for σ-VAE can be seen in likelihood-based anomaly detection, where σ-VAE outperforms σ-AE. Figure 5 compares a reconstruction of a healthy and fractured vertebrae of the same vertebral level. Note the high reconstruction error and a low log-likelihood spatially corresponding to the deformity due to fracture.

4 Conclusions

We presented point-cloud-based auto-encoding architectures for extracting descriptive shape features. Improving their description, we incorporated variance and latent space-modelling capability using specially defined PC specific losses. The former captures the natural variance in the data while the latter regularises the latent space to be continuous. Deploying these networks for the task of unsupervised fracture detection, we achieved an AUC of 76% without using any intensity or textural features. Future work will combine the extracted shape signatures with textural features e.g. bone density and trabecular texture of vertebrae to perform fracture-grade classification.

Acknowledgements. This work is supported by the European Research Council (ERC) under the European Union's 'Horizon 2020' research & innovation programme (GA637164–iBack–ERC–2014–STG). The Quadro P5000 used for this work was donated by NVIDIA Corporation.

References

1. Ingalhalikar, M., et al.: Sex differences in the structural connectome of the human brain. Proc. Natl. Acad. Sci. **111**(2), 823–828 (2014)
2. Shakeri, M., Lombaert, H., Tripathi, S., Kadoury, S.: Deep spectral-based shape features for Alzheimer's disease classification. In: Reuter, M., Wachinger, C., Lombaert, H. (eds.) SeSAMI 2016. LNCS, vol. 10126, pp. 15–24. Springer, Cham (2016). https://doi.org/10.1007/978-3-319-51237-2_2
3. Isensee, F., et al.: Brain tumor segmentation and radiomics survival prediction: contribution to the brats 2017 challenge. arXiv e-prints (2018)
4. Bronstein, M.M., et al.: Geometric deep learning: going beyond euclidean data. IEEE Sig. Process. Mag. **34**(4), 18–42 (2017)
5. Qi, C.R., et al.: PointNet: deep learning on point sets for 3D classification and segmentation. In: CVPR (2017)
6. Gutiérrez-Becker, B., Wachinger, C.: Deep multi-structural shape analysis: application to neuroanatomy. In: Frangi, A.F., Schnabel, J.A., Davatzikos, C., Alberola-López, C., Fichtinger, G. (eds.) MICCAI 2018. LNCS, vol. 11072, pp. 523–531. Springer, Cham (2018). https://doi.org/10.1007/978-3-030-00931-1_60
7. Fan, H., et al.: A point set generation network for 3D object reconstruction from a single image. In: CVPR (2017)
8. Yang, Y., et al.: FoldingNet: point cloud auto-encoder via deep grid deformation. In: CVPR (2018)
9. Baum, T., et al.: Automatic detection of osteoporotic vertebral fractures in routine thoracic and abdominal MDCT. Eur. Radiol. **24**(4), 872–880 (2014)
10. Tomita, N., et al.: Deep neural networks for automatic detection of osteoporotic vertebral fractures on CT scans. Comput. Biol. Med. **98**, 8–15 (2018)
11. Kendall, A., Gal, Y.: What uncertainties do we need in Bayesian deep learning for computer vision? In: NIPS (2017)
12. An, J., Cho, S.: Variational autoencoder based anomaly detection using reconstruction probability. Technical report, SNU Data Mining Center (2015)

Automatically Localizing a Large Set of Spatially Correlated Key Points: A Case Study in Spine Imaging

Alexander Oliver Mader[1,2,3(✉)], Cristian Lorenz[3], Jens von Berg[3],
and Carsten Meyer[1,2,3]

[1] Institute of Computer Science, Kiel University of Applied Sciences, Kiel, Germany
`alexander.o.mader@fh-kiel.de`
[2] Faculty of Engineering, Department of Computer Science,
Kiel University, Kiel, Germany
[3] Department of Digital Imaging, Philips Research, Hamburg, Germany

Abstract. The fully automatic localization of key points in medical images is an important and active area in applied machine learning, with very large sets of key points still being an open problem. To this end, we extend two general state-of-the-art localization approaches to operate on large amounts of key points and evaluate both approaches on a CT spine data set featuring 102 key points. First, we adapt the multi-stage convolutional pose machines neural network architecture to 3D image data with some architectural changes to cope with the large amount of data and key points. Imprecise localizations caused by the inherent downsampling of the network are countered by quadratic interpolation. Second, we extend a common approach—regression tree ensembles spatially regularized by a conditional random field—by a latent scaling variable to explicitly model spinal size variability. Both approaches are evaluated in detail in a 5-fold cross-validation setup in terms of localization accuracy and test time on 157 spine CT images. The best configuration achieves a mean localization error of 4.21 mm over all 102 key points.

Keywords: Key point localization ·
Fully convolutional neural network · Conditional random field · Spine ·
Computed tomography

This work has been financially supported by the Federal Ministry of Education and Research under the grant 03FH013IX5. The liability for the content of this work lies with the authors.

Electronic supplementary material The online version of this chapter (https://doi.org/10.1007/978-3-030-32226-7_43) contains supplementary material, which is available to authorized users.

D. Shen et al. (Eds.): MICCAI 2019, LNCS 11769, pp. 384–392, 2019.
https://doi.org/10.1007/978-3-030-32226-7_43

1   Introduction

Automatic localization of objects of interest is a prerequisite for many medical imaging tasks like image registration, model-based segmentation or plain measurements. Furthermore, it can improve performance of other object-specific approaches (i.e., semantic segmentation) by narrowing down the field of view to the important structures (e.g., in full body scans).

Many approaches have already been proposed to tackle the localization problem. Starting with very simple approaches like the generalized Hough transform, over more elaborate approaches utilizing "classical" machine learning approaches like decision forests [2] to recent dedicated neural network architectures [9]. Early on it was illustrated that the spatial co-occurrence of key points can be exploited to further accelerate the objective performance by using, e.g., Markov networks [3,7] to explicitly model the dependencies between key points. Recently, various convolutional neural network architectures have been proposed that try to exploit the co-occurrence in a model-free way by automatically learning and using the interdependencies [9,10]. Others make specific assumptions, e.g., on a chain-like structure of the key points [6]. However, only few papers address a large number of key points (≥ 100), among them [11], which requires a more rigid structure than the spine.

In this paper, we adapt and extend two general state-of-the-art co-occurrence-exploiting approaches—a recent neural-network-based one and a "classical" one—to cope with large sets of key points (≥ 100) in a reasonable time frame (≤ 60 s test time) on 3D spine CT data. In order to cope with memory problems encountered when localizing such large sets of key points with popular architectures like the V-Net [8], our first approach uses an adaptation of the "convolutional pose machines" neural network architecture [10] (which has much less parameters than the V-Net), motivated by its simplicity and very good performance on 2D non-medical and (very recently) 2D medical trauma data [1]. Here, we adapt it to 3D image data and propose an interpolation step into the continuous image domain based on second order polynomials to compensate for imprecise localizations due to the inherent downsampling of the network. We compare this approach to a second, "classical" framework based on regression tree ensembles spatially regularized by a conditional random field which illustrated good results on various data sets [7]. This approach is extended by a latent scaling variable to tackle spine size variability. We compare both approaches in detail, reporting state-of-the-art results localizing 102 spine-related key points in 157 spine CT scans in a 5-fold cross-validation setup. Furthermore, we show first results for the convolutional pose machine model on a different trauma CT data set without retraining any part of the model, illustrating the transferability of the approach.

2   Method

We apply a state-of-the-art fully convolutional neural network architecture and a classical approach to localize $N = 102$ vertebra key points in spine CT scans.

2.1   3D Convolutional Pose Machines (3D CPM)

The "convolutional pose machines" (CPM) architecture as proposed by Wei et al. [10] is a fully convolutional neural network architecture to regress down-sampled key-point-specific heatmaps. Key concept of this architecture is the stacking of similar prediction modules, where intermediate modules get the image *and* the heatmaps of the previous module in order to solve confusions by looking at the predictions of adjacent key points.

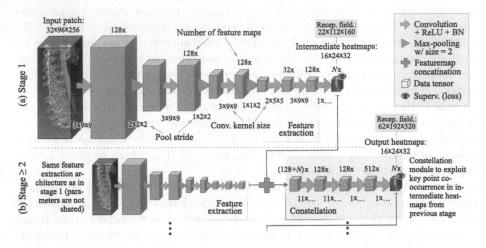

Fig. 1. The proposed network architecture based on "convolutional pose machines" [10] for the localization (by regressing heatmap volumes) of $N = 102$ vertebrae-related key points. Note the missing decoder-path of the network which results in heatmaps downsampled by a factor of $2 \times 4 \times 8$ to $16 \times 24 \times 32$ voxel from an initial patch size of $32 \times 96 \times 256$ voxel.

Here, we extend the 2D approach [1,10] to 3D image data and adapt the network architecture to match the anisotropic resolution ($3 \times 1 \times 1 \text{ mm}^3$/voxel) of the spine CT data set[1]. The resulting architecture is illustrated in Fig. 1. An input patch volume of $32 \times 96 \times 256$ voxel (roughly $10 \times 10 \times 25 \text{ cm}^3$) is used, which is (a) large enough to exploit the co-occurrence of neighboring vertebra key points (see input volume in Fig. 1) and (b) small enough for the model (producing heatmap volumes for 102 key points!) to be fully trainable with at least 3 stages on a GPU with 12 GB of memory. The pooling configurations and kernel sizes are chosen such that the receptive field slightly exceeds the input patch size. The proposed network architecture can be used for different resolutions as well, either by resampling the input (as we did for an unseen trauma CT data set with an average resolution of $0.81 \times 0.81 \times 1.75 \text{ mm}^3$/voxel; see last paragraph

---

[1] Sizes are given as sagittal $\times$ coronal $\times$ axial i.e., 3 mm resolution in medial–lateral direction.

in Sect. 3) or by modifying the input patch size and the filter sizes. At test time, input patches from the test image are extracted using an overlapping (averaged) sliding window approach with a stride of $1/3$ of the input patch size. Note that the image patches could be processed in parallel, further reducing test time below the times reported in Table 1.

From Down-Sampled Heatmap Output to Sub-voxel Predictions. For memory reasons in training, we do not use a decoding (upsampling) path in our network architecture compared to encoder-decoder architectures like the V-Net [8]. Thus, the inherent downsampling by the pooling operations may lead to imprecise localizations. We suggest to efficiently compensate for such errors by applying a fast interpolation technique based on a 3D second order polynomial, since this is the simplest interpolation matching the expected bell-like shape of the heatmap maxima:

$$f(x, y, z) = a_1 x^2 + a_2 y^2 + a_3 z^2 + a_4 xy + a_5 xz + a_6 yz + a_7 x + a_8 y + a_9 z + a_{10}. \quad (1)$$

For each output heatmap, we successively find the maximum and use ordinary least squares to estimate the polynomial coefficients $\mathbf{A} = \{a_i\}$ with the value of the maximum plus the adjacent quantized pixel values as bases. Then, we analytically find the (continuous) position of the maximum of the estimated polynomial. This maximum is discarded if it is outside the local neighborhood.

Training. Proper selection of training samples is crucial for good performance of the trained network. From each training image, we randomly cut 12 input patches of size $32 \times 96 \times 256$ voxel with the constraint to contain at least one key point. Empirically, each resulting input patch contains more than 10 key points, which provides enough co-occurrence clues to be exploited. For each input patch, we create 102 key-point specific target heatmaps placing a Gaussian kernel at the true position of the key points contained in the patch. We use the summation of multiple sum-squared-error (SSE) functions—one for each stage's output mimicking intermediate supervision—as loss function and minimize it using stochastic gradient descent in form of the Adam optimizer [4] over the course of 50 epochs (which resulted in a total training time in our case of 2–3 days with non-optimized code). We refer to this method as "3D CPM" in the following, using only two stages if not stated otherwise.

2.2   CRF-regularized Regression Tree Ensembles (RTEs+CRF)

For comparison with a "classical" (i.e., not neural-network-based), but generic approach we select the method proposed in [7], which uses regression tree ensembles (RTEs) to generate sets of likely positions for each key point, which are then spatially regularized using a conditional random field (CRF). This method has been applied to different applications with only minor modifications including the 26 vertebrae centers in spine CT data [7]. For each key point, an ensemble of regression trees is used to regress voxel-wise pseudo probabilities by evaluating randomized intensity difference patterns of very few voxels taken from a patch centered around the regressed voxel. To prevent confusion between key points and exploit the spatial correlation, a CRF parameterized by some potential functions (unary potentials using the regression values of the ensembles and binary in form of basic spatial statistics, see below) is used to select the most likely set of key point positions. Contrary to the previous method, the spatial correlation between key points is explicitly modelled in the CRF. Formally, we define a function

$$E(\mathbf{X} \mid \Lambda) = \sum_{l=1}^{L} \lambda_l \cdot \phi_l(\mathbf{X}_{\phi_l}) \tag{2}$$

parameterized by L weighted ($\Lambda = \{\lambda_l\}$) potential functions $\phi_l(\cdot)$ that computes the energy for a set of N key point positions $\mathbf{X} = \{\mathbf{x}_1, \ldots, \mathbf{x}_N\}$ with $\mathbf{X}_{\phi_l}$ being the subset of positions whose key points are in ϕ_l's clique. Finding the best set of key point predictions corresponds to the problem of probabilistic graph inference given by $\hat{\mathbf{X}} = \arg \text{mix}_{\mathbf{X}} E(\mathbf{X})$. Since this problem is intractable over the whole image domain for even small numbers of key points, the set of possible positions for each key point is reduced to a set of $n = 100$ local maxima found in the respective ensemble's heatmap.

Size Variability as Latent Variable. A common potential to represent the spatial structure is a binary (i.e., pairwise) Gaussian vector potential. The idea is to model the vector spanned between two key points i and j using a multivariate Gaussian distribution. To better capture the spinal size variability and thus to better characterize deviations from "standard" distances, we introduce a latent scaling variable. Assuming that we estimated the distribution's mean $\boldsymbol{\mu}_{i,j}$ and covariance $\boldsymbol{\Sigma}_{i,j}$ on training data, we can define the potential as

$$\phi_{i,j}^{\text{vec}}(\mathbf{x}_i, \mathbf{x}_j) = -\log \left[g(s \cdot (\mathbf{x}_i - \mathbf{x}_j) \mid \boldsymbol{\mu}_{i,j}, \boldsymbol{\Sigma}_{i,j}) \right], \tag{3}$$

with $g(\cdot)$ being the probability density function of a multivariate Gaussian distribution and s being the latent scaling variable. We use this binary potential (in addition to the unary potentials) to form a tree-structured graph containing the vertebra chain along the foramen with branches towards the vertebral key points (see supplementary material), which allows to perform polynomial time inference in form of belief propagation while providing scaling invariance.

Training. The 102 ensembles—consisting of 32 regression trees each—are trained as described in [7] using a patch size of $67 \times 201 \times 201$ voxel (roughly $20 \times 20 \times 20$ cm^3 to ensure enough local context is seen) and the sufficient statistics are estimated on the training annotations. To estimate the weights Λ of the CRF and also optimize the graph topology, we minimize a max-margin hinge loss

$$L(\Lambda) = \frac{1}{K} \sum_{k=1}^{K} \max(0, m + E(\mathbf{X}_k^+ \mid \Lambda) - E(\mathbf{X}_k^- \mid \Lambda)) \tag{4}$$

on the K training samples using gradient descent in form of the Adam [4] optimizer to increase the difference in energy between the correct positions $\mathbf{X}_k^+$ for sample k and the currently best rated incorrect positions $\mathbf{X}_k^-$, determined by inference using Gibbs sampling starting from the correct positions in each iteration, until the energy difference exceeds a margin $m = 1$ [7]. We carry out the optimization for 100 epochs using a learning rate of 0.01. Note that the ensembles and potentials are trained on the first half of the training images and the CRF weights on the exclusive second half to improve generalization. We refer to this method as "RTEs+CRF" in the following.

Table 1. Results for both methods averaged over the five folds in terms of localization error (Euclidean distance to true position) in mm, localization rate (percentage of correct key points and of fully correct cases; correct if the localization error ≤ 10 mm) and average test time (per case) in seconds.

Method	Localization rate/%		Error/mm		Time/s
	Key points	Cases	Mean	Std. dev.	
3D CPM w/o interp	91.0	49.7	5.86	12.42	45.3
3D CPM	91.1	52.2	4.32	12.66	45.4
3D CPM (3 stages)	91.4	**56.7**	**4.21**	12.51	88.9
RTEs+CRF w/o lat. scale	90.7	49.7	5.95	9.19	**24.8**
RTEs+CRF	91.8	49.7	5.66	9.66	28.0
RTEs+CRF (48 trees)	**92.6**	50.3	5.06	**6.70**	35.9

3 Experiments and Results

We evaluated the proposed methods in a 5-fold subject-based cross-validation setup on 157 spine CT images with an anisotropic resolution of $3 \times 1 \times 1$ mm^3/voxel (see supplementary material for more information). On average, each fold contained 125 training images. For each CT image, a semi-automatic approach was used to generate 102 key point positions, 6 for each of the 17 vertebrae T1 to L5. A model based spine segmentation was performed as described in [5]. The outcome was manually checked for quality, discarding incorrect ones. The triangular mesh model for each vertebra consists of triangles labeled according to their anatomical position, including upper and lower end plate of the vertebral bodies, the foramen, processus spinosus and both processi transversus. Key point positions were calculated as center of mass of the respectively labeled triangles, resulting in 102 key point annotations per CT image (using an in-house data set, since we are not aware of a public CT database with that many key point annotations). All experiments were conducted on the same machine containing an Intel Xeon CPU E5-2650, 512 GB of main memory and an NVIDIA TITAN Xp GPU with 12 GB of memory. Both approaches were implemented in Python using the scientific software stack.

The results for both approaches and the proposed extensions are listed in Table 1. We see that the performance of both approaches and their extensions is comparable with a slight advantage for the 3D CPM with a mean error of 4.32 mm after interpolation (from an initial 5.86 mm prior to the interpolation by taking just an additional 0.1 s), while requiring a 1.5 times longer test time than the RTEs+CRF (i.e., 45.4 s for the 3D CPM against 28.0 s for the RTEs+CRF). The latent scaling of the RTEs+CRF increases the key point localization rate from 90.7% to 91.8%, which is slightly better than the 3D CPM, and improves the mean error to 5.66 mm, which is still behind 3D CPM though. Looking at the localization error histogram depicted in Fig. 2a, we can see that the better localization error (4.32 mm) of the 3D CPM is caused by much more precise correct predictions despite the missing decoder path which is replaced by the quadratic interpolation: the average localization error of correctly localized key points is 1.81 mm for the 3D CPM and 3.58 mm for the RTEs+CRF. If we look how the mis-localizations are distributed over the spine (Fig. 2b), we can see that they are rather homogeneously distributed for the RTEs+CRF except for a slight increase towards the end (from L3 to L5) and more heterogeneously for the 3D CPM. From these observations we can conclude that the 3D CPM architecture is—as commonly assumed of deep networks—better in engineering features to generate accurate predictions, in contrast to the less powerful features used by the regression tree ensembles in the RTEs+CRF. However, the 3D CPM is not as good as the conditional random field in enforcing the global spatial correlation between key points, which is additionally backed by the slighty lower standard deviation of the localization error for the RTEs+CRF (Table 1). This is in line with the qualitative results shown in Fig. 3 in form of typical mis-localizations. The 3D CPM rarely fails to predict a single key point but fails mostly in small sized groups of adjacent key points, whereas the CRF either fails for very small groups (i.e., no good local maximum in the RTE's heatmap) or shifts the whole tree by one vertebra. Interestingly, both methods tend to fail for the same images. See the supplementary material for more illustrated cases.

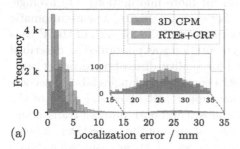 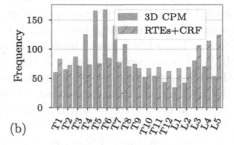

Fig. 2. (a) Histogram of the localization error in mm illustrating that the 3D CPM generates more precise key point predictions. Note the bump around 25 mm caused by vertebral confusions. (b) Number of mis-localization per vertebra illustrating that the CRF is better in enforcing the global spatial model.

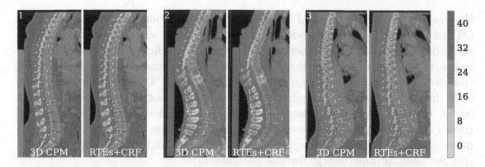

Fig. 3. Illustration of typical errors comparing both approaches side-by-side showing cropped sagittal projections of test images with circles indicating the true position and (possibly invisible) vectors towards the predicted positon (processi transversus ignored due to presentability); the error in mm is color coded.(Color figure online)

To increase the exploitation of the key point co-occurrence of the 3D CPM, we increased the number of stages to 3 (third row in Table 1). As expected, this did improve upon the previous results, but the margin is comparably small given that the test time nearly doubled. To improve the sub-optimal local maxima found in the heatmaps in the RTEs+CRF, we increased the number of regression trees from 32 to 48 in the RTEs+CRF (sixth row in Table 1). As expected, this did improve the key point localization rate (+0.8%) while needing 7.9 s more for testing. The decreased standard deviation of 6.7 mm supports the conclusion that the heatmap generation (RTEs) is the bottleneck of this approach.

Comparing our results to the best published results on the commonly used MICCAI 2014 CSI vertebrae localization challenge CT data set (up to 26 key points), we see that our results of 4.21 mm for the 3D CPM and 5.06 mm for the RTEs+CRF compare favorably to the results by Liao et al. [6] with 6.47 mm while localizing 5 times the amount of key points. First qualitative results (see supplementary material) of applying our trained 3D CPM model on a different spine CT data set (not used in training and with a different average resolution of $0.81 \times 0.81 \times 1.75$ mm^3/voxel, which we resampled to $3 \times 1 \times 1$ mm^3/voxel) featuring trauma cases showed that the conclusions for the 3D CPM still hold, while the RTEs+CRF failed more often due to bad generalization of the RTEs. The RTEs generated incorrect high responses for unseen structures (e.g., the head) which moved the correct position out of scope of the CRF.

4   Conclusions

We extended two state-of-the art fully automatic key point localization methods—a fully convolutional neural network and a classical one—to handle large sets of key points ($\geq$100). A convolutional pose machine architecture was modified (3D CPM) to appropriately define the input patch size and the final receptive field, and "classical" regression tree ensembles regularized by a conditional random field (RTE+CRF) were adjusted for the RTE patch size and the graph structure. Evaluated in a 5-fold cross-validation setup using 157 spine CT images, both approaches successfully localized 102 vertebral key points. We showed that the 3D CPM generated more precise predictions (average localization error of 4.21 mm) than the RTEs+CRF despite the missing decoder path that was compensated for by quadratic interpolation. On the other hand, the CRF has advantages in imposing the global shape model (which is, due to a latent variable, scaling-invariant) resulting in a smaller standard deviation of the localization error, has a lower training and test time and can be interpreted more easily. Note that both approaches are general and do not make domain-specific assumptions (except for size parameters).

References

1. Bier, B., et al.: X-ray-transform invariant anatomical landmark detection for pelvic trauma surgery. In: Frangi, A.F., Schnabel, J.A., Davatzikos, C., Alberola-López, C., Fichtinger, G. (eds.) MICCAI 2018. LNCS, vol. 11073, pp. 55–63. Springer, Cham (2018). https://doi.org/10.1007/978-3-030-00937-3_7
2. Criminisi, A., Shotton, J.: Decision Forests for Computer Vision and Medical Image Analysis. Springer, London (2013). https://doi.org/10.1007/978-1-4471-4929-3
3. Donner, R., Micusik, B., Langs, G., Bischof, H.: Sparse MRF appearance models for fast anatomical structure localisation. In: BMVC, pp. 109.1–109.10 (2007)
4. Kingma, D.P., Ba, J.: Adam: a method for stochastic optimization. In: ICLR (2014)
5. Klinder, T., Ostermann, J., Ehm, M., Franz, A., Kneser, R., Lorenz, C.: Automated model-based vertebra detection, identification, and segmentation in CT images. Med. Image Anal. **13**(3), 471–482 (2009)
6. Liao, H., Mesfin, A., Luo, J.: Joint vertebrae identification and localization in spinal CT images by combining short-and long-range contextual information. IEEE TMI **37**(5), 1266–1275 (2018)
7. Mader, A.O., et al.: Detection and localization of spatially correlated point landmarks in medical images using an automatically learned conditional random field. CVIU **176**, 45–53 (2018)
8. Milletari, F., Navab, N., Ahmadi, S.A.: V-Net: fully convolutional neural networks for volumetric medical image segmentation. In: 3DV, pp. 565–571. IEEE (2016)
9. Payer, C., Štern, D., Bischof, H., Urschler, M.: Regressing heatmaps for multiple landmark localization using CNNs. In: Ourselin, S., Joskowicz, L., Sabuncu, M.R., Unal, G., Wells, W. (eds.) MICCAI 2016. LNCS, vol. 9901, pp. 230–238. Springer, Cham (2016). https://doi.org/10.1007/978-3-319-46723-8_27
10. Wei, S.E., Ramakrishna, V., Kanade, T., Sheikh, Y.: Convolutional pose machines. In: CVPR, pp. 4724–4732 (2016)
11. Zhang, J., Liu, M., Shen, D.: Detecting anatomical landmarks from limited medical imaging data using two-stage task-oriented deep neural networks. IEEE TIP **26**(10), 4753–4764 (2017)

Permutohedral Attention Module
for Efficient Non-local Neural Networks

Samuel Joutard$^{(\boxtimes)}$, Reuben Dorent, Amanda Isaac, Sebastien Ourselin,
Tom Vercauteren, and Marc Modat

School of Biomedical Engineering and Imaging Sciences, King's College London,
London, UK
samuel.joutard@kcl.ac.uk

Abstract. Medical image processing tasks such as segmentation often
require capturing non-local information. As organs, bones, and tissues
share common characteristics such as intensity, shape, and texture, the
contextual information plays a critical role in correctly labeling them.
Segmentation and labeling is now typically done with convolutional neural networks (CNNs) but the context of the CNN is limited by the
receptive field which itself is limited by memory requirements and other
properties. In this paper, we propose a new attention module, that we
call Permutohedral Attention Module (PAM), to efficiently capture non-
local characteristics of the image. The proposed method is both memory and computationally efficient. We provide a GPU implementation of
this module suitable for 3D medical imaging problems. We demonstrate
the efficiency and scalability of our module with the challenging task of
vertebrae segmentation and labeling where context plays a crucial role
because of the very similar appearance of different vertebrae.

Keywords: Non-local neural networks · Attention module ·
Permutohedral Lattice · Vertebrae segmentation

1 Introduction

Convolutional neural networks (CNNs) have become one of the most effective
tools for many medical image processing tasks such as segmentation. However,
working with medical images has its own idiosyncratic challenges. The organs,
tissues or bones can have very similar characteristics, such as intensity, texture,
or shape. As a consequence, the differentiating aspects of each individual structure come from the context and the position of the item of interest in the larger
surroundings. However, naively extracting non-local characteristics of a region
requires much more computation and memory than focusing on its local characteristics. This currently makes using non-local context highly non-trivial in
medical imaging. Hence, an efficient approach to exploit non-local characteristics in deep learning could transform several medical imaging pipelines.

© Springer Nature Switzerland AG 2019
D. Shen et al. (Eds.): MICCAI 2019, LNCS 11769, pp. 393–401, 2019.
https://doi.org/10.1007/978-3-030-32226-7_44

The notion of contextual information is intimately related to the concept of receptive field in deep learning. The receptive field of an output variable corresponds to the region in the input influencing its value. Recent studies on receptive field in CNNs [10] have proven that the receptive field size is sublinear in the number of convolutional layers. In order to improve the receptive fields of a CNN, two main solutions have been adopted: down-sampling layers and dilated convolutions [14]. Use of down-sampling layers efficiently increases the receptive field size but decreases the resolution of the information. Hence, it is not suitable for very granular segmentation in which case dilated convolutions are often preferred [9]. Both of these solutions result in a fixed receptive field, which means that all contextual information in the receptive field will be taken into account whether it is relevant or not. Attention modules have been used to prune irrelevant information in medical imaging [12,15]. Yet, these tools remain suboptimal as they do not allow to capture large scale context. However, the extended self-attention formulation of [13] offers a solution to dynamically adapt the individual receptive field of each output variable to only make use of relevant non-local information. Despite its attractive properties, this formulation of self-attention has not yet been applied to medical images partly because its computational requirements scale as $O(N^2)$ (N is the number of voxels).

In this paper, we propose a new self-attention module called Permutohedral Attention Module (PAM), which makes use of the efficient approximation algorithm of the Permutohedral Lattice [1]. We adapted the algorithm of [1], originally designed to perform denoising, into a trainable self-attention module able to capture and process contextual information. The Permutohedral Lattice algorithm was previously used in a trainable framework in the more general context of sparse high dimensional convolutions for computer vision [7]. The self-attention approach is a suitable compromise for medical image processing in terms of memory and computation between [7] and standard convolutions while preserving most of the model representation capacity increase of [7] to process contextual information. Our module, similarly to the original non-local self-attention mechanism formulation, dynamically adapts the receptive field of each output variable in a learned way while being, in contrast to [13], applicable to medical images as it has low memory requirements, computationally scaling as $O(N)$. We evaluate our module on the challenging task of vertebrae segmentation. Vertebrae segmentation aims to label each individual vertebra and is used in practice as an initial step of various pipelines such as modality fusion, spine surgery planning and surgical guidance. As consecutive vertebrae have very similar local appearance, non-local information is compelling to identify them.

In Sect. 2, we first define self-attention and how it has been used, we then introduce the PAM. In Sect. 3 we first highlight the capability of our module to capture and process contextual information without requiring a deep architecture. Then, we demonstrate its capability to improve state of the art segmentation architectures for vertebrae segmentation.

2   Methods

The Self-attention Mechanism. Self-attention used in deep learning frameworks can be defined as follows: consider a standard deep learning framework where the input $\mathbf{x} = (x_1, ..x_N)$ is processed first by a section of the network we call descriptor network $\mathbf{v}_\psi$, and then by the rest of the network we call prediction network g_θ (ψ and θ are the respective parameter sets). The model predicts $\mathbf{y}$ so that:

$$\mathbf{y} = g_\theta(\mathbf{v}_\psi(\mathbf{x})) \tag{1}$$

We define $A_\phi(.)$ the self-attention mechanism parameterized by ϕ which combines the non-local input descriptors in a learned way. For all input $\mathbf{x}$, $A_\phi(\mathbf{x})$ is a $N \times N$ self-attention matrix where the coefficient $A_\phi(\mathbf{x})_{i,j}$ characterizes the attention of x_i towards x_j. Our framework including an attention mechanism predicts $\mathbf{y}_{att}$:

$$\mathbf{y}_{att} = g_\theta(A_\phi(\mathbf{x}) \cdot \mathbf{v}_\psi(\mathbf{x})) \tag{2}$$

where $\cdot$ represents the matrix multiplication operator. This formulation has two principal strengths; it can increase the receptive field of each output variable up to the whole input, and it can modulate the receptive field of each output variable with respect to the input characteristics. To our knowledge, attention modules in deep learning either compute the entire self-attention matrix on a low dimensional input or use a local attention mechanism that can be seen as a strong approximation of the non-local self-attention formulation. Specifically in the medical imaging context, previous works [11,12,15] implicitly used a simplification of (2) with a diagonal self-attention matrix. This solution can be applied to large images since it scales linearly with the number of voxels but does not help to capture contextual information.

Different implementations of the non-local self-attention matrix are listed in [13]. These can be unified as follows:

$$A_\phi(\mathbf{x}) = [\gamma(\phi_1(x_i)^T \cdot \phi_2(x_j))]_{1 \leq i,j \leq N} \tag{3}$$

where $\phi = (\phi_1, \phi_2)$ is a pair of embedding functions (possibly identities) and γ is typically either identity, exponential or ReLU. Hence, these approaches are impractical to apply to 3D images because the number of interactions to be computed scales as $O(N^2)$.

Permutohedral Attention Module. The proposed PAM relies on a slightly different formulation of the self-attention matrix to align more closely with the formulation of the non-local means filtering algorithm [3] used in the denoising literature. When applied to the set of feature-descriptor pairs $(f_i, v_i)_{i \leq n}$ (where n is the number of variables described), non-local mean gives the set of filtered descriptors:

$$\forall 1 \leq i \leq n, \quad v_i' = \sum_{j=1}^{n} \exp(-||f_i - f_j||_2) v_j \tag{4}$$

Hence:

$$A_\phi(\mathbf{x}) = [\exp(-||f_\phi(x_i) - f_\phi(x_j)||_2)]_{i,j \leq N} \tag{5}$$

is the corresponding attention formulation with f_ϕ a feature extractor network (ϕ its parameter set).

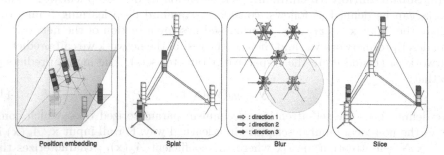

Fig. 1. The features lying in $\mathbb{R}^f$ are embedded in a hyperplane of $\mathbb{R}^{f+1}$ to position each variable. This hyperplane is partitioned in simplices by a mesh called the Permutohedral Lattice. The Splat phase describes the vertices of the Permutohedral Lattice based on the neighbouring variables. The Blur step applies a Gaussian blur along each direction consecutively. Finally, the Slice step re-projects the filtered descriptors from the vertices to the variables.

Avoiding a brute-force computation of (4), we adapted the Permutohedral Lattice approximation algorithm [1] to estimate the self-attention module output $\mathbf{v}'_{\phi,\psi}(\mathbf{x}) = A_\phi(\mathbf{x}) \cdot \mathbf{v}_\psi(\mathbf{x})$ in $O(N)$ against $O(N^2)$ for the original non-local neural network formulations listed in [13]. Learning the parameter sets ϕ and ψ is achieved through back-propagation. Hence, the PAM can be integrated in a deep learning framework to compute self-attention for high dimensional inputs (cf. Sect. 3 for concrete architectures examples). The PAM approximates the proposed attention mechanism in 4 steps: embedding of the features into the Permutohedral Lattice higher dimensional space, Splat, Blur and Slice, as illustrated in Fig. 1. Each of these steps scales linearly in N.

The advantage of this approximation algorithm against other possibilities [2, 5] is that the gradients with respect to the input feature vectors $\mathbf{f}_\phi(\mathbf{x})$ and the descriptor vectors $\mathbf{v}_\psi(\mathbf{x})$ can be expressed using the four steps composing the forward pass and be fully parallelized. Omitting the dependencies in $\mathbf{x}$, ϕ, and ψ, we can express the forward pass as:

$$\mathbf{v}' = \mathcal{S}l(\mathcal{B}(\mathcal{S}(\mathcal{E}(\mathbf{f}), \mathbf{v})), \mathcal{E}(\mathbf{f})) \qquad (6)$$

where $\mathcal{E}$ is the embedding operator, $\mathcal{S}$ is the Splat operator, $\mathcal{B}$ is the Blur operator and $\mathcal{S}l$ is the Slice operator. With the same notations, the backward pass can be expressed as:

$$\frac{\partial L}{\partial \mathbf{v}} = \frac{\partial L}{\partial \mathbf{v}'} \circ \frac{\partial \mathbf{v}'}{\partial \mathbf{v}} = \mathcal{S}l(\tilde{\mathcal{B}}(\mathcal{S}(\mathcal{E}(\mathbf{f}), \frac{\partial L}{\partial \mathbf{v}'})), \mathcal{E}(\mathbf{f})) \qquad (7)$$

$$\frac{\partial L}{\partial f_i} = \frac{\partial L}{\partial \mathbf{v}'} \circ \frac{\partial \mathbf{v}'}{\partial f_i} = E^T \cdot \left[\tilde{\mathcal{B}}\mathcal{S}\mathcal{E}(\mathbf{f}, \frac{\partial L}{\partial \mathbf{v}'})_{\sigma_i^j} \cdot v_i^T + \mathcal{B}\mathcal{S}\mathcal{E}(\mathbf{f}, \mathbf{v})_{\sigma_i^j} \cdot \left(\frac{\partial L}{\partial \mathbf{v}'_i} \right)^T \right]_{j \leq (f+1)} \qquad (8)$$

where L is the loss and $\forall a, b \ \mathcal{BSE}(a, b) = \mathcal{B}(\mathcal{S}(\mathcal{E}(a), b))$ (similarly with $\tilde{\mathcal{BSE}}$). $\tilde{\mathcal{B}}$ is the Gaussian blurring operator where the Gaussian blur is applied in the reverse order in terms of direction of the Lattice. E is the position embedding matrix and σ_i is a permutation computed during $\mathcal{E}$.

3   Experiments

Data. We evaluate the impact of PAM for non-local neural networks for the task of simultaneous segmentation and labeling of vertebrae. We performed our experiment on the CSI 2014 workshop challenge data[1], which consists of 20 CT images. We used all 20 CT images in our framework using a 5-fold cross validation for evaluation. We resampled the data to obtain (1 mm, 1 mm, 3 mm) voxels.

Implementation Details. We implemented the PAM as well as all our pipelines using Pytorch. We optimized our networks with ADAM on $160 \times 160 \times 96$ patches with a fixed learning rate of 0.001 and a batch size of 1. We used the Dice loss as loss function. Our implementation is publicly available[2].

Models. As a preliminary experiment, we consider a specific 6-layer fully convolutional network (referred to as FCN). We design 2 baselines for this shallow setting. FCN is a plain fully convolutional network with a first $(3 \times 3 \times 3)$ convolution with 18 output channels followed by 4 $(3 \times 3 \times 3)$ embedding convolutions with 18 output channels each and a prediction $(1 \times 1 \times 1)$ convolutional layer. Dil.FCN is a similar architecture where we replace each embedding convolution by a dilated block. A dilated block corresponds to 3 $(3 \times 3 \times 3)$ convolutions in parallel with 6 output channels each. Of these 3 convolutions, two have dilated filters (dilatation factor of 2 and 4 respectively). The outputs of a dilated block are then concatenated before the next block. Then, we incorporate in each baseline the PAM (networks are respectively called FCN+PAM and Dil.FCN+PAM) and compare the results of those 4 configurations.

Figure 2 represents the Dil.FCN+PAM architecture. In this figure, we observe that, once we obtain the features $\mathbf{f} = (f_1, ..f_N)$ and descriptors $\mathbf{v} = (v_1, ..v_N)$ to compute attention, we split each feature and descriptor vector in two. Hence we obtain two sets of feature-descriptor pairs $(f_i^0, v_i^0)_{i \leq N}$ and $(f_i^1, v_i^1)_{i \leq N}$ on which we apply the PAM independently. There are two main advantages to doing so. First, it allows us to further reduce computation time and memory footprint. Second, it generates a per-group-of-channel attention map which makes the model more flexible (as a unique attention matrix for all descriptor channels is a particular case of two attention matrix, one for each group of channel). The reason for not splitting the feature-descriptor pairs set into more subsets is because we want a trade-off between the advantages described above and the preservation of relevant features to compute attention.

Then, we consider a 3D U-Net [4] which is one of the most popular architectures for segmentation [6]. We refer to our 3D U-Net simply as U-Net. We

---

[1] http://spineweb.digitalimaginggroup.ca/.

[2] https://github.com/SamuelJoutard/Permutohedral_attention_module.

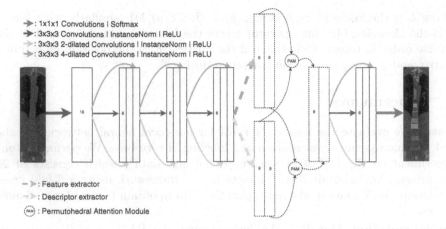

Fig. 2. Dil.FCN+PAM, a shallow architecture including dilated convolutions and PAM. The feature extractor and descriptor extractor are $(1 \times 1 \times 1)$ convolutions. The feature extractor incorporates a mesh of spatial coordinates before applying its convolution, and is followed by a Leaky-ReLU activation function. The number on intermediate results correspond to the number of channels. We call the combination of the dashed elements Permutohedral block.

incorporate the PAM into our U-Net as shown in Fig. 3 and demonstrate that the PAM can also improve architectures which have large receptive fields (we call this network U-PAM-Net). As shown in Fig. 3, we incorporate the PAM at the half-resolution level. Hence, we compute attention for $(2 \times 2 \times 2)$ voxel regions which, in our experiments, led to similar results as computing attention at the voxel level while decreasing computation time and making convergence faster.

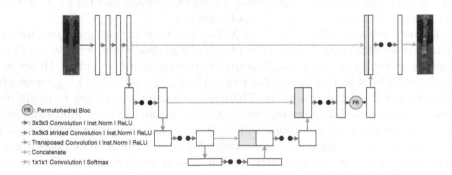

Fig. 3. U-PAM-Net. We make use of the Permutohedral block defined in Fig. 2.

As the PAM introduces a small number of extra parameters, we compensate with additional channels in the first convolution on the architectures without the PAM so that the corresponding networks have either as many as or more degrees of freedom than networks with the PAM integrated.

Results. We measure the performance of the different architectures with the Dice scores. Table 1 shows that the PAM improves performance for all the architectures it was incorporated into. In addition, we highlight that the shallow network Dil.FCN+PAM performs almost as well as the much deeper network 3D U-Net. Indeed, the dilated convolutions manage to describe the voxels using contextual information while the PAM uses those meaningful features to compute voxels interactions. Table 1 also illustrates the limitation of down-sampling layers pointed earlier as U-Net performs poorly on cervical vertebrae which appear very small in our images. U-PAM-Net manages to reach higher accuracy performances than [8], which makes use of a task-specific framework especially tuned to "count" the vertebrae from spine segmentation. While [8] report an accuracy of 81%, our proposed framework obtained 89% using the same evaluation metric and on the same dataset. It should be noted that the training frameworks in terms of test-train split were different for both approaches. Figure 4 shows a representative example of the results we observed.

Table 1. Mean(std) Dice score (%) of the different networks tested

Network	FCN	FCN+PAM	Dil.FCN	Dil.FCN+PAM	U-Net	U-PAM-Net
Full	28(3)	**54**(14)	49(7)	**70**(9)	72(9)	**81**(9)
Cervical	45(30)	**53**(37)	**60**(27)	56(33)	25(38)	**55**(39)
Thoracic	21(3)	**46**(14)	42(10)	**67**(12)	67(13)	**80**(12)
Lumbar	29(4)	**69**(19)	58(8)	**79**(12)	**93**(2)	91(5)

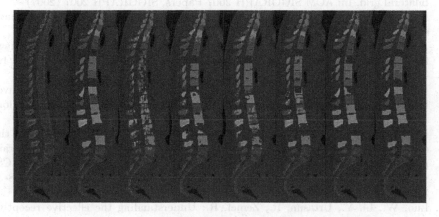

Fig. 4. Example of segmentation obtained by our different networks. In the corresponding order: Input slice, ground truth, FCN, FCN+PAM, Dil.FCN, Dil.FCN+PAM, U-Net, U-PAM-Net.

4   Discussion

In this work, we propose the Permutohedral Attention Module, a computationally efficient attention module to be applied in 3D deep learning framework. The

PAM can be incorporated in any CNN architecture. We demonstrated its ability to efficiently handle non-local information in the context of vertebrae segmentation and presented its potential to reduce networks size in specific tasks. Future work will notably include the investigation of asymmetric attention matrix for feature filtering and the integration of the PAM formulation in path training.

Acknowledgement. We thank E. Molteni, C. Sudre, B. Murray, K. Georgiadis, Z. Eaton-Rosen, M. Ebner for their useful comments. This work is supported by the Wellcome/EPSRC Centre for Medical Engineering [WT 203148/Z/16/Z]. TV is supported by a Medtronic/RAEng Research Chair [RCSRF1819/7/34].

References

1. Adams, A., Baek, J., Davis, M.A.: Fast high-dimensional filtering using the permutohedral lattice. Comput. Graph. Forum **29**, 753–762 (2010)
2. Adams, A., Gelfand, N., Dolson, J., Levoy, M.: Gaussian KD-trees for fast high-dimensional filtering. ACM Trans. Graph. **28**(3), 21:1–21:12 (2009)
3. Buades, A., Coll, B.: A non-local algorithm for image denoising. In: CVPR, pp. 60–65 (2005)
4. Çiçek, Ö., Abdulkadir, A., Lienkamp, S.S., Brox, T., Ronneberger, O.: 3D U-net: learning dense volumetric segmentation from sparse annotation. In: Ourselin, S., Joskowicz, L., Sabuncu, M.R., Unal, G., Wells, W. (eds.) MICCAI 2016. LNCS, vol. 9901, pp. 424–432. Springer, Cham (2016). https://doi.org/10.1007/978-3-319-46723-8_49
5. Chen, J., Paris, S., Durand, F.: Real-time edge-aware image processing with the bilateral grid. In: ACM SIGGRAPH 2007 Papers, SIGGRAPH 2007 (2007)
6. Isensee, F., et al.: nnU-Net: Self-adapting framework for u-net-based medical image segmentation. arXiv preprint arXiv:1809.10486 (2018)
7. Jampani, V., Kiefel, M., Gehler, P.: Learning sparse high dimensional filters: image filtering, dense CRFs and bilateral neural networks (2016). https://doi.org/10.1109/CVPR.2016.482
8. Lessmann, N., van Ginneken, B., de Jong, P.A., Isgum, I.: Iterative fully convolutional neural networks for automatic vertebra segmentation and identification. Med. Image Anal. **53**, 142–155 (2019)
9. Li, W., Wang, G., Fidon, L., Ourselin, S., Cardoso, M.J., Vercauteren, T.: On the compactness, efficiency, and representation of 3D convolutional networks: brain parcellation as a pretext task. In: Niethammer, M., et al. (eds.) IPMI 2017. LNCS, vol. 10265, pp. 348–360. Springer, Cham (2017). https://doi.org/10.1007/978-3-319-59050-9_28
10. Luo, W., Li, Y., Urtasun, R., Zemel, R.: Understanding the effective receptive field in deep convolutional neural networks. In: Advances in Neural Information Processing Systems, vol. 29, pp. 4898–4906 (2016)
11. Roy, A.G., Navab, N., Wachinger, C.: Recalibrating fully convolutional networks with spatial and channel "squeeze and excitation" blocks. IEEE Trans. Med. Imaging **38**(2), 540–549 (2019)
12. Schlemper, J., et al.: Attention gated networks: learning to leverage salient regions in medical images. Med. Image Anal. **53**, 197–207 (2019)

13. Wang, X., Girshick, R.B., Gupta, A., He, K.: Non-local neural networks. In: 2018 IEEE/CVF Conference on Computer Vision and Pattern Recognition, pp. 7794–7803 (2018)
14. Yu, F., Koltun, V.: Multi-scale context aggregation by dilated convolutions. In: International Conference on Learning Representations (ICLR) (2016)
15. Zhang, Z., Xie, Y., Xing, F., McGough, M., Yang, L.: MDNet: a semantically and visually interpretable medical image diagnosis network. In: 2017 IEEE Conference on Computer Vision and Pattern Recognition (CVPR), pp. 3549–3557 (2017)

Improving RetinaNet for CT Lesion Detection with Dense Masks from Weak RECIST Labels

Martin Zlocha, Qi Dou, and Ben Glocker[✉]

Biomedical Image Analysis Group, Imperial College London, London, UK
{martin.zlocha15,qi.dou,b.glocker}@imperial.ac.uk

Abstract. Accurate, automated lesion detection in Computed Tomography (CT) is an important yet challenging task due to the large variation of lesion types, sizes, locations and appearances. Recent work on CT lesion detection employs two-stage region proposal based methods trained with centroid or bounding-box annotations. We propose a highly accurate and efficient one-stage lesion detector, by re-designing a RetinaNet to meet the particular challenges in medical imaging. Specifically, we optimize the anchor configurations using a differential evolution search algorithm. For training, we leverage the response evaluation criteria in solid tumors (RECIST) annotation which are measured in clinical routine. We incorporate dense masks from weak RECIST labels, obtained automatically using GrabCut, into the training objective, which in combination with other advancements yields new state-of-the-art performance. We evaluate our method on the public DeepLesion benchmark, consisting of 32,735 lesions across the body. Our one-stage detector achieves a sensitivity of 90.77% at 4 false positives per image, significantly outperforming the best reported methods by over 5%.

1 Introduction

Detection and localization of abnormalities in Computed Tomography (CT) scans is a critical routine task for radiologists. Accurate, automated detection of suspicious regions could greatly support screening, diagnosis and monitoring of disease progression. Most previous work focuses on a specific type of lesion within a relatively constrained (anatomical) context, such as lymph nodes, lung nodules and brain microbleeds. Recently, Yan et al. [15] pioneered the study of universal lesion detection and introduced today's largest data repository, i.e., the DeepLesion dataset. Detecting diverse types of lesions across the body using one single model is very challenging due to the large variation of lesion types, sizes, locations and heterogeneous appearances. For example, DeepLesion consists of eight types of lesions with diameters ranging from 0.21 to 342.5 mm. In addition, the lesions may appear with limited contrast compared to nearby normal tissue, which further increases the difficulty of detecting subtle signs of disease.

D. Shen et al. (Eds.): MICCAI 2019, LNCS 11769, pp. 402–410, 2019.
https://doi.org/10.1007/978-3-030-32226-7_45

Automated lesion detection has been central in medical image computing. Recent work employs two-stage methods with candidate proposal and false positive reduction steps. State-of-the-art performance on the DeepLesion benchmark has been achieved by Yan et al. [13]. They propose a two-stage, region-based method called 3DCE to effectively incorporate 3D context into 2D regional CNNs. Their method achieves a sensitivity of 85.65% at 4 false positives per image, outperforming the popular detection method of Faster R-CNN [7] on the same dataset. However, their detection sensitivity for small lesions is much lower, which is an important limitation in the critical context of detecting early signs of diseases.

Some recent work take advantage of mask information for improving detection accuracy. Jaeger et al. [4] propose a Retina U-Net, showing that aggregating pixel-wise supervision to train the detector is helpful. Their method shows effectiveness in two scenarios, i.e., lung lesions in CT and breast lesions in MRI. As pixel-wise annotations are tedious and expensive to obtain, Tang et al. [12] generate pseudo masks by fitting ellipses based on the response evaluation criteria in solid tumors (RECIST) [2] diameters. Using a 2D Mask R-CNN [3] with generated lesion masks and other strategies, [12] achieves a sensitivity of 84.38% at 4 false positives per image on DeepLesion dataset. Their pseudo-mask generation procedure relies heavily on the assumption of elliptical geometry of lesions, which may yield imprecise masks limiting the efficacy of dense supervision.

We propose a one-stage detector which directly localizes lesions without the need of candidate region proposals. To meet the specific challenge of detecting small lesions, we revisit the RetinaNet [6] and optimize the feature pyramid scheme and anchor configuration by employing a differential evolution search algorithm. To enhance the model, we leverage high-quality dense masks obtained automatically from weak RECIST labels using GrabCut [8]. Incorporating these generated masks into pixel-wise supervision shows great benefit for training the detector. In addition, we make use of the coherence between lesion mask predictions and bounding-box regressions to calibrate the detector outputs. We further investigate recent strategies for boosting the detection performance, such as integrating attention mechanism into our feature pyramids. We evaluate the contributions of each part using the DeepLesion benchmark, achieving a new state-of-the-art sensitivity of 90.77% at 4 false positives per image, significantly outperforming the currently best performing method 3DCE [13] by over 5%. Our lesion detection system is featured in an online game under spot-the-lesion.com.

2   Improving RetinaNet

An overview of our proposed one-stage lesion detector is illustrated in Fig. 1(a). We first describe the model design before elaborating on how we obtain dense masks from weak RECIST labels and incorporate them into training process. We then show the attention mechanism for further improving detection performance.

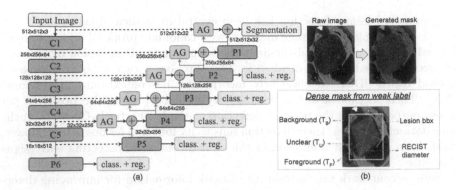

Fig. 1. (a) Overview of our improved RetinaNet, where C is convolution block, P is feature pyramid, AG is attention gate. (b) Automatic dense mask generation from weak RECIST diameters using GrabCut [8].

2.1 Model Design with Optimized Anchor Configuration

The backbone of our approach is a RetinaNet [6], a recent one-stage method for object detection. The use of a focal loss addresses the common problem of class imbalance in detection tasks. The feature pyramids and lateral connections with a top-down architecture [5] are adopted for detecting objects at different scales. This is an important difference with methods such as 3DCE [13], since the feature pyramids can effectively capture information about lesions of varying sizes including very small ones. Our specific network follows the structure of VGG-19 [10]. We also explored ResNet-50 as used originally, but its performance was worse on DeepLesion, which is in line with results reported in [14].

The anchor configuration (i.e., size, aspect ratios and scales) is crucial for the detector, and we find the default settings turn out to be ineffective for detecting lesions of small size and large ratios. We employ a differential evolution search algorithm [11] to optimize configurations of anchors on the validation set. This algorithm iteratively improves a population of candidate solutions with regard to an objective function. New solutions are created by combining existing ones. We aim to find the best anchor settings for 3 scales and 5 ratios. The objective is to maximise the overlap between the lesion bounding-box and the best anchor. We fix one ratio as 1:1, and define other ratios as reciprocal pairs (i.e., if one ratio is $1 : \gamma$ then another is $\gamma : 1$). Thus, we need to optimise only five variables, i.e, two ratio pairs and three scales. When initialising the population of candidate solutions, all scales are bounded to a range of $[0.4, 1.6]$ and the two ratios are respectively bounded in $[1, 2]$ and $[2, 4]$. We obtain optimal scales as 0.425, 0.540 and 0.680, and ratios of 3.27:1, 1.78:1, 1:1, 1:1.78, 1:3.27, which fits objects of small size and large ratios. Anchor sizes remain as (32, 64, 128, 256 and 512). These optimised configurations are then used for training the detector.

2.2 Dense Mask Supervision from Weak RECIST Labels

Although annotations of bounding-boxes are relatively easy to obtain, there are other "weak" labels which are routinely generated in clinical practice, such as RECIST diameters. RECIST is used to track lesion growth, and consists of a pair of diameters to measure the lesion extent (cf. Fig. 1(b)). To leverage this highly valuable information, we automatically generate dense lesion masks from RECIST labels (provided in the DeepLesion dataset) using GrabCut [8]. We initialize a trimap into background (T_B), foreground (T_F) and unclear (T_U) pixels. A segmentation mask is generated based on iterative graph-cuts. Initialization can largely affect the final result, as it defines the Gaussian mixture models capturing the foreground and background intensity distributions.

Cai et al. [1] previously adopt GrabCut to initialise lesion masks of the RECIST-slice for the task of weakly-supervised lesion segmentation in 3D. Their T_B is set as pixels outside the bounding-box defined by RECIST axes, and T_F is obtained by dilation of the diameters. Such an initialisation may be sub-optimal, specifically, for large lesions, where a considerable number of lesion pixels, which are quite certain to belong to foreground, are outside the dilation and omitted in T_F. For small lesions, the dilation has the risk of hard-labelling background pixels into T_F, which cannot be corrected in the optimization.

To achieve a higher-quality masks using GrabCut, we propose a new strategy, as illustrated in Fig. 1(b). We build a quadrilateral by consecutively connecting the four endpoints of the RECIST diameters. A pixel is labelled as foreground if it falls inside the quadrilateral. As most lesions show convex outlines, this is a simple yet reliable strategy. With the annotation of bounding-box provided in the dataset, the pixels outside the box are hard-labelled as background T_B. All remaining pixels are assigned to T_U and estimated through GrabCut.

To exploit these generated dense labels, we add two more upsampling layers (connecting to P2 and P1) and a segmentation prediction layer to the detector. Skip connections are employed by fusing features obtained from C1 (via a 1×1 convolution) and input (via two 3×3 convolutions), as shown in Fig. 1(a). To retain sufficient resolution of feature maps for small lesions, we shift the sub-network operation (i.e., classification and regression) to pyramid levels of P2–P6 from P3–P7. Using dense supervision to help detection task shares the idea with Retina U-Net [4], where we avoid the need for tedious labelling, as our dense masks are automatically generated from labels that are already recorded in clinical routine. Additionally, we leverage the IoU between a bounding-box around the predicted segmentation mask and the directly regressed box (yellow sub-networks in Fig. 1), to calibrate the prediction probability $\tilde{p} = p \times (1 + \mathrm{IoU})$ of a lesion. High coherence between segmentation and detection results indicates high confidence in lesion prediction, and benefits sensitivity at low FP rates.

2.3 Attention Mechanism for Gated Feature Fusion

A recent attention gate (AG) model proposed by Schlemper et al. [9] learns to focus on target structures by producing an attention map. According to this work, this may be beneficial for small, varying structures. We explore AGs to filter feature responses propagated through skip connections and use features upsampled from coarser scale as the gating signal. The AG module only uses 1×1 convolutions and produces a single attention map, which makes it computationally light-weight. The output of AG is the element-wise multiplication of the attention map and the feature map from the skip connection.

Training: We follow the loss used in original RetinaNet for detection, and our segmentation uses focal loss with cross-entropy. We employ the Adam optimizer with a learning rate of 10^{-4} which is reduced during training by a factor of 10 when the mean average precision (mAP) has not improved for 2 consecutive epochs. The batch size is 4 during training. To reduce overfitting, early stopping is used if the mAP has not improved for 4 consecutive epochs on validation.

3 Experiments

3.1 Dataset, Pre-processing, and Augmentation

The public DeepLesion dataset [15] consists of 32,120 axial CT slices from 10,594 studies of 4,427 unique patients. There are $1-3$ lesions in each slice, adding up to 32,735 lesions altogether. For each lesion, there is usually 30 mm of extra slices above and below the key slice to provide contextual information. In most cases, the slices have 1 or 5 mm thickness, but this varies with some being 0.625 or 2 mm. The 2D bounding-boxes and RECIST diameters for lesions are annotated on the key slice. The dataset covers a wide range of lesions from lung, liver, mediastinum (mainly lymph nodes), kidney, pelvis, bone, abdomen and soft tissue. Sizes vary significantly with diameters ranging from 0.21 to 342.5 mm.

We perform lightweight pre-processing where images are resized into 512 × 512 pixels, resulting in a voxel-spacing between 0.175 and 0.977 mm with a mean of 0.802 mm. The Hounsfield units (HU) are clipped into the range of $[-1024, 1050]$. We normalize the intensities to the range of $[-1, 1]$ as input to the network. In our experiments, we use three adjacent slices after resampling to 2 mm thickness. In rare cases where the neighboring slice of the lesion slice is not provided, we duplicate the lesion slice to fill the missing input channels. We use data augmentation where images are flipped in horizontal and vertical directions with 50% chance. We also use random affine transformations with rotation/shearing up to 0.1 radians, and scaling/translation up to 10% of the image size.

3.2 Detection Results on DeepLesion Benchmark

The DeepLesion dataset is provided with splits into 70% for training, 15% for validation, and 15% for testing. Thus, our results can be directly compared with numbers reported in the literature. The current best results have been achieved by Yan et al. [13] and Tang et al. [12]. We also quote their provided baseline performance using popular detection methods, i.e., Faster R-CNN [7] (reported in [13]) and Mask R-CNN [3] (reported in [12]). We further provide the results of our own baseline RetinaNet [6] using its default configuration. A predicted box is regarded as correct if its IoU with a ground truth box is larger than 0.5.

In Table 1, we present the lesion detection sensitivities at different false positives (FP) per image. Our improved RetinaNet consistently outperforms existing methods across all FP rates. Specifically, sensitivity at 4 FPs, which is commonly reported in the literature, we achieve a sensitivity of 90.77%, which is a 5.12% improvement over 3DCE [13] and 6.39% over ULDor [12]. The free-response receiver operating characteristics (FROC) curves of different methods are shown on the left in Fig. 2. We observe that optimized networks for lesion detection are generally better than out-of-the-box detectors, such as Faster R-CNN, Mask R-CNN and RetinaNet. When comparing sensitivity at low FP rates, our improved models perform much better than others, indicating the benefit of task-specific optimization and incorporation of additional mask information.

The sensitivity for detecting different sizes of lesions at 4 FPs are shown on the right in Fig. 2. We divide the lesions into three size groups according to the diameter, following [13] for direct comparison. For small lesions with diameters less than 10 mm, our sensitivity is 88.35% compared to 80% for 3DCE. Using a feature pyramid to retain responses from small lesions together with dense supervision with focal loss seems beneficial for detecting subtle signs of disease. While 3DCE uses richer 3D context, this seems less helpful for small, local structures. Our model works well across all lesion sizes where we improve sensitivity from 87% to 91.73% for lesions of 10–30 mm, and from 84% to 93.02% for lesions larger than 30 mm when compared to 3DCE.

Some visual results are shown in Fig. 3. Average inference time per image is listed in Table 1. Our detection results are obtained using a single network without model ensemble nor test augmentation. Our one-stage detector is highly efficient eliminating the need of generating lesion proposals. The integration of dense supervision and attention mechanism has minimal overhead, taking overall 41 ms per image. Runtimes are reported for 3DCE and Faster R-CNN in [13], but a comparison is only indicative due to different GPUs being used.

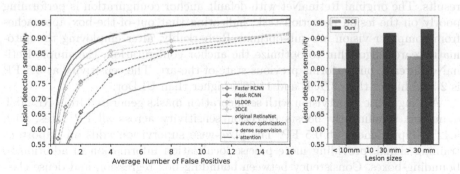

Fig. 2. Left: FROC curves for our improved RetinaNet variants and baselines on DeepLesion dataset. Right: Per lesion size results compared to 3DCE [13].

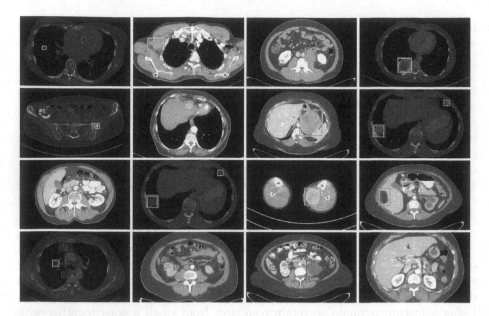

Fig. 3. Visual results for lesion detection at 0.5 FP rate using our improved RetinaNet. The first three columns show different sizes from small to large. The right column shows heatmaps from the segmentation layer overlaid on detections. Yellow boxes are ground truth, green are true positives, red are false positives. Last row shows intriguing failure cases with possibly incorrect ground truth. (Color figure online)

3.3   Contribution of Individual Improvements

We investigate the individual impact of the proposed additions leading to our final improved RetinaNet. In an ablation study, we first evaluate the original RetinaNet [6] with default settings, then incrementally add our improvements, i.e., automatic anchor optimization, dense supervision using lesion masks from weak labels, and attention mechanism. Table 1 and Fig. 2 (left) summarizes these results. The original RetinaNet with default anchor configuration is performing poorly on the lesion detection task, indicating that out-of-the-box approaches from computer vision are sub-optimal. Remarkably, after employing the automatic search algorithm to optimize the anchor configuration, the simple RetinaNet already outperforms previous state-of-the-art. The sensitivity at 0.5 FP is 2.34% higher than 3DCE and 11.96% higher than ULDor.

Adding dense supervision with segmentation masks generated from RECIST diameters significantly boosts detection sensitivity across all FP rates, with 5.42% improvement at 0.5 FP. The pixel-wise supervision adds an important training signal, providing more precise localization information in addition to bounding-boxes. Consistency between bounding-box regression and dense classification helps to reduce false positives. Finally, adding an attention mechanism further improves the performance, achieving a sensitivity of 90.77% at 4 FPs, with an improvement of almost 10% at 0.5 FP over the best reported results.

Table 1. Detection performance of different methods and our ablation study.

Methods	0.5	1	2	4	8	16	Runtime
Faster R-CNN [7]	56.90	67.26	75.57	81.62	85.83	88.74	32 ms
Mask R-CNN [3]	39.82	52.66	65.58	77.73	85.54	91.80	-
ULDor (Tang et al. [12])	52.86	64.80	74.84	84.38	87.17	91.80	-
3DCE (Yan et al. [13])	62.48	73.37	80.70	85.65	89.09	91.06	114 ms
original RetinaNet [6]	45.80	54.17	62.50	69.80	75.34	79.48	28 ms
+ anchor optimization	64.82	74.98	82.29	87.87	92.20	94.90	31 ms
+ dense supervision	70.24	78.28	85.10	90.39	93.81	96.01	39 ms
+ attention gate	**72.15**	**80.07**	**86.40**	**90.77**	**94.09**	**96.32**	41 ms

4 Conclusion

Our improved RetinaNet shows impressive performance on CT lesion detection outperforming state-of-the-art by a significant margin. Interestingly, we could show that by task-specific optimization of an out-of-the-box detector we already achieve results superior than the best reported in the literature. Exploitation of clinically available RECIST annotations bears great promise as large amounts of such training data should be available in many hospitals. With a sensitivity of about 91% at 4 FPs per image, our system may reach clinical readiness. Future work will focus on new applications such as whole-body MRI in oncology.

Acknowledgements. This project has received funding from the European Research Council (ERC) under the European Union's Horizon 2020 research and innovation programme (grant agreement No. 757173, project MIRA, ERC-2017-STG).

References

1. Cai, J., et al.: Accurate weakly-supervised deep lesion segmentation using large-scale clinical annotations. In: Frangi, A.F., Schnabel, J.A., Davatzikos, C., Alberola-López, C., Fichtinger, G. (eds.) MICCAI. LNCS, vol. 11073, pp. 396–404. Springer, Heidelberg (2018). https://doi.org/10.1007/978-3-030-00937-3_46
2. Eisenhauer, E.A., Therasse, P., Bogaerts, J., Schwartz, L.H., et al.: New response evaluation criteria in solid tumours: revised RECIST guideline (version 1.1). Eur. J. Cancer **45**(2), 228–247 (2009)
3. He, K., Gkioxari, G., Dollár, P., Girshick, R.: Mask R-CNN. In: Proceedings of the IEEE International Conference on Computer Vision, pp. 2961–2969 (2017)
4. Jaeger, P.F., et al.: Retina U-Net: Embarrassingly simple exploitation of segmentation supervision for medical object detection. arXiv preprint arXiv:1811.08661 (2018)
5. Lin, T.Y., Dollár, P., Girshick, R., He, K., Hariharan, B., Belongie, S.: Feature pyramid networks for object detection. In: Proceedings of the IEEE Conference on Computer Vision and Pattern Recognition, pp. 2117–2125 (2017)

6. Lin, T.Y., Goyal, P., Girshick, R., He, K., Dollár, P.: Focal loss for dense object detection. In: Proceedings of the IEEE International Conference on Computer Vision, pp. 2980–2988 (2017)
7. Ren, S., He, K., Girshick, R., Sun, J.: Faster R-CNN: towards real-time object detection with region proposal networks. In: Advances in Neural Information Processing Systems, pp. 91–99 (2015)
8. Rother, C., Kolmogorov, V., Blake, A.: GrabCut: interactive foreground extraction using iterated graph cuts. ACM Trans. Graph. **23**, 309–314 (2004)
9. Schlemper, J., et al.: Attention gated networks: learning to leverage salient regions in medical images. Med. Image Anal. **53**, 197–207 (2019)
10. Simonyan, K., Zisserman, A.: Very deep convolutional networks for large-scale image recognition. arXiv preprint arXiv:1409.1556 (2014)
11. Storn, R., Price, K.: Differential evolution–a simple and efficient heuristic for global optimization over continuous spaces. J. Global Opt. **11**(4), 341–359 (1997)
12. Tang, Y., Yan, K., Tang, Y., Liu, J., Xiao, J., Summers, R.M.: ULDor: A universal lesion detector for ct scans with pseudo masks and hard negative example mining. arXiv preprint arXiv:1901.06359 (2019)
13. Yan, K., Bagheri, M., Summers, R.M.: 3D context enhanced region-based convolutional neural network for end-to-end lesion detection. In: Frangi, A.F., Schnabel, J.A., Davatzikos, C., Alberola-López, C., Fichtinger, G. (eds.) MICCAI. LNCS, vol. 11070, pp. 511–519. Springer, Heidelberg (2018). https://doi.org/10.1007/978-3-030-00928-1_58
14. Yan, K., Wang, X., Lu, L., Summers, R.M.: DeepLesion: automated mining of large-scale lesion annotations and universal lesion detection with deep learning. J. Med. Imaging **5**(3), 036501 (2018)
15. Yan, K., et al.: Deep lesion graphs in the wild: relationship learning and organization of significant radiology image findings in a diverse large-scale lesion database. In: Proceedings of the IEEE Conference on Computer Vision and Pattern Recognition, pp. 9261–9270 (2018)

X-ray Imaging

PRSNet: Part Relation and Selection Network for Bone Age Assessment

Yuanfeng Ji[1,2], Hao Chen[1], Dan Lin[3], Xiaohua Wu[1], and Di Lin[2(✉)]

[1] Imsight Medical Technology, Co., Ltd., Shenzhen, China
[2] Shenzhen University, Shenzhen, China
ande.lin1988@gmail.com
[3] Department of Computer Science and Engineering,
The Chinese University of Hong Kong, Sha Tin, Hong Kong SAR, China

Abstract. Bone age is one of the most important indicators for assessing bone's maturity, which can help to interpret human's growth development level and potential progress. In the clinical practice, bone age assessment (BAA) of X-ray images requires the joint consideration of the appearance and location information of hand bones. These kinds of information can be effectively captured by the relation of different anatomical parts of hand bone. Recently developed methods differ mostly in how they model the part relation and choose useful parts for BAA. However, these methods neglect the mining of relationship among different parts, which can help to improve the assessment accuracy. In this paper, we propose a novel part relation module, which accurately discovers the underlying concurrency of parts by using multi-scale context information of deep learning feature representation. Furthermore, based on the part relation, we explore a new part selection module, which comprehensively measures the importance of parts and select the top ranking parts for assisting BAA. We jointly train our part relation and selection modules in an end-to-end way, achieving state-of-the-art performance on the public RSNA 2017 Pediatric Bone Age benchmark dataset and outperforming other competitive methods by a significant margin.

1 Introduction

Bone age assessment (BAA) requires to interpret the maturation of bone, playing an important role in understanding the growth of human. It is utilized in an array of scenarios, such as the diagnosis and treatment of disorder of body. Generally, in clinical diagnosis, radiologists estimate the bone age by using the Graulich-Pyle (G-P) [5] and Tanner-Whitehouse (T-W) methods [12], which rely on expertise at the cost of tremendous time for observing each sample. However, due to the complex pattern of bones, different experts may provide various observations, easily leading to problematic judgements for the down-stream diagnosis and treatment. Thus, recent methods [3,13] incorporate more effective computer-aided system to assist BAA. For example, the BoneXpert [13] diagnosis system

© Springer Nature Switzerland AG 2019
D. Shen et al. (Eds.): MICCAI 2019, LNCS 11769, pp. 413–421, 2019.
https://doi.org/10.1007/978-3-030-32226-7_46

has been approved and applied in various countries. Yet, these systems require too expensive process to generate high-quality images for judging bone ages.

The latest methods [1,6,8,11,14] borrow the success of deep networks in medical image analysis [2,4], and apply deep learning framework in BAA. To address the large variation of bones with respect to positions, sizes and shapes, Pan et al. [6] and Iglovikov et al. [8] partition a bone structure into parts, and select a single part as input to train network individually. It leads to a more focused learning of invariant features, which are discriminative to bone ages. Wu et al. [14] uses the attention module to detect key parts of the hand bone. Bae et al. [1], Larson et al. [9] and Spampinato et al. [11] further extract features on multiple parts to yield richer information. However, the previous methods neglect the relationship between parts of a bone structure, which is important to select useful parts for BAA.

In this paper, we advocate the idea of building relationship between parts of the hand bone and selecting discriminative parts for BAA. Given the hand bone in X-ray images, we propose a *Part Relation Module* which connects strong-correlated parts. It enables the direct communication between parts, embedding more effective context information in part representations. Based on the part relationship, we employ a *Part Selection Module* to harness useful parts for the final estimation of bone age. Note that the part selection is done by self-supervision, without the requirement of heavy labelling effort. More importantly, the relation and selection modules form an end-to-end framework, jointly distilling the features for BAA. This enables our approach to provide more details, i.e., part relation map and part selection results, which are critical to medical analysis. Our method achieves state-of-the-art result on the public benchmark, i.e., RNSA pediatric bone age dataset. It demonstrates the effectiveness of our approach.

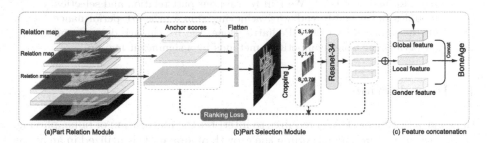

Fig. 1. Our PRSNet consists of the part relation module (a), selection module (b). Finally, we perform the feature concatenation (c) to include global feature, local feature and gender feature for estimating the bone age. (Color figure online)

2   Part Relation Module

Compared to individual parts of the hand bone, part relation provides richer information for understanding the importance of different parts, and yields more accurate information for BAA. But recent methods use independent parts to learn assessment models, which are oblivious to part relations. The latest works compute global representation on the whole image, and implicitly models part relation. However, the whole image is insensitive to positions, sizes and shapes of parts, making it difficult to construct effective representations.

In this paper, we propose the part relation module to discover the useful relationship between parts for BAA. As illustrated in Fig. 1(a), given an X-ray image, we use a CNN to compute different levels of convolutional feature maps (see the blue blocks). Each feature map is used to compute a corresponding relation map for modelling part relation. In the relation map, we produce high responses for strongly-correlated parts of the corresponding hand bone, while suppressing irrelevant regions. At each level, we use the convolutional feature map and the associated relation map to produce the context representation of correlated parts. We use all levels of context representations to provide more detailed information, for precisely scoring parts that have variant spatial and appearance properties.

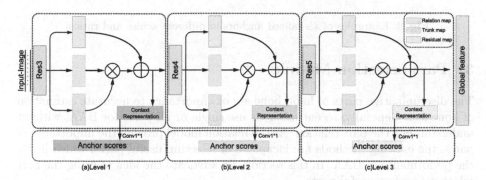

Fig. 2. The architecture of the part relation module. At each level, the convolutional feature map of backbone network undergoes different convolutional operations to yield relation map, trunk map and residual map. The new feature maps are used to compute the context representation, which is fed to estimate anchor scores in the part selection module (see Fig. 3).

More formally, we use a backbone ResNet-34 [7] to produce a set of convolutional feature maps $\{X_i\}$. The feature map X_i is output by the residual block at the ith level. As shown in Fig. 2, we apply different 1×1 convolutional operations on the feature map X_i to produce the relation map R_i, trunk map T_i and residual map D_i, respectively. Then we compute the context representation of correlated parts as:

$$F_i = T_i \cdot \sigma(R_i) + D_i, \qquad (1)$$

where σ is sigmoid activation function. In Eq. (1), we apply the sigmoid activation function to the relation map R_i, yielding an activation map. The new activation map plays as an information adaptor. It scores the part information contained in the trunk map T_i, by respecting the importance of parts. To avoid missing part information during the scoring process, we combine the residual map D_i with the scored part information to form the context representation F_i. As shown in Fig. 2, F_i is fed to the next level for producing the context representation F_{i+1}. Using Eq. 1, we compute context representations $\{F_i\}$ at all levels. Each level of context representation is used for scoring parts for the further selection process, as we will describe below.

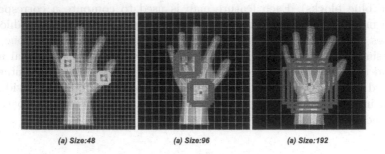

(a) Size:48   (a) Size:96   (a) Size:192

Fig. 3. Examples of visualized anchors in different scales and ratios.

3   Part Selection Module

The discriminative parts of hand bone are of importance to accurate estimation of bone age. Generally, recent methods use single or all parts for BAA, without understanding the part relation. As the relation model provide the importance of parts, the existing methods are incapable of selecting useful parts, which limits the performance of BAA. In this section, we advocate the idea of using the part relation to select useful parts.

We propose a part selection module to select the important parts, which are used to construct the representation for BAA. Given an X-ray image, our part selection module employs a set of anchors $\{A_n\}$ to represent the part candidates for selection. Note that anchors have different sizes and ratios, and span over the entire image to cover potential parts, as illustrated in Fig. 3.

Next, we conduct a scoring process on each anchor, as illustrated in Fig. 1(b). This is done by using different levels of context representations, which are provided by the part relation module, to regress a set of scores $\{S_n\}$ for all anchors. Here, we resort to the convention of object detection [10] and use lower/higher levels of representation to compute scores for smaller/larger anchors. Given the scores for all anchors, we sort the set of scores at all levels, then we employ the non-maximum suppression to eliminating overlapping anchors. and select top-M anchors having highest scores in the image. By following the top-M order of the selected anchors, we crop the corresponding image regions from the X-ray image. These image regions are resized uniformly, and each region is fed to another ResNet-34 for producing a feature vector. We sum all regions' feature vectors as a local feature. Together, we concatenate the local feature F_{local}, global feature F_{global} (i.e., the highest level of context representation) and gender feature F_{gender} (i.e., a one-hot vector) for predicting the bone age (see Fig. 1(c)).

To jointly train the part relation and selection modules, we employ the ranking loss [15] that measures the quality of part relation and selection. As illustrated in Fig. 4, given the selected parts, we associate them with anchor scores. We use each selected part to estimate a bone age, which is compared to the ground-truth age for computing a confidence. Here, the intuition is that the useful part, which has higher anchor score, contributes to the prediction of bone age that is similar to the ground-truth. Thus, the ranking loss for part relation and selection modules is computed as:

$$L_{rank} = \sum_{(i,j)} \mathbb{1}(C_j > C_i) max((1 - S_i - S_j), 0), \qquad (2)$$

where we denote S_i as the anchor score for the ith selected part. Given the ith selected part, C_i is the confidence formulated as:

$$C_i = 1 - \sigma(-|y_i - y^*|), \qquad (3)$$

where σ also means the sigmoid activation function. y_i means the predicted bone age by using the feature vector computed on i^{th} selected part, and y^* is the ground-truth bone age. The confidence measures the difference between the predicted age and the ground-truth age. By using Eq. (2), we compare each pair of parts. In the case where a part has higher anchor score but leads to lower confidence, by comparing to another part, the ranking loss proposes a penalty to guide the training of network.

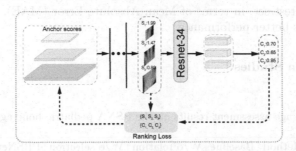

Fig. 4. The ranking loss uses anchor scores and confidences to supervise the network training.

4   Network Training

For network training, we use an objective function, which includes the ranking loss for relation and section module and L2-loss for the final prediction of bone age. The objective function is formulated as:

$$L_{total} = L_{rank} + |\dot{y} - y^*|^2. \qquad (4)$$

We construct PRSNet with the open-source Pytorch toolkit. We use different ResNet-34 models in the part relation and selection modules, respectively. In the part relation module, we employ the layers $res3$, $res4$ and $res5$ of the ResNet-34 model to compute anchor scores and select top-3 anchors over all levels. In the selection module, each anchor is used to extract a feature vector on the corresponding layer ($res3$, $res4$ or $res5$) of another ResNet-34 model. During the network training, we augment X-ray images with conventional strategies, i.e., horizontal flipping, rotation, shifting and scaling. We use SGD to optimize PRSNet, where each mini-batch consists of 16 512×512 images. We set the initial learning rate to 1e−3, and decay the learning rate by 10 after every 25 epochs. We train the network on 2 TITAN XP, for 100 epochs that need 5 hours totally. The BAA process on a testing image requires 20 ms. On average, our PRSNet increases the training/testing time by 10%, in comparison with the baseline network.

5   Experiments

5.1   Dataset and Pre-processing

We evaluate PRSNet on the dataset of RSNA 2017 Pediatric Bone Age Challenge. Totally, this dataset contains 12611 X-ray images for training and 200 images for testing. To reduce noise from background in X-ray images, we conduct a lightweight annotation on 200 images to train a foreground segmentation model. Below, we use the trained segmentation model to remove background and select regions of hand bones for training and testing PRSNet. We report all results on the test set, in terms of Mean Absolute Error (MAE). Smaller score of MAE means better performance.

5.2   Ablation Studies

Table 1. Bone age assessment results on the RSNA pediatric bone age test dataset.

Method	Baseline	W/o relation	W/o selection	PRSNet
MAE	6.52	5.05	5.20	**4.49**

First, we exam the effect on the BBA task by removing the key components of PRSNet, i.e., relation and selection modules. Without these modules, the whole model degrades to the baseline ResNet-34, which yields the score of 6.52 MAE. It lags far behind our full model in terms of BBA accuracy. In Table 1, we test the network without using part relation maps. Here, the part relation module degrades to a basic ResNet-34 model, which yields the score of 5.05 MAE. Comparably, our full model achieves a better score of 4.49 MAE. This is because the relation module provides relevant part information, which is useful for constructing context representation. Next, we disable the part selection module. In this case, we omit the local feature vector and only concatenate the global feature and gender feature for BAA. This model produces a score of 5.20 MAE, which is significantly lower than the result of our full model. Note that hand bone contains useless parts, which embed redundant information to the final feature vector. It demonstrates the effectiveness of our selection module in terms of choosing useful part information (Fig. 5).

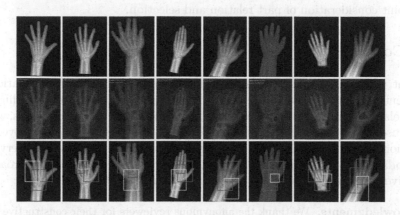

Fig. 5. Visualization of part relation and selection results. Given the input images (fist row), the part relation module produce the relation maps (middle row) and the selection module produces the top-3 anchors (last row).

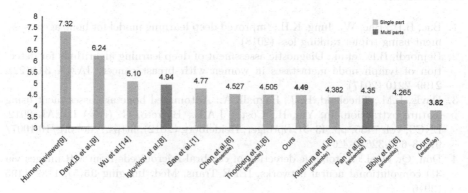

Fig. 6. Comparison with different approaches on the testing set. (Color figure online)

5.3 Comparsion with State-of-the-Arts

In Fig. 6, we compare our PRSNet with state-of-the-art methods in terms of the accuracy of BAA. We divide the compared methods into two groups. In the first group, the methods (marked in yellow) select a single part for BAA. Compared to this kind of methods, our PRSNet yields better performance, since our approach provides richer context information of different parts. In the second group, similar to our approach, the methods (marked in blue) also choose multiple parts for BAA. However, this kind of methods neither model part relation nor select parts according to their importance. Thus, our approach outperforms these methods. For a fair comparison with methods (see [6] in Fig. 6) that ensemble several deep models, we train several PRSNets with different random initializations. We achieve a better result than other methods, demonstrating the effectiveness of our joint consideration of part relation and selection.

6 Conclusion

Recent progress on bone age assessment benefits from context information of different parts. In this paper, we have proposed a novel scheme for modeling the part relation. Our method uses relation maps to activate concurrent parts, which form useful context information. Furthermore, the part relation improves the selection of parts for BAA, and the part selection module provides supervision for updating the relation model. We have demonstrated that our approach is effective and outperforms the state-of-the-art on the public benchmarks.

Acknowledgments. We thank the anonymous reviewers for their constructive comments. This work was supported in part by NSFC (61702338) and Shenzhen Science and Technology Program (No. JCYJ20180507182410327).

References

1. Bae, B.U., Bae, W., Jung, K.H.: Improved deep learning model for bone age assessment using triplet ranking loss (2018)
2. Bejnordi, B.E., et al.: Diagnostic assessment of deep learning algorithms for detection of lymph node metastases in women with breast cancer. JAMA **318**(22), 2199–2210 (2017)
3. Davis, L.M., Theobald, B.-J., Bagnall, A.: Automated bone age assessment using feature extraction. In: Yin, H., Costa, J.A.F., Barreto, G. (eds.) IDEAL 2012. LNCS, vol. 7435, pp. 43–51. Springer, Heidelberg (2012). https://doi.org/10.1007/978-3-642-32639-4_6
4. Dou, Q., et al.: Automatic detection of cerebral microbleeds from MR images via 3D convolutional neural networks. IEEE Trans. Med. Imaging **35**(5), 1182–1195 (2016)
5. Greulich, W.W., Pyle, S.I., Todd, T.W.: Radiographic Atlas of Skeletal Development of the Hand and Wrist, vol. 2. Stanford University Press, Stanford (1959)
6. Halabi, S.S., et al.: The RSNA pediatric bone age machine learning challenge. Radiology **290**(2), 498–503 (2018)
7. He, K., Zhang, X., Ren, S., Sun, J.: Deep residual learning for image recognition. In: Proceedings of the IEEE Conference on Computer Vision and Pattern Recognition, pp. 770–778 (2016)

8. Iglovikov, V.I., Rakhlin, A., Kalinin, A.A., Shvets, A.A.: Paediatric bone age assessment using deep convolutional neural networks. In: Stoyanov, D., et al. (eds.) DLMIA/ML-CDS -2018. LNCS, vol. 11045, pp. 300–308. Springer, Cham (2018). https://doi.org/10.1007/978-3-030-00889-5_34

9. Larson, D.B., Chen, M.C., Lungren, M.P., Halabi, S.S., Stence, N.V., Langlotz, C.P.: Performance of a deep-learning neural network model in assessing skeletal maturity on pediatric hand radiographs. Radiology **287**(1), 313–322 (2017)

10. Lin, T.Y., Dollár, P., Girshick, R., He, K., Hariharan, B., Belongie, S.: Feature pyramid networks for object detection. In: Proceedings of the IEEE Conference on Computer Vision and Pattern Recognition, pp. 2117–2125 (2017)

11. Spampinato, C., Palazzo, S., Giordano, D., Aldinucci, M., Leonardi, R.: Deep learning for automated skeletal bone age assessment in X-ray images. Med. Image Anal. **36**, 41–51 (2017)

12. Tanner, J.M., Whitehouse, R., Cameron, N., Marshall, W., Healy, M., Goldstein, H., et al.: Assessment of Skeletal Maturity and Prediction of Adult Height (TW2 Method), vol. 16. Academic press, London (1975)

13. Thodberg, H.H., Kreiborg, S., Juul, A., Pedersen, K.D.: The BoneXpert method for automated determination of skeletal maturity. IEEE Trans. Med. Imaging **28**(1), 52–66 (2009)

14. Wu, E., et al.: Residual attention based network for hand bone age assessment. arXiv preprint arXiv:1901.05876 (2018)

15. Yang, Z., Luo, T., Wang, D., Hu, Z., Gao, J., Wang, L.: Learning to navigate for fine-grained classification, pp. 420–435 (2018)

Mask Embedding for Realistic High-Resolution Medical Image Synthesis

Yinhao Ren[1], Zhe Zhu[2], Yingzhou Li[3], Dehan Kong[4], Rui Hou[5],
Lars J. Grimm[2], Jeffery R. Marks[6], and Joseph Y. Lo[1,2,5(✉)]

[1] Department of Biomedical Engineering, Duke University, Durham, USA
{yinhao.ren,joseph.lo}@duke.edu
[2] Department of Radiology, Duke University School of Medicine, Durham, USA
{zhe.zhu,lars.grimm}@duke.edu
[3] Department of Mathematics, Duke University, Durham, USA
yinzhou.li@duke.edu
[4] Department of Automation, Beijing Institute of Technology, Beijing, China
dehan.kong@duke.edu
[5] Department of Electrical Engineering, Duke University, Durham, USA
rui.hou@duke.edu
[6] Department of Surgery, Duke University School of Medicine, Durham, USA
jeffery.marks@duke.edu

Abstract. Generative Adversarial Networks (GANs) have found applications in natural image synthesis and begin to show promises generating synthetic medical images. In many cases, the ability to perform controlled image synthesis using masked priors such as shape and size of organs is desired. However, mask-guided image synthesis is challenging due to the pixel level mask constraint. While the few existing mask-guided image generation approaches suffer from the lack of fine-grained texture details, we tackle the issue of mask-guided stochastic image synthesis via mask embedding. Our novel architecture first encodes the input mask as an embedding vector and then inject these embedding into the random latent vector input. The intuition is to classify semantic masks into partitions before feature up-sampling for improved sample space mapping stability. We validate our approach on a large dataset containing 39,778 patients with 443,556 negative screening Full Field Digital Mammography (FFDM) images. Experimental results show that our approach can generate realistic high-resolution (256×512) images with pixel-level mask constraints, and outperform other state-of-the-art approaches.

Keywords: Generative Adversarial Networks · Image synthesis · Mask embedding · Mammogram

---

Electronic supplementary material The online version of this chapter (https://doi.org/10.1007/978-3-030-32226-7_47) contains supplementary material, which is available to authorized users.

D. Shen et al. (Eds.): MICCAI 2019, LNCS 11769, pp. 422–430, 2019.
https://doi.org/10.1007/978-3-030-32226-7_47

1   Introduction

The rapid development of generative models especially on training methodology [1,9] and architecture [10], has led to the significant improvement of resolution and quality of the output images. In the image editing scenario, semantic control of the generated images such as object category and shape is highly desired. Many studies have explored conditional Generative Adversarial Networks (cGANs) [4,12] using class labels (one-hot vectors) [4] and mask labels [8]. Producing highly stochastic outputs as well as capturing the full entropy of the conditional distributions are of a great challenge for current cGANs.

Most cGANs derive from the basic generator–discriminator architecture. By adding conditional information to both the generator and the discriminator, cGANs can control some characteristics of the generated images. The most straightforward way to incorporate class label information is to directly concatenate the label vector with the latent vector in the generator and then to concatenate the conditional information with the latent features in the discriminator [12]. On the other hand, incorporating a pixel-level mask label requires special design of the networks to preserve the fine-grained texture details while satisfying the mask constraint [8].

In this paper we propose a novel approach to improve the generation of realistic high-resolution medical images with semantic control. We use a U-Net [16] style generator that takes both a **latent vector** (Gaussian noise vector) and **semantic mask**. Our generator first perform embedding of the mask input and then concatenate the mask embedding vector to the latent noise vector as the input of the feature projection path. The mask is an image providing constraints and could be an edge map, a segmentation map, a gradient field, etc.

We summarize our contributions as follows:

1. We propose to use mask embedding in semantic cGANs that takes both a mask and a random latent vector as the input. With this novel structure we can generate highly stochastic images with fine-grained details.
2. We apply the proposed approach to a medical image synthesis task, and generated realistic high-resolution images. Specifically we synthesize mammograms with a binary mask that indicates the breast shape. To our best knowledge this is the first work that can generate realistic high-resolution mammograms with semantic control.

2   Motivation

The ability to synthesize FFDM images with cancer lesions in a controlled fashion is greatly desired by the medical imaging machine learning community. Specifically, a mask-guided stochastic generator for medical image data augmentation could potentially yield gains in detection and classification algorithms given the low occupancy of pathology related pixels in most medical imaging modalities. To actually realize this gain, the generator needs to (1) have efficient mechanisms for sample space mapping to majority of the available training images (e.g. Latent Vector); (2) learn joint distribution of semantic inputs and feature realizations (e.g. Mask Embedding). This work represent the first stage for our multi-stage study to synthesize mammogram with lesions. We investigate the feasibility of synthesizing clinically normal FFDM images with mask constraint.

3 Related Work

Medical image synthesis has been a well-motivated research topic for a long time. The ability to generate infinite number of realistic looking medical phantom greatly enables studies such as virtual clinical trials and data augmentation for computer aided diagnosis algorithms.

Recently many studies have been using GANs to synthesize medical images. Those methods can be grouped into unconditioned synthesis [6,13] and conditioned synthesis [3,14,15]. There is also a detailed survey of medical image synthesis using GANs [18]. Note that mammogram synthesis using GANs has been proposed in [11], but their approach focuses on image realism and resolution in the unconditional setting, hence the shape or other morphological characteristics of their synthesized mammograms cannot be controlled.

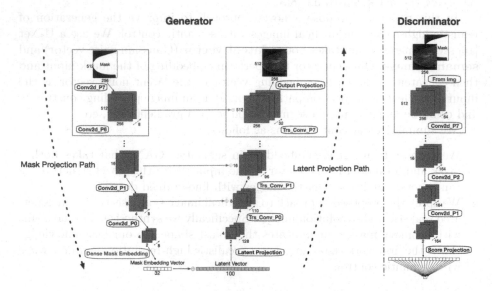

Fig. 1. Proposed architecture with two inputs to the Generator: (1) **Mask** and (2) **Latent Vector**. When doubling the dimension of the networks at beginning of each training phase, layers at the positions indicated by red boxes are newly initialized and faded in as described in the progressive training strategy for GAN [9]; For our without embedding baseline model, the **Dense Mask Embedding Layer** in the generator is removed. The latent vector input is also adjusted to a 132-dimensional vector to maintain the same amount of parameters in the latent projection path for a fair performance comparison. (Color figure online)

4 Network Architecture

The challenge to train an image translation model with latent vector input is to produce latent features that are compatible with the input mask constraint. In other words, the initial latent projection layer could produce features that fall outside the manifold constrained by the semantic mask input in the latent space, resulting in the following deconvolution layers to compensate for this inefficiency, and eventually leading to model capacity reduction. Our solution is to pose an additional constraint on the initially projected features by injecting the mask embedding vector into the input latent vector. This process allows a more efficient initial feature projection that produces latent features that are compatible with the mask input, thus preserving the output image quality.

Our model consists of a generator and a discriminator shown in Fig. 1. The key concept is to perform mask embedding in the generator before the latent feature projection layer to increase the overall feature projection efficiency. The generator follows a U-Net style design that can be divided into the **mask projection** path and the **latent projection** path. The discriminator takes the output of the generator as well as the corresponding mask and produce a probability score.

The input of the generator's mask projection path is a 256×512 mask (a binary image in our case). This mask projection path has 7 convolution layers each with a stride of 2 and depth of 8 features. The output of the mask projection path is a 32-dimensional vector (mask embedding) and is injected into the latent vector as the input of the latent projection layer. The latent vector is a 100-dimensional vector thus the input of the latent projection path is a 132-dimensional vector. Each mask projection feature block (except for the last one) is then concatenated onto the corresponding latent projection feature block to complete the U-Net structure. The initial latent feature block is produced by a dense layer followed by 7 deconvolution layers with stride of 2 and size of 4. The number of kernels of each deconvolution layer starts from 128 and decreases by a factor of 0.8 (rounded to the nearest integer) in each following layer. The output of the projection layer is the synthesized image.

5 Progressive Training

We used the progressive training strategy for GAN [9]. The training was divided into 7 phases. In each phase we doubled the network dimensions and gradually faded in the newly added layer. The model was grown from the resolution of 4×8 to 256×512. We stopped at this resolution due to hardware limitation. We adjusted the batch size and learning rate for each phases so that the standard WGAN-GP [5] converging mechanism can be achieved. We trained our model on three 1080 Ti for approximately a week to reach the maximum resolution. For each phase we train the network until the discriminator loss converges and no further observable improvement is made on the synthesized images. More details can be found in our open sourced implementation.

6 Experiments

6.1 Dataset

We used the mammography dataset collected from our institution. The dataset contains 39,778 negative screening subjects. Each exam has at least 4 images (Craniocaudal view and Mediolateral oblique view for each side of the breast), resulting in 443,556 images in total. The pixel values are truncated and normalized to $[0,1]$ using the window level settings provided by the DICOM header. Each image was padded and resized to 256×512. For each mammography image a binary skin mask is generated using Otsu thresholding, where 1 denotes breast region and 0 denotes background. For comparison against the pix2pix model [8], we extracted the edge map of each mammography images using Sobel filters in both horizontal and vertical direction and then overlay the texture map with the corresponding skin mask.

6.2 Results

Several example results using randomly sampled skin masks and latent vectors are shown in Fig. 2. We compared our proposed model with the pix2pix model and our baseline model without embedding mechanism. Our proposed model generates mammograms with much more realistic texture details.

6.3 Comparison to Pix2Pix Method

We compare the results of our approach with the well-known pix2pix image translation model that takes only semantic mask as input. Results are shown in Fig. 3(c). Due to the image transformation nature of this model, our first approach using a smooth skin mask as the only input failed to generate any meaningful texture details. In order to evaluate the response of pix2pix model to perturbation of mask input, we constructed the texture map as mentioned in Sect. 6.1. Even trained on masks with the prior information of high frequency tissue structures, the standard pix2pix model still under performs our proposed model in terms of fine-grained texture details and variety of parenchymal patterns generated. The pix2pix result lacks stochasticity in which a very limited mapping between mask input space and sample space is possible, thus limiting the output variation. Moreover, the same problem limits training stability since the model is forced to map similar input binary patterns with drastically different realization of tissue structures without having the proper mechanism.

6.4 Comparison to Baseline Method

We explore the effect of mask embedding mechanism by removing the mask embedding layer from our proposed model and training this baseline model from scratch. The design of our baseline model is equivalent to Tub-GAN [19]. The

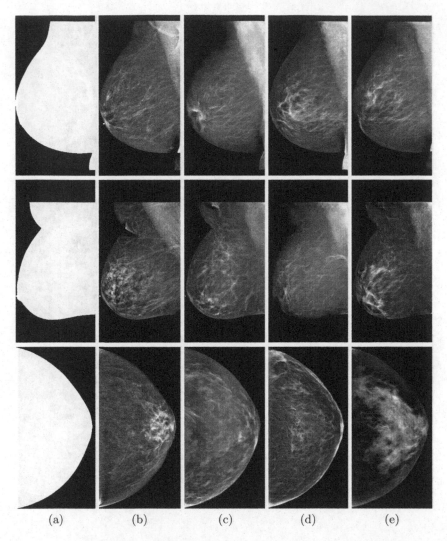

(a)   (b)   (c)   (d)   (e)

Fig. 2. (a) Input mask. (b) Original mammogram. (c), (d), (e) Generated mammograms using our mask embedding approach with different random latent vectors.

latent input vector is adjusted to be 100+32 so that the total number of parameters in the latent projection layer stays the same to our proposed model. The exact same training schedule for our proposed model is repeated. The results are shown in Fig. 3(d). The generated images have more high resolution details compared to pix2pix mode, but lack parenchyma complexity and usually contain obvious artifacts formed during up-sampling. This is an indication of model losing capacity due to the constraint posed by the mask input. A larger collection of comparison images can be found in supplementary material.

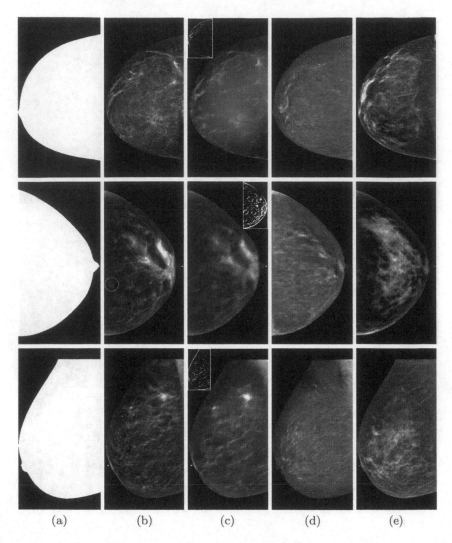

(a)   (b)   (c)   (d)   (e)

Fig. 3. (a) Input mask. (b) Original mammogram. (c) Synthesized mammogram using Pix2Pix. (d) Synthesized mammogram using our approach without mask embedding. (e) Synthesized mammogram using our approach with mask embedding.

6.5   Evaluation

For natural image generation there have been several objective metrics to measure the performance of the generative models such as Inception Score [17], Mode Score [2] and Fréchet Inception Distance [7], in medical image generation however there is no such metric available. Thus we design a reader study and let the expert radiologists assess the realism and quality of the synthesized results.

We randomly picked 50 real breast masks and generated mammograms using the three different approaches: pix2pix, our approach without mask embedding and our approach using mask embedding. All images were presented to readers in random order. Two expert radiologists were asked to rate each mammogram using 5 scores (5: definitely realistic, 4: realistic, 3: neutral, 2: fake, 1: definitely fake). The averaged score for real mammograms, synthesized results using pix2pix, synthesized results using our approach without and **with mask embedding** are 3.78, 1.08, 1.34, **2.38** respectively. Although subjective, these numerical results confirm that our approach with mask embedding provides a considerable improvement in realism.

7   Conclusion

We have proposed to use binary mask constraint to guide image synthesis while preserving output variety and fine-grained texture details. The challenge was to compensate for the generator capacity reduction caused by the pixel-level mask constraint. Our solution is to use mask embedding to further guide the initial projection of latent features to increase the probability of latent features falling within the manifold constrained by the mask. Our approach enables the semantic control of the synthesized mammograms while ensuring the fine-grained texture details are looking realistic. This technique can potentially be applied to other high resolution medical image modalities as well as natural images.

Acknowledgments. This work was supported in part by NIH/NCI U01-CA214183 and U2C-CA233254, and an equipment donation by NVIDIA Corporation.

References

1. Arjovsky, M., Chintala, S., Bottou, L.: Wasserstein generative adversarial networks. In: Precup, D., Teh, Y.W. (eds.) Proceedings of the 34th International Conference on Machine Learning, vol. 70, pp. 214–223 (2017)
2. Che, T., Li, Y., Jacob, A.P., Bengio, Y., Li, W.: Mode regularized generative adversarial networks. CoRR abs/1612.02136 (2016)
3. Costa, P., et al.: End-to-end adversarial retinal image synthesis. IEEE Trans. Med. Imaging **37**(3), 781–791 (2018)
4. Goodfellow, I., et al.: Generative adversarial nets. In: Ghahramani, Z., Welling, M., Cortes, C., Lawrence, N.D., Weinberger, K.Q. (eds.) Advances in Neural Information Processing Systems, vol. 27, pp. 2672–2680 (2014)
5. Gulrajani, I., Ahmed, F., Arjovsky, M., Dumoulin, V., Courville, A.C.: Improved training of Wasserstein GANs. In: Guyon, I., et al. (eds.) Advances in Neural Information Processing Systems, pp. 5767–5777 (2017)
6. Han, C., et al.: GAN-based synthetic brain MR image generation. In: 2018 IEEE 15th International Symposium on Biomedical Imaging (ISBI 2018), pp. 734–738, April 2018. https://doi.org/10.1109/ISBI.2018.8363678
7. Heusel, M., Ramsauer, H., Unterthiner, T., Nessler, B., Klambauer, G., Hochreiter, S.: GANs trained by a two time-scale update rule converge to a Nash equilibrium. CoRR abs/1706.08500 (2017)

8. Isola, P., Zhu, J.Y., Zhou, T., Efros, A.A.: Image-to-image translation with conditional adversarial networks. In: The IEEE Conference on Computer Vision and Pattern Recognition (CVPR), July 2017
9. Karras, T., Aila, T., Laine, S., Lehtinen, J.: Progressive growing of GANs for improved quality, stability, and variation. CoRR abs/1710.10196 (2017)
10. Karras, T., Laine, S., Aila, T.: A style-based generator architecture for generative adversarial networks. CoRR abs/1812.04948 (2018)
11. Korkinof, D., Rijken, T., O'Neill, M., Yearsley, J., Harvey, H., Glocker, B.: High-resolution mammogram synthesis using progressive generative adversarial networks. CoRR abs/1807.03401 (2018)
12. Mirza, M., Osindero, S.: Conditional generative adversarial nets. arXiv e-prints arXiv:1411.1784, November 2014
13. Moradi, M., Madani, A., Karargyris, A., Syeda-Mahmood, T.F.: Chest X-ray generation and data augmentation for cardiovascular abnormality classification, p. 57, March 2018
14. Nie, D., et al.: Medical image synthesis with deep convolutional adversarial networks. IEEE Trans. Biomed. Eng. **65**(12), 2720–2730 (2018)
15. Nie, D., et al.: Medical image synthesis with context-aware generative adversarial networks. In: Descoteaux, M., Maier-Hein, L., Franz, A., Jannin, P., Collins, D.L., Duchesne, S. (eds.) MICCAI 2017. LNCS, vol. 10435, pp. 417–425. Springer, Cham (2017). https://doi.org/10.1007/978-3-319-66179-7_48
16. Ronneberger, O., Fischer, P., Brox, T.: U-net: convolutional networks for biomedical image segmentation. CoRR abs/1505.04597 (2015)
17. Salimans, T., et al.: Improved techniques for training GANs. In: Lee, D.D., Sugiyama, M., Luxburg, U.V., Guyon, I., Garnett, R. (eds.) Advances in Neural Information Processing Systems, vol. 29, pp. 2234–2242 (2016)
18. Yi, X., Walia, E., Babyn, P.: Generative adversarial network in medical imaging: a review. CoRR abs/1809.07294 (2018)
19. Zhao, H., Li, H., Maurer-Stroh, S., Cheng, L.: Synthesizing retinal and neuronal images with generative adversarial nets. Med. Image Anal. **49**, 14–26 (2018)

TUNA-Net: Task-Oriented UNsupervised Adversarial Network for Disease Recognition in Cross-domain Chest X-rays

Yuxing Tang[1(✉)], Youbao Tang[1], Veit Sandfort[1], Jing Xiao[2],
and Ronald M. Summers[1]

[1] National Institutes of Health, Clinical Center, Bethesda, MD, USA
{yuxing.tang,rms}@nih.gov
[2] Ping An Technology Co., Ltd., Shenzhen, China

Abstract. In this work, we exploit the unsupervised domain adaptation problem for radiology image interpretation across domains. Specifically, we study how to adapt the disease recognition model from a labeled source domain to an unlabeled target domain, so as to reduce the effort of labeling each new dataset. To address the shortcoming of cross-domain, unpaired image-to-image translation methods which typically ignore class-specific semantics, we propose a task-driven, discriminatively trained, cycle-consistent generative adversarial network, termed TUNA-Net. It is able to preserve (1) low-level details, (2) high-level semantic information and (3) mid-level feature representation during the image-to-image translation process, to favor the target disease recognition task. The TUNA-Net framework is general and can be readily adapted to other learning tasks. We evaluate the proposed framework on two public chest X-ray datasets for pneumonia recognition. The TUNA-Net model can adapt labeled adult chest X-rays in the source domain such that they appear as if they were drawn from pediatric X-rays in the unlabeled target domain, while preserving the disease semantics. Extensive experiments show the superiority of the proposed method as compared to state-of-the-art unsupervised domain adaptation approaches. Notably, TUNA-Net achieves an AUC of 96.3% for pediatric pneumonia classification, which is very close to that of the supervised approach (98.1%), but without the need for labels on the target domain.

1 Introduction

While deep convolutional neural networks (CNNs) have achieved encouraging results across a number of tasks in the medical imaging domain, they frequently suffer from generalization issues due to source and target domain divergence.

Electronic supplementary material The online version of this chapter (https://doi.org/10.1007/978-3-030-32226-7_48) contains supplementary material, which is available to authorized users.

D. Shen et al. (Eds.): MICCAI 2019, LNCS 11769, pp. 431–440, 2019.
https://doi.org/10.1007/978-3-030-32226-7_48

Examples of such divergence include distribution shift caused by images collected with distinct protocols, from different institutions or patient groups. This can be alleviated by *supervised domain adaptation* (SDA) [2,13], which adapts certain layers of the model that trained with large amounts of well-labeled source data, with additional moderate amounts of labeled target data. However, obtaining abundant labels in each new, unseen domain is a non-trivial and laborious process that relies heavily on skilled clinicians in the majority of clinical applications. Alternatively, *unsupervised domain adaptation* (UDA) [10] aims to mitigate the harmful effects of domain divergence when transferring knowledge from a supervised (labeled) source domain to an unsupervised (unlabeled) target domain. Because of its potential benefits for medical image processing, UDA of deep learning models has attracted many researchers' attention [1,7,12].

Adversarial adaptation methods [5,10] have become increasingly popular with the recent success of generative adversarial networks (GANs) [3] and their variants [14]. In medical imaging, most of the previous work for adversarial adaptation focuses on lesion or organ segmentation [1,7,12,13]. For instance, Kamnitsas *et al.* [7] derive domain-invariant features by an adversarial network for brain lesion segmentation of MR images from two different datasets. GAN-based image-to-image (I2I) translation methods [14] are also widely used to generate medical images cross modalities to help adaptation. For example, Zhang *et al.* [12] segment multiple organs in unlabeled X-ray images with labeled digitally reconstructed radiographs rendered from 3D CT volumes, using I2I translation. Zhang *et al.* [13] improve Cycle-GAN [14] by introducing shape-consistency for CT and MRI cardiovascular 3D image translation to help organ segmentation. Though CT and MR images are not necessarily paired, the shape-consistency loss requires supervision of pixel-wise annotations from both domains. Chen *et al.* [1] preserve semantic structural information of the lungs in chest radiographs (X-rays) for cross-dataset lung segmentation.

All the previous methods deal with limited domain shift or large organs appearing at approximately fixed positions with clear boundaries, or both. Moreover, they do not necessarily preserve **class-specific** semantic information of lesions or abnormalities in the process of distribution alignment. An illustrative example is, when translating an adult X-ray into a pediatric X-ray, there is no guarantee that fine-grained disease content on the original image will be explicitly transferred. The capability of preserving class-specific semantic context across domains is crucial for medical imaging analysis for certain clinically relevant tasks, such as disease classification or detection [8,9]. However, to our best knowledge, solutions to this problem of adversarial adaptation for medical imaging are limited.

In this paper, we present a novel framework to tackle the target task of disease recognition in cross-domain chest X-rays. Specifically, we proposed a task-oriented unsupervised adversarial network (TUNA-Net) for pneumonia (findings on X-rays are airspace opacity, lobar consolidation, or interstitial opacity) recognition in cross-domain X-rays. Two visually discrepant but intrinsically related domains are involved: adult and pediatric chest X-rays. The TUNA-Net consists of a cyclic I2I translation framework with class-aware semantic constraint modules. In the absence of labels from one domain, the proposed model is able to (1) synthesize "radio-realistic" (i.e., a synthesized radiograph that appears anatomically realistic) images with sufficient low-level details across two different domains, (2) preserve high-level class-specific semantic contextual information during translation, (3) regularize learned mid-level features of real and synthetic target domains to be similar, (4) optimize the objective functions simultaneously to generalize to the unlabeled domain. We demonstrate the effectiveness of our approach on two public chest X-ray datasets of sufficient domain shift for pneumonia recognition.

2 Method

2.1 Problem Formulation

In this work, we focus on the problem of unsupervised domain adaptation, where we are given a source domain A with both images X_A (e.g., adult X-rays) and labels Y_A (e.g., normal or pneumonia), and a target domain P with only images X_P (e.g., pediatric X-rays), but no labels. The goal is to learn a classification model $\mathcal{F}$ from images of both domains but with only source labels and predict the labels in the target domain. Note that X_A are naturally unpaired with Y_P as these images are from two different patient populations (adults and children).

A naive baseline method is to learn $\mathcal{F}$ solely from source images and labels, then apply it directly on target domain. While $\mathcal{F}$ performs well on data with similar distribution as the source data, it typically leads to degraded performance on the target data because of domain divergence. To alleviate this effect, we follow previous methods [12–14] to map images from two domains ($X_A \leftrightarrows X_P$) using multi-domain I2I translation with unpaired training data. During translation, we add constraints at different levels to preserve both holistic and fine-grained class-specific image content. Consequently, the model $\mathcal{F}$ learned on the source domain can be well generalized to the target domain. The flowchart of the proposed framework for UDA is shown in Fig. 1.

2.2 Pixel-Level Image-to-image Translation with Unpaired Images

GANs [3] have been widely used for image-to-image translation. Given unpaired images from two domains, we adopt Cycle-GAN [14] to first learn two mappings: $A \to P$ and $P \to A$, with two generators $G_{A \to P}(X_A)$ and $G_{P \to A}(X_P)$, so that discriminators D_P and D_A can not distinguish between real and synthetic images generated by G. For $G_{A \to P}$ and its discriminator D_P, the objective is expressed as the *adversarial learning loss*:

$$\mathcal{L}_{\text{adv}}(G_{A \to P}, D_P) = \mathbb{E}_{x_a \sim X_A}[\log(1 - D_P(G_{A \to P}(x_a)))] + \mathbb{E}_{x_p \sim X_P}[\log D_P(x_p)]. \quad (1)$$

A similar adversarial loss can be designed for mapping $G_{P \to A}$ and its discriminator D_A as well: i.e., $\min_{G_{P \to A}} \max_{D_A} \mathcal{L}_{\text{adv}}(G_{P \to A}, D_A)$.

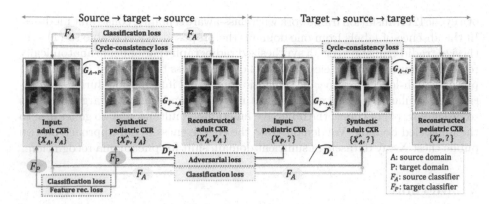

Fig. 1. The framework of TUNA-Net. The question we investigate is whether class-specific semantics can be preserved in an I2I translation framework (*e.g.*, Cycle-GAN [14]) to help domain adaptation, providing disease labels only in source domain (*e.g.*, translate an adult chest X-ray into a pediatric chest X-ray while preserving disease semantics, i.e., normal or pneumonia). In test phase, model $\mathcal{F}_P$ is applied on target pediatric images to make predictions. In this figure, for inputs from both domains, top two examples are normal, bottom two examples are with pneumonia.

To preserve sufficient low-level content information for domain adaptation, we then use the *cycle consistency loss* [14] to force the reconstructed synthetic images x'_a and x'_p to resemble their inputs x_a and x_p:

$$\mathcal{L}_{\text{cyc}}(G_{A \to P}, G_{P \to A}) = \mathbb{E}_{x_a \sim X_A}[\|x'_a - x_a\|_1] + \mathbb{E}_{x_p \sim X_P}[\|x'_p - x_p\|_1], \quad (2)$$

where $x'_a = G_{P \to A}(G_{A \to P}(x_a))$ and $x'_p = G_{A \to P}(G_{P \to A}(x_p))$, $\|\cdot\|_1$ is the l_1 norm.

The generative adversarial training with cycle-consistency enables synthesizing realistic looking radiographs across domains. However, there is no guarantee that high-level semantics would be preserved during translation. For example, when translating an adult X-ray with lung opacities, sometimes it might be converted into a normal pediatric X-ray without opacities, since the disease semantics are not explicitly modelled in the learning process.

2.3   High-Level Class-Specific Semantics Modelling

To preserve high-level class-specific semantic information indicating abnormalities in the image before and after translation, we propose to explicitly model disease labels into the translation framework by incorporating auxiliary classification models with source labels.

A source classification model $\mathcal{F}_A$ is first learned on the labeled source data $A = \{X_A, Y_A\}$ using a cross-entropy loss to classify C categories:

$$\mathcal{L}_{\text{cls}}(\mathcal{F}_A, A) = -\mathbb{E}_{a \sim A} \sum_{c=1}^{C} \mathbb{1}_c \log \left(\sigma(\mathcal{F}_A^{(c)}(x_a)) \right), \quad (3)$$

where σ is the softmax function, $\mathbb{1}_c = 1$ if an input image x_a belongs to class $c \in C$, otherwise $\mathbb{1}_c = 0$. We then enforce the learned $\mathcal{F}_A$ to perform similarly on the reconstructed source data $A' = \{G_{P \to A}(G_{A \to P}(X_A)), Y_A\}$ to minimize $\mathcal{L}_{\text{cls}}(\mathcal{F}_A, A')$. In this way, the high-level class specific content is preserved within the *source* $\to$ *target* $\to$ *source* cycle.

To retain similar semantics within the *target* $\to$ *source* $\to$ *target* cycle in the absence of target labels Y_P, we learn a target classification model $\mathcal{F}_P$ (fine-tuned from $\mathcal{F}_A$) on synthetic target images to minimize $\mathcal{L}_{\text{cls}}(\mathcal{F}_P, \{G_{A \to P}(X_A), Y_A\})$, in the mean time, minimizing $\mathcal{L}_{\text{cls}}(\mathcal{F}_A, \{G_{P \to A}(X_P), \arg\max(\mathcal{F}_P(X_P))\})$, so that classifiers in both domains produce consistent predictions to keep semantic consistency. The total *semantic classification loss* is:

$$\mathcal{L}_{\text{cls}}(\mathcal{F}_A, \mathcal{F}_P) = \mathcal{L}_{\text{cls}}(\mathcal{F}_A, A) + \mathcal{L}_{\text{cls}}(\mathcal{F}_A, A') + \mathcal{L}_{\text{cls}}(\mathcal{F}_P, \{G_{A \to P}(X_A), Y_A\})$$
$$+ \mathcal{L}_{\text{cls}}(\mathcal{F}_A, \{G_{P \to A}(X_P), \arg\max(\mathcal{F}_P(X_P))\}). \tag{4}$$

By modelling disease labels into the translation network, the synthesized images maintain meaningful semantics to favor the target clinically relevant task. For instance, $\mathcal{F}_P$ can be acted as a disease classifier on the target domain.

2.4 Mid-Level Feature Regularization

Inspired by the perceptual loss [6] that encourages image before and after translation to be perceptually similar, we impose *feature reconstruction loss*, to encourage real target image X_P and synthetic target image $G_{(A \to P)}(X_A)$ to be similar in the feature space. Using this feature regularization in training for middle layers of CNNs also tends to generate images that are visually indistinguishable from target domain referring to our experiments. The feature reconstruction loss is the normalized Euclidean distance between feature representations:

$$\mathcal{L}_{\text{feat}}(\mathcal{F}_P) = \sum_i \frac{\|f_i - \hat{f}_i\|_2^2}{H_i W_i C_i}, \tag{5}$$

where i is a convolutional block from target model $\mathcal{F}_P$, and f_i and $\hat{f}_i$ are features maps of size $H_i \times W_i \times C_i$ output by the ith convolutional block.

2.5 Final Objective and Implementation Details

The final objective of TUNA-Net is the sum of adversarial learning losses, cycle-consistency loss, semantic classification loss and feature reconstruction loss:

$$\mathcal{L} = \mathcal{L}_{\text{adv}}(G_{A \to P}, D_P) + \mathcal{L}_{\text{adv}}(G_{P \to A}, D_A)$$
$$+ \lambda \mathcal{L}_{\text{cyc}}(G_{A \to P}, G_{P \to A}) + \mathcal{L}_{\text{cls}}(\mathcal{F}_A, \mathcal{F}_P) + \mathcal{L}_{\text{feat}}(\mathcal{F}_P). \tag{6}$$

Driven by the target task of disease recognition, this corresponds to optimizing the objective for the adapted target model $\mathcal{F}_P$.

We adopt Cycle-GAN [14] for training the I2I translation framework. We use 9 residual blocks [4] for the generator network for an input X-ray image of size 512×512. For source classification networks $\mathcal{F}_A$, we use ImageNet pre-trained ResNet with 18 layers [4] as a trade-off between performance and GPU memory usage. The target classification model $\mathcal{F}_P$ is fine-tuned from the source model $\mathcal{F}_A$ hence has the same network structure with $\mathcal{F}_A$. Feature maps of $conv\_3$ ($56 \times 56 \times 128$) and $conv\_4$ ($28 \times 28 \times 256$) are extracted from $\mathcal{F}_P$ as mid-level feature representations to calculate the reconstruction loss. λ in Eq. 6 is set to 10 as in [14]. All other networks are trained from scratch with a batch size of 1, an initial learning rate of 0.0002 for first 100 epochs and linearly decay to 0 in the next 100 epochs. All the network components are optimized using the Adam solver. The TUNA-Net is implemented using the PyTorch framework. All the experiments are run on a 32 GB NVIDIA Tesla V-100 GPU.

3   Experiments

Material and Settings: We extensively evaluate the proposed TUNA-Net for unsupervised domain adaptation on two public chest X-ray datasets containing normal and pneumonia frontal view X-rays, i.e., an adult chest X-ray dataset used in the RSNA Pneumonia Detection Challenge[1] (a subset of the NIH Chest X-ray 14 [11]) and a pediatric chest X-ray dataset[2] from Guangzhou Women and Children's Medical Center in China. We set the adult dataset as **source** domain and the pediatric dataset as **target** domain. For the adult dataset, we use 6993 normal X-rays and 4659 X-rays with pneumonia. For the pediatric dataset, we use 5232 X-rays (either normal (n = 1349) or abnormal with pneumonia (n = 3883), but labels were removed in our setting) for training and validation. The combined dataset are used to train the adult ⇆ pediatric translation framework. 5-fold cross-validation is performed. Classification performance of the proposed adaptation method is evaluated on a hold-out test of 624 pediatric X-rays (normal: 234, pneumonia: 390) from the target domain.

Reference Methods: Although unsupervised adversarial domain adaptation methods exist in medical imaging field, they are mainly designed for segmentation. Here we compare the performance of our proposed TUNA-Net with the following five relevant reference models:

1. **NoAdapt:** A ResNet-50 [4] CNN trained on adult X-rays is applied to the pediatric X-rays for pneumonia prediction. This serves as a lower bound method.
2. **Cycle-GAN [14]:** Without considering labels indicating diseases in X-rays during I2I translation using [14]. A model trained on labeled real adult X-rays is applied to synthetic adult X-rays generated from pediatric X-rays.

---

[1] https://www.kaggle.com/c/rsna-pneumonia-detection-challenge/data.
[2] https://doi.org/10.17632/rscbjbr9sj.3.

3. **ADDA** [10]: First we train an adult classification network with labeled X-rays. Then we adversarially learn a target encoder CNN such that a domain discriminator is unable to differentiate between the source and target domain. During testing, pediatric images are mapped with the target encoder to the shared feature space of the source adult domain and classified by the adult disease classifier.
4. **CyCADA** [5]: It improves upon ADDA by incorporating cycle consistency at both pixel and feature levels.
5. **Supervised:** We assume that disease labels for target domain are accessible. A supervised model can be trained and tested on labeled target domain. This servers as an upper bound method.

Quantitative Results and Ablation Studies: We calculate the Area Under the Receiver Operating Characteristic Curve (AUC), accuracy (Acc.), sensitivity (Sen.), specificity (Spec.) and F1 score to evaluate the classification performance of our model. The validation set is only used to optimize the threshold using Youden's index (i.e., max(Sen. + Spec. $-$ 1)) for normal versus pneumonia classification. The classification results of our TUNA-Net and reference methods are shown in Table 1. The baseline method without adaptation (NoAdapt) performs poorly on the target task of pediatric pneumonia recognition, though the source classifier excels in pneumonia recognition on adult chest X-rays (AUC = 98.0%). It demonstrates that the gap between the source and target domain are fairly large although they share the same disease labels. Cycle-GAN does not consider disease labels during I2I translation. It generates X-rays without preserving high-level semantics, resulting in many normal adult X-rays converted into pediatric X-rays with opacities on the lungs, or adults with lung opacities converted into normal pediatric X-rays. This hugely decreases the adaptation performance for the classification task, where correct labels are considered to be crucial. Our full TUNA-Net considers high-level class-specific semantics achieves an AUC of

Table 1. Comparison of normal versus pneumonia classification results on the test set of pediatric X-ray dataset.

Model	AUC (%)	Acc. (%)	Sen. (%)	Spec. (%)	F1
NoAdapt	89.3 ± 0.4	82.5 ± 0.3	83.6 ± 0.7	80.8 ± 0.8	0.86 ± 0.02
Cycle-GAN [14]	80.4 ± 2.5	74.2 ± 2.7	76.9 ± 3.3	69.9 ± 2.8	0.76 ± 0.04
ADDA [10]	91.8 ± 0.4	88.1 ± 0.4	88.2 ± 0.5	87.0 ± 0.4	0.89 ± 0.02
CyCADA [5]	93.5 ± 0.5	90.0 ± 0.4	90.4 ± 0.4	89.6 ± 0.5	0.91 ± 0.02
TUNA-Net	$\mathbf{96.3 \pm 0.2}$	$\mathbf{93.1 \pm 0.4}$	$\mathbf{92.9 \pm 0.3}$	$\mathbf{91.1 \pm 0.4}$	$\mathbf{0.93 \pm 0.01}$
(a) w/o feature loss	95.9 ± 0.1	91.9 ± 0.3	91.7 ± 0.3	90.6 ± 0.2	0.92 ± 0.01
(b) w/o $\mathcal{F}_A$ on rec	94.6 ± 0.2	91.3 ± 0.2	91.0 ± 0.3	91.1 ± 0.3	0.92 ± 0.01
(c) w/o $\mathcal{F}_P$, offline	94.1 ± 0.2	90.7 ± 0.2	91.0 ± 0.4	90.5 ± 0.2	0.91 ± 0.01
Supervised	98.1 ± 0.1	96.3 ± 0.1	94.6 ± 0.3	92.8 ± 0.2	0.96 ± 0.01

96.3% with both sensitivity and specificity larger than 91%. It outperforms both ADDA and CyCADA with similar settings. It is also worth noting that the performance of TUNA-Net is very close to that of the supervised model, where labeled training images on the target dataset are available. We ablate different modules in the TUNA-Net to see their influence on the final model: (a) We exclude the feature construction loss in the target classification model; (b) We do not use reconstructed images to retrain the source classification model; (c) We exclude the target classification model $\mathcal{F}_P$ in the training, but use the synthetic images to train it offline. As shown in Table 1, each component contributes to improving the final TUNA-Net. The online end-to-end learning of $\mathcal{F}_P$ with other components is crucial and contributes most to the performance improvement.

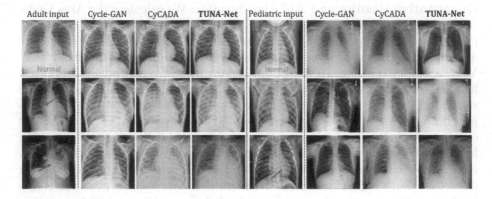

Fig. 2. Qualitative comparison of image-to-image translation. Cycle-GAN is trained without using labels indicating normal or pneumonia, while CyCADA and our TUNA-Net considers labels in source domain in training. Left part shows adult → pediatric, right shows pediatric → adult. The first row shows two normal X-rays as input. The appearances of pneumonia(s) are pointed by arrows. Please refer to supplementary material for higher resolution images.

Qualitative Results: We show some qualitative image-to image translation examples in Fig. 2. Cycle-GAN failed to preserve important semantic information during transfer. CyCADA is able to preserve certain high-level semantics but not as robust as the proposed TUNA-Net. TUNA-Net retains image content of various levels: from low-level content, mid-level features, to high-level semantics. For example, for the bottom left adult input, Cycle-GAN removes the pathology while our TUNA-Net perfectly preserves it. The synthetic X-rays by TUNA-Net are most close to the input source image semantically and to the target domain anatomically.

Discussion: We specifically focused on normal versus pneumonia classification on a cross-domain setting. We showed that the I2I translation framework can be constrained using semantic classification components to preserve class-specific disease content for medical image synthesis. We used two public chest X-ray datasets with sufficient domain shift to demonstrate the ability of our unsupervised domain adaptation method. The domain adaptation from adult to pediatric chest X-rays is natural and intuitive. For example, medical students and radiology residents learn in a similar way: they first learn to read adult chest X-rays, and then they transfer the learned knowledge to pediatric X-rays.

4   Conclusion

In this paper, we investigated how knowledge about class-specific labels can be transferred from a source domain to an unlabeled target domain for unsupervised domain adaptation. Using adversarially learned cross-domain image-to-image translation networks, we found clear evidence that semantic labels could be translated across medical image domains. The proposed TUNA-Net is general and has the potential to be extended to more disease classes (*e.g.*, pneumothorax), other image modalites (such as CT and MRI) and more clinically relevant tasks.

Acknowledgments. This research was supported by the Intramural Research Program of the National Institutes of Health Clinical Center and by the Ping An Technology Co., Ltd. through a Cooperative Research and Development Agreement. The authors thank NVIDIA for GPU donations.

References

1. Chen, C., Dou, Q., Chen, H., Heng, P.-A.: Semantic-aware generative adversarial nets for unsupervised domain adaptation in chest X-ray segmentation. In: Shi, Y., Suk, H.-I., Liu, M. (eds.) MLMI 2018. LNCS, vol. 11046, pp. 143–151. Springer, Cham (2018). https://doi.org/10.1007/978-3-030-00919-9_17
2. Ghafoorian, M., et al.: Transfer learning for domain adaptation in MRI: application in brain lesion segmentation. In: Descoteaux, M., Maier-Hein, L., Franz, A., Jannin, P., Collins, D.L., Duchesne, S. (eds.) MICCAI 2017. LNCS, vol. 10435, pp. 516–524. Springer, Cham (2017). https://doi.org/10.1007/978-3-319-66179-7_59
3. Goodfellow, I., et al.: Generative adversarial nets. In: NIPS (2014)
4. He, K., et al.: Deep residual learning for image recognition. In: CVPR (2016)
5. Hoffman, J., et al.: CyCADA: cycle consistent adversarial domain adaptation. In: ICML (2018)
6. Johnson, J., Alahi, A., Fei-Fei, L.: Perceptual losses for real-time style transfer and super-resolution. In: Leibe, B., Matas, J., Sebe, N., Welling, M. (eds.) ECCV 2016. LNCS, vol. 9906, pp. 694–711. Springer, Cham (2016). https://doi.org/10.1007/978-3-319-46475-6_43
7. Kamnitsas, K., et al.: Unsupervised domain adaptation in brain lesion segmentation with adversarial networks. In: Niethammer, M., et al. (eds.) IPMI 2017. LNCS, vol. 10265, pp. 597–609. Springer, Cham (2017). https://doi.org/10.1007/978-3-319-59050-9_47
8. Tang, Y.X., et al.: Deep adversarial one-class learning for normal and abnormal chest radiograph classification. In: Medical Imaging: CAD (2019)

9. Tang, Y., Wang, X., Harrison, A.P., Lu, L., Xiao, J., Summers, R.M.: Attention-guided curriculum learning for weakly supervised classification and localization of thoracic diseases on chest radiographs. In: Shi, Y., Suk, H.-I., Liu, M. (eds.) MLMI 2018. LNCS, vol. 11046, pp. 249–258. Springer, Cham (2018). https://doi.org/10.1007/978-3-030-00919-9_29
10. Tzeng, E., et al.: Adversarial discriminative domain adaptation. In: CVPR (2017)
11. Wang, X., et al.: ChestX-ray8: hospital-scale chest X-ray database and benchmarks on weakly-supervised classification and localization of common thorax diseases. In: CVPR (2017)
12. Zhang, Y., Miao, S., Mansi, T., Liao, R.: Task driven generative modeling for unsupervised domain adaptation: application to X-ray image segmentation. In: Frangi, A.F., Schnabel, J.A., Davatzikos, C., Alberola-López, C., Fichtinger, G. (eds.) MICCAI 2018. LNCS, vol. 11071, pp. 599–607. Springer, Cham (2018). https://doi.org/10.1007/978-3-030-00934-2_67
13. Zhang, Z., et al.: Translating and segmenting multimodal medical volumes with cycle- and shape-consistency generative adversarial network. In: CVPR (2018)
14. Zhu, J.Y., et al.: Unpaired image-to-image translation using cycle-consistent adversarial networks. In: ICCV (2017)

Misshapen Pelvis Landmark Detection by Spatial Local Correlation Mining for Diagnosing Developmental Dysplasia of the Hip

Chuanbin Liu[1], Hongtao Xie[1(✉)], Sicheng Zhang[2], Jingyuan Xu[1], Jun Sun[2],
and Yongdong Zhang[1]

[1] School of Information Science and Technology,
University of Science and Technology of China, Hefei 230026, China
htxie@ustc.edu.cn
[2] Anhui Provincial Children's Hospital, Hefei 230026, China

Abstract. Developmental dysplasia of the hip (DDH) refers to an abnormal development of the hip joint in infants. Accurately detecting and identifying the pelvis landmarks is a crucial step in the diagnosis of DDH. Due to the temporal diversity and pathological deformity, it is a difficult task to detect the misshapen landmark and diagnose the DDH illness condition for both human expert and computer. Moreover, there is no adequate and public dataset of DDH for research. In this paper, we investigate the spatial local correlation with convolutional neural network (CNN) for misshapen landmark detection. First, we convert the detection of a landmark to the detection of the landmark's local neighborhood patch, which yields effective spatial local correlation for the identification of a landmark. Then, a deep learning based method named FR-DDH network, is proposed for misshapen pelvis landmark detection. It mines the spatial local correlation and detects the best-matched region according to the spatial local correlation. To the end, the landmarks are located at the center of the regions. Besides, a dataset with 9813 pelvis X-ray images is constructed for research in this area, and it will be released for public research. To the best of our knowledge, this is the first attempt to apply deep learning in the diagnosis of DDH. Experimental results show that our approach achieves an excellent precision in landmark location (MAE 1.24 mm) and illness diagnosis over human experts.

Keywords: Developmental dysplasia of the hip · Landmark
detection · Spatial local correlation

1 Introduction

Developmental dysplasia of the hip (DDH) refers to a spectrum of hip joint abnormalities ranging from mild acetabular dysplasia to irreducible hip joint dislocation. It is the most common pediatric hip disorder, affecting 0.16% to

© Springer Nature Switzerland AG 2019
D. Shen et al. (Eds.): MICCAI 2019, LNCS 11769, pp. 441–449, 2019.
https://doi.org/10.1007/978-3-030-32226-7_49

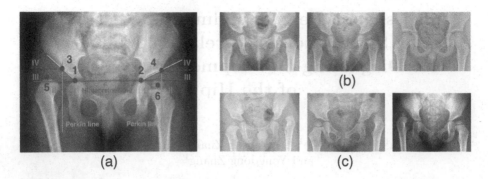

Fig. 1. The diagnosis of developmental dysplasia of the hip. (a) shows the principle of the diagnostic standard, and the key landmarks are: (1) right tri-radiate cartilage center (RTCC), (2) left tri-radiate cartilage center (LTCC), (3) right acetabulum superolateral margin (RASM), (4) left acetabulum superolateral margin (LASM), (5) right femoral head (RFH), (6) left femoral head (LFH). (b) shows the examples of the temporal diversity of DDH. (c) shows the examples of the pathological deformity of DDH.

2.85% of all newborns [1]. The traditional diagnostic methods rely mainly on Xray or Ultrasound images of the pelvis and hip [2,3], and Xray is the primary tool in diagnosing DDH after 6 months of age. Figure 1(a) gives the principle of Xray diagnosis standards. The most important references for Xray DDH diagnosis are the Hilgenreiner's line, the Perkin's line and the femoral head, which are strictly relying on the location of pelvis landmarks. However, the landmarks detection for DDH is a challenging task, because (1) during the different stages of skeleton calcification, the landmarks appear with diversity in shape as Fig. 1(b), (2) different grades of dislocation will lead to varying deformity as Fig. 1(c). The temporal diversity and pathological deformity lead DDH diagnosis a time-consuming and experience-sensitive task for orthopedists. Therefore, it suffers from high inter-exam variability and low accuracy. With the development of machine learning [4,5], to overcome these defects, a series of Computer-Aided Diagnosis (CAD) methods have been proposed [1,6–9].

Related Work: Several CAD methods have been proposed for Xray DDH diagnosis. Bashir et al. [8] propose an edge detection method to measure the acetabular angle from the X-ray images. But the miscalculating *"can result from the incomplete development of femur head for infants less than 6 months"*. Similarly, Sahin et al. [9] present a template-matching method for measuring acetabular angles by finding the obturator foramen. However, patients with *"distorted shape of the obturator foramen are not suitable for this approach"*. Bier et al. [10] put forward a sequential prediction framework to detect pelvic anatomical landmarks. Yet, it exhibits poor robustness and *"is susceptible to scenarios not included in training"*. To sum up, existing methods are inapplicable to deal with the temporal diversity and pathological deformity in DDH.

Recently, Arik et al. [11] propose a convolutional neural network system for cephalometric landmarks detection. To overcome the deformity of pathological cases, an image patch with pre-defined size centered at landmark l is extracted as the local neighborhood. The local neighborhood yields effective spatial local correlation for the identification of a landmark, and CNN exhibits well-suited performance in exploiting spatial local correlation by imposing local connectivity patterns. This method performs a CNN forward pass on each sliding window without sharing computation. Consequently, the training is expensive in space and time, and the landmark detection is slow.

Contribution: The local neighborhood around a landmark yields effective spatial local correlation, which can be strong identification of the landmark. To overcome the temporal diversity and pathological deformity challenge in DDH, in this paper, we convert the detection of a landmark to the detection of the landmark's local neighborhood patch. Then, a deep learning based method named FR-DDH network, is proposed for pelvis landmark detection. It mines the spatial local correlation and detects the best-matched region with CNN. To the end, the landmarks are located at the center of the regions. Besides, a dataset with 9813 pelvis X-ray images is constructed for research in this area, which will be public in the future. To the best of our knowledge, this is the first attempt to apply deep learning in the diagnosis of DDH. Experimental results show that our approach achieves a excellent precision in landmark location (MAE 1.24 mm) and illness diagnosis over human experts.

2 Method

Overall Framework: Figure 2 illustrates the overall FR-DDH framework for Xray DDH diagnosis. The neighbourhood image patch centered at landmark l is extracted as detection target, and FR-DDH is trained to detect the patch from a pelvis image. For an input image, a series of convolutional layers are applied to mine the spatial local correlation and generate the high-dimensional feature map. Then the local neighborhood region proposals are generated by Region Proposal Network (RPN), according to the feature map. Combing the region proposals and the feature map by ROI pooling, FR-DDH predicts the categories of the region and their bounding-box regression offsets, and generates the detection result of each image patch. Finally, the specific landmark is located at the center of the patch, and we get the diagnosis result according to the landmarks.

Local Image Patch Extraction: To detect the landmark l with temporal diversity and pathological deformity, the spatial local correlation around landmark l should be learned from the images in the training set. We extract the $(2N + 1) \times (2N + 1)$ image patch centered at landmark l as the local neighborhood, as Fig. 2 shows, where N is sufficiently large to visually recognize the landmark. Hence, we convert the detection of a landmark to the detection of

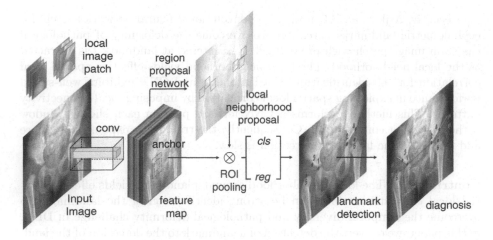

Fig. 2. The framework of our FR-DDH. [Best viewed in color] (Color figure online)

the landmark's local neighbourhood patch, which yields effective spatial local correlation for the identification of a landmark.

Spatial Local Correlation Mining: In FR-DDH, We use ResNet101 with weights trained on ImageNet as feature extraction network. ResNet101 exhibits strong ability in mining spatial local correlation by imposing local connectivity patterns and merging feature map with skip connection. The images are rescaled to $h \times 600 \times 3$ by repeating 3 times to use pretrained weights. The shorter side is rescaled to 600 while the longer side is rescaled to h. After a series of hierarchical *conv*, FR-DDH mines the spatial local correlation and outputs a 2048-D feature map.

Region Proposal and Landmark Detection: Figure 3 illustrates the framework of region proposal and landmark detection of FR-DDH. RPN uses the generated 2048-D feature maps for generating local neighborhood region proposals, each with an objectness score. As proposed by Faster-RCNN [12], we slide a network over the convolutional feature map of the conv5 layer in a sliding-window fashion. This network is fully connected to a spatial window of the convolutional feature map with a 3×3 convolutional layer. Region proposals are relative reference boxes to anchors centered at each sliding window. Each anchor is related with a scale of size 128 and 256 pixels and aspect ratios of $1 : 1$.

Once the local neighborhood region proposal is generated, FR-DDH combines the region proposals and the feature map by ROI pooling. Each proposal is pooled into a fixed-size feature map and then mapped to a feature vector by fully connected layers. Then, each feature vector branches into two sibling output layers: *cls* layer for classifying the categories of local neighborhood, and *reg* layer for regressing the bounding box coordinates. The landmark is finally detected on the center of the local neighborhood region.

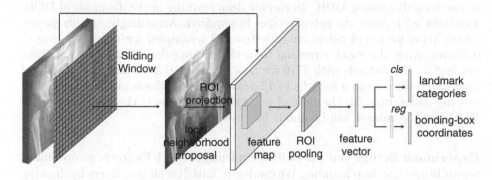

Fig. 3. The framework of Region proposal and landmark detection.

Loss Function for Learning: We minimize an objective function following the multi-task loss in Faster R-CNN [12]. Our loss function for an image is defined as:

$$L\left(\{p_i\}, \{t_i\}\right) = \frac{1}{N_{cls}} \sum_i L_{cls}\left(p_i, p_i^*\right) + \lambda \frac{1}{N_{reg}} \sum_i p_i^* L_{reg}\left(t_i, t_i^*\right) \tag{1}$$

The classification layer *cls* outputs a discrete probability $\{p_i\}(0 \leq i \leq K)$ over $K+1$ (landmarks + background) categories and the regression layer *reg* outputs $\{t_i\}$ bounding-box regression offsets a predicted tuple $t^u = \left(t_x^u, t_y^u, t_w^u, t_h^u\right)$ for class u. Here, i is the index of an anchor in a mini-batch and p_i is the predicted probability of anchor i being an local neighborhood patch. The ground-truth label p_i^* is 1 if the anchor is positive, and is 0 if the anchor is negative. t_i is a vector representing the 4 parameterized coordinates of the predicted bounding box, and t_i^* is ground-truth box associated with a positive anchor.

The classification loss L_{cls} is a log loss over $K + 1$ categories:

$$L_{cls}(p, u) = -\log p_u. \tag{2}$$

The regression loss L_{reg} is a smooth L1 function:

$$\text{smooth}_{L1}(x) = \begin{cases} 0.5x^2 & \text{if } |x| < 1 \\ |x| - 0.5 & \text{otherwise} \end{cases} \tag{3}$$

The term $p_i^* L_{reg}$ means the regression loss is activated only for positive anchors ($p_i^* = 1$) and is disabled otherwise ($p_i^* = 0$). The two terms are normalized with N_{cls}, N_{reg} and a balancing weight λ, which is set to 10.

3 Experiments and Results

Data: We note that there is no public DDH dataset, which seriously limits the research on diagnosing DDH. To employ deep learning in the diagnosis of DDH, a dataset with adequate pelvis images is required. Accordingly, in this paper, 24000 X-ray images of pelvis are collected and resampled with pixel spacing as 0.15 mm. After the strict screening from the orthopedist, 9813 images of them are kept in the dataset, with 7710 for training and 2103 for testing. The age of each case ranges from 3 months to 12 years, and the illness involves normal to terrible dislocation. To the best of our knowledge, this is the first dataset for DDH and the dataset will be public for research[1].

Experiment Setup: Our FR-DDH is implemented with PyTorch, an optimized tensor library for deep learning. We randomly initialize all new layers by drawing weights from a zero-mean Gaussian distribution with standard deviation of 0.01. And the other layers (i.e., the shared convolutional layers) are initialized by ResNet101 pretrained from ImageNet. We use a learning rate of 0.001 for 80k mini-batches, and 0.0001 for the next 30k mini-batches on the dataset. The momentum is set to be 0.9 and the weight decay is set to be 0.0005. The FR-DDH is trained on a Ubuntu workstation with one NVIDIA GeForce 1080Ti GPU, and it takes one day for training the model.

Evaluation Metric: To validate the accuracy of our method, we define the landmark-specific point-to-point error for landmark l as

$$PEL_l = \left(\sum_{i=1}^{n} \|m_{li} - a_{li}\| \right) / n. \tag{4}$$

Here n represents the number of images, m represents the manually labeled landmarks and a represents the automatically identified landmark. The average point-to-point errors (PE) is defined as the average of PEL_l as

$$PE = \sum_{l=1}^{k} \frac{PEL_l}{k} = \sum_{l=1}^{k} \sum_{i=1}^{n} \frac{\|m_{li} - a_{li}\|}{nk}. \tag{5}$$

Here k represents the number of landmarks. We also report the successful detection rate (SDR) which gives the percentage of images for which a landmark l is located within a precision range $z \in \{1.5\,\text{mm}, 2.0\,\text{mm}, 3.0\,\text{mm}\}$ as

$$SDR_l = \# \{i : \|m_{li} - a_{li}\| \leq z\} / n \times 100 \tag{6}$$

---

[1] The dataset, diagnosis method and evaluation code will be released at https://github.com/liuboss1992/FR-DDH.

Result: A series of experiments have been conducted with different scales of local neighborhood patch, where N ranges from 50 to 100. Table 1 shows the relationship between neighborhood region scale N and average point-to-point error PE. In FR-DDH, the $(2N+1) \times (2N+1)$ image patch centered at landmark l is extracted as the local neighborhood. An image patch with small N may not provide adequate spatial local correlation, hence the detection accuracy will be low. Meanwhile, an image patch with oversized N may introduce extraneous information, which will also lead to low accuracy. We achieve the best accuracy with $PE = 1.244\,\text{mm}$ when $N = 80$.

Table 1. Relationship between neighborhood region scale and point-to-point error. For RTCC, LTCC, ..., LFH, please refer to Fig. 1.

PEL_l (pixel)	FR-DDH $N = 50$	FR-DDH $N = 60$	FR-DDH $N = 70$	FR-DDH $N = 80$	FR-DDH $N = 90$	FR-DDH $N = 100$
Average	1.295	1.281	1.277	**1.244**	1.276	1.282
RTCC	1.464	1.518	**1.449**	1.459	1.464	1.459
LTCC	1.569	1.627	1.588	1.601	**1.544**	1.587
RASM	1.170	1.173	**1.104**	1.152	1.172	1.226
LASM	1.277	1.294	1.458	**1.258**	1.331	1.332
RFM	1.069	0.999	**0.953**	0.992	1.013	1.003
LFH	1.223	1.074	1.111	**1.002**	1.130	1.085

As is illustrated in Table 2, we conduct contrast experiment with other baseline for measuring the Acetabular Index. We follow Bashir's work [8] to take absolute error (AE) and average accuracy (AA) as the evaluation metric. Compared with Bashir's work which employs an edge detection approach for landmark detection, our FR-DDH achieves lower error and higher accuracy. In addition, Bashir evaluates its model on only 24 infants. By contrast, our FR-DDH is evaluated on a wider variety of 2000+ infants. The comparison fully shows the reliability and robustness of FR-DDH.

Table 2. Performance on measuring the Acetabular Index.

Method	AE		AA	
	Right	Left	Right	Left
Bashir [8]	3.78°	2.95°	83.60%	85.40%
FR-DDH	**2.32°**	**2.36°**	**87.80%**	**87.20%**

Figure 4 presents the successful detection rate for each landmark of FR-DDH, when $N = 80$. Almost 95% landmarks can be detected within $z = 3\,\text{mm}$, which is a reliable performance for clinical use. With the accurate detection of landmarks, FR-DDH further diagnoses the illness of DDH. Compared with the diagnosis result from domain expert, FR-DDH obtains precision of 92.8% and recall of 97.5%. By contrast, a general doctor obtains precision of 89.9% and recall of 91.5% in our research. FR-DDH achieves excellent performance in illness diagnosis over human experts. The details of the diagnosis code will be released in our provided link.

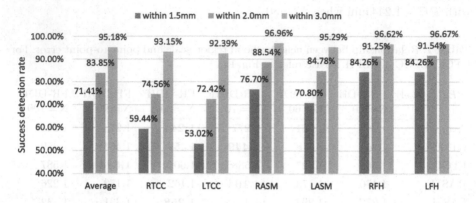

Fig. 4. Success detection rates of each landmark in FR-DDH, when N is set to be 80.

4 Conclusion

This paper puts forward FR-DDH, a novel approach for misshapen pelvis landmarks detection of DDH by mining the spatial local correlation of neighborhood region. The temporal diversity and pathological deformity bring challenges for anatomical landmark detection. We investigate the spatial local correlation for misshapen landmark detection, and convert the detection of a landmark to the detection of the landmark's local neighborhood patch. Besides, a dataset with 9813 pelvis X-ray images is constructed for this task, and it will be released for public research. This work can be an enlightening reference and be generalized for numerous anatomical landmark detection tasks.

Acknowledgements. This work is supported by the Huawei-USTC Joint Innovation Project on Machine Vision Technology (FA2018111122).

References

1. Quader, N., Hodgson, A.J., Mulpuri, K., Cooper, A., Abugharbieh, R.: A 3D femoral head coverage metric for enhanced reliability in diagnosing hip dysplasia. In: Descoteaux, M., Maier-Hein, L., Franz, A., Jannin, P., Collins, D.L., Duchesne, S. (eds.) MICCAI 2017. LNCS, vol. 10433, pp. 100–107. Springer, Cham (2017). https://doi.org/10.1007/978-3-319-66182-7_12

2. Ruiz Santiago, F., et al.: Imaging of hip pain: from radiography to cross-sectional imaging techniques. Radiol. Res. Pract. **2016** (2016)
3. Atweh, L.A., Kan, J.H.: Multimodality imaging of developmental dysplasia of the hip. Pediatr. Radiol. **43**(1), 166–171 (2013)
4. Liu, A.A., Su, Y.T., Nie, W.Z., Kankanhalli, M.: Hierarchical clustering multi-task learning for joint human action grouping and recognition. IEEE Trans. Pattern Anal. Mach. Intell. **39**(1), 102–114 (2016)
5. Xie, H., Yang, D., Sun, N., Chen, Z., Zhang, Y.: Automated pulmonary nodule detection in CT images using deep convolutional neural networks. Pattern Recogn. **85**, 109–119 (2019)
6. Paserin, O., Mulpuri, K., Cooper, A., Hodgson, A.J., Garbi, R.: Real time RNN based 3D ultrasound scan adequacy for developmental dysplasia of the hip. In: Frangi, A.F., Schnabel, J.A., Davatzikos, C., Alberola-López, C., Fichtinger, G. (eds.) MICCAI 2018. LNCS, vol. 11070, pp. 365–373. Springer, Cham (2018). https://doi.org/10.1007/978-3-030-00928-1_42
7. Paserin, O., Mulpuri, K., Cooper, A., Hodgson, A.J., Abugharbieh, R.: Automatic near real-time evaluation of 3D ultrasound scan adequacy for developmental dysplasia of the hip. In: Cardoso, M.J., et al. (eds.) CARE/CLIP -2017. LNCS, vol. 10550, pp. 124–132. Springer, Cham (2017). https://doi.org/10.1007/978-3-319-67543-5_12
8. Al-Bashir, A.K., Al-Abed, M., Sharkh, F.M.A., Kordeya, M.N., Rousan, F.M.: Algorithm for automatic angles measurement and screening for developmental Dysplasia of the Hip (DDH). In: 37th Annual International Conference of the IEEE, EMBC 2015, pp. 6386–6389. IEEE (2015)
9. Sahin, S., Akata, E., Sahin, O., Tuncay, C., Özkan, H.: A novel computer-based method for measuring the acetabular angle on hip radiographs. Acta orthopaedica et traumatologica turcica **51**(2), 155–159 (2017)
10. Bier, B., et al.: X-ray-transform invariant anatomical landmark detection for Pelvic Trauma surgery. In: Frangi, A.F., Schnabel, J.A., Davatzikos, C., Alberola-López, C., Fichtinger, G. (eds.) MICCAI 2018. LNCS, vol. 11073, pp. 55–63. Springer, Cham (2018). https://doi.org/10.1007/978-3-030-00937-3_7
11. Arik, S.Ö., Ibragimov, B., Xing, L.: Fully automated quantitative cephalometry using convolutional neural networks. J. Med. Imaging **4**(1), 014501 (2017)
12. Ren, S., He, K., Girshick, R., Sun, J.: Faster R-CNN: towards real-time object detection with region proposal networks. In: Advances in Neural Information Processing Systems, pp. 91–99 (2015)

Adversarial Policy Gradient for Deep Learning Image Augmentation

Kaiyang Cheng[1,2(✉)], Claudia Iriondo[1,2], Francesco Calivá[2], Justin Krogue[3],
Sharmila Majumdar[2], and Valentina Pedoia[2]

[1] University of California, Berkeley, USA
{victorcheng21,iriondo}@berkeley.edu
[2] Department of Radiology and Biomedical Imaging,
University of California, San Francisco, USA
{francesco.caliva,sharmila.majumdar,valentina.pedoia}@ucsf.edu
[3] University of California, San Francisco, USA
justin.krogue@ucsf.edu

Abstract. The use of semantic segmentation for masking and cropping input images has proven to be a significant aid in medical imaging classification tasks by decreasing the noise and variance of the training dataset. However, implementing this approach with classical methods is challenging: the cost of obtaining a dense segmentation is high, and the precise input area that is most crucial to the classification task is difficult to determine a-priori. We propose a novel joint-training deep reinforcement learning framework for image augmentation. A segmentation network, weakly supervised with policy gradient optimization, acts as an agent, and outputs masks as actions given samples as states, with the goal of maximizing reward signals from the classification network. In this way, the segmentation network learns to mask unimportant imaging features. Our method, Adversarial Policy Gradient Augmentation (APGA), shows promising results on Stanford's MURA dataset and on a hip fracture classification task with an increase in global accuracy of up to 7.33% and improved performance over baseline methods in 9/10 tasks evaluated. We discuss the broad applicability of our joint training strategy to a variety of medical imaging tasks.

Keywords: Deep reinforcement learning · Adversarial training · Semantic segmentation · Image augmentation

1 Introduction

Convolutional neural networks (CNNs) have become an essential part of medical image acquisition, reconstruction, and post-processing pipelines, as this technology significantly improves our ability to detect, study, and predict diseases

Funded by National Institute of Arthritis and Musculoskeletal and Skin Diseases.
K. Cheng and C. Iriondo—These authors contributed equally to this paper.

D. Shen et al. (Eds.): MICCAI 2019, LNCS 11769, pp. 450–458, 2019.
https://doi.org/10.1007/978-3-030-32226-7_50

at scale. In computer-vision, CNNs have achieved above-human performance in natural-object classification tasks [8]. However, in medical imaging, where datasets are limited in size and labels are often uncertain, there is still a significant need for methods that maximize information gain while preventing overfitting. Our work presents a novel reinforcement-learning (RL) based image augmentation framework for medical image classification.

Training data image augmentation imposes image-level regularization on CNNs in order to combat overfitting. Augmentation can include the addition of noise, image transformations such as zooming or cropping, image occlusion, and attention masking [10]. The application of the first three methods is limited as they often rely on domain-knowledge to define the appropriate characteristics and severity of the augmentation. The last method requires dense segmentation masks for the region of interest (ROI). However, ROIs relevant to a classification task may not be known *a-priori*. For instance, when inspecting hip radiographs for bone fracture (Fx), the determination of Fx or no-Fx heavily depends on the location of abnormal signal within the bone and abnormalities from nearby tissues. Our RL image augmentation framework leverages an adversarial reward to weakly supervise a segmentation network and create these ROIs.

Through trial-and-error, reinforcement learning algorithms discover how to maximize their objective or reward R. The careful design of reward functions has enabled the application of RL to multiple medical tasks including landmark detection, automatic view planning, treatment planning, and MR/CT reconstruction. In this work, we present APGA, a joint, reinforcement learning strategy for training of a segmentation network and a classification network, that improves accuracy in the classification task.

2   Methodology

2.1   Improving Classification with Segmentation for Image Masking

The framework has two parts: a classification model with parameters θ_c and a segmentation model with parameters (policy) θ_p.

To mask out the image-level features that are less useful for the classification task, we use the segmentation model to produce the pixel-wise probability p_k of the pixel being useful. We zero out the pixels of the original image with $p_k < 0.5$, and use it for training the classification model, updating θ_c. With the end-goal of improving the classification performance, our method optimizes the segmentation model to evaluate the importance of each image pixel.

2.2   Policy Gradient Training

Following the policy gradient context [11], our segmentation model is seen as a policy in which the image batch is treated as a state s_t, whereas the pixel-wise classification of useful image features is framed as an action a_t. In practice, at each t-th training step, the classification model receives the masked image as the input and outputs a reward signal R_t. To accomplish this, our objective is to maximize the expected reward $J(\theta_p)$ and find the optimal segmentation policy.

$$J(\theta_p) = E_{P(a_t;\theta_p)}[R_t] \tag{1}$$

In Eq. 1, $E_{P(a_t;\theta_p)}$ is the expected reward with respect to the probability of taking an action a_t, when the model has been parameterized with θ_p. The policy is learned through back-propagation, which requires the definition of the gradient of the expected reward with respect to the model parameters. Following the REINFORCE rule presented in [11], the gradient can be defined as

$$\nabla_{\theta_p} J(\theta_p) = E_{P(a_t;\theta_p)}[\nabla_{\theta_p} \log(P(a_t|s_t;\theta_p)) \cdot R_t] \tag{2}$$

The expected reward cannot be estimated and requires approximation. As is common practice in the tractation of policy gradient, we can achieve such approximation using the negative log-likelihood loss, which is differentiable with respect to the model parameters, and can be properly weighted by the reward signal to obtain the segmentation policy loss presented in Eq. 3

$$\mathscr{L} = \mathscr{L}_{BCE}(P(a_t|s_t;\theta_p), a_t) \cdot R_t \tag{3}$$

where $\mathscr{L}_{BCE}$ is the binary cross-entropy loss

$$\mathscr{L}_{BCE}(\widehat{y}, y) = -\frac{1}{N} \sum_{i=1}^{N} y_i \cdot \log(\widehat{y}_i) + (1 - y_i) \cdot \log(1 - \widehat{y}_i) \tag{4}$$

which becomes Eq. 5.

$$\mathscr{L}_{BCE}(P(a_t|s_t;\theta_p), a_t) = -\frac{1}{N} \sum_{i=1}^{N} \Big[a_t \cdot \log(P(a_t|s_t;\theta_p)) \\ + (1 - a_t) \cdot \log(1 - P(a_t|s_t;\theta_p)) \Big]_i \tag{5}$$

By using pixel-wise binary cross entropy, we can achieve preservation of spatial information of the deviation of $P(a_t|s_t)$ from a_t. We then update θ_p by computing $\nabla_{\theta_p}\mathscr{L}$. Consequently, the classification model parameters θ_p are updated with gradient descent by using the cross entropy loss between the classification of the masked image samples and the original target labels. In our experiments, we perform stochastic gradient update for both θ_p and θ_c at each batch step.

2.3   Adversarial Reward

The design of the reward is crucial to the convergence of the segmentation model. Using the change in training loss as a reward, as is done in Neural Architecture Search [12], results in a weak reward signal hardly discernible from the expected changes in loss during training. Similarly, approximating rewards with a critic

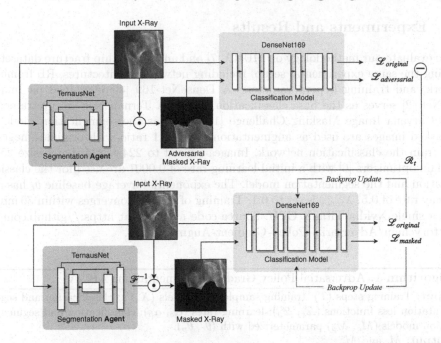

Fig. 1. (top) Adversarial training of segmentation agent and (bottom) training of classification model with original and augmented data

network introduces unnecessary overhead and slows down convergence. We propose a stable adversarial reward R_t. Given pixel-wise feature importance probability $p_k = P(a_t|s_t;\theta_p)$, we zero out the pixels $p_k > 0.5$ to mask-out the features predicted to be of high importance. The original and masked image batches are then fed as inputs to the classification model producing the losses $\mathscr{L}_{original}$ and $\mathscr{L}_{adversarial}$. The reward function is defined as:

$$R_t = \mathscr{L}_{adversarial} - \mathscr{L}_{original} \qquad (6)$$

To reduce the variance of training, a baseline b_t, the exponential moving average of the reward, is included, similarly done in [12]. Intuitively, by erasing the important features we revert the problem and tend to maximize the gain in loss. However, we do not want the segmentation policy to erase all pixels in favor of a gain in R_t, so we penalize the masking of all pixels. Given pixel-wise all zero feature importance a_{zeros} and a weight λ_{zeros} for regularization, the final loss $\mathscr{L}$ is defined as:

$$\mathscr{L} = \mathscr{L}_{BCE}(P(a_t|s_t;\theta_p), a_t) \cdot (R_t - b_t) + \mathscr{L}_{BCE}(P(a_t|s_t;\theta_p), a_{zeros}) \cdot \lambda_{zeros} \qquad (7)$$

The resulting reward signal is strongly related to mask quality, rather than reflecting the stochasticity in training of the classification network (Fig. 1).

3   Experiments and Results

We evaluate our methodology on MURA [7] and an internal hip fracture dataset, using the same experimental setup, including network architectures, RL framework, and training hyperparameters. A DenseNet-169 [4] pretrained on ImageNet [2] serves as the base classification model. A TernausNet [5], pretrained on Carvana Image Masking Challenge [1], serves as the segmentation model. Masked images are used as augmentation in a 1 : 1 ratio with original images to train the classification network. Images resized to 224×224, batch size 25. Adam optimizers [6] with a initial learning rate of 0.0001 are used for the classification and the segmentation model. The exponential average baseline b_t has a decay rate of 0.5. λ_{zeros} is set to 0.1. Training of APGA converges within 30 min on a single Nvidia TitanX GPU. Source code available at https://github.com/victorychain/Adversarial-Policy-Gradient-Augmentation.

Algorithm 1. Adversarial Policy Gradient Augmentation (APGA)

Input: Training steps (T); training samples and labels (X,Y); classification and segmentation loss functions $(\mathscr{L}_c, \mathscr{L}_p)$; learning rates (α_c, α_p); classification and segmentation models (M_c, M_p) parameterized with (θ_c, θ_p).
Output: M_c and M_p

1: Initialize models parameters θ_c and θ_p
2: Train classification model on X to convergence
3: **for** t = 1,..., T **do**
4:     Sample a training batch (x_t, y_t) from the (X, Y) pool
5:     Get classification loss $\mathscr{L}_{original} = \mathscr{L}_c(M_c(x_t), y_t)$
6:     Perform gradient descent update $\theta_c \leftarrow \theta_c - \alpha_c \nabla_{\theta_c} \mathscr{L}_{original}$
7:     Get adversarial action probabilities from the seg network $P_{adversarial} = M_p(x_t)$
8:     Calculate masks of important features $A_{adversarial} = (P_{adversarial} < 0.5)$
9:     Produce masks from segmentation networks and erase the predicted features
       $x_{adversarial} = A_{adversarial} \cdot x_t$
10:    Get adversarial loss $\mathscr{L}_{adversarial} = \mathscr{L}_c(M_c(x_{adversarial}), y_t)$
11:    Calculate reward $R_t = \mathscr{L}_{adversarial} - \mathscr{L}_{original}$
12:    Calculate distances of action probabilities from actions taken $\mathscr{L}_{prob} = \mathscr{L}_p(P_{adversarial}, A_{adversarial})$
13:    Calculate distances of action probabilities from the opposite of undesirable extreme actions (masking all pixels) $\mathscr{L}_{extreme} = \mathscr{L}_p(P_{adversarial}, A_{extreme})$
14:    Calculate adversarial policy gradient loss $\mathscr{L}_{pg} = \mathscr{L}_{prob} \cdot R_t + \mathscr{L}_{extreme}$
15:    Update the segmentation network $\theta_p \leftarrow \theta_p - \alpha_p \nabla_{\theta_p} \mathscr{L}_{pg}$
16:    Produce aiding actions from segmentation network $A_{aid} = M_p(x_t) > 0.5$
17:    Update M_c with the aiding masks $\theta_c \leftarrow \theta_c - \alpha_c \nabla_{\theta_c} \mathscr{L}_c(M_c(A_{aid} \cdot x_t), y_t)$
18: **end for**

Baselines: We benchmark APGA using a DenseNet-169 [4] classifier trained (1) without data augmentation, (2) with cutout [3] augmentation in a 1:1 ratio, and with (3) GradCam [9] derived masks augmentation also in a 1:1 ratio. Cutout augmentation masks out randomly sized patches of the input image while

GradCam masks are produced by discretizing the probability saliency map from
the DenseNet trained without data augmentation. For further comparison, a
segmentation and classification network are trained end-to-end, by propagating
the gradient from the classification loss function through the segmentation network and applying the discretized masks from the segmentation network in the
same update step. Additionally, regularization terms a_{zeros} and λ_{zeros}, a_{ones} and
λ_{ones}, are added to the loss function to prevent all or none masking behavior.
However, end-to-end training was unstable, and the segmentation network pro-
duced all-one or all-zero masks, despite tuning of λ_{zeros} and λ_{ones}. Therefore,
these results were omitted. At its best, the end-to-end network produced all-one
masks and performed the same as the DenseNet trained without augmentation.

3.1   Binary Classification: MURA

The MURA [7] dataset contains 14,863 musculoskeletal studies of elbows, finger,
forearm, hand, humerus, shoulder, and wrist, which contains 9,045 normal and
5,818 abnormal labeled cases. We train the methods on the public training set
and evaluate on the validation set, with global accuracy as the metric. We train
and evaluate separate models on each body part, and train a single model on a
random sample of 100 training images per class to test the performance of our
method under extreme data constraints. The performance on the validation set
is presented in Tables 1 and 2 as average and standard deviation of 5 random
seeds.

Table 1. Classification results (validation accuracy) on MURA.

	DenseNet	DenseNet + Cutout	DenseNet + GradCam	APGA (Ours)
Elbow	82.80 ± 1.10	83.05 ± 0.85	83.18 ± 0.70	**83.26 ± 0.62**
Finger	75.70 ± 1.11	77.66 ± 1.69	76.66 ± 0.83	**77.96 ± 0.19**
Forearm	80.07 ± 1.98	81.80 ± 1.47	79.80 ± 1.70	**83.44 ± 0.53**
Hand	78.35 ± 0.82	78.13 ± 0.86	77.35 ± 1.49	**79.09 ± 1.44**
Humerus	85.69 ± 0.93	85.69 ± 0.79	86.39 ± 1.50	**86.53 ± 0.67**
Shoulder	75.88 ± 0.93	75.77 ± 0.78	**76.80 ± 1.18**	76.59 ± 0.48
Wrist	83.28 ± 0.46	84.04 ± 0.97	82.61 ± 1.19	**84.41 ± 0.54**

Table 2. 100-shot results (validation accuracy) on Elbow in MURA.

	DenseNet	DenseNet + Cutout	DenseNet + GradCam	APGA (Ours)
Elbow	62.68 ± 2.29	64.49 ± 2.77	65.87 ± 1.97	**70.41 ± 2.76**

3.2   Multi-class Classification: Hip Fracture

The Hip Fracture dataset contains 1118 studies with an average patient age of 74.6 years (standard deviation 17.3), and a 62 : 38 female:male ratio. Each study includes a pelvic radiograph, labeled as 1 of 6 classes: No fracture, Intertrochanteric fracture, Displaced femoral neck fracture, Non-displaced femoral neck fracture, Arthroplasty, or ORIF (previous internal fixation). Bounding boxes are manually drawn on each study, resulting in 3034 bounded hips. The images are split by accession number into train:valid:test using a 60 : 25 : 15 split, ensuring no overlap in patients between any of the sets. We train and evaluate separate models on the whole pelvic radiographs and the bounded hip radiographs. Per-image accuracy is used as the metric. The performance on the validation and test set is shown in Table 3.

Table 3. Classification results (validation and test accuracy) on Hip Fx Dataset.

	DenseNet [4]	DenseNet + Cutout	DenseNet + GradCam	APGA (Ours)
Whole Pelvis (val)	59.69 ± 1.64	$\mathbf{62.33 \pm 1.49}$	61.09 ± 0.52	60.46 ± 1.2
Whole Pelvis (test)	51.66 ± 1.32	52.51 ± 2.58	51.92 ± 1.59	$\mathbf{53.38 \pm 2.5}$
Bounded Hip (val)	86.84 ± 0.62	$\mathbf{88.65 \pm 0.89}$	86.51 ± 2.28	87.86 ± 0.99
Bounded Hip (test)	84.53 ± 1.21	85.01 ± 2.58	83.95 ± 2.72	$\mathbf{85.65 \pm 1.53}$

Results: Compared to the baseline, our method achieved higher global accuracy in 9 out of 10 tasks including binary (MURA Table 1) and multi-class (hip Fx Table 3) classification tasks. On average, our method improved MURA validation accuracy by 1.56% and hip validation and testing accuracy by 0.78% and 1.72%

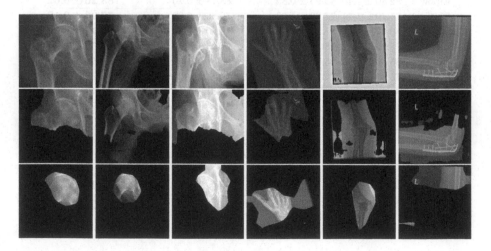

Fig. 2. Example X-Rays (top) and masks created by APGA (middle) and DenseNet+GradCam (bottom) for hip, hand, and elbow.

respectively. The most significant improvement in accuracy over the baseline was 7.33% and it was achieved in a data-constrained condition, reported in Table 2. In this particular experiment, the elbow training data was limited to 100 samples per class. Overall, APGA outperformed baseline methods in 9 out of 10 tasks, and consistently provided higher testing results. Example segmentation masks from the weakly supervised network are shown in Fig. 2. APGA learns to ignore unimportant features in the radiographs, such as anatomy irrelevant to the classification task. APGA masking appears more exploratory in nature compared to saliency based attention masking (DenseNet + GradCam), which contains biases from the converged model.

4 Discussions and Conclusions

We propose a framework, APGA, for producing segmentations to aid medical image classification in a reinforcement learning setting. This framework requires no manual segmentation, which has the benefit of scalability and generalizability. The system is trained online with the goal of improving the performance of the main task, classification. If no improvement is seen, this can be a check for the assumption that masking based augmentation would aid classification, before pursuing more manual work. Marginal improvements should be evidence that APGA has the potential to add valuable information to the training process. The computational overhead in training is justified by those added benefits, and could be eliminated during inference, as the segmentation network can also be used as an inference augmentation technique. This general reinforcement learning with adversarial reward framework could easily be adopted for other medical imaging tasks, involving regression, and segmentation, with different aiding methods, such as bounding box detection, image distortion, and image generation. The reinforcement guided data augmentation has more generalizability compared to traditional data augmentation based on domain knowledge.

References

1. Carvana Image Masking Challenge. https://kaggle.com/c/carvana-image-masking-challenge
2. Deng, J., Dong, W., Socher, R., Li, L.-J., Li, K., Fei-Fei, L.: ImageNet: a large-scale hierarchical image database. In: CVPR 2009 (2009)
3. DeVries, T., Taylor, G.W.: Improved regularization of convolutional neural networks with cutout. arXiv:1708.04552 [cs], August 2017
4. Huang, G., Liu, Z., van der Maaten, L., Weinberger, K.Q.: Densely connected convolutional networks. arXiv:1608.06993 [cs], August 2016
5. Iglovikov, V., Shvets, A.: TernausNet: U-Net with VGG11 encoder pre-trained on ImageNet for image segmentation. arXiv:1801.05746 [cs], January 2018
6. Kingma, D.P., Ba, J.: Adam: a method for stochastic optimization. arXiv:1412.6980 [cs], December 2014
7. Rajpurkar, P., et al.: MURA: large dataset for abnormality detection in musculoskeletal radiographs. arXiv:1712.06957 [physics], December 2017

8. Russakovsky, O., et al.: ImageNet large scale visual recognition challenge. arXiv:1409.0575 [cs], September 2014
9. Selvaraju, R.R., Cogswell, M., Das, A., Vedantam, R., Parikh, D., Batra, D.: Grad-CAM: visual explanations from deep networks via gradient-based localization. arXiv:1610.02391 [cs], October 2016
10. Wallenberg, M., Forssén, P.: Attentional masking for pre-trained deep networks. In: 2017 IEEE/RSJ International Conference on Intelligent Robots and Systems (IROS), pp. 6149–6154, September 2017. https://doi.org/10.1109/IROS.2017.8206516
11. Williams, R.J.: Simple statistical gradient-following algorithms for connectionist reinforcement learning. Mach. Learn. 8(3), 229–256 (1992). https://doi.org/10.1007/BF00992696
12. Zoph, B., Le, Q.V.: Neural architecture search with reinforcement learning. arXiv:1611.01578 [cs], November 2016

Weakly Supervised Universal Fracture Detection in Pelvic X-Rays

Yirui Wang[1]([⊠]), Le Lu[1], Chi-Tung Cheng[2], Dakai Jin[1], Adam P. Harrison[1], Jing Xiao[3], Chien-Hung Liao[2], and Shun Miao[1]

[1] PAII Inc., Bethesda, MD, USA
yiruiwang06@gmail.com
[2] Chang Gung Memorial Hospital, Linkou, Taiwan, ROC
[3] Ping An Technology, Shenzhen, China

Abstract. Hip and pelvic fractures are serious injuries with life-threatening complications. However, diagnostic errors of fractures in pelvic X-rays (PXRs) are very common, driving the demand for computer-aided diagnosis (CAD) solutions. A major challenge lies in the fact that fractures are localized patterns that require localized analyses. Unfortunately, the PXRs residing in hospital picture archiving and communication system do not typically specify region of interests. In this paper, we propose a two-stage hip and pelvic fracture detection method that executes localized fracture classification using weakly supervised ROI mining. The first stage uses a large capacity fully-convolutional network, *i.e.*, deep with high levels of abstraction, in a multiple instance learning setting to automatically mine probable true positive and definite hard negative ROIs from the whole PXR in the training data. The second stage trains a smaller capacity model, *i.e.*, shallower and more generalizable, with the mined ROIs to perform localized analyses to classify fractures. During inference, our method detects hip and pelvic fractures in one pass by chaining the probability outputs of the two stages together. We evaluate our method on 4 410 PXRs, reporting an under the ROC curve value of 0.975, the highest among state-of-the-art fracture detection methods. Moreover, we show that our two-stage approach can perform comparably to human physicians (even outperforming emergency physicians and surgeons), in a preliminary reader study of 23 readers.

Keywords: Fracture classification and localization · Pelvic X-ray · Weakly supervised detection · Cascade two-stage training · Image level labels

Electronic supplementary material The online version of this chapter (https://doi.org/10.1007/978-3-030-32226-7_51) contains supplementary material, which is available to authorized users.

D. Shen et al. (Eds.): MICCAI 2019, LNCS 11769, pp. 459–467, 2019.
https://doi.org/10.1007/978-3-030-32226-7_51

1   Introduction

Hip and pelvic fractures belong to a frequent trauma injury category worldwide [8]. Frontal pelvic X-rays (PXRs) are the standard imaging tool for diagnosing pelvic and hip fractures in the emergency room (ER). However, anatomical complexities and perspective projection distortions contribute to a high rate of diagnostic errors [2] that may delay treatment and increase patient care cost, morbidity, and mortality [10]. As such, an effective PXR computer-aided diagnosis (CAD) approach for *both* pelvic and hip fractures is of high clinical interest, with the aim of reducing diagnostic errors and improving patient outcomes.

Image-level labels are the only supervisory signal typically available in picture archiving and communication system (PACS) data. Thus, a widely adopted formulation for X-ray abnormality detection is a single-stage global classifier [1,3,9,11]. However, for PXRs this approach is challenged by the localized nature of fractures and the complexity of the surrounding anatomical regions. Moreover, such global classifiers can be prone to overfitting, as it is unlikely that a training dataset could capture the combinatorial complexity of configurations of fracture locations, orientations, and background contexts within the whole PXR—this complexity is analogous to similar challenges within computer vision [13]. Indeed, for *hip fractures alone*, Jiménez-Sánchez et al. show that using localized region of interests (ROIs) produces significantly better F1 scores over a global approach [7] and Gale et al. achieve impressive areas under the ROC curve (AUCROCs) of 0.994 by first automatically extracting ROIs centered on the femoral neck [4]. These recent results bolster the argument for concentrating on local fracture patterns.

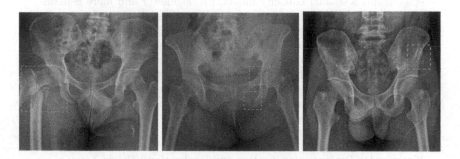

Fig. 1. Example PXR images of hip and pelvic fractures. (**Left**) Hip fracture. (**Middle**) Superior and inferior pubic ramus fracture. (**Right**) Iliac wing fracture.

Nonetheless, the above prior work all only focuses on diagnosing hip fractures and does not attempt to classify the more complex pelvic fractures (fractures in three pelvic bones: the ilium, ischium, and pubis). As Fig. 1 illustrates, the makeup of pelvis fractures is much more complex, as there are a large variety of possible types with very different visual patterns at various locations. In addition,

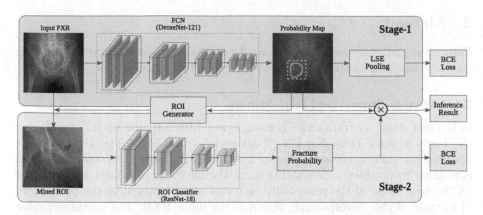

Fig. 2. The proposed two-stage fracture detection system. The first stage uses a large capacity MIL FCN model to perform fracture classification with weakly supervised ROI localization. The second stage uses a smaller capacity model trained with the mined ROIs to perform localized classification. During inference, the two stages are chained together, with the second model applied on the ROIs proposed by the first model, to produce the final estimation.

pelvic bones overlap with the lower abdomen, further confounding image patterns. Finally, unlike hip fractures, which occur at the femoral neck/head, pelvic fractures can occur anywhere on the large pelvis, both increasing the aforementioned image pattern combinatorial complexity and precluding automatic ROI extraction based on anatomy alone, such as was done in prior work [4]. Thus, while using ROI-based classification is even more desirable for pelvic fractures, it is paradoxically more challenging to extract said ROIs.

To bridge this gap, we propose a two-stage weakly supervised ROI mining and subsequent classification method for PXR fracture classification. In the first stage, we train a weakly-supervised, but high capacity, multiple instance learning (MIL) fully-convolutional network (FCN) to mine local probable positive and definite hard negative ROIs. In the second stage, we use the mined ROIs to train a lower capacity network in a fully-supervised setting. During inference, the two networks are chained together to provide a complete classification solution. Experiments use a dataset of 4 410 PXRs, with only image-level labels, that we collected from the PACS of Chang Gung Memorial Hospital. We show that single-stage classifiers, whether low- or high-capacity, are unable to match our two-stage approach. Our chained two-stage method outperforms the best single-stage alternative, with a specificity at recall rate of 95% (S@R95) of 87.6% compared to 80.9%, and corresponding improvements in AUCROCs. Moreover, using an independent reader study of 150 patients, our system achieves an accuracy of 0.907, which is equivalent to 23 physicians. As such, we are the first to tackle automatic PXR pelvis fracture classification and also the first to demonstrate diagnostic performance equivalent to human physicians for *both* hip and pelvic fractures.

2 Method

Figure 2 depicts the overall workflow of our chained two-stage pelvic and hip fracture detection method. We elaborate on the two stages below.

2.1 Weakly-Supervised ROI Mining

In the first stage, we train an FCN using a deep MIL formulation [12], employing the large-capacity DenseNet-121 [6] network as backbone. The DenseNet-121 features are then processed using a 1×1 convolutional layer and a sigmoid activation to produce a probability map. Owing to the localized properties of FCNs, each value of the probability map can be interpreted as the probability of fracture in the corresponding region in the input PXR. The maximum value would then represent the probability of fracture within the entire image. Instead, we use log of the sum of the exponentials (LSE) pooling, which is a differentiable approximation of max pooling, given by

$$LSE(S) = \frac{1}{r} \cdot \log \left[\frac{1}{|S|} \cdot \sum_{(i,j) \in S} \exp\left(r \cdot p_{ij}\right) \right], \tag{1}$$

where $\{p_{ij}\}$ is the probability map, and r is a hyper-parameter controlling the behavior of LSE between max pooling ($r \to \infty$) and average pooling ($r \to 0$). With the pooled global probability, binary cross entropy (BCE) loss is calculated against the image level label, and is used to train the network. While, this formulation has been applied directly for weakly supervised abnormality detection in chest X-rays (CXRs) [12], as we show in our results this approach's performance is limited for hip and pelvic fracture detection. Therefore, we use the FCN as a proposal generator to mine ROIs from the training data.

To mine ROIs from the training data to train a localized classification model, we first create an image-level classifier using $p' = \max_{i,j \in S} p_{ij}$, and select a threshold $\hat{p}$ corresponding to a high sensitivity on the training data (we use 99% in our experiments). We then extract up to $K = 5$ ROIs from each PXR in the training data in every training epoch of the second stage model. Specifically, for PXRs with positive ground-truth image-level labels, i.e., with fracture(s), up to K locations are randomly selected from

$$S' = \{i, j | p_{ij} > \hat{p}\}. \tag{2}$$

These ROIs are labeled as probable fracture positive. For PXRs with negative ground-truth image-level labels, i.e., no fractures, the same ROI extraction strategy selects up to K ROIs. These are considered as definite hard negatives. If there are less than K hard negatives extracted, additional negative ROIs are randomly extracted from the PXR to make up the total. The ROIs produced using the above strategy contains probable positives, hard negatives, and easy negatives. Although this approach adds a degree of label noise due to the probable positive ROI, as we outline in the following, this comes with the added benefits of using a subsequent localized and more generalizable ROI classifier.

2.2 Fracture ROI Classification

In the second stage, we use the ROIs mined from the first stage as training data for a fully supervised localized classification network. Since the positive samples are mostly ROIs around fractures with limited background context, the visual patterns of fractures become more dominant, simplifying the classification task. In addition, the distribution of mined ROIs are heavily weighted toward hard negatives, $i.e.$, false positive regions from the first stage. This concentrates the modeling power of the second-stage classifier on differentiating these difficult/confusing fracture-like patterns. As a result, we are able to train a smaller capacity network, $e.g.$, ResNet-18 [5], to reliably classify the ROIs, which is more generalizable and less prone to overfitting compared to a high-capacity network modeling the entire PXR.

During inference, the two stages are chained together to provide a complete solution. The first stage FCN acts as a proposal generator, and the highest value from the probability map $\{p_{i,j}\}$ is selected, denoted as p_{s1}, along with the corresponding ROI. The second stage classifier is then applied on the proposed ROI to produce a fracture probability score, denoted p_{s2}. The final image-level probability of fracture is computed by multiplying the two probability scores, $p_{s1} \cdot p_{s2}$. As such, we use the second stage classifier as a filter to reject false positives from the first stage.

Hip/Pelvic Fracture Differentiation: Our two-stage method detects hip and pelvic fractures as one class, because the most important goal of PXR CAD is to detect fractures. Using one universal fracture class also helps to prevent the model from picking up co-occurrence relationships between hip/pelvic fractures that may be overly represented from the current training data [13]. In scenarios where hip and pelvic fractures do need to be differentiated, $e.g.$, automatic medical image reporting, an additional classification output node can be added to the second stage model. Similar to the hierarchical classification schemes [3], the new node is trained only on positive fracture ROIs mined in the first stage. Like fracture classification, during inference hip/pelvic fracture differentiation can be obtained in one feed-forward pass of the network.

3 Experiments and Results

We evaluate our framework using PXR images collected from the PACS of Chang Gung Memorial Hospital, corresponding to patients in the trauma registry. We resized all images to 961×961 pixels. The final dataset consisted of 4 410 images, including 2 776 images with fractures (1 975 and 801 hip and pelvic fractures, respectively). Besides this dataset, we also collected an independent PXR dataset, containing 150 cases (50 hip fractures, 50 pelvic fractures, and 50 no findings) for a reader study comparing our approach with that of 23 physicians.

We use ImageNet pre-trained weights to initialize the networks in both stages. The Adam optimizer was used to train both models for 100 epochs with a batch size of 8 and a starting learning rate of 10^{-5} reduced by a factor of 10 upon

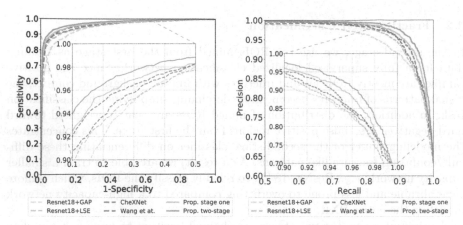

Fig. 3. Comparison of ROC (**left**) and Precision-Recall curve (**right**)

Table 1. Five-fold cross validation of fracture classification on 4 410 PXRs.

Method	AUC	S@R95	R@S95	P@R95
ResNet18-GAP	0.946	0.706	0.786	0.846
ResNet18-LSE	0.956	0.723	0.859	0.851
CheXNet [9]	0.962	0.809	0.870	0.876
Wang *et al.* [11]	0.962	0.752	0.875	0.867
Prop. single-stage	0.968	0.825	0.888	0.903
Prop. two-stage	**0.975**	**0.876**	**0.909**	**0.928**

plateaus. In addition to AUCROC, we measure specificity at recall rate of 95% (S@R95), precision at recall rate of 95% (P@R95) and recall at specificity rate of 95% (R@S95), which help highlight differences in performance under demanding expectations for recall/sensitivity and specificity, respectively.

3.1   Comparison to Prior Work

We evaluate *general fracture* classification performance using five-fold cross-validation with a 70%/10%/20% training, validation, and testing split, respectively. We compare against the single-stage high-capacity approaches of CheXNet [9] and Wang *et al.* [11], both of which use DenseNet-121 as backbones and apply global average pooling (GAP) and LSE pooling, respectively. Note, that unlike our first stage of Sect. 2.1, the pooling is applied to the last feature map. We also compare against the single-stage lower-capacity model of ResNet-18, using both GAP and LSE pooling heads.

Figure 3 and Table 1 quantitatively summarizes these experiments. As can be seen, all lower-capacity models fare relatively poorly, demonstrating the need to use more descriptive models for global PXR interpretation. On the other

Table 2. Algorithm and physician performances in a clinical study on 150 PXRs.

	Accuracy	Hip fracture		Pelvic fracture	
		Sensitivity	Specificity	Sensitivity	Specificity
ER physician	0.881	0.983	0.937	0.813	0.955
Surgeon	0.855	0.931	0.928	0.829	0.932
Orthopedics specialist	0.932	1.000	0.953	0.905	0.990
Radiologist	0.930	0.990	0.965	0.870	0.995
Physician average	0.882	0.962	0.938	0.842	0.953
Our method	0.907	0.960	0.980	0.840	0.960

hand, the first stage of our proposed method achieves an AUCROC of 0.968, compared to the 0.962 achieved by the state-of-the-art single-stage methods [9, 11], demonstrating that our single-stage approach using deep MIL can already outperform prior art. With the second stage, our method was able to further improve the AUCROC to 0.975, the highest among all evaluated methods. This corresponds to improvements of 12.4% (3.4%), 6.7% (3.9%), and 5.1% (2.1%) in S@R95 (R@S95) over Wang *et al.* [11], CheXNet [9], and our single-stage model respectively. These are highly impactful boosts in performance, demonstrating that under high demands of recall and specificity our chained approach can provide drastic improvements.

At our two-stage method achieves a P@R95 of 0.928, measuring 9.7%, 9.0%, 5.9% and 7.0% improvements over the two low-capacity baseline models, ResNet18-GAP and ResNet18-LSE, and two high-capacity baseline models CheXNet [9] and Wang *et al.* [11], respectively. Please note that the actual prevalence of fractures in clinical environments can be lower than our data, which will result in lower precisions for all methods. Nonetheless, the performance ranking would likely to remain, and the improvements of our method over the baselines are expected to be even more significant with a lower prevalence.

In addition, we evaluate the label accuracy of mined probable positive ROIs on 438 PXRs with fracture location annotations, and report a high accuracy of 0.925, demonstrating the effectiveness of the proposed weakly-supervised ROI mining scheme. We also evaluate the hip/pelvic fracture classification performance, and report a high average accuracy of 0.980 over the five-fold cross validation.

3.2   Reader Study

We conduct reader study to compare performance on 150 PXRs with 23 human physicians recruited from the surgical (11), orthopedics (4), ER (6) and radiology (2) departments. For every PXR, physicians were asked to choose from three options: hip fracture, pelvic fracture or no finding. To provide a fair comparison, we used the add-on fracture-type classification output node described in Sect. 2.2, which can differentiate between hip and pelvic fractures, matching the three-class classification performed by the readers.

Table 2 quantitatively summarizes the reader study results. As shown in the results, our method performs comparably to the average physician performance on this dataset, reporting an accuracy of 0.907 compared to 0.882, with higher levels of specificity. Examining the physician specialities in isolation, our method outperforms ER physicians and surgeons, while not performing as well as the orthopedic specialists and radiologists. Of note, is that when trauma patients are sent to the ER, it is common that only ER physicians or surgeons are available to make immediate diagnostic and treatment decisions. As such, the reader study suggests that our approach may be an effective aid for PXR fracture diagnosis in the high-stress ER environment.

4   Conclusion

We introduced a chained two-stage method for universal fracture detection in PXRs, consisting of a weakly supervised fracture ROI mining stage and a localized fracture ROI classification stage. Experiments show that our method can significantly outperform prior works via five-fold cross validation on 4 410 PXRs. Moreover, a preliminary reader study on 150 PXRs involving 23 physicians suggests that our method can perform equivalently to human physicians. Thus, our approach represents an important step forward in automated pelvic and hip fracture diagnosis for ER environments.

References

1. Badgeley, M.A., Zech, J.R., Oakden-Rayner, L., et al.: Deep learning predicts hip fracture using confounding patient and healthcare variables. arXiv:1811.03695 (2018)
2. Chellam, W.: Missed subtle fractures on the trauma-meeting digital projector. Injury **47**(3), 674–676 (2016)
3. Chen, H., Miao, S., Xu, D., Hager, G.D., Harrison, A.P.: Deep hierarchical multi-label classification of chest X-ray images. In: MIDL (2019)
4. Gale, W., Oakden-Rayner, L., Carneiro, G., Bradley, A.P., Palmer, L.J.: Detecting hip fractures with radiologist-level performance using deep neural networks. arXiv:1711.06504 (2017)
5. He, K., Zhang, X., Ren, S., Sun, J.: Deep residual learning for image recognition. In: Proceedings of the IEEE Conference on Computer Vision and Pattern Recognition, pp. 770–778 (2016)
6. Huang, G., Liu, Z., Van Der Maaten, L., Weinberger, K.Q.: Densely connected convolutional networks. In: IEEE CVPR, pp. 4700–4708 (2017)
7. Jiménez-Sánchez, A., et al.: Weakly-supervised localization and classification of proximal femur fractures. arXiv:1809.10692 (2018)
8. Johnell, O., Kanis, J.: An estimate of the worldwide prevalence, mortality and disability associated with hip fracture. Osteoporos. Int. **15**(11), 897–902 (2004)
9. Rajpurkar, P., et al.: CheXNet: radiologist-level pneumonia detection on chest x-rays with deep learning. arXiv preprint arXiv:1711.05225 (2017)

10. Tarrant, S., Hardy, B., Byth, P., Brown, T., Attia, J., Balogh, Z.: Preventable mortality in geriatric hip fracture inpatients. Bone Joint J. **96**(9), 1178–1184 (2014)
11. Wang, X., Peng, Y., Lu, L., Lu, Z., Bagheri, M., Summers, R.M.: ChestX-Ray8: hospital-scale chest x-ray database and benchmarks on weakly-supervised classification and localization of common thorax diseases. In: IEEE CVPR (2017)
12. Yao, L., Prosky, J., Poblenz, E., Covington, B., Lyman, K.: Weakly supervised medical diagnosis and localization from multiple resolutions. arXiv preprint arXiv:1803.07703 (2018)
13. Yuille, A.L., Liu, C.: Deep nets: what have they ever done for vision? CoRR **abs/1805.04025** (2018)

Learning from Suspected Target: Bootstrapping Performance for Breast Cancer Detection in Mammography

Li Xiao[1]([envelope]), Cheng Zhu[1], Junjun Liu[2], Chunlong Luo[1], Peifang Liu[2], and Yi Zhao[1]

[1] Key Laboratory of Intelligent Information Processing,
Advanced Computer Research Center, Institute of Computing Technology,
Chinese Academy of Sciences, Beijing, China
{xiaoli,biozy}@ict.ac.cn
[2] Tianjin Medical University Cancer Institute and Hospital, Tianjin, China
juneliu2010@163.com, cjr.liupeifang@vip.163.com

Abstract. Deep learning object detection algorithm has been widely used in medical image analysis. Currently all the object detection tasks are based on the data annotated with object classes and their bounding boxes. On the other hand, medical images such as mammography usually contain normal regions or objects that are similar to the lesion region, and may be misclassified in the testing stage if they are not taken care of. In this paper, we address such problem by introducing a novel top likelihood loss together with a new sampling procedure to select and train the suspected target regions, as well as proposing a similarity loss to further identify suspected targets from targets. Mean average precision (mAP) according to the predicted targets and specificity, sensitivity, accuracy, AUC values according to classification of patients are adopted for performance comparisons. We firstly test our proposed method on a private dense mammogram dataset. Results show that our proposed method greatly reduce the false positive rate and the specificity is increased by 0.25 on detecting mass type cancer. It is worth mention that dense breast typically has a higher risk for developing breast cancers and also are harder for cancer detection in diagnosis, and our method outperforms a reported result from performance of radiologists. Our method is also validated on the public Digital Database for Screening Mammography (DDSM) dataset, brings significant improvement on mass type cancer detection and outperforms the most state-of-the-art work.

1 Introduction

Deep learning object detection algorithm has been widely used in the task of classifying or detecting objects of natural images [3] and [8], and are receiving

Electronic supplementary material The online version of this chapter (https://doi.org/10.1007/978-3-030-32226-7_52) contains supplementary material, which is available to authorized users.

more and more attentions on its usage in medical image analysis. However, current object detection tasks are all based on the data annotated with object classes and their bounding boxes, those images which are not considered during labeling may contain regions or objects that are similar to the target ones, and may be misclassified in the testing stage. This phenomenon is critical in medical image analysis. For example, as shown in Fig. 1, a healthy mammography may contain benign or normal regions whose features are very similar to a malignant lesion. On the other hand, when doctors perform labeling, they usually search for medical records of patients that are diagnosed as cancer first, and only selected samples are labeled and used for training. As a result, those healthy samples that contain suspected malignant regions are likely to be classified as malignant.

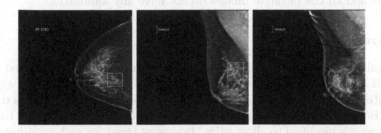

Fig. 1. The image with labeled malignant lesion (left) and healthy images contain unlabeled benign tumor region (middle) or normal region (right) which are suspect to be malignant in vision.

Breast cancer is one of the leading causes of death for women and mammography is the most commonly used modality for screening and early stage detection of breast cancer. Deep learning object detection models have been widely used in classification or detecting cancers of mammography [1,2,7,9]. However, current object detection models can only train well-annotated data, this will cause high false positive rate in practical usage when images with annotated malignant lesions and healthy images with no annotation are mixed together.

In this work, we adapt the region based object detection model to a weakly-supervised learning task that encompasses both images with annotated malignant lesions and healthy images with no annotation. A top likelihood loss together with a new sampling procedure is developed to select and train those suspected target region in healthy images, and a similarity loss is further added to identify the suspected targets from targets. Our model is first validated on a private dense mammogram dataset. By introducing the top likelihood loss and similarity loss, the false positive rate is greatly reduced and the specificity is increased by 25%. It is worth mention that dense breast typically has a higher risk for developing breast cancer and are harder for cancer detection in diagnosis, and our method outperforms the performance of radiologists reported in Giger et al. [4]. Our method is then validated on the public DDSM dataset, brings significant improvement on mass type cancer detection according to all the metrics and also outperforms Al-masni et al. [1], the most state-of-the-art work.

2 Method

In the following, we define a mammography with malignant lesions as a positive image, and those malignant lesions as positive targets or targets. All the other mammography are defined as negative images, including those images contain benign or normal regions that are highly suspect to be malignant (as shown in Fig. 1). And without loss of generality, we called those highly suspected malignant regions as suspected target regions. Within the datasets we used, all the positive targets are annotated with bounding boxes to indicate their precise locations and all the negative images do not have any annotation.

2.1 Architecture

Our detailed network is shown in Fig. 2. The network is developed based on the Faster R-CNN [10], which uses Region Proposal Network (RPN) to generate candidate proposals followed by Fast R-CNN to fine classify and regress the proposals. Both positive and negative images are randomly sorted before training. The network is modified to allow paired images as input for each mini-batch: one is positive with annotations and the other one is negative with no annotation. The positive image is trained with the original Faster R-CNN loss while the RPN loss is replaced by our newly designed top likelihood loss when training

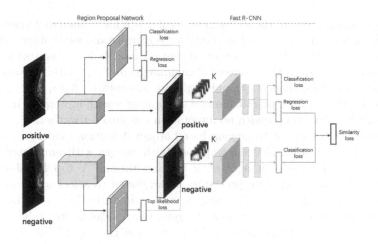

Fig. 2. General architecture of our model. The input contains one positive and one negative image. In the sharing RPN stage, positive images are trained by the original loss and negative images are trained by our proposed top likelihood loss. A similarity loss is also added on the final stage to further identify the positive and negative targets.

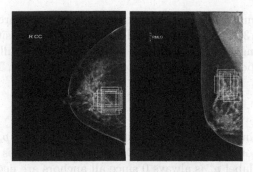

Fig. 3. The sampled anchors (green boxes) for positive image (left) and negative image (right) within a single mini-batch. The red box represents the ground truth target. (Color figure online)

the negative image. A similarity loss is also added on the fc-layers of the Fast R-CNN to better identify features between positive and negative regions.

ResNet101 is adopted as the backbone. The RPN anchors are set as $((4^2, 8^2, 16^2, 32^2, 64^2))$ with aspect ratio as $((\frac{1}{2}, 1, 2))$, which cover most of the target sizes.

2.2 Loss to Discriminate Suspected Target Region

Top Likelihood Loss. When training the negative images, the original RPN loss is replaced by a top likelihood loss to minimize the probability to predict the negative region as positive.

In Faster R-CNN, the RPN anchor is assigned by a binary class label (of being an object or not). The positive label is assigned to two kinds of anchors: (i) the anchor/anchors with the highest Intersection-over-Union (IoU) overlap with a ground-truth box, or (ii) an anchor that has an IoU overlap higher than 0.7 with any ground-truth box. The negative label is assigned to a non-positive anchor if its IoU ratio is lower than 0.3 for all ground-truth boxes. When training the RPN, each mini-batch randomly samples 256 anchors in an image to compute the loss function, where the sampled positive and negative anchors have a ratio of up to 1:1. If there are fewer than 128 positive samples in an image, negative ones will be padded instead.

However, the negative image does not contain any annotation, which means all anchors are negative including those anchors contain suspected targets. It is possible to optimize the loss functions of all anchors, but this will bias towards normal regions since they are dominate. Those suspected target region still likely to be recognized as positive since they don't have enough chance to be trained. To deal with this issue, we propose a top likelihood loss by ranking the scores of all anchors and sample the top 256 anchors to compute the loss function. The anchors with top scores should be more representative for those suspected target regions as the training goes on. On the other hand, as long as those top score anchors get minimized, all anchors are optimized towards negative at the same time. Figure 3 shows the sampled anchors for the positive and negative images within a single mini-batch when training the RPN, all sampled anchors are around the suspected target region for the negative image. The top likelihood loss is defined:

$$L_{tlloss} = \frac{1}{cls} \sum_{i \in (tops\ p_i)} L_{cls}(p_i, p_i^* = 0) \tag{1}$$

Here, i is the index of an anchor in a mini-batch and p_i is the predicted probability of anchor i being an object. Only the top 256 values of p_i are sampled. The ground-truth label p_i^* is always 0 since all anchors are negative. L_{cls} loss is the cross entropy loss, same as the RPN classification loss in Faster R-CNN.

To summarize, the total RPN loss is defined as:

$$L_{rpnloss} = L_{ploss} + L_{nloss} = L_{pclsloss} + \lambda_1 L_{pregloss} + \lambda_2 L_{tlloss} \tag{2}$$

Here the loss for the positive image L_{ploss} is the same that in the original Faster R-CNN, which consists of the classification loss $L_{pclsloss}$ and the regression loss $L_{pregloss}$. The loss L_{nloss} for the negative image only contains the top likelihood loss L_{tlloss}. λ_1, λ_2 are balancing parameters and are set to be 1 in this study.

Similarity Loss. The Fast R-CNN usually takes the top 2000 region proposals from the RPN, for each object proposal a region of interest (RoI) pooling layer extracts a fixed-length feature vector from the feature map. Each feature vector is fed into a sequence of fully connected (fc) layers that finally branch into two sibling output layers: one that produces softmax probability estimates the probabilities of object classes and another layer that outputs a set of four real-valued numbers representing bounding-box positions of the classes.

An essential goal for training the negative image is to make the network better identify highly suspected malignant regions from true malignant lesions. Inspired by the successful use of Siamase loss in face recognition [5], which minimizes a discriminative loss function that drives the similarity metric to be small for pairs of faces from the same person, and large for pairs from different persons. We introduce a similarity loss applied on the softmax probability layer of the classification branch in the Fast R-CNN, aiming at improving the network's ability to discriminate the positive region from negative ones. Specifically, during each mini-batch, we selected the feature vectors of the softmax probability in the classification branch whose label is 1 (target label as the original Faster R-CNN defines) when the network processes the positive image. Those features vectors will then maintain the explicit positive features, we denote the number of the feature vectors as K. When the network processes the negative image, we take the same number of feature vectors generated by the top K score anchors from RPN, and pair them with the selected feature vectors of positive images.

A similarity loss is then obtained from the K paired feature vectors as:

$$L_{simloss}(X_1, X_2) = \frac{1}{K} \sum_{i=1}^{K} sim(X_1^i, X_2^i) \tag{3}$$

where X_1 and X_2 are the feature vectors selected from positive and negative images. sim is the cos-embedding function where $sim(X_1^i, X_2^i) = \frac{X_1^i \cdot X_2^i}{\|X_1^i\|\|X_2^i\|}$. The loss is minimized during training to increase the network's discriminability between the positive and selected negative targets.

The negative image shares the same Fast R-CNN loss as the positive image, but since there is no target, the ground-truth label of all the proposals are 0 and no regression loss occurs. The total Fast R-CNN loss is then summarized as

$$L_{fastloss} = L_{clsloss} + \lambda_3 L_{regloss} + \lambda_4 L_{simloss} , \tag{4}$$

which consists of three terms: the classification loss $L_{clsloss}$, the regression loss $L_{regloss}$, and the similarity loss $L_{simloss}$. λ_3, λ_4 are balancing parameters and are set to be 1 and 0.1 in this study.

2.3 Datasets and Evaluation Metrics

Datasets. To test the effectiveness of our proposed top likelihood loss and similarity loss, we adopted two mammography datasets for evaluation.

(1) Private Dense Mammogram Dataset. A private dense mammogram dataset is collected and labeled from the Tianjin Medical University Cancer Institute and Hospital, which consists 721 patients including 417 healthy ones and 304 sick ones. Mammography includes the cranial cardo (CC) and media lateral oblique (MLO) views for most of the screened breasts. Each patient usually have 4 mammography images (R-CC,R-MLO,L-CC, L-MLO), but a few of them only have unilateral mammography images. A few of the lesions are not labeled due to visual artifacts obscuring the image data, including paddles within magnification views or location markers. There are totally 2908 images with 598 labeled malignant lesions. Noticeably, dense breast has a higher risk in developing breast cancer and are harder for cancer detection based on mammography (AUC of 0.72 according to Giger et al. [4]). Only mammographies with non-specific invasive carcinoma is collected and annotated. The dataset was randomly split to the training and testing set with a ratio of 4:1.

(2) DDSM. The public DDSM dataset [6] is also used to validate our model. Following the work in [1], we selected a set of 600 mammograms of the mass type from DDSM which includes 304 malignant cases and 296 benign cases as the training set. The testing set contains 45 malignant cases and 55 benign cases. All annotations of the benign cases are removed to generate unlabeled negative images.

Evaluation Metrics. Two evaluation metrics are introduced to measure the performances of our model. The first one focus on the performance according to object detection, in which the commonly used mean average precision (mAP) are adopted and measured for the predicted targets. True positive IoU matching threshold is set as 0.5 which is the standard criterion in the PASCAL VOC [3] competition. The second one is based on the clinical criterion, in which the sensitivity, specificity, overall accuracy followed by a ROC curve are adopted and measured according to classification of patients. The predicted box with a confidence probability above 0.5 is treated as a predicted target. The sensitivity, specificity and overall accuracy are defined as:

$$Sensitivity = \frac{TP}{(TP+FN)}, \quad Specificity = \frac{TN}{(TN+FP)}$$

$$Accuracy = \frac{(TP+TN)}{(TP+TN+FP+FN)}$$

$$(5)$$

where TP and FN denote the true positive and false negative patient cases. TN and FP represent the true negative and false positive patient cases.

3   Results and Discussion

Training Details. All images are resized to 512 * 512, the initialization settings of the network are the same as that in the original Faster R-CNN [10]. Each mini-batch contains one positive and one negative image. We employ the Adam optimization method. Learning rate is set to be 0.0001 and is reduced by a factor of 10 every 9 k iterations. The overall training procedure is continued for up to 45 k iterations.

Ablation Study on Private Dataset. Ablation study were performed on the private mammography set with results summarized in Table 1. The ROC curve is plotted in Fig. 4. Both top likelihood loss and similarity loss significantly improves the performances for almost all the metrics. The AUC of the classification can be as high as 0.91, which greatly outperform the AUC (0.72) of radiologists' performance reported in Giger et al. [4]. It is worth mention that the original Faster R-CNN which does not train negative images, results in a low specificity since the high false positive rate caused by misclassifying suspected targets. The specificity is increased by 0.25 after introducing the top likelihood loss. It is also interesting to notice that training on the negative images degrades the performance on true positive targets at some extent, but the similarity loss makes positive targets more distinguishable and improves the sensitivity.

Table 1. Performance of our proposed method on the private dense mammograpm dataset.

	tlloss	simloss	mAP	AUC (%)	Accuracy (%)	Sensitivity(%)	Specificity (%)
Faster R-CNN			0.52	84.07	76.22	96.67	61.45
	✓		0.57	86.96	85.31	83.33	86.75
	✓	✓	0.60	91.10	88.81	91.67	86.75

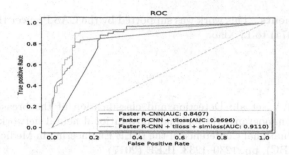

Fig. 4. The ROC curve of our proposed method on the private dataset. Both top likelihood loss (tlloss) and similarity loss (simloss) improve the performance.

Results and Comparisons on DDSM. The performance on the public DDSM dataset is shown in Table 2. We also train the Faster R-CNN with annotated benign cases for comparison. Results show that our proposed model greatly improve the performance according to all the metrics compare to baseline. Especially, the specificity is increased from 0.76 to 0.95. The performance is much better than that in AI-masni et al. [1], the most state-of-the-art work on mass type cancer detection with the same size of training set. Surprisingly, our model also outperforms the baseline even when the annotations of the benign cases are added back for training, with sensitivity increased from 0.87 to 0.91. The increased sensitivity may attribute to that training suspected malignant region makes malignant regions more distinguishable.

Table 2. Performance of our proposed method on the public dataset (DDSM).

	AUC (%)	Accuracy (%)	Sensitivity (%)	Specificity (%)
Faster R-CNN (no annotation on benign)	89.45	81.00	86.67	76.36
Faster R-CNN+tlloss+simloss	94.46	93.00	91.11	94.55
Faster R-CNN (with annotated benign)	92.69	91.00	86.67	94.55
Al-masni et al.	87.74	85.52	93.20	78.00

4   Conclusion

We adapted the region based object detection model to a weakly-supervised learning task that encompasses both images with annotated malignant lesions and healthy images with no annotation. A top likelihood loss together with a new sampling procedure and a similarity loss is distinguish the suspected target from target. The new method demonstrates significant performance improvement in detecting mass type cancer on a private dense mammogram dataset and the public DDSM dataset. We would like to extend this model to other object detection tasks in which normal images contain highly suspected target regions. We would also like to apply the model to detect other type of mammographically visible lesions such as calcifications and architectural distortions.

Acknowledgements. This work was supported by the CAS Pioneer Hundred Talents Program (2017-074) to Li Xiao.

References

1. Al-masni, M.A., et al.: Detection and classification of the breast abnormalities in digital mammograms via regional convolutional neural network. In: 2017 39th Annual International Conference of the IEEE Engineering in Medicine and Biology Society (EMBC), pp. 1230–1233. IEEE (2017)
2. Dhungel, N., Carneiro, G., Bradley, A.P.: A deep learning approach for the analysis of masses in mammograms with minimal user intervention. Med. Image Anal. **37**, 114–128 (2017)
3. Everingham, M., Van Gool, L., Williams, C.K., Winn, J., Zisserman, A.: The pascal visual object classes (VOC) challenge. Int. J. Comput. Vis. **88**(2), 303–338 (2010)
4. Giger, M.L., et al.: Automated breast ultrasound in breast cancer screening of women with dense breasts: reader study of mammography-negative and mammography-positive cancers. AJR Am. J. Roentgenol. **206**(6), 1 (2016)
5. Hadsell, R., Chopra, S., LeCun, Y.: Learning a similarity metric discriminatively, with application to face verification. In: 2005 IEEE Computer Society Conference on Computer Vision and Pattern Recognition, CVPR 2005 (CVPR), vol. 01, pp. 539–546, June 2005. https://doi.org/10.1109/CVPR.2005.202
6. Heath, M., Bowyer, K., Kopans, D., Moore, R., Kegelmeyer, P.: The digital database for screening mammography (2001)
7. Kooi, T., et al.: Large scale deep learning for computer aided detection of mammographic lesions. Med. Image Anal. **35**, 303–312 (2017)
8. Lin, T.Y., et al.: Microsoft COCO: common objects in context. In: Fleet, D., Pajdla, T., Schiele, B., Tuytelaars, T. (eds.) ECCV 2014. LNCS, vol. 8693, pp. 740–755. Springer, Cham (2014). https://doi.org/10.1007/978-3-319-10602-1_48
9. Reiazi, R., Paydar, R., Ardakani, A.A., Etedadialiabadi, M.: Mammography lesion detection using faster R-CNN detector, pp. 111–115, January 2018. https://doi.org/10.5121/csit.2018.80212
10. Ren, S., He, K., Girshick, R., Sun, J.: Faster R-CNN: towards real-time object detection with region proposal networks. In: Advances in Neural Information Processing Systems, pp. 91–99 (2015)

From Unilateral to Bilateral Learning: Detecting Mammogram Masses with Contrasted Bilateral Network

Yuhang Liu[1], Zhen Zhou[2], Shu Zhang[2], Ling Luo[1,3], Qianyi Zhang[1], Fandong Zhang[4], Xiuli Li[1], Yizhou Wang[1,2,5], and Yizhou Yu[1(✉)]

[1] Deepwise AI Lab, Beijing, China
yuyizhou@deepwise.com
[2] Computer Science Department, Peking University, Beijing, China
[3] Beijing University of Posts and Telecommunications, Beijing, China
[4] Center for Data Science, Peking University, Beijing, China
[5] Peng Cheng Laboratory, Shenzhen, China

Abstract. The comparison of bilateral mammogram images is important for finding masses especially in dense breasts. However, most existing mammogram mass detection algorithms only considered unilateral image. In this paper, we propose a deep model called contrasted bilateral network (CBN) to take bilateral information into consideration. In CBN, Mask R-CNN is used as a basic framework, upon which two major modules are developed to exploit the bilateral information: distortion insensitive comparison module and logic guided bilateral module. The former one is designed to be robust to nonrigid distortion of bilateral registration, while the latter one integrates the bilateral domain knowledge of radiologist. Experimental results on DDSM dataset demonstrate that the proposed algorithm achieves the state-of-the-art performance.

Keywords: Mammogram mass · Object detection · Domain knowledge

1 Introduction

Breast cancer is the leading cause of cancer deaths among women worldwide [12]. Early detection and diagnosis is the key to reduce the death rate of breast cancer. Breast mass is one of the most common signs of early breast cancer. Specially, masses differ in shapes, margins, sizes, location and backgrounds. Moreover, in dense breasts, masses may be partially obscured by the gland. Thus, mass detection remains a challenge for both radiologists and Computer-aided detection (CAD) system.

In this paper, we propose a deep network called contrasted bilateral network (CBN) is

---

Y. Liu and Z. Zhou—Equal contribution.

© Springer Nature Switzerland AG 2019
D. Shen et al. (Eds.): MICCAI 2019, LNCS 11769, pp. 477–485, 2019.
https://doi.org/10.1007/978-3-030-32226-7_53

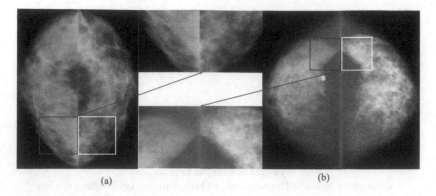

(a)   (b)

Fig. 1. An illustration of identifying masses in mammogram images. (a) and (b) are sampled from DDSM dataset. The mass in (a) is hard to notice with only one lateral image, but obviously asymmetric with the corresponding region in the contralateral image. (b) shows the region may be misclassified as a mass on account of clear boundaries, while the contralateral image presents that both sides are highly symmetrical.

Bilateral information is regarded as important domain knowledge in mass detection. In standard mammographic screening, X-ray images are captured from both two breasts. For each breast, two mammographic views (cranio-caudal and mediolateral oblique views) are taken. Compared with other medical imaging methods, the key factor that disrupts the mammogram reading is the extremely varied glands with high intensity in the background. It is known that both breasts of the same patient tend to have a high degree of symmetry. Radiologists usually take two steps to identify masses. First is to find suspicious regions in one laterality by the details such as texture, shape, margin, location and so on. Then, the symmetric regions in the contralateral image are referred to for further analysis. Figure 1 illustrates the significance of referring to bilateral mammogram images. The mass on Fig. 1(a) is hard to notice with only one lateral image due to interruption of complex gland background. If compared with corresponding region in the contralateral image, the mass can be clearly distinguished since it is asymmetric. As a result, bilateral information helps to improve sensitivity. The region on Fig. 1(b) may be misclassified as a mass on account of clear boundaries and textures, while the contralateral image presents that both sides are highly symmetrical. Consequently, the bilateral analysis helps to remove false positives.

Previous works achieve competitive good performance on mass detection. Tai *et al.* [13] designed an automated mass detection system based on complex handcrafted texture features. Ribli *et al.* [11] attempted to adopt Faster-CNN to detect mammogram masses. However, these approaches only use unilateral image, while bilateral mammogram images containing rich domain knowledge are not explicitly considered.

In this paper, a deep network called contrasted bilateral network (CBN) is proposed for automated mammogram mass detection. Motivated by the domain knowledge that radiologists read mammogram images, we integrate the bilateral information to the model explicitly, and tackle two important problems along the way. To find the corresponding region in the contralateral image, image registration as an image-level solution is firstly applied to map bilateral images into one coordinate system. Moreover, distortion insensitive comparison module is specially designed to tolerate nonrigid distortion of bilateral images. To further boost the performance, we analyze the inherent logic and constraints of the way that radiologists read images, and propose logic guided bilateral module. The overall pipeline can be integrated smoothly to Mask R-CNN framework and trained end-to-end. Experimental results on DDSM public dataset [5] demonstrate that the proposed algorithm has achieved state-of-the art performance.

2   Related Work

The mammogram mass detection methods can be coarsely classified into two categories.

One is traditional methods which use handcrafted features and structures [9]. Tai *et al.* [13] designed an automated mass detection system based on complex handcrafted texture features. However, the model performance is still limited due to a lack of representation ability. Diniz *et al.* [2] attempted to generate proposals by residuals between bilateral images and cascade a classifier to reduce false positives. However, the model cannot be trained end-to-end, namely, the whole pipeline may not be fully optimized since components were separately trained and tuned. Meanwhile, these methods may suffer difficulty in localization, as no refinement on patch proposals is taken in the classification stage.

Another is deep learning based methods. Ribli *et al.* [11] attempted to adopt Faster-CNN to detect mammogram masses. Jung *et al.* [6] proposed a mass detection model based on RetinaNet [7] and achieved comparable or better performance on public and in-house datasets. Dhungel *et al.* [1] detected mass using cascaded deep learning and random forests. Deep learning based methods is powerful, and can learn to extract features automatically. However, the bilateral property regarded as an important domain knowledge, is not explicitly modeled in the model.

3   Methodology

As illustrated in Fig. 2, the CBN uses the state-of-the-art object detection model Mask R-CNN [3] as a basic framework. In order to benefit from bilateral information, we have to address two major concerns: (1) *Where to find the corresponding region in the contralateral image?* (2) *How to contrast the bilateral images?*

We tackle the first problem by image pre-processing and distortion insensitive comparison module in CBN. Meanwhile, the logic guided bilateral module is designed to deal with the second problem. In the following subsections, we describe each step of our approach in detail.

3.1   Pre-processing with Coarse Alignment

We coarsely align the bilateral images via image registration method. It transforms the bilateral images into one coordinate system, in which we can compare the corresponding background surrounding masses. It consists of two major steps:

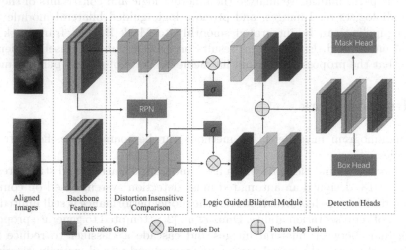

Fig. 2. The architecture of contrasted bilateral network. Bilateral images are coarsely aligned by method in Sect. 3.1. The distortion insensitive comparison module takes ROI aligned features to resist geometric variances, and logic guided bilateral module integrates inherent logic of radiologists reading mammogram images.

Segmentation. Firstly, we performs threshold operation to source image to get breast pre-segment. To reduce the computation cost, the pre-segment mask is zoomed out to one tenth of the original size. Next, we pad three sides of the zoom-out mask (except the side that the breast locate at), and run the flood fill algorithm with seeds starting at the opposite side of the breast. Finally, morphological operations are also used to remove burrs and smooth the boundary.

Image Alignment. After performing breast segmentation on bilateral images, we can firstly get the segments of the breasts. Spontaneously, we crop and get breast regions. Lastly, the contralateral image is zoomed to the same size as the examined image and horizontally flipped.

3.2   Distortion Insensitive Comparison

Coarse alignment in Sect. 3.1 provides an image-level correspondence. However, the geometric deformation is inevitable mainly due to the distortion of the objects and systematic error by image registration method. As a result, it requires the proposed model to tolerate the geometric deformation.

It is intuitive to concatenate the bilateral backbone features and stack convolutional layers on top of them to learn the comparison. However, this kind of method only provides a pix-level correspondence, which is sensitive to geometric variances. Geometric deformation issue remains unsolved.

The key high-level spirit of our distortion insensitive comparison mechanism is to summarize the spatial information of the proposal features. Specifically, proposal-level geometric representations are offered by region proposal network (RPN). RPN filters the backbone features and predicts region proposals with a wide range of scales and aspect ratios. ROI align computes the exact values of the input features at four regularly sampled locations in each ROI bin, and aggregates the result [3]. After ROI align operation, the spatial information is abstracted. Naturally, it's less sensitive to the geometric variances. The distortion insensitive comparison module takes ROI features as input. This connection mode is our particular design to tolerate the geometric variances implicitly.

3.3   Logic Guided Bilateral Module

How to effectively contrast bilateral images? We analyze the inherent logic of the way that radiologists read mammogram images, and conclude the different operations under various circumstances. Let $f_e, f_c \in \mathbf{R}^{C \times WH}$ denote the corresponding region features extracted from the examined breast image and the contralateral image, where C, W and H indicate the channel, spatial width and height of the ROI region. We label $l_* = 1$ as a mass region and $l_* = 0$ as a normal region, where $* \in \{e, c\}$. As shown on Table 1, mass identifying situation analysis and corresponding operations are summarized. "attenuate" and "enhance" mean that f_e should be attenuated or enhanced if given bilateral information, while "ignore" means that our model should ignore f_c signal and focus on f_e only. The table provides a high-level abstraction, and guide the way for the logic guided bilateral design.

Table 1. Mass identifying situation analysis of bilateral images.

f_e	f_c	Operation
0	0	attenuate
1	0	enhance
0	1	ignore
1	1	ignore

Here, we propose an instantiation of analysis above and denote:

$$gate(x) = \sigma(w^T x) \tag{1}$$

$$\sigma(y) = \frac{1}{1 + e^{-y}} \tag{2}$$

Where $x \in \mathbf{R}^n$ denotes input variable, n denotes dimension, and w is learnable weights, σ refers to sigmoid function. Naturally, the situations can be simulated in the following form:

$$f_e^* = gate(w_e^T f_e) \cdot f_e \qquad (3)$$

$$f_c^* = gate(w_c^T f_c) \cdot f_c \qquad (4)$$

$$f_o = tanh(w_o^T [f_e^*, f_c^*]) \qquad (5)$$

Where w_e, w_c and w_o are learnable parameters, and $\cdot$ indicates element-wise product. f_e^* and f_c^* aim to learn the changing according to different situations, while f_o learns to fuse the features. Figure 2 illustrates the detailed connection mode.

4   Experiments

4.1   Datasets and Baselines

We conduct our experiment on the public dataset DDSM [5]. Other datasets [8] are not considered for either insufficient bilateral images or limited mass instances to train deep models. There are 2620 cases in DDSM dataset. The dataset is randomly divided into training, validation and testing sets by 8:1:1.

Faster R-CNN [10] is a solid baseline on object detection task. To exploit the mask supervision for enhanced localization performance, we also employ the Mask R-CNN [3] as a baseline, which is one of the state-of-the art methods on object detection and instance segmentation. ResNet50 [4] is used as the backbone.

Table 2. Proposal evaluations on DDSM dataset (%).

Method	R@0.50	R@1.00	R@2.00	R@3.00	R@4.00
Faster R-CNN	66.10	72.46	78.39	80.50	83.05
Mask R-CNN	64.41	74.58	81.78	85.59	86.86
CBN	**69.07**	**78.81**	**85.59**	**87.71**	**88.98**

4.2   Performance

The performance is evaluated by the recalls at k false positives per image, which is simplified as R@k, where $k \in \{0.5, 1, 2, 3, 4\}$ for all models. The mass is recalled if the IOU (Intersection over Union) is above 0.2 with ground truth bounding box [1].

The detection results are shown in Table 2. We can see that our proposed model outperforms both baseline models. Besides, we visually compare results to indicate how CBN can benefit from bilateral information. As shown in Fig. 3, we can conclude that: (1) CBN effectively improves the sensitivity and localization ability (the first and second rows). (2) The false positives can be reduced by comparing the symmetric regions on bilateral images (the last row).

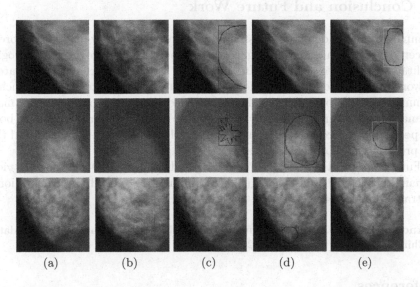

(a)   (b)   (c)   (d)   (e)

Fig. 3. Detection results of CBN. Each row shows a case from DDSM dataset. Column (a)–(c) refer to examined image, contralateral image and ground truth image. Column (d)–(e) present corresponding results by Mask-RCNN and CBN.

Table 3. Ablation study on DDSM dataset (%).

Method	R@0.50	R@1.00	R@2.00	R@3.00	R@4.00
Naive FeatCat	63.98	77.54	83.47	86.44	88.14
CBN w/o LGBM	65.22	75.22	84.48	86.96	88.70
CBN	**69.07**	**78.81**	**85.59**	**87.71**	**88.98**

4.3   Ablation Study

Ablation study is conducted to verify the effectiveness of each module in CBN. As shown in Table 3, we present two variances of CBN: "Naive FeatCat" that directly concatenates the bilateral backbone features before ROI align, "CBN w/o LGBM" that removes logic guided bilateral module of CBN and directly concatenates ROI aligned features, and "CBN" which indicates our proposed model. We draw following conclusions from the results: (1) Feature comparison after the ROI align produces more reliable results; (2) Logic guided bilateral module effectively improves the detection performance.

5   Conclusion and Future Work

Mammogram mass detection is essentially important to early diagnosis of breast cancer. Bilateral information regarded as expert knowledge from radiologists facilitates mass detection task. In this paper, we propose contrasted bilateral network for mammogram mass detection. Geometric consistency issues such as alignment and distortion are explicitly modeled in our approach. Further more, we analyze the inherent logic and propose logic guided bilateral module to boost the performance. Experiment results on DDSM dataset have demonstrated that the proposed method achieves state-of-the-art performance.

Future work will include: (1) integrating multi-view (MLO view and CC view) domain knowledge to the model; (2) exploring more powerful implementation of contrasted modeling.

Acknowledgement. This work is funded by the National Natural Science Foundation of China (Grant No. 61625201, 61527804).

References

1. Dhungel, N., Carneiro, G., Bradley, A.P.: Automated mass detection in mammograms using cascaded deep learning and random forests. In: 2015 International Conference on Digital Image Computing: Techniques and Applications (DICTA), pp. 1–8. IEEE (2015)
2. Diniz, J.O.B., Diniz, P.H.B., Valente, T.L.A., Silva, A.C., de Paiva, A.C., Gattass, M.: Detection of mass regions in mammograms by bilateral analysis adapted to breast density using similarity indexes and convolutional neural networks. Comput. Methods Programs Biomed. **156**, 191–207 (2018)
3. He, K., Gkioxari, G., Dollár, P., Girshick, R.: Mask R-CNN. In: Proceedings of the IEEE International Conference on Computer Vision, pp. 2961–2969 (2017)
4. He, K., Zhang, X., Ren, S., Sun, J.: Deep residual learning for image recognition. In: Proceedings of the IEEE Conference on Computer Vision and Pattern Recognition, pp. 770–778 (2016)
5. Heath, M., Bowyer, K., Kopans, D., Moore, R., Kegelmeyer, W.P.: The digital database for screening mammography. In: Proceedings of the 5th International Workshop on Digital Mammography, pp. 212–218. Medical Physics Publishing (2000)
6. Jung, H., et al.: Detection of masses in mammograms using a one-stage object detector based on a deep convolutional neural network. PloS One **13**(9), e0203355 (2018)

7. Lin, T.Y., Goyal, P., Girshick, R., He, K., Dollár, P.: Focal loss for dense object detection. In: Proceedings of the IEEE International Conference on Computer Vision, pp. 2980–2988 (2017)

8. Moreira, I.C., Amaral, I., Domingues, I., Cardoso, A., Cardoso, M.J., Cardoso, J.S.: INbreast: toward a full-field digital mammographic database. Acad. Radiol. 19(2), 236–248 (2012)

9. Mudigonda, N.R., Rangayyan, R.M., Desautels, J.L.: Detection of breast masses in mammograms by density slicing and texture flow-field analysis. IEEE Trans. Med. Imaging 20(12), 1215–1227 (2001)

10. Ren, S., He, K., Girshick, R., Sun, J.: Faster R-CNN: towards real-time object detection with region proposal networks. In: Advances in Neural Information Processing Systems, pp. 91–99 (2015)

11. Ribli, D., Horváth, A., Unger, Z., Pollner, P., Csabai, I.: Detecting and classifying lesions in mammograms with deep learning. Sci. Rep. 8(1), 4165 (2018)

12. Siegel, R., Ma, J., Zou, Z., Jemal, A.: Cancer statistics, 2014. CA: A Cancer J. Clin. 64(1), 9–29 (2014)

13. Tai, S.C., Chen, Z.S., Tsai, W.T.: An automatic mass detection system in mammograms based on complex texture features. IEEE J. Biomed. Health Inform. 18(2), 618–627 (2014)

Signed Laplacian Deep Learning
with Adversarial Augmentation
for Improved Mammography Diagnosis

Heyi Li[1(✉)], Dongdong Chen[1], William H. Nailon[2], Mike E. Davies[1],
and David I. Laurenson[1]

[1] Institute for Digital Communications, University of Edinburgh, Edinburgh, UK
{Heyi.Li,d.chen,dave.laurenson,mike.davies}@ed.ac.uk
[2] Oncology Physics Department, Edinburgh Cancer Centre,
Western General Hospital, Edinburgh, UK
bill.nailon@luht.scot.nhs.uk

Abstract. Computer-aided breast cancer diagnosis in mammography
is limited by inadequate data and the similarity between benign and
cancerous masses. To address this, we propose a signed graph regularized
deep neural network with adversarial augmentation, named DIAGNET.
Firstly, we use adversarial learning to generate positive and negative
mass-contained mammograms for each mass class. After that, a signed
similarity graph is built upon the expanded data to further highlight the
discrimination. Finally, a deep convolutional neural network is trained
by jointly optimizing the signed graph regularization and classification
loss. Experiments show that the DIAGNET framework outperforms the
state-of-the-art in breast mass diagnosis in mammography.

Keywords: Deep learning · Mammography diagnosis · Adversarial
learning · Graph regularization

1 Introduction

Breast cancer is one of the most frequently diagnosed mortal diseases for women
all over the world [6]. Mammography is extensively applied and computer-aided
diagnosis systems (CADs) are often employed as a second reader. Leveraging
the recent success of deep neural networks on representation learning, deep
learning based CADs [7,11,12,16,17,20] outperform traditional methods, which
rely heavily on handcrafted features. However, two major challenges in mammographic CADs remain (1): limited access to well annotated data [7] and (2): the
similarity between benign and cancerous masses. To alleviate the impact of inadequate data, [7,11,12,20] applied classical geometric transformations for data

---

H. Li and D. Chen—These authors contribute equally to this work.

© Springer Nature Switzerland AG 2019
D. Shen et al. (Eds.): MICCAI 2019, LNCS 11769, pp. 486–494, 2019.
https://doi.org/10.1007/978-3-030-32226-7_54

augmentation (e.g. flips, rotations, random crops etc.), and more recently, [16,17] generated synthetic images on the manifold of real mammograms using adversarial learning [9], which enjoys a powerful ability to learn the unknown underlying distribution. Unfortunately, the following questions remain unanswered: What kind of data augmentation is most helpful for CADs in mammography? How can we alleviate the impact of the similarity between data, i.e., how can we maximize the margin between manifolds with a small difference?

In this paper, we propose a new deep learning framework that improves mammography diagnosis as follows. Firstly, we propose an adversarial data augmentation strategy, in which both positive and negative samples of specific classes are generated in an unsupervised manner, in order to make more distinct boundaries between different classes. After that, we build a signed graph Laplacian over the augmented data to quantitatively capture the geometric structure of data. Finally, we train a deep neural network by jointly optimizing the graph regularization and classification loss, by which the intra-class difference is minimized, and more importantly, the inter-class manifold margin is maximized in the deep representation space. Extensive experiments show that the proposed DIAGNET outperforms the state-of-the-art of breast masses diagnosis in mammography.

2 Preliminary

2.1 Adversarial Learning

Adversarial learning is a technique that attempts to fool models through malicious input [10] and has achieved impressive results in representation learning. The key idea of the success of a Generative Adversarial Network (GAN) is to force the output of the generator to be indistinguishable from the real input [9]. Adversarial training is particularly powerful for image generation, and for learning unknown and complicated distributions from the training data. In this paper, we propose to use adversarial learning to generate off-distribution instances along with on-distribution instances in order to enlarge the medical image data.

2.2 Manifold Learning

In real applications, data typically reside on a low-dimensional manifold embedded into a high-dimensional ambient space [15]. Manifold learning is extensively explored because of its effectiveness for preserving the topological locality, which relies on the assumption that neighbors tend to have the same labels [3]. In this paper, we aim to incorporate graph embedding into a deep neural network as a regularizer in the latent space. In addition, local data manifold structure preservation within the hidden representations in deep neural networks offers the possibility of improving the performance of the classifier [4].

3   Proposed Method

In this section, we formally introduce the details of DIAGNET, which is composed of three steps as shown in Fig. 1: (1) adversarial augmentation, (2) a signed graph Laplacian built upon the augmented data and (3) joint optimization of the classifier loss and signed graph regularizer. We first define the notation applied throughout the paper. Let $\{X, Y\} = \{x_i, y_i\}_{i=1}^n$ be the n mammograms with corresponding labels, where $x_i \in \mathbb{R}^{H \times W}$ is an image sample and $y_i \in \{y_c\}_{c=1}^C$ is the class label. Let $\{X_c, y_c\}$ denote the c-th class data.

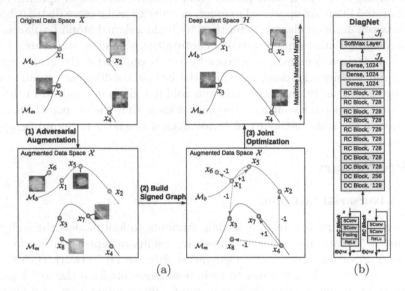

Fig. 1. The proposed DIAGNET for Breast Mass Diagnosis. (a) the framework of the proposed algorithm, which consists of three steps. $\{x_1, x_2\}$ and $\{x_3, x_4\}$ are samples on benign manifold $\mathcal{M}_b$ and malignant manifold $\mathcal{M}_m$ respectively. In the first step, i.e. adversarial data augmentation, positive neighbors $\{x_5, x_7\}$ and negative neighbors $\{x_6, x_8\}$ are generated with (1) and (2) respectively. Then a signed graph is built upon both original and augmented samples as (3). Finally, a joint loss (6) is optimized in the deep latent space, maximizing data manifold margin. (b) The utilized deep network architecture. "DC block" represents a down-sampling convolutional block, "RC block" is a residual convolutional block, and "SConv" is separable convolutions.

3.1   Adversarial Augmentation

As also mentioned in Sect. 1, inadequate data and the similarity between benign and cancerous masses [7] are two main reasons causing high false positives in mammographic CADs. Recently, [1,16,17] employed GANs to create new instances. Even though they generated on-distribution samples that are not separable by discriminators, they ignored the importance of distinguishable but similar instances, which tend to improve the discriminative ability. To overcome this shortcoming, as shown in Fig. 1(a), we propose to use adversarial learning to generate more instances of both *positive neighbors* (i.e. instances on the manifold, e.g. x_5 and x_7) and *negative neighbors* (i.e. instances off the manifold, e.g. x_6 and x_8). Here, there are defined two manifolds: $\mathcal{M}_b$ for benign images and $\mathcal{M}_m$ for malignant images.

In particular, inspired by [19], we generate neighboring instances one by one for a certain data class $\{X_c, y_c\}$, $c = 1, 2, \cdots, C$, where $C = 2$ in this paper. Specifically, both positive and negative neighbors are generated based on the noise corrupted seed points (a number of randomly selected samples in X_c) and they are both close to the original data points. In particular, the positive neighbors X_c^+ are the generated samples that cannot be separated from X_c by a discriminator, while the negative neighbors X_c^- are the ones that can be separated. Finally, the expanded dataset for class c is of the form $\mathcal{X}_c = \{X_c \cup X_c^+ \cup X_c^-\}$, and the whole dataset is $\mathcal{X} = \bigcup_c \mathcal{X}_c$.

Let x be a desired new sample and $P(x; X_c, X_c^+)$ be the probability that x is classified as class c by a discriminator trained on $\{X_c, X_c^+\}$. Similarly $P(x; X_c, X_c^-)$ corresponds to a discriminator trained on $\{X_c, X_c^-\}$. Note that X_c^+ and X_c^- are initialized as empty. In this paper, we trained two SVM classifiers as the discriminators and the corresponding output probability is obtained with logistic sigmoid of the output signed distance. Accordingly, a set of neighboring instances $\{x_t\}_{t=1}^T$ of X_c are iteratively generated. In each iteration t, the discriminator is learned and the weights are updated. After T iterations of training, we select one desired positive neighbor x:

$$\arg\max_x P\left(x; X_c, X_c^+ \cup \{x_t\}_{t=1}^T\right) - \gamma \max\{0, r_1 - \min_{x_i \in X_c^+} d(x, x_i)\}, \quad (1)$$

where $d(\cdot)$ is a distance measure, γ weights the distance regularization, forcing generated points to be different with a minimum distance r_1. Similarly, we select one desired negative neighbor x, with an added distance restriction to force new points to be scattered close to X_c:

$$\arg\min_x P\left(x; X_c, X_c^- \cup \{x_t\}_{t=1}^T\right) + \gamma \max\{0, r_2 - \min_{x_j \in X_c^-} d(x, x_j)\}$$
$$+ \gamma \max\{0, \min_{x_i \in X_c} d(x, x_i) - r_3\}, \quad (2)$$

where the distance regularization forces generated points to acquire a minimum distance r_2 and maximum distance r_3.

3.2   Signed Graph Laplacian Regularizer

Graph embedding trained with distributional context can boost performance in various pattern recognition tasks. In this paper, we aim to incorporate the signed graph Laplacian regularizer [2] to learn a discriminative datum representation $\mathcal{H}(\mathcal{X})$ by a deep neural network, where discriminative here means that the intra-class data manifold structure is preserved in the latent space and the inter-manifold (slightly different) margins are maximized.

Using the supervision of the adversarial augmentation in Sect. 3.1, we build a signed graph upon the expanded data $\mathcal{X}$. Given $\mathcal{X}_c = \{X_c, X_c^+, X_c^-\}$ for class c, and all other classes data $\mathcal{X}_{-c} = \bigcup_{t=1,\cdots,C;t\neq c}\{X_t, X_t^+, X_t^-\}$, for $\forall \boldsymbol{x}_i \in \mathcal{X}_c$, the corresponding elements in the signed graph is built as follows:

$$\phi_{ij} = \begin{cases} +1, & \boldsymbol{x}_j \in \{X_c \cup X_c^+\}_i^{n^+}, \\ -1, & \boldsymbol{x}_j \in \{X_{-c} \cup \mathcal{X}_c^-\}_i^{n^-}, \end{cases} \tag{3}$$

where the $\{\cdot\}_i^{n^+}$ ($\{\cdot\}_i^{n^-}$) denotes the corresponding n^+ (n^-) nearest neighborhood of x_i to approximate the locality of the manifold.

Then, we compute the structure preservation in the deep representation space (directly behind the softmax layer as shown in Fig. 1(b)) $\mathcal{H} = \{h(\boldsymbol{x}_i)\}_{i=1}^N$, where $N = |\mathcal{X}|$. The signed graph Laplacian regularizer is defined as following:

$$\mathcal{J}_g(\mathcal{X}, \varPhi) = \sum_{i,j} \begin{cases} \phi_{ij} \cdot dist(h(\boldsymbol{x}_i), h(\boldsymbol{x}_j)), & \text{if } \phi_{ij} > 0 \\ \max\left(0, m + \phi_{ij} \cdot dist(h(\boldsymbol{x}_i), h(\boldsymbol{x}_j))\right), & \text{if } \phi_{ij} < 0, \end{cases} \tag{4}$$

where $dist(\cdot)$ is a distance metric for the dissimilarity between $h(\boldsymbol{x}_i)$ and $h(\boldsymbol{x}_j)$. It encourages similar examples to be close, and those that are dissimilar to have a distance of at least m each other, where $m > 0$ is a margin.

Note that instead of calculating the manifold embedding by solving an eigenvalue decomposition, we learn the embedding $\mathcal{H}$ by a deep neural network. Specifically, inspired by the depth-wise separable convolutions [5] that are extensively employed to learn mappings with a series of factoring filters, we build stacks of depth-wise separable convolutions with similar topological architecture to that in [5] to learn such deep representations (Fig. 1(b)).

Therefore, by minimizing (4), it is expected that if two connected nodes $\boldsymbol{x}_i$ and $\boldsymbol{x}_j$ are from the same class (i.e. ϕ_{ij} is positive), $h(\boldsymbol{x}_i)$ and $h(\boldsymbol{x}_j)$ are also close to each other, and vice versa. Benefiting from such learned discriminativity, we train a simple softmax classifier to predict the class label, i.e.,

$$\mathcal{J}_l = -\frac{1}{N} \sum_{i=1}^N \sum_{c=1}^C \delta_c(y_i) \log P(y_i \mid \boldsymbol{x}_i; \boldsymbol{\theta}), \tag{5}$$

where $\delta_c(y_i) = 1$ when $y_i = c$, and 0 otherwise; $\boldsymbol{\theta}$ is the parameter set of the neural network.

Finally, by incorporating the signed Laplacian regularizer (4) and the classification loss (5), the total objective of DIAGNET is accordingly defined as:

$$\mathcal{J} = \mathcal{J}_l + \lambda \mathcal{J}_g, \tag{6}$$

where $\lambda \geq 0$ is the regularization trade-off parameter which controls the smoothness of hidden representations.

4 Experiments

4.1 Datasets and ROIs Selection

The DIAGNET is evaluated on the most frequently used full-field digital mammographic dataset, INbreast [13]. 107 mass contained mammograms are divided into a training and a test set containing 80% and 20% of the images respectively. As for ROIs selection, rectangular mass-contained boxes are selected with proportional padding (1.6 times) upon original ROI bounding boxes. The selected ROIs are augmented with flips and further adversarially augmented by 40% more (20% positive neighbors and 20% negative neighbors).

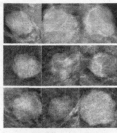 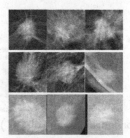

(a) Benign Masses   (b) Malignant Masses

Fig. 2. Generated mammogram examples by proposed adversarial augmentation strategy. The masses in the first row of both (a) and (b) are original data, the second and the third row are generated positive and negative neighbors, respectively.

4.2 Implementation Details

We first solve the proposed adversarial augmentation in (1) and (2) by the derivative-free optimization approach RACOS algorithm [18]. The distance measure $d(\cdot)$ in (1) and (2) is set to be the angular cosine distance because of its superior discriminative information [14]. Let $\rho = \min_{x_i, x_j \in \mathcal{X}_c} d(x_i, x_j)$, then we set the radius parameters $r_1, r_2 = \rho$, and $r_3 = 3 \times \rho$ for $\mathcal{X}_c$. Further $T = 200$ and γ is 10^{-2}.

Secondly, the signed graph is built upon augmented data $\mathcal{X}$. For each graph node, n^+ and n^- in (3) are optimally chosen as 1 and 4 respectively using grid search. In addition, the metric $dist(\cdot)$ in (4) is also the angular cosine distance and m is 1.

Finally, the deep neural network is built with stacks of 3×3 kernel-sized separable convolutional layers. The first three blocks are equipped with increasing feature maps (128, 256, 728) and decreasing spatial squared size (224, 112, 56), and the consecutive seven blocks keep the same feature map with size 28. After global averaging and three fully connected layers of 1024 neurons, a softmax layer is padded for label prediction. Dropout layers with 50% dropout rate and

Table 1. Breast Mass Diagnosis performance comparisons of the proposed DIAGNET and relative state-of-the art methods on INbreast test set.

Methodology	End-to-end	Accuracy	AUC
Domingues *et al.* [8]	✗	89%	N/A
Dhungel *et al.* [7]	✓	91%	0.76
Zhu *et al.* [20]	✓	90%	0.89
Shams *et al.* [16]	✓	93%	0.92
Li *et al.* [11]	✓	88%	0.92
Proposed DIAGNET	✓	**93.4 ± 1.9%**	**0.950 ± 0.02**

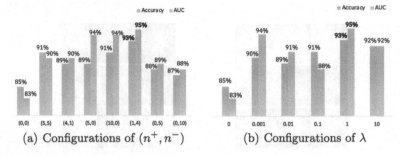

(a) Configurations of (n^+, n^-) (b) Configurations of λ

Fig. 3. Performance of DIAGNET on INBreast with varying parameters. Classification accuracy and AUC score versus (a) different n^+ positive neighbors and n^- negative neighbors and (b) various regularizer parameter λ.

weight decay with l_2 norm rate 10^{-4} are used to prevent over-fitting. Residual skips are added in order to solve the gradient diverging and vanishing problems. The regularization parameter λ in (6) is optimally chosen as 1.

4.3 Results and Analysis

Adversarial Augmentation: To examine the quality of generated images by the proposed adversarial augmentation strategy, we carry out the experiment on the INbreast dataset. Figure 2 visually shows the augmented examples. It can be seen that, for either mass type, the generated positive and negative neighbors are both similar to the original data, but the negative neighbors are more different.

Compare to the State-of-Art: We validate DIAGNET's performance with accuracy and AUC (area under the ROC curve) scores. Table 1 compares the state-of-art algorithms, in which [11] is re-implemented and the results of the remaining ones are taken from the original papers. It shows that, the DIAGNET has achieved the state-of-art with mean accuracy 93.4% and AUC score 0.95. When compared with the second best algorithm [16], the DIAGNET's AUC score is significantly higher with experiments on the whole dataset without any pre-processing, post-processing or transfer learning. In addition, empirical observations show that our model is robust to noise and geometric transforms, and these results are omitted due to the space limitation.

Importance of Signed Graph Laplacian Regularizer: Determining the optimal values of hyper-parameter is a big challenge in deep learning. To explore DIAGNET's performance with different signed graph configurations, the values of n^+ and n^- are first grid searched with fixed regularization parameter $\lambda = 1$, as shown in Fig. 3(a). The best performance occurs when $n^+ = 1$ and $n^- = 4$, which increases at least by 8% the accuracy rate and by 12% the AUC score compared to the baseline (no graph regularization, $n^+, n^- = 0$). This confirms the effectiveness of using the signed graph regularization. In addition, results show that the DIAGNET achieves good performance only when both n^+ and n^- are considered in the corresponding singed graph construction. Figure 3 shows the performances with various values of λ, where the best result occurs at $\lambda = 1$.

5   Conclusions

In this paper, we proposed a DIAGNET for improved mammogram image analysis. By integrating the signed graph regularizer and the adversarial sampling augmentation, DIAGNET works in a simple but effective way to learn discriminative features. Extensive experiments show that our method outperforms state-of-the-art on breast mass diagnosis in mammography.

References

1. Antoniou, A., Storkey, A., Edwards, H.: Data augmentation generative adversarial networks. arXiv preprint arXiv:1711.04340 (2017)
2. Chen, D., Lv, J., Davies, M.E.: Learning discriminative representation with signed Laplacian restricted Boltzmann machine. arXiv preprint arXiv:1808.09389 (2018)
3. Chen, D., Lv, J., Yi, Z.: Unsupervised multi-manifold clustering by learning deep representation. In: Workshops at the 31th AAAI Conference on Artificial Intelligence (AAAI), pp. 385–391 (2017)
4. Chen, D., Lv, J., Yi, Z.: Graph regularized restricted Boltzmann machine. IEEE Trans. Neural Netw. Learn. Syst. **29**(6), 2651–2659 (2018)
5. Chollet, F.: Xception: deep learning with depthwise separable convolutions. In: Proceedings of the IEEE Conference on Computer Vision and Pattern Recognition, pp. 1251–1258 (2017)
6. DeSantis, C., Ma, J., Bryan, L., Jemal, A.: Breast cancer statistics, 2013. CA: Cancer J. Clin. **64**(1), 52–62 (2014)
7. Dhungel, N., Carneiro, G., Bradley, A.P.: The automated learning of deep features for breast mass classification from mammograms. In: Ourselin, S., Joskowicz, L., Sabuncu, M.R., Unal, G., Wells, W. (eds.) MICCAI 2016. LNCS, vol. 9901, pp. 106–114. Springer, Cham (2016). https://doi.org/10.1007/978-3-319-46723-8_13
8. Domingues, I., Sales, E., Cardoso, J., Pereira, W.: INbreast-database masses characterization. In: XXIII CBEB (2012)
9. Goodfellow, I., et al.: Generative adversarial nets. In: Advances in Neural Information Processing Systems, pp. 2672–2680 (2014)

10. Kurakin, A., Goodfellow, I.J., Bengio, S.: Adversarial machine learning at scale (2017)
11. Li, H., Chen, D., Nailon, W.H., Davies, M.E., Laurenson, D.: A deep dual-path network for improved mammogram image processing. In: International Conference on Acoustics, Speech and Signal Processing (2019)
12. Li, H., Chen, D., Nailon, W.H., Davies, M.E., Laurenson, D.: Improved breast mass segmentation in mammograms with conditional residual U-Net. In: Stoyanov, D., et al. (eds.) RAMBO/BIA/TIA-2018. LNCS, vol. 11040, pp. 81–89. Springer, Cham (2018). https://doi.org/10.1007/978-3-030-00946-5_9
13. Moreira, I.C., Amaral, I., Domingues, I., Cardoso, A., Cardoso, M.J., Cardoso, J.S.: INbreast: toward a full-field digital mammographic database. Acad. Radiol. 19(2), 236–248 (2012)
14. Nair, V., Hinton, G.E.: Rectified linear units improve restricted Boltzmann machines. In: Proceedings of the 27th International Conference on Machine Learning, ICML 2010, pp. 807–814 (2010)
15. Seung, H.S., Lee, D.D.: The manifold ways of perception. Science 290(5500), 2268–2269 (2000)
16. Shams, S., Platania, R., Zhang, J., Kim, J., Lee, K., Park, S.-J.: Deep generative breast cancer screening and diagnosis. In: Frangi, A.F., Schnabel, J.A., Davatzikos, C., Alberola-López, C., Fichtinger, G. (eds.) MICCAI 2018. LNCS, vol. 11071, pp. 859–867. Springer, Cham (2018). https://doi.org/10.1007/978-3-030-00934-2_95
17. Wu, E., Wu, K., Cox, D., Lotter, W.: Conditional infilling GANs for data augmentation in mammogram classification. In: Stoyanov, D., et al. (eds.) RAMBO/BIA/TIA -2018. LNCS, vol. 11040, pp. 98–106. Springer, Cham (2018). https://doi.org/10.1007/978-3-030-00946-5_11
18. Yu, Y., Qian, H., Hu, Y.Q.: Derivative-free optimization via classification. In: Thirtieth AAAI Conference on Artificial Intelligence (2016)
19. Yu, Y., Qu, W.Y., Li, N., Guo, Z.: Open-category classification by adversarial sample generation. In: International Joint Conference on Artificial Intelligence (2017)
20. Zhu, W., Lou, Q., Vang, Y.S., Xie, X.: Deep multi-instance networks with sparse label assignment for whole mammogram classification. In: Descoteaux, M., Maier-Hein, L., Franz, A., Jannin, P., Collins, D.L., Duchesne, S. (eds.) MICCAI 2017. LNCS, vol. 10435, pp. 603–611. Springer, Cham (2017). https://doi.org/10.1007/978-3-319-66179-7_69

Uncertainty Measurements for the Reliable Classification of Mammograms

Mickael Tardy[1,2](✉) (iD), Bruno Scheffer[3], and Diana Mateus[1] (iD)

[1] Ecole Centrale de Nantes, LS2N, UMR CNRS 6004, Nantes, France
{mickael.tardy,diana.mateus}@ec-nantes.fr
[2] Hera-MI, SAS, Nantes, France
[3] Institut de cancérologie de l'Ouest, Nantes, France

Abstract. We propose an efficient approach to estimate the uncertainty of deep-neural network classifiers based on the tradeoff of two measurements. The first based on subjective logic and the evidence of soft-max predictions and the second, based the Mahalanobis distance between new and training samples in the embedding space. These measurements require neither modifying, nor retraining, nor multiple testing of the models. We evaluate our methods on different classification tasks including breast cancer risk, breast density, and patch-wise tissue type and considering both an in-house database of 1600 mammographies, as well as on the public INBreast dataset. Throughout the experiments, we show the ability of our method to reject the most evident outliers, and to offer AUC gains of up to 10%, when keeping 60% of most certain samples.

Keywords: Uncertainty · Classification · Deep learning ·
Mammography · Breast cancer

1 Introduction

The risks of erroneous decisions are especially high when developing computer-aided systems for medical decision support. Therefore, there has been a recent interest in measuring the uncertainty of deep-learning-based predictions. In computer vision, the Out-of-distribution (OOD) detection task [5] aims at identifying whether or not a new test image belongs to the train in-distribution (ID) and can thus be classified with certainty. Current OOD benchmarks rely on public datasets that come from distinct data distributions (e.g. MNIST vs. CIFAR). In medical image analysis, the OOD detection is important but challenging because the differences between the data distributions used for training and testing are often subtle, for instance, due to variability in acquisition parameters, machine, or inclusion conditions for the patients. In addition to the in/out distribution

Electronic supplementary material The online version of this chapter (https://doi.org/10.1007/978-3-030-32226-7_55) contains supplementary material, which is available to authorized users.

uncertainty, we are confronted with noisy data (*aleatoric uncertainty*), and a limited knowledge of the underlying phenomena (*model or epistemic uncertainty*), resulting from the scarcity of annotated datasets.

In this work, our goal is to provide a measure of uncertainty allowing us to identify potentially erroneous classifications, whether they come from a data uncertainty or a distribution shift. Similar to [9], the amount of tolerated uncertainty will result in a trade-off between the number of retained images and the level of accuracy. In the quest of generality, we propose combining two uncertainty measurements which neither require modifying the classification model nor re-training it with a modified loss function. The first one, based on subjective logic [6], exploits information from the predicted classification probabilities, while the second, inspired from [2], defines the region within the feature space around the known training data samples which is considered as certain.

We demonstrate the interest of our approach for different breast imaging classification tasks namely, risk assessment (high vs. low risk), breast density stratification according to BI-RADS scores, and glandular vs. conjunctive patch-tissue classification. We evaluate our method on in-house and public datasets [12] and demonstrate that our technique can effectively detect error-prone images while increasing the reliability of the retained predictions (in terms of the accuracy). For the completeness of our study, we also compare to the state-of-the-art methods [4,15]. To the best of our knowledge, we are the first to propose such uncertainty measurements for classification tasks in breast imaging analysis.

Related Work: Usually, for a given sample, a deep learning classifier yields probabilities of belonging to the given classes. Hendrycks et al. [5] established a measure of uncertainty directly from the class probabilities without any further modification or training of the model. Liang et al. [10] pushed this idea forward by proposing an additional adversarial perturbation and soft-max scaling. Similar to [5,10], our first uncertainty measurement also exploits the softmax output but interpreted through the lens of subjective logic [6].

Recently, several approaches have been proposed based on a Bayesian formulation of the uncertainty. Bayesian networks are well suited for isolating different sources of uncertainty but have an inherent high complexity. Approximations like Monte-Carlo dropout [4] have been leveraged to propose practical uncertainty estimates [7] which has been successfully used in different classification and segmentation tasks [1,3,13]. These methods, however, require the modification of the training to include dropout layers (if not present) and multiple runs during the test. Also, following a Bayesian approach, several recent works model the output of a deep network with a Dirichlet distribution [11,15]. By designing uncertainty-aware loss functions and through variational optimization, these approaches allow extracting uncertainty measurements from a unique run. However, they are still not generalizable to pre-trained models.

The third line of approaches [2,8] uses the Mahalanobis distance in the feature space (produced by the network embedding) to define a region of certainty and evaluate how far a new sample is from the known dataset. Considering the above state-of-the-art techniques and fixing as objective the practicality of implementation, we propose an efficient yet affordable method to measure the uncertainty, which combines a subjective logic interpretation of the soft-max outputs as well as the Mahalanobis Distance.

2   Methods

Let $\mathcal{X} = \{\mathbf{x}_i, \mathbf{y}_i\}_{i=1}^N$ be a training dataset composed of images $\mathbf{x}_i$ and class labels $\mathbf{y}_i \in \{\mathcal{C}_k\}_{k=1}^K$. Consider a classifier h that assigns to an input $\mathbf{x}_i$ a class proba-bility vector $\hat{\mathbf{p}} = h(\mathbf{x}_i)$, where $p_{ik} \in \hat{\mathbf{p}}_i$ denotes the probability of $\mathbf{x}_i$ to belong to class $\mathcal{C}_k$. Then, suppose the classifier can be decomposed into two steps, where the first computes a feature representation $\mathbf{z}_i = g(\mathbf{x}_i)$ and the second, estimates the class probabilities $\hat{\mathbf{p}} = f(\mathbf{z}_i)$. The classifier can be a deep neural network trained end-to-end, where the $g(\cdot)$ corresponds to the penultimate layer and $f(\cdot)$ stands for the soft-max. Our goal is to determine an uncertainty measurement v for each prediction of h. By defining a tolerated amount of uncertainty th_v we should be able to detect and put aside uncertain test samples while increasing the expected performance of the classifier.

In this work, we consider a combination of two uncertainty measurements $v = [u, D_\mathrm{m}]$. First, a prediction uncertainty $u(\mathbf{p}) : \mathbf{p} \mapsto \mathbb{R}$, based on the infor-mation contained from the probabilistic predictions. Second, a data closeness measurement $D_\mathrm{m}(\mathbf{z}) : \mathbf{z} \mapsto \mathbb{R}$ following a Mahalanobis approach [2] that mea-sures the distance D_m of a sample to the training distribution cluster.

The **prediction uncertainty** u builds on recent works interpreting the maximum predicted probability [5], or the entropy of the probabilistic predic-tions [11,13] as a measure of uncertainty. However, inspired from [15] we rely on Subjective Logic [6], a formalization of Dempster-Shafer evidence theory to facilitate a direct interpretation of the uncertainty values. While Malinin et.al. [11] argue that the Dirichlet Loss function is required to induce a meaningful notion of uncertainty, we show as in [5], that the output of a classifier network trained with a soft-max layer and a cross-entropy loss still has practical value for uncertainty estimation. Formally, for K classes we have:

$$u + \sum_{k=1}^K b_k = 1, \quad b_k = \frac{e_k}{S}, \quad u = \frac{K}{S}, \quad S = \sum_{k-1}^K (e_k + 1), \tag{1}$$

where u is the sought uncertainty, b_k is the belief for the class k and e_k is the evidence provided by the network for the class k. Having $e_k + 1 = \exp^{f(x)}$ we obtain the uncertainty estimate:

$$u(\mathbf{x}) = \frac{K}{\sum_{k=1}^K \exp^{f(\mathbf{x})}} \tag{2}$$

The use of subjective logic requires particular attention to the logits' scale. From Eq. 1 we have $u \in [0,1]$, with $u_{max} = 1$ corresponding to the case with no evidence. With Eq. 2 and the logits $f(\mathbf{x}) \in [-\infty, +\infty]$, we may have com-putational issues for large values of $f(x)$. To avoid this phenomenon, logits are rescaled, or saturated for instance to $\exp(f(\mathbf{x})) \in [0, 2 \cdot 10^{12}]$.

The second considered uncertainty measurement is the **Mahalanobis distance** [2] calculated from a given sample to the known distribution, as:

$$D_M(\mathbf{x}) = \sqrt{(g(\mathbf{x}) - \mu)^T \Sigma^{(-1)} (g(\mathbf{x}) - \mu)}, \qquad (3)$$

where $g(\mathbf{x})$ is the output of the model's penultimate layer for a sample $\mathbf{x}$, μ and Σ are the mean and the covariance matrix of the cluster of all points in the training dataset $\mathcal{X}$, once mapped to the embedding space through function $g()$.

Although the entropy and related measurements on the posterior probabilities are well-known to be related uncertainty, we have observed that the Mahalanobis distance brings a complementary aspect especially related to out-of-distribution cases [2]. For instance, when a classifier trained on breast images (ID) is fed with outliers from a flower dataset (OOD), we see that the rejection criterion based on the Mahalanobis distance is quite effective (See Fig. 1-left). In a situation where we artificially generate a linear transition from an ID patch to an OOD patch (Fig. 1-right) for a binary classification problem[1], we observe a similar behavior. The efficiency of the uncertainty u is obvious at the middle of the transition corresponding to a mix between an ID and the OOD patch. However, the uncertainty fails to rise after this point to indicate that the prediction of the pure OOD patch is wrong. In contrast, the Mahalanobis distance is more representative towards the OOD patch indicating an uncertain prediction.

Following the potential complementarity of the two estimates, we propose to simultaneously consider thresholds on both uncertainty measures, in order to reject uncertain predictions using $u > th_u$ as well as data points that are too far from the certain ID region $D_M > th_D$.

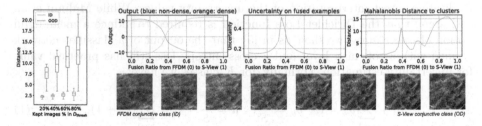

Fig. 1. Left: Toy example with OOD coming from the Flowers database **Right**: prediction probabilities (output) and variation of the uncertainty u and distance D_m measurements for the linear transition between an ID and an OOD patches.

3   Experimental Validation

To evaluate the performance of our method, we performed experiments targeting three mammography image analysis problems: risk classification, breast density

---

[1] Model and patches from the $TissueCLS_{raw}$ experiment described in Sect. 3.

classification, and a patch-wise tissue characterization task. For the three problems, we study the performance of the classifiers while changing uncertainty tolerance thresholds and thus the ratio of test images kept. In particular, (i) we show the precision at several cut-off values of the ratio of kept images (90%, 60%); (ii) we study the AUC and AUCPR of the predictions, and (iii) we analyze the statistics of u and D_M in the retained ID and OOD samples (see Fig. 4).

RiskCLS. We devise this experiment intending to show the generality and performance of our method on public models and databases. We focus on the image-wise risk classification according to Assessment Categories (ACR), where ACR1-2 stand for low-risk (negative) and ACR4-6 represent high risk (positive) cases. To create a basis for comparison, we rely on the VGG-based CNN model from [16], pre-trained on the DDSM (Digital Database for Screening Mammography) database. As in [16], we perform fine-tuning of the model using a second open dataset (INBreast) [12] taking 80 images for fine-tuning and keeping 305 for validation. We evaluate our method with ($RiskCLS_{tune}$) and without the fine-tuning ($RiskCLS_{init}$) step to show the behavior of the uncertainty measurements for the samples from the shifted INBreast distribution, either when it is completely or only partially unknown.

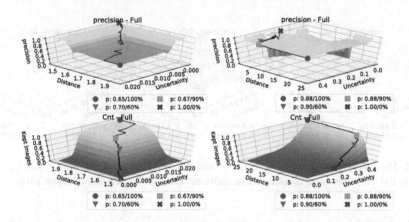

Fig. 2. Precision and ratio of kept images in the u and D_M space: without ($RiskCLS_{init}$, on the left) and with ($RiskCLS_{tune}$, on the right) fine-tuning. The legends list the precision associated to different cut-offs of the kept image ratio. (Color figure online)

In Fig. 2 we show the precision (top) and ratio of images kept (bottom) for different values of uncertainty th_u and distance thresholds th_D. We also plot in black the optimal path for the studied test dataset (thresholds that maximize the precision for a decreasing ratio of images kept) and highlight the performance at several cut-off points (colored shapes).

We observe the increase of precision between $RiskCLS_{init}$ and $RiskCLS_{tune}$ models (0.65 vs. 0.88) with 100% of the data produced by the fine-tuning step.

By retaining only the 60% most certain predictions, the performance increases respectively by +5% and +2%. Note that without fine-tuning both uncertainty measurements are equally important for defining the optimal performance path. The effect of the Mahalanobis distance is reduced with fine-tuning since the shape of the distribution cluster changes and, thus, the distances of test samples towards the center of the cluster become shorter.

DensityCLS. The second experiment targets the 4-class image-wise classification of breast density based on the 4th edition of BI-RADS. The goals here are (i) to evaluate our approach when dealing with multi-class classification and (ii) to challenge it with the real-life scenario of images from a distribution shift caused by images from different manufacturers. We use the VGG-based model from [14]. The in-house training set consists of 1232 images from a Planmed Nuance Excel (PNE) mammography system. For validation, we rely on 370 PNE images as well as on 370 images from Siemens MammoNovation (INBreast [12]).

In Fig. 3, we evaluate the precision for the full test set, as well as for the ID and OOD parts separately. For the ID dataset, a significant performance improvement (+8%) is obtained retaining 60% of the data. However, for the OOD dataset, without any fine-tuning, the performance is low despite the uncertainty checks. This result shows the limits of our method for subtle distribution shifts.

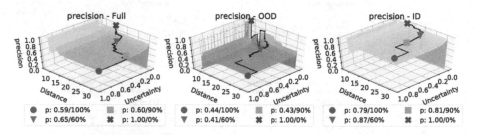

Fig. 3. Precision of kept images in the u and D_M spaces for the $DenseCLS_{raw}$. The legends list the precision associated to different cut-offs of the kept image ratio.

TissueCLS. Our final experiment is focused on the patch-wise classification of image-patches into dense and non-dense tissues. The goal of this experiment is twofold: (i) to measure the effect of a distribution shift between native 2D Full-Field Digital Mammography (FFDM) images and 2D views synthesized from 3D tomosynthesis acquisitions, which is of great clinical interest; (ii) to compare our method to state-of-the-art approaches. For the training, we used a dataset of patches from FFDM images (pixel spacing $50\,\mu$m). For validation, the ID patches came from FFDM images and OOD patches from S-View images (pixel spacing $98\,\mu$m).

Figure 4-left shows the smooth improvement of the ROC curves for a decreasing amount of kept images selected with optimal th_u and th_D. When analyzing the actual values of u and D_M on the ID and OOD samples separately (Fig. 4-right), we see that the threshold on Mahalanobis distance is more critical for the first rejected samples (from 100% up to 70%) while the effect of the uncertainty comes after (from 70%), illustrating once more their complementarity.

Finally, we compare our approach against two state-of-the-art methods using the same network architecture in all three experiments. The first consists of an MC dropout approach [4], that adds dropout layers to the existing model and keeps them active during test time to collect the variance of the predictions over different runs (here 10). The variance is then used as the uncertainty measurement. The second method results from training the same model with the Dirichlet distribution loss function from [15]. From the results reported in Table 1, we see that our approach is very competitive, while neither requiring model changes nor additional training. Gal's method [4] performs better at baseline (100%) due to the dropout training, but it is at most comparable when considering uncertainty sample pruning (90% and 60%) while requiring redesign, retraining, and multiple test runs. We also note that softmax probabilistic predictions (u_{prob}) and the entropy (u_{entr}) may be used as uncertainty alternatives with similar results. However, Subjective Logic (Eq. 1) remains competitive with the advantage of yielding directly interpretable uncertainty and belief values.

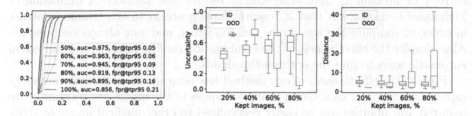

Fig. 4. TissueCLS experiment. **Left**: ROC curves with kept images ratio, AUC and FPR@TPR95, **Right**: statistics of u and D_M among the retained samples, for an increasing amount of kept images.

Table 1. Precision, AUC and AUCPR of different models on the thresholded datasets. Cut-offs of 100%, 90%, 60% images are reported.

Model	Precision			AUC			AUCPR		
	100%	90%	60%	100%	90%	60%	100%	90%	60%
Gal [4]	0.74	0.75	0.81	**0.89**	0.89	0.87	**0.87**	0.84	0.72
Sensoy [15]	0.87	0.89	0.93	0.87	0.90	0.93	0.81	0.82	0.83
Ours $u_{prob} + D_M$	**0.89**	**0.90**	**0.94**	0.88	**0.90**	**0.96**	0.81	**0.84**	**0.90**
Ours $u_{entr} + D_M$	**0.89**	**0.90**	**0.95**	0.88	**0.91**	**0.96**	0.81	**0.84**	**0.91**
Ours $u_{SL} + D_M$	**0.89**	**0.90**	**0.95**	0.86	**0.90**	**0.96**	0.75	0.81	**0.91**

4   Discussion and Conclusion

In the context of mammography image classification problems, we have studied the problem of uncertainty measurement, aiming to define a method capable of differentiating certain from uncertain predictions, and thus increasing the safety of CAD system suggestions. Uncertainty measurements based on the probability predictions and the Mahalanobis distance have been shown to be effective tools towards this end.

With the proposed combination of the two measurements we have demonstrated that it is possible to detect evident out-of-distribution samples (as the flowers) while achieving more moderate improvements of performance for subtle forms of distribution shift (e.g. scanned films vs FFDM or FFDM of different manufacturers). In these cases, our method deployed on a validation dataset may be useful to detect the effectiveness of augmentation and fine-tuning strategies when dealing with small datasets.

With respect to the uncertainty measure based on the probabilistic predictions, the scale of the logits used for the estimate u is worthy of attention: when using subjective logic a rescaling may be needed. However, we showed, that entropy or probability may yield similar results (see Table 1). A limitation of Mahalanobis distance is that it requires having access to the training dataset in order to compute the covariance matrix, which may not always be possible. Also, despite the effectiveness of the combination further research is required on automatic ways to find the optimal thresholds.

Finally, the effectiveness of our method has been shown in several mammography classification tasks. Given that no changes in the model nor retraining are required, our findings can be easily generalized to other medical image analysis problems confronted to uncertainties coming from the data but also from the distribution shifts.

References

1. Bragman, F.J.S., et al.: Uncertainty in multitask learning: joint representations for probabilistic MR-only radiotherapy planning. In: Frangi, A.F., Schnabel, J.A., Davatzikos, C., Alberola-López, C., Fichtinger, G. (eds.) MICCAI 2018. LNCS, vol. 11073, pp. 3–11. Springer, Cham (2018). https://doi.org/10.1007/978-3-030-00937-3_1
2. Denouden, T., Salay, R., Czarnecki, K., Abdelzad, V., Phan, B., Vernekar, S.: Improving reconstruction autoencoder out-of-distribution detection with mahalanobis distance. CoRR abs/1812.02765 (2018)
3. Eaton-Rosen, Z., Bragman, F., Bisdas, S., Ourselin, S., Cardoso, M.J.: Towards safe deep learning: accurately quantifying biomarker uncertainty in neural network predictions. In: Frangi, A.F., Schnabel, J.A., Davatzikos, C., Alberola-López, C., Fichtinger, G. (eds.) MICCAI 2018. LNCS, vol. 11070, pp. 691–699. Springer, Cham (2018). https://doi.org/10.1007/978-3-030-00928-1_78
4. Gal, Y., Ghahramani, Z.: Dropout as a Bayesian approximation: representing model uncertainty in deep learning. In: International Conference on Machine Learning, pp. 1050–1059 (2016)

5. Hendrycks, D., Gimpel, K.: A baseline for detecting misclassified and out-of-distribution examples in neural networks. CoRR abs/1610.02136 (2016)
6. Jøsang, A.: Subjective Logic: A Formalism for Reasoning Under Uncertainty. Springer (2018, Incorporated)
7. Kendall, A., Gal, Y.: What uncertainties do we need in Bayesian deep learning for computer vision? In: Guyon, I., et al. (eds.) Advances in Neural Information Processing Systems 30, pp. 5574–5584. Curran Associates, Inc. (2017)
8. Lee, K., Lee, K., Lee, H., Shin, J.: A simple unified framework for detecting out-of-distribution samples and adversarial attacks. In: Bengio, S., Wallach, H., Larochelle, H., Grauman, K., Cesa-Bianchi, N., Garnett, R. (eds.) Advances in Neural Information Processing Systems 31, pp. 7167–7177. Curran Associates, Inc. (2018)
9. Leibig, C., Allken, V., Ayhan, M.S., Berens, P., Wahl, S.: Leveraging uncertainty information from deep neural networks for disease detection. Sci. Rep. **7**(1), 17816 (2017)
10. Liang, S., Li, Y., Srikant, R.: Principled detection of out-of-distribution examples in neural networks. CoRR abs/1706.02690 (2017)
11. Malinin, A., Gales, M.: Predictive uncertainty estimation via prior networks. In: Bengio, S., Wallach, H., Larochelle, H., Grauman, K., Cesa-Bianchi, N., Garnett, R. (eds.) Advances in Neural Information Processing Systems 31, pp. 7047–7058. Curran Associates, Inc. (2018)
12. Moreira, I.C., Amaral, I., Domingues, I., Cardoso, A., Cardoso, M.J., Cardoso, J.S.: INbreast: toward a full-field digital mammographic database. Acad. Radiol. **19**(2), 236–248 (2012)
13. Nair, T., Precup, D., Arnold, D.L., Arbel, T.: Exploring uncertainty measures in deep networks for multiple sclerosis lesion detection and segmentation. In: Frangi, A.F., Schnabel, J.A., Davatzikos, C., Alberola-López, C., Fichtinger, G. (eds.) Medical Image Computing and Computer Assisted Intervention - MICCAI 2018, pp. 655–663. Springer International Publishing, Cham (2018). https://doi.org/10.1007/978-3-030-00928-1_74
14. Ribli, D., Horváth, A., Unger, Z., Pollner, P., Csabai, I.: Detecting and classifying lesions in mammograms with deep learning. Sci. Rep. **8**(1), 4165 (2018)
15. Sensoy, M., Kaplan, L., Kandemir, M.: Evidential deep learning to quantify classification uncertainty. In: Bengio, S., Wallach, H., Larochelle, H., Grauman, K., Cesa-Bianchi, N., Garnett, R. (eds.) Advances in Neural Information Processing Systems 31, pp. 3183–3193. Curran Associates, Inc. (2018)
16. Shen, L.: End-to-end training for whole image breast cancer diagnosis using an all convolutional design. arXiv preprint arXiv:1708.09427, November 2017

GraphX^{NET} – Chest X-Ray Classification Under Extreme Minimal Supervision

Angelica I. Aviles-Rivero[1(✉)], Nicolas Papadakis[2], Ruoteng Li[3], Philip Sellars[1], Qingnan Fan[4], Robby T. Tan[3,5], and Carola-Bibiane Schönlieb[1]

[1] DPMMS and DAMPT, Faculty of Mathematics,
University of Cambridge, Cambridge, UK
{ai323,ps644,cbs31}@cam.ac.uk
[2] CNRS, Universite de Bordeaux, Talence, France
nicolas.papadakis@math.u-bordeaux.fr
[3] National University of Singapore, Singapore, Singapore
liruoteng@u.nus.edu
[4] Stanford University, Stanford, USA
fqnchina@gmail.com
[5] Yale-NUS College, Singapore, Singapore
robby.tan@yale-nus.edu.sg

Abstract. The task of classifying X-ray data is a problem of both theoretical and clinical interest. Whilst supervised deep learning methods rely upon huge amounts of labelled data, the critical problem of achieving a good classification accuracy when an extremely small amount of labelled data is available has yet to be tackled. In this work, we introduce a novel semi-supervised framework for X-ray classification which is based on a graph-based optimisation model. To the best of our knowledge, this is the first method that exploits graph-based semi-supervised learning for X-ray data classification. Furthermore, we introduce a new multiclass classification functional with carefully selected class priors which allows for a smooth solution that strengthens the synergy between the limited number of labels and the huge amount of unlabelled data. We demonstrate, through a set of numerical and visual experiments, that our method produces highly competitive results on the ChestX-ray14 data set whilst drastically reducing the need for annotated data.

Keywords: Semi-supervised learning · Classification · Chest X-Ray · Graphs · Transductive learning

1 Introduction

The Chest X-Ray (CXR) is the most commonly performed x-ray examination which captures details of the lungs, heart, bones and blood vessels. CXRs play a critical role in diagnosing and monitoring conditions such as pneumonia, heart

---

A.I. Aviles-Rivero and N. Papadakis—Equal Contribution.

D. Shen et al. (Eds.): MICCAI 2019, LNCS 11769, pp. 504–512, 2019.
https://doi.org/10.1007/978-3-030-32226-7_56

problems and lung cancer. However, it remains one of the most complex imaging studies to interpret [10]. The effectiveness and accuracy of the interpretation heavily relies on the radiologist's expertise and still there is a substantial clinical error on the outcome [4]. Furthermore, the requirement of human expertise increases the finical cost and time required for evaluation. Therefore, there is a clear need for fast automated evaluations of CXRs.

CXR classification has been widely addressed by the community, yet it remains an open problem. Early developments were based in handcrafted classification e.g. [16]. However, this set of algorithmic approaches require particular modelling hypothesis to be met (e.g. texture, geometry, intensity), which may not be feasible to fulfill in practice. Due to the incredible results produced by deep learning in the field of computer vision, there has been a rush to apply deep learning architectures to the classification of CXRs [1,17,19], which have shown promising results. The majority of these methods utilise deep convolutional neural network with architectures such as ResNet [12], due to the success of these architectures in computer vision classification tasks. Several training methods have been considered including: pre-trained networks, fine tuned networks and networks trained from scratch on X-ray data e.g. [1,17,19].

However, a major drawback of these techniques is the high dependence on a large corpus of labelled data. Particularly in the medical domain, this might be a strong assumption for a solution, as annotated data contains strong human bias. Although there has been a huge effort in the community to mitigate this drawback by providing datasets such as ChestX-ray14, the has annotations but is far from being a definite expression of ground truth [14]. Therefore, by using supervised learning techniques one allows the labelling error and uncertainty to adversely effect the classification output of our machine learn framework. To tackle both the effect of human bias and the limited amount of labelled data, we propose using the power of semi-supervised learning and graph representations.

Our Contributions. We propose a novel semi-supervised graph-based framework called GraphX^{NET}. Our contributions are: (1) *a new multi-class classification functional with carefully chosen class priors*. Our framework is based on the normalised and non-smooth $p = 1$ Laplacian. (2) We demonstrate that our novel framework learns to accurately classify CXRs, with a performance comparable to state-of-the-art deep learning techniques, whilst using an extremely smaller amount of labelled data. (3) This work also represents the first time that graph representations have been used for X-ray classification.

2   GraphX^{NET} Framework for X-Ray Data Classification.

Our approach is motivated by a central problem in medical imaging which is the lack of reliable quality annotated data. Although, transfer learning [1] or Generative Adversarial Networks [15] somewhat mitigate this problem, they fail to account for the mismatch between expert annotation and ground truth annotation created by human bias and uncertainty. With this motivation in mind, we propose, for the first time, using a semi-supervised framework, call GraphX^{NET} (see Fig. 1 for illustration).

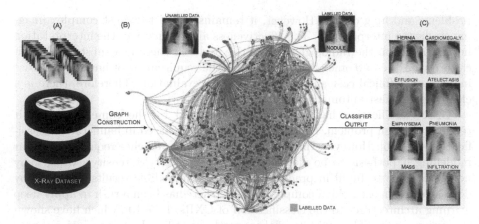

Fig. 1. Overview of our proposed GraphX^{NET} method. We exploit both labeled and unlabeled data to produce high classification accuracy. In this framework, we aim to propagate labels for the unlabeled data with minimal supervision.

Data Representation with Graphs. Although there are different methods for representing data including conventional grid form. In this work, we motivate the use of graph data representations as follows. Firstly, graphs are a natural representation for groups of images where each node represents an individual image. Secondly, given that graph based methods seek to find smooth solutions to the created embedding, they are able to correct for initially mislabelled samples. Lastly, graph has strong and mathematical properties such as sparseness which allows for fast computation.

We represent a given dataset as an undirected weighted graph $\mathcal{G} = (\mathcal{V}, \mathcal{E}, W)$ compromising a set of n nodes $\mathcal{V}$ which are connected by a set of edges $\mathcal{E}$ with weights $w_{ij} = S(i, j) \geq 0$ that correspond to some similarity measure S between the features of nodes $i \in \mathcal{V}$ and $j \in \mathcal{V}$, $w_{ij} = 0$ if $(i, j) \notin \mathcal{E}$; and functions $u \in \mathbb{R}^n$. Our setting is based on the normalised graph p-Laplacian, which reads:

$$\Delta_p(u) = \sum_{i,j} w_{ij} \left\| \frac{u_i}{d_i^{1/p}} - \frac{u_j}{d_j^{1/p}} \right\|^p, \quad \text{with } p \geq 1 \text{ and } d_i = \sum_j w_{ij} > 0, \quad (1)$$

where d_i is the degree of node i. The eigenfunctions of the graph Laplacian operator give interesting understanding of the substructures of the graph. Eigenfunctions of a normalised graph Laplacian for $p = 2$ have been successfully used in different applications such as in [2,7,8].

Learning to Classify Under Extreme Minimal Supervision. However, unlike those works, our framework has a different aim which is to solely obtain classification estimates on the unlabeled samples. That is, to perform a node classification task on $\mathcal{G}$ with L available classes, given an extremely small amount of labelled nodes x_i. More precisely, given a small amount of labeled data $\{(x_i, y_i)\}_{i=1}^l$ with provided labels $\mathcal{L} = \{1, .., L\}$ and $\{y_i\}_{i=1}^l \in \mathcal{L}$ and a large amount of unlabelled data $\{x_k\}_{k=l+1}^n$, we seek to infer a function $f : \mathcal{X}^n \mapsto \mathcal{Y}^n$ such that f gets a good estimate for $\{x_k\}_{k=l+1}^n$.

Although several works have explored this learning style, either from a pure machine learning perspective e.g. [20] or a medical imaging perspective e.g. [18], these methods seek to only approximate $p \to 1$ in the graph Laplacian. However, recent developments on machine learning showed that the use of the unnormalised (i.e. without the re-scaling by the node degrees in (1)) and non smooth $p = 1$ Laplacian, related to total variation, can achieve better performance [5].

To mitigate these current drawbacks in the literature, we propose a novel semi-supervised framework, GraphX**NET**, based on the normalised and non smooth $p = 1$ Laplacian in (1). The function can then be rewritten as: $\Delta_1(u) = |WD^{-1}u|$, where W is the weight matrix w_{ij} and D the diagonal matrix containing the degrees d_i. To this end, we generalise the unsupervised binary normalised graph method of [9] to a semi-supervised multi-class graph approach. To this aim, our algorithmic approach is as follows.

For each class, $k = 1 \cdots L$, we consider a variable u^k that has values for all nodes of the graph. For all unlabeled nodes $i > l$, the L variables are then coupled with the constraints that for all nodes i: $\sum_{k=1}^L u_i^k = 0, \forall i > l$. This simple coupling indeed leads to faster projection algorithms than simplex [3,11] or non convex orthogonality constraints between u^k's [8]. We assume that a set of annotated nodes $\mathcal{I}_k \subset \{1 \cdots l\}$ are available for each class k: $y_i = k \in \mathcal{L}$ for all $i \in \mathcal{I}_k$. Taking a small parameter $\epsilon > 0$, we therefore constrain that:

$$\begin{cases} u_i^k \geq \epsilon & \text{if } i \in \mathcal{I}_k \\ u_i^{k'} \leq -\epsilon & \text{if } i \in \mathcal{I}_k \text{ and } k' \neq k. \end{cases} \tag{2}$$

This information is then used in an iterative PDE process with a time parameter t, in which we seek to minimise the sum of normalised ratios $\sum_k \frac{\Delta_1(u^k)}{|u^k|}$. Denoting $\mathbf{u} = [u^1, \cdots u^L]$ and a time step $\Delta t > 0$. Then formally, we seek to minimise:

$$\mathbf{u}^{(t+1)} = \underset{\mathbf{u}}{\operatorname{argmin}} \frac{\|\mathbf{u} - \mathbf{u}^{(t)}\|^2}{2\Delta t} + \sum_{k=1}^L \left(\Delta_1(u^k) - \frac{\Delta_1(u^{k,(t)})}{|u^{k,(t)}|} \langle \operatorname{sign}(u^{k,(t)}), u^k \rangle \right),$$

$$(3)$$

under the set of previously described coupling and data (2) constraints. Following [9,13], a final shifting $u^{k,(t+1)} = u^{k,(t+1)} - \operatorname{median}(u^{k,(t+1)})$ and a normalisation $\mathbf{u}^{(t+1)} = \mathbf{u}^{(t+1)}/\|\mathbf{u}^{(t+1)}\|$ are necessary at the end of each iteration to prevent from converging to trivial solutions.

When a unique u^k is considered, the scheme iteratively decreases the ratio $\frac{\Delta_1(u^{k,(t)})}{|u^{k,(t)}|}$ since $\langle \operatorname{sign}(u^{k,(t)}), u^{k,(t)} \rangle = |u^{k,(t)}|$, so that the solution $u^{k,(t+1)}$ of (3) necessarily satisfies:

$$\Delta_1(u^{k,(t+1)}) \leq \frac{\Delta_1(u^{k,(t)})}{|u^{k,(t)}|} \langle \operatorname{sign}(u^{k,(t)}), u^{k,(t+1)} \rangle \leq \frac{\Delta_1(u^{k,(t)})}{|u^{k,(t)}|} |u^{k,(t+1)}|. \tag{4}$$

As noticed in [9], the scheme makes $u^{k,(t)}$ converge to a bivalued function that naturally segment the graph. As L variables are coupled, the final labelling of a node i is chosen from the variable u_i^k with the highest value: $y_i = \underset{k}{\mathrm{argmax}}\ u_i^k$.

Optimisation Scheme. For each time step t, the problem (3) is solved at successive time steps using the accelerated primal dual algorithm of [6]. Denoting as $\mathbf{v} = \mathbf{u}^{(t)}$ the current estimation and initialising $\mathbf{u}_0 = \tilde{\mathbf{u}}_0 = \mathbf{v}$, $z_0^k = WD{-}1u_0^k$, the algorithm to obtain $\mathbf{u}^{(t+1)}$ with an iterative sequence $\mathbf{u}_\ell$ indexed by ℓ reads:

$$
\begin{cases}
z_{\ell+1}^k = z_\ell^k + \sigma_\ell W D^{-1}\tilde{u}_\ell^k \\
z_{\ell+1}^k = \dfrac{z_{\ell+1}^k}{\max(1,|z_{\ell+1}^k|)} \\
u_{\ell+1}^k = \dfrac{u_\ell^k + \tau_\ell \Delta t\left(\frac{\Delta_1(v^k)}{|v^k|}\mathrm{sign}(v^k)+D^{-1}Wz_{\ell+1}^k\right)}{1+\tau_\ell \Delta t} \\
u_{\ell+1}^k = \mathrm{Proj}_C(u_{\ell+1}^k) \\
\gamma_\ell = 1/\sqrt{1+\tau_\ell/\Delta t}, \ \tau_{\ell+1} = \tau_\ell \gamma_\ell, \ \sigma_{\ell+1} = \sigma_\ell/\gamma_\ell \\
\tilde{u}_{\ell+1}^k = u^k + \gamma_\ell(\tilde{u}^{k+1} - u^k),
\end{cases}
$$

where the projection onto the set of constraints C combining the coupled constraint and (2) reads pointwise:

$$
\mathrm{Proj}_C(u_i^k) = \begin{cases}
\max(u_i^k, \epsilon) & \text{if } i \in \mathcal{I}_k \\
\min(u_i^k, -\epsilon) & \text{if } i \in \mathcal{I}_{k'} \text{ and } k' \neq k. \\
u_i^k - \frac{1}{L}\sum_{k'} u_i^{k'} & \text{if } i > l.
\end{cases} \tag{5}
$$

For positive parameters σ_0 and τ_0 satisfying $\sigma\tau < 4$, such process makes $\mathbf{u}_\ell$ converges to $\mathbf{u}^{(t+1)}$, the solution of (3).

3 Experimental Results

This section is devoted to describe in detail the set of experiments that we conducted to validate our GraphX$^{\mathbf{NET}}$ approach.

Data Description. We evaluate our approach using the ChestX-ray14 [17] dataset, which is composed of $112,120$ frontal chest view X-ray with size of 1024×1024. The dataset is composed of 14 classes (pathologies). All measurements were taken from this dataset.

Evaluation Methodology. We validate our theory as follows. Firstly, we visualise the graphical construction and classification tasks of our graph-based semi-supervised framework. Secondly, the main part of the evaluation is to compare our GraphX$^{\mathbf{NET}}$ to the state-of-the-art methods on X-ray classification. We compare ours against two deep learning techniques: WANG17 [17] and YAO18 [19]. To evaluate the classifier output quality of the compared approaches, we performed a ROC analysis using the area under the curve (AUC) per pathology along with their average. Finally, beside the official split, we perform a comparison with random partitions on ChestX-ray8 using WANG17 [17] as baseline.

Results and Discussion. Firstly, we start by giving some insight into our approach with some visualisations shown in Fig. 2. The left side of the figure shows two graphs in which the first one illustrates the initial state of the graph created after computing the feature distances between the given X-ray data while the second one shows the graph after computing (3). The colours on the graph indicates an images belonging to a particular class. The right side shows few sample graph label output, that were correctly classified, of our approach.

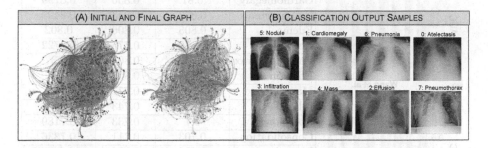

Fig. 2. Graphical Construction and Classification: (A) shows the graphical representation of the ChestX-ray14 dataset, where in the final classified graph, each colour represents a different class and (B) demonstrates examples of correct classifications produced by our framework. (Color figure online)

To evaluate the performance of our approach, we compared it against state of the art Deep Learning approaches, namely WANG17 [17] and YAO18 [19]. To the best of our knowledge, there are no semi-supervised learning method, for X-ray classification, that we can compare against. Therefore, we set as our baseline WANG17 and YAO18. Table 1 shows the AUC results of the compared approaches where overall our approach outperformed the other methods across most pathology. Even though YAO18 performs better in some classes, a clear advantage of our approach over these two baselines is that while their approach rely in a huge percentage of data, 70%, we were able to report a better average AUC result with only 20% of the data.

Moreover, due to the semi-supervised nature of the GraphX^{NET} framework, the classification output is very stable with respect to changes in the partition of the dataset. In the plots next to Table 1, we tested the AUC of both the GraphX^{NET} framework and WANG17 [17] using three different random data partitions, including the partition suggested by Wang. The Wang method is very sensitive to changes in the partition due to the face that supervised methods are heavily reliant on the training set being representative. However, there is minimal change in the performance of GraphX^{NET} over the three different partitions as the underlying graphical representation is invariant to the partition.

For more detailed analysis of this dependency on the portioning and to further support the advantage of our GraphX^{NET}, in Table 2, we compare the AUC produced by GraphX^{NET} against WANG17 using a random split over ChestX-ray8. We find that GraphX^{NET} produces a more accurate classification using 5%

Table 1. Comparison of the classification accuracy of GraphX^{NET} against two state-of-the-art deep learning method, Wang et al. [17] and Yao et al. [19]. Here we report the AUC measure over all 14 pathology classes along with the overall average. Plots on the left side highlight the sensitivity of the AUC for each class when changing the data partition of the data set (using 15% for training)

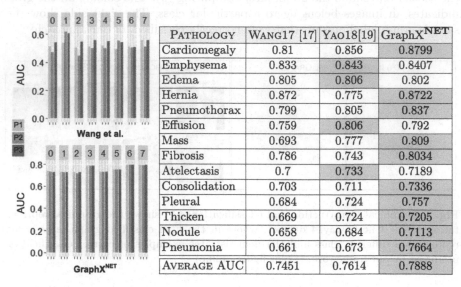

Pathology	Wang17 [17]	Yao18[19]	GraphX^{NET}
Cardiomegaly	0.81	0.856	0.8799
Emphysema	0.833	0.843	0.8407
Edema	0.805	0.806	0.802
Hernia	0.872	0.775	0.8722
Pneumothorax	0.799	0.805	0.837
Effusion	0.759	0.806	0.792
Mass	0.693	0.777	0.809
Fibrosis	0.786	0.743	0.8034
Atelectasis	0.7	0.733	0.7189
Consolidation	0.703	0.711	0.7336
Pleural	0.684	0.724	0.757
Thicken	0.669	0.724	0.7205
Nodule	0.658	0.684	0.7113
Pneumonia	0.661	0.673	0.7664
Average AUC	0.7451	0.7614	0.7888

of the data labels than the WANG17 method does using 70% of the data labels. Furthermore, as we feed GraphX^{NET} more of the data labels, the classification

Table 2. Comparison of the classification accuracy of GraphX^{NET} against a state-of-the-art deep learning method by Wang et al. [17]. We give the average AUC measure over all eight classes using different amounts of labelled data. Additionally, we give a class by class comparison between the two methods using 70% of the labelled data for the Wang method and 20% for GraphX^{NET}.

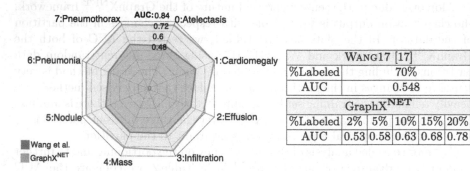

Wang17 [17]				
%Labeled	70%			
AUC	0.548			

GraphX^{NET}				
%Labeled	2%	5%	10%	15%	20%
AUC	0.53	0.58	0.63	0.68	0.78

accuracy increases and becomes competitive against other the deep learning framework of that YAO18 [19] whilst using a far smaller amount of data labels.

4   Conclusion

In this work, we tackled the problem of X-ray classification and introduced a novel semi-supervised framework based on a graph-based optimisation model, which is the first method that exploits graph-based semi-supervised learning for X-ray data classification. We also introduced a new multi-class classification functional with carefully selected class priors that allows for a smooth solution. We demonstrated that our method produces highly competitive results on the ChestX-ray14 data set whilst drastically reducing the need for annotated data.

Acknowledgments. AIAI is supported by the CMIH, University of Cambridge. NP is supported by the European Union's Horizon 2020 research and innovation programme under the Marie Skłodowska-Curie grant No 777826. CBS acknowledges Leverhulme Trust (Breaking the non-convexity barrier), the Philip Leverhulme Prize, the EPSRC grants EP/M00483X/1 and EP/N014588/1, the European Union Horizon 2020, the Marie Skodowska-Curie grant 777826 NoMADS and 691070 CHiPS, the CCIMI and the Alan Turing Institute.

References

1. Bar, Y., Diamant, I., Wolf, L., Lieberman, S., Konen, E., Greenspan, H.: Chest pathology detection using deep learning with non-medical training. In: International Symposium on Biomedical Imaging (ISBI), pp. 294–297 (2015)
2. Belkin, M., Niyogi, P.: Laplacian eigenmaps for dimensionality reduction and data representation. Neural Comput. **15**, 1373–1396 (2003)
3. Bresson, X., Laurent, T., Uminsky, D., Von Brecht, J.: Multiclass total variation clustering. In: Advances in Neural Information Processing Systems (2013)
4. Bruno, M.A., Walker, E.A., Abujudeh, H.H.: Understanding and confronting our mistakes: the epidemiology of error in radiology and strategies for error reduction. Radiographics **35**(6), 1668–1676 (2015)
5. Bühler, T., Hein, M.: Spectral clustering based on the graph p-Laplacian. In: International Conference on Machine Learning (ICML) (2009)
6. Chambolle, A., Pock, T.: A first-order primal-dual algorithm for convex problems with applications to imaging. J. Math. Imaging Vis. **40**, 120–145 (2011)
7. Chen, H., Li, K., Zhu, D.E.A.: Inferring group-wise consistent multimodal brain networks via multi-view spectral clustering. IEEE Trans. Med. Imaging (TMI) **32**, 1576–1586 (2013)
8. Dodero, L., Gozzi, A., Liska, A., Murino, V., Sona, D.: Group-wise functional community detection through joint laplacian diagonalization. In: Golland, P., Hata, N., Barillot, C., Hornegger, J., Howe, R. (eds.) MICCAI 2014. LNCS, vol. 8674, pp. 708–715. Springer, Cham (2014). https://doi.org/10.1007/978-3-319-10470-6_88
9. Feld, T.M., Aujol, J.F., Gilboa, G., Papadakis, N.: Rayleigh quotient minimization for absolutely one-homogeneous functionals. Inverse Prob. **35**, 064003 (2019)
10. Folio, L.R.: Chest Imaging: An Algorithmic Approach to Learning. Springer, New York (2012). https://doi.org/10.1007/978-1-4614-1317-2

11. Gao, Y., Adeli-M., E., Kim, M., Giannakopoulos, P., Haller, S., Shen, D.: Medical image retrieval using multi-graph learning for MCI diagnostic assistance. In: Navab, N., Hornegger, J., Wells, W.M., Frangi, A.F. (eds.) MICCAI 2015. LNCS, vol. 9350, pp. 86–93. Springer, Cham (2015). https://doi.org/10.1007/978-3-319-24571-3_11
12. He, K., Zhang, X., Ren, S., Sun, J.: Deep residual learning for image recognition. In: IEEE Conference on Computer Vision and Pattern Recognition (CVPR) (2016)
13. Hein, M., Setzer, S., Jost, L., Rangapuram, S.S.: The total variation on hypergraphs-learning on hypergraphs revisited. In: Advances in Neural Information Processing Systems (2013)
14. Kohli, M.D., Summers, R.M., Geis, J.R.: Medical image data and datasets in the era of machine learning-whitepaper from the 2016 C-MIMI meeting dataset session. J. Digit. Imaging **30**, 392–399 (2017)
15. Moradi, E., Pepe, A., Alzheimer's Disease Neuroimaging Initiative et al.: Machine learning framework for early MRI-based Alzheimer's conversion prediction in MCI subjects. Neuroimage **104**, 398–412 (2015)
16. Toriwaki, J.I., Suenaga, Y., Negoro, T., Fukumura, T.: Pattern recognition of chest x-ray images. Comput. Graph. Image Process. **2**, 252–271 (1973)
17. Wang, X., Peng, Y., Lu, L., Lu, Z., Bagheri, M., Summers, R.M.: ChestX-Ray8: hospital-scale chest x-ray database and benchmarks on weakly-supervised classification and localization of common thorax diseases. In: IEEE Conference on Computer Vision and Pattern Recognition (CVPR), pp. 2097–2106 (2017)
18. Wang, Z., et al.: Progressive graph-based transductive learning for multi-modal classification of brain disorder disease. In: Ourselin, S., Joskowicz, L., Sabuncu, M.R., Unal, G., Wells, W. (eds.) MICCAI 2016. LNCS, vol. 9900, pp. 291–299. Springer, Cham (2016). https://doi.org/10.1007/978-3-319-46720-7_34
19. Yao, L., Prosky, J., Poblenz, E., Covington, B., Lyman, K.: Weakly supervised medical diagnosis and localization from multiple resolutions. arXiv preprint arXiv:1803.07703 (2018)
20. Zhu, X., Ghahramani, Z., Lafferty, J.D.: Semi-supervised learning using Gaussian fields and harmonic functions. In: International conference on Machine learning (ICML), pp. 912–919 (2003)

3DFPN-HS²: 3D Feature Pyramid Network Based High Sensitivity and Specificity Pulmonary Nodule Detection

Jingya Liu[1], Liangliang Cao[2,3], Oguz Akin[4], and Yingli Tian[1(✉)]

[1] The City College of New York, New York, NY 10031, USA
ytian@ccny.cuny.edu
[2] UMass CICS, Amherst, MA 01002, USA
[3] Google AI, New York, NY 10011, USA
[4] Memorial Sloan Kettering Cancer Center, New York, NY 10065, USA

Abstract. Accurate detection of pulmonary nodules with high sensitivity and specificity is essential for automatic lung cancer diagnosis from CT scans. Although many deep learning-based algorithms make great progress for improving the accuracy of nodule detection, the high false positive rate is still a challenging problem which limited the automatic diagnosis in routine clinical practice. In this paper, we propose a novel pulmonary nodule detection framework based on a 3D Feature Pyramid Network (3DFPN) to improve the sensitivity of nodule detection by employing multi-scale features to increase the resolution of nodules, as well as a parallel top-down path to transit the high-level semantic features to complement low-level general features. Furthermore, a High Sensitivity and Specificity (HS²) network is introduced to eliminate the falsely detected nodule candidates by tracking the appearance changes in continuous CT slices of each nodule candidate. The proposed framework is evaluated on the public Lung Nodule Analysis (LUNA16) challenge dataset. Our method is able to accurately detect lung nodules at high sensitivity and specificity and achieves 90.4% sensitivity with 1/8 false positive per scan which outperforms the state-of-the-art results 15.6%.

Keywords: Lung nodule detection · False positive reduction · CT · Deep learning

1 Introduction

Lung cancer is one of the leading cancer killers around the world which makes the study of lung cancer diagnosis eminently crucial. Computer-aided diagnosis

Electronic supplementary material The online version of this chapter (https://doi.org/10.1007/978-3-030-32226-7_57) contains supplementary material, which is available to authorized users.

© Springer Nature Switzerland AG 2019
D. Shen et al. (Eds.): MICCAI 2019, LNCS 11769, pp. 513–521, 2019.
https://doi.org/10.1007/978-3-030-32226-7_57

(CAD) systems provide assistance for radiologists to accelerate the diagnosing process. Many efforts [3,6,11] have been made for lung nodule detection by generalizing the recent powerful deep detection models in computer vision. Although these efforts made good progress in accurately detecting pulmonary nodules from CT scans, the false positive rate is still very high which limits the real application in routine clinical practice. For example, most of the previous work [3,6,9,11] obtained less than 75% sensitivity with 1/8 false positives per scan. To get sensitivity scores as high as 95.8%, these models would bear about eight false positives, which prevent their use in routine clinical practice.

We believe two main challenges prevent the existing models from accurate lung nodule detection. (1) Some normal tissues have similar morphological appearances as nodules in CT images which cause high false positives by wrongly detecting these tissues as nodules. (2) The high discrepancy of the volume between nodules and the whole CT scan may cause missing detection of real nodules. For example, the volume of a nodule with 10 mm size in the diameter only occupied 0.059% of the volume of whole CT scan (in average 213 × 293 pixels with 281 slices). Furthermore, the size of pulmonary nodules can vary by as much as 10 times. For example, nodules in diameter can range from 3 mm to 30 mm in LUNA16 dataset. Therefore, it is particularly crucial for designing methods which can detect small volume nodules from large volume CT scans as well as to differentiate nodules from tissues with similar appearances in CT images.

To address the above two challenges, this paper attempts to integrate the most recent progress in computer vision as well as the domain expert knowledge in medical imaging. Motivated by the-state-of the-art image detector using 2D Feature Pyramid Network (FPN) [7], we develop a 3D feature pyramid network (3DFPN) for small nodule detection by appending the low-level high-resolution features to the high-level strong semantic features and a multi-scale feature prediction guarantees the wide-scale nodule detection. In addition, we carefully analyze the difference between nodules and the tissues where are wrongly detected as nodule candidates, and find that although they look similar on single CT slice, their spatial variances within continuous CT slices are distributed differently. This unique insight motivates us to design a novel refinement network, based on the location history image in the continuous CT slices. The final model benefits from both the powerful deep network and medical imaging insights, and reduces a significant amount of the previous false detected nodule candidates. Our model achieves a 90.4% sensitivity at 1/8 false positive per scan which significantly outperforms the state-of-the-art method 15.6%.

2   Our Method

As shown in Fig. 1, the input of our lung nodule detection framework is a whole 3D volume of CT scan which is fed into a 3D Feature Pyramid ConvNet (3DFPN) to detect the 3D locations of nodule candidates. After the nodule candidates are detected, we crop a 3D cube region centered with the candidate and develop a High Sensitivity and Specificity (HS^2) network to further recognize whether the detected nodule candidates are real nodules or false detected tissues which effectively reduces false positives. In this framework, the 3DFPN benefits from the progress of state-of-the-art deep learning, and the HS^2 network benefits from the insight of medical images. We will discuss them respectively.

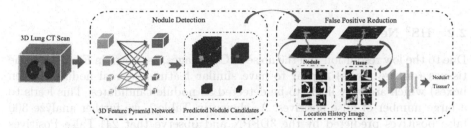

Fig. 1. The proposed 3DFPN-HS^2 framework of high sensitivity and specificity lung nodule detection by combining a 3D Feature Pyramid ConvNet (3DFPN) with an HS^2 network. A whole CT scan is fed into the 3DFPN to predict nodule candidates. For the detected nodule candidates, the HS^2 network eliminates the miss-predicted normal tissues based on the location variance within continuous CT slices. More detailed structure of the proposed 3DFPN network can be found in the supplementary document.

2.1 3D Feature Pyramid ConvNet

The recent progress in computer vision suggests feature pyramid networks (FPNs) are good at detect objects at different scales [7]. However, traditional FPNs are designed for 2D images. Here, we propose a 3DFPN network to detect 3D locations of lung nodules from 3D CT volumetric scans. Different than [7] which only concatenates the upper-level features in feature pyramid, we use a dense pyramid network to integrate both the low-level high-resolution features as well as high-level high-semantic features, which enriches the location details and strong semantics for nodule detection. Table 1 highlights the main differences between 2DFPN and our 3DFPN.

Table 1. Comparison between 2DFPN [7] and our proposed 3DFPN. We take 3D volume as input and the feature pyramid layers are integrated with lateral connections of all the high-level and low-level features.

Method	Input 3D volume	Lateral connections	Integrate upper layer	Integrate lower layer	Upsample higher layer	Downsample lower layer
2DFPN [7]	No	✓	✓		✓	
3DFPN	✓	✓	✓	✓	✓	✓

The bottom-up network extracts features from the convolution layer 2–5, refer as C2, C3, C4, C5, is followed by a convolution layer with kernel size

$1 \times 1 \times 1$ to convert feature channels with the same number of channels. The feature pyramid network contains four layers, as P2, P3, P4, P5, which integrates the low-level features by a max pooling layer and the downsampled high-level features by deconvolution. 3DFPN predicts location with four parameters as $[x, y, z, d]$, where $[x, y]$ as the spatial coordinates at each CT slices, z as CT slice number, and d as nodule diameter and a confidence score for each candidate.

2.2   HS² Network

Due to the low resolution and the noise of CT images, as shown in Fig. 2(a), some tissues (orange boxes) appear to have similar features as real nodules (green boxes) which are very likely to be detected as nodule candidates. This leads to a large number of false positives. As shown in Table 2, we further analyze 300 false positives predicted by the 3DFPN and observe that 241 False Positives (FPs) are caused by the high similarity of tissues (80.3%), 33 of them are caused by inaccurate size detection, and 26 FPs are due to the inaccurate location detection.

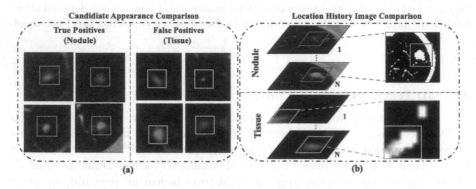

Fig. 2. The proposed Location History Images (LHI) to distinguish tissues and nodules from the predicted nodule candidates. (a) Similar appearance of true nodules (green boxes) and false detected tissues (orange boxes). (b) The orientations of the location variances for nodules and tissues are presented differently in LHIs. True nodules generally have a circular region which indicates the spatial changes with either a brighter center (when nodule sizes in following CT slices are smaller) or a darker center (when nodule sizes in following CT slices are bigger). On the other hand, the location variance for false detected tissues usually tends to change in certain directions such as a gradually changed trajectory line. (Color figure online)

It is crucial to obtain a major difference to distinguish similar tissues from nodules for false positive reduction. By observing the continues slices, we discover that for tissues, the orientation of the location changes could be tracked in certain patterns, while the variance of true nodules tends to expand outside the contour or diminishing to the center at continuous CT slices. For instance, Fig. 2(b) shows

Table 2. Statistic analysis for false positive nodule candidates.

	Tissue	Inaccurate size	Inaccurate location
Percentage	80.3%	11%	8.7%

nodules and tissues in the appearance of continuous slides. For a gray-scale value of each pixel represents the closest change of the pixel in the region of nodules within a series of CT slices, with the gray value orthogonal to the movement, we obtain the location variance of the candidates.

Inspired by Motion History Image (MHI) [2,10], we define the Location History Image (LHI) as f. By given any pixel location (x, y) on a CT slice s, $f(x, y, s)$ represents the intensity value of LHI within $(1, \tau)$ slice. The LHI is fed to a HS^2 (high sensitivity and specificity) network which is a feed-forward neural network with 2 convolution layers followed by 3 fully connected layers. The outputs of the HS^2 network are refined predicted labels of true nodules and tissues. Sensitivity is defined as a ratio of true positives over the total number of true positives and false negatives. Specificity is the ratio of true negatives over the total number of the true negatives and false positives.

The intensity of LHI is calculated as in Eq. (1):

$$f(x, y, s) = \begin{cases} \tau & if \ \psi(x, y, s) = 1 \\ max(0, f(x, y, s-1) - 1) & otherwise \end{cases} \quad (1)$$

where the update function $\psi(x, y, s)$ given by the spatial differentiation of the pixel intensity of two continuous CT slices. The algorithm has the following steps. (1) If $|I(x, y, s) - I(x, y, s-1)|$ is larger than a threshold, $\psi(x, y, s) = 1$, otherwise, $\psi(x, y, s) = 0$. (2) For the current slice, if $\psi(x, y, s) = 1$, $f = \tau$. Otherwise, if $f(x, y, s)$ is not zero, it is attenuated with a gradient of 1. If $f(x, y, s)$ equals zero, then remains as zero. (3) Repeat steps (1) and (2) until all the slices are processed. Therefore, the location variance among continues CT slices and their change patterns can be effectively represented by our proposed LHIs.

3   Experimental Results and Discussions

3.1   Dataset and Evaluation

The performance of the proposed framework is evaluated on the most popular LUNA16 challenge dataset [1] which consists of 1186 nodules in the size between 3–30 mm from 888 CT scans and agreed by at least 3 out of 4 radiologists. It is divided into 10 subsets. In order to conduct a fair comparison with other methods, we follow the same process to conduct cross validations by using 9 subsets for training and the remaining 1 subset for testing, then obtain the final results by averaging the 10 experiments. Data augment is applied by flipping and resizing the CT scans. Same as other methods, the Free-Response Receiver Operating Characteristic (FROC) analysis [8] and Competition Performance

Metric (CPM) of detection sensitivity and the corresponding false positives at $1/8, 1/4, 1/2, 1, 2, 4, 8$ per scan are employed to measure the performance. The CPM score is calculated by the average of sensitivity for all the levels of false positives per scan.

3.2   Experimental Results

Experimental Settings. The framework takes the whole CT scan as input, while volume at $96 \times 96 \times 96$ pixels is selected by a sliding window method as the input of the 3DFPN network. This size is selected based on experiments which is bigger enough to contain the whole nodule even when it is with the largest size (about 30 mm). The anchor sizes employed in our 3DFPN to obtain the candidate regions from feature maps are $[3^3, 5^3, 10^3, 15^3, 20^3, 25^3, 30^3]$ pixels. For all the anchors, the corresponding regions obtained from all the 3D feature map levels are gathered to predict the position of nodules.

In the training phase, the regions with an Intersection-over-Union (IoU) threshold to the ground-truth regions less than 0.02 are referred to negative samples and greater than 0.4 are positive samples. The samples in between are ignored to avoid the positive and negative samples similarity. A classification layer is used to predict a confidence score for the candidate class and a region regression layer is applied to learn the offset between the position of region proposals and the ground-truth. We adopt Smooth $L1$ loss [5] and binary cross entropy loss (BCE-loss) for location regression and classification score respectively. In the testing, for each region proposal, a confidence score is calculated by the classification layer. The proposals with a probability larger than 0.1 are chosen as nodule candidates. Non-maximum suppression is further applied to eliminate the multiple predicted candidates for one nodule.

The two convolution layers of the HS^2 network are set to $(1, 30)$, $(30, 50)$ dimensions and followed by three fully connected layers with the channel sizes of $(2048, 1024, 512)$. The cross entropy loss is applied for classification during the training. Image patches aligned with each predicted nodule candidate region but

Table 3. FROC Performance comparison with the state-of-the-arts: sensitivity (recall) and the corresponding false positives at $1/8, 1/4, 1/2, 1, 2, 4, 8$ per scan. Our 3DFPN-HS^2 method achieves the best performance (with >90% sensitivity) at all false positive levels and significantly outperforms others especially at the low false positive levels $(1/8$ and $1/4)$.

Methods	1/8	1/4	1/2	1	2	4	8	CPM score
Dou et al. [4]	0.659	0.745	0.819	0.865	0.906	0.933	0.946	0.839
Zhu et al. [11]	0.692	0.769	0.824	0.865	0.893	0.917	0.933	0.842
Wang et al. [9]	0.676	0.776	0.879	0.949	0.958	0.958	0.958	0.878
Ding et al. [3]	0.748	0.853	0.887	0.922	0.938	0.944	0.946	0.891
Khosravan et al. [6]	0.709	0.836	0.921	0.953	0.953	0.953	0.953	0.897
3DFPN (Ours)	**0.848**	**0.876**	**0.905**	**0.933**	**0.943**	**0.957**	**0.970**	**0.919**
3DFPN-HS^2 (Ours)	**0.904**	**0.914**	**0.933**	**0.957**	**0.971**	**0.971**	**0.971**	**0.952**

with twice size (in both x and y directions) are selected from 11 continuous CT slices (5 slices before and after the current slice of nodule candidate respectively). The LHI of these patches is extracted and resized to 48 × 48 pixels as the input of the HS² network.

In the training, the learning rate starts from 0.01 and decreases to 1/10 for every 500 epochs. Total of 2,000 epochs is conducted for the framework. The average prediction time for a whole CT scan is about 0.53 min/scan on a server with one GeForce GTX 1080 GPU using Pytorch 2.7.

Comparison with Other Methods. Table 3 shows the FROC evaluation results with $(1/8, 1/4, 1/2, 1, 2, 4, 8)$ false positive levels of our proposed method compared with state-of-the-art methods. The highlighted numbers in the table indicate the best performance within each column. All the methods are tested on LUNA16 dataset followed the same FROC evaluation. As shown in the table, our framework outperforms 5.5% average sensitivity than the best result of other methods. In addition, the proposed framework achieves the best performance at every FP level. As previously mentioned, the CAD system is not only required a high sensitivity, but also a high specificity. Table 3 demonstrates that the false positives are greatly reduced by the proposed HS² network. 3DFPN-HS² obtains a highest 97.14% sensitivity at 2 FPs per scan. In addition, for the FP of 1/8, 1/4, and 1/2 per scan, the proposed framework still remains a high sensitivity above 90%. The experimental results show that 3DFPN-HS² reaches a state-of-the-art performance for high sensitivity and specificity lung nodule detection.

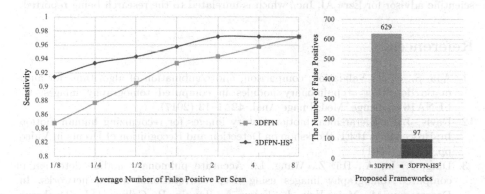

Fig. 3. Left: Comparison between the proposed 3DFPN and 3DFPN-HS² (with High Sensitivity and Specificity network for false positive reduction.) 3DFPN-HS² greatly improves the performance of the 3DFPN at all the FP levels. Right: The number of false positives is reduced from 629 to 97 for a total of 88 CT scans with the confidence score above 0 after the HS² network is applied. More visualized detection results are provided in the supplementary document. (Color figure online)

Effectiveness of HS² for FP Reduction. Two experiments are conducted to demonstrate the advantages of HS² network. As shown in Fig. 3(a), compared with 3DFPN without the HS^2 network, the result of 3DFPN-HS^2 with the false positive reduction is increased more than 5% at 1/8 FP level. In addition, the numbers of FPs with (blue bar) and without (orange bar) HS^2 network for all the predicted nodule candidates from a total of 88 CT scans (subset 9) are further compared in Fig. 3(b). By applying HS^2, the 3DFPN-HS^2 is able to distinguish the falsely detected tissues from true nodules, therefore significantly reduces FPs by 84.5%. It is worth noting that our proposed 3DFPN without HS^2 network still achieves 97% at 8 FPs per scan and 91.9% CPM, which surpasses other state-of-the-art methods (see Table 3).

4   Conclusion

In this paper, we have proposed an effective framework 3DFPN-HS^2 by employing a 3D feature pyramid network with local and global feature enrichment for small volume and multi-scale nodule detection. HS^2 network is introduced to reduce false positives based on the different patterns of location variance for nodules and tissues in continuous CT slices. The proposed framework significantly outperforms the state-of-the-art methods and has achieved high sensitivity and specificity which has a great potential in routine clinical practice.

Acknowledgements. This material is based upon work supported by the National Science Foundation under award number IIS-1400802 and Memorial Sloan Kettering Cancer Center Support Grant/Core Grant P30 CA008748. Oguz Akin, MD serves as a scientific advisor for Ezra AI, Inc., which is unrelated to the research being reported.

References

1. Aaa, S., et al.: Validation, comparison, and combination of algorithms for automatic detection of pulmonary nodules in computed tomography images: the LUNA16 challenge. Med. Image Anal. **42**, 1–13 (2017)
2. Davis, J.W.: Hierarchical motion history images for recognizing human motion. In: Proceedings IEEE Workshop on Detection and Recognition of Events in Video, pp. 39–46 (2001)
3. Ding, J., Li, A., Hu, Z., Wang, L.: Accurate pulmonary nodule detection in computed tomography images using deep convolutional neural networks. In: Descoteaux, M., Maier-Hein, L., Franz, A., Jannin, P., Collins, D.L., Duchesne, S. (eds.) MICCAI 2017. LNCS, vol. 10435, pp. 559–567. Springer, Cham (2017). https://doi.org/10.1007/978-3-319-66179-7_64
4. Dou, Q., Chen, H., Jin, Y., Lin, H., Qin, J., Heng, P.-A.: Automated pulmonary nodule detection via 3D ConvNets with online sample filtering and hybrid-loss residual learning. In: Descoteaux, M., Maier-Hein, L., Franz, A., Jannin, P., Collins, D.L., Duchesne, S. (eds.) MICCAI 2017. LNCS, vol. 10435, pp. 630–638. Springer, Cham (2017). https://doi.org/10.1007/978-3-319-66179-7_72
5. Girshick, R.: Fast R-CNN. In: Proceedings of the IEEE International Conference on Computer Vision, pp. 1440–1448 (2015)

6. Khosravan, N., Bagci, U.: *S4ND*: single-shot single-scale lung nodule detection. In: Frangi, A.F., Schnabel, J.A., Davatzikos, C., Alberola-López, C., Fichtinger, G. (eds.) MICCAI 2018. LNCS, vol. 11071, pp. 794–802. Springer, Cham (2018). https://doi.org/10.1007/978-3-030-00934-2_88

7. Lin, T.Y., Dollár, P., Girshick, R., He, K., Hariharan, B., Belongie, S.: Feature pyramid networks for object detection. In: Proceedings of the IEEE Conference on Computer Vision and Pattern Recognition, pp. 2117–2125 (2017)

8. Setio, A.A., et al.: Pulmonary nodule detection in CT images: false positive reduction using multi-view convolutional networks. IEEE Trans. Med. Imaging **35**(5), 1160–1169 (2016)

9. Wang, B., Qi, G., Tang, S., Zhang, L., Deng, L., Zhang, Y.: Automated pulmonary nodule detection: high sensitivity with few candidates. In: Frangi, A.F., Schnabel, J.A., Davatzikos, C., Alberola-López, C., Fichtinger, G. (eds.) MICCAI 2018. LNCS, vol. 11071, pp. 759–767. Springer, Cham (2018). https://doi.org/10.1007/978-3-030-00934-2_84

10. Yang, X., Zhang, C., Tian, Y.: Recognizing actions using depth motion maps-based histograms of oriented gradients. In: Proceedings of the 20th ACM International Conference on Multimedia, pp. 1057–1060 (2012)

11. Zhu, W., Liu, C., Fan, W., Xie, X.: DeepLung: deep 3D dual path nets for automated pulmonary nodule detection and classification. In: 2018 IEEE Winter Conference on Applications of Computer Vision (WACV), pp. 673–681 (2018)

Automated Detection and Type Classification of Central Venous Catheters in Chest X-Rays

Vaishnavi Subramanian[1,2], Hongzhi Wang[1(✉)], Joy T. Wu[1], Ken C. L. Wong[1], Arjun Sharma[1], and Tanveer Syeda-Mahmood[1]

[1] IBM Research, Almaden Research Center, San Jose, CA, USA
hongzhiw@us.ibm.com
[2] University of Illinois Urbana-Champaign, Urbana, IL, USA

Abstract. Central venous catheters (CVCs) are commonly used in critical care settings for monitoring body functions and administering medications. They are often described in radiology reports by referring to their presence, identity and placement. In this paper, we address the problem of automatic detection of their presence and identity through automated segmentation using deep learning networks and classification based on their intersection with previously learned shape priors from clinician annotations of CVCs. The results not only outperform existing methods of catheter detection achieving 85.2% accuracy at 91.6% precision, but also enable high precision (95.2%) classification of catheter types on a large dataset of over 10,000 chest X-rays, presenting a robust and practical solution to this problem.

Keywords: Chest X-rays · Catheters · Classification · Segmentation · U-Net

1 Introduction

Central venous catheters (CVCs) are commonly used in critical care settings and surgeries to monitor a patient's heart function and deliver medications close to the heart. These are inserted centrally or peripherally through the jugular, subclavian or brachial veins and advanced towards the heart through the venous system, most often blindly. Portable anterior-posterior (AP) chest X-Rays (CXRs) obtained after the CVC placements are used to rule out malpositioning and complications. The interpretation of the CXRs is currently done manually after loading these into the hospital's electronic systems.

With the advancement of deep learning approaches to anatomical findings in chest X-rays, it is conceivable that radiology reports may be produced automatically in the future, which would considerably expedite the clinical workflow. However, any such report, particularly for in-hospital settings, will need to mention the presence of the CVC, its type such as internal jugular (IJ) or peripherally

© Springer Nature Switzerland AG 2019
D. Shen et al. (Eds.): MICCAI 2019, LNCS 11769, pp. 522–530, 2019.
https://doi.org/10.1007/978-3-030-32226-7_58

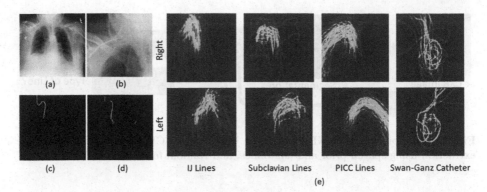

Fig. 1. Example of central venous catheters (CVCs) and collection of annotations: (a) original CXR where the CVC is barely visible, (b) enlarged region of interest focusing on the CVC, (c) manual CVC annotation, (d) segmentation produced by U-Net (e) The pixel-wise overlay of manual annotations for four common types of CVCs, which are used to construct spatial priors.

inserted central catheter (PICC), and any problems with their positioning and insertions. Different types of CVCs also have slightly different optimal tip locations. Automated detection and recognition of CVCs through direct whole image based recognition approaches is unlikely to yield good results as it is difficult to learn discriminative features from these thin tubular structures that occupy less than 1% of the footprint in the overall image, as shown in Fig. 1(a–d). Hence most methods have focused on local extraction of these structures.

There is vast literature using conventional medical image processing on the detection of catheters both in angiography imaging and chest X-rays. Recent work, however, has applied deep learning for the detection of the presence of the catheters and their tips. In [1], the detection of tip location for PICC lines was attempted. In CXR fluoroscopy images, the sequence information was used to aid automatic segmentation of catheters [2] based on the U-Net [3]. An approach recently proposed [4] for segmentation employs scale-recurrent neural networks on synthetic catheters in pediatric data. Existing approaches result in partial detection using the deep learning stages with post-processing steps to complete the contours, have been tested on smaller datasets or on synthetic datasets. Their robustness to variations on real, large datasets still needs to be determined. Further, while existing methods aim for either segmentation and detection of a specific CVC type or its placement, the general task of identifying the type of CVC shown in adult chest X-rays has not been attempted, to our knowledge.

In this paper, we simultaneously address the detection and classification of the CVC type on a large public CXR dataset. Specifically, we can detect and distinguish between four common types of CVCs, namely, peripherally inserted central catheters (PICC), internal jugular (IJ), subclavian and Swan-Ganz catheters. Our main idea is to augment the detection of catheters with the

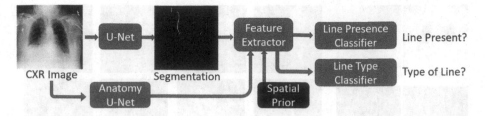

Fig. 2. Our workflow for CXR comprising U-Net based CVC segmentation, feature extraction using spatial prior and anatomies, and random forest based classifiers.

introduction of shape priors generated from clinician segmentation of catheters to focus on relevant regions for classification.

Recognizing the identity of the catheters can be a challenge since different CVCs have different contours depending on the origin of insertion and how far they go into the body. However, after annotation of these catheters on hundreds of AP chest X-rays by our clinicians, we discovered that the shape spanned by the various CVC insertion approaches still have a surprisingly distinctive signature and proximity patterns to known anatomical structures as shown in Fig. 1(e). Since the type of CVCs can be easily recognized visually by the insertion approaches, in this paper, we exploit this information to both confirm the presence of CVCs as well as recognize their identity. Specifically, we first detect the presence of CVCs using prior annotations of these structures through a deep learning segmentation network based on U-Net [3,5] to approximately identify potential fragments of CVCs if present. We then develop features exploiting the segmentation within regional priors and their relation to key anatomical features. The features are then classified into the respective labels of CVCs using random forests. By utilizing the spatial priors, we demonstrate that the complete delineation of the CVC is not required for recognizing either its presence or type. We demonstrate that our features are superior to features extracted by deep learning methods such as VGG16 and DenseNet [6,7] in a comparative study for this problem. Therefore, our approach is a hybrid combination of automatic feature learning for initial candidate CVC regions with high precision custom features for recognizing the identity of the CVCs based on prior knowledge, in the form of shape priors, within a conventional machine learning classifier.

2   Method

We now describe our hybrid approach to detecting the presence of CVCs and the classification of their types in AP chest X-ray images, shown in Fig. 2.

2.1   Segmentation of CVC Using Modified U-Net

To identify regions of interest, we adapted the commonly used U-Net [3] for CVC segmentation. While the original loss function works well for large structures, because CVCs are small structures, we used the exponential logarithmic loss function proposed recently [5] to address the highly imbalanced label sizes. When the CXR has no CVC of interest, the segmentation output is a blank image, representing no interesting region.

2.2 Feature Extraction

Given the segmentation of possible CVCs in the CXR from the U-Net, we design image processing features describing the segmentation, its relation to prior knowledge of CVC contours, and its relation to key anatomical features of the chest as below. These describe the overall properties of the potential CVCs, even if the initial detected region is imperfect.

Spatial Prior for Each Class: To obtain shape priors, our clinicians annotated the contours of CVCs in hundreds of training images. The CVCs are traced from their anatomical origin of insertion to their tip to give contours that are reflective for different types of CVCs. We averaged the manual annotations per-pixel for each class (Fig. 1(e)) and blurred them spatially to obtain signature spatial priors for each of the CVC classes: left/right PICC, IJ, subclavian and Swan-Ganz catheters as shown in Fig. 1(e).

We then performed a pixel-wise multiplication of the segmentation output with the prior for each class and characterized this overlap using an n-bin intensity histogram, and histogram of oriented gradients (HoG) features for each class. This informs us how well a CVC segmentation aligns with priors of particular CVC classes.

Relation to Anatomical Features: We extracted the segmentation of chest anatomical structures including the clavicles, lungs, heart and mediastinum using an independent U-Net again trained on clinician annotations. We obtained the Euclidean distance distributions of the segmentation relative to the center of these different chest anatomies. These provide contextual information and distinguish confusing classes such as PICC and subclavian lines.

Size and Shape Properties: We also characterized the shape and size properties of the positive regions of segmentation: the area, length and width characterize the overall presence/absence of CVCs, the histogram of oriented gradients (HoG) describe the shape contours which are crucial for type classification since different CVC types have different shape signatures, as shown in Fig. 1(e).

2.3 Classification Using Random Forests

The extracted features are used for classification on the presence of CVCs, and identifying the type of CVCs. We employ a random forest (RF) for each task. The first RF yields a binary presence/absence label, and the second provides a multi-label output, with 4 indicators, one for each type of CVC: PICC, IJ, subclavian and Swan-Ganz.

We chose the current architecture after experimenting with different end-to-end deep learning architectures. Feeding spatial priors and anatomical segmentation as additional channels into a VGG-like network failed to learn distinguishing relations. For our specific problem characterized by small area footprint, long and indistinguishable tubular structures with uneven sample sizes, random forests were found to have better generalization.

3 Experiments and Results

3.1 Data

We worked with the NIH dataset comprising of 112,000 CXRs [8]. A subset of these were labelled and annotated for different tasks:

CVC Segmentation - Pixel Level Annotation: A random sample of 1500 AP CXRs was selected from the NIH dataset. The CXRs with CVCs were annotated at the pixel level, to provide annotations for 359 IJ lines, 78 subclavian lines, 277 PICC lines, and 32 Swan-Ganz catheters, yielding a total of 608 annotated images of size 512×512. The remaining images have no lines. An overlay of the different annotations, based on CVC types, is shown in Fig. 1(e).

CVC Presence - Whole Image Level Annotation: A subset of 3000 images was chosen from the NIH dataset, which a radiologist labeled globally for presence of external medical devices. This resulted in 2381 CXRs with some device present, and 619 CXRs with an absence of any device. Since devices are usually associated with catheters, this label extends to CVC presence.

CVC Type - Whole Image Level Annotation: A subset of around 16,000 CXRs was sampled from the NIH dataset and a group of radiologists reported on these using a semi-structured template, where one section was dedicated for device reporting. A recently proposed NLP sentence clustering algorithm [9] was applied to the device section and a sentence from each resultant cluster was validated manually by two clinicians to derive the global labels for the presence of different CVCs.

This resulted in 10,746 CXRs with at least one type of externally inserted catheter, with 4249 PICC lines, 1651 IJ lines, 201 subclavian lines, 192 Swan-Ganz catheters, and 4453 CXRs with other catheters including airway and drainage tubes. The related dataset has been released as part of the MICCAI 2019 Multimodal Learning for Clinical Decision Support (ML-CDS) Challenge.

3.2 U-Net Segmentation

We trained a U-Net for identifying the lines as discussed in Sect. 2.1, treating the all clinician annotated CVCs as belonging to a positive class without specific distinction on CVC type. We split the pixel-level annotated images into 80% training and 20% validation. We trained the U-Net until convergence using the

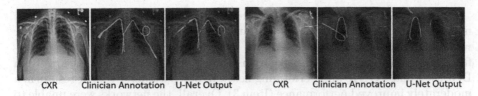

CXR   Clinician Annotation   U-Net Output   CXR   Clinician Annotation   U-Net Output

Fig. 3. Some example CXR images, overlay of clinician annotations of CVCs, and overlay of U-Net segmentations on the original CXR.

Adam optimizer with learning rate of $5e^{-5}$ and the exponential loss with the best-performing weights ($w_{Dice} = 0.8$ and $w_{Cross} = 0.2$) from [5].

Some segmentation results are shown in Fig. 3. We observe that sections of the CVCs are missed in some cases, and there are false positives in some confusing areas of the CXRs.

We evaluate the quality of our segmentation by computing the extent of overlap between the ground truth annotations and the U-Net segmentation output on the held-out set. Since CVCs are thin structures, for reliable overlap estimation between automatic and manual CVC segmentation, we enlarged the binary manual segmentations via a dilation operation. With the radius of 2-pixel dilation, 75% cases have >50% overlap and 84% cases have >40% overlap and a 5-pixel dilation radius resulted in 80% and 90% cases with greater than 50% and 40% overlap, respectively.

Table 1. Results for CVC detection (P: Precision, R: Recall, Acc: Acccuracy, AUC: Area under ROC, DN: DenseNet, VGG: VGG16, SP: spatial prior). Best values for each column are in bold.

Method	P	R	Acc	AUC	Method	P	R	Acc	AUC
1. DN	20.0	20.0	20.0	50.0	8. Seg-VGG-RF	80.2	95.0	78.2	53.6
2. VGG	20.0	20.0	20.0	50.0	9. + CXR	79.2	97.2	79.8	49.8
3. DN+VGG	81.6	95.0	75.3	63.0	10. Mask-DN-RF	84.0	92.4	79.4	62.0
4. DN-RF	79.4	**98.8**	78.8	50.2	11. Mask-VGG-RF	84.2	91.6	79.6	62.8
5. VGG-RF	79.4	98.0	78.4	50.0	12. Seg-SP-RF (Ours)	89.6	89.6	83.8	75.0
6. Seg-DN-RF	80.0	95.8	77.8	58.6	13. + HoG (Ours)	91.4	89.4	**85.2**	78.8
7. + CXR	79.6	97.2	78.4	51.4	14. + Anatomy (Ours)	**91.6**	89.6	**85.2**	**79.4**

3.3 CVC Presence Identification

We next focus on the task of identifying CVC presence in CXRs. We performed a 5-fold cross-validation using a 60-20-20 split for training-validation-testing using the 3000 CXRs labeled for device presence. The classifier outputs a binary label indicating the presence of at least one CVC in the CXR (label: 1), or the absence of any CVCs (label: 0). Results for this task are presented in Table 1. The parameters (number of trees, and depth of trees) for all random forests were chosen with hyper-parameter tuning for validation performance, for each fold.

To set the baseline, we trained state-of-the-art VGG16 [6] and DenseNet [7] networks for the classification task directly on the CXRs, fine-tuning their weights pre-trained on ImageNet. We observed that this yields poor classifiers, with less than 50% accuracy (Items 1–2). Concatenating the features from DenseNet and VGG16 and performing heavy hyper-parameter tuning results in a moderately improved performance (Item 3). Overall, the networks were unable to recognize the discriminative regions and performed poorly, due to the small area footprint, long tubular structures that blend into the background, and uneven sample sizes. Thus, in further experiments, we treated the ImageNet pre-trained neural networks as feature extractors, feeding the pre-final layer outputs to random forest (RF) classifiers, henceforth abbreviated NN-RF. Using the original CXR as input to the NN-RF improved accuracy, while the area under ROC (AUC) still remained at 50% (Items 4–5).

Next, we processed all the CXRs through the U-Net generating segmentation images. We fed combinations of the segmentation (Seg) and the original CXR image to NN-RFs: Seg alone (Items 6, 8), Seg with CXR as one of the image channels (Items 7, 9) and the original CXR masked to zero out the lowest values of the segmentation output to create a masked CXR image focused on regions of potential CVCs (Items 10–11). These showed considerable improvements in the AUC, while the other metrics (precision, recall, F-score and accuracy) remained primarily unchanged.

Finally, we extracted the image-processing features describing the size, shape, likelihood based on CVC spatial priors, and relation to chest anatomical elements, as presented in Sect. 2.2. The simplest set of features comprising the spatial prior information itself yielded a 12% increase in AUC (Item 12). The further addition of size and HoG shape features (Item 13) and anatomical relation information (Item 14) improved the classifier performance further, giving 85.2% accuracy at a precision of 91.6% and a recall of 89.6%.

3.4   CVC Type Identification

For the classification problem of identifying the type of CVC present, we again perform a 5-fold cross-validation using a 60-20-20 split for training-validation-testing. We used the 10,746 CXRs which have at least one catheter. We report the support-weighted average performance metrics, and the precision and recall for each CVC type in Table 2 using the different methods presented for CVC presence identification (except for DenseNet+VGG concatenation).

As in the previous classification problem, pre-trained DenseNet and VGG16 are unable to perform well (Item 1–2), though treating these as feature extractors for a RF classification improves performance substantially (Item 3–4). Utilizing the features extracted from fine-tuned VGG performs similarly achieving an average 79.6% precision, 49.2% recall and 59.5% accuracy, while DenseNet performs worse. Segmentations and CXRs input to the networks for feature extraction marginally improve the average accuracy and AUC (Item 5–10), leaving the other metrics unchanged. The image-processing based features perform the best (Item 11–13), reaching an average classification accuracy of 78.2% at a precision of 95.2%. Our method also achieves lower metric variation as brought out by the standard deviation values of the average accuracy.

From our best-performing classifier (Item 13), it can be observed that recall for CVCs other than PICC is under 50%. This reveals that the RF classifier performs best on PICC lines, primarily due to the fact that PICC lines make up about 40% of the CVC images while having the simplest contours. More complex contours like the Swan-Ganz are under-represented and comprise only 2% of all CVCs, and make the task challenging. This could be overcome by obtaining more data for these classes. Some example CXRs with the U-Net output, and the final class prediction are presented in Fig. 4. It can be observed that our approach identifies the type of CVC correctly despite the incomplete segmentations from the U-Net. Our method can also handle the presence of multiple CVCs in the same CXR.

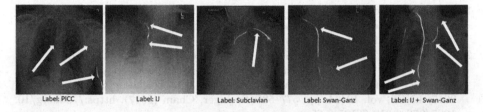

Label: PICC   Label: IJ   Label: Subclavian   Label: Swan-Ganz   Label: IJ + Swan-Ganz

Fig. 4. Some examples of CXRs with U-Net output overlayed. Despite the incomplete segmentation by the U-Net, our method correctly labels each of the catheters.

Table 2. Results for CVC type identification (Mean ± standard deviation, P: Precision, R: Recall, AUC: Area under ROC, DN: DenseNet, SP: spatial prior). Best values for each column are in bold. Our algorithm: rows 11–13.

Method	PICC P	PICC R	IJ P	IJ R	SC P	SC R	SG P	SG R	Weighted average P	R	Accuracy	AUC
1. DN	34.6	11.6	13.2	22.2	0.0	0.0	2.6	51.4	34.2	20.4	20.0 ± 0.71	51.0 ± 1.00
2. VGG	36.6	2.8	16.6	8.8	1.2	16.8	2.8	6.2	36.0	27.6	28.0 ± 0.00	48.6 ± 0.89
3. DN-RF	78.4	55.0	96.6	32.4	100.0	33.8	100.0	25.8	84.6	47.4	66.2 ± 1.10	67.0 ± 0.71
4. VGG-RF	77.2	54.6	96.4	32.2	100.0	33.2	100.0	25.8	83.8	47.2	65.6 ± 0.89	66.8 ± 0.84
5. Seg-DN-RF	77.4	64.8	84.2	38.2	100.0	33.2	100.0	24.6	80.8	55.4	68.6 ± 0.89	68.6 ± 0.89
6. +CXR	78.2	52.2	98.2	33.2	100.0	33.8	100.0	25.2	85.0	45.8	65.4 ± 1.14	66.8 ± 0.45
7. Seg-VGG-RF	76.4	63.8	82.4	37.6	100.0	32.6	100.0	25.8	79.2	54.8	67.4 ± 0.55	68.2 ± 0.84
8. +CXR	76.2	52.6	96.2	32.8	100.0	33.2	100.0	23.8	83.2	45.8	64.8 ± 1.30	66.6 ± 0.55
9. Mask-DN-RF	75.6	60.0	88.6	35.6	100.0	33.8	100.0	25.2	80.6	51.6	66.6 ± 0.89	67.8 ± 0.45
10. Mask-VGG-RF	74.6	58.0	87.2	34.8	100.0	33.8	100.0	25.2	79.2	50.2	65.4 ± 1.14	67.2 ± 0.84
11. Seg-SP-RF	88.6	75.4	95.8	33.4	100.0	31.6	100.0	25.8	91.2	61.6	75.6 ± 0.55	70.0 ± 0.71
12. + HoG	93.0	78.8	99.0	32.4	100.0	33.2	100.0	25.8	95.2	**63.8**	78.2 ± 0.84	70.8 ± 0.84
13. + Anatomy	**93.0**	**78.8**	**99.6**	32.2	100.0	**33.8**	100.0	25.8	**95.6**	63.6	**78.4 ± 0.55**	**71.0 ± 0.71**

4   Conclusions

In this paper, we have addressed, for the first time, the detection and classification of central venous catheters in chest X-rays. Due to the small footprint of these devices, it is difficult for deep learning networks to detect these structures based on whole image input. Our method presents a robust solution to this problem by using deep learning for an approximate segmentation of these structures followed by conventional machine learning on features from these regions incorporating spatial priors from distribution atlases extracted from CXR images. Techniques to better incorporate handcrafted features, including anatomical features and spatial priors, into neural networks will be explored in the future.

References

1. Lee, H., Mansouri, M., Tajmir, S., Lev, M.H., Do, S.: A deep-learning system for fully-automated peripherally inserted central catheter (PICC) tip detection. J. Digital Imaging **31**, 393–402 (2017)
2. Ambrosini, P., Ruijters, D., Niessen, W.J., Moelker, A., van Walsum, T.: Fully automatic and real-time catheter segmentation in x-ray fluoroscopy. In: Descoteaux, M., Maier-Hein, L., Franz, A., Jannin, P., Collins, D.L., Duchesne, S. (eds.) MICCAI 2017. LNCS, vol. 10434, pp. 577–585. Springer, Cham (2017). https://doi.org/10.1007/978-3-319-66185-8_65
3. Ronneberger, O., Fischer, P., Brox, T.: U-Net: convolutional networks for biomedical image segmentation. In: Navab, N., Hornegger, J., Wells, W.M., Frangi, A.F. (eds.) MICCAI 2015. LNCS, vol. 9351, pp. 234–241. Springer, Cham (2015). https://doi.org/10.1007/978-3-319-24574-4_28
4. Yi, X., Adams, S., Babyn, P., Elnajmi, A.: Automatic catheter and tube detection in pediatric x-ray images using a scale-recurrent network and synthetic data. J. Digital Imaging 1–10 (2019)
5. Wong, K.C.L., Moradi, M., Tang, H., Syeda-Mahmood, T.: 3D segmentation with exponential logarithmic loss for highly unbalanced object sizes. In: Frangi, A.F., Schnabel, J.A., Davatzikos, C., Alberola-López, C., Fichtinger, G. (eds.) MICCAI 2018. LNCS, vol. 11072, pp. 612–619. Springer, Cham (2018). https://doi.org/10.1007/978-3-030-00931-1_70
6. Simonyan, K., Zisserman, A.: Very deep convolutional networks for large-scale image recognition. arXiv preprint arXiv:1409.1556 (2014)
7. Huang, G., Liu, Z., Van Der Maaten, L., Weinberger, K.Q.: Densely connected convolutional networks. In: CVPR (2017)
8. Wang, X., Peng, Y., Lu, L., Lu, Z., Bagheri, M., Summers, R.M.: ChestX-ray8: hospital-scale chest X-ray database and benchmarks on weakly-supervised classification and localization of common thorax diseases. In: 2017 IEEE Conference on Computer Vision and Pattern Recognition (CVPR), pp. 3462–3471. IEEE (2017)
9. Syeda-Mahmood, T.F., et al.: Building a benchmark dataset and classifiers for sentence-level findings in AP chest X-rays. CoRR abs/1906.09336 (2019). http://arxiv.org/abs/1906.09336

Hand Pose Estimation for Pediatric Bone Age Assessment

María Escobar[1(✉)], Cristina González[1], Felipe Torres[1], Laura Daza[1],
Gustavo Triana[2], and Pablo Arbeláez[1]

[1] Universidad de los Andes, Bogotá, Colombia
{mc.escobar11,ci.gonzalez10,f.torres11,la.daza10,
pa.arbelaez}@uniandes.edu.co
[2] Fundación Santa Fe de Bogotá, Bogotá, Colombia

Abstract. We present a new experimental framework for the task of
Bone Age Assessment (BAA) based on a local analysis of anatomical Regions Of Interest (ROIs) of hand radiographs. For this purpose,
we introduce the Radiological Hand Pose Estimation (RHPE) Dataset,
composed of 6,288 hand radiographs from a population that is different from the currently available BAA datasets. We provide Bone Age
groundtruths annotated by two expert radiologists as well as bounding
boxes and keypoints denoting anatomical ROIs annotated by multiple
trained subjects. In addition to RHPE, we provide bounding boxes and
ROIs annotations for the publicly available BAA dataset by the Radiological Society of North America (RSNA) [9]. We propose a new experimental framework with hand detection and hand pose estimation as
new tasks to extract local information for BAA methods. Thanks to its
fine-grained and precisely localized annotations, our dataset will allow to
exploit local information to push forward automated BAA algorithms.
Additionally, we conduct experiments with state-of-the-art methods in
each of the new tasks. Our proposed model, named BoNet, leverages
local information and significantly outperforms state-of-the-art methods
in BAA. We provide the RHPE dataset with the corresponding annotations, as well as the trained models, the source code for BoNet and the
additional annotations created for the RSNA dataset.

Keywords: Bone Age Assessment · Computer aided diagnosis · Hand
radiograph · Regions Of Interest

1 Introduction

Bone age is a quantification of the skeletal development of children. This measurement differs from chronological age as it goes from 0 to 20 years, while

---

M. Escobar and C. González—Both authors contributed equally to this work.

Electronic supplementary material The online version of this chapter (https://
doi.org/10.1007/978-3-030-32226-7_59) contains supplementary material, which is
available to authorized users.

© Springer Nature Switzerland AG 2019
D. Shen et al. (Eds.): MICCAI 2019, LNCS 11769, pp. 531–539, 2019.
https://doi.org/10.1007/978-3-030-32226-7_59

varying according to gender, age and ethnicity. Bone Age Assessment (BAA) is performed by radiologists and pediatricians to diagnose growth disorders or to determine the final adult height of a child [17]. This evaluation is commonly accomplished through visual inspection of ossification patterns in a radiograph of the non-dominant hand and wrist. The most commonly used manual methods are Greulich and Pyle (G&P) [8] and Tanner and Whitehouse (TW2) [17]. In G&P the entire hand is classified into a stage, while in TW2 it is divided into 20 Regions Of Interest (ROIs) that are analyzed individually to estimate the patient's bone age. As a result, TW2 is more precise because it makes a *local analysis* of the hand. However, both manual approaches are prone to intra and inter observer errors due to the level of expertise of the radiologist or possible variations in the radiograph.

To improve the accuracy of BAA, there has been a growing interest in the development of automated methods. The commercial software BoneXpert [18], created in 2009 by Hans Henrik Thodberg and Sven Kreiborg, is currently used in clinical settings. This tool performs BAA based on edge detection and active appearance models [2] to generate candidates and make comparisons according to G&P and TW2. However, the method was developed using patients from a Danish cohort, therefore the reliability is not guaranteed when assessing data from other countries.

Recently, the Radiological Society of North America (RSNA) created a BAA dataset for the 2017 Boneage Pediatric Challenge [9]. The RSNA Challenge encouraged the development of several deep learning and machine learning approaches to accurately perform BAA [9]. The winners of the challenge achieved a Mean Absolute Difference (MAD) of 4.26 months over the test set [1]. Similarly, most top-performing methods used shallower neural networks to extract features from the entire image. Other methods uniformly extracted overlapping patches or first segmented the bones to localize the analysis, obtaining 4.35 and 4.50 MAD, respectively [9]. Similarly, [12] developed an approach to focus on the carpal bones, the metacarpal and proximal phalanges, achieving 4.97 MAD.

Although some of the approaches above build explicitly on local information when assessing bone age, existing BAA datasets [3,6,7,9] provide only bone age annotations at the image level, and hence they are not designed to exploit the information of anatomical ROIs. A suitable approach for identifying ROIs in the hand is through hand pose estimation. This task has been studied in the context of 3D hand models directed towards human computer interaction, virtual reality and augmented reality applications [4,5]. In this work, we propose a 2D framework focused on radiological hand pose estimation as a new task, enabling various medical applications in this field.

We present the Radiological Hand Pose Estimation (RHPE) dataset containing 6,288 images of hand radiographs from a population with different characteristics than the currently available datasets, ensuring a high variability for a better model generalization. In addition to the new dataset, we introduce hand detection and hand pose estimation as new tasks to extract local information from images. To establish a robust framework, we collect manually annotated keypoints for anatomical ROIs and bounding boxes of each hand radiograph. An example of our annotations is presented in Fig. 1. We also provide bounding boxes and keypoint annotations for the RSNA dataset. We evaluate the performance of state-of-the-art methods on our proposed tasks on both RSNA and RHPE datasets, and we propose a new local approach to BAA called BoNet that significantly outperforms all existing approaches. Additionally, we prove that both datasets are complementary and can be combined to create a robust benchmark with a better model generalization, regardless of the population's characteristics.

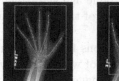

Fig. 1. Different examples of our keypoint and bounding box annotations. We provide groundtruth for hand detection and hand pose estimation for both RHPE and RSNA datasets.

Our main contributions can be summarized as follows:

1. We introduce RHPE, a new dataset from a diverse population, and create a new benchmark for the development of BAA methods.
2. We provide the first manually annotated bounding boxes and keypoints in the RSNA and RHPE datasets. These annotations enable a new experimental framework including hand detection and hand pose estimation as tasks for the extraction of local information from hand radiographs.
3. We present BoNet, a novel CNN architecture that leverages anatomical ROIs to perform BAA. BoNet significantly outperforms all state-of-the-art methods on the RSNA and RHPE datasets.

To ensure reproducibility of our results and to promote further research on BAA, we provide the RHPE dataset and the corresponding annotations for train and validation, as well as the trained models, the source code for BoNet and the additional annotations created for the RSNA dataset [9]. We also deploy a server for automated evaluation of the test set.[1]

2   Radiological Hand Pose Estimation Dataset

2.1   Dataset Description

We collect the RHPE data from a population that is different from the ones in the currently available datasets for BAA. The database comprises images of

---

[1] https://biomedicalcomputervision.uniandes.edu.co/.

radiographs taken from left and right hands of both male and female patients between 0 and 240 months of age (0–20 years), with bone age annotations made by two expert radiologists for each patient. The dataset is composed of 6,288 images divided into 3 sets: 5,492 for training, 716 for validation and 80 for testing, maintaining the proportion of images used in each split of the RSNA dataset. 54% of the dataset corresponds to female patients and 46% to male patients. This division has the same proportions as the RSNA dataset and the Gaussian distribution of bone age on our dataset and on the RSNA dataset is approximately the same, centered around 126 months of age. A similar bone age distribution between the datasets suggests that they are compatible and can be used to study the influence of ethnicity on bone age assessment algorithms. See supplementary material for a further analysis of the similarities and differences of both datasets.

We gather anatomical landmark annotations from 96 trained subjects. For each image, the subject is shown an example of where the keypoints should be located. We obtain multiple annotations per image and perform outlier rejection by identifying the annotations that are 2 standard deviations away from the mean. From this procedure, we obtain at least 4 annotations per image made by different trained subjects. With 17 keypoints per hand radiograph, this accounts for more than 1.3 million annotated keypoints. These annotations correspond to the proximal, middle and distal phalanges, the carpal bones, and the distal radius and ulna. For compatibility, we store all our annotations using the MS-COCO [13] format. For the detection groundtruth, we include the upper-left coordinates, width and height of the bounding box that encloses the hand.

2.2 Tasks

Hand Detection. The goal of hand detection is to determine the location of a specific hand in the image. The importance of including detection as a task in our dataset lies in the fact that the images in RHPE include both hands and it is necessary to isolate the non-dominant hand for the assessment. For evaluation, we use the same standard metrics as in MS-COCO for object detection: mean Average Precision (mAP) and mean Average Recall (mAR) at Intersection over Union (IoU) thresholds @[.50 : .05 : .95].

Hand Pose Estimation. In this task, the objective is to estimate the position of anatomical ROIs in the hand radiograph. For the evaluation of hand pose estimation algorithms, we use the mAP and mAR at Object Keypoint Similarity (OKS) [13] @[.50 : .05 : .95]. It is worth noting that the evaluation code used in MS-COCO only takes into account instances that were accurately detected. To obtain a more realistic assessment of performance, we modify this metric to consider the effect of every image regardless of the detection mAR@[.5:.05:.95]. Additionally, the standard deviation σ_i with respect to object scale s varies significantly for different keypoints. In full-sized images, our σ penalizes any keypoint estimation 10 pixels away or more from the mean location. See supplementary material for additional information.

Bone Age Assessment. In the BAA task, we aim at estimating bone age in months for a given hand radiograph. To evaluate the performance, we use the same metric as in the RSNA 2017 Pediatric Bone Age Challenge: the Mean Absolute Distance (MAD) between the groundtruth values and the model's predictions. We evaluate our performance on the RSNA dataset using the challenge evaluation server.

2.3 Baselines

Hand Detection. As baseline for the hand detection task, we use Faster R-CNN [15] with an ImageNet pre-trained model and ResNet-50 [11] as backbone. This widely used object detector consists of a network that generates and scores object proposals. We train the Faster R-CNN [15] method for 5,000 iterations with a constant learning rate of 2.5×10^{-3} using the implementation released in [14].

Hand Pose Estimation. To address hand pose estimation, we build on the recent state-of-the-art architecture proposed by Xiao *et al.* in [19] for human pose estimation. This model consists of an encoder-decoder based on deconvolutional layers added on a backbone network. We train the model initialized on ImageNet with ResNet-50 as backbone [11] using the suggested training parameters for 20 epochs.

Bone Age Assessment. As baseline for the BAA task, we re-implement the method proposed by the winners of the RSNA 2017 Pediatric Bone Age Challenge. However, our inference differs from that method because [1] used an ensemble of the best models at inference while we use only a single model. This model uses an Inception-V3 [16] architecture combined with a network to include gender information, and adds two 1000-neuron densely connected layers to produce the final prediction. For the baseline, we train the model for 150 epochs, using Adam optimizer with an initial learning rate of 3×10^{-3}.

3 BoNet

Inspired by the way physicians perform BAA, we introduce a method that leverages local information to accurately address this task. For this purpose, we first locate the hand and find the anatomical ROIs. Afterwards, we create attention maps by generating a Gaussian distribution around each anatomical landmark. Our network, which we call BoNet, takes as input both the X-ray image and the attention map, and extracts high-level visual features from them using two independent pathways. We then combine these features from both pathways through a mixed Inception module and follow the suggestion in [1] to include gender information. Finally, after two fully-connected layers, BoNet regresses to the bone age using an L1 loss. See supplementary material for additional information. Figure 2 illustrates an overview of the complete method. To train BoNet, we start from our BAA baseline's weights. We use Adam optimizer with an initial learning rate of 1×10^{-4} over 50 epochs and reduce the learning rate by a factor of 0.1 once a loss plateau is reached.

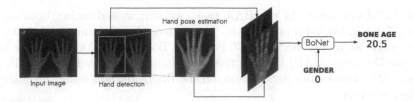

Fig. 2. Overview of the pipeline used in BoNet. The original image goes through hand detection and hand pose estimation to identify ROIs. Then we use as input for BoNet the cropped image, the heatmap and the gender for BAA.

4   Experiments

Hand Detection. For this task, we evaluate the performance of our baseline method on the RSNA and RHPE datasets. Since the RHPE dataset contains both left and right hands on the image, we evaluate the detection of the left one, statistically assuming that it is the non-dominant hand [10]. Table 1 shows the results obtained in the validation split for both datasets. The performance of Faster R-CNN given by the mAP and the mAR at different IoU thresholds (@[.5:.05:.95]) is considerably high. Specifically, the mAP@[.75] indicates an excellent localization of the detections. This behaviour is appropriate considering that detecting the bounding box of the hand is the first step towards using local information for BAA. Consequently, precision and recall in hand detection will significantly affect the performance of BAA. The errors in finding bounding boxes can be associated to the detection of false positives contained inside the annotation bounding box and to the low IoU of most true positives. Since the RHPE dataset contains both left and right hands in the image, the hand detection task is more complex than for the RSNA dataset.

Table 1. Results of the hand detection task in the validation split for the RSNA and RHPE datasets using our baseline.

	mAP@[.5,.95] (%)	mAP@[.5] (%)	mAP@[.75] (%)	mAR@[.5,.95] (%)
RSNA	93.7	99.0	98.9	96.1
RHPE	90.1	96.9	96.9	93.1

Hand Pose Estimation. With the aim of determining the relevance of bounding box detection for hand pose estimation, we use the datasets separately following three modalities: full image of the radiograph, image cropped with groundtruth bounding boxes and image cropped with detected bounding boxes. In the RHPE dataset we consider *full image* as the left half of the radiograph to only include the non-dominant hand. The results obtained for the validation set are reported in Table 2. The results prove that, for both datasets, the performance of the hand pose estimation task is considerably affected by the input used. Thus, we establish the upper bound for this task by using the groundtruth bounding boxes. Consequently, the performance of our predicted bounding boxes is lower than using groundtruth information since it depends on the results from the hand detection task. In contrast, the full image includes noise associated with background, tags and other artifacts in the radiograph, hence it obtains the lowest precision. The low performance in the full image setup show that it is necessary to use as input for this task a bounding box of the hand radiograph.

Table 2. Comparison of results in the validation set of RSNA [9] and RHPE datasets using our baseline for the hand pose estimation task.

		mAP@[.5,.95] (%)	mAP@[.5] (%)	mAP@[.75] (%)	mAR@[.5,.95] (%)
RSNA	Full image	73.0	96.3	90.0	77.6
	Groundtruth bounding boxes	**81.4**	**97.8**	**96.8**	**84.1**
	Detected bounding boxes	80.8	94.1	93.2	83.0
RHPE	Full image	53.1	91.2	60.1	59.3
	Groundtruth bounding boxes	**81.4**	**97.8**	**96.8**	**84.1**
	Detected bounding boxes	80.8	94.1	93.2	83.0

Bone Age Assessment. We design three sets of experiments to study the effect of training on different data. The first set uses only RSNA, the second one uses only RHPE, and the third one combines both datasets. For each set we assess the importance of local information by training on whole and cropped images. We use the training and the validation splits during the training stage and evaluate our results on the test split. The results shown on Table 3 demonstrate that hand detection is beneficial for accurate bone age assessment. Additionally, we

Table 3. BAA results on the RSNA and RHPE test sets.

Experiment		MAD	
Training on RSNA	Baseline (full image)	4.45	
	BoNet (full image)	4.37	
	Baseline + cropped image	4.20	
	BoNet + cropped image	**4.14**	
Training on RHPE	Baseline (full image)	8.57	
	BoNet (full image)	7.78	
	Baseline + cropped image	8.05	
	BoNet + cropped image	**7.60**	
Training on RSNA + RHPE	Baseline (full image)	RSNA	RHPE
	Baseline + cropped image	4.41	8.25
	BoNet + cropped image	4.09	7.99
		3.85	**6.86**

observe that BoNet leverages effectively local information, achieving a significant improvement in performance over the re-implementation of state-of-the-art which is our baseline with full image. We also find that combining both datasets during training produces better results than training on a single dataset. These results indicate that increasing and diversifying the data is beneficial for model generalization. Regarding the time complexity of the algorithm, the final model using BoNet and cropped images takes 0.079 s per image on inference, making it a suitable choice for a future real time implementation.

5   Conclusions

We introduce the Radiological Hand Pose Estimation Dataset as a benchmark for the development of robust methods for BAA, hand detection and hand pose estimation in radiological images as a way of exploiting local information as done by physicians in current clinical practice. For each task, we propose an experimental framework and validate state-of-the-art methods as baselines. Our results prove that the use of local information is beneficial for BAA. We also develop BoNet, a new method based on exploiting local information that outperforms the state-of-the-art method that exploit only global information. The RHPE Dataset and its associated resources will push the envelope further in the development of robust BAA automated methods with better generalization regardless of the population's characteristics.

Acknowledgments. This project was partially funded by Colciencias grant 841-2017. The authors thank Edgar Margffoy-Tuay for his support in developing the annotation server and the students of IBIO-3470 at Uniandes for their help as annotators.

References

1. Cicero, M., Bilbily, A.: Machine learning and the future of radiology: how we won the 2017 RSNA ML challenge (2017)
2. Cootes, T.F., Edwards, G.J., Taylor, C.J.: Active appearance models. IEEE Trans. Pattern Anal. Mach. Intell. (TPAMI) **23**, 681–685 (2001). https://doi.org/10.1109/34.927467
3. Gaskin, C.M., Kahn, M.M.S.L., Bertozzi, J.C., Bunch, P.M.: Skeletal Development of the Hand and Wrist: A Radiographic Atlas and Digital Bone Age Companion. Oxford University Press, Oxford (2011)
4. Ge, L., Cai, Y., Weng, J., Yuan, J.: Hand PointNet: 3D hand pose estimation using point sets. In: IEEE Conference on Computer Vision and Pattern Recognition (CVPR), pp. 8417–8426 (2018)
5. Ge, L., Ren, Z., Yuan, J.: Point-to-point regression pointnet for 3D hand pose estimation. In: Ferrari, V., Hebert, M., Sminchisescu, C., Weiss, Y. (eds.) ECCV 2018. LNCS, vol. 11217, pp. 489–505. Springer, Cham (2018). https://doi.org/10.1007/978-3-030-01261-8_29
6. Gertych, A., Zhang, A., Sayre, J., Pospiech-Kurkowska, S., Huang, H.: Bone age assessment of children using a digital hand atlas. Comput. Med. Imaging Graph. **31**(4–5), 322–331 (2007)

7. Gilsanz, V., Ratib, O.: Hand Bone Age: A Digital Atlas of Skeletal Maturity. Springer, Heidelberg (2005)
8. Greulich, W.W., Pyle, S.I., Todd, T.W.: Radiographic Atlas of Skeletal Development of the Hand and Wrist, vol. 2. Stanford University Press, Palo Alto (1959)
9. Halabi, S.S., Prevedello, L.M., et al.: The RSNA pediatric bone age machine learning challenge. Radiology 290(2), 498–503 (2019)
10. Hardyck, C., Petrinovich, L.F.: Left-handedness. Psychol. Bull. 84(3), 385 (1977)
11. He, K., Zhang, X., Ren, S., Sun, J.: Deep residual learning for image recognition. In: Proceedings of the IEEE Conference on Computer Vision and Pattern Recognition, pp. 770–778 (2016)
12. Iglovikov, V.I., Rakhlin, A., Kalinin, A.A., Shvets, A.A.: Paediatric bone age assessment using deep convolutional neural networks. In: Stoyanov, D., et al. (eds.) DLMIA/ML-CDS -2018. LNCS, vol. 11045, pp. 300–308. Springer, Cham (2018). https://doi.org/10.1007/978-3-030-00889-5_34
13. Lin, T.-Y., et al.: Microsoft COCO: common objects in context. In: Fleet, D., Pajdla, T., Schiele, B., Tuytelaars, T. (eds.) ECCV 2014. LNCS, vol. 8693, pp. 740–755. Springer, Cham (2014). https://doi.org/10.1007/978-3-319-10602-1_48
14. Massa, F., Girshick, R.: maskrcnn-benchmark: fast, modular reference implementation of Instance Segmentation and Object Detection algorithms in PyTorch (2018)
15. Ren, S., He, K., Girshick, R., Sun, J.: Faster R-CNN: towards real-time object detection with region proposal networks. In: Advances in Neural Information Processing Systems (NIPS), pp. 91–99 (2015)
16. Szegedy, C., Vanhoucke, V., Ioffe, S., Shlens, J., Wojna, Z.: Rethinking the inception architecture for computer vision. In: 2016 IEEE Conference on Computer Vision and Pattern Recognition, CVPR 2016, Las Vegas, NV, USA, 27–30 June 2016, pp. 2818–2826 (2016). https://doi.org/10.1109/CVPR.2016.308
17. Tanner, J., Whitehouse, R., Marshall, W., Carter, B.: Prediction of adult height from height, bone age, and occurrence of menarche, at ages 4 to 16 with allowance for midparent height. Arch. Dis. Child. 50(1), 14–26 (1975)
18. Thodberg, H., Kreiborg, S., Juul, A., Pedersen, K.: The BoneXpert method for automated determination of skeletal maturity. IEEE Trans. Med. Imaging 28(1), 52–66 (2009). https://doi.org/10.1109/tmi.2008.926067
19. Xiao, B., Wu, H., Wei, Y.: Simple Baselines for Human Pose Estimation and Tracking. In: Ferrari, V., Hebert, M., Sminchisescu, C., Weiss, Y. (eds.) ECCV 2018. LNCS, vol. 11210, pp. 472–487. Springer, Cham (2018). https://doi.org/10.1007/978-3-030-01231-1_29

An Attention-Guided Deep Regression Model for Landmark Detection in Cephalograms

Zhusi Zhong[1], Jie Li[1], Zhenxi Zhang[1], Zhicheng Jiao[2], and Xinbo Gao[1(✉)]

[1] School of Electronic Engineering, Xidian University, Xi'an 710071, China
xbgao@mail.xidian.edu.cn
[2] Department of Radiology and BRIC, University of North Carolina at Chapel Hill, Chapel Hill, NC 27599, USA

Abstract. Cephalometric tracing method is usually used in orthodontic diagnosis and treatment planning. In this paper, we propose a deep learning based framework to automatically detect anatomical landmarks in cephalometric X-ray images. We train the deep encoder-decoder model for landmark detection, which combines global landmark configuration with local high-resolution feature responses. The proposed framework is based on a 2-stage u-net, regressing the multi-channel heatmaps for landmark detection. In this framework, we embed attention mechanism with global stage heatmaps, guiding the local stage inferring, to regress the local heatmap patches in a high resolution. Besides, an Expansive Exploration strategy is applied to improve robustness while inferring, expanding the searching scope without increasing model complexity. We have evaluated the proposed framework in the most widely-used public dataset of landmark detection in cephalometric X-ray images. With less computation and manually tuning, the proposed framework achieves state-of-the-art results.

Keywords: Landmark detection · Deep learning · Heatmap regression · Attention mechanism · 2D X-ray cephalometric analysis

1 Introduction

Cephalometric analysis is a standard tool to quantitatively analyze the human skull and mandible, usually used in maxillofacial surgeries and orthodontic treatments. Cephalometric evaluation is based on some anatomical landmarks on the skull and surrounding soft tissue. Although newer techniques such as cone beam computed tomography (CBCT) begin to apply, due to the high price, the traditional 2D longitudinal section X-ray image of human head is still the most widely used in the cephalometric analysis. No matter which kind of data modality is adopted, the landmarks are still annotated manually, which remains a time-consuming work for an experienced doctor. Moreover, the manual annotation is extremely subjective to observer variability. Because the 2D X-ray images are the projection of the spatial structure which contains anatomical differences across organizations with individual difference, the automatic detection is a challenging problem. Despite the challenges, the identification of the skeletal structure contained in cephalograms is the key to the automatic detection.

© Springer Nature Switzerland AG 2019
D. Shen et al. (Eds.): MICCAI 2019, LNCS 11769, pp. 540–548, 2019.
https://doi.org/10.1007/978-3-030-32226-7_60

Therefore, an automatic annotation method would release orthodontists from the time-consuming work and especially avoid the observation errors. Our study concentrates on detecting the widely used 19 landmarks from the 2D radiograph automatically.

Related work: More recently, the automatic landmark detection was held as a Grand Challenge at ISBI 2015. The organizers provided the dataset [1] and published the benchmark of the dental radiography analysis algorithms [2]. Ibragimov et al. [3] computerized cephalometry by game-strategy with a shape-based model, Lindner et al. [4] won first place with Random Forest regression-voting method. After that, Lindner et al. [5] expanded their experiments with 4-fold cross-validation on all the data and presented the results with comprehensive experimental analysis.

Deep learning methods have achieved great success in the field of medical image analysis [6–9]. The cascade and hierarchy are the basic idea to improve performance from coarse to fine. Lee et al. [10] applied deep learning method to cephalometric landmark detection for the first time. They trained 38 independent CNN structures to regress the 19 landmarks' x- and y-coordinate variables separately. As most of the existing landmark detection methods, they need to train a number of models to refine each point on a small scale one by one, which demands massive but inefficient computation.

Different from the traditional coordinate regression methods, deep encoder-decoder methods, such as u-net [11] and fully convolutional networks (FCN) [12], achieve the goal with target transform. In medical landmark detection, by regressing heatmaps for landmarks simultaneously instead of absolute landmark coordinates, Payer et al. [13] transformed the coordinate regression problem to a pixel regression problem and simplified the procedure with multi-layer cascaded deep neural networks. These pixel-to-pixel heatmap regression methods are intrinsically more suitable for landmark detection, they extract the location information from X-ray images, with less divide between data forms than coordinate.

Contribution: In this paper, we propose a novel deep learning framework for automatically locating the anatomical landmarks in 2D cephalometric radiographs. The proposed method regress heatmaps of landmarks from coarse to fine in 2 stages, informing global configuration as well as accurately describing local appearance. The Attention-Guide mechanism connects the coarse-to-fine stages, which is similar to [14] but our Attention-Guide mechanism makes effect on several regions simultaneously. The high efficiency of our framework owes to these strategies: (i) our patch-based strategy optimizes the utilization of convolution kernels, to learn the informative feature around landmarks; (ii) the proposed Attention-Guide mechanism acts as an information extractor while inferring and minimizes the proposal region of sliding-window; (iii) with our Expansive Exploration strategy, the framework infers in a large scope, refining local heatmaps without increasing model complexity. The stage-wise training process makes our framework trainable.

542   Z. Zhong et al.

2 Method

Overall Framework: As shown in Fig. 1, the overall framework for landmark detection includes 2 stages, regressing 20-channel heatmaps of landmarks from coarse to fine. The two stages share the same u-net structure (Fig. 1c), but they are assigned with different learning scopes. Stage 1 trains the u-net with the global field, as "global stage", regressing the global heatmaps H_G as landmark configuration. Stage 2 is assigned as "local stage", with patch-based u-net model. Guided by the coarse attention from H_G, local stage searches in the proposal regions, regressing the heatmap patches H_P in a high resolution. As shown in Fig. 2, the Expansive Exploration strategy refines each landmark by multiple inference. The predicted coordinates are obtained as the locations of highlights in first 19 channels of heatmaps H_M, which is merged from H_P.

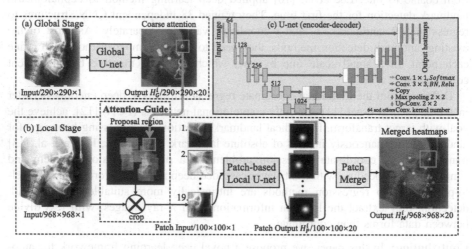

Fig. 1. Overall framework of the Attention-Guided deep regression model. (a) Global stage is shown at the top left. (b) Local stage embedded with Attention-Guide is shown in bottom. (c) We illustrate the u-net as encoder-decoder for global u-net and patch-based local u-net.

Target Transform: Inspired by [13], we convert the coordinate regression to a heatmap regression task. First of all, we represent the abstract coordinates L of 19 landmarks as the 20-channel concrete heatmaps H. We model each landmark as a channel heatmap with a 2D Gaussian distribution centered at the landmark. The distribution is normalized to a range of 0 to 1 and the Standard Deviation σ depends the size of distribution. The Correlation Coefficient ρ is 0, to make sure the shape of distributions is circular:

$$G(x,y) = exp\left[-\frac{1}{2\sigma^2}\left((x-\mu_1)^2 + (y-\mu_2)^2\right)\right] \tag{1}$$

where (μ_1, μ_2) is the center of the distribution. In the circular area of one channel, the pixel values indicate appearing probability of the landmark, so that the distributions can contain the uncertainty which involved in the landmark locations. However, the distributions are much smaller than the outside areas which represent negative class for a channel. We handle this class-imbalance problem similar to [15]. We apply the classification approach to estimate a shared background channel additionally. So that, the 20-channel heatmaps H, which represent classes separately, are described as follow:

$$H^i(x,y) = \begin{cases} exp\left[-\frac{1}{2\sigma^2}\left((x-x_i)^2+(y-y_i)^2\right)\right], & i = 1, 2, \ldots, 19 \\ 1 - \sum_{j=1}^{19} H^j(x,y), & i = 20 \end{cases} \quad (2)$$

where heatmap H^i denotes a channel whose distribution is located at the position of landmark $L_i = (x_i, y_i)$, while i is in the range of 1 to 19. And the last channel of heatmaps H^{20} represents the shared background, to ensure the sum of all 20 classes probabilities is 1 for each pixel. The specific variable σ is different at stages according to target distribution size. The coordinate regression problem is transformed to a pixel classification task, which achieves goal by regressing the 20-channel heatmaps H.

Global Stage and Pixel Regression: The global stage takes the entire images as input, and informs the underlying global landmark configuration. We train a modified u-net (Fig. 1c) as the backbone model, followed by a SoftMax activation layer to separate pixel classes probability in channels. Limited by the computational capabilities and the learning ability of the neural network, we have to scale the training data to small size. The output is the 20-channel heatmaps H_G, as shown in Fig. 1a (right). The channel-wise highlights indicate the high appearing probability of landmarks. Some areas overlap together on the schematic, it is actually due to compress multi-channel distributions of close landmarks into a plane.

Although, the large size of distributions limits the accuracy of prediction. The convolution kernels cannot distinguish subtle features from low resolution data, and the network cannot regress heatmaps with the small distributions. Besides, the prediction errors increase as sizing back to the original scale. So, we take those highlights on H_G as the coarse attention for local stage, and design a patch-based structure to narrow the learning scope, in order to process data and feature maps in a higher resolution.

Local stage and Attention-Guided inference: The local stage with patch-based u-net, guided by the coarse attention, focuses on learning local appearance around landmarks. The patch-based u-net shares the same structure with global stage. But it is trained with the small image patches, which is sampled around ground-truth labels L_{GT} randomly. The local stage learns to regress multi-channel heatmap patches H_P with smaller Gaussian distributions than global stage. So, the local stage u-net informs the high-resolution local features and has better distinguishing ability than the global stage. Our patch-based strategy optimizes the efficiency of local training process, avoiding the negative impact of the areas without landmarks.

The Attention-Guide mechanism is embedded in the local stage inference. We firstly resolve the 19 coarse coordinates which are obtained as the maximum in the first 19 channels of H_G. We set the coarse locations as center of the proposal regions. As shown in Fig. 1b (center), the proposal regions guide the patch selection, by cropping patches in the input image at the corresponding places. Combining with the patch-based strategy, the Attention-Guide acts as an information extractor for local stage, to minimize the proposal region of sliding-window. Local stage takes these image patches as input, regressing 19 heatmap patches H_P. Then H_P are normalized and merged to the complete heatmaps H_M. As shown in Fig. 1b (right), H_M gather highlights in the small points, those in the overlap regions are refined to smaller and more precise. The 19 predicted coordinates L_P are obtained as the locations of highlights in the first 19 channels of H_M. The details are described in the experimental section.

Expansive Exploration: The small searching scope of local stage obtains most of landmarks successfully, but the coarse stage dose not guarantee that all landmarks are detected in the proposal regions. To increase the robustness, we propose the Expansive Exploration strategy for the Attention-Guided inference at the local stage, similarly to the overlap-tile strategy in [11]. As shown in Fig. 2, we enlarge the sampling scope and fix the relative position for multiple inference. The expansive proposal regions are the expanded squares centered at coarse locations. The image patches are inputted to local u-net separately, expanding search scope without expansion of the network structure. Overlap margin is controlled by the expand parameter $\varepsilon \in (1,2)$.

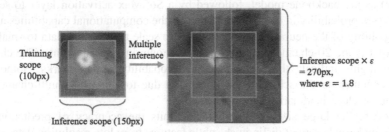

Fig. 2. Expansive exploration strategy for local inferring. We firstly enlarge the single inference scope to 150 px (the training scope is 100 px), then apply stack searching with fix relative position. 4 regions overlap each other with margin to be a big square, and 1 region places in the center of the expanded square. Here we set the expand parameter ε to 1.8.

Heatmap Regression Loss: Considering the class-imbalance problem, which means the areas as negative class are much larger than those of landmarks, and the small size of distribution target, we add a combination of binary cross-entropy loss (BCE loss) and focal loss [16] as the loss function to balance the cost of background and targets, which is described as follows:

$$L\left(H,\widehat{H}\right) = -\frac{1}{N}\sum_{b=1}^{N}\left(\frac{1}{2}\cdot H\cdot log\widehat{H} + \frac{1}{2}\cdot \alpha_t \cdot (1-H_t)^{\gamma}\cdot log H_t\right),$$

$$where\, H_t = \begin{cases} \widehat{H} & if\, H > 0.01 \\ 1-\widehat{H} & otherwise \end{cases}$$

where $\widehat{H}$ and H denote the predicted heatmaps and the ground-truth heatmaps generated from L_{GT}, and N indicates the batch size. The BCE loss plays a major role in evaluating the areas with most background. Then the focal loss tends to mainly finetune the target regions in Gaussian distributions after 60 epochs in our experiments.

3 Experiments

This study includes the widely-used public dataset from the Grand Challenge. The dataset contains 400 dental X-ray cephalometric images and the 2 sets of annotations with 19 landmarks from 2 experienced doctors. The data is divided into 3 sets, 150 images for training data, 150 images for Test 1 data and 100 images for Test 2 data. The resolution of images was 1935 × 2400 pixels with a pixel spacing of 0.1 mm. We crop the images to squares (1935 × 1935px) and the annotated y-axis coordinates are subtracted by 465, as shown in Fig. 3c.

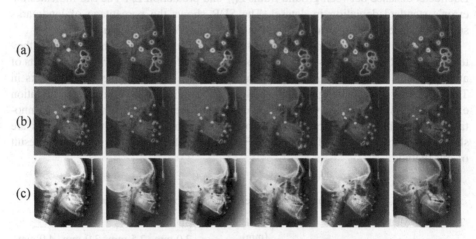

Fig. 3. Examples of prediction on testing X-ray images. (a) 1st row shows the channel-compressed H_G. (b) 2nd row shows the channel-compressed H_M. (c) 3rd row shows the predicted landmarks (red) transformed from H_M, and the ground truths (green). (Color figure online)

For global stage training, we scale the cropped images and the coordinates by 0.15 times. The global heatmaps H_G are the same size as the scaled images. The Gaussian distributions of H_G are 40-pixel width which are 267-pixel width in the original scale. The global u-net takes the scaled images as input, and it learns to regress the 20-channel coarse heatmaps H_G. The channel-compressed results are shown in Fig. 3a.

For local stage training, we down-sample image data by 0.5 times. The original entire heatmaps are as large as the scaled image, with 30-pixel width distribution, whose original width is 60 pixels. The patch-based u-net is trained by randomly sampling an image patch (100 × 100px) around one landmark a time, to regress the correspond 20-channel heatmap patches H_P cropped from the entire heatmaps. Through numbers of training epochs, the sampler randomly travers all landmarks. The two-stage networks are trained separately with our Heatmap Regression Loss.

While inferring, the patch selection is guided by the coarse attention with our Expansive Exploration strategy. The expansive H_P of each landmark are merged to the H_M by placing at the corresponding location in the expansive proposal regions. In H_M, we assume there is no landmark out of patches, so the pixel values of these areas are 0. For overlapping areas, we average the pixel values to raise robustness, receding the artifacts (fake shadow). The first 19 channels of H_M are normalized to a range of 0 to 1 each channel separately, then pass a filter with threshold of 0.5 to reduce the artifacts whose pixel values are less than 0.5. The final 19 coordinates L_P are the mean positions of nonzero pixels each channel separately, they represent the centers of the distributions with high possible of the landmarks.

The mean radial error (MRE, in mm) and the successful detection rate (SDR, in %) are the evaluation indexes of the Grand Challenge. The MRE is defined by $MRE = \left(\sum_{i=1}^{n} R_i\right)/n$ where n indicates the number of data and R indicates the Euclidean distance between ground truths L_{GT} and prediction L_P. The Std indicates the error's standard deviation in dataset. The SDR shows the percentage of landmarks successfully detected in a range of 2.0 mm, 2.5 mm, 3.0 mm, 4 mm.

We have evaluated the proposed method on 2 experiments. In the challenge, they tested on Test1 data and Test 2 data independently, and took the average of two sets of annotations as the ground truth. The comparisons are shown in the first 2 blocks in Table 1. After the challenge, Lindner et al. [5] applied the 4-fold cross-validation experiments on the dataset with all 400 cases, and the ground truths were the annotations from the senior doctor. We follow experiments settings and the results are shown in the third block in Table 1. The Fig. 4 shows the 4-fold cross-validation result of our method.

Table 1. Comparison on proposed deep regression model with other approaches

Test data	Method	MRE ± Std (mm)	SDR (%)			
			2.0 mm	2.5 mm	3.0 mm	4.0 mm
Test 1 data	Ibragimov et al. [3]	1.84 ± 1.76	71.70	77.40	81.90	88.00
	Lindner et al. [4]	1.67 ± 1.65	74.95	80.28	84.56	89.68
	Ours (stage 1)	1.90 ± 1.17	62.41	75.63	83.82	93.72
	Ours (stage 2 no expand)	1.22 ± 1.42	85.38	91.19	94.21	97.27
	Ours	**1.12 ± 0.88**	**86.91**	**91.82**	**94.88**	**97.90**
Test 2 data	Ibragimov et al. [2]		62.74	70.47	76.53	85.11
	Lindner et al. [2]	1.92 ± 1.24	66.11	72.00	77.63	87.42
	Ours (stage 1)	2.28 ± 1.72	52.53	66.00	77.58	89.53
	Ours (stage 2 no expand)	1.53 ± 1.42	74.42	82.42	88.11	94.63
	Ours	**1.42 ± 0.84**	**76.00**	**82.90**	**88.74**	**94.32**
4-fold cross.	Lindner et al. [5]	**1.20 ± 0.06**	84.70	89.38	92.62	96.30
	Ours	1.22 ± 2.45	**86.06**	**90.84**	**94.04**	**97.28**

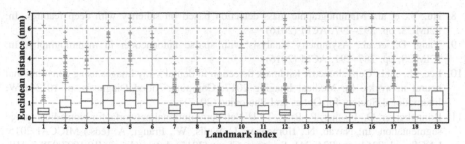

Fig. 4. Boxplot of Euclidean distances between predicted landmarks L_P and ground truths L_{GT}.

4 Conclusion

Our deep learning framework achieves good performance in detecting anatomical landmarks in cephalometric X-ray images. In our framework, the landmark detection task transforms to classification of image pixel. The Attention-Guide and the Expansive Exploitation strategy make sure that the searching scopes is smaller and data resolution is higher with minimum information redundancy. The data augmentation is embedded in the random sampling to avoid overfitting. Our model with higher efficiency but less manual tuning achieves a state-of-the-art result on automatic landmark detection in cephalometric radiograph. Moreover, the encoder-decoder structure which we apply with u-net, is easily transferred to any other model with better performance. And our deep regression model is easily generalized to other landmark detection tasks.

Acknowledgement. This work was supported in part by the National Natural Science Foundation of China under Grant 61671339, 61432014 and 61772402, and in part by National High-Level Talents Special Support Program of China under Grant CS31117200001.

References

1. Ching-Wei, W., et al.: Evaluation and comparison of anatomical landmark detection methods for cephalometric X-ray images: a grand challenge. IEEE TMI **34**, 1890–1900 (2015)
2. Wang, C.W., et al.: A benchmark for comparison of dental radiography analysis algorithms. Med. Image Anal. **31**, 63 (2016)
3. Ibragimov, B., et al.: Computerized cephalometry by game theory with shape-and appearance-based landmark refinement. In: ISBI (2015)
4. Lindner, C., et al.: Fully automatic cephalometric evaluation using random forest regression-voting. In: ISBI (2015)
5. Lindner, C., et al.: Fully automatic system for accurate localisation and analysis of cephalometric landmarks in lateral cephalograms. Sci. Rep. **6**, 33581 (2016)
6. Jiao, Z., et al.: A deep feature based framework for breast masses classification. Neurocomputing **197**, 221–231 (2016)
7. Jiao, Z., et al.: Deep convolutional neural networks for mental load classification based on EEG data. Pattern Recogn. **76**, 582–595 (2018)

8. Hu, Y., et al.: Mammographic mass detection based on saliency with deep features. In: ICIMCS, pp. 292–297. ACM (2016)
9. Yang, D., et al.: Asymmetry Analysis with sparse autoencoder in mammography. In: ICIMCS, pp. 287–291. ACM (2016)
10. Lee, H., et al.: Cephalometric landmark detection in dental x-ray images using convolutional neural networks. In: Medical Imaging 2017: Computer-Aided Diagnosis, p. 101341 W. International Society for Optics and Photonics (2017)
11. Ronneberger, O., Fischer, P., Brox, T.: U-Net: convolutional networks for biomedical image segmentation. In: Navab, N., Hornegger, J., Wells, W., Frangi, A. (eds.) MICCAI 2015. LNCS, vol. 9351, pp. 234–241. Springer, Cham (2015). https://doi.org/10.1007/978-3-319-24574-4_28
12. Long, J., et al.: Fully convolutional networks for semantic segmentation. In: CVPR, pp. 3431–3440 (2015)
13. Payer, C., Štern, D., Bischof, H., Urschler, M.: Regressing heatmaps for multiple landmark localization using CNNs. In: Ourselin, S., Joskowicz, L., Sabuncu, M., Unal, G., Wells, W. (eds.) MICCAI 2016. LNCS, vol. 9901, pp. 230–238. Springer, Cham (2016). https://doi.org/10.1007/978-3-319-46723-8_27
14. Guan, Q., et al.: Diagnose like a radiologist: attention guided convolutional neural network for thorax disease classification. arXiv preprint arXiv:1801.09927 (2018)
15. Tuysuzoglu, A., Tan, J., Eissa, K., Kiraly, A.P., Diallo, M., Kamen, A.: Deep adversarial context-aware landmark detection for ultrasound imaging. In: Frangi, A., Schnabel, J., Davatzikos, C., Alberola-López, C., Fichtinger, G. (eds.) MICCAI 2018. LNCS, vol. 11073, pp. 151–158. Springer, Cham (2018). https://doi.org/10.1007/978-3-030-00937-3_18
16. Lin, T.-Y., et al.: Focal loss for dense object detection. In: ICCV, pp. 2980–2988 (2017)

Learning-Based X-Ray Image Denoising Utilizing Model-Based Image Simulations

Sai Gokul Hariharan[1,2]([✉]) [ID], Christian Kaethner[2] [ID], Norbert Strobel[2,3] [ID],
Markus Kowarschik[1,2] [ID], Shadi Albarqouni[1] [ID], Rebecca Fahrig[2,4] [ID],
and Nassir Navab[1,5] [ID]

[1] Computer Aided Medical Procedures,
Technische Universität München, Munich, Germany
saigokul.hariharan@tum.de
[2] Siemens Healthineers AG, Advanced Therapies, Forchheim, Germany
[3] Fakultät für Elektrotechnik, Hochschule für angewandte Wissenschaften
Würzburg-Schweinfurt, Schweinfurt, Germany
[4] Pattern Recognition Lab,
Friedrich-Alexander-Universität Erlangen-Nürnberg, Erlangen, Germany
[5] Whiting School of Engineering, Johns Hopkins University, Baltimore, USA

Abstract. X-ray guidance is an integral part of interventional procedures, but the exposure to ionizing radiation poses a non-negligible threat
to patients and clinical staff. Unfortunately, a reduction in the X-ray dose
results in a lower signal-to-noise ratio, which may impair the quality of
X-ray images. To ensure an acceptable image quality while keeping the
X-ray dose as low as possible, it is common practice to use denoising techniques. However, at very low dose levels, the application of conventional
denoising techniques may lead to undesirable artifacts or oversmoothing.
On the other hand, supervised learning techniques have outperformed
conventional techniques in producing suitable results, provided aligned
pairs of associated high- and low-dose X-ray images are available. Unfortunately, it is neither acceptable nor possible to acquire such image pairs
during a clinical intervention. To enable the use of learning-based methods for the denoising of X-ray images, we propose a novel strategy that
involves the use of model-based simulations of low-dose X-ray images during the training phase. We utilize a data-driven normalization step that
increases the robustness of the proposed approach to varying amounts
of signal-dependent noise associated with different X-ray image acquisition protocols. A quantitative and qualitative analysis based on clinical
and phantom data shows that the proposed strategy outperforms well-
established conventional X-ray image denoising methods. It also indicates that the proposed approach allows for a significant dose reduction
without sacrificing important image information.

Keywords: Low-dose X-ray image denoising · Deep learning · Noise
simulation

© Springer Nature Switzerland AG 2019
D. Shen et al. (Eds.): MICCAI 2019, LNCS 11769, pp. 549–557, 2019.
https://doi.org/10.1007/978-3-030-32226-7_61

1   Introduction

X-ray guidance during interventional procedures has gained immense importance in the recent past. Since X-ray imaging involves ionizing radiation, the medical benefits are accompanied by health risks. Even though the X-ray radiation dose could be lowered to reduce them, it would also lower the image quality and may result in images that are clinically unacceptable. To preserve the required image quality at lower dose levels, sophisticated denoising techniques can be used. Noise reduction has been an important requirement not only for medical images, but also for optical images. Among others, block matching 3D (BM3D) [3] and denoising based on weighted nuclear norm minimization (WNNM) [4] are well-engineered patch-based approaches that combine non-local self similarity with transform-based processing to provide a significant noise reduction. Though BM3D has been developed about a decade ago, it is still considered to be one of the most effective methods [2,13]. However, as these methods rely on solving a complex optimization problem [13], applying them in real-time is non-trivial.

Deep learning-based denoising techniques have been applied to optical images [13] and medical images, e.g., fluoroscopic X-ray images [10]. Unfortunately, such methods require pairs of noise-free and noisy images. Acquiring such image pairs in a clinical setting is close to impossible due to the associated increase in ionizing radiation and patient motion. Fortunately, Lehtinen et al. [9] have recently shown that deep learning-based denoising techniques can be designed by training networks with pairs of spatially aligned noisy instances of images alone. However, even acquiring such pairs may be difficult in a clinical scenario. In principle, the need for aligned image pairs could be overcome by resorting to generative adversarial networks that make use of a cycle consistency loss [8]. However, high-dose X-ray images would again be needed, which may not be available. Since the results of the method are at the most as good as the high-quality images used for training [8], the lack of appropriate data is a limiting factor.

In this work, we propose a strategy that overcomes the above mentioned issues. It involves the training of a denoising neural network using different instances of simulated low-dose X-ray images. Since we desire an approach that is suitable for denoising X-ray images acquired at different dose levels, we introduce a model-based and data-driven normalization step. The normalization removes the dependency of the trained network on different amounts of signal-dependent noise in the input images acquired at different dose levels. To the best of our knowledge, this is the first work that has shown the benefits of considering an imaging model when designing learning-based X-ray image denoising algorithms.

2   Materials and Methods

Depending on the imaging system and the situation, X-ray images can be corrupted by different amounts and types of noise, e.g., quantum noise, electronic noise and quantization noise. Moreover, the signal-to-noise-ratio is directly proportional to the radiation dose used. Based on these characteristics, we have designed a learning-based method to denoise X-ray images.

2.1 X-Ray Imaging Model

The transformation of the received X-ray quanta collected at a flat-panel detector to a gray value in an image involves a series of steps, namely the absorption of the X-rays in the scintillator as well as the generation, coupling and integration of the optical photons by evenly spaced photo-diodes [11]. It can be assumed that this process follows a linear model [12]. Thus, the observed noise-corrupted gray value $y \in \mathbb{R}^{M \times N}$ at row r and column c can be represented as

$$y[r,c] = \beta \cdot x[r,c] + g + n[r,c], \tag{1}$$

where $x \in \mathbb{R}^{M \times N}$, $n \in \mathbb{R}^{M \times N}$, β and g represent the charges (corrupted by quantum noise) at the photo-diodes, the electronic noise with standard deviation (STD) σ_n, the overall system gain and the (constant) system offset, respectively. The (mixed) noise variance of a detector pixel's gray value can be expressed as

$$\sigma_y^2[r,c] = \alpha \cdot (\bar{y}[r,c] - g) + \sigma_n^2, \tag{2}$$

a line with slope α and y-intercept σ_n^2. $\bar{y}[r,c]$ denotes the mean (noise-free) value of $y[r,c]$ and the parameter α depends on the gain mode of the detector [12]. The imaging parameters α and σ_n^2 can, for example, be obtained from the system specifications or using calibration measurements [11]. Once known, they can be taken into account to perform a noise variance stabilization (NVS) based on the generalized Anscombe transform (GAT) as suggested in [5,6]:

$$y'[r,c] = t(y[r,c]) = \frac{2}{\alpha}\sqrt{\alpha \cdot y[r,c] + \frac{3}{8}\alpha^2 - \alpha \cdot g + \sigma_n^2}. \tag{3}$$

The resulting pixel values $y'[r,c]$ have signal-independent noise with unit variance.

2.2 Denoising of Low-Dose X-Ray Images

The learning process involves the transformation of noise-corrupted instances of an image (or a region) into another [9], where the different instances have the same underlying noise statistics. In order to get two such noise-corrupted instances, we have relied on realistic simulations of low-dose images y_{l_1} and y_{l_2} from a standard-dose X-ray image y_s. In the first step, y_s is scaled down – such that its gray value range matches the gray value range of a corresponding low-dose image – to obtain $y_{s \to l}$. Then, to simulate a low-dose image y_l from $y_{s \to l}$, signal-dependent and signal-independent noise need to be added [1]. We have simulated the signal-independent electronic noise as additive white Gaussian noise (AWGN) $\eta_e[r,c]$ in the image domain [1]. Since the gray values of $y_{s \to l}$

are not noise-free, we have simulated the signal-dependent quantum noise by adding filtered AWGN (correlated noise) $\eta_q[r, c]$ in the GAT domain [7]. Filtered AWGN is used to include the influence of the detector blur on quantum noise. The process is described by

$$y_l[r, c] = t^{-1}(t(y_{s \to l}[r, c] + k_q * \eta_q[r, c])) + \eta_e[r, c], \tag{4}$$

where $t^{-1}(.)$ represents the inverse GAT. The filtering kernel k_q and the noise components η_q and η_e can be derived from the system's modulation transfer function and noise power spectrum. As mentioned earlier, we have performed an NVS on y_{l_1} and y_{l_2} as per Eq. 3 to obtain y'_{l_1} and y'_{l_2}, respectively. Similarly, $y_{s \to l}$ can be normalized using the imaging parameters associated with y_{l_1} to get $y'_{s \to l}$. From y'_{l_1}, y'_{l_2} and $y'_{s \to l}$, we randomly select regions of size $K \times K$ around a particular location (e.g, around $[r, c]$) to get $l'_1 \in \mathbb{R}^{K \times K}$, $l'_2 \in \mathbb{R}^{K \times K}$ and $s' \in \mathbb{R}^{K \times K}$, respectively. Since X-ray images are always corrupted by some amount of noise, s' can be expressed as:

$$s'[r, c] = \bar{s}'[r, c] + \eta_{s \to l}[r, c], \tag{5}$$

where $\bar{s}'[r, c]$ is the noise-free version of $s'[r, c]$ and $\eta_{s \to l}[r, c]$ is the filtered white Gaussian noise component (associated with $s'[r, c]$ in the GAT domain) with STD $\sigma_{s \to l}$. Similarly, l'_1 and l'_2 can be expressed as:

$$
\begin{aligned}
l'_1[r, c] &= \bar{s}'[r, c] + \eta_{s \to l}[r, c] + \eta_1[r, c] = \bar{s}'[r, c] + \eta_{l_1}[r, c], \\
l'_2[r, c] &= \bar{s}'[r, c] + \eta_{s \to l}[r, c] + \eta_2[r, c] = \bar{s}'[r, c] + \eta_{l_2}[r, c],
\end{aligned}
\tag{6}
$$

where, η_1 and η_2 are noise matrices with filtered AWGN of STD $\sqrt{1 - \sigma_{s \to l}^2}$ and the STD of noise in η_{l_1} and η_{l_2} is 1.

The network $D(l'_1, \theta)$ is then trained with P randomly chosen pairs of noisy regions $\{l_1'^{(i)}, l_2'^{(i)}\}_{i=1}^P$ based on minimizing the function

$$l(\theta) = \frac{1}{P} \sum_{i=1}^P \left\| \left(D(l_1'^{(i)}, \theta) - l_2'^{(i)} \right) \right\|_2 = \frac{1}{P} \sum_{i=1}^P \left\| \left(l_1'^{(i)} + R(l_1'^{(i)}, \theta) - l_2'^{(i)} \right) \right\|_2, \tag{7}$$

where θ represents the parameters of D and the output of $D(l'_1, \theta)$ has been rewritten as $l'_1 + R(l'_1, \theta)$ ($R(l'_1, \theta) \in \mathbb{R}^{K \times K}$ is the difference between the output and the input of the network). Using Eqs. 6, 7 can be rewritten as

$$
\begin{aligned}
l(\theta) &= \frac{1}{P} \sum_{i=1}^P \left\| \left(\bar{s}'^{(i)} + \eta_{l_1}^{(i)} + R(l_1'^{(i)}, \theta) - (\bar{s}'^{(i)} + \eta_{l_2}^{(i)}) \right) \right\|_2 \\
&= \frac{1}{P} \sum_{i=1}^P \left\| \left(\eta_{l_1}^{(i)} + R(l_1'^{(i)}, \theta) - \eta_{l_2}^{(i)} \right) \right\|_2.
\end{aligned}
\tag{8}
$$

Due to the use of a large amount of simulations, the random nature of noise and the dependency of the output of the network mainly on l'_1 (and its independence from l_2'), it is not possible for the network to result in $R(l_1', \theta) = \eta_{l_2} - \eta_{l_1}$ to reach an average minimum loss of 0. On the other hand, it may be possible to obtain $R(l_1', \theta) \sim -\eta_{l_1}$, which would result in an average loss of around 1 as STD of noise in $\eta_{l_1} \sim 1$. This implies that the best possible solution to Eq. 8 is the generation of a noise-free region.

Since the proposed method involves pairs of low-dose images as input, we have referred to it as L2L (low2low as analogy to noise2noise [9]). As an alternative, l_2' can also be replaced by s' in Eq. 7, which would result in the convergence of the average loss to $\sigma_{\eta_{s \to l}}$. We have referred to this approach as L2H (low2high).

2.3 Material

In terms of the network architecture, we have used the U-Net architecture and the training strategy proposed in [9]. To train networks for the different denoising approaches, we have made use of 1200 unprocessed clinical X-ray images ($M = N = 896$) acquired at 100% of the standard X-ray dose and simulated X-ray images corresponding to 25% and 30% of the standard X-ray dose. We have trained the networks (one network for each approach) for 1000 epochs using quadratic regions of width $K = 128$. Then, we have evaluated the trained networks on 4475 clinical X-ray images (2425 at 25% and 2050 at 30% of the standard X-ray dose) and 400 X-ray images of 4 different anthropomorphic phantoms (200 at 25% and 200 at 30% of the standard X-ray dose). To show the impact of using an NVS, we have presented the results of the networks trained for L2L and L2H with and without an NVS. As a benchmark, we have also compared the results of the learning-based approaches with those of WNNM [4] and BM3D [3]. Since these methods have been designed specifically for AWGN, we have applied an NVS (Eq. 3) before using them. For the phantom images, quantitative analyses have been performed with respect to peak signal-to-noise-ratio (PSNR), structural similarity index (SSIM) and contrast-to-noise ratio (CNR). Noise-free ground-truth (GT) images have been generated by temporally averaging 500 noisy static images. Since it is not possible to acquire a GT for clinical images, we have performed a quantitative evaluation using CNR alone. In addition, a blind qualitative evaluation of fifteen scenes by six independent X-ray image quality experts has been conducted.

3   Results

In Fig. 1, we have presented the input as well as the processed regions of interest (ROIs) of an angiographic head phantom acquired at 30% of the standard X-ray dose. It can be seen that, even after applying an NVS, BM3D has resulted in noticeable artifacts (Fig. 1d) and WNNM has yielded a comparatively blurred output (Fig. 1e). The learning-based approaches, L2L as well as L2H, have also resulted in mild artifacts when an NVS is not used (Fig. 1f and g). However, combining these approaches with an NVS has improved their performance significantly (Fig. 1h and i). In particular, L2L with an NVS (Fig. 1i) has achieved a superior denoising performance compared to the other methods. Moreover, the result of L2L with NVS (Fig. 1i) is more similar to its noise-free counterpart (Fig. 1a) and also less noisy compared to the corresponding unprocessed standard-dose ROI (Fig. 1b). In Fig. 2, it can be seen that for the clinical images acquired at 30% of the standard-dose the results are in accordance with those from the phantom study. Since the use of L2L has resulted in less artifacts when compared to L2H in the phantom study, we have focused on L2L for this comparison.

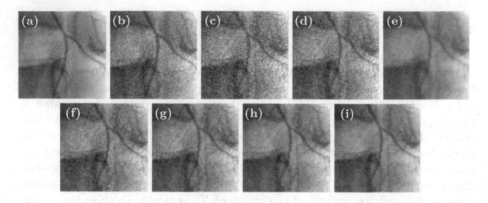

Fig. 1. Visualization of X-ray acquisitions (selected ROI) of an angiographic head phantom: (a) GT, (b) standard-dose, (c) 30% standard-dose and the results of processing (c) using: (d) BM3D with NVS (e) WNNM with NVS, (f) L2H without NVS, (g) L2L without NVS, (h) L2H with NVS and (i) L2L with NVS.

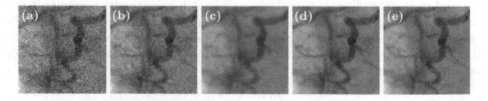

Fig. 2. Visualization of selected ROIs of an angiographic sequence acquired at 30% of the standard dose level: (a) input, (b) BM3D with NVS (c) WNNM with NVS, (d) L2L without NVS and (e) L2L with NVS.

In Table 1, we have presented the results of the quantitative analyses for the X-ray images acquired at 25% and 30% of the standard dose level. It can be observed that all the methods have resulted in a substantial improvement over the input. The learning-based approaches L2L and L2H have performed better when an NVS is involved. In fact, L2L with NVS has outperformed the other methods with respect to mean PSNR and SSIM. On the other hand, WNNM with NVS has resulted in a mean CNR that is even higher than that of the GT images indicating that the resulting images have been oversmoothed. These findings support the visual analysis.

The result of the experts' evaluation presented in Fig. 3 indicates that the learning-based approaches outperform BM3D and WNNM. Even though WNNM has obtained high scores for denoising performance and freedom from artifacts, it has received low scores for sharpness and realistic appearance. On an average, L2L with NVS has been found to produce visually superior results that are well denoised, sharp, artifact-free and most importantly realistic.

4   Discussion and Conclusion

We have presented a learning-based denoising approach that uses an imaging model to generate training data as well as to normalize the input data. Since the well established patch-based denoising techniques BM3D [3] and WNNM [4] have been designed to produce smooth images, they underperform on low-dose X-ray images corrupted by high amounts of noise – even when used with an NVS.

Table 1. Quantitative evaluation of the denoising methods. The mean values for the different metrics are presented and the values closest to GT are highlighted.

Dose	Category	Metric	Input	BM3D NVS	WNNM NVS	L2H	L2L	L2H NVS	L2L NVS	GT
25%	Phantom	PSNR	25.69	29.92	32.54	30.28	30.67	31.70	**32.63**	Inf
		SSIM	0.927	0.971	0.984	0.973	0.975	0.980	**0.985**	1
		CNR	16.39	45.84	84.72	36.98	38.92	40.90	**52.16**	58.69
	Clinical	CNR	15.81	43.96	94.57	34.83	35.70	36.12	46.02	-
30%	Phantom	PSNR	26.75	30.93	33.06	31.26	31.66	32.65	**33.65**	Inf
		SSIM	0.941	0.977	0.985	0.978	0.980	0.984	**0.988**	1
		CNR	18.75	50.99	119.86	39.92	41.98	44.36	**57.07**	63.59
	Clinical	CNR	17.25	42.63	83.58	35.71	36.55	37.01	45.67	-

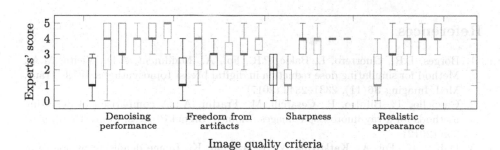

Fig. 3. Qualitative evaluation of BM3D with NVS (black), WNNM with NVS (cyan), L2H without NVS (blue), L2L without NVS (green), L2H with NVS (red) and L2L with NVS (brown), where 0 is the worst and 5 is the best possible score. (Color figure online)

The learning-based approaches L2L and L2H (irrespective of whether an NVS is used) have produced visually superior results for low-dose X-ray images when compared to BM3D and WNNM. A possible explanation could be the use of a sufficiently large amount of realistic training data that is usually important for learning the required features. Furthermore, a significant gain in the performance of both L2L and L2H can be achieved when the data is normalized using an NVS. This is due to the fact that the system gain is not consistent across different dose levels. Moreover, if the presence of signal-dependent noise is not taken into account, denoising may result in an uneven smoothing across different gray values thereby producing artifacts. Therefore, the proposed strategy of applying an NVS prior to the training as well as during the application not only avoids such artifacts, but also makes the network robust to different dose levels. This reiterates the fact that considering simple noise models, such as a Gaussian noise model [10], to simulate training data may not always be a suitable strategy. Since L2L makes use of pairs of low-dose simulations, the network is exposed to more instances of noisy data when compared to L2H. This factors into a marginal improvement of L2L over the latter. In addition, the method results in an image quality that is superior to that of the standard-dose images used for training. This indicates that unlike [8], the performance of the method is not limited by the quality of the data used during the training phase.

Finally, quantitative and qualitative evaluations with respect to the images used in the study suggest that the proposed approach allows for a significant dose reduction without sacrificing important image information. However, more experiments are needed to thoroughly analyze the dose saving potential of the proposed method. A further reduction in the dose may be difficult to achieve in practice using spatial denoising alone as ultra low-dose images can be severely corrupted by detector artifacts. In such cases, it would be necessary to include temporal information to achieve an optimal denoising performance.

Acknowledgement and Disclaimer. This work was supported by Siemens Healthineers AG. The concepts and results presented in this paper are based on research and are not commercially available.

References

1. Borges, L.R., Guerrero, I., Bakic, P.R., Foi, A., Maidment, A.D., Vieira, M.A.: Method for simulating dose reduction in digital breast tomosynthesis. IEEE Trans. Med. Imaging **36**(11), 2331–2342 (2017)
2. Cerciello, T., Bifulco, P., Cesarelli, M., Fratini, A.: A comparison of denoising methods for x-ray fluoroscopic images. Biomed. Signal Process. Control **7**(6), 550–559 (2012)
3. Dabov, K., Foi, A., Katkovnik, V., Egiazarian, K.: Image denoising by sparse 3-D transform-domain collaborative filtering. IEEE Trans. Image Process. **16**(8), 2080–2095 (2007)
4. Gu, S., Zhang, L., Zuo, W., Feng, X.: Weighted nuclear norm minimization with application to image denoising. In: Proceedings of IEEE Conference on Computer Vision and Pattern Recognition, pp. 2862–2869 (2014)

5. Hariharan, S.G., et al.: Preliminary results of DSA denoising based on a weighted low-rank approach using an advanced neurovascular replication system. Int. J. Comput. Assist. Radiol. Surg. **14**(7), 1117–1126 (2019)
6. Hariharan, S.G., et al.: A photon recycling approach to the denoising of ultra-low dose x-ray sequences. Int. J. Comput. Assist. Radiol. Surg. **13**(6), 847–854 (2018)
7. Hariharan, S.G., Strobel, N., Kaethner, C., Kowarschik, M., Fahrig, R., Navab, N.: An analytical approach for the simulation of realistic low-dose fluoroscopic images. Int. J. Comput. Assist. Radiol. Surg. **14**, 601–610 (2019)
8. Kang, E., Koo, H.J., Yang, D.H., Seo, J.B., Ye, J.C.: Cycle-consistent adversarial denoising network for multiphase coronary CT angiography. Med. Phys. **46**(2), 550–562 (2019)
9. Lehtinen, J., et al.: Noise2Noise: learning image restoration without clean data. In: Proceedings of International Conference on Machone Learning, pp. 2965–2974 (2018)
10. Matviychuk, Y., et al.: Learning a multiscale patch-based representation for image denoising in x-ray fluoroscopy. In: Proceedings of International Conference on Image Processing, pp. 2330–2334 (2016)
11. Siewerdsen, J., et al.: Empirical and theoretical investigation of the noise performance of indirect detection, active matrix flat-panel imagers (AMFPIs) for diagnostic radiology. Med. Phys. **24**(1), 71–89 (1997)
12. Yang, K., Huang, S.Y., Packard, N.J., Boone, J.M.: Noise variance analysis using a flat panel x-ray detector: a method for additive noise assessment with application to breast CT applications. Med. Phys. **37**(7), 3527–3537 (2010)
13. Zhang, K., Zuo, W., Chen, Y., Meng, D., Zhang, L.: Beyond a gaussian denoiser: residual learning of deep CNN for image denoising. IEEE Trans. Image Process. **26**(7), 3142–3155 (2017)

LVC-Net: Medical Image Segmentation with Noisy Label Based on Local Visual Cues

Yucheng Shu[✉], Xiao Wu, and Weisheng Li

Chongqing University of Posts and Telecommunications, Chongqing 400065, China
{shuyc,liws}@cqupt.edu.cn, wxwsx1997@gmail.com

Abstract. CNN-based deep architecture has been successfully applied to medical image semantic segmentation task because of its effective feature learning mechanism. However, due to the lack of semantic guidance, such supervised learning model may be susceptible to annotation noise. In order to address this problem, we propose a novel medical image segmentation algorithm based on automatic label error correction. Firstly, local visual saliency regions, namely the Local Visual Cues (LVCs), are captured from low-level feature channels. Then, a deformable spatial transformation module is integrated into our LVC-Net to build visual connections between the predictions and LVCs. By combining noisy labels with image LVCs, a novel loss function is proposed based on their intrinsic spatial relationship. Our method can effectively suppress the influence of label noise by utilizing potential visual guidance during the learning process, thereby generate better semantic segmentation results. Comparative experiment on hip x-ray image segmentation task demonstrate that our algorithm achieves significant improvement over state-of-the-arts in the presences of noisy label.

1 Introduction

Semantic segmentation plays an important role in the field of medical image analysis and understanding. By extracting the visual homogeneous regions within the image, it can provide useful information to many visual tasks, such as medical image recognition, medical image registration, medical image reconstruction, etc.

With the theoretical development of machine learning techniques, most state-of-the-art methods were proposed to utilize the feature learning mechanism of deep neural networks and have shown promising medical image segmentation results [1–3]. Among them, Fully Convolutional Networks (FCN) [4] and U-Net [5] are most popular methods in this field. FCN define a skip architecture that combines semantic information from a coarse layer with appearance information from a fine layer to produce detailed segmentations. In an encoder-decoder fashion, U-Net consists of a contracting path to capture context and a symmetric expanding path that enables precise localization. Since then, more and more medical segmentation methods are proposed based on these fundamental

© Springer Nature Switzerland AG 2019
D. Shen et al. (Eds.): MICCAI 2019, LNCS 11769, pp. 558–566, 2019.
https://doi.org/10.1007/978-3-030-32226-7_62

architectures. SegNet [6] uses pooling indices computed in the max-pooling step of the corresponding encoder to perform non-linear upsampling. Alom, etc. [7] propose a Recurrent Residual Convolutional Neural Network based on U-Net model. Compared to equivalent models, this method, also known as R2U-net, shows superior performance on many medical segmentation tasks.

To sum up, the skip-connections used in such methods can directly forward low level information to the backend of network such that the segmentation accuracy can be greatly improved. Yet its effectiveness highly depends on the quality of annotations. Prior work [8] shows that neural networks have such a strong capability to converge even if the training data is inaccurate. Therefore if the annotation is greatly contaminated, the real and effective features may not be necessarily learned. In such cases, especially when the learning model is built upon a label-dependent supervised framework, there is no guarantee that the algorithm could spontaneously discover useful visual cues to fight against wrong annotations and eventually reach real optima. To address this problem, Lu, etc. [9] proposes a sparse learning model to directly and explicitly detect noisy labels in a superpixel setting. Khoreva, etc. [10] design a weakly supervised learning technique to acquire semantic label from bounding box detection annotations. More recently, a new image boundary generation framework, namely STEAL [11], is proposed to learn more accurate semantic boundaries from noisy annotations by enforcing maximum response along the normal edge direction.

Therefore, in order to acquire meaningful segmentations under the influence of label noisy, it is essential to conduct weak-supervised learning by integrating useful prior information that sterns directly from the images. In this paper, we present a novel medical image segmentation algorithm, namely the LVC-Net, to deal with the label noise. Firstly, since the front-end of network is relatively less affected by supervised signals, we propose to capture local visual saliency features, called Local Visual Cues (LVCs), from low-level convolutional channels. Then we further integrate an deformable spatial transformation module into our encoder-decoder network, to provide extra freedom for local receptive fields so that the network could spontaneously establish visual connections between the predictions and LVCs during the learning process. Finally, a novel loss function is proposed to build effective regularizations for the noisy label, the LVCs, and the deformable modules. Comparative experiment on hip x-ray image segmentation task demonstrate that our algorithm achieves significant improvement over baselines in the presences of noisy label.

2   Method

2.1   Overview

In our framework, we employ the classic U-Net as our basic build block. The encoder-decoder net is built based on traditional convolutional layer, max-pooling layer, and up-sampling layer. Note that these basic operational layers can be easily transformed into modern recurrent or residual version as proposed

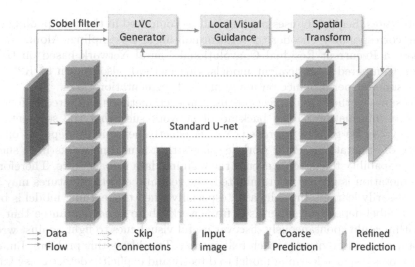

Fig. 1. The framework of LVC-Net

in [7]. As shown in Fig. 1, the whole layout consists 3 parts: the U-Net module, the LVC generator, and the spatial transform module. We use a multi-loss function to guide the learning behavior of our network. Detailed information is shown in the following sections.

2.2   Local Visual Cues

As discussed above, in supervised deep learning architecture, the annotation plays an essential role as it is the only training criterion that the learning algorithms have to trust. Although low-level features fed by the skip-connection may bring meaningful influences to the high-level "decision-making" branch, once the labels are badly corrupted, the neural networks still have the capability to converge or even over-fit the wrong training data [8]. In medical image segmentation tasks, the algorithms are often required to output detailed pixel-level segmentation results, but if the annotations are not trustworthy, it may bring a great challenge to most existing supervised methods. And because of the complexity and diversity of medical images, the label-generating work can be both tricky and onerous, thus the label noise of medical image is much of a practical and urgent issue.

It is a common observation that during the learning process, the front-end of network may less affected by supervised signals, thus can be used to generate detailed image features like the method proposed in [12]. Inspired by this work, we propose to capture local visual saliency features, called Local Visual Cues (LVCs), from low-level convolutional channels.

Specifically, the homogeneous pixels can be clustered into one class because of their visual and semantic similarity, thus one of the most important low-level visual cue for segmentation task is the inter-class boundaries, or image edges. To fully utilize the deep network and learn class-specific LVCs, we first use generic image filters such as Sobel operator to generate the initial coarse ground truth. By incorporating frond-end channels, prediction results and the initial edge ground truth, the LVC generation loss is proposed to calculate the cross-entropy at every pixel as:

$$LVC_{loss} = \begin{cases} P(s) \cdot y_s \cdot \log{(y_i)} & \rho \leq y_i \leq 1 \\ (1 - P(s)) \cdot (1 - y_s) \cdot \log{(1 - y_i)} & 0 \leq y_i < \rho \end{cases} \tag{1}$$

where y_i is the output of LVC generator, $P(s)$ is the intensity ratio of Sobel signals in each initial edge ground truth mask, y_s represents the class weight, and ρ is set to a typical value of 0.5. Then, a regularization term is proposed to punish LVCs that are away from prediction boundaries. Relative spatial computations will be introduced in following section. All the computations mentioned above are preformed in a differentiable manner such that the network is able to learn and preserve useful low-level visual cues to compensate weak predictions wherever label noise appears. The LVC generator and the segmentation framework are trained alternately to have a better segmentation performance.

2.3   Spatial Transformation Based on Visual Guidance

After the extraction of LVCs, the segmentation net is able to perform classification base on both noisy annotations and the local visual cues. However, the direct computation of the pixel-wise loss is rather discrete that the LVCs may be suppressed and may cause spatial discontinuous. In order to provide extra freedom for local receptive fields so that the network could spontaneously establish visual connections between the predictions and LVCs during the learning process, we propose a spatial transform module to navigate the classification boundaries away from wrong labels.

As shown in Fig. 2, the proposed spatial transform module consists of two parts. By multiply the network prediction and LVC responses with a coordinate template, the position of local visual attentions is acquired as the visual guidance. Then we perform a spatial convolution step to get 2-dimensional offsets for each pixel. To update the predictions, we create a parameterized sampling grid to cultivate spatial calculation into a differentiable way. Based on the offset between each pixel and visual attentions centers, a regularization loss is proposed to control the deformation ability of the network. Eventually, the classification probability of each pixel could be re-assigned accordingly.

Local Visual Guidance. We generate a coordinate template by using 2D convolution with 1×1 kernel to get a the full sized coordinate mask:

$$R = \{(x, y) | 0 \leq x \leq W, 0 \leq y \leq H, (x, y) \in \mathbb{N} \times \mathbb{N}\} \tag{2}$$

Then, the location of local visual attention centers is calculated based on the network prediction and LVC responses. By using Eq. (3), the values of prediction

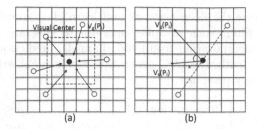

Fig. 2. The spatial transformation based on local visual guidance. (a) Local Visual Guidance acquisition. (b) Spatial sampling offsets. Dotted line indicates the classification boundary.

and LVCs are both taken into account, and that the network is able to estimate probabilistic centers of local visual attention.

$$\text{center}(p_i) = \frac{1}{|N(p_i)|} \sum_{j \in N(p_i)} Y(p_j) L(p_j) R(p_j) \tag{3}$$

where $Y(p_j)$ is the network prediction, $L(p_j)$ is the LVC responses, $R(p_j)$ is the coordinate mask value of p_j, $N(p_i)$ is a convolutional window, which forms a local receptive filed to investigate the relative intensity of the prediction an LVCs. If the network failed to generate correct predictions because of the label noise, the LVC in that region will take over and provide guidance for the segmentation by:

$$V_g(p_i) = [R(p_i) - \text{center}(p_i)]_{x,y} \tag{4}$$

in which V_g is the local visual guidance for each pixel to re-sample classification probability accordingly.

Spatial Sampling Offsets. In order to have a better generalization ability and transformation freedom, an adaptive spatial transform model is proposed so that the segmentation sampling offsets can be inferred based on different local visual information. We adopt the spatial-convolution and sampling method proposed in [13], which applying convolution layers to learn adaptive spatial transformation. At each pixel, a offset $V_s(p_i)$ will be generated by the spatial transformation module, and then spatial sampling parameters can be learned by using the L2 regularization between sampling offsets and the local visual guidance:

$$G_{loss} = \|V_g(p_i) - V_s(p_i)\|^2 \tag{5}$$

Then the original segmentation prediction can be re-sampled based on offsets that associated with LVCs and noisy labels.

$$S(p_i) = \sum_{j \in N(p_i)} \phi(V_s(p_j)) w(Y(p_j)) \tag{6}$$

where ϕ is the standard network sampling function, and w is the local intensity weighting function.

2.4   LVC-Net Losses

The final prediction of the network is made by integrating three losses: (1) LVC-generation loss LVC_{loss}, (2) LVC-guidance loss G_{loss}, and (3) LVC-segmentation loss S_{loss}. During training stage, this losses can be trained successively to shape the final segmentation LVC-Net.

As mentioned above, we propose Local Visual Cues to provide extra visual regularizations to fight against bad annotations. Once the LVCs are obtained, the original pixel-wise segmentation loss can be re-written as:

$$S_{loss} = -\left[y_s \log \widehat{y} - y_s \log (1 - \widehat{y})\right] - \left[y_G \log \widehat{y} + (1 - y_G) \log (1 - \widehat{y})\right] \quad (7)$$

where S_{loss} is the LVC-segmentation loss. The predictions will be dynamically affected by both label masks y_G and LVC masks y_s. Therefore, the final LVC-Net is able to spontaneously discover local visual information, and attempt to compensate weak predictions wherever label noise appears based on a spatial transformation mechanism.

3   Experiment

We conduct comparative experiments with FCN and U-Net on hip X-ray image data set. The convolution layer is initialized by default setup, and we use stochastic gradient descent with the learning rate of 10^{-4}. All the networks are trained for same 1200 epochs on a Nvidia Tesla v100 GPU.

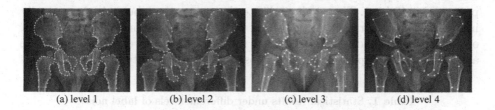

(a) level 1   (b) level 2   (c) level 3   (d) level 4

Fig. 3. Label noise from level 1 to level 4

Data Preparation and Evaluation Metric. COCO format is used to build our dataset that contains images and mask annotations. The size of all training and testing image is normalized to [128, 128], and the total number of images in each set is 1464 and 366, respectively. As show in Fig. 3, for each training image, we manually generated 4 groups of annotations by Labelme with the label noise form level 1 up to level 4 (higher level indicates coarser annotations). The label quality of ground truth in testing dataset is equivalent to level 1. We trained all the networks (FCN, U-Net, LVC-Net) for each label group, and evaluated the segmentation performance accordingly. The evaluation metric we use is segmentation precession, recall and the mIoU. We performed 5 rounds of evaluation. In each round, 50 images were randomly selected, and mean evaluation metrics were calculated. Experimental results are presented in the following section.

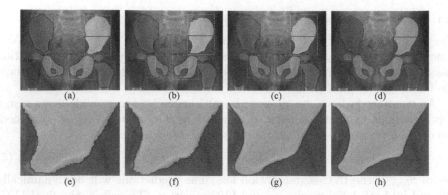

Fig. 4. Segmentation examples. The first row is the result of different algorithms on the entire X-ray image, the second row shows detailed results within the red squares. (a)(e) FCN, (b)(f) U-Net, (c)(g) LVC-Net, (d)(h) Ground truth (Color figure online)

Results. Some segmentation results are presented in Fig. 4 in which all the nets were trained in the level 3 noisy dataset for same epochs. As clearly shown in this picture, compared to other networks, our LVC-Net is capable of discovering more accurate edges of left ilium bone under the guidance of local visual cues generated directly from the image. In contrast, the segmentation precision of FCN and U-Net are greatly affected by bad annotations. More statistical results are presented in Table 1. The results indicate that when the label noise is gradually increased, the performance of FCN and U-Net drops at a faster rate. However, our proposed method remains relatively robust at higher level of label noise. We also did module experiments on proposed methods, results demonstrate that

Table 1. Statistical results under different levels of label noise

Noise level	Methods	Precision	Recall	mIoU
Level 1	FCN	0.894	0.924	0.831
Level 1	U-Net	0.912	**0.955**	0.874
Level 1	LVC-Net	**0.951**	0.929	**0.886**
Level 2	FCN	0.811	0.878	0.770
Level 2	U-Net	0.835	0.883	0.804
Level 2	LVC-Net	**0.915**	**0.906**	**0.836**
Level 3	FCN	0.784	0.816	0.731
Level 3	U-Net	0.790	0.828	0.772
Level 3	LVC-Net	**0.902**	**0.859**	**0.810**
Level 4	FCN	0.652	0.704	0.620
Level 4	U-Net	0.664	0.728	0.690
Level 4	LVC-Net	**0.815**	**0.796**	**0.738**

our proposed LVC-generation module and LVC-based spatial transform module is able to generate meaningful visual information and further improver the medical image segmentation performance. And because of the space limitation, all experiment results will be presented in our extended journal version.

4 Conclusion

In this paper, we introduced a novel medical image segmentation network based on Local Visual Cues. Firstly, the LVC generator is proposed to capture local visual saliency features from low-level convolutional channels. Then, a deformable spatial transformation module is integrated into our LVC-Net to provide extra freedom for the network to build visual connections between the predictions and LVCs during the learning process. The multi-loss function is proposed to build effective regularizations. Experiments on hip medical image data sets indicated that the proposed method can effectively suppress the influence of label noise, thus outperformed the state-of-the-art on segmentation tasks.

Acknowledgments. This research was funded in part by National Key R&D Program of China 2016YFC1000307-3, National Natural Science Foundation of China 61801068 & 61906024, Natural Science Foundation of Chongqing cstc2016jcyjA0407, Scientific and Technological Research Program of Chongqing Education Commission KJ1600419. The authors would like to thank Prof. Guoxin Nan for providing the data.

References

1. Yu, C., Wang, J., Peng, C., Gao, C., Gang, Y., Sang, N.: Learning a discriminative feature network for semantic segmentation. In: IEEE Conference on Computer Vision and Pattern Recognition, pp. 1857–1866 (2018)
2. Kaul, C., Manandhar, S., Pears, N.: FocusNet: an attention-based fully convolutional network for medical image segmentation. arXiv preprint arXiv:1902.03091 (2019)
3. Milletari, F., Navab, N., Ahmadi, S.-A.: V-net: fully convolutional neural networks for volumetric medical image segmentation. In: 2016 Fourth International Conference on 3D Vision (3DV), pp. 565–571 (2016)
4. Long, J., Shelhamer, E., Darrell, T.: Fully convolutional networks for semantic segmentation. In: IEEE Conference on Computer Vision and Pattern Recognition, pp. 3431–3440 (2015)
5. Ronneberger, O., Fischer, P., Brox, T.: U-Net: convolutional networks for biomedical image segmentation. In: Navab, N., Hornegger, J., Wells, W.M., Frangi, A.F. (eds.) MICCAI 2015. LNCS, vol. 9351, pp. 234–241. Springer, Cham (2015). https://doi.org/10.1007/978-3-319-24574-4_28
6. Badrinarayanan, V., Kendall, A., Cipolla, R.: SegNet: a deep convolutional encoder-decoder architecture for image segmentation. IEEE Trans. Pattern Anal. Mach. Intell. **39**(12), 2481–2495 (2017)
7. Alom, M.Z., Hasan, M., Yakopcic, C., Taha, T.M., Asari, V.K.: Recurrent residual convolutional neural network based on U-net (R2U-net) for medical image segmentation. arXiv preprint arXiv:1802.06955 (2018)

8. Zhang, C., Bengio, S., Hardt, M., Recht, B., Vinyals, O.: Understanding deep learning requires rethinking generalization. arXiv preprint arXiv:1611.03530 (2016)
9. Lu, Z., Fu, Z., Xiang, T., Han, P., Wang, L., Gao, X.: Learning from weak and noisy labels for semantic segmentation. IEEE Trans. Pattern Anal. Mach. Intell. **39**(3), 486–500 (2016)
10. Khoreva, A., Benenson, R., Hosang, J., Hein, M., Schiele, B.: Simple does it: weakly supervised instance and semantic segmentation. In: IEEE Conference on Computer Vision and Pattern Recognition, pp. 876–885 (2017)
11. Acuna, D., Kar, A., Fidler, S.: Devil is in the edges: learning semantic boundaries from noisy annotations. In: IEEE Conference on Computer Vision and Pattern Recognition, pp. 11075–11083 (2019)
12. Liu, Y., Cheng, M., Hu, X., Wang K., Bai, X.: Richer convolutional features for edge detection. In: IEEE Conference on Computer Vision and Pattern Recognition, Honolulu, pp. 5872–5881 (2017)
13. Dai, J., et al.: Deformable convolutional networks. In: IEEE International Conference on Computer Vision, pp. 764–773 (2017)

Cone-Beam Computed Tomography (CBCT) Segmentation by Adversarial Learning Domain Adaptation

Xiaoqian Jia[1,2], Sicheng Wang[1,3], Xiao Liang[1], Anjali Balagopal[1],
Dan Nguyen[1], Ming Yang[1], Zhangyang Wang[3], Jim Xiuquan Ji[2],
Xiaoning Qian[2], and Steve Jiang[1(✉)]

[1] Medical Artificial Intelligence and Automation Laboratory,
Department of Radiation Oncology,
University of Texas Southwestern, Dallas, USA
Steve.Jiang@UTSouthwestern.edu
[2] Department of Electrical and Computer Engineering,
Texas A&M University, College Station, USA
[3] Department of Computer Science and Engineering,
Texas A&M University, College Station, USA

Abstract. Cone-beam computed tomography (CBCT) is increasingly
used in radiotherapy for patient alignment and adaptive therapy where
organ segmentation and target delineation are often required. However,
due to the poor image quality, low soft tissue contrast, as well as the difficulty in acquiring segmentation labels on CBCT images, developing effective segmentation methods on CBCT has been a challenge. In this paper,
we propose a deep model for segmenting organs in CBCT images without requiring labelled training CBCT images. By taking advantage of the
available segmented computed tomography (CT) images, our adversarial
learning domain adaptation method aims to synthesize CBCT images
from CT images. Then the segmentation labels of the CT images can
help train a deep segmentation network for CBCT images, using both
CTs with labels and CBCTs without labels. Our adversarial learning
domain adaptation is integrated with the CBCT segmentation network
training with the designed loss functions. The synthesized CBCT images
by pixel-level domain adaptation best capture the critical image features that help achieve accurate CBCT segmentation. Our experiments
on the bladder images from Radiation Oncology clinics have shown that
our CBCT segmentation with adversarial learning domain adaptation
significantly improves segmentation accuracy compared to the existing
methods without doing domain adaptation from CT to CBCT.

Keywords: CBCT segmentation · CycleGAN · Domain adaptation

1 Introduction

Cancer radiotherapy often takes several weeks. During the process, patient's
anatomy may change significantly and the initially optimized treatment plan

© Springer Nature Switzerland AG 2019
D. Shen et al. (Eds.): MICCAI 2019, LNCS 11769, pp. 567–575, 2019.
https://doi.org/10.1007/978-3-030-32226-7_63

may become sub-optimal, leading to degraded treatment outcome. One way to address this problem is adaptive radiation therapy (ART), where the treatment plan is re-optimized using the updated patient anatomy right before the treatment on a particular treatment day. Cone-beam computed tomography (CBCT), the most widely available 3D imaging modality on modern linacs, is often used for ART re-planning, whose efficacy depends on accurate segmentation of the organs and treatment target(s) in CBCT images. Unlike segmentation in CT images, where the image quality is much better and the segmentation labels are readily available from the routine treatments, accurate segmentation in CBCT images is far more challenging. For CBCT, labels are not part of routine clinical work, and therefore are not available in a supervised learning setting.

Unsupervised domain adaptation has been intensively studied to enable deep networks to achieve competitive performance on unlabeled data for the new domain (**target**), only with annotated data from the **source** domain. We adopt the same idea for CBCT segmentation without labelled data for model training based on the CyCADA framework [4]. CyCADA enables task-driven adversarial learning by combining domain adaptation using CycleGAN [8] with image classification or segmentation as the ultimate goal. Specifically, CycleGAN is constituted by two generative adversarial networks (GANs) [2] to transfer images between domains through a consistency loss function, requiring no paired data when training. The integration of adversarial domain adaptation and task-driven adversarial learning in CyCADA can capture both pixel-level and feature-level domain invariant representations and therefore better helps the ultimate task. This idea has been applied to medical image analysis in [7], for synthesizing unpaired head and neck MR and CT images.

In this paper, we develop such an integrated framework, as illustrated in Fig. 1, for CBCT segmentation without labelled data. First, we apply Cycle-GAN for pixel-level domain adaptation to generate synthesized CBCT (sCBCT) images from CT images with the anatomical structures inherited from CT images. Thus, the available segmentation masks of CT images can help train a reliable segmentation model. With this segmentation as a pre-trained model, the adversarial learning is then implemented. For sCBCT, we can derive supervised segmentation as described. To further improve segmentation by adversarial learning, we generate segmentation masks for both CBCT and sCBCT images and plug them into a "feature" discriminator to capture the domain differences for CBCT (target) and CT (source). Such adversarial learning will integrate domain adaptation and segmentation to help both tasks for accurate "unsupervised" CBCT segmentation. To summarize, our main contributions are: (1) We adapt the CyCADA framework for CBCT segmentation without using labelled data for training. (2) We extend CycleGAN to transfer CT images into CBCT domain and apply adversarial learning to perform domain adaptation between CT and CBCT, specifically designed for the segmentation task.

2 Methods

In this section, we introduce the proposed adversarial domain adaptation guided image segmentation network. As illustrated in Fig. 1, our network consists of two critical modules: adversarial domain adaptation and deep segmentation. These two modules are intertwined with the segmentation module designed to provide necessary anatomical details as the feedback to help better guide the synthesis of CBCT images from training CT images in adversarial domain adaptation.

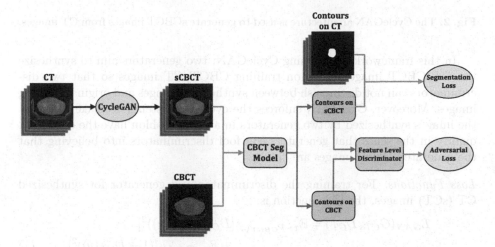

Fig. 1. Workflow of our proposed method, which generates synthetic CBCT from CT, and does the adversarial learning based on segmentation

2.1 Adversarial Learning Domain Adaptation

We first introduce the adversarial domain adaptation module based on Cycle-GAN. The key idea here is to develop a generative model for effective synthesis of CBCT images with inherited CT image segmentation labels so that labeled CT images can be used for CBCT segmentation training.

In our implementation of CycleGAN for adversarial domain adaptation (in Fig. 2), CycleGAN has two generators G_{CT} and G_{CBCT}, which synthesize CT and CBCT images respectively. The synthesized images will be judged by two corresponding discriminators D_{CT} and D_{CBCT}. During the training, the synthesized images will be compared to the corresponding CT images in the source domain and CBCT images in the target domain. The generators also derive the "CycleCT" and "CycleCBCT" images from the synthesized images in a cyclic fashion. These images will also be compared to the original CT and CBCT images to achieve "cyclic consistent" domain adaptation.

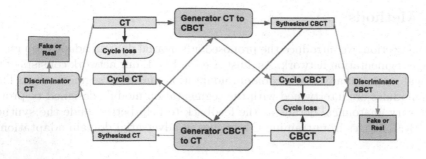

Fig. 2. The CycleGAN architecture is used to generate sCBCT images from CT images.

In this framework, by training CycleGAN, two generators aim to synthesize the CT/CBCT images based on training CBCT/CT images so that two discriminators can not distinguish between synthesized images and original training images. Moreover, CycleGAN enforces the cyclic consistency to make sure that the images synthesized by two generators in a cyclic fashion have the consistent quality in the sense that generators can fool discriminators into believing that the generated "fake" images are "real".

Loss Functions. For training the discriminator and generator for synthesized CT (sCT) images, the loss function is:

$$L_{GAN}(G_{CT}, D_{CT}) = \mathbb{E}_{x \sim \mathcal{P}_{CBCT}(x)}[D_{CT}(G_{CT}(x))^2]$$
$$+ \mathbb{E}_{y \sim \mathcal{P}_{CT}(y)}[(1 - D_{CT}(y))^2], \quad (1)$$

where $\mathcal{P}_{CT}$ and $\mathcal{P}_{CBCT}$ are the sets of unpaired input training CT and CBCT images. Again, the generator G_{CT} aims to generate sCT images that are similar to the input CT images; and D_{CT} aims to distinguish between sCT images and original input CT images $\mathcal{P}_{CT}$. Similarly, for the synthesized CBCT (sCBCT) branch in Fig. 2 (top), we have the corresponding MSE-based adversarial learning loss:

$$L_{GAN}(G_{CBCT}, D_{CBCT}) = \mathbb{E}_{y \sim \mathcal{P}_{CT}(y)}[D_{CBCT}(G_{CBCT}(y))^2]$$
$$+ \mathbb{E}_{x \sim \mathcal{P}_{CBCT}(x)}[1 - D_{CBCT}(x))^2]. \quad (2)$$

To guarantee the high-quality domain adaptation, an additional cycle consistency loss [8] is imposed to have the reconstructed image in a cyclic fashion become identical to the original input training images. This is done by imposing an $\mathcal{L}_1$ difference on the reconstruction error, given as:

$$L_{cycle}(G_{CT}, G_{CBCT}) = \mathbb{E}_{y \sim \mathcal{P}_{CT}(y)}[\|(G_{CT}(G_{CBCT}(y)) - y)\|_1]$$
$$+ \mathbb{E}_{x \sim \mathcal{P}_{CBCT}(x)}[\|(G_{CBCT}(G_{CT}(x)) - x)\|_1]. \quad (3)$$

Furthermore, an identity loss is added:

$$L_{identity}(G_{CT}, G_{CBCT}) = \mathbb{E}_{y \sim \mathcal{P}_{CT}(y)}[\|(G_{CT}(y) - y)\|_1]$$
$$+ \mathbb{E}_{x \sim \mathcal{P}_{CBCT}(x)}[\|(G_{CBCT}(x) - x)\|_1], \quad (4)$$

leading to the final total loss function:

$$L_{cyclegan} = L_{GAN}(G_{CT}, D_{CT}) + L_{GAN}(G_{CBCT}, D_{CBCT})$$
$$+ \lambda_{cycle}L_{cycle}(G_{CT}, G_{CBCT}) + \lambda_{id}L_{identity}(G_{CT}, G_{CBCT}), \quad (5)$$

where λ_{cycle} and λ_{id} controls the relative importance of the L_{cycle} and $L_{identity}$. Notice the symmetry of the designed loss functions to have the cyclic consistency guarantee for better quality adversarial domain adaptation. For CBCT segmentation, we focus on the sCBCT branch on the top of Fig. 2. When the training reaches an optimum with respect to the total loss function, we hope that from the source CT images, we can generate sCBCT images whose representations are similar to those of the target CBCT images so that they can be used to train an effective CBCT segmentation network.

Network Architecture. In our implementation, we choose the generator network architecture to be the U-net [6] for end-to-end pixel-level image transformation, as similarly adopted in the original CycleGAN [8], where the inputs and outputs of the U-net are $512 \times 512 \times 1$ images. For discriminators, a 142×142 PatchGAN [5] is applied to output the $32 \times 32 \times 1$ feature maps for discriminating the synthesized and original training images. All layers of these networks utilize instance normalization and LeakyReLU (rate $= 0.2$) activation functions, except that the last layers of the generators and discriminators use 'tanh' and linear activation functions, respectively.

2.2 Deep Segmentation via Adversarial Learning

Adversarial domain adaptation module feeds sCBCT images into the deep segmentation module. Specifically, the deep segmentation network can be pre-trained using sCBCT images with their inherited segmentation masks of original CT images. However, due to the domain shift between CT and CBCT, the CT segmentation masks may not work properly for training the segmentation network in CBCT domain. Thus, the segmentation module is designed to deploy both sCBCT and CBCT images as inputs, creating the corresponding output segmentation maps. Then, a feature (segmentation) discriminator D_{feat} is integrated to determine whether the segmentation maps are from CT or CBCT domains (Fig. 1). The segmentation networks can be considered as the corresponding generators of segmentation maps in GAN. When two generators can produce segmentation maps to fool D_{feat} so that the corresponding sCBCT segmentation maps and CBCT maps are indistinguishable, we achieve a good segmentation network for CBCT images. Through this operation, the segmentation network can learn more info about target domain (CBCT) via adversarial learning, and predict on target images more reliably even without any label.

Loss Functions. The segmentation network is denoted as *Seg*. To overcome the unbalanced in medical image masks, loss function is chosen as DSC (Dice

---

sililarity coefficient):

$$L_{seg} = 1 - \frac{2Y_{CT}Y_{map} + a}{Y_{CT} + Y_{map} + a}, \tag{6}$$

where Y_{CT} is the CT segmentation mask (Ground Truth), Y_{map} is the output of the deep model. The smoothing term a ensures the stability of the loss function by avoiding potential numerical issues when the denominator becomes 0.

As shown in Fig. 1, D_{feat} aims to distinguish the segmentation maps of two domains. The loss function of D_{feat} is given as:

$$L_{adv} = \mathbb{E}_{x \sim P_{CBCT}(x)}[D_{feat}(Seg(x))^2] + \mathbb{E}_{z \sim P_{sCBCT}(z)}[(1 - D_{feat}(Seg(z)))^2], \tag{7}$$

where P_{CBCT}, P_{sCBCT} are the sets of input CBCT and sCBCT images. Finally, we establish the total loss function:

$$L_{feat} = L_{adv} + \lambda_{seg}L_{seg}. \tag{8}$$

Network Architecture. In the segmentation module, the Resnet50 [3] block is built in the encoder part of U-net [6] as the basic architecture. Again, we choose PatchGAN [5] as a discriminator with receptive field size 70×70. The network consists of 5 convolutional layers with 4×4 kernel size and stride of 2, except for the last one layers with convolution stride of 1. The numbers of feature maps are $32, 64, 128, 256, 1$ for each layer, respectively. For the first four layers, each convolutional layer is followed by a leaky ReLU with rate $= 0.2$ and an instance normalization layer. Through the integration of adversarial domain adaptation and segmentation modules, the available CT images with segmentation masks as well as CBCT images are taken the best advantage of when training for CBCT segmentation. In the training, we first train D_{feat} until the accuracy reaches an accuracy threshold $\mathcal{R}$ (initial setting is 0.6). Next, we train the segmentation part until get a reliable module for CBCT.

3   Experiments

3.1   Data

Collected data from 90 patients, for each patient, we select one planning CT and 5 CBCTs to perform the CycleGAN training. The pixel spacing of CT and CBCT are normalized into 1×1, where the thickness is 3 mm. All slices are cropped into 512×512 resolution. Each CBCT study has 88 slices, and each CT study has about 220 slices, while we crop CT into 88 slices which focus on bladder and prostate portion. The HU value range for CT is $[-1000, 3500]$, and that for CBCT is $[-1000, 7000]$. All the image HU values are normalized to $(-1, 1)$ range for training and validation. Due to the fact that segmentation masks of CBCT slices are not available, we use manual segmentations to validate the proposed method as the ground truth.

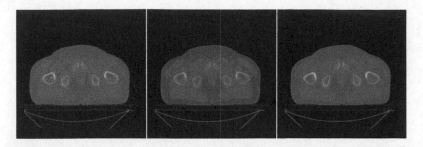

Fig. 3. Domain adaptation between CT and CBCT: from left to right are: raw CT, sCBCT, reconstructed CT

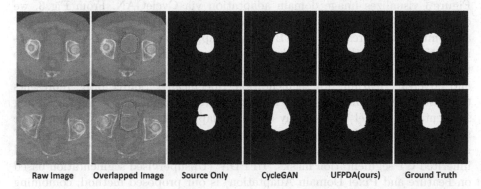

Raw Image   Overlapped Image   Source Only   CycleGAN   UFPDA(ours)   Ground Truth

Fig. 4. Visual comparison of segmentation results by different methods. From left to right: raw CBCT image, overlapped image, segmentation by 'Source only' (yellow in Overlapped Image), 'CycleGAN' (blue) and UFPDA (red), Ground tuth (light blue). (Color figure online)

Table 1. Sensitivity analysis from λ_{seg} 1 to 10

λ_{seg}	1	2	3	4	5	6	7	8	9	10
DSC (%)	82.3	**83.6**	80.3	80.8	79.3	80.1	80.7	78.9	80.8	79.9

3.2 Implementation Details

The networks are implemented and trained using Keras [1] on a PC with an NVIDIA Tesla K80 dual-GPU. For CycleGAN [8], the following hyper-parameters are set for training the module: the batch size is set to 1 with ADAM for optimization at the learning rate 0.003 with scheduled decay rate at 0.005; $\beta_1 = 0.9$ and the epoch number $= 50$. For the CycleGAN loss, we set $\lambda_{cycle} = 10$, $\lambda_{id} = 5$. For feature-level adversarial learning in the segmentation module, we have explored different loss weight λ_{seg} settings during training. For segmentation, we first train U-net with the Resnet50 backbones on both CT and sCBCT datasets. Owing to data imbalance and memory limits, we crop the images into 256×256.

Table 2. Performance comparison for CBCT bladder segmentation

Method	Pixel	Feature	DSC (%)
Source only	No	No	70.1
CycleGAN	Yes	No	75.8
UFPDA (ours)	Yes	Yes	**83.6**

3.3 Evaluation

We have evaluated our algorithms on 7 patients' CBCT, with 676 slices in total. Figure 3 visualizes image domain adaptation via CycleGAN. From Fig. 3, we can see the sCBCT has higher noise and lower contrast while it keeps the CT anatomical structures with the CBCT image appearance. Figure 4 shows the segmentation maps by different methods and ground truth. In Fig. 4, we can observe the improvement by our approach integrating cycle-consistent domain adaption and adversary learning for segmentation. Specifically, 'Source only' represents the results by segmenting CBCT images directly using the CT pre-training segmentation model without any domain adaptation. 'CycleGAN' denotes the results by using CycleGAN for pixel-level domain adaptation to generate sCBCT images and then train the segmentation network using only sCBCT images and inherited CT segmentation masks. 'UFPDA' (Unsupervised segmentation based on Feature and Pixel Domain Adaptation) is our proposed method, combining the pixel-level domain adaptation and feature-level adversarial learning. Table 1 shows the comparison of sensitivity analysis. With $\lambda_{seg} = 2$, we achieve the best segmentation performance with DSC 83.6%.

Table 2 shows the DSC of ablation studies. As shown in Fig. 4 and Table 2, our proposed method (UFPDA) improves CBCT segmentation performance by about 7.8% for the DSC score, compared to the naive implementation of CycleGAN to synthesize CBCT images.

4 Conclusions

In this paper, we proposed a method combining the cycle-consistent domain adaptation and adversarial learning for unsupervised CBCT image segmentation. The method can generate CBCT segmentation without the need for labelled CBCT data for training. In our studies using 90 clinical bladder CBCT datasets, our method enables training with both CT and CBCT images and improves the DSC score by about 13.6% as compared with the segmentation model trained only with CT images. The proposed method can be extended to other applications where existing segmentation labels can be transferred to the datasets in new domains.

References

1. Chollet, F.: et al.: Keras. https://keras.io (2015)
2. Goodfellow, I., et al.: Generative adversarial nets. In: NIPS, Sherjil Ozair (2014)
3. He, K., Zhang, X., Ren, S., Sun, J.: Deep residual learning for image recognition. In: CVPR, pp. 770–778 (2016)
4. Hoffman, J., et al.: CyCADA: cycle consistent adversarial domain adaptation. In: ICML (2018)
5. Isola, P., Zhu, J.-Y., Zhou, T., Efros, A.A.: Image-to-image translation with conditional adversarial networks. In: CVPR, pp. 5967–5976 (2017)
6. Ronneberger, O., Fischer, P., Brox, T.: U-Net: convolutional networks for biomedical image segmentation. In: Navab, N., Hornegger, J., Wells, W.M., Frangi, A.F. (eds.) MICCAI 2015. LNCS, vol. 9351, pp. 234–241. Springer, Cham (2015). https://doi.org/10.1007/978-3-319-24574-4_28
7. Yang, H., et al.: Unpaired brain MR-to-CT synthesis using a structure-constrained CycleGAN. CoRR (2018)
8. Zhu, J.-Y., et al.: Unpaired image-to-image translation using cycle-consistent adversarial networkss. In: ICCV (2017)

Pick-and-Learn: Automatic Quality Evaluation for Noisy-Labeled Image Segmentation

Haidong Zhu[1], Jialin Shi[1], and Ji Wu[1,2(✉)]

[1] Department of Electronic Engineering, Tsinghua University, Beijing, China
{zhuhd15,shi-jl16}@mails.tsinghua.edu.cn
[2] Institute for Precision Medicine, Tsinghua University, Beijing, China
wuji_ee@mail.tsinghua.edu.cn

Abstract. Deep learning methods have achieved promising performance in many areas, but they are still struggling with noisy-labeled images during the training process. Considering that the annotation quality indispensably relies on great expertise, the problem is even more crucial in the medical image domain. How to eliminate the disturbance from noisy labels for segmentation tasks without further annotations is still a significant challenge. In this paper, we introduce our label quality evaluation strategy for deep neural networks automatically assessing the quality of each label, which is not explicitly provided, and training on clean-annotated ones. We propose a solution for network automatically evaluating the relative quality of the labels in the training set and using good ones to tune the network parameters. We also design an overfitting control module to let the network maximally learn from the precise annotations during the training process. Experiments on the public biomedical image segmentation dataset have proved the method outperforms baseline methods and retains both high accuracy and good generalization at different noise levels.

Keywords: Image segmentation · Noisy labels · Quality evaluation

1 Introduction

Researchers have witnessed the significant improvement of many visual understanding tasks based on deep learning methods [1–3] in the past few years, but the community is still struggling to get a massive amount of clean and precise labels to train a good model. Noisy-labeled images can seriously damage the performance of the deep neural networks [4]. For example, the computer-aided image segmentation for nodes and organs will directly help doctors and surgeons to understand, diagnose and perform the operation. But low-accuracy segmentation model trained on noisy labels, like examples shown in Fig. 1, will severely

---

H. Zhu and J. Shi contributed equally to this work.

© Springer Nature Switzerland AG 2019
D. Shen et al. (Eds.): MICCAI 2019, LNCS 11769, pp. 576–584, 2019.
https://doi.org/10.1007/978-3-030-32226-7_64

impact the result and can lead to more serious misunderstandings during the surgery. High-quality annotations for the data require the accumulation of years of knowledge and experience, which directly conflicts with the need for the great need of data.

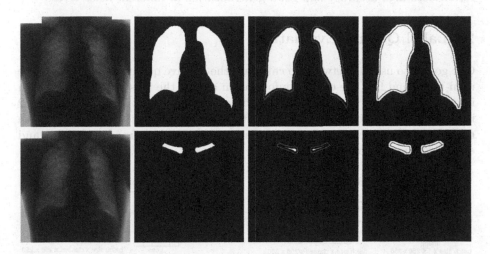

Fig. 1. Two examples of noisy labels in the segmentation problem. Images in the second row are the clean-annotated ground-truth. The third and fourth columns show two types of noisy labels: dilation and erosion. Correct segmentation boundaries are shown in red. (Color figure online)

Compared with the solutions for low-quality images, noisy labels are more difficult to deal with if no further annotation for quality is available. Most approaches for low-quality annotations are designed for the classification tasks [5–11]. For example, based on the distribution of the noise, Goldberger et al. [5] and Patrini et al. [6] relied on the relationship between clean data and noisy data to improve the performance. This needs strong reliability of the predicted distribution of the data. Veit et al. [9] focused on tuning the network on clean data before adding noisy data, which needed extra human annotations. Xue et al. [11] and Jiang et al. [7] showed the improvement by clustering and using the reweighted loss in the final stage, but they ignored the inner-connection between the input images and annotations. In addition, all the methods described above showed improvement in image classification, but none of them can be applied to the segmentation task.

In this paper, we introduce a label quality evaluation strategy to assess the quality of annotations for model training. Based on the conflict between noisy labels and consistency in clean-labeled samples, the method can be applied to segmentation tasks for images with noisy labels. Specifically, we apply this method on biomedical image segmentation task. With the predicted quality score for each sample in the mini-batch, the network re-weights the loss to tune the network. This work makes two main contributions: first, a novel automatic quality evaluation module inspired by the relationship between labels and inputs; and second, an overfitting control module to ensure enough trainable samples and avoid overfitting. Experiments on the public dataset prove the method can retain both high accuracy and good generalization at different noise levels.

2   Label Quality Evaluation

Our goal is to use the network to calculate the relative quality score in the same mini-batch and find the conflict information among the noisy labels. With such information, the network can distinguish noisy labels from the good ones. Fig. 2 illustrates our proposed network structure. Our network is composed of three modules, a feature extraction module, a quality awareness module (QAM) and an overfitting control module (OCM).

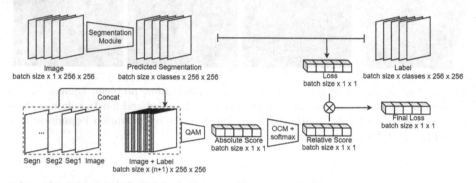

Fig. 2. The end-to-end architecture of our proposed label quality evaluation strategy. The segmentation module is the CNN structure module for generating segmentation. The quality awareness module (QAM) is a CNN structure network taking the concatenation of the image and its labels, marked as Segn in the image, as input, and running parallelly with the segmentation module. To re-weight the samples in the same mini-batch, the quality awareness module and the overfitting control module (OCM) generate a score for each input annotation, followed by a softmax layer and the multiplication between it and the loss generated by segmentation module. The final loss will be summed up and backpropagated to tune the segmentation and quality awareness modules together.

2.1   Quality Awareness Module (QAM)

One significant modification in our architecture is the quality awareness module, which runs parallelly with the segmentation module to calculate the weight value. During the training process, the predicted segmentation for the noisy-labeled samples might have a higher loss compared with well-annotated ones.

Different noise types and noise levels among the noisy-labeled samples can confuse the network and show a slower speed of loss descent. In this regard, the quality awareness module is proposed to evaluate the potential quality of the labels. During the training process, the quality awareness module supervises the descending speed of the losses in the same mini-batch. After re-weighting the losses, the segmentation module backpropagates based on the re-weighted loss and focuses more on those with the higher weight, while the quality awareness module backpropagates on the same loss.

More specifically, let x_i be the ith input image in the training set and y_i be its annotation. L_i is the ith loss calculated by the segmentation module in the mini-batch with N samples. We use the VGG [1] based network $\Theta(\cdot)$ in the experiment and change the number of input channel to $n + 1$, where n is the number of segmentation classes, to take both image and labels as input. Also, we replace the final layer as a one-channel average pooling layer to assess the weight for each sample in the mini-batch. A softmax layer is followed to rescale all the score to $[0, 1]$. Instead of naively using the average value of the loss to backpropagate, the final loss is calculated as

$$Loss = \sum_{i=1,...,N} \Theta(x_i, y_i) \cdot L_i$$

$$s.t. \sum_{i=1,...,N} \Theta(x_i, y_i) = 1, 0 \le \Theta(x_i, y_i) \le 1 \tag{1}$$

to distinguish different quality of the labels.

2.2 Overfitting Control Module (OCM)

Although the quality awareness module can separate clean-annotated labels from the noisy ones, it can cause serious overfitting problems as well, since the loss can further decrease if the quality awareness module has a larger weight on a small subset with clear-labeled samples. Also, if the quality awareness module makes mistakes during the training process, the relative weight of this sample can be too small or too big for the network to correct. In this regard, we add an extra restriction between the quality awareness module and the softmax layer to limit the relative ratio of the output quality score. We use the function

$$\Phi(t) = \lambda tanh(t) \tag{2}$$

as the new score instead of the absolute quality score t produced by quality awareness module. This will rescale the output score from $(-\infty, \infty)$ to $(-\lambda, \lambda)$. After processed by the overfitting control module and the softmax layer, the maximum possible ratio of two relative scores in the same mini-batch decrease from ∞ to $e^{2\lambda}$. This ensures that after multiplying the score with the loss, the quality awareness module will not fully ignore any sample in the same mini-batch or ignore clean labels while making mistakes in the early quality evaluation.

3   Experiments and Results

In this section, we conducted experiments on a publicly available medical dataset to demonstrate the effectiveness of the label quality evaluation network. We compared our method with the supervised segmentation network without the QAM or OCM modules on different noise levels respectively. We also made a comparison to show the effect of different modules on the performance.

3.1   Dataset

We employed a public segmentation medical image dataset JSRT [12] for the experiments. The JSRT dataset contains 247 images and three types of organ structures: heart, clavicles, and lungs. Specifically, each image contains both left and right lungs as well as left and right clavicles. Each image is a 2D grayscale image with 1024×1024 pixels. We randomly split the data into training (165 images) and testing (82 images) subsets in experiments.

3.2   Implementation Details

We used the PyTorch in our experiments, and selected the structure of UNet [3] for the segmentation network. We resized the input image to 256×256 pixels and set the hyperparameter $\lambda = 2$ in the OCM empirically. In order to generate noisy-labeled images with different types and levels of noises, we randomly selected 0%, 25%, 50% and 75% samples from the training set and further randomly eroded or dilated them with $1 \leq n_i \leq 8$ and $5 \leq n_i \leq 13$ pixels. We empirically set the learning rate as 0.0001, and the batch size was fixed to 32 in the experiments.

3.3   Quantitative Results

In this subsection, we compared our strategies with existing state-of-the-art methods on different levels of noises firstly. Then we conducted ablation experiments to investigate the effectiveness of QAM and OCM. Finally, we evaluated the effectiveness and capabilities of picking clean-labeled samples by using the label quality assessment strategy. In the experiments, we used Dice value

$$Dice = \frac{2 \times V_{pred} \cap V_{gt}}{V_{pred} + V_{gt}} \tag{3}$$

as our evaluation criteria, where V_{pred} represents the segmentation area of prediction and V_{gt} is the area of annotation.

Comparison with Baseline Methods. We conducted the experiments on the datasets described in the previous section. We trained the network on the training set with different levels of noisy labels and tested on clean labels. Table 1 illustrates the experimental results with and without the label quality evaluation strategy. On clean-annotated dataset, both these methods have high accuracy in

Table 1. Results on JSRT dataset

Noise percentage	Noise level	Strategy	Lungs	Heart	Clavicles	Average
No noise	-	Baseline	0.943	0.941	0.862	0.915
No noise	-	QAM	0.939	0.923	0.831	0.898
No noise	-	QAM+OCM	0.941	0.940	0.852	0.911
25% noise	$1 \leq n_i \leq 8$	Baseline	0.868	0.888	0.538	0.765
25% noise	$1 \leq n_i \leq 8$	QAM	0.925	0.926	0.748	0.866
25% noise	$1 \leq n_i \leq 8$	QAM+OCM	0.936	0.925	0.823	0.895
50% noise	$1 \leq n_i \leq 8$	Baseline	0.873	0.884	0.539	0.765
50% noise	$1 \leq n_i \leq 8$	QAM	0.922	0.925	0.726	0.857
50% noise	$1 \leq n_i \leq 8$	QAM+OCM	0.936	0.929	0.828	0.898
75% noise	$1 \leq n_i \leq 8$	Baseline	0.820	0.828	0.512	0.720
75% noise	$1 \leq n_i \leq 8$	QAM	0.898	0.825	0.536	0.753
75% noise	$1 \leq n_i \leq 8$	QAM+OCM	0.937	0.939	0.809	0.895
25% noise	$5 \leq n_i \leq 13$	Baseline	0.865	0.857	0.422	0.715
25% noise	$5 \leq n_i \leq 13$	QAM	0.893	0.835	0.615	0.781
25% noise	$5 \leq n_i \leq 13$	QAM+OCM	0.935	0.935	0.801	0.890
50% noise	$5 \leq n_i \leq 13$	Baseline	0.755	0.807	0.393	0.652
50% noise	$5 \leq n_i \leq 13$	QAM	0.828	0.853	0.491	0.714
50% noise	$5 \leq n_i \leq 13$	QAM+OCM	0.942	0.942	0.853	0.912
75% noise	$5 \leq n_i \leq 13$	Baseline	0.745	0.738	0.381	0.621
75% noise	$5 \leq n_i \leq 13$	QAM	0.770	0.772	0.366	0.636
75% noise	$5 \leq n_i \leq 13$	QAM+OCM	0.938	0.937	0.801	0.892

all three segmentation tasks. But as the noise level increases both in the area and ratio, the segmentation performance for the baseline method decreases sharply. The results for smaller anatomical structures, such as clavicles, suffer terribly. However, when adding the modules of quality awareness and overfitting control, the segmentation network can recover and even retain its high accuracy. We observe that the performance of our method is comparable to the model trained on clean datasets. Figure 3 shows the average class accuracy and loss curves of the network on the noisy-labeled datasets with different noise levels. Compared with high loss values without adding the modules, the quality awareness network can find out the relative better examples and show lower loss during training.

Effect of Overfitting Control Module. We also evaluated the influence of the overfitting control module in the experiment. The quality awareness module without overfitting control shows smaller training loss on the training set on all noise levels, but the test score is below the result of the experiments with the overfitting control module. When noise level increases, the final test accuracy for segmentation network is relatively high at some noise levels, but it performs badly and is extremely unstable. For example, for clavicles, when 75% of the labels are noisy-labeled, and $5 \leq n_i \leq 13$, the segmentation accuracy without the overfitting control module decreases from 0.862 to 0.366, which is even worse compared with baseline method, but with such strategy, the network can still keep a 0.801 segmentation accuracy. The network with the overfitting control module consistently retains its high accuracy when the noise level increases and shows a stable and competitive result. Experiment results demonstrate that without overfitting control module, the network suffers severe overfitting and will lose its ability in generalization.

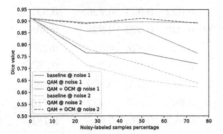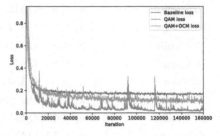

Fig. 3. Average class accuracy and loss plots of different noise levels on JSRT. Noise 1 and noise 2 represent $1 \leq n_i \leq 8$ and $5 \leq n_i \leq 13$ respectively. Loss curves belong to models trained on the training set with 50% of labels dilated or eroded 8 to 13 pixels.

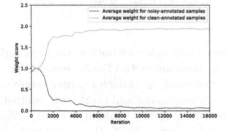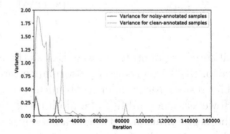

Fig. 4. Relative weights and variances for clean and noisy-labeled data.

Evaluating the Selecting Policy. We evaluated the performance of the label quality evaluation strategy during the training process. At different steps, we calculated the average weight of the noisy-labeled data and clean data. We tested the network on the dataset with 50% of its mini-batch are $5 \leq n_i \leq 13$ pixels dilated or eroded from its correct annotation. Figure 4 shows the analysis. At the beginning of the training, the network cannot separate between these two types of data. However, the relative score given to the clean samples gradually goes higher, and the ratio between good samples and noisy-labeled samples got larger, showing that quality awareness module can pick out some of the clean-labeled samples first. As training goes further, the variance value of the weight decreases, indicating that quality evaluation strategy can gradually find a consistent criteria of picking clean annotated samples and gradually increase its recall rate. The network can find out bad samples very quickly, and with the overfitting control module, it can gradually find more clean annotated samples for training. The weight value for the samples with same quality is getting more and more stable.

4 Conclution

In this paper, we have proposed a method to tune the segmentation network on noisy-labeled datasets called label quality evaluation strategy, which consists of three parts: segmentation module, quality awareness module, and overfitting control module. Quality awareness module can evaluate the relative quality of the labels in the mini-batch and re-weight them, and the overfitting control module can retain the generalization of the network. Compared with models without this method, our quality awareness model keeps high segmentation accuracy when the noise level increases. We have presented and analyzed the efficiency and necessity of these two modules. Experimental results on the benchmark dataset demonstrate that our quality awareness network outperforms other methods on segmentation tasks and achieves very competitive results on the noisy-labels dataset with the state-of-the-art supervised methods trained on clean-annotated data.

Acknowledgement. This work is supported by the National Key Research and Development Program of China (No. 2018YFC0116800).

References

1. Simonyan, K., Zisserman, A.: Very deep convolutional networks for large-scale image recognition. arXiv preprint arXiv:1409.1556 (2014)
2. He, K., Zhang, X., Ren, S., Sun, J.: Deep residual learning for image recognition. In: Proceedings of the IEEE Conference on Computer Vision and Pattern Recognition, pp. 770–778 (2016)
3. Ronneberger, O., Fischer, P., Brox, T.: U-Net: convolutional networks for biomedical image segmentation. In: Navab, N., Hornegger, J., Wells, W.M., Frangi, A.F. (eds.) MICCAI 2015. LNCS, vol. 9351, pp. 234–241. Springer, Cham (2015). https://doi.org/10.1007/978-3-319-24574-4_28
4. Zhang, C., Bengio, S., Hardt, M., Recht, B., Vinyals, O.: Understanding deep learning requires rethinking generalization. In: ICLR (2017)
5. Goldberger, J., Ben-Reuven, E.: Training deep neural-networks using a noise adaptation layer (2016)
6. Patrini, G., Rozza, A., Krishna Menon, A., Nock, R., Qu, L.: Making deep neural networks robust to label noise: a loss correction approach. In: Proceedings of the IEEE Conference on Computer Vision and Pattern Recognition, pp. 1944–1952 (2017)

7. Jiang, L., Zhou, Z., Leung, T., Li, L.J., Fei-Fei, L.: MentorNet: regularizing very deep neural networks on corrupted labels. arXiv preprint arXiv:1712.05055, April 2017

8. Tanaka, D., Ikami, D., Yamasaki, T., Aizawa, K.: Joint optimization framework for learning with noisy labels. In: Proceedings of the IEEE Conference on Computer Vision and Pattern Recognition, pp. 5552–5560 (2018)

9. Veit, A., Alldrin, N., Chechik, G., Krasin, I., Gupta, A., Belongie, S.: Learning from noisy large-scale datasets with minimal supervision. In: Proceedings of the IEEE Conference on Computer Vision and Pattern Recognition, pp. 839–847 (2017)

10. Dgani, Y., Greenspan, H., Goldberger, J.: Training a neural network based on unreliable human annotation of medical images. In: 2018 IEEE 15th International Symposium on Biomedical Imaging (ISBI 2018), pp. 39–42. IEEE, April 2018

11. Xue, C., Dou, Q., Shi, X., Chen, H., Heng, P.A.: Robust learning at noisy labeled medical images: applied to skin lesion classification. arXiv preprint arXiv:1901.07759 (2019)

12. Shiraishi, J., et al.: Development of a digital image database for chest radiographs with and without a lung nodule: receiver operating characteristic analysis of radiologists' detection of pulmonary nodules. AJR **174**, 71–74 (2000)

Anatomical Priors for Image Segmentation via Post-processing with Denoising Autoencoders

Agostina J. Larrazabal, Cesar Martinez, and Enzo Ferrante(✉)

Research Institute for Signals, Systems and Computational Intelligence, sinc(i),
FICH-UNL/CONICET, Santa Fe, Argentina
eferrante@sinc.unl.edu.ar

Abstract. Deep convolutional neural networks (CNN) proved to be highly accurate to perform anatomical segmentation of medical images. However, some of the most popular CNN architectures for image segmentation still rely on post-processing strategies (e.g. Conditional Random Fields) to incorporate connectivity constraints into the resulting masks. These post-processing steps are based on the assumption that objects are usually continuous and therefore nearby pixels should be assigned the same object label. Even if it is a valid assumption in general, these methods do not offer a straightforward way to incorporate more complex priors like convexity or arbitrary shape restrictions.

In this work we propose Post-DAE, a post-processing method based on denoising autoencoders (DAE) trained using only segmentation masks. We learn a low-dimensional space of anatomically plausible segmentations, and use it as a post-processing step to impose shape constraints on the resulting masks obtained with arbitrary segmentation methods. Our approach is independent of image modality and intensity information since it employs only segmentation masks for training. This enables the use of anatomical segmentations that do not need to be paired with intensity images, making the approach very flexible. Our experimental results on anatomical segmentation of X-ray images show that Post-DAE can improve the quality of noisy and incorrect segmentation masks obtained with a variety of standard methods, by bringing them back to a feasible space, with almost no extra computational time.

Keywords: Anatomical segmentation · Autoencoders · Convolutional neural networks · Learning representations · Post-processing

1 Introduction

Segmentation of anatomical structures is a fundamental task for biomedical image analysis. It constitutes the first step in several medical procedures such

Electronic supplementary material The online version of this chapter (https://doi.org/10.1007/978-3-030-32226-7_65) contains supplementary material, which is available to authorized users.

© Springer Nature Switzerland AG 2019
D. Shen et al. (Eds.): MICCAI 2019, LNCS 11769, pp. 585–593, 2019.
https://doi.org/10.1007/978-3-030-32226-7_65

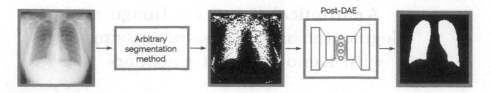

Fig. 1. Post-DAE works as a post-processing step and improves the anatomical plausability of segmentation masks obtained with arbitrary methods.

as shape analysis for population studies, computed assisted diagnosis and automatic radiotherapy planning, among many others. The accuracy and anatomical plausibility of these segmentations is therefore of paramount importance, since it will necessarily influence the overall quality of such procedures.

During the last years, convolutional neural networks (CNNs) proved to be highly accurate to perform segmentation in biomedical images [1–3]. One of the tricks that enables the use of CNNs in large images (by reducing the number of learned parameters) is known as parameter sharing scheme. The assumption behind this idea is that, at every layer, shared parameters are used to learn new representations of the input data along the whole image. These parameters (also referred as weights or kernels) are successively convoluted with the input data resulting in more abstract representations. This trick is especially useful for tasks like image classification, where invariance to translation is a desired property since objects may appear in any location. However, in case of anatomical structures in medical images where their location tend to be highly regular, this property leads to incorrect predictions in areas with similar intensities when enough contextual information is not considered. Shape and topology tend also to be preserved in anatomical images of the same type. However, as discussed in [4], the pixel-level predictions of most CNN architectures are not designed to account for higher-order topological properties.

Before the advent of CNNs, other classical learning based segmentation methods were popular for this task (e.g. Random Forest (RF) [5]), some of which are still being used specially when the amount of annotated data is not enough to train deep CNNs. The pixel-level predictions of these approaches are also influenced by image patches of fixed size. In these cases, handcrafted features are extracted from image patches and used to train a classifier, which predicts the class corresponding to the central pixel in that patch. These methods suffer from the same limitations related to the lack of shape and topological information discussed before.

In this work, we introduce Post-DAE (post-processing with denoising autoencoders), a post-processing method which produces anatomically plausible segmentations by improving pixel-level predictions coming from arbitrary classifiers (e.g. CNNs or RF), incorporating shape and topological priors. We employ Denoising Autoencoders (DAE) to learn compact and non-linear representations of anatomical structures, using only segmentation masks. This model is then applied as a post-processing method for image segmentation, bringing arbitrary and potentially erroneous segmentation masks into an anatomically plausible space (see Fig. 1).

Contributions. Our contributions are 3-fold: (i) we show, for the first time, that DAE can be used as an independent post-processing step to correct problematic and non-anatomically plausible masks produced by arbitrary segmentation methods; (ii) we design a method that can be trained using segmentation-only datasets or anatomical masks coming from arbitrary image modalities, since the DAE is trained using only segmentation masks, and no intensity information is required during learning; (iii) we validate Post-DAE in the context of lung segmentation in X-ray images, bench-marking with other classical post-processing method and showing its robustness by improving segmentation masks coming from both, CNN and RF-based classifiers.

Related Works. One popular strategy to incorporate prior knowledge about shape and topology into medical image segmentation is to modify the loss used to train the model. The work of [4] incorporates high-order regularization through a topology aware loss function. The main disadvantage is that such loss function is constructed ad-hoc for every dataset, requiring the user to manually specify the topological relations between the semantic classes through a topological validity table. More similar to our work are those by [6,7], where an autoencoder (AE) is used to learn lower dimensional representations of image anatomy. The AE is used to define a loss term that imposes anatomical constraints during training. The main disadvantage of these approaches is that they can only be used during training of CNN architectures. Other methods like RF-based segmentation can not be improved through this technique. On the contrary, our method post-processes arbitrary segmentation masks. Therefore, it can be used to improve results obtained with any segmentation method, even those methods which do not rely on an explicit training phase (e.g. level-sets methods).

Post-processing methods have also been considered in the literature. In [3], the output CNN scores are considered as unary potentials of a Markov random field (MRF) energy minimization problem, where spatial homogeneity is propagated through pairwise relations. Similarly, [2] uses a fully connected conditional random field (CRF) as post-processing step. However, as stated by [2], finding a global set of parameters for the graphical models which can consistently improve the segmentation of all classes remains a challenging problem. Moreover, these methods do not incorporate shape priors. Instead, they are based on the assumption that objects are usually continuous and therefore nearby pixels (or pixels with similar appearence) should be assigned the same object label. Conversely, our post-processing method makes use of a DAE to impose shape priors, transforming any segmentation mask into an anatomically plausible one.

2   Anatomical Priors for Image Segmentation via Post-processing with DAE

Problem Statement. Given a dataset of unpaired anatomical segmentation masks $\mathcal{D}_\mathcal{A} = \{S_i^A\}_{0 \le i \le |\mathcal{D}_\mathcal{A}|}$ (unpaired in the sense that no corresponding intensity image associated to the segmentation mask is required) we aim at learning

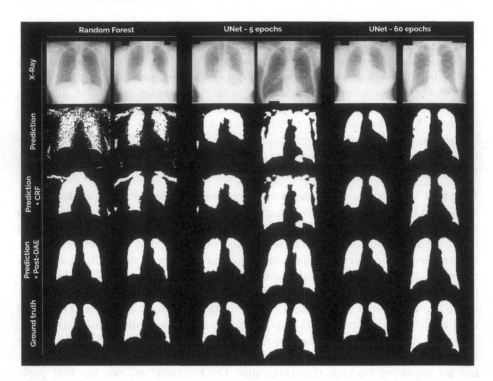

Fig. 2. Predictions obtained with three different methods: Random Forest, UNet trained for 5 epochs and until convergence. Rows from top to bottom: (i) X-Ray image; (ii) original mask obtained with the corresponding method; (iii) mask post-processed with a fully connected CRF; (iv) mask post-processed with the proposed Post-DAE method; and (v) ground-truth.

a model that can bring segmentations $\mathcal{D}_\mathcal{P} = \{S_i^P\}_{0 \leq i \leq |\mathcal{D}_\mathcal{P}|}$ predicted by arbitrary classifiers P into an anatomically feasible space. We stress the fact that our method works as a post-processing step in the space of segmentations, making it independent of the predictor, image intensities and modality. We employ denoising autoencoders (DAE) to learn such model.

Denoising Autoencoders. DAEs are neural networks designed to reconstruct a clean input from a corrupted version of it [8]. In our case, they will be used to reconstruct anatomically plausible segmentation masks from corrupted or erroneous ones. The standard architecture for an autoencoder follows an encoder-decoder scheme (see the Sup. Mat. for a detailed description of the architecture used in this work). The encoder $f_{enc}(S_i)$ is a mapping that transforms the input into a hidden representation h. In our case, it consists of successive non-linearities, pooling and convolutional layers, with a final fully connected layer that concentrates all information into a low dimensional code h. This code is then feed into the decoder $f_{dec}(h)$, which maps it back to the original input dimensions through a series of up-convolutions and non-linearities. The output of $f_{dec}(h)$ has the same size than the input S_i.

The model is called *denosing* autoenconder because a degradation function ϕ is used to degrade the ground-truth segmentation masks, producing noisy segmentations $\hat{S}_i = \phi(S_i)$ used for training. The model is trained to minimize the reconstruction error measured by a loss function based on the Dice coefficient (DSC), a metric used to compare the quality of predicted segmentations with respect to the ground-truth (we refer the reader to [9] for a complete description of the Dice loss):

$$\mathcal{L}_{DAE}(S_i) = DSC(S_i, f_{dec}(f_{enc}(\phi(S_i)))). \tag{1}$$

The dimensionality of the learned representation $h = f_{enc}(S_i)$ is much lower than the input, producing a bottleneck effect which forces the code h to retain as much information as possible about the input. In that way, minimizing the reconstruction error amounts to maximizing a lower bound on the mutual information between input S_i and the learnt representation h [8].

Mask Degradation Strategy. The masks used to train the DAE were artificially degraded during training to simulate erroneous segmentations. To this end, we randomly apply the following degradation functions $\phi(S_i)$ to the ground truth masks S_i: (i) addition and removal of random geometric shapes (circles, ellipses, lines and rectangles) to simulate over and under segmentations; (ii) morphological operations (e.g. erosion, dilation, etc.) with variable kernels to perform more subtle mask modifications and (iii) random swapping of foreground-background labels in the pixels close to the mask borders.

Note that, even if the proposed degradation strategy does not represent the distribution of masks generated by a particular classifier, it worked well in practice when post-processing both, random forest and U-Net masks. However, better results could be obtained if we know the classifier beforehand, by feeding the predicted segmentation masks while training the DAE.

Post-processing with DAEs. The proposed method is rooted in the so-called manifold assumption [10], which states that natural high dimensional data (like anatomical segmentation masks) concentrate close to a non-linear low-dimensional manifold. We learn such low-dimensional anatomically plausible manifold using the aforementioned DAE. Then, given a segmentation mask S_i^P obtained with an arbitrary predictor P (e.g. CNN or RF), we project it into that manifold using f_{enc} and reconstruct the corresponding anatomically feasible mask with f_{dec}. Unlike other methods like [6,7] which incorporate the anatomical priors while training the segmentation network, we choose to make it a post-processing step. In that way, we achieve independence with respect to the initial predictor, and enable improvement for arbitrary segmentation methods.

Our hypothesis (empirically validated by the following experiments) is that those masks which are far from the anatomical space, will be mapped to a similar, but anatomically plausible segmentation. Meanwhile, masks which are anatomically correct, will be mapped to themselves, incurring in almost no modification.

3 Experiments and Discussion

Database Description. We benchmark the proposed method in the context of lung segmentation in X-Ray images, using the Japanese Society of Radiological Technology (JSRT) database [11]. JSRT is a public database containing 247 PA chest X-ray images with expert segmentation masks, of 2048×2048 pixels and isotropic spacing of 0.175 mm/pixel, which are downsampled to 1024×1024 in our experiments. Lungs present high variability among subjects, making the representation learning task especially challenging. Note that we did not perform any pre-processing regarding image alignment. We divide the database in 3 folds considering 70% for training, 10% for validation and 20% for testing. The same folds were used to train the U-Net, Random Forest and Post-DAE methods.

Post-processing with DAE. Post-DAE receives a 1024×1024 binary segmentation as input. The network was trained to minimize the Dice loss function using Adam Optimizer. We employed learning rate 0.0001; batch size of 15 and 150 epochs.

Post-processing with CRF. We compare Post-DAE with the SOA post-processing method based on a fully connected CRF [12]. The CRF is used to impose connectivity constraints to a given segmentation, based on the assumption that objects are usually continuous and nearby pixels with similar appearance should be assigned the same object label. We use an efficient implementation of a dense CRF[1] that can handle large pixel neighbourhoods in reasonable inference times. Differently from our method which uses only binary segmentations for post-processing, the CRF incorporates intensity information from the original images. Therefore, it has to be re-adjusted depending on the image properties of every dataset. Instead, our method is trained once and can be used independently of the image properties. Note that we do not compare Post-DAE with other methods like [6,7] which incorporate anatomical priors while training the segmentation method itself, since these are not post-processing strategies.

Baseline Segmentation Methods. We train two different models which produce segmentation masks of various qualities to benchmark our post-processing method. The first model is a CNN based on UNet architecture [1] (see the Sup. Mat. for a detailed description of the architecture and the training parameters such as optimizer, learning rate, etc.). The UNet was implemented in Keras and trained in GPU using a Dice loss function. To evaluate the effect of Post-DAE in different masks, we save the UNet model every 5 epochs during training, and predict segmentation masks for the test fold using all these models. The second method is a RF classifier trained using intensity and texture features. We used Haralick [13] features which are based on gray level co-ocurrency in

---

[1] We used the public implementation available at https://github.com/lucasb-eyer/pydensecrf with Potts compatibility function and hand-tuned parameters $\theta_\alpha = 17$, $\theta_\beta = 3$, $\theta_\gamma = 3$ chosen using the validation fold. See the implementation website for more details about the aforementioned parameters.

image patches. We adopted a public implementation available online with default parameters[2] which produces acceptable segmentation masks.

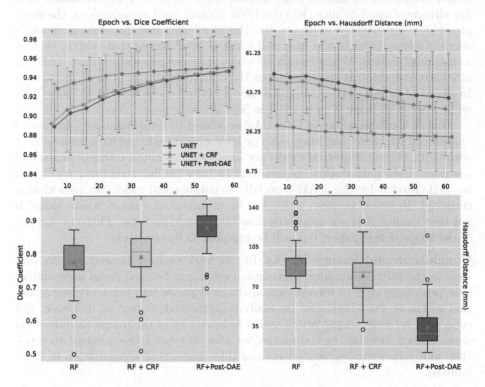

Fig. 3. Quantitative evaluation of the proposed method. We compare Post-DAE with the classic fully-connected CRF [12] adopted as post-processing step by many segmentation methods like [2]. Top row shows mean and standard deviation for post-processing UNet predictions on the test fold at different training stages (from 5 epochs to convergence). We use Dice coefficient and Hausdorff distance to measure the segmentation quality. Bottom row show results for post-processing the Random Forest predictions. The symbol ∗ indicates that Post-DAE outperforms the other methods (no post-processing and CRF) with statistical significance (p-value < 0.05 according to Wilcoxon test). The green triangle in the box indicates the mean value. (Color figure online)

Results and Discussion. Figure 2 shows some visual examples while Fig. 3 summarizes the quantitative results (see the video in the Sup. Mat. for more visual results). Both figures show the consistent improvement that can be obtained using Post-DAE as a post-processing step, specially in low quality segmentation masks like those obtained by the RF model and the UNet trained for

---

[2] The source code and a complete description of the method is publicly available online at: https://github.com/dgriffiths3/ml_segmentation.

only 5 epochs. In these cases, substantial improvements are obtained in terms of Dice coefficient and Hausdorff distance, by bringing the erroneous segmentation masks into an anatomically feasible space. In case of segmentations that are already of good quality (like the UNet trained until convergence), the postprocessing significantly improves the Hausdorff distance, by erasing spurious segmentations (holes in the lung and small isolated blobs) that remain even in well trained models. When compared with CRF post-processing, Post-DAE significantly outperforms the baseline in the context of anatomical segmentation. In terms of running time, the CRF model takes 1.3 s in a Intel i7-7700 CPU, while Post-DAE takes 0.7 s in a Titan Xp GPU.

One of the limitations of Post-DAE is related to data regularity. In case of anatomical structures like lung, heart or liver, even if we found high inter-subject variability, the segmentation masks are somehow uniform in terms of shape and topology. Even pathological organs tend to have similar structure, which can be well-encoded by the DAE (specially if pathological cases are seen during training). However, in other cases like brain lesions or tumors where shape is not that regular, it is not clear how Post-DAE would perform. This case lies out of the scope of this paper, but will be explored as future work.

Conclusions and Future Works. In this work we have showed, for the first time in the MIC community, that autoencoders can be used as an independent post-processing step to incorporate anatomical priors into arbitrary segmentation methods. Post-DAE can be easily implemented, is fast at inference, can cope with arbitrary shape priors and is independent of the image modality and segmentation method. In the future, we plan to extend this method to muti-class and volumetric segmentation cases (like anatomical segmentation in brain images).

Acknowledgments. EF is beneficiary of an AXA Research Fund grant. The authors gratefully acknowledge NVIDIA Corporation with the donation of the Titan Xp GPU used for this research, and the support of UNL (CAID-PIC-50420150100098LI) and ANPCyT (PICT 2016-0651).

References

1. Ronneberger, O., Fischer, P., Brox, T.: U-Net: convolutional networks for biomedical image segmentation. In: Navab, N., Hornegger, J., Wells, W.M., Frangi, A.F. (eds.) MICCAI 2015. LNCS, vol. 9351, pp. 234–241. Springer, Cham (2015). https://doi.org/10.1007/978-3-319-24574-4_28
2. Kamnitsas, K., et al.: Efficient multi-scale 3d CNN with fully connected CRF for accurate brain lesion segmentation. Med. Image Anal. **36**, 61–78 (2017)
3. Shakeri, M., et al.: Sub-cortical brain structure segmentation using F-CNN's. In: Proceedings of ISBI (2016)
4. BenTaieb, A., Hamarneh, G.: Topology aware fully convolutional networks for histology gland segmentation. In: Proceedings of MICCAI (2016)
5. Breiman, L.: Random forests. Mach. Learn. **45**(1), 5–32 (2001)
6. Oktay, O., et al.: Anatomically constrained neural networks (ACNNs): application to cardiac image enhancement and segmentation. IEEE TMI **37**(2), 384–395 (2018)

7. Ravishankar, H., et al.: Learning and incorporating shape models for semantic segmentation. In: Proceedings of MICCAI (2017)
8. Vincent, P., et al.: Stacked denoising autoencoders: Learning useful representations in a deep network with a local denoising criterion. JMLR **11**, 3371–3408 (2010)
9. Milletari, F., Navab, N., Ahmadi, S.A.: V-Net: fully convolutional neural networks for volumetric medical image segmentation. In: Proceedings of Fourth International Conference on 3D Vision (3DV) (2016)
10. Chapelle, O., Scholkopf, B., Zien, A.: Semi-Supervised Learning. MIT Press, Cambridge (2009)
11. Shiraishi, J., et al.: Development of a digital image database for chest radiographs with and without a lung nodule: receiver operating characteristic analysis of radiologists' detection of pulmonary nodules. Am. J. Roentgenol. **174**(1), 71–74 (2000)
12. Krähenbühl, P., Koltun, V.: Efficient inference in fully connected CRFs with Gaussian edge potentials. In: Proceedings of Nips (2011)
13. Haralick, R.M., Shanmugam, K., et al.: Textural features for image classification. IEEE Trans. Syst. Man Cybern. **6**, 610–621 (1973)

Simultaneous Lung Field Detection and Segmentation for Pediatric Chest Radiographs

Wei Zhang[1], Guanbin Li[1], Fuyu Wang[1], Longjiang E[2], Yizhou Yu[3],
Liang Lin[1], and Huiying Liang[2]([✉])

[1] Sun Yat-sen University, Guangzhou, Guangdong, China
[2] Institute of Pediatrics, Guangzhou Women and Children's Medical Center,
Guangzhou Medical University, Guangzhou, Guangdong, China
lianghuiying@hotmail.com
[3] Deepwise AI Lab, Beijing, China

Abstract. Accurate lung field segmentation (LFS) method is highly demanded in computer-aid diagnosis (CAD) system. However, LFS in pediatric CXR images has received few attention due to the lack of publicly available dataset and the challenges caused by their unique characteristics, such as great variations of the size, location and orientation of lungs. To fill this gap, this paper for the first time presents a simultaneous lung field detection and segmentation framework for pediatric CXR images. Our framework, called SDSLung Net, is a multi-tasking convolutional neural network architecture tailor-made for X-ray images with relatively weak appearance feature but abundant spatial rules and structural information. It is adapted from a Mask R-CNN framework [1] by incorporating a newly designed Organ Structure-Aware Encoding layer in the backbone network for more accurate spatial variation and structural representation, in parallel with a deeply supervised fully convolutional network based segmentation branch for precise lung field segmentation inside detected bounding box. Moreover, we also constructed a new and so far the largest pediatric CXR dataset with pixelwise lung field annotations. Experimental results demonstrate that our proposed SDSLung is capable of achieving significantly superior performance over state-of-the-art LFS methods on our large-scale pediatric CXR dataset and also achieving extremely competitive results on adults' CXR dataset.

Keywords: Pediatric CXR images · Lung field segmentation · Segmentation · Detection

1 Introduction

With the potential to reduce the workloads of radiologists and facilite appropriate treatments, Computer-Aid Diagnosis (CAD) for Chest X-ray (CXR) images has long been desired, especially in pediatrics where the increasing shortage of radiologists has been widely noticed. In CAD systems, lung field segmentation

© Springer Nature Switzerland AG 2019
D. Shen et al. (Eds.): MICCAI 2019, LNCS 11769, pp. 594–602, 2019.
https://doi.org/10.1007/978-3-030-32226-7_66

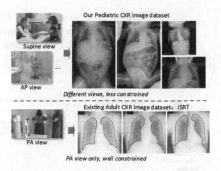

Fig. 1. An illustration of the difference between our pediatric CXR image dataset and existing adults' CXR image dataset. The lung field segmentation results of our framework and the ground-truth are shown in red and green curves, respectively. As can be observed, our framework produces high quality lung field segmentation results on both datasets. (Color figure online)

(LFS) which precisely recognizes lung fields acts as a crucial role for intelligent diagnosis, e.g. pediatric atelectasis analysis. Unfortunately, the existing LFS study did not pay sufficient attention to pediatric CXR images. Besides the inherent difficulties in conventional CXR images, pediatric CXR images also features significant variations in terms of sizes, positions and orientations of lung fields, making the LFS significantly more challenging than in conventional adults' CXR images. Examples are shown in Fig. 1. Although numbers of LFS methods have been proposed based on publicly available JSRT dataset [2] and MC dataset [3], they are limited in handling pediatric CXR images due to the lack of precise lung field positioning. Moreover, existing LFS datasets only contain adults' CXR images which are filmed under standard posterior-antero (PA) view such that accurate lung field localization is less discussed in existing LFS studies. Therefore, to deal with aforementioned difficulties of LFS in pediatric CXR images, novel LFS methods that can simultaneously perform lung field detection and mask segmentation inside detected regions are particularly demanded.

To fill this gap, in this paper, we present a novel simultaneous lung field detection and segmentation framework for pediatric CXR images. Simultaneous object detection and segmentation (SDS) [4], also known as instance level object segmentation [1,5,6], is an important research topic in the field of computer vision, which aims at accurately detecting and segmenting generic objects of some specific categories in natural scenes. Although the goal of LFS appears to be consistent with SDS, borrowing the techniques of SDS to LFS is non-trivial due to the following reasons: first, compared with SDS models developed for natural scenes, SDS models for CXR images is expected to be simple in classification part (only left and right lung are considered) but demand more precise segmentation of lung fields to serve as important cues for diagnosis. Second, there exist inherent differences between natural images and CXR images – natural images are rich in color and texture information while CXR images are in gray-scale with lower contrast and fewer textures. Most importantly, SDS models developed for natural

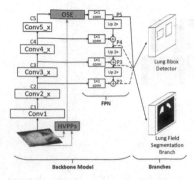

Fig. 2. The overall framework of
our proposed *SDSLung Net*.

Table 1. A comparison between our newly collected Pediatric CXR Dataset and existing publicly available LFS datasets. Our dataset is significantly larger than existing datasets.

Dataset	# CXR	View	Age	gt Mask
JSRT	247	PA	4–89 years old	✓
MC	138	PA	16–84 years old	✓
Ours	**733**	**PA, Supine, etc.**	1 day–14 years old	✓

images solely rely on Deep Convolutional Neural Networks (DCNNs) to extract
feature representations, in which the anatomical structure of lung fields in CXR
images is not well utilized. Inspired by Mask R-CNN [1], an elegant end-to-end
neural network framework for object instance segmentation, we propose to adapt
it for lung field segmentation in CXR images by addressing the aforementioned
issues. We conduct comprehensive experiments on a newly constructed and so-far
the largest pediatric LFS dataset, demonstrating state-of-the-art performance.
Moreover, our proposed framework achieves extremely competitive results on
adults' CXR dataset.

Pediatric CXR Dataset. We collaborate with one Women and Children's
Hospital and collect 733 pediatric CXR images from their daily clinical practice.
According to pediatric clinical requirements, the collected CXR images are filmed
under different views, such as supine antero-posterior (AP) and posterior-antero
(PA). The collected CXR images are densely sampled from the age range of 1 day
to over 10 years old, in which the appearance of lungs manifests more variations
compared with other age ranges. We invite experienced pediatric radiologists to
manually segment the lung field for each CXR image.

A comparison between our newly collected Pediatric CXR Dataset and existing publicly available LFS datasets is shown in Table 1.

2   SDSLung Net

As illustrated in Fig. 2, the framework of *SDSLung Net*, which is adapted from
Mask-RCNN, contains two branches: one bounding box detector that localizes
two lungs in CXR images and a segmentation branch that aims at precisely
masking out the lung region inside each detected lung box. Both of the two
branches share the same backbone model, in which a newly proposed *Organ
Structure-Aware Encoding* (OSE) layer is integrated with vanilla ResNet [7].
Inspired by the common practice in modern object detection and instance segmentation frameworks [1,8], we add a top-down path with lateral connections
in the form of the Feature Pyramid Network (FPN) [8], connected to the top of

ResNet-OSE, to take full account of multi-scale deep features (P5 to P2) while performing detection and segmentation inference.

Organ Structure-Aware Encoding. Based on the observation of the horizontal and vertical regular structural relationships between the lung fields and the surrounding torso region, we introduce scanning operations in OSE layer. As shown in Fig. 3(a), *(i)* there exists certain column-wise and row-wise regularity in the gray-scale patterns across lung fields; *(ii)* the ups and downs in horizontal and vertical projections contain useful cues for distinguishing body and background as well as the localization of lung fields. We rely on Recurrent Neural Networks (RNN) to capture anatomical structure around lung fields across the torso region, since fully convolutional layers are not adept at modeling such long-range dependencies. Specifically, we adopt ReNet [9,10] which is composed of 4 Gated Recurrent Units (GRUs) that perform horizontal and vertical sweeps respectively. The architecture of OSE layer is depicted in Fig. 4. Next, we further introduce global image information in the scanning process to enhance the feature representation of the backbone network. Traditionally, horizontal and vertical projection profiles (HVPPs) [11] are wildly adopted to probing the distribution of patterns in simple gray-scale images, such as text lines in handwriting samples and lung fields in high-contrast PA CXR images. We propose to incorporate HVPPs into the scanning process to serve as image-level cues. Formally, the horizontal projection profile l^h and vertical projection profile l^v are defined as:

$$l_j^h = \frac{1}{H} \sum_{i=1}^{H} s_{i,j}, \quad l_i^v = \frac{1}{W} \sum_{j=1}^{W} s_{i,j} \tag{1}$$

Where H, W denotes the height, width of the input gray-scale CXR image. $s_{i,j}$ denotes the gray-scale value of pixel located at i, j. One example of HVPPs is shown in Fig. 3. To make the projection profiles compact, l^h and l^v are downsampled to an uniform dimension of 128×1. We subsequently make use of the downsampled HVPP vectors by feeding them to GRUs.

Each OSE layer takes as input the raw input image or the feature activation of one intermediate layer. Formally, we denote the input tensor by $X = x_{i,j} \in \mathbb{R}^{H' \times W' \times C}$ where H', W' and C denotes the height, width and the number of channels, respectively. In order to perform the sweeps in orthogonal directions efficiently, we divide the input tensor X into a grid, which consists of $I \times J$ non-overlapping patches $P = \{p_{i,j}\}$, where each patch $p_{i,j} \in \mathbb{R}^{\in H_p \times W_p \times C}$. We first sweep horizontally from left to right and right to left with two GRUs $f^{\rightarrow}$ and $f^{\leftarrow}$. For the sweeps working alone row j in the grid, every time step each GRUs takes as input the next non-overlapping patch $p_{i,j}$ as well as the downsampled vertical projection profile l^v, producing horizontally encoded feature $o_{i,j}^{\rightarrow}$ (or $o_{i,j}^{\leftarrow}$) and updates its hidden states $z_{i-1,j}^{\rightarrow}$ (or $z_{i+1,j}^{\leftarrow}$):

$$o_{i,j}^{\rightarrow} = f^{\rightarrow}(z_{i-1,j}^{\rightarrow}, \{p_{i,j}, l^v\}), \quad for\ i = 1, ...I$$
$$o_{i,j}^{\leftarrow} = f^{\leftarrow}(z_{i+1,j}^{\leftarrow}, \{p_{i,j}, l^v\}), \quad for\ i = I, ...1 \tag{2}$$

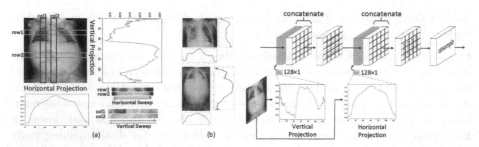

Fig. 3. (a) is an illustration of our observations regarding the anatomical structure of torso in CXR images. (b) provides two more examples of the horizontal and vertical projections.

Fig. 4. The architecture of OSE layer.

Once the two GRUs have processed all rows in the grid of X, the horizontally encoded features $o_{i,j}^{\rightarrow}$ and $o_{i,j}^{\leftarrow}$ are concatenated to obtain a horizontal organ structure-aware feature representation $O^{\leftrightarrow}$, where $O^{\leftrightarrow} \in \mathbb{R}^{\in H_p \times W_p \times 2U}$. U denotes the dimension of encoded feature $o_{i,j}^{\rightarrow}$ (or $o_{i,j}^{\leftarrow}$) emitted by one directional GRUs at each step. Similarly, column-wise bidirectional sweeps are then performed vertically on $O^{\leftrightarrow}$ as well as the downsampled horizontal projection profile l^h using another pair of GRUs $f^{\downarrow}$ and $f^{\uparrow}$. We concatenate $o_{i,j}^{\downarrow}$ and $o_{i,j}^{\uparrow}$ to obtain a composite feature map. Finally, we upsample the obtained feature representation to the same size as the input of OSE layer, allowing the OSE layer can be integrated at any stage of CNN architecture. We found that with one OSE layer inserted between the encoding and decoding stages, the whole pipeline reaches the best performance. The framework of our proposed *SDSLung Net* is illustrated in Fig. 2.

Lung Field Detector. To reduce the redundancy in CNN architecture, we cut out the classification part in Mask-rcnn which is originally designed for multiple object categories in natural scenes. Moreover, instead of using the anchor boxes in [1,12] with hand-picked aspect ratios, we consider the prior knowledge of aspect ratio of lungs to generate better anchor boxes for lung field detection. Specifically, we run k-means clustering on the training set lung field bounding boxes with the following distance metric:

$$d(box, centroid) = 1 - IOU(box, centroid). \tag{3}$$

Where the *box* and *centroid* denote the bounding box and current clustering centroid box, respectively.

Segmentation with Spatial Refinement. As the boundary precision is one of the key requirements in LFS, we propose a two-step architecture in lung field segmentation branch. In the first step, we obtain initial mask predictions using fully convolutional layers that work on low-resolution and fixed-size feature maps, then in the second step a multi-scale refinement sub-network is adopted to obtain high resolution segmentation results. In this refinement sub-network, we cast the architecture of HED [13] which features multi-scale representation and deep supervisions for spatial refinement. Besides, to include context information, we extend the size of each detected bounding box by a factor of 1.5. Then, the region inside the extended bounding box is cropped from the input image and concatenated with the initial mask prediction to form the input of the refinement sub-network. We apply deep supervisions on both of the initial mask and refined result.

Multi-task Loss. During the training phase, we define a multi-task loss that account for the lung detection and segmentation branches.

$$L = L_{obj} + L_{reg} + L_{seg}. \tag{4}$$

Following the objective functions in Faster-RCNN [12], we define an objectness loss L_{obj} over two classes (lung fields or not).

$$L_{obj} = -(\frac{1}{N_P} \sum_{i \in P} log(b_i) + \frac{1}{N_N} \sum_{j \in N} log(1 - b_j)), \tag{5}$$

where N_p and N_N denote the number of positive and negative anchors respectively with a ratio of 1:3. The regression loss accounts for predicting the offsets of lung field bounding boxes and is activated only for positive anchors $b_i^* = 1$:

$$L_{reg} = \frac{1}{N_{reg}} \sum_i b_i^* R(t_i - t_i^*), \tag{6}$$

where $t_i = (t_x^i, t_y^i, t_w^i, t_h^i)$ is the vector of offsets for bounding box i. R is the robust loss function (smooth L_1) defined in [14].

$$L_{seg} = -\frac{1}{N_{seg}} \sum_{s \in 1,2} (\sum_i (w_i log p_i^s + (1 - w_i) log(1 - p_i^s))),$$

We adopt a cross-entropy loss for the lung field segmentation branch, in which p_i^s is the predicted probability of pixel i belonging to lung field in the initial mask prediction or in the output of the refinement sub-network. The binary value $w_i = 1$ indicates that the groundtruth of pixel i belongs to lung field, otherwise $w_i = 0$. N_{seg} is the total number of pixels inside the detected bounding box.

3   Experiments

Implementation Details. We randomly select 489 CXR images from aforementioned pediatric CXR dataset as the training data and use the remaining 244 CXR images for testing. Our implementation is based on Tensorflow and each experiment runs on a Nvidia GTX1080 GPU. The input of refinement sub-network are scaled to $512 \times 320 \times 4$, in which the first 3 channels represent the cropped image and the rest 1 channel being the initial mask prediction. The architecture of the refinement sub-network is the same as in [13] except the input layer is modified to tolerate 4 channel's input. During the inference phase, we run the lung field detection branch to obtain 1000 box proposals. Subsequently, the lung field segmentation branch is performed on the 100 highest scoring boxes. Our training is conducted for 120 epochs in total with a learning rate of 0.001. We set the weight decay to 0.0001 and the momentum to 0.9.

Evaluation Metrics. We conduct quantitative evaluations using three commonly used metrics in previous LFS studies: *The Jaccard Similarity Coefficient*(JSC), *Dice's Coefficient*(DC) and *Average Contour Distance*(ACD). The detailed definitions of these metrics can be found in [15].

Table 2. Comparison with state-of-the-art LFS methods on our Pediatric CXR Dataset.

Method	JSC	DC
[15]	0.677±0.171	0.794±0.137
[16]	0.864±0.092	0.924±0.063
SDSLung Net	**0.901±0.062**	**0.947±0.038**

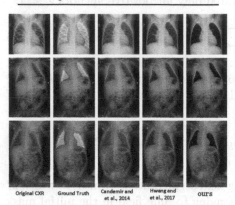

Original CXR | Ground Truth | Candemir and et al., 2014 | Hwang and et al., 2017 | ours

Fig. 5. A visual comparison between results of the proposed *SDSLung Net* and state-of-the-art LFS methods. Note our proposed SDS framework is also able to predict the bounding box of each lung field. Here, we only show the segmented mask for a better visualization.

Table 3. Comparison with state-of-the-art LFS methods on JSRT Dataset. Without the need of cumbersome network-wise training [16] *stage*3, the performance of the proposed *SDSLung Net* is almost equal to the state-of-the-art.

Method	JSC	DC	ACD
[17]	0.949 ± 0.020	-	1.62 ± 0.66
[15]	0.945 ± 0.015	0.967 ± 0.08	1.321 ± 0.316
[18]	0.947 ± 0.004	-	-
[19]	0.950	0.973	-
[16] *stage*1	0.950 ± 0.023	0.974 ± 0.012	1.347 ± 0.919
[16] *stage*3	**0.961 ± 0.015**	**0.980 ± 0.008**	1.237 ± 0.702
SDSLung Net	**0.961± 0.019**	**0.980±0.010**	1.261±0.242

Table 4. Performances of the proposed *SDSLung Net* by choosing different architectures for the backbone model. Note in all kinds of above settings, FPN is adopted while the refinement sub-network is not included. Note ResNet101 here denotes exactly the same backbone as in Mask-RCNN.

Backbone model	JSC	DC
ResNet101(Mask-rcnn)	0.856±0.020	0.923±0.002
ResNet18	0.868±0.015	0.905±0.030
ResNet18+OSE (w/o HVPPs)	0.880±0.007	0.936±0.014
ResNet18+OSE (w/HVPPs)	**0.884±0.061**	**0.937±0.037**

Comparisons Against Leading Methods. We compare the proposed *SDSLung Net* against two state-of-the-art LFS methods [15,16] on our newly collected pediatric CXR dataset. The quantitative comparison results are listed in Table 2. With the ability of simultaneous detection and segmentation, our method significantly outperform previous state-of-the-arts on the challenging pediatric CXR dataset. Besides, to test the adaptability of the proposed *SDSLung Net* to adults' CXR images, we also compare against state-of-the-art LFS methods on JSRT dataset. Results are listed in Table 3. As can be seen, our results significantly outperforms most of the leading methods. Moreover, we note *SDSLung Net* is able to achieve almost equal performance with [16] *stage3* which is obtained by repeating 3 stages of the network-wise training. Next, we provide a visual comparison in Fig. 5. As can be seen, our framework is able to predict satisfying results for difficult pediatric CXR images, surpassing previous state-of-the-art LFS methods.

The Effectiveness of Organ Structure-Aware Encoding. From the results listed in Table 4, we can observe 1.2% improvement in JSC gained by the RNN-based organ structure-aware encoding. By introducing HVPPs, another 0.4% improvement in JSC can be obtained.

4 Conclusions

In this paper, we present *SDSLung Net*, which is the first simultaneous lung field detection and segmentation framework for CXR images. We also introduce a novel Organ Structure-Aware Encoding layer as well as a multi-scale refinement sub-network, which allow the proposed *SDSLung Net* to achieve the state-of-the-art performance on both pediatric and adults' CXR dataset.

References

1. He, K., Gkioxari, G., Dollár, P., Girshick, R.: Mask R-CNN. In: Proceedings of the IEEE International Conference on Computer Vision, pp. 2961–2969 (2017)
2. Shiraishi, J., et al.: Development of a digital image database for chest radiographs with and without a lung nodule: receiver operating characteristic analysis of radiologists' detection of pulmonary nodules. Am. J. Roentgenol. **174**(1), 71–74 (2000)
3. Jaeger, S., et al.: Two public chest x-ray datasets for computer-aided screening of pulmonary diseases. Quant. Imaging Med. Surg. **4**(6), 475 (2014)
4. Hariharan, B., Arbeláez, P., Girshick, R., Malik, J.: Simultaneous detection and segmentation. In: Fleet, D., Pajdla, T., Schiele, B., Tuytelaars, T. (eds.) ECCV 2014. LNCS, vol. 8695, pp. 297–312. Springer, Cham (2014). https://doi.org/10.1007/978-3-319-10584-0_20
5. Pinheiro, P.O., Dollár, P.: Learning to segment object candidates. In: NIPS, pp. 1990–1998 (2015)
6. Dai, J., He, K., Li, Y., Ren, S., Sun, J.: Instance-sensitive fully convolutional networks. In: Leibe, B., Matas, J., Sebe, N., Welling, M. (eds.) ECCV 2016. LNCS, vol. 9910, pp. 534–549. Springer, Cham (2016). https://doi.org/10.1007/978-3-319-46466-4_32
7. He, K., et al.: Deep residual learning for image recognition. In: CVPR, pp. 770–778 (2016)

8. Lin, T.Y., Dollár, P., Girshick, R., He, K., Hariharan, B., Belongie, S.: Feature pyramid networks for object detection. In: Proceedings of the IEEE Conference on Computer Vision and Pattern Recognition, pp. 2117–2125 (2017)
9. Visin, F., et al.: ReNet: a recurrent neural network based alternative to convolutional networks. arXiv preprint arXiv:1505.00393 (2015)
10. Visin, F., et al.: ReSeg: a recurrent neural network-based model for semantic segmentation. In: CVPR Workshops, pp. 41–48 (2016)
11. Semmlow, J.L., et al.: Biosignal and Medical Image Processing. CRC Press, Boca Raton (2014)
12. Ren, S., et al.: Faster R-CNN: towards real-time object detection with region proposal networks. In: NIPS, pp. 91–99 (2015)
13. Xie, S., Tu, Z.: Holistically-nested edge detection. In: ICCV, pp. 1395–1403 (2015)
14. Girshick, R.: Fast R-CNN. In: ICCV, pp. 1440–1448 (2015)
15. Candemir, S., et al.: Lung segmentation in chest radiographs using anatomical atlases with nonrigid registration. IEEE Trans. Med. Imaging 33(2), 577–590 (2014)
16. Hwang, S., Park, S.: Accurate lung segmentation via network-wise training of convolutional networks. In: Cardoso, M.J., et al. (eds.) DLMIA/ML-CDS -2017. LNCS, vol. 10553, pp. 92–99. Springer, Cham (2017). https://doi.org/10.1007/978-3-319-67558-9_11
17. Van Ginneken, B., et al.: Segmentation of anatomical structures in chest radiographs using supervised methods: a comparative study on a public database. Med. Image Anal. 10(1), 19–40 (2006)
18. Dai, W., et al.: Scan: structure correcting adversarial network for chest x-rays organ segmentation. arXiv preprint arXiv:1703.08770 (2017)
19. Novikov, A.A., Lenis, D., Major, D., Hladvka, J., Wimmer, M., Bühler, K.: Fully convolutional architectures for multiclass segmentation in chest radiographs. IEEE Trans. Med. Imaging 37(8), 1865–1876 (2018)

Deep Esophageal Clinical Target Volume Delineation Using Encoded 3D Spatial Context of Tumors, Lymph Nodes, and Organs At Risk

Dakai Jin[1(✉)], Dazhou Guo[1], Tsung-Ying Ho[2(✉)], Adam P. Harrison[1], Jing Xiao[3], Chen-kan Tseng[2], and Le Lu[1]

[1] PAII Inc., Bethesda, MD, USA
jindakai376@paii-labs.com
[2] Chang Gung Memorial Hospital, Linkou, Taiwan, ROC
tyho@cgmh.org.tw
[3] Ping An Technology, Shenzhen, China

Abstract. Clinical target volume (CTV) delineation from radiotherapy computed tomography (RTCT) images is used to define the treatment areas containing the gross tumor volume (GTV) and/or sub-clinical malignant disease for radiotherapy (RT). High intra- and inter-user variability makes this a particularly difficult task for esophageal cancer. This motivates automated solutions, which is the aim of our work. Because CTV delineation is highly context-dependent—it must encompass the GTV and regional lymph nodes (LNs) while also avoiding excessive exposure to the organs at risk (OARs)—we formulate it as a deep contextual appearance-based problem using encoded spatial contexts of these anatomical structures. This allows the deep network to better learn from and emulate the margin- and appearance-based delineation performed by human physicians. Additionally, we develop domain-specific data augmentation to inject robustness to our system. Finally, we show that a simple 3D progressive holistically nested network (PHNN), which avoids computationally heavy decoding paths while still aggregating features at different levels of context, can outperform more complicated networks. Cross-validated experiments on a dataset of 135 esophageal cancer patients demonstrate that our encoded spatial context approach can produce concrete performance improvements, with an average Dice score of $83.9 \pm 5.4\%$ and an average surface distance of $4.2 \pm 2.7\,\mathrm{mm}$, representing improvements of 3.8% and $2.4\,\mathrm{mm}$, respectively, over the state-of-the-art approach.

1 Introduction

Esophageal cancer ranks the sixth in global cancer mortality [1]. As it is usually diagnosed at rather late stage [18], radiotherapy (RT) is a cornerstone of treatment. Delineating the 3D clinical target volume (CTV) on a radiotherapy computed tomography (RTCT) scan is a key challenge in RT planning. As

© Springer Nature Switzerland AG 2019
D. Shen et al. (Eds.): MICCAI 2019, LNCS 11769, pp. 603–612, 2019.
https://doi.org/10.1007/978-3-030-32226-7_67

Fig. 1 illustrates, the CTV should spatially encompass, with a mixture of predefined and judgment-based margins, primary tumor(s), *i.e.*, the gross tumor volume (GTV), regional lymph nodes (LNs) and sub-clinical disease regions, while simultaneously limiting radiation exposure to organs at risk (OARs) [2].

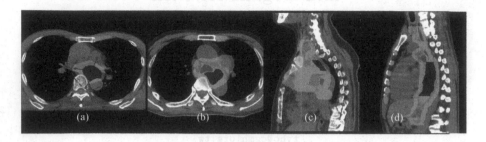

Fig. 1. Esophageal cancer CTV delineation, where red, yellow, and cyan indicate the GTV, regional LNs and CTV, respectively. (a) shows that the CTV is not a uniform margin expansion (brown-dotted line) from the GTV, while (b)–(d) shows how delineation becomes more complicated when regional LNs are present. (c) and (d) also depict wide and long examples of esophageal CTV, respectively. (Color figure online)

Esophageal clinical target volume (CTV) delineation is uniquely challenging because tumors may potentially spread along the entire esophagus and metastasize up to the neck or down to the upper abdomen LNs. Current clinical protocols rely on manual CTV delineation, which is very time and labor consuming and is subject to high inter- and intra-observer variability [12]. This motivates automated approaches to the CTV delineation.

Deep convolutional neural networks (CNNs) have achieved notable successes in segmenting semantic objects, such as organs and tumors, in medical imaging [4,6–10]. However, to the best of our knowledge, no prior work, CNN-based or not, has addressed esophageal cancer CTV segmentation. Works on CTV segmentation of other cancer types mostly operate based on the RTCT appearance alone [14,15]. As shown in Fig. 1, CTV delineation depends on the radiation oncologist's visual judgment of both the appearance *and* the spatial configuration of the GTV, LNs, and OARs, suggesting that only considering the RTCT makes the problem ill-posed. Supporting this, Cardenas *et al.* recently showed that considering the GTV and LN binary masks together with the RTCT can boost oropharyngeal CTV delineation performance [3]. However, the OARs were not considered in their work. Moreover, binary masks do not explicitly provide distances to the model. Yet CTV delineation is highly driven by distance-based margins to other anatomical structures of interest, and it is difficult to see how regular CNNs could capture these precise distance relationships with binary masks alone.

Our work fills this gap by introducing a spatial-context encoded deep CTV delineation framework. Instead of expecting the CNN to learn distance-based margins from the GTV, LN, and OAR binary masks, we provide the CTV delineation network with the 3D signed distance transform maps (SDMs) [16] of these structures. Specifically, we include the SDMs of the GTV, LNs, lung, heart, and spinal canal with the original RTCT volume as inputs to the network. From a clinical perspective, this allows the CNN to emulate the oncologist's manual delineation, which uses the distances of GTV and LNs vs. the OARs as a key constraint in determining CTV boundaries. To improve robustness, we randomly choose manually and automatically generated organ at risk OAR SDMs during training, while augmenting the GTV and LNs SDMs with the domain-specific jittering. We adopt a 3D progressive holistically nested network (PHNN) [6] to serve as our delineation model, which enjoys the benefits of strong abstraction capacities and multi-scale feature fusion with a light-weighted decoding path. We extensively evaluate our approach using a 3-fold cross-validated dataset of 135 esophageal cancer patients. Since we are the first to tackle automated esophageal cancer CTV delineation, we compare against previous CTV delineation methods for other cancers [3,15], using the 3D PHNN as the delineation model. When comparing against pure appearance-based [15] and binary-mask-based [3] solutions, we show that our approach provides improvements of 10% and 3.8% in Dice score, respectively, with analogous improvements in Hausdorff distance (HD) and average surface distance (ASD). Moreover, we also show that PHNN is responsible for providing improvements of 1% in Dice score and 0.4 mm reduction in ASD over a 3D U-Net model [4].

2   Methods

CTV delineation in RT planning is essentially a margin expansion process, starting from observable tumorous regions (GTV and regional LNs) and extending into the neighboring regions by considering the possible tumor spread margins and distances to nearby healthy OARs. Figure 2 depicts an overview of our method, which consists of four major modularized components: (1) segmentation of prerequisite regions; (2) SDM computation; (3) domain-specific data augmentation; and (4) a 3D PHNN to execute the CTV delineation.

2.1   Prerequisite Region Segmentation

To provide spatial context/distance of the anatomical structures of interest, we must first know their boundaries. We assume that manual segmentations for the esophageal GTV and regional LNs are available. However, we do not make this assumption for the OARs. Indeed, missing organ at risk (OAR) segmentations (~ 20%) is common in our dataset. For the OARs, we consider three major organs: the lung, heart, and spinal canal, since most esophageal CTVs are closely integrated with these organs. Using the available organ labels, we trained a 2D

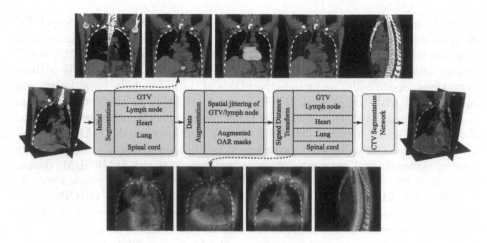

Fig. 2. Overall workflow of our spatial context encoded CTV delineation framework. The top and bottom rows depict different masks and SDMs, respectively, overlayed on the RTCT. From left to right are the GTV, LNs, heart, lung, and spinal canal. The GTV and LNs share a combined SDM.

PHNN [6] to segment the OARs, considering its robust performance in pathological lung segmentation and its computational efficiency. Examples of automatic OAR segmentation are illustrated in the first row in Fig. 2 and validation Dice score for the lung, heart and spinal canal were 97%, 95% and 78%, respectively, in our dataset.

2.2 SDM Computation

To encode the spatial context with respect to the GTV, regional LNs, and OARs, we compute signed distance transform maps (SDMs) for each. The SDM is generated from a binary image, where the value in each voxel measures the distance to the closest object boundary. Voxels inside and outside the boundary have positive and negative values, respectively. More formally, let $\mathcal{O}_i$ denote a binary mask, where $i \in \{\text{GTV+LNs, lung, heart, spinal canal}\}$ and let $\Gamma(\cdot)$ be a function that computes boundary voxels of a binary image. The SDM value at a voxel p with respect to $\mathcal{O}_i$ is computed as

$$\text{SDM}_{\Gamma(\mathcal{O}_i)}(p) = \begin{cases} \min\limits_{q \in \Gamma(\mathcal{O}_i)} d(p,q) & \text{if} \quad p \notin \mathcal{O}_i \\ -\min\limits_{q \in \Gamma(\mathcal{O}_i)} d(p,q) & \text{if} \quad p \in \mathcal{O}_i \end{cases}, \tag{1}$$

where $d(p,q)$ is a distance measure from p to q. We choose to use Euclidean distance in our work and use Maurer *et al.*'s efficient algorithm [13] to compute the SDMs. The bottom row in Fig. 2 depicts example SDMs for the combined GTV and LNs and the other 3 OARs. Note that we compute SDMs separately for each of the three OARs, meaning we can capture each organ's influence on the CTV. Providing the SDMs of the GTV, LNs, and OARs to the deep convolutional neural network (CNN) allows it to more easily infer the distance-based margins to these anatomical structures, better emulating the oncologist's CTV inference process.

2.3 Domain-Specific Data Augmentation

We adopt specialized data augmentations to increase the robustness of the training and harden our network to noise in the prerequisite segmentations. Specifically, two types of data augmentation are carried out. (1) We calculate the GTV and LNs SDMs from both the manual annotations and also spatially jittered versions of those annotations. We jitter each GTV and lymph node (LN) component by random shift within $4 \times 4 \times 4\,mm^3$, mimicking that in practice 4 mm average distance error represents the state-of-the art performance in esophageal GTV segmentation [8,17]. (2) We calculate SDMs of the OARs using both the manual annotations and the automatic segmentations from Sect. 2.1. Combined, these augmentations lead to four possible combinations, which we randomly choose between during every training epoch. This increases model robustness and also allows the system to be effectively deployed in practice by using SDMs of the automatically segmented OARs, helping to alleviate the labor involved.

2.4 CTV Delineation Network

To use 3D CNNs in medical imaging, one has to strike a balance between choosing the appropriate image size covering enough context and the GPU memory. The symmetric encoder-decoder segmentation networks, e.g., 3D U-Net [4], are computationally heavy and memory-consuming since half of its computation is consumed on the decoding path, which may not always be needed for all 3D segmentation tasks. To alleviate the computational/memory burden, we adopt a 3D version of PHNN [6] as our CTV delineation network, which is able to fuse different levels of features using parameter-less deep supervision. We keep the first 4 convolutional blocks and adapt it to 3D as our network structure. As we demonstrate in the experiments, the 3D PHNN is not only able to achieve reasonable improvement over the 3D U-Net but requires 3 times less GPU memory.

3 Experiments and Results

To evaluate the performance of our esophageal CTV delineation framework, we collected from 135 anonymized RTCTs of esophageal cancer patients undergoing RT. Each RTCT is accompanied by a CTV mask annotated by an experienced oncologist, based on a previously segmented GTV, regional LNs, and OARs. The average RTCT size is $512 \times 512 \times 250$ voxels with the average resolution of $1.05 \times 1.05 \times 2.6\,mm$.

608   D. Jin et al.

Training Data Sampling: We first resample all the CT and SDM images to a fixed resolution of $1.0 \times 1.0 \times 2.5$ mm, from which we extract $96 \times 96 \times 64$ training volume of interest (VOI) patches in two manners: (1) To ensure enough VOIs with positive CTV content, we randomly extract VOIs centered within the CTV mask. (2) To obtain sufficient negative examples, we randomly sample ~ 20 VOIs from the whole volume. This results in on average 80 VOIs per patient. We further augment the training data by applying random rotations of $\pm 10°$ in the x-y plane.

Implementation Details: The Adam solver [11] is used to optimize all segmentation models with a momentum of 0.99 and a weight decay of 0.005 for 30 epochs. We use the Dice loss for training. For testing, we use 3D sliding windows with sub-volumes of $96 \times 96 \times 64$ and strides of $64 \times 64 \times 32$ voxels. The probability maps of sub-volumes are aggregated to obtain the whole volume prediction taking on average 6–7 s to process one input volume using a Titan-V GPU.

Comparison Setup and Metrics: We use 3-fold cross-validation, separated at the patient level, to evaluate performance of our approach and the competitor methods. We compare against setups using only the CT appearance information [14,15] and setups using the CT with binary GTV/LN masks [3]. Finally, we also compare against setups using the CT + GTV/LN SDMs, which does not consider the OARs. We compare these setups using the 3D PHNN. For the 3D U-Net [4], we compared against the setup using the computed tomography (CT) appearance information. We evaluate the performance using the metrics of Dice score, ASD and HD.

Table 1. Quantitative results for the esophageal cancer CTV delineation.

Models	Setups	Dice	HD (mm)	ASD (mm)
U-Net	CT	0.739±0.126	69.5±42.7	10.1±9.4
	CT + GTV/LN/OAR SDMs	0.829±0.061	36.9±23.8	4.6±3.0
PHNN	CT	0.739±0.117	68.5±43.8	10.6±9.2
	CT + GTV/LN masks	0.801±0.075	56.3±35.4	6.6±5.3
	CT + GTV/LN SDMs	0.816±0.067	44.7±25.1	5.4±4.1
	CT + GTV/LN/OAR SDMs	**0.839±0.054**	**35.4±23.7**	**4.2±2.7**
	CT + GTV/LN/OAR SDMs*	0.823±0.059	43.6±26.4	5.1±3.3

*The last, starred row represents performance when using automatically generated OAR SDMs.

Results: Table 1 outlines the quantitative comparisons of the different model setups and choices. As can be seen, methods based on pure CT appearance, seen in prior art [14,15], exhibits the worst performance. This is because inferring distance-based margins from appearance alone is too hard of a task for CNNs. Focusing on the PHNN performance, when adding the binary GTV and LN

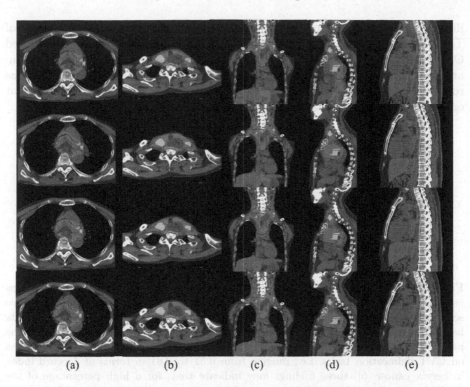

(a) (b) (c) (d) (e)

Fig. 3. Qualitative illustration of esophageal CTV delineation using different PHNN setups. Red, yellow and cyan represent the GTV, LN and predicted CTV regions, respectively. The purple line indicates the ground truth CTV boundary. The 1st and 2nd rows show examples from setups using pure RTCT [15] and when adding GTV/LN binary masks [3], respectively. The 3rd and 4th row show examples when adding GTV/LN SDMs and our proposed GTV/LN/OAR SDMs, respectively. (a) and (d) demonstrate that the pure RTCT setups fail to include the regional LNs, while (c) to (e) depict severe over-segmentations. While these errors are partially addressed using the GTV/LN mask setup, it still suffers from inaccurate CTV boundaries (a–c) or over coverage of normal regions (d, e). These issues are much better addressed by our proposed method. (Color figure online)

masks as contextual information [3], the performance increases considerably from 0.739 ± 0.117 to 0.801 ± 0.075 in Dice score. When using the SDM encoded spatial context of GTV/LN, PHNN further improves the Dice score and ASD by 1.5% and 1.2 mm, respectively, confirming the value of using the distance information for esophageal CTV delineation. Finally, when the OAR SDMs are included, *i.e.*, our proposed framework, PHNN achieves the best performance reaching 0.839 ± 0.054 Dice score and 4.2 ± 2.7 mm ASD, with a reduction of 9.3 mm in HD as compared to the next best PHNN result. Figure 4 depicts cumulative histograms of the Dice score and ASD, visually illustrating the distribution of improvements in the CTV delineation performance. Figure 3 shows some qualitative examples illustrating these performance improvements. Interestingly, as the last row of Table 1 shows, when using SDMs computed from the automatically segmented OARs for testing, the performance compares favorably to the best configuration, and outperforms all other configurations. This indicates that our method remains robust to noise within the OAR SDMs and also that our approach is not reliant on manual OAR masks for good performance, increasing its practical value.

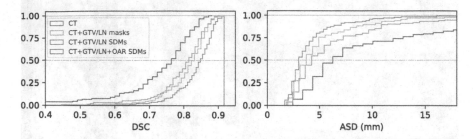

Fig. 4. Cumulative histograms of the CTV delineation performance under 4 setups using 3D PHNN on cross-validated 135 patients. The left and right depict the Dice score and ASD results, respectively. From the results, we observe that > 77% patients have Dice score ≥ 0.80, and > 55% patients have Dice score ≥ 0.85 by using the proposed method (shown in red). Since there are often large inter-observer variations on CVT delineation tasks, $i.e.$, ranging from 0.51 to 0.81 in terms of Jaccard index in cervix cancer [5], these findings may indicate that, for a high percentage of the studied patient population, little to no additional manual revision is needed on the automatically delineated CTVs. (Color figure online)

We also compare the 3D PHNN network performance with that of 3D U-Net [4] when using the CT appearance based setup and the proposed whole framework. As Table 1 demonstrates, when using the whole pipeline PHNN outperforms U-Net by 1% dice score. Although PHNN has similar performance against U-Net when using only the CT appearance information, the GPU memory consumption is roughly 3 times less than that of the U-Net. These results indicate that for esophageal CTV delineation, a CNN equipped with strong encoding capacity and a light-weight decoding path can be as good as (or even superior to) a heavier network with a symmetric decoding path.

4   Conclusion

We introduced a spatial-context encoded deep esophageal CTV delineation framework designed to produce superior margin-based CTV boundaries. Our system encodes spatial context by computing the SDMs of the GTV, LNs and OARs and feeds them together with the RTCT image into a 3D deep CNN. Analogous to clinical practice, this allows the system to consider both appearance and distance-based information for delineation. Additionally, we also developed domain-specific data augmentation and adopted a 3D PHNN to further improve robustness. Using extensive three-fold cross-validation, we demonstrated that our spatial-context encoded approach can outperform state-of-the-art CTV alternatives by wide margins in Dice score, HD, and ASD. As we are the first to address automated esophageal CTV delineation, our method represents an important step forward for this important problem.

References

1. Bray, F., Ferlay, J., et al.: Global cancer statistics 2018: Globocan estimates of incidence and mortality worldwide for 36 cancers in 185 countries. CA a Cancer J. Clin. **68**(6), 394–424 (2018)
2. Burnet, N.G., Thomas, S.J., Burton, K.E., Jefferies, S.J.: Defining the tumour and target volumes for radiotherapy. Cancer Imaging **4**(2), 153 (2004)
3. Cardenas, C.E., Anderson, B.M., et al.: Auto-delineation of oropharyngeal clinical target volumes using 3D convolutional neural networks. Phys. Med. Biol. **63**(21), 215026 (2018)
4. Çiçek, Ö., Abdulkadir, A., Lienkamp, S.S., Brox, T., Ronneberger, O.: 3D U-Net: learning dense volumetric segmentation from sparse annotation. In: Ourselin, S., Joskowicz, L., Sabuncu, M.R., Unal, G., Wells, W. (eds.) MICCAI 2016. LNCS, vol. 9901, pp. 424–432. Springer, Cham (2016). https://doi.org/10.1007/978-3-319-46723-8_49
5. Eminowicz, G., McCormack, M.: Variability of clinical target volume delineation for definitive radiotherapy in cervix cancer. Radiother. Oncol. **117**(3), 542–547 (2015)
6. Harrison, A.P., Xu, Z., George, K., Lu, L., Summers, R.M., Mollura, D.J.: Progressive and multi-path holistically nested neural networks for pathological lung segmentation from CT images. In: Descoteaux, M., Maier-Hein, L., Franz, A., Jannin, P., Collins, D.L., Duchesne, S. (eds.) MICCAI 2017. LNCS, vol. 10435, pp. 621–629. Springer, Cham (2017). https://doi.org/10.1007/978-3-319-66179-7_71
7. Heinrich, M.P., Oktay, O., Bouteldja, N.: OBELISK-Net: fewer layers to solve 3D multi-organ segmentation with sparse deformable convolutions. Med. Image Anal. **54**, 1–9 (2019)
8. Jin, D., Guo, D., Ho, T.Y., et al.: Accurate esophageal gross tumor volume segmentation in pet/ct using two-stream chained 3d deep network fusion. In: Shen, D., et al. (eds.) MICCAI 2019. LNCS, vol. 11765, pp. 182–191. Springer. Cham (2019)
9. Jin, D., Xu, Z., Harrison, A.P., George, K., Mollura, D.J.: 3D convolutional neural networks with graph refinement for airway segmentation using incomplete data labels. In: Wang, Q., Shi, Y., Suk, H.-I., Suzuki, K. (eds.) MLMI 2017. LNCS, vol. 10541, pp. 141–149. Springer, Cham (2017). https://doi.org/10.1007/978-3-319-67389-9_17
10. Jin, D., Xu, Z., Tang, Y., Harrison, A.P., Mollura, D.J.: CT-realistic lung nodule simulation from 3D conditional generative adversarial networks for robust lung segmentation. In: Frangi, A.F., Schnabel, J.A., Davatzikos, C., Alberola-López, C., Fichtinger, G. (eds.) MICCAI 2018. LNCS, vol. 11071, pp. 732–740. Springer, Cham (2018). https://doi.org/10.1007/978-3-030-00934-2_81
11. Kingma, D.P., Ba, J.: Adam: a method for stochastic optimization. arXiv:1412.6980 (2014)
12. Louie, A.V., Rodrigues, G., et al.: Inter-observer and intra-observer reliability for lung cancer target volume delineation in the 4D-CT era. Radiother. Oncol. **95**(2), 166–171 (2010)

13. Maurer Jr., C.R., Qi, R., Raghavan, V.: A linear time algorithm for computing exact euclidean distance transforms of binary images in arbitrary dimensions. IEEE Trans. Pattern Anal. Mach. Intell. **25**(2), 265–270 (2003)
14. Men, K., Dai, J., Li, Y.: Automatic segmentation of the clinical target volume and organs at risk in the planning ct for rectal cancer using deep dilated convolutional neural networks. Med. Phys. **44**(12), 6377–6389 (2017)
15. Men, K., Zhang, T., et al.: Fully automatic and robust segmentation of the clinical target volume for radiotherapy of breast cancer using big data and deep learning. Physica Med. **50**, 13–19 (2018)
16. Sethian, J.: A fast marching level set method for monotonically advancing fronts. Proc. Natl. Acad. Sci. **93**(4), 1591–1595 (1996)
17. Yousefi, S., et al.: Esophageal gross tumor volume segmentation using a 3D convolutional neural network. In: Frangi, A.F., Schnabel, J.A., Davatzikos, C., Alberola-López, C., Fichtinger, G. (eds.) MICCAI 2018. LNCS, vol. 11073, pp. 343–351. Springer, Cham (2018). https://doi.org/10.1007/978-3-030-00937-3_40
18. Zhang, Y.: Epidemiology of esophageal cancer. World J. Gastroenterol. WJG **19**(34), 5598 (2013)

Weakly Supervised Segmentation Framework with Uncertainty: A Study on Pneumothorax Segmentation in Chest X-ray

Xi Ouyang[1,2], Zhong Xue[1], Yiqiang Zhan[1], Xiang Sean Zhou[1], Qingfeng Wang[3], Ying Zhou[4], Qian Wang[2], and Jie-Zhi Cheng[1(✉)]

[1] Shanghai United Imaging Intelligence Co., Ltd., Shanghai, China
jiezhi.zheng@united-imaging.com
[2] Institute for Medical Imaging Technology, School of Biomedical Engineering,
Shanghai Jiao Tong University, Shanghai, China
wang.qian@sjtu.edu.cn
[3] School of Computer Science and Technology,
Southwest University of Science and Technology, Mianyang, China
[4] Radiology Department, Mianyang Central Hospital, Mianyang, China

Abstract. Pneumothorax is a critical abnormality that shall be treated with higher priority, and hence a computerized triage scheme is needed. A deep-learning-based framework to automatically segment the pneumothorax in chest X-rays is developed to support the realization of a triage system. Since a large number of pixel-level annotations is commonly needed but difficult to obtain for deep learning model, we propose a weakly supervised framework that allows partial training data to be weakly annotated with only image-level labels. We employ the attention masks derived from an image-level classification model as the pixel-level masks for those weakly-annotated data. Because the attention masks are rough and may have errors, we further develop a spatial label smoothing regularization technique to explore the uncertainty for the incorrectness of the attention masks in the training of segmentation model. Experimental results show that the proposed weakly supervised segmentation algorithm relieves the need of well-annotated data and yield satisfactory performance on the pneumothorax segmentation.

Keywords: Pneumothorax · Weakly supervised segmentation · Spatial label smoothing regularization

1 Introduction

Pneumothorax is a lung abnormality with air leaking into the space between the lung and chest wall. It can be caused by chest injury or trauma, certain medi-

Electronic supplementary material The online version of this chapter (https://doi.org/10.1007/978-3-030-32226-7_68) contains supplementary material, which is available to authorized users.

D. Shen et al. (Eds.): MICCAI 2019, LNCS 11769, pp. 613–621, 2019.
https://doi.org/10.1007/978-3-030-32226-7_68

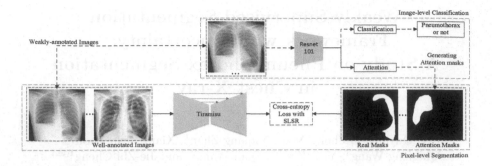

Fig. 1. Training process of our weakly supervised segmentation method. In the testing stage, only the segmentation model is used.

cal procedures, damage from underlying lung disease, or sometimes no obvious reason [12]. The most common imaging tool for the diagnosis of pneumothorax is chest X-ray (CXR). Large pneumothorax can be fatal as air compression may cause significant impairment to circulation and respiration. Accordingly, large pneumothorax shall be classified as a critical abnormality that requires immediate treatment, as shown in the latest computerized CXR triage study [1].

Since the diagnosis and treatment of critical pneumothorax are directly related to the size of pneumothorax area, segmenting pneumothorax accurately rather than image-level classification, is needed for the triage of CXR. However, as shown in a previous study [5], the performance of pneumothorax diagnosis in CXR is highly dependent on the physicians experience, implying that the pixel-level annotations with good quality is difficult to obtain and can be very limited. On the other hand, large image-level annotations can be relatively easy to access with the text analysis techniques on radiological reports [9]. Motivated by this, we propose a weakly supervised learning approach that aims to ease the requirement of annotating all training data in pixel level. Specifically, we allow parts of training data to be weakly annotated with only image-level labels, i.e., pneumothorax or not.

In the literature, to boost the localization of abnormalities, Li et al. [7] developed an end-to-end deep multi-instance network to identify image-level abnormalities with annotated bounding boxes. Yan et al. [10] introduced a weakly-supervised deep learning framework for abnormality identification and localization. Cai et al. [2] further proposed an attention mining strategy to improve identification performance. However, these studies focused on providing rough heatmaps to indicate abnormal regions. However, the precise pixel-level segmentation results, can not be acquired through these methods.

To get better synergy between the well- and weakly-annotated data, our approach employs the spatial label smoothing regularization (SLSR) technique to leverage the network-generated attention masks from the weakly-annotated data. Specifically, we realize the proposed method in two stages, see Fig. 1. First, an image-level classification (pneumothorax or not) model is implemented to obtain the attention masks. The attention masks from this classification model

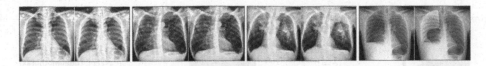

Fig. 2. Several pneumothorax cases. Blue masks indicate the pneumothorax regions labeled by an experienced radiologist. Inter-subject variations, as well as the variety of pneuothorax degree, location, and shape, can be observed. The last case is hydropneumothorax with pleural effusion and pneumothorax. (Color figure online)

may roughly suggest the pneumothorax regions from the weakly-annotated data. Second, an image segmentation model is designed to use both well- and weakly-annotated data, where the attention masks for weakly-annotated data are incorporated. Since the attention masks do not delineate the exact pneumothorax regions and may have some errors, we employ the SLSR technique to consider the uncertainty for the incorrectness of the attention masks during the training process of the segmentation model. The label smoothing regularization technique addresses label corruption issue by treating labels as probability variables with slightly numerical perturbation, and is proved to be robust to noisy labels [13]. Our experimental results show that our method can improve the performance of the segmentation model with both well- and weakly-annotated data. The contribution of this paper can be two-fold. First, a novel weakly supervised framework is proposed to equip the deep learning segmentation with the capability of learning with well- and weakly-annotated data. Second, we demonstrate the effectiveness of the weakly supervised framework on the pneumothorax segmentation problem in CXR images. As shown in Fig. 2, the pneumothorax segmentation is difficult as several issues such as inter-subject variations, the variety of pneumothorax degree, location and shape, need to be addressed. The pneumothorax segmentation can help identify critical cases and expedite the treatment process.

2 Methodology

As shown in Fig. 1, the proposed weakly supervised approach consists of two steps: (1) image-level classification that generates attention masks at the same time; (2) pixel-level segmentation with SLSR that leverages attention masks. The details will be elaborated as follows.

2.1 Image-Level Classification

Image-level classification for our task (pneumothorax or not) is carried out with Resnet101 model [11]. The attention mining method, Guided Attention Inference Network (GAIN) [6], is performed to generate the attention masks. The sizes of the obtained attention masks are 1/8 of the input sizes, and they are further resized via bilinear interpolation to fit the requirement for the pixel-level segmentation model.

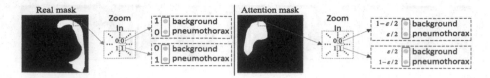

Fig. 3. Perturbation on one-hot label distribution. into the probabilistic domain. For the left real mask, the label is either 1 or 0, whereas labels in the right attention mask are perturbed with ε.

2.2   Pixel-Level Segmentation

The SLSR technique is developed to leverage the attention masks of the weakly-annotated data for better performance and mitigate the problem of less accessibility of well-annotated data. Since the attention masks simply capture rough pneumothorax regions and may have some errors, we explore the uncertainty of attention masks by numerically perturbing one-hot label distribution into the probabilistic domain as shown in Fig. 3. Specifically, let $k \in \{0, 1\}$ be the object classes, where class 0 stands for background and 1 for pneumothorax class.

Assuming that label prior distribution is uniform, the ground-truth label distribution with the consideration of potential label corruption in each pixel $PIX_{i,j}$ (i and j refer to the row and column indices, respectively) is defined as:

$$q_{i,j}(k) = \begin{cases} \frac{\varepsilon}{2}, & k \neq y_{i,j} \\ 1-\varepsilon+\frac{\varepsilon}{2}, & k = y_{i,j} \end{cases} = \begin{cases} \frac{\varepsilon}{2}, & k \neq y_{i,j} \\ 1-\frac{\varepsilon}{2}, & k = y_{i,j}, \end{cases} \tag{1}$$

where $y_{i,j}$ is the ground-truth class of the pixel $PIX_{i,j}$, and ε is the perturbing parameter. The uncertainty for an attention mask can be categorized into two types: all-class and ground-truth uncertainty. The all-class uncertainty suggests that each pixel in an attention mask has equal potential to be either pneumothorax or background with the probability of $\varepsilon/2$. The ground-truth uncertainty specifies that the pneumothorax region in an attention mask may have errors and the corresponding probabilities of the pixels are perturbed with ε.

Assuming $p_{i,j}(k)$ is the predicted probability of class k from the network, it comes from the softmax function after the final convolutional layer in the segmentation task. With the Eq. 1, the cross-entropy loss of the pixel $PIX_{i,j}$ can be further computed as:

$$l_{i,j} = -\sum_{k=0}^{1} \log(p_{i,j}(k))q_{i,j}(k) = -(1-\varepsilon)\log(p_{i,j}(y_{i,j})) - \frac{\varepsilon}{2}\sum_{k=0}^{1}\log(p_{i,j}(k)). \tag{2}$$

Accordingly, the loss function for a weakly-annotated image with the attention mask is the summation of $l_{i,j}$ in all the pixels (H and W are height and width of the input image), which is defined as:

$$l = \sum_{i=1}^{H}\sum_{j=1}^{W} l_{i,j} = -(1-\varepsilon)\sum_{i=1}^{H}\sum_{j=1}^{W}\log(p_{i,j}(y_{i,j})) - \frac{\varepsilon}{2}\sum_{k=0}^{1}\sum_{i=1}^{H}\sum_{j=1}^{W}\log(p_{i,j}(k)). \tag{3}$$

Since the training data are comprised of well- and weakly-annotated data, we further introduce a variable of indicator, z, to specify if the data is well or weakly annotated. Meanwhile, referring to Eq. 3, the first term is only effective in the foreground class whereas the second term considers both foreground and background classes. Since in most cases the number of background pixels is significantly larger than the number of the foreground, we implement a weighting factor to soothe the pixel sample imbalance issue. Specifically, the loss function is further defined as:

$$
\begin{aligned}
l_{SLSR} = & -(1 - z \cdot \varepsilon) \sum_{i=1}^{H} \sum_{j=1}^{W} \log(p_{i,j}(y_{i,j})) \\
& - z \sum_{k=0}^{1} \left\{ (1 + \sum_{i=1}^{H} \sum_{j=1}^{W} I(k = y_{i,j})) \cdot \frac{\varepsilon}{2HW} \cdot \sum_{i=1}^{H} \sum_{j=1}^{W} \log(p_{i,j}(k)) \right\},
\end{aligned}
\tag{4}
$$

where $I(k = y_{i,j})$ is an indicator function to calculate the ground-truth pixel number for k-th class. For a well-annotated image sample, we set $z = 0$, while $z = 1$ for weakly-annotated image sample. With the implementation of Eq. 4, the pixel-level segmentation model can be trained with well- and weakly-annotated data, and still attain satisfactory performance.

3 Experiments

3.1 Dataset

Totally, 5400 frontal-view chest X-ray images are collected from the Mianyang Central Hospital, Mianyang, Sichuan, China, with IRB approval. Specifically, 3400 images were diagnosed with pneumothorax, whereas the 2000 images are normal cases. 800 pneumothorax images are well-annotated with pixel-level ground-truth masks by an experienced radiologist and the remaining 2600 pneumothorax images only have the image-level labels. The 800 well-annotated data and 2000 normal cases are randomly and evenly split into 2 groups for training and testing. Therefore, the total number of testing data is 1400, whereas the number of available data for training is 4000.

3.2 Experimental Settings

For the segmentation network, three state-of-the-art (SOTA) networks: U-Net [8], LinkNet [3], and Tiramisu [4] are implemented. For Tiramisu, the specific FCDenseNet67 is employed. For all three models, Adam optimization method is employed and the value of momentum is set as 0.9. The learning rate is initiated with 0.0001 and will be gradually degraded by a factor of 0.1 every 100 epochs. The size of network inputs is 256×256. For U-Net and LinkNet, we set the batch size as 32, whereas the batch size of Tiramisu model is set as 5. The perturbing parameter ε is set to 0.1.

Table 1. Performance of different the SOTA models, and Tiramisu achieves the best performance.

	U-Net	LinkNet	Tiramisu
IoU	0.515	0.572	0.640

Table 2. Performance w.r.t. different pneumothorax degrees.

	Small	Medium	Large
IoU	0.257	0.584	0.771

3.3   Experimental Results

Results of SOTA Networks. In this experiment, we aim to illustrate the performance limitation of the SOTA networks on the pneumothorax segmentation problem. Specifically, the training data for segmentation, i.e. 400 well-annotated and 1000 normal CXR images, is employed to train the three SOTA networks. The results of the SOTA networks on the 1400 testing data with the IoU (intersection over union) metrics are shown in Table 1. As can be found, the Tiramisu model achieves the best performance with 0.640 of IoU value. Accordingly, the pneumothorax segmentation problem is quite difficult. To further investigate the factor of pneumothorax severity on the segmentation efficacy, the 400 pneumothorax cases are further divided into three groups of small, medium and large, based on the collapse ratios that meet the criteria of $<= 0.10$, 0.10–0.30, and $>= 0.30$, respectively. The collapse ratio of the pneumothorax region against the lung field is one of the common quantitative metrics for the measure of pneumothorax severity. The small, medium, and large groups comprise of 156, 142, and 102 cases, respectively. The performance of the Tiramisu model on the three groups is shown in Table 2. Since the IoU is very sensitive to object size, the IoU value for the small group is not very high. Small pneumothorax is usually less critical as large pneumothorax, and sometimes may heal on its own.

Efficacy of the SLSR. In this experiment, the efficacy of the SLSR on the weakly supervised framework is illustrated. Referring to Table 1, we here only consider the Tiramisu model. The image-level classification model (GAIN) is firstly trained with the 2600 weakly-annotated pneumothorax and 1000 normal images to obtain the attention masks. We use this model to generate attention masks for all test images, and take these results as segmentation prediction and get the IoU value (0.128), which serves the baseline of only using image-level annotations. Afterward, the segmentation models are trained with different experimental settings of ratios between well- and weakly-annotated data. Specifically, we set 4 groups of experiments that include 100, 200, 300, and 400 well-annotated pneumothorax cases. For each group, we firstly train a Tiramisu model using the selected well-annotated pneumothorax cases and 1000 normal images. Then, we also add the selected well-annotated cases to retrain the GAIN model, which can help to improve the quality of generated attention masks. Finally, we consider several experiments with adding 0, 200, 400, and 800 weakly-annotated pneumothorax cases to train the Tiramisu models with SLSR loss (Eq. 4).

The experimental results are shown in Table 2. As can be found, more involvement of well-annotated data will improve the segmentation performance. Mean-

Table 3. The results with different combinations of well- and weakly-annotated data. The column "Test" the IoU performance of the entire testing data, whereas the columns "Small", "Medium" and "Large" are the IoU performances of the dataset with three groups of severity, respectively.

Data	Small	Medium	Large	Test
only image-level annotations	0.051	0.124	0.231	0.128
100 well-annotated cases*	0.129	0.443	0.613	0.495*
+ 200 weakly-annotated cases	0.180	0.501	0.677	**0.536**
+ 400 weakly-annotated cases	0.184	0.482	0.661	0.526
+ 800 weakly-annotated cases	0.138	0.456	0.647	0.501
200 well-annotated cases*	0.198	0.488	0.702	0.545*
+ 200 weakly-annotated cases	0.226	0.538	0.768	**0.615**
+ 400 weakly-annotated cases	0.237	0.527	0.734	0.590
+ 800 weakly-annotated cases	0.205	0.480	0.704	0.558
300 well-annotated cases*	0.224	0.551	0.768	0.611*
+ 200 weakly-annotated cases	0.265	0.563	0.774	**0.637**
+ 400 weakly-annotated cases	0.250	0.561	0.760	0.627
+ 800 weakly-annotated cases	0.240	0.559	0.751	0.614
400 well-annotated cases*	0.257	0.584	0.771	0.640*
+ 200 weakly-annotated cases	0.291	0.600	0.782	0.655
+ 400 weakly-annotated cases	0.278	0.616	0.804	**0.669**
+ 800 weakly-annotated cases	0.262	0.593	0.768	0.648

while, for each group of experiments, it can be observed from Table 2 that if the numbers of weakly- and well-annotated data are close, the best synergy can be achieved. In particular, for the case of adding of 200 weakly-annotated data to the 300 well-annotated group, the best segmentation performance such as 0.637 IoU can be achieved, which is close to 0.640 IoU achieved by the Tiramisu model in the SOTA experiment. Meanwhile, the models with 200–800 weakly-annotated data in the 400 well-annotated group can outperform the model with only 400 well-annotated data, whereas the best performance can be achieved by the model with 400 weakly-annotated data and 400 well-annotated data (0.669 IoU). We also conduct an experiment for the setting of ε with the results given in Table 4, where $\varepsilon = 0$ equals to the vanilla cross-entropy loss. We can see the setting of $\varepsilon = 0.1$ can achieve the best performance.

Visualization Results. The intermediate results of three testing data with the different degree of pneumothorax severity are shown in Fig. 4. As can be found, the segmentation results with only 200 well-annotated data (without including weakly-annotated data) are not very promising. However, with the inclusion of more well-annotated data and even number of weakly-annotated data, better performance can be achieved. Meanwhile, the attention maps of classification

Table 4. Results of different settings for ε value.

	200 well + 200 weakly				400 well + 400 weakly			
	$\varepsilon = 0$	$\varepsilon = 0.1$	$\varepsilon = 0.3$	$\varepsilon = 0.5$	$\varepsilon = 0$	$\varepsilon = 0.1$	$\varepsilon = 0.3$	$\varepsilon = 0.5$
IoU	0.544	0.615	0.611	0.526	0.632	0.669	0.663	0.639

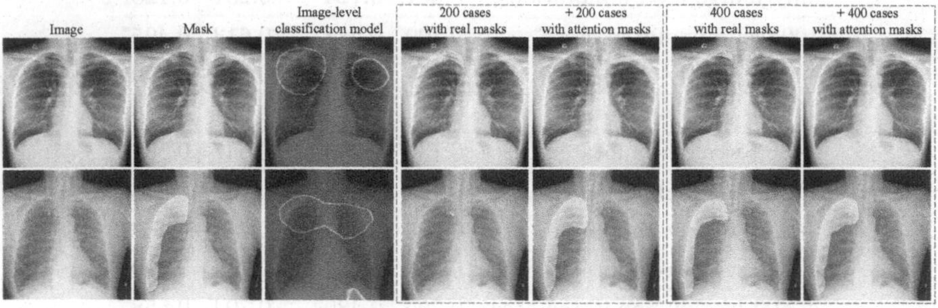

Fig. 4. Visualization of results.

model with image-level annotations are also shown in Fig. 4. The attention maps are very rough and have too many errors to precisely segment and measure the pneumothorax for the application of CXR triage. More examples can be found in supplementary materials.

4   Conclusion

A novel spatial label smoothing regularization method has been developed to explore the uncertainty of weakly-annotated data in the weakly supervised segmentation framework. As can be observed in Table 3 and Fig. 4, the proposed method can relieve the need for well-annotated data by achieving competitive performance. The proposed method has been evaluated on the difficult pneumothorax segmentation problem in CXR images with extensive experiments.

Acknowledgement. This work was partially supported by the National Key Research and Development Program of China (2018YFC0116400), STCSM grants (19QC1400600, 17411953300), and the Shanghai Municipal Commission of Economy and Informatization (2017RGZN01026).

References

1. Annarumma, M., Withey, S.J., Bakewell, R.J., Pesce, E., Goh, V., Montana, G.: Automated triaging of adult chest radiographs with deep artificial neural networks. Radiology **291**, 180921 (2019)
2. Cai, J., Lu, L., Harrison, A.P., Shi, X., Chen, P., Yang, L.: Iterative attention mining for weakly supervised thoracic disease pattern localization in chest X-Rays.

In: Frangi, A.F., Schnabel, J.A., Davatzikos, C., Alberola-López, C., Fichtinger, G. (eds.) MICCAI 2018. LNCS, vol. 11071, pp. 589–598. Springer, Cham (2018). https://doi.org/10.1007/978-3-030-00934-2_66

3. Chaurasia, A., Culurciello, E.: LinkNet: exploiting encoder representations for efficient semantic segmentation. In: 2017 IEEE Visual Communications and Image Processing (VCIP), pp. 1–4. IEEE (2017)

4. Jégou, S., Drozdzal, M., Vazquez, D., Romero, A., Bengio, Y.: The one hundred layers tiramisu: fully convolutional densenets for semantic segmentation. In: 2017 IEEE Conference on Computer Vision and Pattern Recognition Workshops (CVPRW), pp. 1175–1183. IEEE (2017)

5. Kelly, B.S., Rainford, L.A., Darcy, S.P., Kavanagh, E.C., Toomey, R.J.: The development of expertise in radiology: in chest radiograph interpretation,"expert" search pattern may predate "expert" levels of diagnostic accuracy for pneumothorax identification. Radiology 280(1), 252–260 (2016)

6. Li, K., Wu, Z., Peng, K.C., Ernst, J., Fu, Y.: Tell me where to look: guided attention inference network. arXiv preprint arXiv:1802.10171 (2018)

7. Li, Z., et al.: Thoracic disease identification and localization with limited supervision. arXiv preprint arXiv:1711.06373 (2017)

8. Ronneberger, O., Fischer, P., Brox, T.: U-Net: convolutional networks for biomedical image segmentation. In: Navab, N., Hornegger, J., Wells, W.M., Frangi, A.F. (eds.) MICCAI 2015. LNCS, vol. 9351, pp. 234–241. Springer, Cham (2015). https://doi.org/10.1007/978-3-319-24574-4_28

9. Wang, X., Peng, Y., Lu, L., Lu, Z., Bagheri, M., Summers, R.M.: ChestX-ray8: Hospital-scale chest X-ray database and benchmarks on weakly-supervised classification and localization of common thorax diseases. In: Proceedings of the IEEE Conference on Computer Vision and Pattern Recognition, pp. 2097–2106 (2017)

10. Yan, C., Yao, J., Li, R., Xu, Z., Huang, J.: Weakly supervised deep learning for thoracic disease classification and localization on chest x-rays. In: Proceedings of the 2018 ACM International Conference on Bioinformatics, Computational Biology, and Health Informatics, pp. 103–110. ACM (2018)

11. Yu, F., Koltun, V., Funkhouser, T.: Dilated residual networks. In: Proceedings of the IEEE Conference on Computer Vision and Pattern Recognition, pp. 472–480 (2017)

12. Zarogoulidis, P., et al.: Pneumothorax: from definition to diagnosis and treatment. J. Thorac. Dis. 6(Suppl 4), S372 (2014)

13. Zheng, Z., Zheng, L., Yang, Y.: Unlabeled samples generated by GAN improve the person re-identification baseline in vitro. In: Proceedings of the IEEE International Conference on Computer Vision, pp. 3754–3762 (2017)

Multi-task Localization and Segmentation for X-Ray Guided Planning in Knee Surgery

Florian Kordon[1,2,3](✉), Peter Fischer[1,2], Maxim Privalov[4],
Benedict Swartman[4], Marc Schnetzke[4], Jochen Franke[4], Ruxandra Lasowski[3],
Andreas Maier[1], and Holger Kunze[2]

[1] Pattern Recognition Lab, Department of Computer Science,
Friedrich-Alexander-Universität Erlangen-Nürnberg, Erlangen, Germany
florian.kordon@fau.de
[2] Advanced Therapies, Siemens Healthcare GmbH, Forchheim, Germany
[3] Faculty of Digital Media, Hochschule Furtwangen, Furtwangen, Germany
[4] Department for Trauma and Orthopaedic Surgery,
BG Trauma Center Ludwigshafen, Ludwigshafen, Germany

Abstract. X-ray based measurement and guidance are commonly used tools in orthopaedic surgery to facilitate a minimally invasive workflow. Typically, a surgical planning is first performed using knowledge of bone morphology and anatomical landmarks. Information about bone location then serves as a prior for registration during overlay of the planning on intra-operative X-ray images. Performing these steps manually however is prone to intra-rater/inter-rater variability and increases task complexity for the surgeon. To remedy these issues, we propose an automatic framework for planning and subsequent overlay. We evaluate it on the example of femoral drill site planning for medial patellofemoral ligament reconstruction surgery. A deep multi-task stacked hourglass network is trained on 149 conventional lateral X-ray images to jointly localize two femoral landmarks, to predict a region of interest for the posterior femoral cortex tangent line, and to perform semantic segmentation of the femur, patella, tibia, and fibula with adaptive task complexity weighting. On 38 clinical test images the framework achieves a median localization error of 1.50 mm for the femoral drill site and mean IOU scores of 0.99, 0.97, 0.98, and 0.96 for the femur, patella, tibia, and fibula respectively. The demonstrated approach consistently performs surgical planning at expert-level precision without the need for manual correction.

Keywords: Landmark localization · Multi-label bone segmentation · MPFL · X-ray guidance · Orthopaedics · Surgical planning

1 Introduction

In orthopaedics, X-ray imaging is frequently used to facilitate planning and operative guidance for surgical interventions. By capturing patient-specific characteristics and contextual information prior to and during the procedure, such

© Springer Nature Switzerland AG 2019
D. Shen et al. (Eds.): MICCAI 2019, LNCS 11769, pp. 622–630, 2019.
https://doi.org/10.1007/978-3-030-32226-7_69

image-based tools benefit a more reliable and minimally invasive workflow at reduced risk for the patient. To this end, typical assessment involves geometric measurements of patient anatomy, verification of correct positioning of surgical tools and implants, as well as navigational guidance with help of anatomical landmarks and bone morphology. In current clinical practice, several methodologies have been established which leverage this toolset to standardize routine procedures. One example is the Schoettle planning methodology for reconstruction surgery of a ruptured medial patellofemoral ligament (MPFL) [8]. To restore the anatomically correct biomechanics and to forestall recurrent injuries, the optimal fixation area on the femur is approximated by the Schoettle Point, which can be derived from several osseous landmarks (Fig. 1). Unfortunately, execution of such a methodology faces several clinical and technical challenges [5,9]. First, many orthopaedic surgeries target anatomical regions which are not directly inferable from the image but rely on auxiliary structures derived from anatomical landmarks, leading to inter-rater and intra-rater differences. Secondly, the overlay of the planning result on subsequent intra-operational images requires registration to compensate for motion which should be restricted to the anatomical region of interest (ROI), in the case of MPFL, the femoral bone. And lastly, manual intra-operational planning and interaction with a guidance application in a sterile setting are disruptive in the doctor's surgical workflow.

Using MPFL reconstruction as an example, we present a framework which allows fully-automatic localization of anatomical landmarks, semantic segmentation of bone structures, and prediction of ROIs for geometric line features on X-ray images. Building upon the ideas of [1], we exploit recent advances in sequential deep learning architectures in form of deep stacked hourglass networks (SHGN) [7] to refine predictions based on the learned residual information between the ground truth and intermediate estimates. We propose an extension to a multi-task learning approach to incorporate cross-task information for an enriched and more general feature set, which proved to be beneficial in X-ray

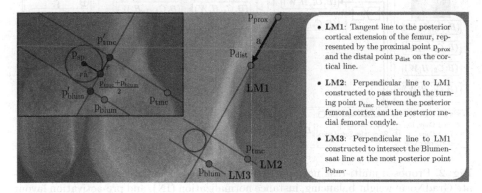

Fig. 1. Approximation of the Schoettle Point p_{sp} [8] as the center of the inner circle of three lines. These lines can be derived from osseous landmarks on a lateral radiograph.

based segmentation tasks [2]. To automatically weight the single task loss terms,
our framework introduces a novel adaption of gradient normalization [3] for
stacked network architectures by integrating it with a deeply supervised optimization scheme. We evaluate this approach for femoral attachment site planning
in MPFL reconstruction surgery which is a clinically relevant and common procedure. We demonstrate expert-level performance of our proposed solution with
a comprehensive evaluation including clinical data and an inter-rater study with
multiple surgeons. The achieved results enable direct integration into the operative workflow and in almost all cases allow the number of manual planning steps
to be limited to the confirmation of the planning proposal, so that the surgeon
can remain sterile throughout the procedure.

2 Methods

2.1 Multi-task Stacked Hourglass Network

A SHGN is a multi-stage convolutional network architecture which sequentially
arranges $l = 1, 2, ..., L$ symmetrical Fully Convolutional Networks referred to as
hourglass modules (HG) [7]. By cascaded inference, several iterations of bottom-
up and top-down processing of data and features are performed to capture and
combine the input morphology at various scales and abstraction levels. At the
end of the expanding path of each HG, features are fed into an additional bottleneck residual unit before being distributed for individual task processing. For
each task $t = 1, 2, ..., T$ we introduce a separate prediction module to facilitate
task-specific discriminative power, allow for intermediate estimates, and exploit
iterative refinement by reinjection (Fig. 2).

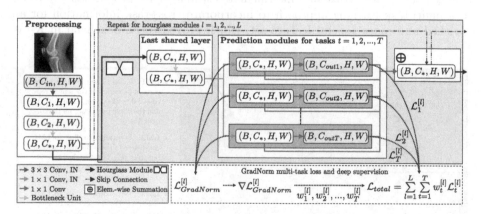

Fig. 2. Proposed multi-task network based on the SHGN architecture with intermediate GradNorm weight balancing, instance normalization (IN), and pre-activation layout
for residual bottleneck units [3,4,7]. Here, $C_{in} = 1$, $C_1 = 64$, $C_2 = 128$, and $C_* = 256$.

Weighted Multi-label Segmentation Loss. X-ray images are superimposition projections, which leads to ambiguities in class assignment for overlapping bones with similar imaging characteristics. Instead of using multinomial pixel-wise classification, we therefor define bone segmentation as a multi-class/multi-label problem and perform separate binomial classifications for each bone in the target region to allow a pixel to be assigned multiple labels. We further exploit this multi-label information to penalize errors in overlap regions, which we derive by a characteristic function $g_{bij} = [\sum_c y_{bcij} > 1]$ and incorporate into the loss function with scaling factor β. y corresponds to a 4th-order tensor (B, C, H, W), where the task-specific ground truth maps are stacked along C. Each tensor element is indexed with $b \in [1, B]$, $c \in [1, C]$, $i \in [1, H]$, and $j \in [1, W]$ where B, C, H, W mark batch, channel, height, and width dimensions. The resulting segmentation loss for prediction $\hat{y}^{[l]}$ with sigmoid nonlinearity σ computes by

$$\mathcal{L}_{\text{seg}}^{[l]} = \frac{1}{BHW} \sum_{(b,c,i,j)} (1+\beta g_{bij}) \Big[-y\log\Big(\sigma\big(\hat{y}^{[l]}\big)\Big) - (1-y)\log\Big(1-\sigma\big(\hat{y}^{[l]}\big)\Big) \Big]_{bcij}. \quad (1)$$

Landmark and Region of Interest Loss. Landmarks and ROIs are represented as heat-maps, which encode the localization likelihood as a spatial intensity distribution. For landmark ground truth, a 2D unnormalized Gaussian with a standard deviation of 6 pixels is centered on the annotated position. Likewise, the line's ROI ground truth is derived by placing equidistant pseudo landmarks along the ground truth cortical line. For loss calculation, heat-map matching is performed as

$$\mathcal{L}_{\{lm,roi\}}^{[l]} = \frac{1}{BCHW} \sum_{(b,c,i,j)} \Big(\hat{y}_{bcij}^{[l]} - y_{bcij}\Big)^2. \quad (2)$$

We derive landmark positions by performing the arg max operation on the predicted likelihood scores. For the posterior femoral cortex tangent line LM1 (Fig. 1), we mask the femur segmentation outline with the predicted ROI and discard features with a likelihood below 0.5 prior to a least squares regression.

Task Weighting and Total Loss. We utilize deep supervision to ease gradient flow across multiple stages of the SHGN and to facilitate faster training. For this purpose, individual task losses are calculated and summed up for both intermediate and final HGs to form a single loss value. To respect imbalanced task difficulties and to avoid overfitting to only a subset of tasks, we use gradient normalization (GradNorm) and adapt it to a deeply supervised setting [3]. Grad-Norm generally tackles task imbalance by reducing the variance across the tasks' training rates. For this purpose, task-specific loss weighting factors are learned by jointly reducing an additional multi-task loss function on the basis of gradient magnitudes to adaptively adjust the gradient norm at each update step [3]. The GradNorm weights for each supervised HG are based on the last shared bottleneck layer before branching off to the prediction modules (Fig. 2). The resulting balanced loss is given by $\mathcal{L}_{total} = \sum_{l=1}^{L} w_{seg}^{[l]} \mathcal{L}_{seg}^{[l]} + w_{lm}^{[l]} \mathcal{L}_{lm}^{[l]} + w_{roi}^{[l]} \mathcal{L}_{roi}^{[l]}$.

2.2   Dataset and Training Procedures

Training and validation data consists of 185 lateral X-ray projections of the knee joint acquired prior to reconstruction surgery. The data was split with ratio 0.8/0.2 for training and validation (149/36 images). For evaluation, 38 separate test images with standardized measuring spheres of 30 mm diameter were used. Annotation of the ground truth landmark positions and line reference points on training and validation images was performed by one orthopaedic surgeon with an interactive proprietary tool (Fig. 1). To allow for an estimate on inter-rater variability, annotation on the test data was extended to three orthopaedic surgeons from the same hospital. Ground truth segmentation masks for the femur, patella, tibia, and fibula were created by the first author. A basic set of data augmentations (rotation, scaling, horizontal flipping) as well as linear contrast scaling with a probability of $p = 0.5$ each were applied during training. After augmentation, the variably sized images were zero-padded to square spatial dimensions and subsequently downsampled to a resolution of 256×256 pixels.

We devise a multi-task SHGN with $L = 4$ HGs and introduce instance normalization layers for approximate contrast invariance and to smooth the optimization landscape [6]. We consider $T = 3$ tasks and hence construct three prediction modules at the end of each HG. The network was implemented with PyTorch (v0.4.1) and trained on a NVIDIA Quadro P5000 over 250 epochs with batch size 2. The network parameters and GradNorm task weights were optimized with RMSProp at learning rates of 0.00025 and 0.025 respectively. The learning rate for network parameters was halved every 60 epochs. Based on prior hyper-parameter optimization, GradNorm's asymmetry hyper-parameter was set to $\alpha = 1$ at each HG, and the penalizing weight factor for multi-label segmentation was assigned to $\beta = 0.6$.

3   Evaluation

Bone Segmentation. The model consistently yields high overlap- and contour-based metric results and successfully delineates all target bone structures (Table 1). Qualitative assessment indicates successful disambiguation in overlapping areas, in narrow interarticular joint spaces, and in low-contrast regions (Fig. 3). Also, uncommon image characteristics like osteophytes along joint contours as well as aberrant lateral projections are resolved with high precision. However, subpar performance is observed for the fibula due to the proximal part being mostly overlapped by the tibia with seemingly no intensity shifts. Likewise, wrongful assignment of spherical markers to the tibia or the femur leads to high contour distances.

Line and Landmark Localization. Predictions for the landmarks p_{blum} and p_{tmc} are spatially precise with median Euclidean distance (ED) errors of 1.18, $\text{CI}_{80\%}[0.99, 1.74]$ mm and 2.14, $\text{CI}_{80\%}[1.71, 2.63]$ mm respectively (Fig. 3). In general, it can be observed that localization of p_{tmc} is less robust due to its

Table 1. Segmentation performance on 38 test images for all bones in target region.

Anatomy	Mean IOU (Mean ± STD)	Average surface distance (Mean ± STD) (mm)	Hausdorff distance (Mean ± STD) (mm)
Femur	0.99 ± 0.01	0.12 ± 0.61	2.96 ± 7.51
Patella	0.97 ± 0.02	0.02 ± 0.02	0.62 ± 0.56
Tibia	0.98 ± 0.02	0.23 ± 0.85	3.76 ± 10.77
Fibula	0.96 ± 0.02	0.14 ± 0.68	2.38 ± 5.41

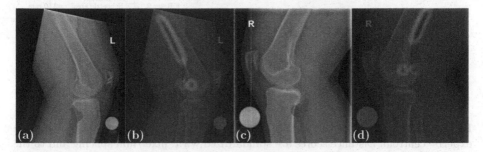

Fig. 3. Automatic results for multi-task segmentation (a, c) and localization (b, d). In (a), false-positive assignment of a spherical marker to the tibia is observed.

dependence on true-lateral imaging. Slight deviations from a true-lateral projection lead to non-overlapping femoral epicondyles, which necessitates three-dimensional reasoning and compensation for correct spatial positioning. For measuring the alignment of the cortical extension line, ED of the ground truth points p_{prox} and p_{dist} to the predicted line are averaged, yielding a median score of 0.62, $CI_{80\%}[0.48, 0.79]$ mm.

Adaptive Task Weighting. The learned GradNorm task weights generally reduce the segmentation training rate across all modules in exchange for increased landmark and ROI loss contributions (Fig. 4). With advanced training time, balancing slightly converges which indicates harmonization of the task-specific loss magnitudes and gradients. Especially in early HGs, optimization towards a single task is observed.

Inter-rater Analysis and Automatic Planning. The observed inter-rater EDs of the constructed Schoettle Points are generally within a circular confidence area with radius $r = 2.50$ mm, which describes an anatomically correct femoral MPFL insertion site [8]. In comparison, automatic plannings are equally reliable and can reduce variability caused by differences in planning strategy between expert raters (Table 2, Fig. 5). However, morphological variations of the femoral cortex or a too short predicted line ROI frequently lead to slight anterior shifting. Likewise, projection of individual ED errors onto the longitudinal and

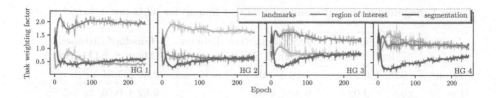

Fig. 4. Development of GradNorm task weights for each HG during training.

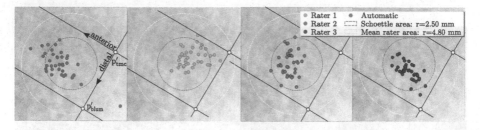

Fig. 5. Visualization of errors between individually planned Schoettle Points and the experts' centroid. Distance scores are standardized w.r.t. pixel/mm spacing and to the mean orientation of LM1 based on expert annotations. Per image, all results are visually aligned to a reference planning, whose Schoettle Point corresponds to this centroid. For comparison with the original Schoettle area of $r = 2.50$ mm, the average confidence circle as planned by the experts (bounded by LM1, LM2 and LM3) is overlayed.

Table 2. Inter-rater variability and comparison with proposed automatic planning. The median ED at 80% confidence level (mm) between raters is reported for full dataset and subset of images agreed to be suitable for surgical planning by all raters.

First rater	Second rater	Schoettle point (38/38 test images)	Schoettle point (29/38 suitable test images)
1	2	2.35, [1.94, 2.85]	2.68, [2.09, 3.13]
1	3	2.31, [1.91, 2.79]	2.49, [1.91, 2.95]
2	3	1.67, [1.37, 2.22]	1.62, [1.07, 2.12]
Autom.	1	2.41, [1.97, 2.99]	2.64, [1.64, 3.10]
Autom.	2 (gr. truth training)	1.46, [1.00, 1.85]	1.33, [0.91, 1.59]
Autom.	3	1.61, [1.45, 1.87]	1.56, [1.27, 1.73]
Autom.	Expert centroid	1.50, [1.41, 2.07]	1.41, [1.28, 1.52]

anteroposterior axes indicates an error tendency towards the anterior direction, which underlines difficulties in correct assessment of the femoral bow (Fig. 5).

4   Discussion and Conclusion

We proposed an automatic framework for joint prediction of segmentations and heatmaps for spatial localization of landmarks and line features. On the example of MPFL reconstruction surgery, we could show that we can facilitate surgical planning by providing planning proposals at expert-rater precision. We see limitations in that the proposed method was only trained and tested on pre-operational, conventional X-ray images which depict a large portion of the femoral shaft and typically have high contrast. For seamless integration into a clinical workflow with subsequent overlay of the planning result on live images, the framework performance must be evaluated on fluoroscopic image data. This modality however imposes additional difficulties onto automated prediction by superimposed surgical tools and by greater overall heterogeneity in image characteristics and acquisition settings. This could partially by solved by overlay of simulated tools and implants in the image domain during training, which showed to increase robustness of learning-based algorithms [6].

As shown in this work, planning methods like the Schoettle methodology might also inherently tolerate variability in assessment strategy and typically cannot be securely validated due to absence of anatomical ground truth. An automatic solution should therefor utilize an adequate encoding of this variability to alleviate overfitting to a certain type of annotation strategy by a single rater. Furthermore, while we experience satisfactory results in estimating a line by masking segmentation contour features, such cross-task coupling introduces additional failure points in the planning pipeline. As for estimation of the posterior femoral cortex, strongly curved femoral shafts allow an anterior shift of the fitted line, which is directly conditioned by the longitudinal extends of the predicted ROI. To this end, we aim to look at ways to derive confidence estimates for each task and to keep the number of interdependent tasks at a reasonable level. In future work, we also seek to adapt our approach to different anatomies by exploiting the highly generalizable concept of heat-map matching for a direct representation of arbitrarily shaped features.

Disclaimer. The methods and information presented here are based on research and are not commercially available.

References

1. Bier, B., et al.: X-ray-transform invariant anatomical landmark detection for pelvic trauma surgery. In: Frangi, A.F., Schnabel, J.A., Davatzikos, C., Alberola-López, C., Fichtinger, G. (eds.) Medical Image Computing and Computer Assisted Intervention - MICCAI 2018. LNCS, vol. 11073, pp. 55–63. Springer, Cham (2018)
2. Breininger, K., et al.: Multiple device segmentation for fluoroscopic imaging using multi-task learning. In: Stoyanov, D., et al. (eds.) LABELS/CVII/STENT -2018. LNCS, vol. 11043, pp. 19–27. Springer, Cham (2018). https://doi.org/10.1007/978-3-030-01364-6_3
3. Chen, Z., Badrinarayanan, V., Lee, C., Rabinovich, A.: Gradnorm: Gradient normalization for adaptive loss balancing in deep multitask networks. In: Proceedings of International Conference Machine Learning, pp. 793–802 (2018)
4. He, K., Zhang, X., Ren, S., Sun, J.: Identity mappings in deep residual networks. In: Leibe, B., Matas, J., Sebe, N., Welling, M. (eds.) ECCV 2016. LNCS, vol. 9908, pp. 630–645. Springer, Cham (2016). https://doi.org/10.1007/978-3-319-46493-0_38

5. Joskowicz, L., Hazan, E.J.: Computer aided orthopaedic surgery: Incremental shift or paradigm change? Med. Image Anal. **33**, 84–90 (2016)
6. Kordon, F., Lasowski, R., Swartman, B., Franke, J., Fischer, P., Kunze, H.: Improved X-ray bone segmentation by normalization and augmentation strategies. In: Handels, H., Deserno, T., Maier, A., Maier-Hein, K., Palm, C., Tolxdorff, T. (eds.) Bildverarbeitung für die Medizin 2019. I, pp. 104–109. Springer, Wiesbaden (2019). https://doi.org/10.1007/978-3-658-25326-4_24
7. Newell, A., Yang, K., Deng, J.: Stacked hourglass networks for human pose estimation. In: Leibe, B., Matas, J., Sebe, N., Welling, M. (eds.) Computer Vision - European Conference on Computer Vision 2016, pp. 483–499. Springer, Cham (2016)
8. Schöttle, P.B., Schmeling, A., Rosenstiel, N., Weiler, A.: Radiographic landmarks for femoral tunnel placement in medial patellofemoral ligament reconstruction. Am. J. Sports Med. **35**(5), 801–804 (2007)
9. Székely, G., Nolte, L.P.: Image guidance in orthopaedics and traumatology: a historical perspective. Med. Image Anal. **33**, 79–83 (2016)

Towards Fully Automatic X-Ray to CT Registration

Javier Esteban[1]([✉]), Matthias Grimm[1], Mathias Unberath[2], Guillaume Zahnd[1], and Nassir Navab[1,3]

[1] Computer Aided Medical Procedures, Technische Universität München, Boltzmannstraße 3, 85748 Garching bei München, Germany
javier.esteban@tum.de, grimmma@in.tum.de
[2] Laboratory for Computational Sensing + Robotics, Johns Hopkins University, 3400 North Charles Street, Baltimore, MD 21218, USA
[3] Computer Aided Medical Procedures, Johns Hopkins University, 3400 North Charles Street, Baltimore, MD 21218, USA

Abstract. The main challenge preventing a fully-automatic X-ray to CT registration is an initialization scheme that brings the X-ray pose within the capture range of existing intensity-based registration methods. By providing such an automatic initialization, the present study introduces the first end-to-end fully-automatic registration framework. A network is first trained once on artificial X-rays to extract 2D landmarks resulting from the projection of CT-labels. A patient-specific refinement scheme is then carried out: candidate points detected from a new set of artificial X-rays are back-projected onto the patient CT and merged into a refined meaningful set of landmarks used for network re-training. This network-landmarks combination is finally exploited for intraoperative pose-initialization with a runtime of 102 ms. Evaluated on 6 pelvis anatomies (486 images in total), the mean Target Registration Error was 15.0 ± 7.3 mm. When used to initialize the BOBYQA optimizer with normalized cross-correlation, the average ($\pm$ STD) projection distance was 3.4 ± 2.3 mm, and the registration success rate (projection distance < 2.5% of the detector width) greater than 97%.

Keywords: X-ray to CT Registration · Projective geometry · Neural network · Patient-specific training

1 Introduction

Registration deals with the problem of finding the optimal transformation from one coordinate space to another. Within a medical context, registration plays a crucial role to match preoperative and intraoperative data. Preoperative images,

J. Esteban and M. Grimm-Contributed equally to this work.
This work was supported by the German Federal Ministry of Research and Education (FKZ: 13GW0236B) and a GPU Grant from Nvidia.

D. Shen et al. (Eds.): MICCAI 2019, LNCS 11769, pp. 631–639, 2019.
https://doi.org/10.1007/978-3-030-32226-7_70

such as CT scans, are usually captured days before the actual surgery to execute surgical planning, while intraoperative images, such as X-ray, are used for live navigation and monitoring. Without registration, surgeons must rely on their experience to perform a mental mapping between pre- and intraoperative images. Therefore, automatic registration is important to facilitate the surgical workflow, reduce the mental load, and potentially improve the clinical outcome.

Effective initialization is usually considered as the Achilles' heel of most registration approaches. Considering two images $\{I_1, I_2\}$ and a given registration method $\mathcal{R}$, if I_1 and I_2 originally have a substantially different pose (namely, a great discrepancy in their relative rotation and translation within six degrees of freedom, 6DoF), the subsequent operation of spatial alignment $\mathcal{R}(I_1, I_2)$ is likely to fail. For this reason, the notion of *capture range* is used to describe the maximum initial displacement from which $\mathcal{R}$ is able to provide an accurate result [5]. Initialization can then be defined as estimating a transformation matrix $\mathcal{T} = [\mathbf{R}|\mathbf{T}]$ (i.e. rotation, translation) such that $\mathcal{T}(I_1)$ falls in the capture range of $\mathcal{R}$, thus enabling the end-to-end operation $\mathcal{R}(\mathcal{T}(I_1), I_2)$ to provide a correct spatial alignment between I_1 and I_2. Although marker-based registration approaches (i.e. relying on a set of external fiducial targets) are known for their relative agnosticism to initialization due to their higher built-in robustness, this family of methods suffers from other drawbacks: bone-implanted markers require an additional invasive surgical procedure, whereas skin-attached markers are prone to deformation and yield a lower accuracy [5]. For purely image-based registration methods—such as intensity-based or feature-based approaches—to perform accurately, providing a correct initialization is indeed crucial.

Although registration methodologies are now well established, the challenge of providing a robust initialization towards enabling registration convergence remains an open problem. An approach based on the projection-slice theorem and phase correlation was put forward [2]. Despite the fact that good results were achieved, the authors report severe limitations: running time not suited for intraoperative use, and geometric discrepancy between the theoretical parallel-beam and the actual cone-beam. A regression technique was designed to deal with arbitrary motion and to predict slice transformations relative to a learned canonical atlas coordinate system [3]. The applicability of that scheme is however constrained by the relatively poor resulting accuracy. A different strategy relying on a specific initialization framework via several coarse segmentations was proposed [6]. A potential drawback of this method is that the initialization step is based upon a third-party segmentation scheme that shall be provided by the user. An original approach was recently introduced to automatically detect anatomical landmarks in 2D X-ray images, thus enabling to determine the transformation $\mathcal{T}$ with respect to the corresponding 3D CT volume [1]. Nevertheless, this method is hindered by two limitations: (1) the original 3D CT landmarks must be manually annotated for each new patient, which is a tedious and analyst-dependant task, and (2) the landmark model is pre-generated from a set of patients and may therefore not fully capture patient-specific anatomical details when applied intraoperatively.

The aim of the present work is to propose a method to estimate the initial rigid transformation $\mathcal{T}$ between a preoperative 3D CT volume and intraoperative 2D X-ray images. The main contribution is a patient-specific landmark-refinement scheme based on deep learning and projective geometry. Addressing the limitations mentioned above, the framework is fully automatic, falls in the capture range of standard registration methods, and its runtime is compatible with intraoperative applications. The proposed method is fully integrated into an end-to-end registration scheme, where the provided initial pose can be directly and automatically exploited by standard registration techniques. Validation is performed on pelvis anatomy in the context of trauma surgery.

2   Methods

A schematic representation of the proposed method is shown in Fig. 1. The framework consists of three main phases, as described hereafter.

Phase 1—Network Pre-training: This phase is run only once and for all. Here, a convolutional neural network $\mathbb{N}$ is trained to detect a set of $\Omega = 23$ anatomical landmarks $\mathcal{M} = [m_1, m_2, \ldots, m_\Omega]$ on X-ray images, similar to a method introduced by another group [1]. The training data for $\mathbb{N}$ consists of synthetically generated X-ray images from a collection of manually annotated CT volumes from 13 patients from the NIH Cancer Imaging Archive [7] (referred to as the "pre-training set"). Twelve patients were used for training and one for validation. Landmark locations were chosen such that they correspond to clinically meaningful and clearly identifiable points [1]. X-rays were generated with a commercially available Digitally Reconstructed Radiograph (DRR) generator[1]. For each CT, a total of 3,456 X-rays were generated, covering a wide range of poses (Translation: ± 15 mm along $\{x, y, z\}$ (where x is medial/lateral, y is anterior/posterior, z is cranial/caudal); Rotation: $\pm 35°$ around x, $\pm 15°$ around y, and $\pm 45°$ around z). Values were sampled evenly along those dimensions, with 6 rotation samples around z, 3 rotation samples around x and y, and 4 translation samples along x, y, and z. Ground truth landmarks for the training were obtained by projecting the points m_ω from CT to X-ray, knowing the DRR pose. The network $\mathbb{N}$ corresponds to a previously introduced architecture [9]. Training was carried out with the Adam optimizer for 4 epochs until convergence was reached, with a learning rate of 0.00001 and a batch size of 1 [1].

Phase 2—Automatic Patient-Specific Landmarks Extraction: This phase is the main contribution of the present work. A patient-specific CT volume, referred to as CT_{pat}, is processed in three steps, as described below.

Phase 2.a—Ray Back-Projection: X-ray images are synthetically generated from CT_{pat} using the DRR generator, covering $K = 90$ poses (Translation: ± 15 mm along z; Rotation: $\pm 15°$ around x, $\pm 40°$ around z). Equidistantly-spaced samples were chosen: 10 rotation samples around z, 3 rotation samples

---

[1] ImFusion GmbH, Munich, Germany (https://www.imfusion.de).

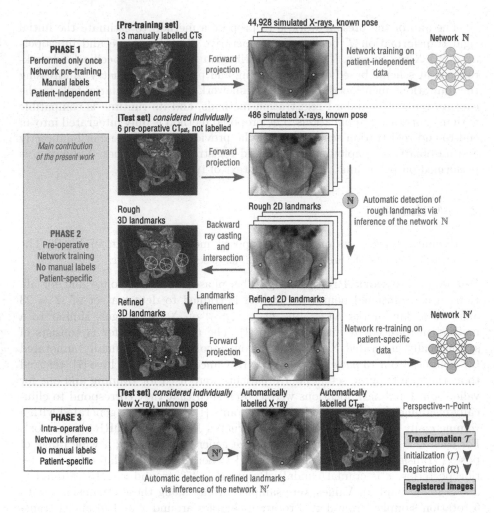

Fig. 1. Schematic representation of the global framework. For clarity purpose, only three landmarks out of 23 are depicted.

around x, and 3 translation samples along z. The network $\mathbb{N}$ is then applied to detect the rough locations of the landmarks $\mathcal{M}$. The known geometry of all the generated X-ray images is exploited to back-project each point m_ω onto a series of rays r_ω^k, with $k = [1, 2, \ldots, K]$ (Fig. 2). Each ray r_ω^k passes through the detected location of m_ω in the image and the camera center of the projection.

Phase* 2.b—*Landmark Refinement: Due to the prediction inaccuracy inherent to the network $\mathbb{N}$, the set of 3D rays r_ω^k resulting from a given landmark m_ω do not perfectly intersect on the same point (Fig. 2). To cope with this lack of precision, a set of refined landmarks $\mathcal{M}' = [m_1', m_2', \ldots, m_\Omega']$ is generated, respecting the two following criteria: each new landmark m_ω' shall (1) stay as close as

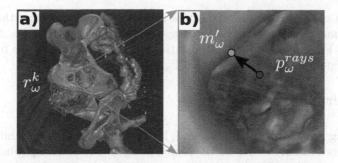

Fig. 2. Landmark refinement, applied here to a single landmark m_ω. (a) Set of back-projected rays (r_ω^k). (b) Determination of the barycenter (p_ω^{rays}) via robust ray intersection, and projection to the bone surface (m_ω').

possible to the barycenter of the intersection of all the rays r_ω^k, and (2) be located on the bone surface. The rationale of this refinement operation is to ensure that the final landmarks m_ω' describe meaningful local anatomical regions, thus facilitating learning and registration. This approach is independently conducted for all landmarks, and is described hereafter for a single landmark m_ω'.

First, the point p_ω^{rays}, corresponding to the rough barycenter of the intersection of all rays r_ω^k, is determined (Fig. 2a–b). For two given rays $\{r_\omega^{k_1}, r_\omega^{k_2}\}$, the closest equidistant point $p_\omega^{k_1,k_2}$ is calculated. A constant threshold $\tau = 6$ mm is used to discard candidate points when two rays are too far apart. The coordinates of p_ω^{rays} are defined as the median x, y, and z coordinates of all valid $p_\omega^{k_1,k_2}$ points.

Then, the point m_ω' corresponding to the projection of p_ω^{rays} onto the bone surface is determined (Fig. 2b). The volume CT_{pat} is first thresholded (Hounsfield units in $[200, 500]$ are mapped to one—bone, all other values are mapped to zero—background). A contour detection scheme is then applied to the thresholded image [8]. The point m_ω' is finally determined via a sphere-growing scheme centered on p_ω^{rays} to find the closest point on the bone surface.

Phase 2.c—Patient-Specific Re-training: Since the landmark sets $\mathcal{M}$ and $\mathcal{M}'$ do not necessarily describe the same real-world points, network re-training is necessary. The network $\mathbb{N}'$ is therefore generated to detect the refined landmarks $\mathcal{M}'$. The weights of $\mathbb{N}'$ are initialized with the weights of $\mathbb{N}$. To enable patient-specific re-training, the synthetic DRR X-rays are only generated from CT_{pat} (as opposed to from the collection of 13 patients used during phase (1)). Thus generated X-ray poses are similar to those used during the training of $\mathbb{N}$. Validation is carried out with 10% of randomly selected poses.

Phase 3—Intraoperative Registration: Here, the transformation matrix $\mathcal{T}$ is computed, to define the rough initial 6DoF alignment of any new X-ray image, as an input for a given registration method $\mathcal{R}$. An unknown X-ray pose (i.e. previously unseen during phases 1-2) is generated from CT_{pat}. First, the network $\mathbb{N}'$ is applied to fully-automatically infer the landmarks $\mathcal{M}'$ on the X-ray image.

Then, $\mathcal{T}$ is computed via a Perspective-n-Point scheme [4], using the detected X-ray landmarks together with the corresponding CT_{pat} landmarks determined in phase 2. Finally, this rough initialization $\mathcal{T}$ is exploited by a fine registration $\mathcal{R}$ to accurately match the X-ray to CT_{pat}, as detailed in Sect. 3.

3   Experiments and Results

Evaluating the Initialization $\mathcal{T}(\mathbf{I}_1)$: The accuracy of the initialization method was evaluated with DRR X-ray images. Pre-training (phase 1) was applied on 13 patient CTs (i.e. the training set). Landmark refinement (phase 2) was performed individually on 6 new CTs, each from a different and previously unseen patient (referred to as the "test set"). Patient-specific re-training was carried out for 4 epochs. Initial transformation ($\mathcal{T}$, phase 3) was computed for 81 X-ray poses per CT (Fig. 3a). Ground-truth poses (GT) were evenly sampled using 9 samples for the rotation around the z axis (range: $\pm 40°$) and 3 samples for both translation along z (range: top to bottom of the pelvis) and rotation around y (range: $\pm 15°$). Special care was taken so that these poses were previously unseen during pre-training or validation. First, the Target Registration Error (TRE) was assessed by computing the pairwise distance between landmarks resulting from $\mathcal{T}$ and GT. A fair evaluation was conducted by using the set $\mathcal{M}$, since these points are different from those used for training and pose estimation (i.e. $\mathcal{M}'$). Then, the C-Arm pose was investigated by comparing the camera centers resulting from $\mathcal{T}$ and GT (Fig. 3b). The translational error was computed via the Euclidean distance between the two camera centers, measured in CT_{pat} coordinate space. The rotational error was computed as the absolute angle of the axis-angle representation of $\mathbf{R}_{\mathcal{T}}\mathbf{R}_{\mathrm{GT}}^{T}$.

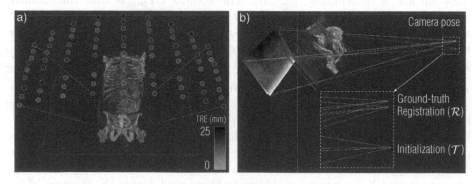

Fig. 3. (a) Mean post-initialization TRE for all the 6 test patients, in relation to the 81 applied camera poses. (b) Representative example for one single X-ray, showing the cone-beam geometry for ground truth, initialization $\mathcal{T}$, and final registration $\mathcal{R}$.

Evaluating the Subsequent Registration $\mathcal{R}(\mathcal{T}(\mathbf{I}_1), \mathbf{I}_2)$: The applicability of the proposed initialization method $\mathcal{T}$ was investigated by determining whether the resulting error was within the capture range of a registration method $\mathcal{R}$. An intensity-based registration algorithm using the widely established BOBYQA optimizer was applied to the initialized poses $T(\mathbf{I}_1)$ on the entire test set. Both normalized cross-correlation (NCC) and local normalized cross-correlation (LNCC) similarity metrics were independently assessed. The registration error was computed as the average pairwise projection distance between the landmark set $\mathcal{M}$ resulting from $\mathcal{R}$ and GT. Registration success was empirically defined as a mean projection distance smaller than 2.5% of the detector width (i.e. <9.7 mm).

Imaging Parameters: For the X-ray C-Arm geometry: 1200 mm source-to-detector distance; 700 mm source iso-center; $384 \times 300\,\mathrm{mm}^2$ detector size; and $1.6\,\mathrm{mm}^2$ isotropic pixel size. For the CT: $0.82\,\mathrm{mm}^3$ isotropic voxel size.

Results: The results of the evaluation of the initialization $T(\mathbf{I}_1)$ are detailed in Fig. 4. The average ($\pm$ STD) TRE over all patients and all poses was $15.0 \pm 7.3\,\mathrm{mm}$ (Fig. 3—no substantial difference was found between patients). As for the results of the final registration $\mathcal{R}\big(T(\mathbf{I}_1), \mathbf{I}_2\big)$, the registration algorithm was successful on 472/486 and 450/486 cases with the NCC and LNCC metrics, respectively (Fig. 5). In successful operations, the average ($\pm$ STD) projection distance error was $3.4 \pm 2.3\,\mathrm{mm}$ and $2.2 \pm 1.6\,\mathrm{mm}$ for NCC and LNCC, respectively. The execution time on a workstation (Core i7 9700K, 8 GB RAM, Nvidia Titan XP) was 102 ms for the intra-operative initialization (Fig. 1, phase 3) and 40 min per CT for the offline DRR generation required for patient-specific re-training (phase 2.c).

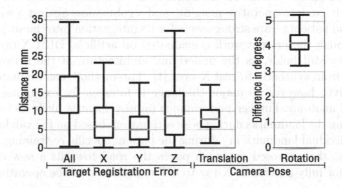

Fig. 4. Evaluation of the accuracy of the initialization method T on a total of 486 images (81 X-rays poses for all 6 previously unseen patients CTs of the test set). Here, X, Y, Z correspond to camera-coordinate axes.

4   Discussion and Conclusion

A framework was introduced to enable X-ray to CT registration without any user interaction required. The focus of this study is a patient-specific initialization

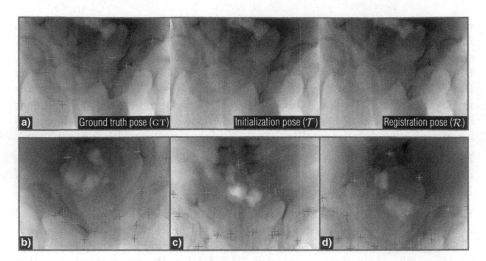

Fig. 5. Evaluation of the initialization method $\mathcal{T}$ when combined with the BOBYQA optimizer for end-to-end registration. Four different patients and poses are displayed. The green and red crosses indicate ground truth (GT) and registered ($\mathcal{R}$) location of the landmarks $\mathcal{M}$, respectively. (a–c) Representative cases. (d) Failure case. (Color figure online)

scheme that can be coupled to standard intensity-based registration methods. The fully-automatic nature of the framework—combined with a runtime compatible with live intraoperative imaging, and a robustness against a wide variety of poses and patients—are strong assets for its integration into the surgical workflow. Although the present work is evaluated on artificial DRR X-rays, clinical applicability still holds, as the underlying architecture of the network $\mathbb{N}$ can generalize from synthetic to real X-rays [1]. The method was evaluated for the human pelvis, however no major challenge is foreseen for extending it to any other rigid anatomy. Further performance improvement is likely to be achieved by weighting the landmarks during pose estimation, based on the validation error of each individual landmark m'_ω during the patient specific re-training (phase 2). Concluding, the proposed approach paves the road towards a new end-to-end paradigm for fully-automatic X-ray to CT registration in the operating room.

References

1. Bier, B., et al.: X-ray-transform invariant anatomical landmark detection for pelvic trauma surgery. In: Frangi, A.F., Schnabel, J.A., Davatzikos, C., Alberola-López, C., Fichtinger, G. (eds.) MICCAI 2018. LNCS, vol. 11073, pp. 55–63. Springer, Cham (2018). https://doi.org/10.1007/978-3-030-00937-3_7
2. Van der Bom, M.J., et al.: Robust initialization of 2D–3D image registration using the projection-slice theorem and phase correlation. Med. Phys. **37**(4), 1884–1892 (2010)

3. Hou, B., et al.: Predicting slice-to-volume transformation in presence of arbitrary subject motion. In: Descoteaux, M., Maier-Hein, L., Franz, A., Jannin, P., Collins, D.L., Duchesne, S. (eds.) MICCAI 2017. LNCS, vol. 10434, pp. 296–304. Springer, Cham (2017). https://doi.org/10.1007/978-3-319-66185-8_34

4. Li, S., Xu, C., Xie, M.: A robust O(n) solution to the perspective-n-point problem. IEEE Trans. Pat. Anal. Mach. Intel. **34**(7), 1444–1450 (2012)

5. Markelj, P., Tomaževič, D., Likar, B., Pernuš, F.: A review of 3D/2D registration methods for image-guided interventions. Med. Im. Anal. **16**(3), 642–661 (2012)

6. Rackerseder, J., Baust, M., Göbl, R., Navab, N., Hennersperger, C.: Initialize globally before acting locally: enabling landmark-free 3D US to MRI registration. In: Frangi, A.F., Schnabel, J.A., Davatzikos, C., Alberola-López, C., Fichtinger, G. (eds.) MICCAI 2018. LNCS, vol. 11070, pp. 827–835. Springer, Cham (2018). https://doi.org/10.1007/978-3-030-00928-1_93

7. Roth, H.R., et al.: A new 2.5 D representation for lymph node detection in CT. The Cancer Imaging Archive (2015)

8. Suzuki, S., Abe, K.: Topological structural analysis of digitized binary images by border following. Comput. Vis. Graph. Image Process. **30**(1), 32–46 (1985)

9. Wei, S.E., Ramakrishna, V., Kanade, T., Sheikh, Y.: Convolutional pose machines. In: IEEE Conference on Computer Vision and Pattern Recognition, pp. 4724–4732 (2016)

Adaptive Image-Feature Learning for Disease Classification Using Inductive Graph Networks

Hendrik Burwinkel[1(✉)], Anees Kazi[1], Gerome Vivar[2], Shadi Albarqouni[1],
Guillaume Zahnd[1], Nassir Navab[1,3], and Seyed-Ahmad Ahmadi[2]

[1] Computer Aided Medical Procedures, Technische Universität München,
Boltzmannstraße 3, 85748 Garching bei München, Germany
hendrik.burwinkel@tum.de
[2] German Center for Vertigo and Balance Disorders, Ludwig-Maximilians Universität
München, Marchioninistr. 15, 81377 München, Germany
[3] Computer Aided Medical Procedures, Johns Hopkins University,
3400 North Charles Street, Baltimore, MD 21218, USA

Abstract. Recently, Geometric Deep Learning (GDL) has been introduced as a novel and versatile framework for computer-aided disease classification. GDL uses patient meta-information such as age and gender to model patient cohort relations in a graph structure. Concepts from graph signal processing are leveraged to learn the optimal mapping of multi-modal features, e.g. from images to disease classes. Related studies so far have considered image features that are extracted in a pre-processing step. We hypothesize that such an approach prevents the network from optimizing feature representations towards achieving the best performance in the graph network. We propose a new network architecture that exploits an inductive end-to-end learning approach for disease classification, where filters from both the CNN and the graph are trained jointly. We validate this architecture against state-of-the-art inductive graph networks and demonstrate significantly improved classification scores on a modified MNIST toy dataset, as well as comparable classification results with higher stability on a chest X-ray image dataset. Additionally, we explain how the structural information of the graph affects both the image filters and the feature learning.

Keywords: Graph convolutional networks · Representation learning · Disease classification

1 Introduction

In the past few years, the potential of data processing with Geometric Deep Learning (GDL) on non-Euclidian data structures has been demonstrated by a large body of work [1,2,6–8]. One uprising application, which is also the subject of this work, lies in the field of computer-aided disease classification (CAD),

© Springer Nature Switzerland AG 2019
D. Shen et al. (Eds.): MICCAI 2019, LNCS 11769, pp. 640–648, 2019.
https://doi.org/10.1007/978-3-030-32226-7_71

where the usage of patient meta-information is leveraged to build a graph system of meaningful patient inter-relations [5,8]. These patient relations allow e.g. an improved classification of image data, which enables the prediction of a disease. This is achieved by using various forms of graph signal processing for the training of localized graph filters, where patients are modeled as vertices in the graph, and images as feature vectors. One family of approaches [1,6,8] are graph spectral methods, which utilize the normalized graph Laplacian L to perform a Fourier transform in order to find optimal filters in the frequency domain. A major drawback of spectral methods is the limitation of their learned representation to the graph they are trained on. Therefore, their transductive approach requires a retraining for every new graph system, making them difficult to use for a direct application on newly received patient data. We therefore focus on non-spectral methods, which overcome this limitation by working on local graph structures, mimicking the standard convolution operation on the spatial relations of a graph node. The concept relevant for this work are composition-based spatial methods that use multiple consecutive layers to update the vertex representation. Hamilton et al. presented GraphSage [3], which samples a fixed number of neighbors of a vertex and aggregates them to receive an updated representation of the feature vector in every layer. This inductive approach allows the successive processing of every vertex of the graph. The system however did not define a preference of which neighboring feature representations are most relevant for the update. We thus focus on and adapt Graph Attention Networks (GAT) in this work. GAT was introduced by [10] and leverages an attention mechanism to learn this importance measure in order to optimize the representation learning.

Regarding CAD systems, in [8] a GDL-approach for disease classification was proposed, modeling patient similarities through meta-information and performing patient classification in the ABIDE and ADNI datasets using Graph Convolutional Networks (GCN). In 2018, self-attention was used in [5] to optimize the usage of meta-information in the TADPOLE dataset. Both methodologies used pre-learned features in their approach. Since we are evaluating our method on chest X-ray images, we are also mentioning related works out of this field. In 2017, Wang et al. [11] proposed a new chest X-ray database, known as "ChestX-ray8", which contains 108,948 frontal view X-ray images of 32,717 unique patients for eight different disease classifications and performed multi-label disease classification and localisation using class activation mapping [12]. In [4], disease classification was realized on three chest X-ray datasets using standard deep convolutional networks, localizing activations with occlusion mapping. CheXNet [9], a DenseNet of 121-layers, was used for classification of all 14 diseases for the NIH ChestX-ray 14 dataset, with an emphasis on pneumonia. All the works relied on standard CNN approaches and did not leverage any non-imaging information.

Contributions. Although GDL approaches used for CAD showed promising performance, two major drawbacks are present in the methodologies developed so far. First, it is necessary to extract the features in a pre-processing step, which results in additional effort. Second, a potentially not optimized feature representation for the usage inside the graph system is learned. To address these limitations we propose CNNGAT, a novel method that yields an inductive end-to-end approach for both learning an optimized feature representation and performing the graph convolutions during training time. Additionally, the introduced concept leverages inter-class connections to specifically improve the performance on instances from classes which are more difficult to distinguish. To the best of our knowledge this is the first work that combines the training of the CNN and the graph network to obtain optimized feature representations. We evaluate our proposed method on the ChestX-ray 14 [9] and a modified MNIST dataset.

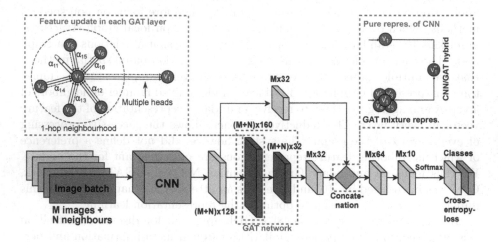

Fig. 1. CNNGAT for a classification of 10 classes. An image batch of M images and N neighboring images is loaded and processed by the CNN. The extracted features are passed through the GAT layers. Then, only the M main batch representations resulting from the GAT network and CNN are concatenated and used to perform the final classification and loss backpropagation.

2 Methodology

2.1 Explanation of the Proposed Model

General Framework. Our proposed network CNNGAT performs the classification of images represented as 2D intensity arrays $\mathbf{X}$ using non-imaging meta-information in an inductive end-to-end approach. It tries to optimize the objective function $f(\mathbf{X}, G(\mathbf{V}, \mathbf{E})) : \mathbf{X} \rightarrow \mathbf{Y}$, where $G(\mathbf{V}, \mathbf{E})$ is a graph with vertices $\mathbf{V}$ containing a feature representation of every image $\boldsymbol{x}_i$ and binary edges $\mathbf{E}$ as connections between the vertices and $\mathbf{Y}$ as set of classes. The whole set of feature representations for every vertex $\boldsymbol{v}_i$ of the graph is therefore defined as:

$\mathbf{V} = \{\boldsymbol{v}_1, \boldsymbol{v}_2, ..., \boldsymbol{v}_N\}, \boldsymbol{v}_i \in \mathbb{R}^F$, where F is the dimension of the representation. The edges $\mathbf{E}$ are created based on non-imaging information belonging to every image $\boldsymbol{x}_i$. The CNN extracts a feature representation of image $\boldsymbol{x}_i$ and distributes it to the corresponding vertex $\boldsymbol{v}_i$. Subsequently, the obtained representation is processed by two consecutive GAT layers. The resulting representation is concatenated with the initial one of the CNN to perform the final prediction (Fig. 1).

Neighborhood Concept. A GAT layer updates the feature representation $\boldsymbol{v}_i$ based on the ones of neighboring vertices. Therefore, it requires that a neighborhood of images is processed together with $\boldsymbol{x}_i$. Since the general size of image datasets prohibits the use of all neighbors for a vertex $\boldsymbol{v}_i \in \mathbf{V}$, different from [10], only a fixed sub-sample of size n of all vertices $\boldsymbol{v}_j$ with $e_{ij} \in \mathbf{E}$ is considered as neighborhood N_i of $\boldsymbol{v}_i$. If for a vertex $\boldsymbol{v}_i$, the size n of the neighborhood cannot be reached, a random selection of N_i is used multiple times until the amount n of vertices is achieved. As described in [3], this procedure has the advantage of setting the computational effort of the network to a fixed amount.

GAT Layer. To achieve a higher representation of $\boldsymbol{v}_i \in \mathbb{R}^F$ with new dimension F', a shared learnable linear transformation $\mathbf{W} \in \mathbb{R}^{F' \times F}$ is applied to $\boldsymbol{v}_i$ and its considered neighbors $\boldsymbol{v}_j \in N_i$. Then, a shared attention mechanism a that consists of a single-layer feed-forward network is used to obtain the attention coefficient α, representing how important $\boldsymbol{v}_j$ is for the update of $\boldsymbol{v}_i$ and computed as $a(\mathbf{W}\boldsymbol{v}_i, \mathbf{W}\boldsymbol{v}_j) = \boldsymbol{a}^T[\mathbf{W}\boldsymbol{v}_i||\mathbf{W}\boldsymbol{v}_j]$, with the concatenation (symbolized as $[\,||\,]$) of $\mathbf{W}\boldsymbol{v}_i$ and $\mathbf{W}\boldsymbol{v}_j$ and $\boldsymbol{a} \in \mathbb{R}^{2F'}$. After activating the calculated attention using the activation $\sigma = $ LeakyReLU, the softmax function is applied for all $\boldsymbol{v}_j \in N_i$ to obtain normalized and easily comparable attention coefficients α:

$$\alpha_{ij} = \frac{\exp(\sigma(\boldsymbol{a}^T([\mathbf{W}\boldsymbol{v}_i||\mathbf{W}\boldsymbol{v}_j])))}{\sum_{r \in N_i} \exp(\sigma(\boldsymbol{a}^T[\mathbf{W}\boldsymbol{v}_i||\mathbf{W}\boldsymbol{v}_r]))} \tag{1}$$

Every attention coefficient is multiplied with the feature representation $\mathbf{W}\boldsymbol{v}_j$ and added up to obtain the new representation $\boldsymbol{v}'_i$. To stabilize the representation, this procedure is repeated multiple times with individual $\mathbf{W}^k$, called heads, performing the same attention mechanism for a vertex $\boldsymbol{v}_i$. The representations $\boldsymbol{v}'_i$ are concatenated (represented as $||$), yielding the new feature representation:

$$\boldsymbol{v}'_i = ||_{k=1}^K \sigma \left(\sum_{j \in N_i} \alpha_{ij}^k \mathbf{W}^k \boldsymbol{v}_j \right), \tag{2}$$

where α_{ij}^k is the attention coefficient of head k for the vertices $\boldsymbol{v}_i$ and $\boldsymbol{v}_j$, and K is the number of heads [10].

CNN/GAT Hybrid. The initial representation $\boldsymbol{v}_i$ is processed at the same time in a skip connection using a single-layer feed-forward network $\mathbf{W}_{skip}$. The output of the layer is activated using LeakyReLU and then concatenated with the output of the graph attention network $\boldsymbol{v}'_i$ to receive the hybrid representation $\boldsymbol{v}''_i = [\boldsymbol{v}_i||\boldsymbol{v}'_i]$. This strategy enables both the initial representation of the CNN and the altered representation after neighborhood interaction to be used for the prediction, leveraging both information. After a final activation, a last single-layer feed-forward network is used to map the concatenated vector to the class output and apply a softmax function. The gradients are backpropagated through the whole network, updating not only the graph network but also the CNN, and therefore updating the feature extraction in every iteration.

2.2 Motivation of Skip Connection for CNN/GAT Hybrid

Two concepts motivate the concatenation of the representations extracted from the CNN and the GAT. First, the skip connection allows a direct gradient propagation to the CNN, thus fortifying a proper filter learning. More importantly, the combination of both outputs enables a comparison of the pure feature extraction of the CNN and the "impure" feature representation after its interaction with the neighborhood (Fig. 1 top right). The individual connectivity of instances from a class to other classes in the graph can yield an additional unique contribution to the feature representation after the feature aggregation process of GAT, if these inter-class connections are different for every class. Especially for classes usually difficult to distinguish, this individual contribution of feature representations from other instances significantly improves the classification performance on these classes since their originally similar feature representations are altered and more distinct compared to their initial representation transported by the skip-connection. Therefore, the interesting and unintuitive observation is obtained that inter-class connections can be highly beneficiary in the used setup.

3 Experiments

3.1 Datasets

First, a modified version of the MNIST dataset is used to prove the concept of the proposed method. MNIST consists of 70,000 handwritten digits from 0 to 9. Only the lower half of every image is used as image input, while the upper half is processed for the creation of the affinity graph. The objective is to show the improved classification of classes difficult to distinguish like 3 and 5 due to their identical lower shape. Following the inter-class setup explained in Sect. 2.2, we additionally take into account the digit 6, which shows a similarity to only the number 5 in the upper half. We therefore create a subset of 6,000 images of the numbers 3, 5 and 6 for training and 2,860 images for testing.

Secondly, we adapt the approach to the task of disease classification on the NIH ChestX-ray14 dataset. The dataset consists of 112,120 labelled X-ray images, containing one or more of 14 different diseases, with substantial imbalance for some classes. 16,000 single-label images of the eight diseases suggested by [11] are taken into consideration to obtain a potentially clearer patient cohort system.

3.2 Experimental Setup

Affinity Graph Construction. For MNIST, the construction of the affinity graph is based on the upper half of the image. As a metric, the $l1$-distance of the flattened image intensity vectors is used. If the distance between the two image vectors v_1 and v_2 is below the threshold θ, the edge is established. The best threshold was found with $\theta = 0.1$ for the average pixel intensity difference on an intensity scale from 0 to 1. Then, to analyze the proposed network and to prove that the obtained improvement is related to the previously described meaningful inter-class connections, three additional settings are used: (1) random edges, (2) edges based on label information, and (3) edges based on labels including the helpful inter-class connection between 5 and 6. It has to be stated that the usage of label information is just used here to prove the concept of the network.

For the NIH chest X-ray dataset, the accessible meta-information is used to create the affinity graph. Here, we are following the current state of the art introduced by [8] to leverage an age and gender difference metric. After performing an analysis of the statistics of the age and gender distribution with respect to the patients' diseases, we connect subjects in our experiments if at least one of the following three conditions is fulfilled for two patients P_1 and P_2:

(1) patient id_{P_1} = patient id_{P_2}
(2) $gender_{P_1} = gender_{P_2}$ and $|age_{P_1} - age_{P_2}| \leq 1y$
(3) $gender_{P_1} \neq gender_{P_2}$ and $age_{P_1} = age_{P_2}$

Network Setup. We create three baselines and one alternative method to analyze the different aspects of CNNGAT. To show the improved learning of feature representations we compare against the performance of a simple CNN, the normal GAT network on pre-learned features by the CNN (RawGAT), and our CNNGAT with pre-learnt features instead of end-to-end training (SkipGAT). To validate the hybrid approach we compare against our end-to-end CNNGAT network without using skip connections (EndGAT).

Feature Extraction. For MNIST, the CNNGAT was trained with a simple CNN containing two convolutional layers (32 and 64 channels). For the NIH dataset, AlexNet was used to easily prevent overfitting on the 16,000 images.

Parameters. The following parameters were chosen:

MNIST: 60 features as GAT input, 2 GAT layers (30 and 10 units), 5 heads, dropout: 0.3, neighbors: 4, weight decay: 5e-3, lr: 0.02, lr $\times$ 0.3 every 20 epochs.

NIH: 60 features as GAT input, 2 GAT layers (30 and 32 units), 5 heads, dropout: 0.3, neighbors: 4, weight decay: 5e-3, lr: 0.01, lr $\times$ 0.3 every 30 epochs.

3.3 Modified MNIST Dataset

The results on the above described MNIST toy dataset shown in Table 1 indicate that the CNNGAT is indeed improving the classification by using the inter-class connections for numbers 5 and 6. Using pre-trained features in the proposed network approach (SkipGAT) diminishes the performance of the system, showing the value of adaptive feature learning. Also the approach without Skip-Connection (EndGAT) is significantly outperformed (Wilcoxon signed-rank test, significance level $p < 0.05$). To give further evidence that the features are learned in a more robust way, we perform a shifted occlusion for 1000 random images. A occluding window is slid across the image and after prediction is performed, the probability of the correct class in the softmax function is recorded for every position. One example is shown in Fig. 2(a–d) for an instance of the number 3. It is visible that the classification is significantly more stable compared to the other networks, also stated in Table 1.

For the second setting of graph edges described in Sect. 3.2, the lower part of Table 1 clearly shows that the presence of meaningful inter-class connections is leading to top-level performance even outperforming a clean label graph.

Table 1. Performance on MNIST dataset. Aff. shows which affinity mechanism was used: $\theta = $ll-distance, L = labels, CL = labels with connection between 5 and 6. P-val is reported against CNNGAT. Occ. shows average correct class probability of softmax function for occlusion shift. O. p-val shows p-value compared to CNNGAT.

Network	Aff.	Accuracy	Lowest class acc	p-val	Occ.	O. p-val
CNN	/	0.822 ± 0.005	0.69 ± 0.049	10e-5	0.69	0.0
RawGAT	θ	0.794 ± 0.003	0.450 ± 0.008	10e-5	/	/
SkipGAT	θ	0.829 ± 0.014	0.538 ± 0.066	10e-5	0.68	0.0
EndGAT	θ	0.881 ± 0.016	0.780 ± 0.087	10e-4	/	/
CNNGAT	θ	$\mathbf{0.911 \pm 0.005}$	$\mathbf{0.810 \pm 0.035}$	/	**0.81**	/
CNNGAT	Rand	0.816 ± 0.004	0.613 ± 0.052	/		
CNNGAT	L	0.980 ± 0.036	0.956 ± 0.079	/		
CNNGAT	**CL**	$\mathbf{0.992 \pm 0.001}$	$\mathbf{0.989 \pm 0.003}$	/		

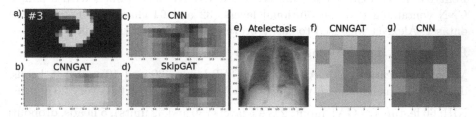

Fig. 2. Left: (a) MNIST number 3. (b–d) Occlusion shift on (a) with 7×7 window and stride length (SL) 1. Color bar corresponds to probability in softmax function for correct class when occ. is performed in that image region, the brighter the higher the probability (bright yellow: highest achieved probability for compared occlusions). **Right:** (e) Atelectasis. (f–g) Occ. shift on (e) with 50×50 window and SL 50. (Color figure online)

3.4 NIH ChestX-Ray 14 Dataset

Table 2 shows the results on the ChestX-ray 14 dataset. The CNNGAT had a slightly better performance than the used CNN, but the improvement is not significant. The absence of the effects seen on the MNIST dataset are addressed in the discussion. The occlusion shift analysis however shows that the classification is stabilized by the graph (Fig. 2 right). The probability of predicting the correct class under occlusion is significantly higher compared to the raw CNN (Table 2).

Table 2. Performance of CNN and CNNGAT on the described NIH ChestX-ray 14 dataset for 16,000 images. The column setting is identical to Table 1.

Network	Aff.	Accuracy	Lowest class acc	p-val	Occ.	O. p-val
CNN	/	0.429 ± 0.015	0.144 ± 0.102	0.109	0.27	2.6e-5
CNNGAT	meta	**0.437 ± 0.014**	0.086 ± 0.070	/	**0.30**	/

4 Discussion and Conclusion

The results on the MNIST dataset follow the expectation of the network performance. Only when training the CNN and GAT end-to-end, optimized performance is reached. Especially the comparison to SkipGAT, which is identical to CNNGAT except its pre-learned features, states the importance of the feature learning during training time. Additionally, the fact that the EndGAT setting is significantly outperformed fortifies the usage of the CNN/GAT hybrid approach. This behaviour was not clearly reproducible on the ChestX-ray 14 dataset. After performing a statistical analysis on the data distributions we hypothesize that the available meta-information was not relevant enough to build the required patient cohorts. Generating an artificial meaningful graph on the dataset showed the expected clear performance improvement.

We have proposed a new methodology to train a CNN and GAT network end-to-end and used their output in a hybrid approach to leverage both advanced feature learning and inter-class feature representations. The experiments clearly showed the superiority of the approach under the constraint that a meaningful graph can be created. In future work, the network architecture can be further optimized by e.g. including a learning mechanism for the adjacency system. With an automatized graph creation the necessity of finding meaningful meta-information is erased what makes the network applicable in a more general way.

Acknowledgements. The study was supported by the Carl Zeiss Meditec AG in Oberkochen, Germany, and the German Federal Ministry of Education and Research (BMBF) in connection with the foundation of the German Center for Vertigo and Balance Disorders (DSGZ) (grant number 01 EO 0901). Further, we thank NVIDIA Corporation for the sponsoring of a Titan V GPU.

References

1. Bronstein, M.M., Bruna, J., LeCun, Y., Szlam, A., Vandergheynst, P.: Geometric deep learning: going beyond Euclidean data. IEEE Sig. Process. Mag. **34**(4), 18–42 (2017)
2. Defferrard, M., Bresson, X., Vandergheynst, P.: Convolutional neural networks on graphs with fast localized spectral filtering. NIPS (2016)
3. Hamilton, W.L., Ying, R., Leskovec, J.: Inductive representation learning on large graphs. NIPS (2017)
4. Islam, M.T., Aowal, M.A., Minhaz, A.T., Ashraf, K.: Abnormality detection and localization in chest X-rays using deep convolutional neural networks (2017). http://arxiv.org/abs/1705.09850
5. Kazi, A., Krishna, S.A., Shekarforoush, S., Kortuem, K., Albarqouni, S., Navab, N.: Self-attention equipped graph convolutions for disease prediction. ISBI (2019)
6. Kipf, T.N., Welling, M.: Semi-supervised classification with graph convolutional networks. ICLR (2017)
7. Monti, F., Boscaini, D., Masci, J., Rodola, E., Svoboda, J., Bronstein, M.: Geo. deep learning on graphs and manifolds using mixture model CNNs. CVPR (2017)
8. Parisot, S., et al.: Spectral graph convolutions for population-based disease prediction. In: Descoteaux, M., Maier-Hein, L., Franz, A., Jannin, P., Collins, D.L., Duchesne, S. (eds.) MICCAI 2017. LNCS, vol. 10435, pp. 177–185. Springer, Cham (2017). https://doi.org/10.1007/978-3-319-66179-7_21
9. Rajpurkar, P., et al.: CheXNet: radiologist-level pneumonia detection on chest X-rays with deep learning (2017). http://arxiv.org/abs/1711.05225
10. Velickovic, P., Cucurull, G., Casanova, A., Romero, A., Lio, P., Bengio, Y.: Graph attention networks. ICLR (2018)
11. Wang, X., Peng, Y., Lu, L., Lu, Z., Bagheri, M., Summers, R.M.: ChestX-Ray8: hospital-scale chest X-ray database and benchmarks on weakly-supervised classification and localization of common thorax diseases. CVPR (2017)
12. Zhou, B., Khosla, A., Lapedriza, A., Oliva, A., Torralba, A.: Learning deep features for discriminative localization. CVPR (2016)

How to Learn from Unlabeled Volume Data: Self-supervised 3D Context Feature Learning

Maximilian Blendowski[1]([⊠]) [iD], Hannes Nickisch[2] [iD], and Mattias P. Heinrich[1] [iD]

[1] Institute of Medical Informatics, University of Lübeck, Lübeck, Germany
{blendowski,heinrich}@imi.uni-luebeck.de
[2] Philips Research Hamburg, Hamburg, Germany

Abstract. The vast majority of 3D medical images lacks detailed image-based expert annotations. The ongoing advances of deep convolutional neural networks clearly demonstrate the benefit of supervised learning to successfully extract relevant anatomical information and aid image-based analysis and interventions, but it heavily relies on labeled data. Self-supervised learning, that requires no expert labels, provides an appealing way to discover data-inherent patterns and leverage anatomical information freely available from medical images themselves. In this work, we propose a new approach to train effective convolutional feature extractors based on a new concept of image-intrinsic spatial offset relations with an auxiliary heatmap regression loss. The learned features successfully capture semantic, anatomical information and enable state-of-the-art accuracy for a k-NN based one-shot segmentation task without any subsequent fine-tuning.

Keywords: Self-supervised learning · Volumetric image segmentation

1 Introduction and Related Work

Deep learning with convolutional networks (DCNN) has become a powerful and versatile tool for a large variety of medical image analysis tasks. DCNNs stand out with their ability to learn informative features that are robust to artifacts or noise and which do not rely on hand-crafted feature engineering and explicit domain knowledge. However, up to date, nearly all deep networks require large datasets with strong supervision through expert annotations. In contrast to computer vision, tasks where layman can cost-effectively label abundantly available images at low cost are rare in medical imaging [7].

Thus, a large fully-annotated high-quality training corpus is rarely available in medical imaging, which triggered research to relax this assumption in various ways. Weak labels can enable registration tasks [4], noisy labels allow for classification tasks [9], a few labels suffice for segmentation tasks [10] and transfer learning on data from a different domain [11] can be used to detect lung nodules.

© Springer Nature Switzerland AG 2019
D. Shen et al. (Eds.): MICCAI 2019, LNCS 11769, pp. 649–657, 2019.
https://doi.org/10.1007/978-3-030-32226-7_72

In the quest to – ultimately – use unlabeled data for learning, the computer vision community recently explored *self-supervision*, a form of unsupervised learning, where auxiliary tasks are derived from unlabeled data enabling a machine to extract visual knowledge. These auxiliary tasks are usually easy to verify but require a certain degree of image understanding. Prominent examples are hole filling (inpainting), the prediction of spatial neighborhood relations of image patches [2], the colorization of grayscale images [15] or a combination of a number of them [3].

Applications of self-supervision to medical imaging range from leveraging follow up scans in spine MRI [6] over surrogate supervision used for segmentation from only a fraction of the labels [12] to unsupervised learning employed for image registration [14]. Our work is closely related to the context prediction of neighbouring patches introduced by Doersch et al. [2], which demonstrated the capabilities of using spatial relations (e.g. top/bottom, left/right) that already are inherently given as auxiliary task to pretrain feature extractors in natural, two-dimensional images. The large variety of details and presence of multiple relational objects in natural 2D images enabled them to learn CNNs that extract

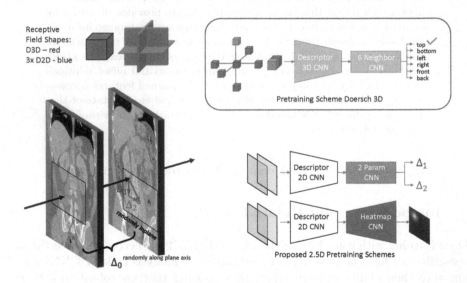

Fig. 1. Top left: inspired by [2] and extended to 3D, DOERSCH uses a cubic receptive field, while our proposed method uses three intersecting planar volumes (2.5D). Top right: DOERSCH ■ predicts the spatial arrangement of two cubic image subvolumes inside a 6 neighborhood as auxiliary task to pretrain *Descriptor 3D CNN*. Bottom left - our approach: per axis predict small continuous-valued offsets (Δ_1, Δ_2) between the centers of disjoint planar volumes that are Δ_0 apart in order to pretrain *Descriptor 2D CNN*. Bottom right: Different ways to implement the auxiliary offset prediction task. (1) REG2D ■: Direct regression of both parameters with fully connected layers in *2 Param CNN*. (2) HEATMAP ■: Regressing (Δ_1, Δ_2)-heatmaps using transposed convolutions in *Heatmap CNN*. (Color figure online)

semantically meaningful descriptors. To ensure a sufficiently demanding self-supervision task, the image patches cannot have any overlap and must also contain recognizable object parts. When considering volumetric medical scans (CT, MRI) there exists a conflicting relation between an increasing size of the patch for the CNN (equivalently its receptive field), which is necessary to capture enough spatial information for an expressive feature learning and a suitable difficulty of the auxiliary task: i.e. the learning task can become too easy, when the receptive field grows, because neighboring subvolumes are likely to contain easily identifiable structures, e.g. body borders ('body border problem').

As illustrated in the upper part of Fig. 1, the *Doersch*-inspired pre-training scheme randomly extracts two 3D subvolumes (red box and green box) from within a six neighbourhood of a considered scan. Both intensity patches are fed into a Siamese convolutional network that yields one feature vector each. These are concatenated and used within a conventional fully-connected network to predict the spatial relation of the two patches as a categorical six-class task.

2   Methods

We strongly believe that a simple extension of a spatial patch-based context prediction to 3D does not fully exploit the potential of self-supervised pre-training for medical scans. Consequently, we introduce a novel method that is inspired by the work of Doersch et al. [2], but aims to overcome the trade-off between the receptive field limitations imposed by unsuitable pretext problems.

Contributions: (1) We propose a new scheme to appropriately leverage spatial information in 3D scans by predicting orthogonal offsets of two large planar patches that are extracted with a small intermediate gap and enables the use of more flexible auxiliary tasks. (2) We use an auxiliary decoder network for 2D heatmap regression that increases the robustness of this offset computation.

2.1   Self-supervised Feature Learning

The lower part of Fig. 1 illustrates the basic ideas of our work that introduces a new unsupervised pre-training scheme based on spatial cues. Instead of relying on cubical patches (as done in [2]), we propose to extract two nearly planar 2.5D subvolumes along the main imaging axis (e.g. the coronal plane in Fig. 1, approx. $117 \times 97 \times 9$ mm) with a fixed spatial offset of Δ_0, chosen large enough so that no overlap exists. The anchor patch (green box) is extracted around the voxel of interest in the first slice, while the second patch (yellow box) is randomly shifted in its position along the normal (inplane) direction with continuously drawn offsets (Δ_1, Δ_2) (purple and blue). Since the second slice shares *no* obvious spatial hints (e.g. continuing lines) with the anchor patch, we are no longer limited to few discrete neighbourhood relations and can consider a greater variability of displaced patches. In essence, compared to [2], shrinking the cubical patches along one dimension allows us to avoid the 'body border problem': due to the unknown offset Δ_0, we are able to present diverse image pairs to our networks that provide a sufficiently large receptive field (2D, perpendicular to the Δ_0 offset axis) to inherently learn anatomical information. As before a Siamese convolutional architecture (denoted as *Descriptor 2D CNN* (D2D-CNN)) is trained to extract vector-valued descriptors for both patches individually. While the cross entropy (CE-loss) for a six-class prediction was a natural choice as loss function for the *Doersch*-inspired 3D pre-training method, we propose to formulate our continuous offset approach as the following auxiliary learning task: Predict the two offset parameters (Δ_1, Δ_2) with heatmap regression (seen to provide a more informative gradient flow in [8]) using an expanding decoder network with transposed convolutions.

The proposed planar patch offset prediction is not limited to a certain axis of a 3D volume and hence three separate D2D-CNN networks are trained in parallel. The final descriptor for a voxel positioned at the intersection of each of the three planar subvolumes is obtained by simply concatenating the output of all three D2D-CNNs. For the sake of a clear notation, we assume all image axes to be normalized to $[-1, 1]$, i.e. with a side length of 2 in the following.

Details on Heatmap ∎ Network Training[1]: We train our proposed 2.5D feature extractor D2D-CNNs (1 per axis) paired with one *Heatmap CNN* each. Following the scheme visually presented in the lower part of Fig. 1, we sample a near planar subvolume represented as a 3-channel 2D image for each axis. These slices have dimensions of 3×42^2 with side lengths 0.8, a depth of 0.05 in the normal direction and form the input of the feature CNN. The anchor slice's central position within the scan is uniformly drawn from $[-0.5, 0.5]^3$. The second subvolume is sampled so that it is displaced by at least $\Delta_0 = 0.125$ and up to $\Delta_0 = 0.25$ in normal direction. This perpendicular offset is *not used* during the training process. The inplane offset parameters (Δ_1, Δ_2) that are the target of the auxiliary learning task are uniformly drawn from $\pm[0.25, 0.3]^2$ in the beginning and up to $\pm[0, 0.7]^2$ at the end of the training process. Enforcing offsets of at least ± 0.25 initially accelerates the context learning. The MSE-loss between the network's predicted heatmaps and the ground truth was used as a penalty term. The heatmap is obtained from the offsets using

$$heat_{gt}(i, j, \Delta_1, \Delta_2) = 10 \cdot e^{-15 \cdot \left[(i/9 - \Delta_1)^2 + (j/9 - \Delta_2)^2\right]}$$

with $(i, j) \in \{-9, -8, ..., +8, +9\}^2$, yielding 19×19 sized images. The final 2.5D descriptors for both methods result from the concatenation of all 3 D2D-CNNs (axial, coronal and sagittal axes).

Implementation of the Comparitive 3D Doersch ∎ Approach: We combine a 3D convolutional network (D3D-CNN) as feature extractor with a six-class prediction network *6 Neighbor CNN* as a straight-forward 3D extension of [2]. The 6 possible neighbouring relations define the auxiliary task trained with a

---

[1] Code and pre-trained networks as well as detailed data preprocessing steps to enable reproducibility can be found at https://github.com/multimodallearning/miccai19_self_supervision.

CE-loss. We extract an anchor 3D subvolume of 25^3 voxels as cubes with side-length 0.4 - its center is again uniformly sampled in $[-0.5, 0.5]^3$ within the image volume in order to be positioned inside the patient's body. As partner, we randomly sample one of its 6 neighboring subvolumes and add jitter to its center coordinates to avoid e.g. line continuation hints [2].

Table 1. Network Architectures. Building blocks of our architectures are abbreviated as follows: (1) $\mathrm{Conv}\langle TP\rangle(c_{in}, c_{out}, kernel, dilation) \stackrel{\wedge}{=} \langle\mathrm{Transposed}\rangle\mathrm{Convolution}$, (2) $\mathrm{MP}(kernel, stride) \stackrel{\wedge}{=} \mathrm{MaxPooling}$, (3) $\mathrm{GN} \stackrel{\wedge}{=} \mathrm{GroupNorm}$, (4) $\mathrm{LR} \stackrel{\wedge}{=} \mathrm{LeakyReLU}$, 5.) $\mathrm{interp}(width, height) \stackrel{\wedge}{=}$ upscaling to the specified dimensionality

CNN	D2D	2 Param	Heatmap	D3D	6 Neighbor
Input	image data	D2D features	D2D features	image data	D3D features
Layer 1	Conv(3,32,3,1) MP(2,2),GN,LR	Conv(128,128,1,1) GN,LR	Conv(128,64,1,1) GN,LR	Conv(1,16,5,1) GN,LR	Conv(384,64,1,1) GN,LR
Layer 2	Conv(32,32,3,1) MP(2,2),GN,LR	Conv(128,64,1,1) GN,LR	Conv(64,32,1,1) GN,LR	Conv(16,32,3,2) GN,LR	Conv(64,64,1,1) GN,LR
Layer 3	Conv(32,32,3,1) GN,LR	Conv(64,32,1,1) GN,LR	Conv(32,16,1,1) GN,LR	Conv(32,32,3,2) GN,LR	Conv(64,32,1,1) GN,LR
Layer 4	Conv(32,64,3,1) GN,LR	Conv(32,2,1,1) —	ConvTP(16,16,5,1) GN,LR Conv(16,16,3,1) GN,LR interp(11x11)	Conv(32,32,3,2) GN,LR	Conv(32,6,1,1) —
Layer 5	Conv(64,64,3,1) GN,LR		ConvTP(16,16,5,1) GN,LR Conv(16,8,3,1) GN,LR	Conv(32,32,3,1) GN,LR	
Layer 6	Conv(64,64,3,1) GN,LR		ConvTP(8,4,5,1) GN,LR interp(19x19)	Conv(32,32,5,1) GN,LR	
Layer 7	Conv(64,64,3,1) GN,LR		Conv(4,1,1,1) —	Conv(32,192,3,1) GN,LR	
(x,y,z,c)-in	(42,42,1,3)	(1,1,1,128)	(1,1,1,128)	(25,25,25,1)	(1,1,1,192)
(x,y,z,c)-out	(1,1,1,64)	(1,1,1,2)	(19,19,1,1)	(1,1,1,192)	(1,1,1,6)
# params	139.744	27.138	28.189	393.392	31.238

3 Experiments and Results

To evaluate our contributions, we compare the two self-supervised pre-training schemes on a few-shot CT segmentation task with respect to Dice scores.

Dataset: We perform experiments on the VISCERAL Anatomy3 data [13] using the contrast-enhanced thoracoabdominal scans (training: 63 unlabeled silver-corpus scans, testing: 19 expert labeled scans; leaving out corrupted scans). After resampling to isotropic voxels of size $1.5\,\mathrm{mm}^3$, we crop all images to roughly the same region containing 6 target structures (liver, spleen, left/right kidney, left/right psoas major muscle) - yielding image sizes of $243 \times 176 \times 293$ (LR-AP-SI).

Training: In general, we share the same setting for the two compared self-supervision pre-training schemes. Using an Adam optimizer with an initial learning rate of $5 \cdot 10^{-5}$ and a batchsize of 8, we train each method on 800,000 random batches. Each method outputs a feature descriptor of length 192 per position. Details with respect to the network architectures of the different approaches can

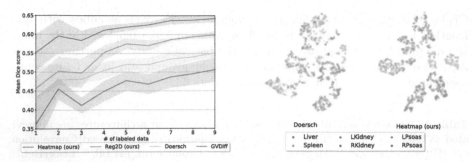

Fig. 2. *Left*: Mean Dice scores for different methods over an increasingly number of labeled testdata. *Right*: t-SNE plots visualizing the more clearly separated feature descriptor clusters for our proposed HEATMAP ■ method compared to DOERSCH ■. (Color figure online)

be found in Table 1. Note that all CNN for descriptor extraction have ≈ 400 k parameters, have comparably powerful auxiliary task CNNs and are trained as Siamese networks.

In addition to the two self-supervised learning approaches presented in Sect. 2 we consider two additional baselines in our experiments and an ablation study to our proposed HEATMAP ■ method.

Xavier2D: In order to assess the necessity to train the D2D-CNNs in the first place, we also extract 2.5D descriptors with network weights initialized by the Xavier method and without any subsequent training.

GVDiff ■: As comparison to 'classical' hand-crafted methods, we extract grey-value difference features (cf. [1]) with a 3D random pattern sampled from a Gaussian distribution with standard deviation 0.4 - i.e. comparable to the receptive fields of the CNN-based methods.

Reg2D ■: To examine the influence of the heatmap approach, we alter our proposed auxiliary learning task to a direct regression of the displacements (Δ_1, Δ_2). In contrast to combining the D2D-CNNs with *Heatmap CNNs*, we use the L1-Loss as penalty to train *2 Param* CNNs that do not reconstruct any spatial information and only operate on the 1D descriptor signals (see Table 1 for architectural details).

3.1   Results

We evaluate all 5 extracted descriptors on 19 datasets, with manual expert annotations. We perform two-fold cross validation (splits: 1–10, 11–19) and examine the influence of an increasing number of labeled datasets (one-shot, 2, 3, ..., 9). We predict the organ label at every 4th voxel (192,720 positions per image) - based on an approximate k-Nearest Neighbor (kNN) search using the Vantage Point Forest Method introduced in [5] with $k = 21$ and 15 trees - and compute the resulting Dice as indirect measure of descriptor expressiveness. Note, that

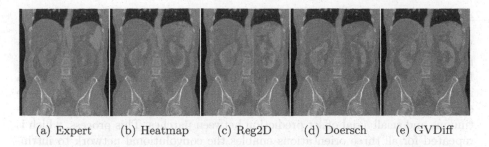

(a) Expert   (b) Heatmap   (c) Reg2D   (d) Doersch   (e) GVDiff

Fig. 3. Segmentation visualization of different approaches for a 2D slice of a patient.

we do *not* employ any finetuning strategies to this segmentation task that would require additional GPU-DCNN-training hours - instead building & evaluating the kNN-Forests takes only a few seconds per scan.

Table 2 provides the mean scores for all 6 considered organ structures given a labeled patient database of size 9. Qualitative results with respect to the organ segmentation task are shown in Fig. 3 for a 2D slice of a patient. Figure 2 (left) shows the mean Dice scores over all organ structures for all patients and folds with an increasing number of available labeled datasets for the kNN classification. Overall, our proposed the HEATMAP-approach performs best and achieves a one-shot segmentation accuracy of ≈ 55% average Dice score. Our alternative approach REG2D achieves the second highest accuracy and also outperforms DOERSCH, the straight-forward 3D extension of [2]. With both auxiliary task implementations, our proposed new 2.5D scheme demonstrates its usefulness as self-supervised pre-training scheme for 3D image data. Interestingly, we also outperform [10], which proposed a sophisticated dual CNN architecture specifically designed for one-shot segmentation and achieved 52.6% Dice accuracy on the same dataset.

Visualizing the extracted features using an unsupervised t-SNE embedding from the same foreground positions in Fig. 2 (right) (no labels provided during training) shows the discovery of very clean and separable clusters for individual structures using our HEATMAP method compared to DOERSCH - supporting our hypothesis that leveraging a larger context is of great importance in self-supervised learning.

Table 2. Mean Dice scores in % over all folds with 9 labeled test images.

Experiment	Liver	Spleen	LKidney	RKidney	LPsoas	RPsoas	Mean
HEATMAP (ours)	85.3	65.7	66.3	53.5	50.4	65.6	**64.2 ± 2.9**
REG2D (ours)	81.4	54.0	63.4	51.0	49.0	60.9	60.0 ± 2.9
DOERSCH	76.9	43.0	59.0	51.2	49.1	52.3	55.2 ± 3.1
GVDIFF	80.7	58.2	54.5	43.0	29.0	37.1	50.4 ± 5.0
XAVIER	70.1	28.3	17.2	3.3	24.5	27.1	28.4 ± 1.0

4 Conclusion

We have presented a novel self-supervised pre-training strategy to effectively leverage inherent 3D information from abundant unlabeled medical volumes. Inspired by the method proposed in [2] for 2D natural images, we designed a new context prediction task that takes explicit advantage of the third image dimension and uses nearly planar subvolumes to train an auxiliary task for continuous and small axial offset prediction between patches. This process, which is repeated for all three orientations enables the convolutional network to intrinsically encode anatomical cues into expressive, pre-trained descriptors. When evaluating our scheme with its extracted features within a few-shot kNN-based organ segmentation task and without any supervised refinement, we obtain a large increase of Dice scores from 55.2% to 65.6% compared to the 3D extension of [2]. Despite the fact that we only trained with spatial relations and perform no fine-tuning, we also achieve state-of-the-art results in accuracy for one-shot-segmentation on a public abdominal CT dataset. In future work a more extensive investigation of the influence of network architectures, including convolution filter hyperparameters will be considered. In addition the use of arbitrarily oriented 2D stacks could further enhance the method and many more medical applications, e.g. image registration could benefit from these pre-trained descriptors.

Acknowledgements. This work was supported by the German Research Foundation (DFG) under grant number 320997906 (HE 7364/2-1). We gratefully acknowledge the support of the NVIDIA Corporation with their GPU donations for this research.

References

1. Calonder, M., Lepetit, V., Strecha, C., Fua, P.: BRIEF: binary robust independent elementary features. In: Daniilidis, K., Maragos, P., Paragios, N. (eds.) ECCV 2010. LNCS, vol. 6314, pp. 778–792. Springer, Heidelberg (2010). https://doi.org/10.1007/978-3-642-15561-1_56
2. Doersch, C., Gupta, A., Efros, A.A.: Unsupervised visual representation learning by context prediction. In: ICCV (2015)
3. Doersch, C., Zisserman, A.: Multi-task self-supervised visual learning. In: ICCV (2017)
4. Ferrante, E., Dokania, P.K., Silva, R.M., Paragios, N.: Weakly-supervised learning of metric aggregations for deformable image registration. IEEE J. Biomed. Health Inform. (2018)
5. Heinrich, M.P., Blendowski, M.: Multi-organ segmentation using vantage point forests and binary context features. In: Ourselin, S., Joskowicz, L., Sabuncu, M.R., Unal, G., Wells, W. (eds.) MICCAI 2016. LNCS, vol. 9901, pp. 598–606. Springer, Cham (2016). https://doi.org/10.1007/978-3-319-46723-8_69
6. Jamaludin, A., Kadir, T., Zisserman, A.: Self-supervised learning for spinal MRIs. In: DLMIA (2017)
7. Maier-Hein, L., et al.: Crowd-algorithm collaboration for large-scale endoscopic image annotation with confidence. In: Ourselin, S., Joskowicz, L., Sabuncu, M.R., Unal, G., Wells, W. (eds.) MICCAI 2016. LNCS, vol. 9901, pp. 616–623. Springer, Cham (2016). https://doi.org/10.1007/978-3-319-46723-8_71

8. Payer, C., Štern, D., Bischof, H., Urschler, M.: Regressing heatmaps for multiple landmark localization using CNNs. In: Ourselin, S., Joskowicz, L., Sabuncu, M.R., Unal, G., Wells, W. (eds.) MICCAI 2016. LNCS, vol. 9901, pp. 230–238. Springer, Cham (2016). https://doi.org/10.1007/978-3-319-46723-8_27

9. Reed, S., Lee, H., Anguelov, D., Szegedy, C., Erhan, D., Rabinovich, A.: Training deep neural networks on noisy labels with bootstrapping. ICLR workshop (2015)

10. Roy, A.G., Siddiqui, S., Pölsterl, S., Navab, N., Wachinger, C.: 'squeeze & excite' guided few-shot segmentation of volumetric images. arXiv:1902.01314 (2019)

11. Shin, H.C., et al.: Deep convolutional neural networks for computer-aided detection: CNN architectures, dataset characteristics and transfer learning. IEEE Trans. Med. Imaging 35(5), 1285–1298 (2016)

12. Tajbakhsh, N., et al.: Surrogate supervision for medical image analysis: Effective deep learning from limited quantities of labeled data. In: ISBI (2019)

13. Jimenez-del Toro, O., et al.: Cloud-based evaluation of anatomical structure segmentation and landmark detection algorithms: visceral anatomy benchmarks. IEEE Trans. Med. Imaging 35(11), 2459–2475 (2016)

14. de Vos, B.D., Berendsen, F.F., Viergever, M.A., Sokooti, H., Staring, M., Išgum, I.: A deep learning framework for unsupervised affine and deformable image registration. Med. Image Anal. 52, 128–143 (2019)

15. Zhang, R., Isola, P., Efros, A.A.: Colorful image colorization. In: Leibe, B., Matas, J., Sebe, N., Welling, M. (eds.) ECCV 2016. LNCS, vol. 9907, pp. 649–666. Springer, Cham (2016). https://doi.org/10.1007/978-3-319-46487-9_40

Probabilistic Radiomics: Ambiguous Diagnosis with Controllable Shape Analysis

Jiancheng Yang[1,2,3], Rongyao Fang[1], Bingbing Ni[1,2,3](✉),
Yamin Li[1], Yi Xu[1], and Linguo Li[1]

[1] Shanghai Jiao Tong University, Shanghai, China
nibingbing@sjtu.edu.cn
[2] MoE Key Lab of Artificial Intelligence, AI Institute,
Shanghai Jiao Tong University, Shanghai, China
[3] Shanghai Institute for Advanced Communication and Data Science,
Shanghai, China

Abstract. Radiomics analysis has achieved great success in recent years. However, conventional Radiomics analysis suffers from insufficiently expressive hand-crafted features. Recently, emerging deep learning techniques, e.g., convolutional neural networks (CNNs), dominate recent research in Computer-Aided Diagnosis (CADx). Unfortunately, as black-box predictors, we argue that CNNs are "diagnosing" voxels (or pixels), rather than lesions; in other words, visual saliency from a trained CNN is not necessarily concentrated on the lesions. On the other hand, classification in clinical applications suffers from inherent ambiguities: radiologists may produce diverse diagnosis on challenging cases. To this end, we propose a controllable and explainable *Probabilistic Radiomics* framework, by combining the Radiomics analysis and probabilistic deep learning. In our framework, 3D CNN feature is extracted upon lesion region only, then encoded into lesion representation, by a controllable Non-local Shape Analysis Module (NSAM) based on self-attention. Inspired from variational auto-encoders (VAEs), an Ambiguity PriorNet is used to approximate the ambiguity distribution over human experts. The final diagnosis is obtained by combining the ambiguity prior sample and lesion representation, and the whole network named *DenseSharp*[+] is end-to-end trainable. We apply the proposed method on lung nodule diagnosis on LIDC-IDRI database to validate its effectiveness.

Keywords: Radiomics · Deep learning · Attention · Computer-Aided Diagnosis (CADx) · Explainable Artificial Intelligence (XAI)

J. Yang. and R. Fang are contributed equally.

Electronic supplementary material The online version of this chapter (https://doi.org/10.1007/978-3-030-32226-7_73) contains supplementary material, which is available to authorized users.

1   Introduction

Medical images are more than pictures [2]. Mining hidden information using image analysis techniques is referred as *Radiomics* analysis, which raises numerous research attention in clinical decision making. Conventional Radiomics analysis follows the pipeline: (1) manual/automatic delineation of volumes of interest (VOIs); (2) image processing and feature extraction (e.g., SIFT, wavelet); (3) machine learning to associate features and target variables. These hand-craft features are named "Radiomics". Though powerful and successful, emerging deep learning techniques indicate that hand-crafted features could be hardly comparable with end-to-end deep representations given enough data [12].

Deep learning[1] provides a strong alternative to learn representation from raw voxels (or pixels) in an end-to-end fashion. Convolutional neural networks (CNNs) have achieved great success in medical image analysis, though they are classifying **voxels, rather than lesions**. In other words, there is no guarantee that black-box CNNs correctly learn evidence from lesions, especially with limited supervision. We illustrate several failures in Appendix Fig. A.1, by checking the Class Activation Maps (CAMs) [13] from a 3D DenseNet [4,12] on lung nodule malignancy classification. These failures make the predictions given by CNNs unreliable. In contrast, Radiomics analysis is more controllable and transparent for users than black-box deep learning.

On the other hand, classification in clinical applications suffers from inherent ambiguities; on challenging cases, experienced radiologists may produce diverse diagnosis. Though a "ground truth" to eliminate ambiguity could be obtained through a more sophisticated examination (e.g., biopsy) theoretically, this information may be unavailable from imaging only. Discriminative training procedure biases the model towards the mean values rather than ambiguity distribution.

To address these issues, we propose a controllable and explainable *Probabilistic Radiomics* framework. A *DenseSharp* Network [11] is used as a backbone, which is a multi-task 3D CNN on learning classification and segmentation developed from 3D DenseNet [4,12]. Point clouds, named *feature clouds*, extracted from manual-labeled or predicted VOIs on CNN feature maps are regarded as lesion representations. To enable non-local shape analysis, we further introduce self-attention [8,10] to learn representations from the feature clouds. To capture label ambiguity, an Ambiguity PriorNet is used to approximate the ambiguity distribution over expert labels, inspired by Variational Auto-Encoders (VAEs) [7]. By combining the ambiguity prior sample and lesion representation, the final decision is controllable (by lesion VOI) and probabilistic, which mimics the decision process of human radiologists. Please refer to Appendix Fig. A.2 for comparison among conventional Radiomics analysis, deep learning and Probabilistic Radiomics. On LIDC-IDRI [1] database, we validate the effectiveness of our methodology on lung nodule characterization from CT scans.

---

[1] We refer to deep learning in a narrow sense, i.e., applying CNNs directly on the medical image analysis problems.

The key contributions of this paper are threefold: (1) We propose a novel viewpoint to regard deep representations from lesions on medical images as point clouds (i.e., feature clouds), and develop a Non-local Shape Analysis Module (NSAM) to end-to-end learn representations from feature clouds (rather than voxels); (2) We explicitly model the diagnosis ambiguity within a probabilistic and controllable approach, which mimics the decision process of human radiologists; (3) The whole network named $DenseSharp^+$ is end-to-end trainable.

2 Materials and Methods

2.1 Task and Dataset

Lung cancer is the leading cause of cancer-related mortality worldwide. Early diagnosis of lung cancer with LDCT is an effective way to reduce the related death. In this study, we address the lung nodule malignancy classification problem to explore the performance of the proposed Probabilistic Radiomics method.

We use LIDC-IDRI [1] dataset, one of the largest publicly available databases for lung cancer screening. There are 2,635 nodules from 1,018 CT scans in the dataset, where nodules with diameters $\geq 3\,\text{mm}$ are annotated by at most 4 radiologists. For malignancy classification, rating mode ranges from "1" (highly benign) to "5" (highly malignant), while "3" means undefined/uncertain rating. Besides, each radiologist delineates a VOI for a lesion. Empirically, the malignancy labels and segmentation VOIs are diverse for many instances in the dataset. Prior studies [5,14] define a unique binary label for each instance by voting, we instead treat these labels with **ambiguity**, with all the **5 classes**. We called the whole dataset with 2,635 nodules as $HighAmbig$ (high ambiguous) dataset. To fairly compare the model performance, a $LowAmbig$ (low ambiguous) dataset is constructed, with a similar nodule inclusion criteria to prior studies [5,14]: (1) the CT slice thickness $\leq 3\,\text{mm}$, (2) annotated by at least 3 radiologists, and (3) the average rating $\neq$ "3". The remaining nodules with average ratings $\leq$ "3" are defined as benign, or malignant otherwise, resulting in 656 benign and 527 malignant.

We pre-process the data as follows: CT are resampled into $1\,\text{mm} \times 1\,\text{mm} \times 1\,\text{mm}$. The voxel intensity is normalized to $[-1, 1)$ from the Hounsfield unit (HU), by $I = \lfloor \frac{I_{HU}+1024}{400+1024} \times 255 \rfloor / 128 - 1$. Each data sample is a voxel with a size of $32\,\text{mm} \times 32\,\text{mm} \times 32\,\text{mm}$. For simplicity, only single-scale inputs are used.

2.2 Non-local Shape Analysis Module (NSAM)

In our study, we use a CNN (DenseSharp [11] specifically) for extracting representations of nodules. Instead of a typical Global Pooling to derive the final classification, we use the lesion VOIs (manually annotated/automatically predicted) to crop the lesion features into point clouds [10], namely *feature clouds*, for subsequent processing. Inspired by self-attention transformer [8,10], we develop a Non-local Shape Analysis Module (NSAM) to consume the feature clouds.

Define $X \in \mathbb{R}^{N \times c}$ as a feature cloud, X is a permutation-invariant and size-varying set. We figure out that self-attention is well suitable for set; besides, it enables non-local representation learning. We use scaled dot-product attention,

$$Attn(X) = softmax(XX^T/\sqrt{c}) \cdot \sigma(X), \tag{1}$$

where σ is an activation function (e.g., ELU in our study).

Multi-head attention [8] is proved to be effective in attention mechanism, where a scaled dot-product attention is applied multiple times on linear transformed input with various weights. The $NSAM$ is a variant of multi-head attention, by sharing the linear transformation weights in the K, Q, V-formation [8]. Define g as the number of heads and $c_g = c/g$, the inputs are transformed by the weight $W_g \in \mathbb{R}^{c \times c_g}$ multiple times, before feeding into a scaled dot-product attention module. We further use skip connections [3] to ease the optimization.

$$NSAM(X) = concat\{Attn(X_i)|X_i = XW_i\}_{i=1,..,g} + X. \tag{2}$$

The whole shape analysis module is a stack of L-layer $NSAM$ ($L = 3$, $c = 256$ in this study). The features are subsequently fed into a global average pooling with multi-layer perceptron to obtain a single representation for a lesion VOI.

2.3 Ambiguity PriorNet

To deal with the ambiguous labels, we model the final decision as ambiguity prior distribution over the human experts. Inspired from Variational Auto-Encoders (VAEs) [7], a probabilistic module with a similar structure as 3D DenseNet backbone, named Ambiguity PriorNet (APN), is introduced to model the probabilistic component. APN produces (μ, σ), which controls a Gaussian distribution $N(\mu, \sigma)$ to serve as the ambiguity prior on malignancy labels and segmentation for human experts. To enable the gradient back-propagation, a reparameterization trick [7] is applied to draw a prior sample f_{Ambig} from $N(\mu, \sigma)$.

$$f_{Ambig}(x) = \sigma x + \mu, x \in N(0, 1). \tag{3}$$

In subsequent modules, the prior sample f_{Ambig} is concatenated with lesion representations to produce ambiguous malignancy labels and segmentation.

2.4 *DenseSharp*$^+$ Network Architecture

The proposed $DenseSharp^+$ Network (Fig. 1) is based on $DenseSharp$ Networks [11], which is a multi-task 3D DenseNet [4,12] with classification and segmentation heads. The $DenseSharp$ Network uses a light-weight head for segmentation, which enables a top-down supervision for learning where the lesions are. At each resolution level ($32 \times 32 \times 32$, $16 \times 16 \times 16$ and $8 \times 8 \times 8$), dense blocks with 3D convolution and Batch Normalization [6] are repeated [3, 8, 4] times before each down-sampling. Bottleneck ($B = 4$), compression ($C = 2$) and growth rate $k = 32$ are used following the setting in the $DenseSharp$ paper [11].

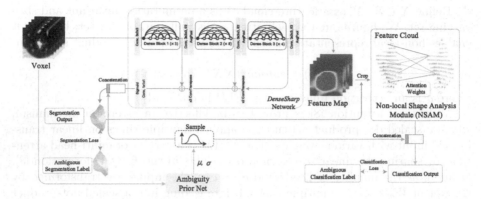

Fig. 1. *DenseSharp*$^+$ **Network Architecture.** A *DenseSharp*$^+$ Network is mainly a *DenseSharp* Network followed by a Non-local Shape Analysis Module (NSAM). *DenseSharp* is a deep 3D CNN based on DenseNet, with a classification head and segmentation head for multi-task learning. We use the feature maps from the classification head, cropped by manual/automatic segmentation, as *feature clouds*, rather than the raw feature maps, for the subsequent NSAM to consume. The NSAM use self-attention to associate non-local spatial information. An Ambiguity PriorNet conditional on the voxel inputs produces prior samples, which is concatenated with the classification and segmentation head to make their outputs probabilistic. Note the whole *DenseSharp*$^+$ Network is end-to-end trainable, with multi-task classification and segmentation loss.

The feature maps outputted by the last convolution layer of classification head is upsampled (trilinear interpolation), and then cropped by the lesion segmentation into feature clouds which are consumed by NSAM (Sect. 2.2). Either manual or automatic segmentation by the segmentation head could be used as the lesion segmentation to generate the feature clouds. Although NSAM is able to process size-varying inputs, due to the GPU memory constraint, we sample up to $N^{\mathrm{max}} = 1,024$ points from the feature cloud with sampling strategy Φ. For the manual segmentation, the sampling strategy Φ is random sampling. For the predicted segmentation $\hat{y}_{seg}$, we first estimate the volume by $\hat{v} = \sum \hat{y}_{seg}$. We then sample the $K = \lfloor \hat{v} \rfloor$ points with top-K output scores from the segmentation head. If $N \leq N^{\mathrm{max}}$, all points in the feature cloud are selected.

A DenseNet conditional on the voxel inputs (with a half parameter size of *DenseSharp*) is used as Ambiguity PriorNet (APN), which outputs 6-dimension prior samples to concatenate onto the classification and segmentation heads, to make their outputs probabilistic. Ideally, one prior sample encodes one "human expert", controlling the classification and segmentation results simultaneously.

2.5   Training and Inference

The *DenseSharp*$^+$ Networks is trained with two different schemes individually in order to better evaluate the probabilistic capability of the model. The first scheme trains on the *LowAmbig* dataset (see Sect. 2.1). This scheme denotes as *LowAmbig* (low ambiguous) training scheme. The second scheme trains the model on the whole labeled dataset, which denotes as *HighAmbig* (high ambiguous) training scheme. In both training schemes, unlike prior studies [5,14] with a unique label on each voxel, we randomly select one of the four experts and the corresponding 5-class malignancy label and segmentation during training.

For training the multi-task neural networks, a cross entropy loss for classification and a dice loss for segmentation are used. The loss weights for classification and segmentation are set as 1 and 0.2, respectively. Online data augmentation is applied on the voxels, including rotation, flipping and shifting within $[-1, 1]$ on a random axis. We use Adam optimizer to train the whole *DenseSharp*$^+$ end-to-end with a batch size of 128 and a learning rate of 0.001 for 150 epochs.

For simplicity, feature maps from the *DenseSharp* are cropped by predicted segmentation to feed into NSAM for training and inference. However, if the prediction segmentation volume is less than 10, the model refuses to use it to classify the nodule. In this case, it is not counted in classification loss during training, and is ignored during the evaluation on classification.

3   Experiments

Our *DenseSharp*$^+$ Network is trained to classify ambiguous labels of 5 malignancy modes from 4 radiologists. N prior samples ($N = 10$ in our experiments) are obtained from the reparameterized conditional Gaussian distribution of the Ambiguous PriorNet. Hence, each tested voxel corresponds to N 5-way outputs. In order to compare with prior studies quantitatively, the corresponding binary classification outputs are computed using Eq. 4.

$$(p_1, p_2, p_4, p_5) = \frac{1}{N} \sum_{i=1}^{N} \text{Softmax}(l_1^i, l_2^i, l_4^i, l_5^i),$$

$$p_b = p_1 + p_2, \quad p_m = p_4 + p_5,$$

(4)

where $l_1^i, l_2^i, l_4^i, l_5^i$ denote the ith logit outputs in the N samples of mode 1, 2, 4, and 5 from 5-mode classification. Note mode 3 is ignored in the evaluation since it defines "uncertain" diagnosis.

We evaluate the performance of all models via test AUC and accuracy on *LowAmbig* LIDC-IDRI dataset (see Sect. 2.1) with 5-fold cross validation method. It is worth noting that only *LowAmbig* voxels are evaluated in all our experiments, since the binary labels for data in *HighAmbig* are not trivially defined.

Table 1 shows the performance of our models and baselines[2]. It is noticeable that 3D DenseNet reveals a comparable performance with 3D DPN [14]. The *DenseSharp*$^+$ network with *HighAmbig* training scheme outperforms the one with *LowAmbig* training scheme. The *HighAmbig DenseSharp*$^+$ is trained

---

[2] Note that all counterparts use (sightly) different evaluation protocols.

Table 1. AUC and accuracy of DenseNet, *DenseSharp*, *DenseSharp*[+], and prior studies. The performance of our models is evaluated on *LowAmbig* LIDC-IDRI [1] dataset (see Sect. 2.1) with 5-fold cross validation.

Method	AUC	Accuracy (%)
3D DPN [14]	–	88.28
3D DPN ensemble [14]	–	90.44
3D CNN w. MTL [5]	–	80.08
3D CNN w. sparse MTL [5]	–	91.26
3D DenseNet (our implementation)	0.9218	87.82
DenseSharp [11] (our implementation)	0.9393	89.26
DenseSharp[+] (LowAmbig)	0.9480	90.87
DenseSharp[+] (HighAmbig)	**0.9566**	**91.52**

on an ambiguous dataset with a larger scale, resulting in a better performance than that of *LowAmbig DenseSharp*[+], which shows an excellent ability to learn from the ambiguous data distribution. The performance of *HighAmbig* trained *DenseSharp*[+] is also better than 3D DPN ensemble [14] and 3D CNN w. sparse MTL [5]. Notably, compared with other methods, we adopt a coarser dataset pre-processing strategy and a simpler evaluation setting. For instance, both counter-parts [5,14] use 10-fold cross validation, with more training samples than 5-fold in our study. The 3D DPN [14] only evaluates its performance on the overlapping nodules with LUNA16 dataset, which are easier to classify. The sparse MTL [5] resamples voxels at a higher resolution (spacing of 0.5 mm), besides the CNN is pre-trained on large-scale video dataset, rather than randomly initialized.

As for the segmentation output of *DenseSharp*[+], the average segmentation dice coefficient is 0.7625 on *LowAmbig* LIDC-IDRI with 5-fold cross validation. The segmentation output is of good quality with such a light-weight segmentation head. Due to the probabilistic segmentation output, *DenseSharp*[+] with automatic segmentation refuses to classify the nodules whose predicted volume is less than 10; 73 nodules are refused by *HighAmbig*-trained *DenseSharp*[+].

For further evaluation of probabilistic property of *DenseSharp*[+] model, we compute the mean standard deviation of softmax outputs as a diversity metric, derived from the softmax outputs of all the tested voxels (Eq. 5),

$$\mathrm{DIV} = \frac{1}{5} \sum_{i=1}^{5} \mathrm{Std}_{j=1...N}(p_{ij}),$$ (5)

in which p_{ij} is the softmax output of malignancy mode i and j^{th} sample of Gaussian distribution from one voxel. $\mathrm{Std}(\cdot)$ is the standard deviation operation. The distribution of DIV from all the tested voxels reflects the probabilistic output variance of *DenseSharp*[+] Networks. Figure 2 shows the DIV distribution of all the tested voxels. The two highlight samples show that the classification predictions from the model mimic the ambiguous labels from different experts.

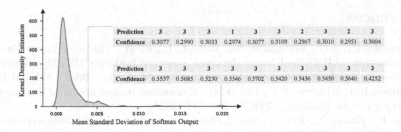

Fig. 2. The diversity metric (DIV) distribution of all tested voxels. The two highlight examples show that the output of $DenseSharp^+$ model varies as the prior sample varies, thanks to its probabilistic property.

Moreover, thanks to the explicit modeling, only voxels in lesions are counted, the visual saliency maps produced by the $DenseSharp^+$ is highly calibrated with the nodules. Please refer to Appendix Fig. A.3 for illustration.

4 Conclusion and Further Work

In this study, a Probabilistic Radiomics framework is proposed, which is well-performing, controllable and explainable in Computer-Aided Diagnosis (CADx). The proposed method is more expressive than conventional Radiomics analysis, more controllable and explainable than conventional deep learning approaches. Moreover, we explicitly model the ambiguity of the classification with a probabilistic approach. However, there are still limitations to make the Probabilistic Radiomics an *omics*-level approach (e.g., genomics, proteomics, immunomics).

Compared to other "omics" approaches, Radiomics is generally less reproducible [2]. Perturbations (e.g., rotations, different imaging parameters, adversarial attacks) on the images/point clouds [9] could introduce large variances to the outputs. Besides, the data-hungriness issue makes current MIC research a Sisyphean challenge; model learning on a certain task is non-trivial to transfer to another task. A more generalizable representation learning is the key to this problem, (probably) following a route of self-supervised learning and meta-learning. We will explore the robustness, transferability, and reproducibility of Probabilistic Radiomics in the future study.

Acknowledgment. This work was supported by National Science Foundation of China (U1611461, 61502301, 61521062). This work was supported by SJTU-UCLA Joint Center for Machine Perception and Inference, China's Thousand Youth Talents Plan, STCSM 17511105401, 18DZ2270700 and MoE Key Lab of Artificial Intelligence, AI Institute, Shanghai Jiao Tong University, China. This work was also jointly supported by SJTU-Minivision joint research grant.

References

1. Armato III, S.G., McLennan, G., Bidaut, L., et al.: The lung image database consortium (LIDC) and image database resource initiative (IDRI): a completed reference database of lung nodules on CT scans. Med. Phys. **38**(2), 915–931 (2011)
2. Gillies, R.J., Kinahan, P.E., Hricak, H.: Radiomics: images are more than pictures, they are data. Radiology **278**(2), 563–577 (2015)
3. He, K., Zhang, X., Ren, S., Sun, J.: Deep residual learning for image recognition. In: CVPR, pp. 770–778 (2016)
4. Huang, G., Liu, Z., Van Der Maaten, L., Weinberger, K.Q.: Densely connected convolutional networks. In: CVPR, vol. 1, p. 3 (2017)
5. Hussein, S., Cao, K., Song, Q., Bagci, U.: Risk stratification of lung nodules using 3D CNN-based multi-task learning. In: Niethammer, M., Styner, M., Aylward, S., Zhu, H., Oguz, I., Yap, P.-T., Shen, D. (eds.) IPMI 2017. LNCS, vol. 10265, pp. 249–260. Springer, Cham (2017). https://doi.org/10.1007/978-3-319-59050-9_20
6. Ioffe, S., Szegedy, C.: Batch normalization: accelerating deep network training by reducing internal covariate shift. In: ICML (2015)
7. Kingma, D.P., Welling, M.: Auto-encoding variational bayes. In: ICLR (2014)
8. Vaswani, A., Shazeer, N., Parmar, N., et al.: Attention is all you need. In: NIPS, pp. 5998–6008 (2017)
9. Yang, J., Zhang, Q., Fang, R., Ni, B., Liu, J., Tian, Q.: Adversarial attack and defense on point sets. arXiv preprint arXiv:1902.10899 (2019)
10. Yang, J., Zhang, Q., Ni, B., et al.: Modeling point clouds with self-attention and gumbel subset sampling. In: CVPR, pp. 3323–3332 (2019)
11. Zhao, W., Yang, J., et al.: 3D deep learning from ct scans predicts tumorinvasiveness of subcentimeter pulmonary adenocarcinomas. Cancer Res. **78**(24), 6881–6889 (2018)
12. Zhao, W., Yang, J., et al.: Toward automatic prediction of EGFR mutation status in pulmonary adenocarcinoma with 3d deep learning. Cancer Med. (2019)
13. Zhou, B., Khosla, A., Lapedriza, A., Oliva, A., Torralba, A.: Learning deep features for discriminative localization. In: CVPR, pp. 2921–2929 (2016)
14. Zhu, W., Liu, C., Fan, W., Xie, X.: Deeplung: 3D deep convolutional nets for automated pulmonary nodule detection and classification. In: WACV (2017)

Extract Bone Parts Without Human Prior: End-to-end Convolutional Neural Network for Pediatric Bone Age Assessment

Chuanbin Liu[1], Hongtao Xie[1(✉)], Yizhi Liu[2], Zhengjun Zha[1], Fanchao Lin[1], and Yongdong Zhang[1]

[1] School of Information Science and Technology,
University of Science and Technology of China, Hefei 230026, China
htxie@ustc.edu.cn
[2] Hunan University of Science and Technology, Xiangtan 411201, China

Abstract. Pediatric bone age assessment (BAA) is a common clinical practice to investigate endocrinology, genetic and growth disorders of children. The morphological characters of different specific bone parts, such as wrist and phalanx, have important reference significance in BAA. Previous deep learning approaches can be divided into two branches, (1) the single-stage structure ignores the attention on specific bone parts, thus it can be trained end-to-end but suffers from low accuracy, (2) the multi-stage structure extracts the bone parts with human prior, thus it exhibits high accuracy but suffers from model generalization and resource consumption problem. To enable an end-to-end training method extracting discriminative bone parts automatically without human prior, in this paper, we propose a novel single-stage Attention-Recognition Convolutional Neural Network (AR-CNN). The AR-CNN consists of one attention agent for discriminative bone parts proposing and one recognition agent for feature learning and age assessment. The attention agent can discover and extract bone parts automatically, meanwhile the recognition agent can learn the features from the proposing bone parts and assess the bone age. Furthermore, the assessment result will be fed back to attention agent for the optimization of bone parts extracting. Therefore, the two agents can reinforce each other mutually and the overall network can be trained end-to-end without human prior. To the best of our knowledge, this is the first end-to-end structure to extract bone parts for BAA without segmentation, detection and human prior. Experimental results show that our approach achieves state-of-the-art accuracy on the public RSNA datasets with mean absolute error(MAE) of 4.38 months.

Keywords: Bone age assessment · Deep learning · Object detection

1 Introduction

Pediatric bone age assessment (BAA) is a common clinical practice to investigate endocrinology, genetic and growth disorders of children [1,2]. Based on

© Springer Nature Switzerland AG 2019
D. Shen et al. (Eds.): MICCAI 2019, LNCS 11769, pp. 667–675, 2019.
https://doi.org/10.1007/978-3-030-32226-7_74

the discrepancy between the reading of the bone age and the chronological age, physicians can make accurate diagnoses of abnormal development in children. Currently, the left-hand X-ray image is widely used for assessing the bone age, and the morphological characters of different specific bone parts, such as wrist and phalanx, have important reference significance in BAA. There are a series of popular standards of BAA, i.e., the Greulich and Pyle (G&P) standard and the Tanner-Whitehouse (TW) standard, which extract a different set of specific bone part as regions of interest (ROIs) for assessment. Taking different standard as the reference, conventional manual assessment methods mainly rely on personal experience and opinion of the clinicians, which show some intrinsic limitations with low efficiency, unstable accuracy, and expensive time-consuming. Recent years, benefitting from a huge amount of data, deep learning methods have achieved impressive success [3–5] and a series of deep learning approaches have been proposed for BAA.

Related Work: The deep learning methods for bone age assessment can be divided into two categories: The first single-stage structure adopts an end-to-end learning method [6–8], where the entire image is taken as input to a convolutional neural network (CNN) and predicts the bone age directly. Larson et al. [8] take ResNet50 as the backbone to output a probability score for each month. Spampinato et al. [7] design a customized six-layer network with one deformation layer for age regression. Their models can be trained end-to-end, but ignore the attention on the specific bone parts as regions of interest. Consequently, the precision is limited. Moreover, it is confusing to visualize and interpret the results to clinicians [9].

The second category uses a multi-stage structure with image preprocessing and human prior knowledge [9–12], segmenting the hands out from original radiography, detecting and extracting the bone parts with human prior knowledge, then generating the prediction result. Iglovikov et al. [11] segment the hands out from radiography by U-Net and then crop out the carpal bones, metacarpals and proximal phalanges for ensemble regression. Wang et al. [10] detect the distal radius and ulna areas from the hand by Faster-RCNN to estimate the bone age. The multi-stage structure with human prior brings improvement in accuracy, as well as a series of limitations [7]: (1) the visual features identified by domain experts may not suitable for automated methods, and the strict human prior limits the generalization of deep learning. (2) it requires extra labels and algorithms in detection and segmentation, which brings additional costs. (3) it cannot be trained end-to-end and has high complexity and time expenditure.

Contribution: To combine the advantages of single-stage structure and multi-stage structure, specifically, to enable an end-to-end training method extracting discriminative bone parts automatically without human prior, in this paper, we propose a novel single-stage Attention-Recognition Convolutional Neural Network (AR-CNN) for bone age assessment. As shown in Fig. 1, the AR-CNN consists of one attention agent for discriminative bone parts proposing and one

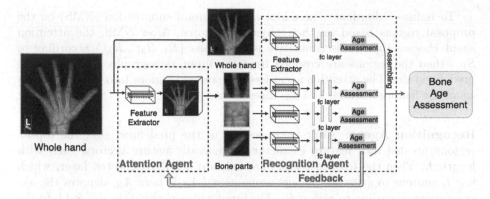

Fig. 1. The framework of AR-CNN.

recognition agent for feature learning and age assessment. The attention agent can discover and extract the discriminative bone parts automatically without human prior knowledge. Meanwhile the recognition agent can learn the features from the proposing ROIs and assess the bone age. Furthermore, the assessment result in recognition agent will be fed back to attention agent for the optimization of bone parts extracting. To the best of our knowledge, this is the first end-to-end structure to discover and extract bone parts for bone age assessment without any segmentation, detection and human prior.

2   Method

Overall Framework: Figure 1 illustrates the overall AR-CNN framework for bone age assessment. The attention agent takes the entire hand image as input and produces the proposal of discriminative bone parts as ROIs. These regions are cropped from the input radiography and fed into the recognition agent. The recognition agent learns the features from these bone parts as well as the input image, and produces the corresponding assessment results. Meanwhile, the assessment results are fed back to attention agent for optimization. To the end, it assembles all the assessment results and makes a final prediction.

Attention Agent: It has been proven by weakly-supervised object detection [13], that the higher-layer activation maps of a CNN for classification, can indicate the location of the discriminative parts. Therefore, the detection of an object can be realized even without bounding box annotations. Inspired by this idea, the attention agent of AR-CNN employs a Region Proposal Network (RPN) [14] to detect the discriminative bone parts without human prior.

Specifically, the RPN takes the radiography as input and produces a list of rectangle regions $\{R'_1, R'_2, ...R'_A\}$, each with an objectness score $S_{R'_i}$ of the region. Here we resize the input radiography X with the size of 448, and choose anchors with scales of $\{48, 96, 192\}$ and ratios of $\{1:1, 3:2, 2:3\}$.

To reduce redundancy, we adopt non-maximum suppression (NMS) on the proposal regions based on their objectness scores. After NMS, the attention agent chooses top-M discriminative part regions $\{R_1, R_2, ...R_M\}$ according to S_{R_i}, then the regions are cropped from the input radiography and resized to predefined size. The attention agent feeds the resized regions into the recognition agent for feature learning and age assessment.

Recognition Agent: After being resized to the predefined size, the top-M regions are fed into feature extractor to generate feature vectors, each with length L. Then the feature vectors are fed into a fully-connected layer, which has L neurons to generate the age assessment $\{A_{R_i}\}$, here A_{R_i} denotes the age assessment according to region R_i. The input radiography X is also fed into the recognition agent and we generate its prediction as A_X. To further leverage the benefit of part feature ensemble, we concatenate the feature vectors of the input radiography and the top-K ($K \leq M$) regions. The concatenated feature vector, denoted as C, is fed into a fully-connected layer, which has $L(K+1)$ neurons, to generate the assessment A_C. Then we average A_C, A_X, $\{A_{R_1}, A_{R_2}, ..., A_{R_K}\}$ and get the assembling age assessment A_{asb} as Eq. 1.

$$A_{asb} = \frac{1}{K+2}\{A_C + A_X + \sum_{i=1}^{K} A_{R_i}\} \tag{1}$$

Feedback: In AR-CNN, a feedback flow is established from recognition agent to attention agent. The absolute deviation of the extracted regions $\{D_{R_1}, D_{R_2}, ...D_{R_M}\}$ between assessment and ground-truth A_{gt} will be fed back to the attention agent for optimization.

An accurate attention agent means that, if a region R_i is predicted with high objectness score S_{R_i} in the attention agent, it will get low absolute deviation D_{R_i} to ground-truth age A_{gt} in the recognition agent, as in Eq. 2.

$$D_{R_i} < D_{R_j} \quad if \quad S_{R_i} > S_{R_j} \tag{2}$$

Accordingly, an optimization strategy for attention agent can be set up, and the discriminative bone parts can be extracted without human prior.

Loss Function and Optimization: The strategy of optimizing attention agent is to make $\{S_{R_1}, S_{R_2}, ..., S_{R_M}\}$ and $\{-D_{R_1}, -D_{R_2}, ..., -D_{R_M}\}$ have the same order. Hence the attention agent loss function L_{att} is defined as a pairwise ranking loss in Eq. 3. The function ϕ is hinge loss function $\phi(x) = max\{1-x, 0\}$ in our experiment.

$$L_{att} = \sum_{s=i}^{M-1} \sum_{j=s+1, D_{R_i} > D_{R_j}}^{M} \phi\left(S_{R_i} - S_{R_j}\right) \tag{3}$$

Since the recognition agent can be viewed as an assemblage of multiple regressor. Its loss function L_{cls} can be defined as the sum of the total regression loss in Eq. 4. $\mathcal{R}$ denotes the regression loss, and we employ L1 loss as regression loss in our approach.

$$L_{cls} = \mathcal{R}(C) + \mathcal{R}(X) + \sum_{i=1}^{M} \mathcal{R}(R_i) \tag{4}$$

The total loss of our MAR-CNN is defined as below:

$$L_{total} = L_{cls} + L_{att} = \sum_{s=i}^{M-1} \sum_{j=s+1, D_{R_i} > D_{R_j}}^{M} \phi\left(S_{R_i} - S_{R_j}\right) + D_c + D_X + \sum_{i=1}^{M} D_{R_i} \tag{5}$$

3   Experiments and Results

Data: We run experiments on the RSNA Pediatric Bone Age Challenge dataset[1], which consists of 12611 images for training, 1425 images for validation and 200 images for testing. And the ground-truth age ranges from 0 to 18 years. The Mean Absolute Error(MAE) between predicted age and ground-truth age on test set is the final evaluation standard for models performance.

Experiment Setup: We use Pytorch to implement AR-CNN and the algorithm are trained separately for male and female. The input hand radiography and extracted bone parts are resized to 448×448 and 224×224 respectively. ResNet50 is chosen as the backbone. We fix $M = 6$ in attention agent and the comparative experiments are carried out where K ranges from 1 to 4. Our AR-CNN is trained on a Ubuntu workstation with eight NVIDIA GeForce 1080Ti GPU, and the code and pre-trained model will be released for public research[2].

Result: We first make ablation study on hyper-parameter K, which means the recognition agent takes K bone parts for age assessment. Table 1 compares the MAE of male with different K. As we can see, with the increasing of K, the MAE reduces at the beginning. We obtain the best accuracy of 4.32 months when $K = 3$, then the MAE gets increased. This phenomenon indicates that, we do not need undue bone parts for assessment, which will bring misleading by introducing the less discriminative bone parts. Hence, extracting three specific bone parts is enough in AR-CNN.

With $K = 3$, the recognition agent takes the input radiography X, three bone parts R_1, R_2, R_3 and their contacted feature C for assembling age assessment. As we can see in Table 2, the MAE according to X are 5.76 and 6.20 months for males and females, respectively. The contacted feature C can reduce the MAEs

---

[1]   http://rsnachallenges.cloudapp.net/competitions/4.
[2]   https://github.com/liuboss1992/AR-CNN.

Table 1. Ablation study on hyper-parameter K.

Hyper-parameter K	1	2	3	4
MAE (months)	5.87	5.45	**4.32**	7.43

Table 2. Ablation study on assembling age assessment.

Unit	X	C	R_1	R_2	R_3	Assembling
MAE (male)	5.76	4.99	5.55	5.59	6.03	**4.32**
MAE (female)	6.20	5.46	6.58	6.31	7.04	**4.44**

to 4.99 and 5.46 months. Furthermore, when we take the bone parts R_i into assembling, the MAEs can be reduced to 4.32 and 4.44 months. This indicates the important reference significance of specific bone parts in BAA.

Table 3 compares AR-CNN with other state-of-art methods. Typically, the multi-stage method [9, 11] can achieve better accuracy than the single-stage ones [7,8], since it employs human prior to focus on specific bone parts. Iglovikov et al. [11] segment the hands out from radiography by U-Net and then crop out the carpal bones, metacarpals and proximal phalanges for assessment. Thus, they achieve impressive accuracy. Human prior brings improvement in accuracy, however, it can limit the generalization. AR-CNN can extract the discriminative bone parts without human prior knowledge, and is free of segmentation or detection. Experimental results show that AR-CNN achieves the best accuracy with MAE of 4.38 months over all the methods. This indicates that, the human prior is not a one-size-fits-all reference for deep learning in BAA task.

Table 3. Comparison results with the state-of-art methods. *RSNA.* represents the experiment which is performed on RSNA dataset.

Method	Human [8]	Spampinato [7]	Larson [8]	Iglovikov [11]	Ren [9]	Our AR-CNN
Stage		Single-stage	Single-stage	Multi-stage	Multi-stage	Single-stage
RSNA.	✓		✓	✓	✓	✓
MAE	7.32	9.12	6.24	4.97	5.20	**4.38**

Analysis and Visualization: Figure 2 shows the assessment result and deviation on test set. From Fig. 2(a) we can see, our assessment result keeps strong consistency with the actual age. Meanwhile, from Fig. 2(b) we can see, the absolute deviation of our model is controlled within 20 months.

Moreover, visualization experiments are carried out to observe the extraction result of discriminative bone parts. We highlight the extracted bone parts in attention agent with colored bounding box on the input images. As shown in Fig. 3, our attention agent mostly extracts the carpal bones and proximal phalanges as the discriminative parts, which keeps consistent with human prior

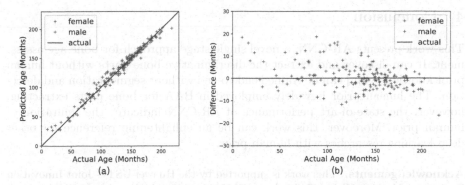

Fig. 2. Statistical results of our AR-CNN in bone age assessment. (a) shows the relationship between actual age and predicted age. (b) shows the relationship between actual age and deviation. [Best viewed in color] (Color figure online)

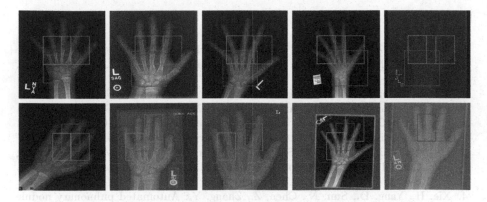

Fig. 3. Visualization experiments for bone parts extraction. The first row shows the results of female, and the second row shows the results of male. [Best viewed in color] (Color figure online)

knowledge. This indicates that AR-CNN can learn and establish correct knowledge without human prior. Meanwhile, AR-CNN embodies discrepant attention within gender, which differs from human prior. The carpal and the proximal phalanges are extracted for female, by contrast, the proximal phalanges of the index finger, middle finger and ring finger are usually separately extracted for male. This suggests that some of the human prior currently employed by clinicians might not be consummate. AR-CNN can slip the leash of human knowledge, and it could be a suggestion for a new clinical standard. In addition, AR-CNN presents stable performance with different rotation, scaling ratio and contrast ratio. This illustrates the strong reliability and expansibility of our approach.

4   Conclusion

This work presents AR-CNN, a novel single-stage approach for bone age assessment. It can discover and extract the discriminative bone parts without human prior knowledge, and can be trained end-to-end without segmentation and detection. The human prior is widely employed in BAA for bone parts extracting, however, the state-of-art performance of AR-CNN indicates the limitation of human prior. Moreover, this work can be an enlightening reference for other deep learning researches with human prior.

Acknowledgements. This work is supported by the Huawei-USTC Joint Innovation Project on Machine Vision Technology (FA2018111122). And we would like to thank Brain-inspired Technology Corporation (http://www.leinao.ai/) for its calculation support.

References

1. Gertych, A., Zhang, A., Sayre, J., Pospiech-Kurkowska, S., Huang, H.K.: Bone age assessment of children using a digital hand atlas. Comput. Med. Imaging Graph. **31**(4–5), 322–331 (2007)
2. Stern, D., Ebner, T., Bischof, H., Grassegger, S., Ehammer, T., Urschler, M.: Fully automatic bone age estimation from left hand MR images. In: Golland, P., Hata, N., Barillot, C., Hornegger, J., Howe, R. (eds.) MICCAI 2014. LNCS, vol. 8674, pp. 220–227. Springer, Cham (2014). https://doi.org/10.1007/978-3-319-10470-6_28
3. Liu, A.A., Xu, N., Nie, W.Z., Su, Y.T., Wong, Y., Kankanhalli, M.: Benchmarking a multimodal and multiview and interactive dataset for human action recognition. IEEE Trans. Cybern. **47**(7), 1781–1794 (2016)
4. Xie, H., Yang, D., Sun, N., Chen, Z., Zhang, Y.: Automated pulmonary nodule detection in ct images using deep convolutional neural networks. Pattern Recogn. **85**, 109–119 (2019)
5. Min, S., Chen, X., Zha, Z.J., Wu, F., Zhang, Y.: A two-stream mutual attention network for semi-supervised biomedical segmentation with noisy labels. In: AAAI 2019 (2018)
6. Mutasa, S., Chang, P.D., Ruzal-Shapiro, C., Ayyala, R.: MABAL: a novel deep-learning architecture for machine-assisted bone age labeling. J. Digit. Imaging **31**(4), 513–519 (2018)
7. Spampinato, C., Palazzo, S., Giordano, D., Aldinucci, M., Leonardi, R.: Deep learning for automated skeletal bone age assessment in X-ray images. Med. Image Anal. **36**, 41–51 (2017). https://doi.org/10.1016/j.media.2016.10.010
8. Larson, D.B., Chen, M.C., Lungren, M.P., Halabi, S.S., Stence, N.V., Langlotz, C.P.: Performance of a deep-learning neural network model in assessing skeletal maturity on pediatric hand radiographs. Radiology **287**(1), 313–322 (2018)
9. Ren, X., Li, T., Wang, Q.: Regression convolutional neural network for automated pediatric bone age assessment from hand radiograph. IEEE J. Biomed. Health Inform. **pp**(c), 1 (2018)
10. Wang, S., Shen, Y., Zeng, D., Hu, Y.: Bone age assessment using convolutional neural networks. In: 2018 International Conference on Artificial Intelligence and Big Data (ICAIBD), pp. 175–178. IEEE (2018)

11. Iglovikov, V.I., Rakhlin, A., Kalinin, A.A., Shvets, A.A.: Paediatric bone age assessment using deep convolutional neural networks. In: Stoyanov, D., et al. (eds.) DLMIA/ML-CDS -2018. LNCS, vol. 11045, pp. 300–308. Springer, Cham (2018). https://doi.org/10.1007/978-3-030-00889-5_34

12. Hao, P., Chen, Y., Chokuwa, S., Wu, F., Bai, C.: Skeletal bone age assessment based on deep convolutional neural networks. In: Hong, R., Cheng, W.-H., Yamasaki, T., Wang, M., Ngo, C.-W. (eds.) PCM 2018. LNCS, vol. 11165, pp. 408–417. Springer, Cham (2018). https://doi.org/10.1007/978-3-030-00767-6_38

13. Singh, K.K., Lee, Y.J.: Hide-and-seek: forcing a network to be meticulous for weakly-supervised object and action localization. In: ICCV, pp. 3544–3553. IEEE (2017)

14. Ren, S., He, K., Girshick, R., Sun, J.: Faster R-CNN: towards real-time object detection with region proposal networks. In: Advances in neural information processing systems, pp. 91–99 (2015)

Quantifying and Leveraging Classification Uncertainty for Chest Radiograph Assessment

Florin C. Ghesu[1]([✉]), Bogdan Georgescu[1], Eli Gibson[1], Sebastian Guendel[1], Mannudeep K. Kalra[2,3], Ramandeep Singh[2,3], Subba R. Digumarthy[2,3], Sasa Grbic[1], and Dorin Comaniciu[1]

[1] Digital Technology and Innovation, Siemens Healthineers, Princeton, NJ, USA
`florin.ghesu@siemens-healthineers.com`
[2] Department of Radiology, Massachusetts General Hospital, Boston, MA, USA
[3] Harvard Medical School, Boston, MA, USA

Abstract. The interpretation of chest radiographs is an essential task for the detection of thoracic diseases and abnormalities. However, it is a challenging problem with high inter-rater variability and inherent ambiguity due to inconclusive evidence in the data, limited data quality or subjective definitions of disease appearance. Current deep learning solutions for chest radiograph abnormality classification are typically limited to providing probabilistic predictions, relying on the capacity of learning models to adapt to the high degree of label noise and become robust to the enumerated causal factors. In practice, however, this leads to overconfident systems with poor generalization on unseen data. To account for this, we propose an automatic system that learns not only the probabilistic estimate on the presence of an abnormality, but also an explicit uncertainty measure which captures the confidence of the system in the predicted output. We argue that explicitly learning the classification uncertainty as an additional measure to the predicted output, is essential to account for the inherent variability characteristic of this data. Experiments were conducted on two datasets of chest radiographs of over 85,000 patients. Sample rejection based on the predicted uncertainty can significantly improve the ROC-AUC, e.g., by 8% to 0.91 with an expected rejection rate of under 25%. Eliminating training samples using uncertainty-driven bootstrapping, enables a significant increase in robustness and accuracy. In addition, we present a multi-reader study showing that the predictive uncertainty is indicative of reader errors.

1 Introduction

The interpretation of chest radiographs is an essential task in the practice of a radiologist, enabling the early detection of thoracic diseases [9,12]. To accelerate and improve the assessment of the continuously increasing number of radiographs, several deep learning solutions have been recently proposed for the automatic classification of radiographic findings [4,12,13]. Due to large variations in

© Springer Nature Switzerland AG 2019
D. Shen et al. (Eds.): MICCAI 2019, LNCS 11769, pp. 676–684, 2019.
https://doi.org/10.1007/978-3-030-32226-7_75

image quality or subjective definitions of disease appearance, there is a large inter-rate variability which leads to a high degree of label noise [9]. Modeling this variability when designing an automatic system for assessing this type of data is essential; an aspect which was not considered in previous work.

Using principles of information theory and subjective logic [6] based on the Dempster-Shafer framework for modeling of evidence [1], we present a method for training a system that generates both an image-level label and a classification uncertainty measure. We evaluate this system for classification of abnormalities on chest radiographs. The main contributions of this paper include:

1. describing a system for jointly learning classification probabilities and classification uncertainty in a parametric model;
2. proposing uncertainty-driven bootstrapping as a means to filter training samples with highest predictive uncertainty to improve robustness and accuracy;
3. comparing methods for generating stochastic classifications to model classification uncertainty;
4. presenting an application of this system to identify cases with uncertain classification, yielding more accurate classification on the remaining cases;
5. showing that the uncertainty measure can distinguish radiographs with correct and incorrect labels according to a multi-radiologist-consensus study.

2 Background and Motivation

2.1 Machine Learning for the Assessment of Chest Radiographs

The open access to the ChestX-Ray8 dataset [12] of chest radiographs has led to a series of recent publications that propose machine learning based systems for disease classification. With this dataset, Wang et al. [12] also report a first performance baseline of a deep neural network at an average area under receiver operating characteristic curve (ROC-AUC) of 0.75. These results have been further improved by using multi-scale image analysis [13], or by actively focusing the attention of the network on the most relevant sub-regions of the lungs [3]. State-of-the-art results on the official split of the ChestX-Ray8 dataset are reported in [4] (avg. ROC-AUC of 0.81), using a location-aware dense neural network. In light of these contributions, a recent study compares the performance of such an AI system and 9 practicing radiologists [9]. While the study indicates that the system can surpass human performance, it also highlights the high variability among different expert radiologists for the reading of chest radiographs. The reported average specificity of the readers is very high (over 95%), with an average sensitivity of $50\% \pm 8\%$. With such a large inter-rater variability, one may ask: How can real 'ground truth' data be obtained? Does the label noise affect the training? Current solutions do not consider this variability, which leads to models with overconfident predictions and limited generalization.

Principles of Uncertainty Estimation: One way to handle this challenge is to explicitly estimate the classification uncertainty from the data. Recent methods for uncertainty estimation in the context of deep learning rely on Bayesian estimation theory [8] or ensembles [7] and demonstrate increased robustness to out-of-distribution data. However, these approaches come with significant computational limitations; associated with the high complexity of sampling parameter spaces of deep models for Bayesian risk estimation; or associated with the challenge of managing ensembles of deep models. Sensoy et al. [10] propose an efficient alternative based on the theory of subjective logic [6], training a deep neural network to estimate the sample uncertainty based on observed data.

3   Proposed Method

Following the work of Sensoy et al. [10] based on the Dempster-Shafer theory of evidence [1], we apply principles of subjective logic [6] to derive a binary classification model that can support the joint estimation of per-class probabilities $(\hat{p}_+; \hat{p}_-)$ and predictive uncertainty $\hat{u}$. In this context, a decisional framework is defined through the assignment of so called belief masses from evidence collected from observed data to individual attributes, e.g., membership to a class [1,6]. Let us denote b^+ and b^- the belief values for the positive and negative class, respectively. The uncertainty mass u is defined as: $u = 1 - b^+ - b^-$, where $b^+ = e^+/E$ and $b^- = e^-/E$ with $e^+; e^- \geq 0$ denoting the per-class collected evidence and total evidence $E = e^+ + e^- + 2$. For binary classification, we propose to model the distribution of such evidence values using the beta distribution, defined by two parameters α and β as: $f(x; \alpha, \beta) = \frac{\Gamma(\alpha+\beta)}{\Gamma(\alpha)\Gamma(\beta)} x^{\alpha-1}(1-x)^{\beta-1}$, where Γ denotes the gamma function and $\alpha, \beta > 1$ with $\alpha = e^+ + 1$ and $\beta = e^- + 1$. In this context, the per-class probabilities can be derived as $p^+ = \alpha/E$ and $p^- = \beta/E$. Figure 1 visualizes the beta distribution for different α, β values.

A training dataset is provided: $\mathcal{D} = \{I_k, y_k\}_{k=1}^{N}$, composed of N pairs of images I_k with class assignment $y_k \in \{0, 1\}$. To estimate the per-class evidence values from the observed data, a deep neural network parametrized by θ can be applied, with: $[e_k^+, e_k^-] = \mathcal{R}(I_k; \theta)$, where $\mathcal{R}$ denotes the network response function. Using maximum likelihood estimation, one can learn the network parameters $\hat{\theta}$ by optimizing the Bayes risk of the class predictor p_k with a beta prior distribution:

$$\mathcal{L}_k^{data} = \int \|y_k - p_k\|^2 \frac{\Gamma(\alpha+\beta)}{\Gamma(\alpha)\Gamma(\beta)} p_k^{\alpha-1}(1-p_k)^{\beta-1} dp_k, \qquad (1)$$

where $k \in \{1, \ldots, N\}$ denotes the index of the training example from dataset $\mathcal{D}$, p_k the predicted probability on the training sample k, and $\mathcal{L}_k^{data}$ defines the goodness of fit. Using linearity properties of the expectation, Eq. 1 becomes:

$$\mathcal{L}_k^{data} = (y_k - \hat{p}_k^+)^2 + (1 - y_k - \hat{p}_k^-)^2 + \frac{\hat{p}_k^+(1 - \hat{p}_k^+) + \hat{p}_k^-(1 - \hat{p}_k^-)}{E_k + 1}, \qquad (2)$$

where $\hat{p}_k^+$ and $\hat{p}_k^-$ denote the network's probabilistic prediction. The first two terms measure the goodness of fit, and the last term encodes the variance of the prediction [10].

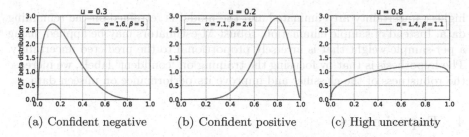

(a) Confident negative   (b) Confident positive   (c) High uncertainty

Fig. 1. Probability density function of the beta distribution: example parameters (α, β) modeling confident and uncertain predictions.

To ensure a high uncertainty value for data samples for which the gathered evidence is not conclusive for an accurate classification, an additional regularization term $\mathcal{L}_k^{reg}$ is added to the loss. Using information theory, this term is defined as the relative entropy, i.e., the Kullback-Leibler divergence, between the beta distributed prior term and the beta distribution with total uncertainty $(\alpha, \beta = 1)$. In this way, cost deviations from the total uncertainty state, i.e., $u = 1$, which do not contribute to the data fit are accounted for [10]. With the additional term, the total cost becomes $\mathcal{L} = \sum_{k=1}^{N} \mathcal{L}_k$ with:

$$\mathcal{L}_k = \mathcal{L}_k^{data} + \lambda \, \mathrm{KL}\left(f(\hat{p}_k; \tilde{\alpha}_k, \tilde{\beta}_k) \| f(\hat{p}_k; \langle 1, 1 \rangle) \right), \tag{3}$$

where $\lambda \geq 0$, $\hat{p}_k = \hat{p}_k^+$, with $(\tilde{\alpha}_k, \tilde{\beta}_k) = (1, \beta_k)$ for $y_k = 0$ and $(\tilde{\alpha}_k, \tilde{\beta}_k) = (\alpha_k, 1)$ for $y_k = 1$. Removing additive constants and using properties of the logarithm function, one can simplify the regularization term to the following:

$$\mathcal{L}_k^{reg} = \log \frac{\Gamma(\tilde{\alpha}_k + \tilde{\beta}_k)}{\Gamma(\tilde{\alpha}_k)\Gamma(\tilde{\beta}_k)} + \sum_{x \in \{\tilde{\alpha}_k, \tilde{\beta}_k\}} (x - 1)\left(\psi(x) - \psi(\tilde{\alpha}_k + \tilde{\beta}_k) \right), \tag{4}$$

where ψ denotes the digamma function and $k \in \{1, \ldots, N\}$. Using stochastic gradient descent, the total loss $\mathcal{L}$ is optimized on the training set $\mathcal{D}$.

Sampling the Data Distribution: An important requirement to ensure training stability and to learn a robust estimation of evidence values is an adequate sampling of the data distribution. We empirically found dropout [11] to be a simple and very effective strategy to address this problem. In practice, dropout emulates an ensemble model combination driven by the random deactivation of neurons. Alternatively, one may use an explicit ensemble of M models $\{\theta_k\}_{k=1}^{M}$, each trained independently. Following the principles of deep ensembles [7], the per-class evidence can be computed from the ensemble estimates $\{e^{(k)}\}_{k=1}^{M}$ via averaging. In our work, we found dropout to be as effective as deep ensembles.

Uncertainty-driven Bootstrapping: Given the predictive uncertainty measure $\hat{u}$, we propose a simple and effective algorithm for filtering the training set with the target of reducing label noise. A fraction of training samples with highest uncertainty are eliminated and the model is retrained on the remaining data. Instead of sample elimination, robust M-estimators may be applied, using a per-sample weight that is inversely proportional to the predicted uncertainty. The hypothesis is that by focusing the training on 'confident' labels, we increase the robustness of the classifier and improve its performance on unseen data.

4   Experiments

Dataset and Setup: The evaluation is based on two datasets, the ChestX-Ray8 [12] and PLCO [2]. Both datasets provide a series of AP/PA chest radiographs with binary labels on the presence of different radiological findings, e.g., granuloma, pleural effusion, or consolidation. The ChestX-Ray8 dataset contains 112,120 images from 30,805 patients, covering 14 findings extracted from radiological reports using natural language processing (NLP) [12]. In contrast, the PLCO dataset was constructed as part of a screening trial, containing 185,421 images from 56,071 patients and covering 12 different abnormalities.

For performance comparison, we selected location-aware dense networks [4] as baseline. This method achieves state-of-the-art results on this problem, with a reported average ROC-AUC of **0.81** (significantly higher than that of competing methods: 0.75 [12] and 0.77 [13]) on the official split of the ChestX-Ray8 dataset and a ROC-AUC of **0.88** on the official split of the PLCO dataset. To evaluate our method, we identified testing subsets with higher confidence labels from multi-radiologist studies. For PLCO, we randomly selected 565 test images and had 2 board-certified expert radiologists read the images – updating the labels to the majority vote of the 3 opinions (incl. the original label). For ChestX-Ray8, a subset of 689 test images was randomly selected and read by 4 board-certified radiologists. The final label was decided following a consensus discussion. For both datasets, the remaining data was split at patient level in 90% training and 10% validation. All images were rescaled to 256×256 using bilinear interpolation.

System Training: We constructed our learning model from the DenseNet-121 architecture [5]. A dropout layer with a dropout rate of 0.5 was inserted after the last convolutional layer. We also investigated the benefits of using deep ensembles to improve the sampling ($M = 5$ models trained on random subsets of 80% of the training data; we refer to this with the keyword [**ens**]). A fully connected layer with ReLU activation units maps to the two outputs α and β. We used a systematic grid search to find the optimal configuration of training meta-parameters: learning rate (10^{-4}), regularization factor ($\lambda = 1$; decayed to 0.1 and 0.001 after 1/3, respectively 2/3 of the epochs), training epochs (around 12, using an early stop strategy with a patience of 3 epochs) and a batch size of 128. The low number of epochs is explained by the large size of the dataset.

Uncertainty-driven Sample Rejection: Given a model trained for the assessment of an arbitrary finding, one can directly estimate the prediction uncertainty $\hat{u} = 2/(\alpha + \beta) \in [0, 1]$. This is an additional measure to the predicted probability,

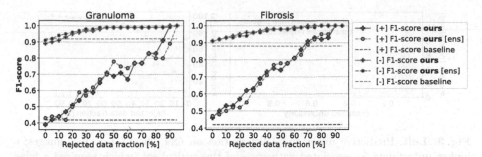

Fig. 2. Evolution of the F1-scores for the positive (+) and negative (−) classes relative to the sample rejection threshold - determined using the estimated uncertainty. We show the performance for granuloma and fibrosis based on the PLCO dataset [2]. The baseline (horizontal dashed lines) is determined using the method from [4] (working point at max. average of per-class F1 scores). Decision threshold for our method is fixed at 0.5.

Table 1. Comparison between the reference method [4] and several versions of our method calibrated at sample rejection rates of 0%, 10%, 25% and 50% (based on the PLCO dataset [2]). Lesion refers to lesions of the bones or soft tissue.

| Finding | ROC-AUC | | | | |
	Guendel et al. [4]	Ours [0%]	Ours [10%]	Ours [25%]	Ours [50%]
Granuloma	0.83	0.85	0.87	**0.90**	**0.92**
Fibrosis	0.87	0.88	0.90	**0.92**	**0.94**
Scaring	0.82	0.81	0.84	**0.89**	**0.93**
Lesion	0.82	0.83	0.86	**0.88**	**0.90**
Cardiac Ab	0.93	0.94	0.95	**0.96**	**0.97**
Average	0.85	0.86	0.89	**0.91**	**0.93**

with increased values on out-of-distribution cases under the given model. One can use this measure for sample rejection, i.e., set a threshold u_t and steer the system to not output its prediction on all cases with an expected uncertainty larger than u_t. Instead, these cases are labeled with the message *"Do not know for sure; process case manually"*. In practice this leads to a significant increase in accuracy compared to the state-of-the-art on the remaining cases, as reported in Table 1 and Fig. 2. For example, for the identification of granuloma, a rejection rate of 25% leads to an increase of over 20% in the micro-average F1 score. On the same abnormality, a 50% rejection rate leads to a F1 score over 0.99 for the prediction of negative cases. We found no significant difference in average performance when using ensembles (see Fig. 2).

System versus Reader Uncertainty: To provide an insight into the meaning of the uncertainty measure and its correlation with the difficulty of cases, we evaluated our system on the detection of pleural effusion (excess accumulation

682   F. C. Ghesu et al.

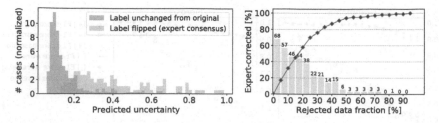

Fig. 3. Left: Predictive uncertainty distribution on 689 ChestX-Ray test images; a higher uncertainty is associated with cases of the critical set, which required a label correction according to expert committee. **Right**: Plot showing the capacity of the algorithm to eliminate cases from the critical set via sample rejection. Bars indicate the percentage of critical cases for each batch of 5% rejected cases.

of fluid in the pleural cavity) based on the ChestX-Ray8 dataset. In particular, we analyzed the test set of 689 cases that were relabeled using an expert committee of 4 experts. We defined a so called *critical set*, that contains only cases for which the label was changed after the expert reevaluation. According to the committee, this set contained not only easy examples for which probably the NLP algorithm has failed to properly extract the correct labels from the radiographic report; but also difficult cases for which the evidence of effusion was very subtle. In Fig. 3 (left), we empirically show that the uncertainty estimates of our algorithm correlate with the committee's decision to change the label. Specifically, for unchanged cases, our algorithm displayed very low uncertainty estimates (average 0.16) at an average AUC of 0.976 (rejection rate of 0%). In contrast, on cases in the critical set, the algorithm showed higher uncertainties distributed between 0.1 and the maximum value of 1 (average 0.41). This indicates the ability of the algorithm to recognize the cases where annotation errors occurred in the first place (through NLP or human reader error). In Fig. 3 (right) we show how cases of the critical set can be effectively filtered out using sample rejection. Qualitative examples are shown in Fig. 4.

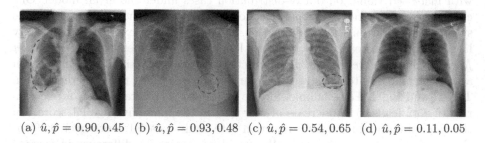

(a) $\hat{u}, \hat{p} = 0.90, 0.45$ (b) $\hat{u}, \hat{p} = 0.93, 0.48$ (c) $\hat{u}, \hat{p} = 0.54, 0.65$ (d) $\hat{u}, \hat{p} = 0.11, 0.05$

Fig. 4. ChestX-Ray8 test images assessed for pleural effusion ($\hat{u}$: est. uncertainty, $\hat{p}$: output probability; with affected regions circled in red). Figures 4a, 4b and 4c show positive cases of the critical set with high predictive uncertainty – possibly explained by the atypical appearance of accumulated fluid in 4a, and poor quality of image 4b. Figure 4d shows a high confidence case with no pleural effusion. (Color figure online)

Uncertainty-driven Bootstrapping: We also investigated the benefit of using bootstrapping based on the uncertainty measure on the example of plural effusion (ChestX-Ray8). We report performance as $[AUC;\ F1\text{-}score$ (pos. class); $F1\text{-}score$ (neg. class)]. After training our method, the baseline performance was measured at $[0.89; 0.60; 0.92]$ on testing. We then eliminated 5%, 10% and 15% of training samples with highest uncertainty, and retrained in each case on the remaining data. The metrics improved to $[0.90; 0.68; 0.92]_{5\%}$, $[0.91; 0.67; 0.94]_{10\%}$ and $[\mathbf{0.93; 0.69; 0.94}]_{15\%}$ on the test set. This is a significant increase, demonstrating the potential of this strategy to improve the robustness to label noise.

5   Conclusion

In conclusion, this paper presents an effective method for the joint estimation of class probabilities and classification uncertainty in the context of chest radiograph assessment. Extensive experiments on two large datasets demonstrate a significant accuracy increase if sample rejection is performed based on the estimated uncertainty measure. In addition, we highlight the capacity of the system to distinguish radiographs with correct and incorrect labels according to a multi-radiologist-consensus user study, using the uncertainty measure only.

The authors thank the National Cancer Institute for access to NCI's data collected by the Prostate, Lung, Colorectal and Ovarian (PLCO) Cancer Screening Trial. The statements contained herein are solely those of the authors and do not represent or imply concurrence or endorsement by NCI.

Disclaimer. The concepts and information presented in this paper are based on research results that are not commercially available.

References

1. Dempster, A.P.: A generalization of bayesian inference. J. Royal Stat. Soc.: Ser. B (Methodol.) **30**(2), 205–232 (1968)
2. Gohagan, J.K., Prorok, P.C., Hayes, R.B., Kramer, B.S.: The prostate, lung, colorectal and ovarian (PLCO) cancer screening trial of the National Cancer Institute: history, organization, and status. Control. Clin. Trials **21**(6), 251–272 (2000)
3. Guan, Q., Huang, Y., Zhong, Z., Zheng, Z., Zheng, L., Yang, Y.: Diagnose like a radiologist: attention guided convolutional neural network for thorax disease classification. arXiv:1801.09927 (2018)
4. Guendel, S., et al.: Learning to recognize abnormalities in chest X-rays with location-aware dense networks. arXiv:1803.04565 (2018)
5. Huang, G., Liu, Z., v. d. Maaten, L., Weinberger, K.Q.: Densely connected convolutional networks. In: CVPR, pp. 2261–2269 (2017)
6. Jøsang, A.: Subjective Logic: A Formalism for Reasoning Under Uncertainty, 1st edn. Springer, Heidelberg (2016). https://doi.org/10.1007/978-3-319-42337-1
7. Lakshminarayanan, B., Pritzel, A., Blundell, C.: Simple and scalable predictive uncertainty estimation using deep ensembles. In: NIPS, pp. 6402–6413 (2017)
8. Molchanov, D., Ashukha, A., Vetrov, D.: Variational dropout sparsifies deep neural networks. In: ICML, pp. 2498–2507 (2017)

9. Rajpurkar, P., et al.: Deep learning for chest radiograph diagnosis: a retrospective comparison of the CheXNeXt algorithm to practicing radiologists. PLoS Med. **15**(11), e1002686 (2018)
10. Sensoy, M., Kaplan, L., Kandemir, M.: Evidential deep learning to quantify classification uncertainty. In: NIPS, pp. 3179–3189 (2018)
11. Srivastava, N., Hinton, G., Krizhevsky, A., Sutskever, I., Salakhutdinov, R.: Dropout: a simple way to prevent neural networks from overfitting. JMLR **15**(1), 1929–1958 (2014)
12. Wang, X., Peng, Y., Lu, L., Lu, Z., Bagheri, M., Summers, R.: ChestX-Ray8: hospital-scale chest X-ray database and benchmarks on weakly-supervised classification and localization of common thorax diseases. In: CVPR, pp. 3462–3471 (2017)
13. Yao, L., Prosky, J., Poblenz, E., Covington, B., Lyman, K.: Weakly supervised medical diagnosis and localization from multiple resolutions. arXiv:1803.07703 (2018)

Adversarial Regression Training for Visualizing the Progression of Chronic Obstructive Pulmonary Disease with Chest X-Rays

Ricardo Bigolin Lanfredi[1]([×]) [iD], Joyce D. Schroeder[2] [iD], Clement Vachet[1] [iD], and Tolga Tasdizen[1] [iD]

[1] Scientific Computing and Imaging Institute, University of Utah, Salt Lake City, UT 84112, USA
ricbl@sci.utah.edu

[2] Department of Radiology and Imaging Sciences, University of Utah, Salt Lake City, UT 84112, USA

Abstract. Knowledge of what spatial elements of medical images deep learning methods use as evidence is important for model interpretability, trustiness, and validation. There is a lack of such techniques for models in regression tasks. We propose a method, called visualization for regression with a generative adversarial network (VR-GAN), for formulating adversarial training specifically for datasets containing regression target values characterizing disease severity. We use a conditional generative adversarial network where the generator attempts to learn to shift the output of a regressor through creating disease effect maps that are added to the original images. Meanwhile, the regressor is trained to predict the original regression value for the modified images. A model trained with this technique learns to provide visualization for how the image would appear at different stages of the disease. We analyze our method in a dataset of chest x-rays associated with pulmonary function tests, used for diagnosing chronic obstructive pulmonary disease (COPD). For validation, we compute the difference of two registered x-rays of the same patient at different time points and correlate it to the generated disease effect map. The proposed method outperforms a technique based on classification and provides realistic-looking images, making modifications to images following what radiologists usually observe for this disease. Implementation code is available at https://github.com/ricbl/vrgan.

Keywords: COPD · Chest x-ray · Regression interpretation · Visual attribution · Adversarial training · Disease effect · VR-GAN

1 Introduction

Methods of visual attribution in deep learning applied to computer vision are useful for understanding what regions of an image models are using [1]. These

© Springer Nature Switzerland AG 2019
D. Shen et al. (Eds.): MICCAI 2019, LNCS 11769, pp. 685–693, 2019.
https://doi.org/10.1007/978-3-030-32226-7_76

methods improve a model's interpretability, help in building user trust and validate if the model is using the evidence humans would expect it to use for its task. They have been mostly used to explain models in classification tasks. A common way of formulating the problem of visual attribution is by asking "What regions of the image are weighted positively in the decision to output this class?". This question is not suitable for regression tasks, for which we propose to ask "What would this image look like if it had this other regression value?".

To answer the proposed question, we draw from conditional generative adversarial networks (GANs) [10] and image-to-image GANs [7], both of which have been shown to model complex non-linear relations between conditional labels, input images, and generated images. We hypothesize that using the regression target value for training a visual attribution model with the proposed novel loss will improve the visualization when compared to a similar formulation that only uses classification labels since it does not lose the information of a continuous regression target value by imposing a set of classes. We name our method visualization for regression with a generative adversarial network (VR-GAN).

We study our model in the context of how a value characterizing chronic obstructive pulmonary disease (COPD) is related to changes in x-ray images. COPD is defined by pulmonary function tests (PFTs) [8]. A PFT measures forced expiratory volume in one second (FEV_1), which is the volume of air a patient can exhale in one second, and forced vital capacity (FVC), which is the total volume of air a patient can exhale. A patient with FEV_1/FVC ratio lower than 0.7 is diagnosed to have COPD.

Radiology provides a few clues that can be used for raising suspicion of COPD directly from an x-ray [4]. There is a higher chance of COPD when diaphragms are low and flat, corresponding to high lung volumes, and when the lung tissue presents low-attenuation (dark, or lucent), corresponding to emphysema, air trapping or vascular pruning. We show that our model highlights low and flat diaphragm and added lucency. Our method is, to the best of our knowledge, the first data-driven approach to model disease effects of COPD on chest x-rays.

1.1   Related Work

One way to visualize evidence of a class using deep learning is to perform backpropagation of the outputs of a trained classifier [1]. In [11], for example, a model is trained to predict the presence of 14 diseases in chest x-rays, and class activation maps [15] are used to show what regions of the x-rays have a larger influence on the classifier's decision. However, as shown in [2], these methods suffer from low resolution or from highlighting limited regions of the original images.

In [2], researchers visualize what brain MRIs of patients with mild cognitive impairment would look like if they developed Alzheimer's disease, generating disease effect maps. To solve problems with other visualization methods, they propose an adversarial setup. A generator is trained to modify an input image which fools a discriminator. The modifications the generator outputs are used as visualization of evidence of one class. This setup inspires our method. However, instead of classification labels, we use regression values and a novel loss function.

There have been other works on generating visual attribution for regression. In [13], Seah et al. start by training a GAN on a large dataset of frontal x-rays, and then train an encoder that maps from an x-ray to its latent space vector. Finally, Seah et al. train a small model for regression that receives the latent vector of the images from a smaller dataset and outputs a value which is used for diagnosing congestive heart failure. To interpret their model, they backpropagate through the small regression model, taking steps in the latent space to reach the threshold of diagnosis, and generate the image associated with the new diagnosis.

The loss function we provide for this task is similar to the cost function provided in [14]. Unlike our formulation, [14] models adversarial attackers and defenders in a game theoretic sense and arrives at an optimal solution for the defenders, using only linear models and applying it to simple features datasets. In [3], Bazrafkan et al. propose a method for training GANs conditioned in a continuous regression value. However, the model has a discriminator in parallel with the regressor, it is not used for visual attribution, and the used loss function is different than the one we propose.

2   Method

2.1   Problem Definition

We want to generate what an image would look like for different levels of a regression target value, without changing the rest of the content of the image. To formalize this mathematically, we can model an image as $x = f(y, z)$, where x is a dependent variable representing an image, y is an independent variable that determines an aspect of x, and z another independent variable representing the rest of the content. In our application, x is an x-ray image, y is the value from a PFT of the same patient taken contemporaneously to the chest x-ray approximating the severity of COPD for that patient, and z represents factors such as patient anatomy unrelated to COPD and position of the body at the moment the x-ray was taken.

We want to construct a model that, given an image x associated with a value y and a content z, can generate an image x' conditioned on the same z, but on a different value y'. By doing this, we can visualize what impacts the change of y to y' has on the image. Similar to [2], we formulate the modified image as

$$x' = \Delta x + x = G(x, y', y) + x, \tag{1}$$

where G is a conditional generator, and Δx is a difference map or a disease effect map. By summing Δx to x, the task of G is made easier, since G only has to model the impact of changing y to y', and the content z should be already in x.

2.2   Loss Function

Figure 1 shows the loss terms that are defined in this section and how the modules are connected for training a VR-GAN. We start by defining a regressor R that

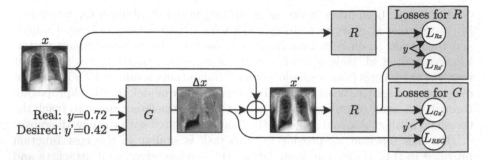

Fig. 1. Overall model architecture for training with the proposed adversarial loss. The losses L_{Rx}, $L_{Rx'}$ and $L_{Gx'}$ are $L1$ regression losses, and L_{REG} is an $L1$ norm penalty.

has the task to, given an image x, predict its y value. We start building our loss function by defining a term, which is used to optimize only the weights of R, to assure R can perform the task of regression over the original dataset:

$$L_{Rx} = L_{Rx}(x, y) = \|R(x) - y\|_{L1}. \tag{2}$$

The regressor is used to assess how close to having y' an image x' is. We also define a term, which is used to optimize only the weights of G, to make G learn to create a map Δx that, when added to the original image, changes the output of R to a certain value y':

$$L_{Gx'} = L_{Gx'}(\Delta x + x, y') = \|R(G(x, y', y) + x) - y'\|_{L1}. \tag{3}$$

Training a model using only these two terms would lead to an R that does not depend on G, and, consequently, to a G that can modify the output of R in simple and unexpressive ways, similar to noisy adversarial examples [5]. We define an adversarial term, which is used to optimize the weights of R, to make R learn to output the same value as the original image for the modified image:

$$L_{Rx'} = L_{Rx'}(\Delta x + x, y) = \|R(G(x, y', y) + x) - y\|_{L1}. \tag{4}$$

As G learns trivial or unrealistic modifications to images, R learns to ignore them due to Eq. (4), forcing the generator to create more meaningful Δx. This game between G and R should reach an equilibrium where G produces images that are realistic and induces the desired output from R. At this point, R should not be able to find modifications to ignore, being unable to output the original y. In our formulation, R replaces a discriminator from a traditional GAN.

We define another loss term to assure that G only generates what is needed to modify the label from y to y' and does not modify regions that would alter z. An $L1$ penalty is used over the difference map to enforce sparsity:

$$L_{REG} = L_{REG}(\Delta x) = \|\Delta x\|_{L1}. \tag{5}$$

Intuitively, when the modifications generated by G are unrealistic and ignored by R, not having any impact to the term defined in Eq. (3), the norm penalty defined in Eq. (5) should enforce their removal from the disease effect map.

The complete optimization problem is defined as

$$G^* = \operatorname*{argmin}_{G}(\lambda_{Gx'}L_{Gx'} + \lambda_{REG}L_{REG}), R^* = \operatorname*{argmin}_{R}(\lambda_{Rx'}L_{Rx'} + \lambda_{Rx}L_{Rx}), \quad (6)$$

where the λ's are hyperparameters. Optimizations are performed alternatingly.

3   Experiments

We used a U-Net [12] as G. The conditioning inputs y and y', together with their difference, were normalized and concatenated to the U-Net bottleneck layer (Fig. 1). For R, we used a Resnet-18 [6], pretrained on ImageNet and with the output changed to a single linear value. We froze the batch normalization parameters in R, as in [2]. Since R depends on the supervision from the original regression task, it will only be able to learn to output values in the range of the original y. Therefore, during training we sampled y' from the same distribution as y. The hyperparameters were chosen as $\lambda_{Gx'} = 0.3$, $\lambda_{REG} = 0.03$, $\lambda_{Rx} = 1.0$, $\lambda_{Rx'} = 0.3$, using validation over the toy dataset presented in Sect. 3.1. The same set of hyperparameters were used for the x-ray dataset and were not sensitive to change of dataset. Adam [9] was used as the optimizer, with a learning rate of 10^{-4}. To prevent overfitting, early stopping was used.

We employed the VA-GAN method presented in [2] as a baseline, since it is a classification version of our method[1]. We used $\lambda = 10^2$ and gradient penalty with a factor of 10, as in [2]. Baseline optimizers and models were the same as the ones described for our model.

We compared the results visually to check if they agreed with radiologists' expectations. For quantitative validation, we used the normalized cross-correlation between the generated Δx map and the expected Δx map, averaged over the test set. Each result is given with its mean and its standard deviation over 5 tests, with training initialized using distinct random seeds.

3.1   Toy Dataset

To test our model, we generated images of squares, superimposed with a Gaussian filtered white noise and with a resolution of 224×224. An example is presented in Fig. 2(a). The side length of the square is proportional to a regression target y that follows a Weibull distribution with a shape parameter of 7 and a scale parameter of 0.75. The class threshold for our baseline model [2] was set at 0.7. It was trained to receive images of big squares ($y \geq 0.7$), and output a difference map that made that square small ($y < 0.7$). We generated 10,000

---

[1] Our implementations of VA-GAN and VR-GAN extends code from github.com/orobix/Visual-Feature-Attribution-Using-Wasserstein-GANs-Pytorch.

images for training. Since we generated the images, we could evaluate with perfect ground truth for Δx. We evaluated using input examples where $y \geq 0.7$ and sampling $y' < 0.7$ from the Weibull distribution. This resulted in 5,325 images for validation and 5,424 images for testing.

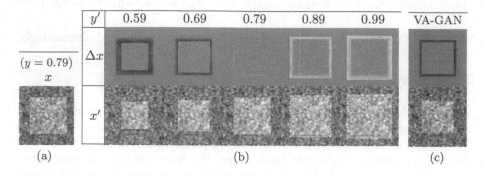

Fig. 2. Results on a test example from the toy dataset. **Top:** difference maps Δx. **Bottom:** images of squares, x or x'. (a) Original image x, with square size $y = 0.79$. (b) VR-GAN result for several desired square side lengths y'. (c) VA-GAN result.

Examples of difference maps and modified versions of the original image for a few levels of the desired square side length are presented in Fig. 2(b). While the baseline presents a fixed modification for an image, shown in Fig. 2(c), and can only generate smaller squares, our method can generate different levels of change for the map, and also generate both bigger and smaller squares. The baseline [2], using VA-GAN, obtained a score of 0.780 ± 0.007 for the normalized cross-correlation, while our method, VR-GAN obtained a score of 0.853 ± 0.014.

3.2 Visualizing the Progression of COPD

We gathered a dataset of patients that had a chest x-ray exam and a PFT within 30 days of each other at the University of Utah Hospital from 2012 to 2017. This study was performed under an approved Institutional Review Board process[2] by our institution. Data was transferred from the hospital PACS system to a HIPAA-compliant protected environment. Orthanc[3] was used for data de-identification by removing protected health information. Lung transplants patients were excluded, and only posterior-anterior (PA) x-rays were used. PFTs were only associated with their closest x-ray exam and vice-versa. For validation and testing, all subjects with at least one case without COPD (used as original image x) and one case with COPD (used as desired modified image x') were selected, using COPD presence as defined by PFTs. This setup was chosen because the trained baseline model can only handle transitions from no disease

---

[2] IRB_00104019, PI: Schroeder MD.

[3] orthanc-server.com.

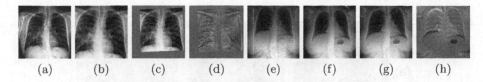

(a)   (b)   (c)   (d)   (e)   (f)   (g)   (h)

Fig. 3. Examples of results of the alignment. **(a)** and **(e)**: Reference images without COPD. **(b)** and **(f)**: Images to align, with COPD. **(c)** and **(g)**: Aligned images. **(d)** and **(h)**: Difference between reference and aligned images, used as Δx ground truth.

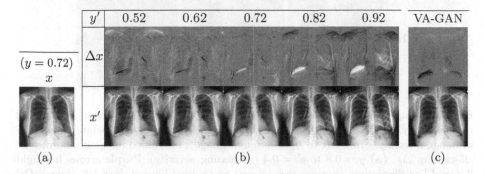

(a)   (b)   (c)

Fig. 4. Results on a test example of the COPD dataset. **Top:** disease effect maps Δx. **Bottom:** chest x-rays, x or x'. **(a)** Original image x, with FEV_1/FVC (y) 0.72. **(b)** VR-GAN results for several desired FEV_1/FVC (y'). The lower this value, the more severe the disease. **(c)** VA-GAN results.

to disease. For each of these subjects, we used all combinations of pair of cases with distinct diagnoses. The average time between paired exams was 17 months. We used 3,414 images for training, 208 pair of images for validation and 587 pair of images for testing. Images were cropped to a centered square, resized to 256×256 and randomly cropped to 224×224. We equalized their histogram and normalized their individual intensity range to $[-1,1]$. We used FEV_1/FVC as the regression target value y. To generate ground truth disease effect maps, we aligned two x-rays of the same patient, using an affine registration employing the pystackreg library[4], and subtracted them. Examples are shown in Fig. 3.

Disease effect maps and modified images for both methods are presented in Fig. 4. Note that our method can modify images to increase and decrease severity by any desired amount in contrast to [2], which can only be trained to modify the classification of images in a single direction. In Fig. 5, we show images generated using VR-GAN which highlight the height and flatness of diaphragm and show changes in the level of lung lucency, features that radiologists use as evidence for COPD on chest x-rays. Small changes in the cardiac contour are consistent with the accommodation of a shift in lung volume. Using normalized cross-correlation, VA-GAN obtained a score of 0.012 ± 0.015, while VR-GAN obtained a score of

---

[4] bitbucket.org/glichtner/pystackreg.

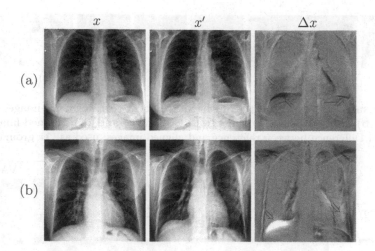

Fig. 5. Examples of disease effects that correspond with visual feature changes expected radiologically. In Δx, gray represents no change, black a decrease and white an increase in image intensity. From left to right: original image x, modified image x' and disease effect map Δx. **(a)** $y = 0.8$ to $y' = 0.4$ (increasing severity). Purple arrows highlight flat and low diaphragm (bottom two arrows) and added lucency (top left arrow). **(b)** $y = 0.37$ to $y' = 0.8$ (decreasing severity). Purple arrows highlight high and curved diaphragm (left arrow) and reduced lucency (right arrow). (Color figure online)

0.127 ± 0.017. The low correlation scores may result from imperfect alignments with affine transformations and potential changes between x-ray pairs unrelated to COPD. However, our method still obtained a significantly better score.

4   Conclusion

We introduced a visual attribution method for datasets with regression target values and validated it for a toy task and for chest x-rays associated with PFTs, assessing the impact of COPD in the images. We demonstrated significant improvement in the disease effect maps generated by a model trained with adversarial regression when compared to a baseline trained using classification labels. Furthermore, the generated disease effect maps highlighted regions that agree with radiologists' expectations and produced realistic images.

References

1. Ancona, M., Ceolini, E., Öztireli, C., Gross, M.: Towards better understanding of gradient-based attribution methods for deep neural networks. In: ICLR (2018)
2. Baumgartner, C.F., Koch, L.M., Tezcan, K.C., Ang, J.X.: Visual feature attribution using Wasserstein GANs. In: CVPR (2018)
3. Bazrafkan, S., Corcoran, P.: Versatile auxiliary regressor with generative adversarial network (VAR+GAN). arXiv preprint arXiv:1805.10864 (2018)

4. Foster, W.L., et al.: The emphysemas: radiologic-pathologic correlations. Radiographics **13**(2), 311–328 (1993)
5. Goodfellow, I., Shlens, J., Szegedy, C.: Explaining and harnessing adversarial examples. In: ICLR (2015)
6. He, K., et al.: Deep residual learning for image recognition. In: CVPR (2016)
7. Isola, P., Zhu, J., Zhou, T., Efros, A.A.: Image-to-image translation with conditional adversarial networks. In: CVPR (2017)
8. Johnson, J.D., Theurer, W.M.: A stepwise approach to the interpretation of pulmonary function tests. Am. Fam. Phys. **89**(5), 359–66 (2014)
9. Kingma, D.P., Ba, J.: Adam: a method for stochastic optimization. In: ICLR (2015)
10. Mirza, M., Osindero, S.: Conditional generative adversarial nets. CoRR abs/1411.1784 (2014)
11. Rajpurkar, P., Irvin, J., et al.: Chexnet: Radiologist-level pneumonia detection on chest x-rays with deep learning. CoRR abs/1711.05225 (2017)
12. Ronneberger, O., Fischer, P., Brox, T.: U-Net: convolutional networks for biomedical image segmentation. In: MICCAI (2015)
13. Seah, J.C.Y., et al.: Chest radiographs in congestive heart failure: visualizing neural network learning. Radiology **290**(2), 514–522 (2019)
14. Tong, L., et al.: Adversarial regression with multiple learners. In: ICML (2018)
15. Zhou, B., Khosla, A., Lapedriza, À., Oliva, A., Torralba, A.: Learning deep features for discriminative localization. In: CVPR (2016)

Medical-based Deep Curriculum Learning for Improved Fracture Classification

Amelia Jiménez-Sánchez[1]([✉])(iD), Diana Mateus[2], Sonja Kirchhoff[3,4],
Chlodwig Kirchhoff[4], Peter Biberthaler[4], Nassir Navab[5],
Miguel A. González Ballester[1,6], and Gemma Piella[1](iD)

[1] BCN MedTech, DTIC, Pompeu Fabra University, Barcelona, Spain
amelia.jimenez@upf.edu
[2] Ecole Centrale de Nantes, LS2N, UMR CNRS 6004, Nantes, France
[3] Institute of Clinical Radiology, LMU München, Munich, Germany
[4] Department of Trauma Surgery, Klinikum rechts der Isar,
Technische Universität München, Munich, Germany
[5] Computer Aided Medical Procedures,
Technische Universität München, Munich, Germany
[6] ICREA, Barcelona, Spain

Abstract. Current deep-learning based methods do not easily integrate to clinical protocols, neither take full advantage of medical knowledge. In this work, we propose and compare several strategies relying on curriculum learning, to support the classification of proximal femur fracture from X-ray images, a challenging problem as reflected by existing intra- and inter-expert disagreement. Our strategies are derived from knowledge such as medical decision trees and inconsistencies in the annotations of multiple experts, which allows us to assign a degree of difficulty to each training sample. We demonstrate that if we start learning "easy" examples and move towards "hard", the model can reach a better performance, even with fewer data. The evaluation is performed on the classification of a clinical dataset of about 1000 X-ray images. Our results show that, compared to class-uniform and random strategies, the proposed medical knowledge-based curriculum, performs up to 15% better in terms of accuracy, achieving the performance of experienced trauma surgeons.

Keywords: Curriculum learning · Multi-label classification · Bone fractures · Computer-aided diagnosis · Medical decision trees

1 Introduction

In a typical educational system, learning relies on a curriculum that introduces new concepts building upon previously acquired ones. The rationale behind, is

Electronic supplementary material The online version of this chapter (https://doi.org/10.1007/978-3-030-32226-7_77) contains supplementary material, which is available to authorized users.

that humans and animals learn better when information is presented in a meaningful way rather than randomly. Bringing these ideas from cognitive science, Elman [1] proposed the *starting small* concept, to train neural networks that learn the grammatical structure of complex sentences. The networks were only able to solve the task when starting with a small sample size, highlighting the importance of systematic and gradual learning. Bengio *et al.* [2] made the formal connection between machine learning and starting small, demonstrating a boost in performance by combining *curriculum learning* (CL) with neural networks on two toy examples: shape recognition and language modeling. In the medical image analysis community, the idea of exploiting CL with deep learning has only recently been explored [3–5]. Even though these techniques have been successful in applications such as image segmentation or computer-aided diagnosis, they remain agnostic of clinical standards and medical protocols.

Our goal is to fill the gap between machine learning algorithms and clinical practice by introducing medical knowledge integrated in a CL strategy. Current applications of CL to medical images focus on gradually increasing context in segmentation, whereas active learning approaches aim for reducing annotation efforts. Our focus is on the integration of knowledge, extracted from medical guidelines, directly from expert recommendations, or from ambiguities in their annotations, to ease the training of convolutional neural networks (CNNs). Similar in spirit, [5] integrates, as part of a more complex method for disease localization, a curriculum derived from clinical reports, extracted by natural language processing.

We restrict our study to the classification of proximal femur fractures according to the AO standard [6]. Some example X-ray images with their corresponding category are depicted in Fig. 1. This kind of fracture represents a notable problem in our society, especially in the elderly population, having a direct socioeconomic repercussion [7]. Early detection and classification of such fractures are essential for guiding appropriate treatment and intervention. However, several years of training are needed, and inter-reader agreement ranges between 66–71% for trauma surgery residents and experienced trauma surgeons, respectively [8]. A similar classification problem was recently addressed in [9], where the focus was on the use of attention methods to improve fracture classification.

We explore the potential of curriculum learning to design three medical-based data schedulers that control the training sequence every epoch. Results on multilabel fracture classification show that by using our curriculum approaches, F_1-score can be improved up to 15%, outperforming two baselines: without curriculum (random) and uniform-class reordering. Our proposed medical data schedulers, on restricted training data, outperform also the baselines having access to the entire training set. Furthermore, we reach a comparable performance to those of experienced trauma surgeons.

2   Related Work

Curriculum learning's main hypothesis is that the order in which samples are presented to an iterative optimizer is important, as it can drastically change

A1   A2   A3   B1   B2   B3   Healthy

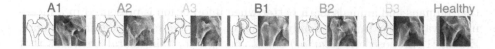

Fig. 1. AO standard and example radiographs.

the outcome (*i.e.* which local-minima is found). Bengio *et al.* [2] showed that a significant improvement in the generalization of the machine learning algorithm could be achieved when samples were presented from "easy" to "hard", where the "hardness" of the samples was determined by some heuristic or a human expert. Similar to Bengio *et al.*, we propose a series of heuristics to infer the hardness level of the training samples, but taking as guiding principles medical knowledge in the form of standards, such as the AO [6], or disagreement between experts.

There is little prior work in CL for medical image analysis. Maicas *et al.* [4] proposed to emulate how radiologists learn based on a set of increasing difficulty tasks. A combination of meta-learning and teacher-student curriculum learning allowed them to improve the selection of the tasks to achieve a boosted detection of malignancy cases in breast screening. For medical image segmentation, [3] also demonstrated that gradually increasing the difficulty of the task benefits the performance. A pseudo-curriculum approach was employed for segmentation of brain tumors and multiple sclerosis lesions in magnetic resonance (MR) images. Training starts from an easy scenario, where learning can be done from multi-modal MR images, and after a few warm-up epochs some of the modalities are randomly dropped.

Novel variants of curriculum learning include self-paced learning, where the curriculum is automated. Such approach has been used to tackle imbalance in the segmentation of lung nodules in computed tomography images [10]. Instead of relying on prior medical knowledge, their approach updates the curriculum with respect to the model parameters' change, letting the learner focus on knowledge near the decision frontier, where examples are neither too easy nor too hard. Self-paced learning and active learning were used in [11] to reduce annotation efforts. Though related, active learning has a different motivation than our work, as it focuses on retrieving examples from an unlabeled pool aiming to achieve a better performance with fewer labeled data. In our study, we restrict to the original concept of CL aiming to ease the learning process and improve the classification performance with the medical-based data schedulers.

3   Methods

We tackle multiclass image classification problems where an image x_i needs to be assigned to a discrete class label $y_i \in \{y_1, y_2, \ldots, y_M\}$. Let us consider the training set $\{\mathcal{X}, \mathcal{Y}\}$ composed of N element pairs, and assume training is performed in mini-batches of size B for a total of E epochs. We address the problem by training a CNN with stochastic gradient descent (SGD) along with CL, favoring

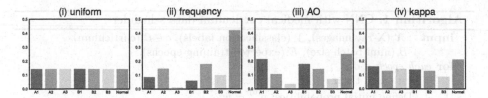

Fig. 2. Initial probabilities $p^{(0)}$ for our medical-based curriculums: **(i)** **uniform**: samples are selected according to a uniform class-distribution. **(ii)** **frequency**: proportional to their original frequency in the dataset. **(iii)** **AO**: probabilities are assigned based on the difficulty of the AO classes. **(iv)** **kappa**: intra-rater Cohen's kappa coefficient to define the probabilities.

easier examples at the beginning of the training while solving the non-convex optimization in the long term. A curriculum $c \in \mathcal{C}$ induces a bias in the order of presenting samples to the optimizer. The bias reflects a notion of "hardness", which in this work depends upon different forms of prior medical knowledge. In practice, any of the curriculums is implemented by assigning a probability to each training pair, such that simpler cases have higher probabilities of being selected first. Over different rounds, the probabilities are updated according to a scheduler to reach a uniform distribution at the end.

Initially, each image $x_i \in \mathcal{X}$ is assigned a curriculum probability $p_i^{(0)}$, here defined according to medical knowledge (see Eq. 3 for practical definitions of $p_i^{(0)}$). At the beginning of every epoch, the training set $\{\mathcal{X}, \mathcal{Y}\}$ is permuted to $\{\mathcal{X}, \mathcal{Y}\}^c$ using a reordering function $f^{(e)}$. This mapping results from sampling the training set according to the probabilities at the current epoch $p^{(e)}$. Mini-batches are then formed from $\{\mathcal{X}, \mathcal{Y}\}^c$ and the probabilities are decayed towards a uniform distribution [2], based on the following function [12]:

$$q_i^{(e)} = p_i^{(e-1)} \cdot \exp(-cn_i^2/10) \quad \forall e > 0, \tag{1}$$

$$p_i^{(e)} = \frac{q_i^{(e)}}{\sum_{i=1}^N q_i^{(e)}}, \tag{2}$$

where cn_i is a counter that is incremented when sample i is selected. The process for training a CNN with our medical curriculum data scheduler is summarized in Algorithm 1.

The proposed CL method is demonstrated on the classification of proximal femur fractures according to the AO system. In this standard, the first level of distinction differentiates fractures of type "A", located in the trochanteric region, from type "B" found in the femoral neck. Further subdivision of classes A and B depends on the specific location of the fracture and its morphology, *i.e.* the number of fragments and their arrangement. We target the fine-grained classification to distinguish 6 types of fracture (A1-A3, B1-B3) plus the non-fracture case, *i.e.* a 7-class problem, as shown in Fig. 1.

Algorithm 1: CNN with medical curriculum data scheduler

---

input : $\mathcal{X}$ (X-ray images), $\mathcal{Y}$ (classification labels), $c \in \mathcal{C}$ (curriculum)
$\phantom{\textbf{input} :\ }$ B (mini-batch size), E (expected training epochs)
for *each epoch e* **do**
$\quad$ **if** *first epoch* **then**
$\quad\quad|$ Define initial probabilities: $p_i^{(0)} = w_m^c$;
$\quad$ **else**
$\quad\quad|$ Update probabilities with Eqs. (1–2);
$\quad$ **end**
$\quad$ Get reordering function $f^{(e)}$ by sampling $\{\mathcal{X}, \mathcal{Y}\}$ according to $p^{(e)}$
$\quad$ Permute training set $f^{(e)} : \{\mathcal{X}, \mathcal{Y}\} \mapsto \{\mathcal{X}, \mathcal{Y}\}^c$;
$\quad$ **for** *each training round* **do**
$\quad\quad|$ Get the **next** mini-batch from $\{\mathcal{X}, \mathcal{Y}\}^c : \{x_b, y_b\}_{b=1}^{B}$;
$\quad\quad|$ Calculate cross-entropy loss $\mathcal{L}(y_b, \hat{y}_b)$;
$\quad\quad|$ Compute gradients and update model weights;
$\quad$ **end**
end

The curriculum probabilities of each of the classes are given by:

$$p^{(0)}(y_i = m) = w_m^c, \tag{3}$$

where $m \in [1, 2, \ldots, M]$ serves as index of the classes, and w_m^c is defined according to $c \in \mathcal{C} = \{\text{uniform}, \text{frequency}, \text{AO}, \text{kappa}\}$:

c : **uniform** (see Fig. 2-(i)): all classes are treated equally, *i.e.*,

$$w_m = 1/M. \tag{4}$$

c : **frequency** (see Fig. 2-(ii)): classes are assigned a probability equal to their original frequency of appearance in the dataset,

$$w_m = \frac{1}{N} \sum_{i=1}^{N} \delta_{y_i, m}, \tag{5}$$

where δ is the indicator function equal to one when $y_i = m$, and 0 otherwise.

c : **AO** (see Fig. 2-(iii)): an experienced radiologist ranked the difficulty of the classes in the following order $v = [\text{A3}, \text{B3}, \text{A2}, \text{B2}, \text{B1}, \text{A1}, \text{non-fracture}]$ from hardest to easiest. As a naive approach, we consider the categories equally spaced and use the rank index k, such that:

$$w_m = \frac{k}{\sum_{m=1}^{M} m}. \tag{6}$$

c : **kappa** (see Fig. 2-(iv)): Cohen's kappa statistic is used to measure the agreement of clinical experts on the classification between two readings. Basically, kappa quantifies the ratio between the observed and chance agreement. Here, each class is assigned a probability proportional to the intra-reader agreement found by a committee of experts.

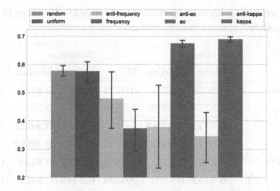

Fig. 3. Mean F_1-score and variance over 10 runs on the 7-way classification of the different curriculum strategies, together with their corresponding anti-curriculum, and compared against random and uniform-curriculum.

4 Experimental Validation

Dataset. Our in-house dataset consists of anonymized X-rays of the hip and pelvis collected at the trauma surgery department of the Rechts der Isar Hospital in Munich. The studies contain lateral view and anterior-posterior images. The latter, which involved both femora, were parted into two, resulting into additional non-fracture examples. The dataset consists of 327 type-A, 453 type-B fractures and 567 non-fracture cases. Subtypes of the fracture classes are highly unbalanced, reflecting the incidence of the different fracture types, as depicted in Fig. 2-(ii). To address this problem, offline data augmentation techniques such as translation, scaling and rotation were used. The dataset was split patient-wise into three parts with the ratio 70% : 10% : 20% to build respectively the training, validation and test sets. We employ a test distribution that is balanced between fracture type-A, type-B and non-fracture. All evaluations below are based on the weighted F_1-score, which takes into account the unbalanced class-distribution using as weights the support of each class.

Clinical experts provided along with the classification (based on the AO standard) a square region of interest (ROI) around the femur. ROIs were downsampled to 224 × 224 px to fit into the proposed architecture.

Implementation Details. We used a ResNet-50 [13] pretrained on the Imagenet dataset. The architecture and curriculums were implemented with TensorFlow[1] and ran on an Nvidia Titan XP GPU. All models were run for 50 epochs with cross-entropy loss, in mini-batches of 64 samples and saved at minimum validation loss. SGD with a momentum of 0.9 was used as optimizer. Early stop was implemented if there was no improvement in the last 20 epochs. 70% dropout was used in the fully-connected layer. Initial learning rate was set to 1×10^{-3} and decayed by 10 every 15 epochs.

---

[1] https://www.tensorflow.org/

Table 1. Classification results over 10 runs. The highlighted indices in bold correspond to the best two models.

F_1-score	7 classes			3 classes		
	Mean	Median	SD	Mean	Median	SD
Random	0.5662	0.5731	0.0423	0.8063	0.8171	0.0337
Uniform	0.5757	0.5923	0.0590	0.8011	0.7971	0.0399
AO	0.6757	**0.6783**	0.0197	0.8651	**0.8657**	0.0172
Kappa	0.6893	**0.6900**	0.0150	0.8623	**0.8657**	0.0146
AO - 60%	0.6325	0.6188	0.0302	0.8457	0.8486	0.0191
Kappa - 60%	0.6352	0.6500	0.0398	0.8446	0.8457	0.0222

4.1   Results

We evaluate our proposed medical curriculum data schedulers in which difficulty is gradually increased ($\mathcal{C}$: easy → hard) by comparing them against two baseline approaches: random permutations and class-uniform reordering. Besides, we discuss their performance with respect to the opposite strategies in which difficulty is decreased, and we refer to as anti-curriculum (anti-$\mathcal{C}$: hard → easy).

Figure 3 presents the results over 10 runs of the 7-class classification problem. Firstly, we find a similar performance between randomly shuffling the training data and learning with a uniform-curriculum, with a mean (median) F_1-score of 0.57 (0.57) and 0.58 (0.59), respectively. Secondly, we found that the sequence of the samples presented in each epoch has a significant effect in the classification, *i.e.* there is a clear difference between curriculum and anti-curriculum strategies. Interestingly, our experiments suggest that, in the case of the frequency-curriculum, the easy scenario is the class-imbalance, which agrees with results reported in [14]. The behaviour could also be related to the high imbalance in the original distribution and the offline augmentation. Finally, our two explicit medical AO- and kappa-curriculums boost the median F_1-score by approximately 15% when compared against the baselines. The differences were found statistically significant (Suppl. Material). Moreover, our proposed schedulers help to reduce variance over the runs.

By aggregating the posterior probability distribution obtained from our model, we can evaluate a 3-class problem, *i.e.* transform the predictions to "A", "B" and "non-fracture". Although, we did not provide any supervision regarding the 3-class problem while training the CNN, we obtain a median F_1-score of 0.87 for AO- and kappa-curriculums, outperforming state-of-the-art results [9], and about 7% better than random and uniform (0.82, 0.80). This means that mispredictions are usually within the same fracture type.

Our dataset size is typical for medical applications. An additional experiment was performed, under a restricted amount of balanced training data (only using 60%), to investigate the performance of our medical-based data schedulers under reduced amounts of annotated data. Our AO- and kappa-curriculums performed even better than the baselines using all data (see Table 1).

Analyzing the training and validation loss curves while learning, we observed that random and uniform-curriculum converged smoothly and fast, whereas our proposed medical-based data schedulers were "noisier" in the first epochs. We hypothesize that the curriculum might lead to a better exploration of the weights during the first epochs.

5   Conclusions

We have shown that the integration of medical knowledge is useful for the design of data schedulers by means of CL. Although we have focused on the AO standard and the multi-class proximal femur fracture problem, our work could be exploited in other applications where medical decision trees are available, such as grading malignancy of tumors, as well as whenever inter-expert agreement is available. As future work, we plan to explore the combination of our medical curriculum data schedulers with uncertainty of the model, and investigate which samples play a more significant role in the decision boundary.

Acknowledgments. This project has received funding from the European Union's Horizon 2020 research and innovation programme under the Marie Skłodowska-Curie grant agreement No. 713673 and by the Spanish Ministry of Economy [MDM-2015-0502]. A. Jiménez-Sánchez has received financial support through the "la Caixa" Foundation (ID Q5850017D), fellowship code: LCF/BQ/IN17/11620013. D. Mateus has received funding from Nantes Métropole and the European Regional Development, Pays de la Loire, under the Connect Talent scheme. Authors thank Nvidia for the donation of a GPU.

References

1. Elman, J.L.: Learning and development in neural networks: the importance of starting small. Cognition 48(1), 71–99 (1993)
2. Bengio, Y., Louradour, J., Collobert, R., Weston, J.: Curriculum learning. In: Proceedings of the 26th Annual International Conference on Machine Learning ICML 2009, pp. 41–48. ACM, New York (2009)
3. Havaei, M., Guizard, N., Chapados, N., Bengio, Y.: HeMIS: hetero-modal image segmentation. In: Ourselin, S., Joskowicz, L., Sabuncu, M.R., Unal, G., Wells, W. (eds.) MICCAI 2016. LNCS, vol. 9901, pp. 469–477. Springer, Cham (2016). https://doi.org/10.1007/978-3-319-46723-8_54
4. Maicas, G., Bradley, A.P., Nascimento, J.C., Reid, I., Carneiro, G.: Training medical image analysis systems like radiologists. In: Frangi, A.F., Schnabel, J.A., Davatzikos, C., Alberola-López, C., Fichtinger, G. (eds.) MICCAI 2018. LNCS, vol. 11070, pp. 546–554. Springer, Cham (2018). https://doi.org/10.1007/978-3-030-00928-1_62
5. Tang, Y., Wang, X., Harrison, A.P., Lu, L., Xiao, J., Summers, R.M.: Attention-guided curriculum learning for weakly supervised classification and localization of thoracic diseases on chest radiographs. In: Shi, Y., Suk, H.-I., Liu, M. (eds.) MLMI

2018. LNCS, vol. 11046, pp. 249–258. Springer, Cham (2018). https://doi.org/10.1007/978-3-030-00919-9_29

6. Kellam, J.F., Meinberg, E.G., Agel, J., Karam, M.D., Roberts, C.S.: Introduction. J. Orthop. Trauma **32**, S1–S10 (2018)

7. Moran, C.G., Wenn, R.T., Sikand, M., Taylor, A.M.: Early mortality after hip fracture: is delay before surgery important? JBJS **87**(3), 483–489 (2005)

8. van Embden, D., Rhemrev, S., Meylaerts, S., Roukema, G.: The comparison of two classifications for trochanteric femur fractures: the AO/ASIF classification and the Jensen classification. Injury **41**(4), 377–381 (2010)

9. Kazi, A., Albarqouni, S., Sanchez, A.J., Kirchhoff, S., Biberthaler, P., Navab, N., Mateus, D.: Automatic classification of proximal femur fractures based on attention models. In: Wang, Q., Shi, Y., Suk, H.-I., Suzuki, K. (eds.) MLMI 2017. LNCS, vol. 10541, pp. 70–78. Springer, Cham (2017). https://doi.org/10.1007/978-3-319-67389-9_9

10. Jesson, A., Guizard, N., Ghalehjegh, S.H., Goblot, D., Soudan, F., Chapados, N.: CASED: curriculum adaptive sampling for extreme data imbalance. In: Descoteaux, M., Maier-Hein, L., Franz, A., Jannin, P., Collins, D.L., Duchesne, S. (eds.) MICCAI 2017. LNCS, vol. 10435, pp. 639–646. Springer, Cham (2017). https://doi.org/10.1007/978-3-319-66179-7_73

11. Wang, W., Lu, Y., Wu, B., Chen, T., Chen, D.Z., Wu, J.: Deep active self-paced learning for accurate pulmonary nodule segmentation. In: Frangi, A.F., Schnabel, J.A., Davatzikos, C., Alberola-López, C., Fichtinger, G. (eds.) MICCAI 2018. LNCS, vol. 11071, pp. 723–731. Springer, Cham (2018). https://doi.org/10.1007/978-3-030-00934-2_80

12. Ren, Z., Dong, D., Li, H., Chen, C.: Self-paced prioritized curriculum learning with coverage penalty in deep reinforcement learning. IEEE Trans. Neural Netw. Learn. Syst. **29**(6), 2216–2226 (2018). https://ieeexplore.ieee.org/document/8278851

13. He, K., Zhang, X., Ren, S., Sun, J.: Deep residual learning for image recognition. In: 2016 IEEE Conference on Computer Vision and Pattern Recognition (CVPR), pp. 770–778 (2016)

14. Wang, Y., Gan, W., Wu, W., Yan, J.: Dynamic curriculum learning for imbalanced data classification. CoRR abs/1901.06783 (2019)

Realistic Breast Mass Generation
Through BIRADS Category

Hakmin Lee[1], Seong Tae Kim[2], Jae-Hyeok Lee[1],
and Yong Man Ro[1(✉)]

[1] Image and Video Systems Lab, School of Electrical Engineering, KAIST,
Daejeon, Republic of Korea
ymro@kaist.ac.kr
[2] Computer Aided Medical Procedures, Technical University of Munich,
Munich, Germany

Abstract. Generating realistic breast masses is a highly important task because the large-size database of annotated breast masses is scarcely available. In this study, a novel realistic breast mass generation framework using the characteristics of the breast mass (i.e. BIRADS category) has been devised. For that purpose, the visual-semantic BIRADS description for characterizing breast masses is embedded into the deep network. The visual-semantic description is encoded together with image features and used to generate the realistic masses according the visual-semantic description. To verify the effectiveness of the proposed method, two public mammogram datasets were used. Qualitative and quantitative experimental results have shown that the realistic breast masses could be generated according to the BIRADS category.

Keywords: Lesion generation · BIRADS description · Generative adversarial network

1 Introduction

Generating realistic breast masses is a highly important task in a data-driven mass analysis such as deep learning approach because the large-size database of annotated breast masses is scarcely available. Collecting large-scale mammograms and the annotation of breast masses on mammograms are time-consuming and expensive tasks. Recently, a few research efforts have been devoted to developing lesion generation methods with generative models [1, 2]. However, these studies also induces additional efforts to annotate the characteristics of generated lesions for real-world applications such as computer-aided diagnosis and educating radiologist residents. If the lesions could be generated with respect to the predefined conditions which doctors are looking for, it would be much easier to use the generated lesions in real-world.

In this study, a new realistic breast mass generation method using breast imaging reporting and data system (BIRADS) description has been devised. The BIRADS is the standardized terminology to record characteristics of breast cancer [3]. By generating the breast masses according to the BIRADS, the data collection problem in the medical domain can be resolved. The main contribution of this paper is summarized as

© Springer Nature Switzerland AG 2019
D. Shen et al. (Eds.): MICCAI 2019, LNCS 11769, pp. 703–711, 2019.
https://doi.org/10.1007/978-3-030-32226-7_78

followings: (1) A new framework for generating realistic breast masses using BIRADS description has been devised. For the purpose of a realistic breast mass generation, BIRADS description is embedded into the deep network. The deep network is learned by the adversarial learning scheme to be able to change the characteristics of breast masses. (2) Comprehensive experiments have been conducted to verify the effectiveness of the proposed generation method in both qualitative and quantitative ways. Experimental results showed that the proposed method could generate various types of realistic breast masses according to the BIRADS description.

2 Realistic Breast Mass Generation According to BIRADS

2.1 Overview of Proposed Breast Mass Generation

Overall deep network framework of the proposed method for synthesizing masses is shown in Fig. 1. As shown in Fig. 1, the proposed method is based upon conditional generative adversarial networks (GAN) [4] mapping from the seed image (real mass) and a target BIRADS description (margin, shape, or malignancy). Our deep network framework consists of three networks: BIRADS description embedding network, mass generator network (G) and discriminator network (D). Details and learning procedure for the overall deep network are described in the following subsections.

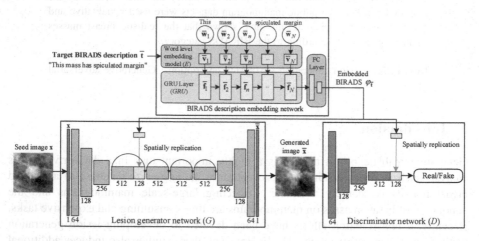

Fig. 1. Overall framework of the proposed method for synthesizing lesions according to BIRADS descriptions

2.2 BIRADS Description Embedding Network

The BIRADS description embedding network is constructed by a gated recurrent unit (GRU) network that encodes the target BIRADS description. The BIRADS description embedded vector is combined with the image features at the same semantic level in the lesion generator network and the discriminator network. The target BIRADS description sentence ($\bar{t}$) is firstly divided into each word level $\bar{t} = \{\bar{w}_1, \ldots, \bar{w}_n, \ldots, \bar{w}_{N_w}\}$ where N_w denotes the number of words in the BIRADS description sentence. Each word is converted into word vectors through a pretrained word level embedding model [5]. To extract the BIRADS description embedded vector, the GRU network-based text encoder [6] is employed. The output of the last step in the GRU network $\bar{f}_N$ is encoded by two fully-connected layers into the same semantic level as the image. Then, the visual-semantic BIRADS description embedded vector $\varphi_{\bar{t}}$ is combined with image features in the lesion generator network and discriminator network (please see Fig. 1).

2.3   Lesion Generator Network with BIRADS Description

To synthesize the mass with respect to the visual-semantic BIRADS description, the proposed lesion generator network is designed based on an encoder-decoder network with residual blocks. The lesion generator network takes an input seed image $\mathbf{x} \in \Re^{M \times M}$ and the BIRADS description embedded vector $\varphi_{\bar{t}}$. More specifically, the encoder is a convolutional neural network (CNN) that encodes seed image into image feature representation. After that, the BIRADS description embedded vector $\varphi_{\bar{t}}$ is spatially replicated to be concatenated with the encoded image features along the channel dimension. The encoded image features combined with BIRADS description embedded vector are fed into several residual blocks. The residual blocks consist of the 3×3 size of convolutions with stride 1. Finally, the decoders consist of several up-sampling layers that convert latent feature representations into the generated image $\bar{x} \in \Re^{M \times M}$. In other words, the generated image is calculated as $\bar{x} = G(\mathbf{x}, \varphi_{\bar{t}})$ where $G(\cdot)$ denotes the lesion generator network in Fig. 1. The residual blocks could help the generator network to learn the identity function, which makes the generated image retains similar breast background of the source image. As a result, the realistic mass is generated on the background of realistic breast tissue by changing the characteristic according to the target BIRADS category.

2.4   Discriminator Network with BIRADS Description

The discriminator network distinguishes generated image and real image with the BIRADS description embedded vector. Like the encoder of the mass generator network, the image is encoded to feature representations. The encoded feature is concatenated with the spatially replicated the BIRADS description embedded vector $\varphi_{\bar{t}}$. The concatenated features are processed by two convolutional layers to calculate final probabilities of being real mass or fake mass. A leaky ReLU activation is performed for all layers except the output layer and batch normalization is applied to all layers except the first and last layer.

2.5   Learning Strategy of Proposed Breast Mass Generation Network

In this session, we explain the learning strategy for the proposed method for generating realistic masses. The loss function for learning the lesion generator network (G) is defined as

$$L_G = E_{\mathbf{x},\hat{\mathbf{t}} \sim p_{data}} log(1 - D(G(\mathbf{x}, \varphi_{\hat{\mathbf{t}}}), \varphi_{\hat{\mathbf{t}}})). \tag{1}$$

The loss functions encourage generated image to fit the distribution of real data p_{data}. To explain the loss function for learning the discriminator network, we define some notations. Let $\mathbf{t}$ and $\hat{\mathbf{t}}$ denote the original BIRADS description of seed image and misaligned BIRADS description, respectively. The misaligned BIRADS description is defined as the description with incorrect ordering. For example, "Spiculated this mass has margin" is one of the mismatching BIRADS descriptions from the original BIRADS description "This mass has spiculated margin". The loss function for learning the discriminator network (D) is defined as

$$L_D = E_{\mathbf{x},\mathbf{t} \sim p_{data}} log(1 - D(\mathbf{x}, \varphi_{\mathbf{t}})) + E_{\mathbf{x},\hat{\mathbf{t}} \sim p_{data}} logD(\mathbf{x}, \varphi_{\hat{\mathbf{t}}}) \\ + E_{\mathbf{x},\hat{\mathbf{t}} \sim p_{data}} logD(G(\mathbf{x}, \varphi_{\hat{\mathbf{t}}}), \varphi_{\hat{\mathbf{t}}}). \tag{2}$$

The overall network is trained to alternatively minimize Eqs. (1) and (2). During alternative training, the lesion generative network (G) and the discriminator network (D) are improved.

3   Experiments and Results

3.1   Dataset

For evaluating the proposed method, we used the publicly available DDSM dataset [7] and INbreast dataset [8]. The mammograms scanned by Howtek 960 were selected from DDSM dataset for the experiments. A total of 1,088 regions of interests (ROIs) were cropped based on the radiologist's annotations. 454 ROIs were malignant masses and 634 ROIs were benign masses. INbreast is a full-filled digital mammographic dataset which contains 115 cases with 410 images. 116 images contain benign or malignant masses. For evaluating the proposed method 20% of the dataset was set aside as test data and the remaining 80% of the dataset was used for training in both datasets. The size of the seed image was resized to 64×64 in both datasets.

In the DDSM dataset, the BIRADS categories of the margin (circumscribed, obscured, microlobulated, ill-defined, and speculated) and the shape (round, oval, lobulated, irregular, and architectural distortion) were used. We formed six descriptions per mass. The BIRADS description was formed by expressing margin alone, shape alone, or both margin and shape together [9]. For example, for a mass with spiculated margin and irregular shape characteristic, six descriptions were formed as follows.

The descriptions for margin alone are "This mass has a spiculated margin" and "A mass with spiculated margin". The descriptions for shape alone are "This mass has an irregular shape" and "A mass with irregular shape". The descriptions for both margin and shape together are, "This mass has a spiculated margin and irregular shape" and "A mass with spiculated margin and irregular shape".

In the INbreast dataset, the BIRADS assessment category was used in this study. In other words, the BIRADS assessment categories of 2 and 3 were defined as benign and the categories of 4, 5, and 6 were defined as malignant. We used a description according to the BIRADS assessment category provided in this database. For example, for BIRADS assessment category provided in this database. For example, for BIRADS assessment category of 5, the example description was "This mass is highly suggestive of malignancy". In addition, we also used additional sentences based on a BIRADS assessment categorization. For example, for category 2 and 3, example description was "This mass is benign".

3.2 Implementation Detail

Each encoder and decoder of the lesion generative network composed of convolution layers with a filter size of 4×4. Except for the first and last layer, the ReLU activation and the batch normalization are applied after all convolutional layers in all encoder and decoder network. After the first convolution layer, give stride 2 to reduce the feature size of each layer. The discriminator network has the same structure as the generator's encoder. The output of the GRU network was a 300-dimensional vector. The output of the GRU network was processed by the two fully-connected layers which have 300 and 128 neurons, respectively.

3.3 Qualitative Results on Generated Lesions

Figure 2 shows the qualitative results on the INbreast dataset. The benign masses were used as seed images and the description for the malignant mass generation was used. As shown in the figure, the spiculated patterns were generated from the benign masses according to the description regarding the malignant while keeping similar breast tissue backgrounds.

To show that the generated masses are realistic, the real masses and the generated masses from DDSM dataset are represented in Fig. 3. As shown in the figure, the generated masses are visually similar to the real masses and it is not distinguishable compared with real masses. As shown in the figure, the proposed method could generate realistic masses according to the target BIRADS. In order to verify the effectiveness of the proposed method, comparative experiments have been conducted on DDSM dataset. Figure 4 shows the comparison of generated images for validating the effectiveness of the proposed BIRADS embedding. For comparison, the one-hot label vector, which was popularly used in GAN [10], was used for conditioning the target BIRADS. As shown in the figure, by using the visual-semantic BIRADS embedding, the proposed generation method could have an ability to understand the relations between visual-semantic BIRADS and the mass images.

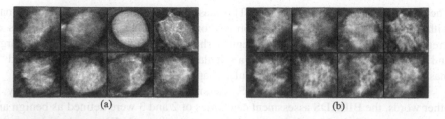

Fig. 2. Qualitative results on the INbreast dataset. (a) Seed images (real benign masses). (b) Malignant masses generated from (a) by "This mass is malignant".

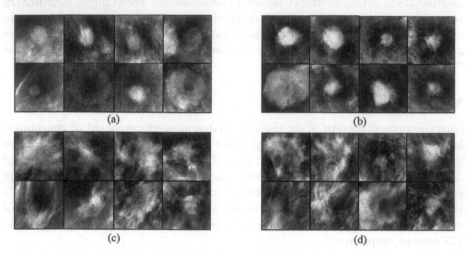

Fig. 3. Comparisons of generated masses and original masses. (a) Real masses with the round shape. (b) Masses generated by the target BIRADS description of "This mass has round shape". (c) Real masses with the irregular shape. (d) Masses generated by the target BIRADS description of "This mass has irregular shape".

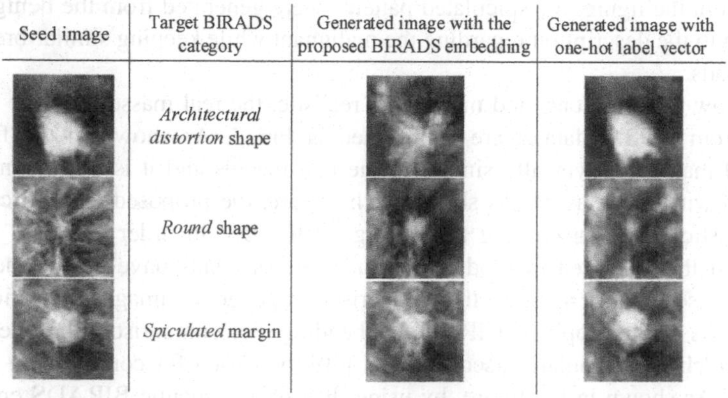

Seed image	Target BIRADS category	Generated image with the proposed BIRADS embedding	Generated image with one-hot label vector
	Architectural distortion shape		
	Round shape		
	Spiculated margin		

Fig. 4. Comparison of generated masses. The first column shows the seed images. The second column shows the target BIRADS category. The third column shows generated images with the proposed BIRADS embedding. The fourth column shows generated images with the one-hot label vector.

3.4   Quantitative Evaluation on Generated Lesions

To quantitatively evaluate the proposed method, we measured the spiculation and the circularity on the DDSM dataset. For evaluating the spiculation of generated masses, a spiculation score [11] was calculated from the generated masses. Table 1 shows the average spiculation scores of masses calculated from the real spiculated masses, the generated spiculated masses, and the real circumscribed masses. The generated speculated masses were obtained from the seed image with circumscribed margin (which is not speculated). As shown in the table, the difference of the average spiculation score between real spiculated masses and the generated spiculated masses were not statistically significant ($p = 0.485$) in Wilcoxon signed-rank tests). Moreover real circumscribed was significantly lower than the speculation score of the generated spiculated masses ($p = 0.013$). In other words, the original masses were changed to have realistic and distinct spiculated margin.

The circularity is a representative feature for characterizing benign masses because the benign masses could be represented with a round or oval shape. The benign masses also have smooth and circumscribed margins [12]. Table 2 shows circularity calculated from the real spiculated masses, the generated circumscribed masses, and the real circumscribed masses. As shown in the result, the circularity of the generated circumscribed masses was similar to the real circumscribed masses (i.e. the difference was not statistically significant). Moreover, the difference of the circularity between the generated circumscribed masses and the real speculated masses was statistically significant. Table 3 also shows the circularity calculated from real irregular masses, the generated round masses, and real round masses. As shown in the result, the circularity of the generated round masses was similar to the real round masses (i.e. the difference was not statistically significant).

Table 1. Spiculation score for the real circumscribed masses, the generated spiculated masses, and the real spiculated masses.

Mass types	Spiculation score (mean ± standard deviation)	Statistical analysis	
		Compared to	p-value
Real spiculated masses	5.912 ± 0.525	Generated spiculated	0.485
Generated spiculated masses	5.849 ± 0.610	Real circumscribed	0.013
Real circumscribed masses	4.772 ± 0.621	–	–

Table 2. Circularity calculated from the real spiculated masses, the generated circumscribed masses, and the real circumscribed masses.

Mass types	Circularity (mean ± standard deviation)	Statistical analysis	
		Compared to	p-value
Real circumscribed masses	0.712 ± 0.257	Generated circumscribed	0.421
Generated circumscribed masses	0.673 ± 0.117	Real spiculated	0.037
Real spiculated masses	0.582 ± 0.128	–	–

710   H. Lee et al.

Table 3. Circularity calculated from real irregular masses, the generated round masses, and real round masses.

Mass types	Circularity (mean ± standard deviation)	Statistical analysis	
		Compared to	p-value
Real round masses	0.842 ± 0.183	Generated round	0.551
Generated round masses	0.813 ± 0.122	Real irregular	0.014
Real irregular masses	0.685 ± 0.129	–	–

4 Conclusions

In this study, the new realistic breast mass generation method using the BIRADS category has been proposed. The proposed method could generate the breast masses according to the BIRADS category. For that purpose, the visual-semantic BIRADS description for characterizing breast masses was embedded and encoded together with image features in the generator. To effectively learn the deep network for generating realistic breast masses, the visual-semantic BIRADS description was also embedded in the discriminator network with adversarial learning scheme. By the comparative experiments, the effectiveness of the proposed generation method was validated. Experimental results showed that the proposed method could generate various realistic breast masses according to the visual-semantic BIRADS description. As a future work, the proposed approach will be investigated in more various applications. By removing additional efforts to annotate the characteristics of masses, it is expected that the proposed method could be used for training the radiologists and computer-aided diagnosis model.

Acknowledgements. This work was supported by Institute for Information & communications Technology Planning & Evaluation (IITP) grant funded by the Korea government (MSIT) (No. 2017-0-01779, A machine learning and statistical inference framework for explainable artificial intelligence).

References

1. Chuquicusma, M.J., et al.: How to fool radiologists with generative adversarial networks? A visual turing test for lung cancer diagnosis. In: IEEE 15th International Symposium on Biomedical Imaging. IEEE (2018)
2. Frid-Adar, M., et al.: Synthetic data augmentation using GAN for improved liver lesion classification. In: IEEE 15th International Symposium on Biomedical Imaging. IEEE (2018)
3. D'Orsi, C.J.: ACR BI-RADS atlas: breast imaging reporting and data system. 2013. American College of Radiology (2013)
4. Goodfellow, I., et al.: Generative adversarial nets. In: Advances in Neural Information Processing Systems (2014)
5. Bojanowski, P., et al.: Enriching word vectors with subword information. Trans. Assoc. Comput. Linguist. **5**, 135–146 (2017)

6. Chung, J., et al.: Empirical evaluation of gated recurrent neural networks on sequence modeling. In: NIPS 2014 Workshop on Deep Learning (2014)
7. Heath, M., et al.: The digital database for screening mammography. In: Proceedings of the 5th International Workshop on Digital Mammography. Medical Physics Publishing (2000)
8. Moreira, I.C., et al.: Inbreast: toward a full-field digital mammographic database. Acad. Radiol. **19**(2), 236–248 (2012)
9. Reed, S., et al.: Learning deep representations of fine-grained visual descriptions. In: Proceedings of the IEEE Conference on Computer Vision and Pattern Recognition (2016)
10. Chen, X., et al.: Infogan: interpretable representation learning by information maximizing generative adversarial nets. In: Advances in Neural Information Processing Systems (2016)
11. Karssemeijer, N., te Brake, G.M.: Detection of stellate distortions in mammograms. IEEE Trans. Med. Imaging **15**(5), 611–619 (1996)
12. Chan, H.P., et al.: Characterization of masses in digital breast tomosynthesis: Comparison of machine learning in projection views and reconstructed slices. Med. Phys. **37**(7Part1), 3576–3586 (2010)

Learning from Longitudinal Mammography Studies

Shaked Perek[✉], Lior Ness, Mika Amit, Ella Barkan, and Guy Amit

IBM Research, Haifa University, Mount Carmel, 31905 Haifa, Israel
{shaked.perek,lior.ness,mika.amit,ella,guyam}@il.ibm.com

Abstract. When reading imaging studies, radiologists often compare the acquired images to one or more prior studies of the patient. Machine learning algorithms that assist in identifying abnormalities in medical images usually do not analyze prior images. This work describes a deep-learning classification framework for mammography studies, which incorporates prior image information using four approaches: (1) late fusion of prediction scores; (2) early fusion of input layers; (3) feature fusion combining a convolutional neural network (CNN) and gradient boosting trees; and (4) feature fusion using CNN and long-short term memory (LSTM) architecture. We demonstrate the advantages and limitations of each approach and compare their performance in identifying biopsy-proven malignancies in mammography screening studies. On an evaluation cohort of 439 patients, adding prior studies to the analysis improved the diagnostic performance of the classification framework. The CNN-LSTM architecture achieved the highest area under the ROC curve of 0.88, with sensitivity and specificity of 0.87 and 0.78, respectively. The methods that were trained using information from prior studies achieved better results than the baseline classifier, with up to 45% reduction in false-positive rate at the same sensitivity. The major advantage of the CNN-LSTM approach is in its flexibility and scalability; it allows to use the same network to classify sequences of multiple priors with variable length. The study demonstrates that longitudinal analysis of images can potentially improve the ability of machine learning algorithms to accurately and reliably interpret imaging studies, thus providing value to the radiology community.

Keywords: Deep learning · Longitudinal analysis · Breast imaging

1 Introduction

Comparing the current imaging study to a previous reference is common practice in diagnostic radiology. In breast mammography, where suspicious findings may be very subtle, it is well-established that comparison to one or more prior studies improves the accuracy of cancer detection [4,13] (Fig. 1). Mammography is a widely-used modality for breast cancer screening, which has contributed to the reduction in mortality rates [10]. However, as the volumes of mammography

© Springer Nature Switzerland AG 2019
D. Shen et al. (Eds.): MICCAI 2019, LNCS 11769, pp. 712–720, 2019.
https://doi.org/10.1007/978-3-030-32226-7_79

studies increase, the shortage of trained breast radiologists promotes the incorporation of automated tools in the diagnostic workflow [1]. AI-based technology has recently shown promising preliminary results in the automated classification of mammograms. Previous methods demonstrated the potential of using inter-image relations within a single study, such as the relations between different viewpoints or between left and right breasts [3,11]. In this work, we explore methods for using images from prior studies to improve the accuracy of the classification algorithm.

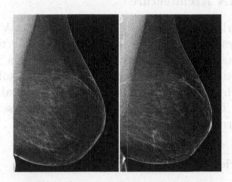

Fig. 1. Example of a pair of a current (right) and prior (left) mediolateral-oblique mammograms of a patient with developing asymmetry in the right breast (red circle), diagnosed by breast biopsy as invasive ductal carcinoma. (Color figure online)

Automatic analysis of longitudinal medical image data was previously attempted by Santeramo et al. [14], who used a Long Short Term Memory (LSTM) network to analyze temporal context from a series of chest x-rays. In the field of mammography, Kooi et al. [6] proposed a Region-of-Interest (ROI) based solution, where aligned patches from different time points are compared to each other. While the latter approach showed a marginal improvement over using a single exam, it relied on explicit lesion detection and therefore required locally-annotated data. Our proposed solutions use only global (per-image) annotations, which are more readily available, as they can be extracted from radiology reports.

In this paper, our contribution consists of comparing four methods for longitudinal analysis of mammograms studies using deep learning. These include: (1) late fusion of prediction scores (2) early fusion of input layers (3) feature fusion combining a CNN and gradient boosting trees; and (4) feature fusion using LSTM cells. We use a large mammography dataset consisting of several providers and manufacturers. We evaluate our methods as part of an image classification system that separates studies with malignant findings from those with benign or no findings. Our system learns using image-level labels, and does not require lesion-specific annotation. We report the performance of each method, and discuss the advantages and limitations of each method, alongside its applicability to other use cases of longitudinal image analysis.

2   Methods

We use a convolutional neural network (CNN) for feature extraction and base-line prediction of a severity score per image, to quantify the level of suspicious abnormality. We also process matched pairs of images, of the same breast side and viewpoint, from the current and prior studies and evaluate four different data fusion approaches.

2.1   Baseline CNN Architecture

The baseline network is a customized Inception-ResNet-V2 architecture [16], whose input is a grayscale image resized to 2048×1024. The network is composed of 14 Inception-Resnet blocks that are concatenated to a global max pooling (GMP) layer followed by two fully connected layers and a softmax layer (Fig. 2). The features of each image are extracted after the global max pooling layer (Fig. 2 green layer). The output of the softmax layer is a severity score S. This network will be referred to as GMP from hereon.

2.2   Fusion of Prior Studies

Late Fusion of Prediction Scores. We used the GMP network to predict severity scores S^c and S^p for the current and prior image, respectively (Fig. 2a). A final score for a pair of images is calculated by $S_{LF} = average(S^c, S^p)$.

Early Fusion of Input Images. We modified the input layer of the GMP to take an input tensor of size $2048 \times 1024 \times 2$, where the current and prior images were two concatenated channels. As a preprocessing step, we aligned the two images by finding an affine transformation between the binary masks of the breasts. The dimensions of the filters in the first convolutional layer were adjusted accordingly, while the rest of network's architecture remained intact. In cases without a matching prior study, or in cases where the image registration was poor, we duplicated the current image as the second channel. We denote the early fusion score output score by S_{EF}.

Feature Fusion by Gradient Boosting Trees. We concatenated the extracted feature vectors F^c and F^p of the current and prior images into a 1×786 vector, and trained a gradient boosting decision tree model to predict a severity score S_{GB} (Fig. 3a). In cases where a prior study is missing, we used zero-padding to achieve the desired vector size. Gradient boosting is an ensemble technique, which trains multiple tree models in a gradual, additive and sequential manner. We used the Extreme Gradient Boosting (XGBoost) implementation [2].

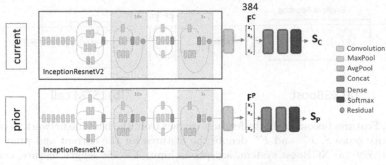

(a) Late fusion of current and prior images

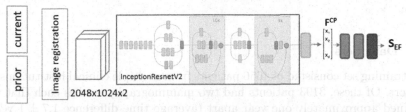

(b) Early fusion of current and prior images

Fig. 2. Network architectures. (a) The baseline network (GMP) composed of Inception-ResNet blocks and a global max pooling layer (green), which outputs a feature vector F^x. This feature is used for feature fusion and for predicting a severity score S. (b) The same architecture with a two-channel input, obtained from registration and concatenation of the current and prior images (Color figure online)

Feature Fusion by LSTM. A Long Short-Term Memory (LSTM) [5] cell has the ability to learn and remember past information using its three gates: input, output, and forget. This network has the advantage of accepting a variable length input, which enables us to test the potential benefit of using multiple priors of the same patient. We used three LSTM cells, with hidden units $[256, 128, 64]$ followed by a fully connected layer to return the final score S_{LSTM} (Fig. 3b) for a pair of current and prior image features.

2.3   Patient Classification

A patient typically has four images per mammography study, with two projections for each breast. For a patient with N consecutive studies, we denote the fused scores of the temporal image sequence by $\{S_N^{RCC}, S_N^{RMLO}, S_N^{LCC}, S_N^{LMLO}\}$. We calculated a severity score per patient by:

$$S = max(average(S_N^{RCC}, S_N^{RMLO}), average(S_N^{LCC}, S_N^{LMLO})) \qquad (1)$$

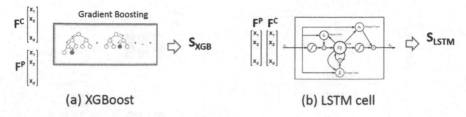

(a) XGBoost   (b) LSTM cell

Fig. 3. Features fusion, using the features extract from the baseline network to calculate a severity score S. F^C and F^P denote the features for the current and prior images, respectively. (a) XGBoost system, accepts as input 1×786 length feature, consisting of the two concatenated features. (b) an LSTM cell. In this work we used three LSTM cells, with hidden units $[256, 128, 64]$ and input features from the current and prior image.

2.4 Data Sets

The training set consisted of 4656 patients from multiple clinical institutions and vendors. Of these, 3193 patients had two mammography studies each that were obtained approximately one year apart (average time difference 1.7 ± 1 years). The remaining 1463 patients, which had a single study, were added in order to enrich the set with more biopsy-proven cases. The evaluation set contained 439 unseen patients from a different clinical institution. The ground truth labels were determined for each patient based on the BI-RADS category [15] of the latest study and the follow-up outcome. Patients were labeled as 'Normal' if they had a low screening BI-RADS (1 or 2) for at least two years after the last examination, and were not referred for breast biopsy. Patients with high screening BI-RADS (0, 4 or 5) that underwent breast biopsy within a year, were labeled 'Malignant' or 'Benign', based on the pathology report of the biopsied breasts. By this ground-truth definition, the prior studies of all patients were labeled 'Normal'. The distribution of ground truth categories in the training and evaluation cohorts are given in Table 1.

Table 1. Number of patients from each class in the training and testing dataset

	Patients	Normal	Benign	Malignant
Training set 1 (with priors)	3193	2265	795	133
Training set 2 (without priors)	1463	305	601	557
Evaluation set	439	337	55	47

2.5 Experiments

We trained the baseline CNN classifier using images of a single study per patient, without prior studies. The various fusion models were trained using pairs of images from matching current and prior studies. The ground-truth label of the pair was determined by the label of the current study. We trained the CNN models on an IBM PowerAI machine with Nvidia Tesla-V100-16G GPU, and used an Adam optimizer with a learning rate of 10^{-4}. The duration of a typical training epoch was approximately one hour. The diagnostic performance of each method was measured using the area under the receiver operating characteristics curve (AUROC), and the specificity achieved at a human-level sensitivity of 0.87 [8]. Confidence intervals of 95% were estimated by bootstrapping with 10000 repetitions. The statistical significance of the differences between each classifier and the baseline was estimated using McNemar's 2-tailed test [9].

3   Results

The baseline classifier, which did not use prior studies, achieved AUROC of 0.82 on the evaluation set, with a specificity of 0.60 at sensitivity 0.87. Classification of the prior studies alone, using the patient's ground-truth labels, was not discriminative, with low AUROC of 0.61. Incorporating the prediction scores of the prior studies by late fusion approach did not improve the accuracy, and showed a slight decrease compared to the baseline (Table 2). Early fusion of the prior and current images as two input channels increased the AUROC to 0.84 and the specificity to 0.64, without statistical significance ($P = 0.08$ compared to baseline). The improvement obtained by gradient boosting fusion was more significant (AUROC 0.86, specificity 0.77, $P < 1e-6$). The LSTM network further improved the performance, with AUROC of 0.88 and 0.78 specificity at sensitivity 0.87. The ROC curves of the five classifiers are given in Fig. 4.

Table 2. Results for all models, AUROC and specificity at sensitivity of 0.87, with 95% confidence interval (CI) displayed in brackets

	AUROC [CI]	SPC@SEN 0.87 [CI]
Baseline	0.82 [0.755–0.874]	0.60 [0.382–0.768]
Baseline Late Fusion	0.80 [0.732–0.855]	0.56 [0.413–0.717]
2 Channels Early Fusion	0.84 [0.789–0.889]	0.64 [0.563–0.814]
XGBoost	0.86 [0.805–0.917]	0.77* [0.519–0.853]
LSTM	0.88 [0.825–0.93]	0.78* [0.552–0.912]

*$P < 1e-6$ compared to baseline

4   Discussion

Deep learning algorithms have been reported to achieve high performance in mammogram classification tasks [6,7,12,17]. Nevertheless, the current algorithms are still inferior to the average human radiologist on real-world data.

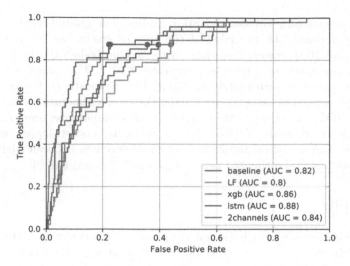

Fig. 4. ROC curve of each model; Blue is the baseline network evaluated on current images, Orange is the late fusion (LF) between current and prior images; Green is gradient boost (xgb), red is LSTM and purple is the two channel inputs. The markers on each curve indicate the operation point of sensitivity 0.87 (Color figure online)

One explanation for this remaining gap is that radiologists incorporate additional information into their case analysis process, such as non-image clinical features and comparisons to prior studies. We addressed the latter by allowing our algorithms to analyze both current and prior studies. Most publications in this field have not used prior images, hence an exact performance comparison is not feasible. The reported AUROC values for cancer classification range from 0.79 to 0.95 on various datasets. Our AUROC with and without priors were 0.82 and 0.88, respectively, which unlike related work [6] reflects a significant benefit from using prior studies. The benefit is also clear from the reduction of the false-positive rate by 45% from 0.40 to 0.22 (at sensitivity 0.87). An advantage of our approach is that it only requires a global label per breast, rather than costly local delineation of the lesions. Our results suggest that separate classification of the prior and current images is insufficient; an improvement was achieved only when the classification algorithms were trained on fused information from both images. The training architecture that provided the highest performance was LSTM, trained on CNN-extracted features. The LSTM-based solution is also scalable for analyzing a sequence of multiple priors, which was not part of the current work. The early fusion approach was inferior to gradient boosting and LSTM, as the capacity of the network to learn from the combined pair of images is limited to the first convolution layer. This approach is also limited by the computational cost of the preprocessing step, which requires image registration. Although the size of the evaluation set used in this work was relatively small, it consists of unseen studies obtained from a different institution than those providing the training data. The small number of positive studies leads to wider confidence intervals, as shown in Table 2. We intend to validate our preliminary observations on a much larger evaluation set. An additional future enhancement to this work is to simultaneously train the CNN and LSTM components, to allow joint optimization of the entire classification architecture. Furthermore, by incorporating a region-detection algorithm, we can compare the current and prior suspicious regions locally, rather than using implicit whole-image comparison, which may be less robust. In addition, clinical data can be incorporated into the pipeline to improve classification. Finally, we can also evaluate the effect of using multiple prior studies in the training set. In conclusion, incorporating prior mammography studies in a deep learning analysis framework can improve the classification performance, as well as strengthen the confidence of the radiologists in the reliability of decision support technology.

References

1. Austin, C., Rijken, T., et al.: The role of deep learning in breast screening. Curr. Breast Cancer Rep. **11**, 17–22 (2019)
2. Chen, T., Guestrin, C.: XGBoost: a scalable tree boosting system. J. Assoc. Phys. India **42**(8), 785–794 (2016)
3. Geras, K.J., Wolfson, S., et al.: High-resolution breast cancer screening with multi-view deep convolutional neural networks, pp. 1–9 (2017)
4. Hayward, J.H., Ray, K.M., et al.: Improving screening mammography outcomes through comparison with multiple prior mammograms. AJR Am. J. Roentgenol. **207**(4), 918–924 (2016)
5. Hochreiter, S., Urgen Schmidhuber, J.: LTSM. Neural Comput. **9**(8), 1735–1780 (1997)
6. Kooi, T., Karssemeijer, N.: Classifying symmetrical differences and temporal change in mammography using deep neural networks, pp. 1–18 (2017)
7. Kyono, T., Gilbert, F.J., van der Schaar, M.: MAMMO: a deep learning solution for facilitating radiologist-machine collaboration in breast cancer diagnosis (2018)
8. Lehman, C.D., Arao, R.F., et al.: National performance benchmarks for modern screening digital mammography: update from the breast cancer surveillance consortium. Radiology **283**(1), 49–58 (2017)
9. McNemar, Q.: Note on the sampling error of the difference between correlated proportions or percentages. Psychometrika **12**(2), 153–157 (1947)
10. Myers, E.R., Moorman, P., et al.: Benefits and harms of breast cancer screening. JAMA **314**(15), 1615 (2015)
11. Perek, S., Hazan, A., Barkan, E., Akselrod-Ballin, A.: Siamese network for dual-view mammography mass matching. In: Stoyanov, D., et al. (eds.) RAMBO/BIA/TIA -2018. LNCS, vol. 11040, pp. 55–63. Springer, Cham (2018). https://doi.org/10.1007/978-3-030-00946-5_6
12. Ribli, D., Horváth, A., et al.: Detecting and classifying lesions in mammograms with Deep Learning. Sci. Rep. **8**(1), 4165 (2018)
13. Roelofs, A.A.J., Karssemeijer, N., et al.: Importance of comparison of current and prior mammograms in breast cancer screening. Radiology **242**(1), 70–77 (2007)
14. Santeramo, R., Withey, S., Montana, G.: Longitudinal detection of radiological abnormalities with time-modulated LSTM. In: Stoyanov, D., et al. (eds.) DLMIA/ML-CDS -2018. LNCS, vol. 11045, pp. 326–333. Springer, Cham (2018). https://doi.org/10.1007/978-3-030-00889-5_37

720   S. Perek et al.

15. Sickles, E.A., d'Orsi, C.J., Bassett, L.W., et al.: ACR BI-RADS® mammography. In: ACR BI-RADS® Atlas, Breast Imaging Reporting and Data System. American College of Radiology, Reston (2013)
16. Szegedy, C., Ioffe, S., et al.: Inception-v4, Inception-ResNet and the impact of residual connections on learning (2016)
17. Wu, N., Phang, J., et al.: Deep neural networks improve radiologists' performance in breast cancer screening (2019)

Automatic Radiology Report Generation Based on Multi-view Image Fusion and Medical Concept Enrichment

Jianbo Yuan[1(✉)], Haofu Liao[1], Rui Luo[2], and Jiebo Luo[1]

[1] Department of Computer Science, University of Rochester, Rochester, USA
{jyuan10,hliao6,jluo}@cs.rochester.edu
[2] Futurewei Technologies, Inc., Bellevue, WA 98004, USA
rui.luo@futurewei.com

Abstract. Generating radiology reports is time-consuming and requires extensive expertise in practice. Therefore, reliable automatic radiology report generation is highly desired to alleviate the workload. Although deep learning techniques have been successfully applied to image classification and image captioning tasks, radiology report generation remains challenging in regards to understanding and linking complicated medical visual contents with accurate natural language descriptions. In addition, the data scales of open-access datasets that contain paired medical images and reports remain very limited. To cope with these practical challenges, we propose a generative encoder-decoder model and focus on chest x-ray images and reports with the following improvements. First, we pretrain the encoder with a large number of chest x-ray images to accurately recognize 14 common radiographic observations, while taking advantage of the multi-view images by enforcing the cross-view consistency. Second, we synthesize multi-view visual features based on a sentence-level attention mechanism in a late fusion fashion. In addition, in order to enrich the decoder with descriptive semantics and enforce the correctness of the deterministic medical-related contents such as mentions of organs or diagnoses, we extract medical concepts based on the radiology reports in the training data and fine-tune the encoder to extract the most frequent medical concepts from the x-ray images. Such concepts are fused with each decoding step by a word-level attention model. The experimental results conducted on the Indiana University Chest X-Ray dataset demonstrate that the proposed model achieves the state-of-the-art performance compared with other baseline approaches.

1 Introduction

Medical images are widely used in clinical decision-making. For example, chest x-ray images are used for diagnosing pneumonia and pleural effusion. The interpretation of medical images requires extensive expertise and is prone to human errors. Considering the demands of accurately interpreting medical images in

© Springer Nature Switzerland AG 2019
D. Shen et al. (Eds.): MICCAI 2019, LNCS 11769, pp. 721–729, 2019.
https://doi.org/10.1007/978-3-030-32226-7_80

large amounts within short times, an automatic medical imaging report generation model can be helpful to alleviate the labor intensity involved in the task. In this work, we aim to propose a novel medical imaging report generation model focusing on radiology. To be more specific, the inputs of the proposed framework are chest x-ray images under different views (frontal and lateral) based on which radiology reports are generated accordingly. Radiology reports contain information summarized by radiologists and are important for further diagnosis and follow-up recommendations.

The problem setting is similar to image captioning, where the objective is to generate descriptions for natural images. Most existing studies apply similar structures including an encoder based on convolutional neural networks (CNN), and a decoder based on recurrent neural networks (RNN) [11] which captures the temporal information and is widely used in natural language processing (NLP). Attention models have been applied in captioning to connect the visual contents and semantics selectively [13]. More recently, studies on radiology report generation have shown promising results. To handle paragraph-level generation, a hierarchical LSTM decoder has been applied to generate medical imaging reports [6] incorporating with visual and tag attentions. Xue *et al.* build an iterative decoder with visual attentions to enforce the coherence between sentences [14]. Li *et al.* propose a retrieval model based on extracted disease graphs for medical report generation [7]. Medical report generation is different from image captioning in that: (1) data in medical and clinical domains is often limited in scales and thus it is difficult to obtain robust models for reasoning; (2) medical reports are paragraphs other than sentences as in image captioning, where conventional RNN decoders such as long short-term memory (LSTM) have issues of gradient vanishing; and (3) generating medical reports requires higher precision when used in practice, especially on medical-related contents, such as disease diagnosis.

We choose the widely used Indiana University Chest X-ray radiology report dataset (IU-RR) [1] for this task. In most cases, radiology reports contain descriptive findings in the form of paragraphs, and conclusive impressions in one or a few sentences. To address the challenges mentioned above, we aim to improve both the encoder and decoder in the following aspects:

First, we construct a multi-task scheme consisting of chest x-ray image classification and report generation. This strategy has been shown to be successful because the encoder is enforced to learn radiology-related features for decoding [6]. Since the data scale of IU-RR is small, encoder pretraining is important in order to obtain a robust performance. Different from previous studies using ImageNet which is collected for general-purposed object recognition, we pretrain with large scale chest x-ray images from the same domain, namely CheXpert [5], to better capture domain specific image features for decoding. Second, most of previous studies using chest x-ray images for disease classification and report generation consider the frontal and lateral images from *the same* patient as *two* independent cases [6,12]. We argue that lateral images contain complementary information to frontal images in the process of interpreting medical images. Such multi-view features should be synthesized selectively other than contributing

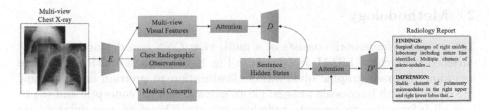

Fig. 1. Overall framework of the proposed encoder and decoder with attentions. E, D, and D' denote the encoder, sentence decoder, and word decoder, respectively.

equally (concatenate, mean or sum) to the final results. Moreover, it is likely to generate inconsistent results for the same patient based on images from different views. We propose to synthesize multi-view information by applying a sentence-level attention model, and enforce the encoder to extract consistent features with a cross-view consistency (CVC) loss.

From the decoder side, we use hierarchical LSTM (sentence and word level LSTM) to generate radiology reports. RNN decoders tend to memorize word distributions and patterns which frequently occur in the training data, and thus might produce inaccurate results when the target contents have not been observed, or when multiple patterns share similar distributions given the previous contents. Such limitations significantly hinders the credibility of machine-generated results in practical use, since incorrect medical-related contents can be very misleading. For example, generating "left-sided pleural effusion" while the ground truth is "right-sided pleural effusion". In addition, the source visual contents stay too far from the targeted word decoder in hierarchical LSTM which makes the generation process more difficult. To address such issues, we explore the semantics conveyed in the textual contents and apply them directly to the word decoder. We first extract frequent medical concepts based on the radiology reports and fine-tune the encoder to recognize such concepts. The obtained medical concepts contain explicit information to accurately generate deterministic medical-related contents, such as diagnosis, locations, and observations.

The main contributions of our work are summarized as follows: (1) to the best of our knowledge, we are the first to employ the latest CheXpert dataset to obtain a more robust encoder for radiology report generation; (2) we selectively incorporate multi-view visual contents with sentence-level attentions and enforce the consistency between different views; (3) we extract and apply medical concepts to the decoder with word-level attentions to enhance the correctness of the medical-related contents; (4) our integrated framework outperforms the state-of-the-art baselines in the experiments, and (5) we visualize uncertain radiographic observations predicted by the encoder to provide an added benefit to direct more expert attention to such uncertainties for further analysis in practice.

2   Methodology

The proposed framework consists of a multi-view CNN encoder and a concept enriched hierarchical LSTM decoder as in Fig. 1. We apply a multi-task scheme including: (1) radiographic observation classification to pretrain and fine-tune the encoder with large-scale images; (2) to extract medical concepts; and (3) to fuse all information to generate radiology reports. Therefore, two datasets are used in this work: CheXpert [5], a large collection of chest x-ray images under 14 common chest radiographic observations to pretrain the image encoder, and Indiana University Chest X-ray [1] containing full radiology reports but in a considerably smaller scale for training and evaluating the report generation task.

2.1   Image Encoder

The encoder uses Resnet-152 [4] as the backbone and extracts visual features for predicting chest radiologic observations and radiology report generation.

Chest Radiographic Observations: The task is formulated as a multi-label classification with 14 common radiographic observations following [5] including: *enlarged cardiom, cardiomegaly, lung opacity, lung lesion, edema, consolidation, pneumonia, atelectasis, pneumothorax, pleural effusion, pleural other, fracture, support devices,* and *no finding.* Compared with previous studies using pretrained encoders based on ImageNet [6,14], pretraining with images from the same domain yields better results. We add one full-connected layer as classifier and compute the binary cross entropy (BCE) loss. Additionally, we consider both frontal and lateral images of one patient as one input pair and enforce the prediction consistencies under different views by a mean square error (MSE) loss over the multi-view encoder outputs. The loss function is thus defined in Eq. 1 where $y_{i,j}$ is the j-th ground truth entry ($j \in [1,14]$)) of the i-th sample ($i \in (1,N)$), the frontal view and lateral view prediction are denoted as $\hat{y}_{i_f}$ and $\hat{y}_{i_l}$. The encoder outputs global features after average-pooling, and local features $\mathbf{v} \in \mathbb{R}^{k \times d_v}$ from the last CNN block where k denotes the number of local regions and d_v denotes the dimension.

$$\mathcal{L}_I = - \sum_{v \in \{f,l\}} \sum_{i,j} \left[y_{i,j} \log \hat{y}^v_{i,j} + (1 - y_{i,j}) \log \left(1 - \hat{y}^v_{i,j} \right) \right] + \lambda \sum_i \left(y_{i_f} - y_{i_l} \right)^2 \quad (1)$$

Medical Concepts: The textual reports contain descriptive information related to the visual contents which have not yet been explored by existing models. In IU-RR, Medical text indexer (MTI) can be potentially used in a similar manner [6]. However, MTIs are sometimes noisy and not normalized. Therefore, we use Semrep[1] to extract *normalized* medical concepts that frequently occur in the training reports. We empirically set the minimal occurrences as 80 and obtained 69 medical concepts for a decent detection accuracy. We fix the pretrained image encoder, and add another fully connected layer on top as the concept classifier.

---

[1] https://semrep.nlm.nih.gov/.

2.2 Hierarchical Decoder

Since conventional RNN decoder is not suitable for paragraph generation, we apply a hierarchical decoder, which has been widely used in paragraph encoding and decoding, to generate radiology reports. The decoder contains two layers: a sentence LSTM decoder that outputs sentence hidden states, and a word LSTM decoder which decodes the sentence hidden states into natural languages. In this way, reports are generated sentence-by-sentence.

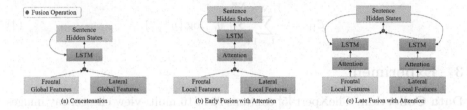

Fig. 2. Different fusion schemes for multi-view image features.

Sentence Decoder with Attentions: The sentence decoder is fed with visual features extracted from the encoder, and generates sentence hidden states. Since we have both frontal and lateral features, the selection of fusion schemes is important. As show in Fig. 2, we propose and compare three fusion schemes: an intuitive solution is to directly concatenate the features from both views; early fusion where the concatenated features are selectively attended by the previous hidden state; and late fusion which fuses the hidden states by two decoders after visual-sentence attentions. To generate sentence hidden state $\mathbf{h}_{t_s}$ at time step $t_s \in (1, N^s)$, we compute the visual attention weights α_i with Eq. 2, where v_m is the m-th local feature, and $\mathbf{W}_a$, $\mathbf{W}_v$ and $\mathbf{W}_s$ are weight matrices.

$$\mathbf{a}_i = \mathbf{W}_a \left[\tanh\left(\mathbf{W}_v \mathbf{v_i} + \mathbf{W}_s \mathbf{h}_{t_s-1}\right)\right], \quad \alpha_i = softmax(\mathbf{a}_i) \tag{2}$$

By leveraging all the local regions, the attended local feature is thus calculated as $v_{att} = \sum_{m=1}^{k} \alpha_{i,m} v_m$, and is concatenated with the previous hidden state to be fed into the sentence LSTM for computing the current hidden state $\mathbf{h}_{t_s}$.

Word Decoder with Attentions: Incorporated with the obtained medical concepts, the sentence hidden states are used as inputs to the word LSTM decoder. For each word decoding step, the previous word hidden state $\hat{\mathbf{h}}_{t_w}$ for time step $t_w \in (1, N_{t_s}^w)$ is used to generate the word distribution over the vocabulary and output the word with the highest score. The embedding $\mathbf{w}_{t_w}$ of the predicted word $\hat{w}_{t_w}$ is then fused with medical concepts in order to generate the next word hidden state. Given the medical concept embeddings $\mathbf{c} \in \mathbb{R}^{n \times d_c}$ for p medical concepts for the i-th sample, and the predicted concept distributions

$\hat{y}_i^c$, the attention weights over all medical concepts at time step t_w is defined in Eq. 3 where $\mathbf{W}_{a^c}$, $\mathbf{W}_c$, and $\mathbf{W}_w$ are the weight matrices to be learned.

$$\mathbf{a}_i^c = \mathbf{W}_{a^c}\left[\tanh\left(\hat{y}_i^c\mathbf{W}_c\mathbf{c} + \mathbf{W}_w\hat{\mathbf{h}}_{t_w-1}\right)\right], \quad \alpha_i^c = softmax(\mathbf{a}_i^c) \qquad (3)$$

Similar to visual attention model, the attended medical concept feature is calculated as $c_{att} = \sum_{n=1}^{p}\alpha_{j,n}^c c_n$, and is concatenated with the previous word embedding to generate the next word. We use cross entropy loss $\mathcal{L}_W$ given the predicted word distribution $\hat{y}^w{}_{t_w}$ and the ground truth $y_{t_w}^w$ using Eq. 4.

$$\mathcal{L}_W = -\sum_{t_s=1}^{N^s}\sum_{t_w=1}^{N_{t_s}^w} y_{t_w}^w \log\left(\hat{y}^w{}_{t_w}\right) \qquad (4)$$

3 Experiment

Data Collection: CheXpert [5] contains 224,316 multi-view chest x-ray images from 65,240 patients of 14 common radiographic observations. The observations are generated using NLP tools from the radiology reports labeled as positive, negative, and uncertain. We inherited and visualized the uncertain predictions to address more expert attention for practical use. An alternative dataset is ChestX-ray14 [12]. We chose to use CheXpert because its labeler is reported to be more reliable as compared with ChestX-ray14 [5].

Since neither of the aforementioned datasets released radiology reports, we use IU-RR [1] for evaluating radiology report generation. For preprocessing, we first removed samples without multi-view images, and concatenated the "findings" and "impression" sections because in some forms all contents are either in the "findings" or "impression" section with the other left blank. We filtered out the reports with less than 3 sentences. In the end, we obtained 3,074 samples with multi-view images of which 20% (615 samples/1,330 images) are used for testing, and the 80% (2459 samples/4,918 images) are used for training and validation. For encoder fine-tuning, we extract the same 14 labels as [5] on IU-RR. For report parsing, we converted the texts to tokens, and added "⟨start⟩" and "⟨end⟩" to the beginning and end of each sentence, respectively. Low frequency (less than 3 occurrences) words were dropped, and textual errors were replaced with "⟨unk⟩" which are caused by being falsely recognized as confidential information during the original data de-identification of IU-RR.

Table 1. Average ROC-AUC (avg-AUC) on radiographic observation classification.

Metrics	Base	ImgNet	CX	CX+CVC	CX+CVC+F
avg-AUC	0.727	0.731	0.747	0.751	**0.764**

Chest Radiographic Observations: We conducted extensive experiments on the encoder regarding two factors: how to properly pretrain and fine-tune the encoder, and how to leverage the multi-view information. The classification results on radiographic observations are shown in Table 1. In general, pretraining with ImageNet (ImgNet) performs marginally better than models without pretraining (Base), and encoders pretrained by CheXpert (CX) performs the best, indicating that pretraining with large scale data in the same domain helps. Enforcing cross-view consistency (CX+CVC) also improves the results. We obtained the best result by fusing multi-view predictions with max operation (CX+CVC+F).

Table 2. Evaluations of generated radiology reports.

Methods	BLEU-1	BLEU-2	BLEU-3	BLEU-4	METEOR	ROUGE
Vis-Att [13]	0.399	0.251	0.168	0.118	0.167	0.323
MM-Att [14]	0.464	0.358	0.270	0.195	0.274	0.366
KERP [7]	0.482	0.325	0.226	0.162	–	0.339
Co-Att [6]	0.517	**0.386**	0.306	0.247	0.217	0.447
(Ours) MvH	0.478	0.334	0.277	0.191	0.265	0.318
(Ours) MvH+AttE	0.483	0.337	0.285	0.228	0.282	0.335
(Ours) MvH+AttL	0.488	0.357	0.296	0.246	0.313	0.351
(Ours) MvH+AttL+MC	**0.529**	0.372	**0.315**	**0.255**	**0.343**	**0.453**
(Ours) MvH+AttL+MC*	0.649	0.500	0.413	0.303	0.418	0.496

Radiology Report Generation: The evaluation metrics we use are BLEU [9], METEOR [2], and ROUGE [8] scores, all of which are widely used in image captioning and machine translation tasks. We compared the proposed model with several state-of-the-art baselines: (1) a visual attention based image captioning model (Vis-Att) [13]; (2) radiology report generation models, including a hierarchical decoder with co-attention (Co-Att) [6], multimodal generative model with visual attention (MM-Att) [14], and knowledge-drive retrieval based report generation (KERP) [7]; and (3) the proposed multi-view encoder with hierarchical decoder (MvH) model, the base model with visual attentions and early fusion (MvH+AttE), MvH with late fusion fashion (MvH+AttL), and the combination of late fusion with medical concepts (MvH+AttL+MC). MvH+AttL+MC* is an oracle run based on *ground-truth* medical concepts and considered as the upper bound of the improvement caused by applying medical concepts. As shown in Table 2, our proposed models generally outperform the state-of-the-art baselines. Compared with MvH, multi-view feature fusions by attentions (AttE and AttL) yield better results. Applying medical concepts significantly improve the performance especially on Meteors because the recalls rise with more semantical information provided directly to the word decoder, and Meteor weights more on recalls over precisions. However, the improvement is subject to prediction errors on medical concepts, indicating that a better encoder would benefit the whole model by a large margin as shown in MvH+AttL+MC*.

Discussion: As Fig. 3 shows, AttL (and other baseline models) have difficulties generating abnormalities and locations because there is no explicit abnormal information involved in word-level decoding compared with our proposed model. Not all the predicted medical concepts would necessarily appear in the generated reports. On the other hand, the prediction errors from the encoder propagate, such as predicting "right" instead of "right lung", and affect the generated reports, suggesting a more accurate encoder is beneficial. Moreover, since there are no constraints on the sentence decoder during the training, it is likely to generate similar hidden states for our model. In this case, a stacked attention mechanism would be beneficial for forcing the decoder to focus on different image sub-regions. In addition, we observe that it is difficult for our model to generate unseen sentences and sometimes there are syntax errors. Such errors are due to the limited corpus scale of IU-RR, and we expect by exploring unpaired textual data for pretraining the decoder would address such limitations [3].

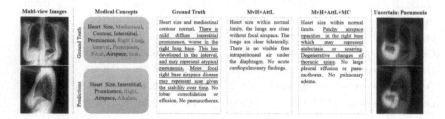

Fig. 3. An example report generated by the proposed model. The medical concepts marked red are false (positive/negative) predictions. The underlined sentences are abnormality descriptions. Uncertain predictions are visualized using Grad-cam [10]. (Color figure online)

4   Conclusions

In this paper, we present a novel encoder-decoder model for radiology report generation. The proposed model takes advantage of multi-view information in radiology by applying visual attentions in a late fusion fashion, and enriches the semantics involved in the hierarchical LSTM decoder with medical concepts. Consequently, both the visual and textual contents have been better exploited to achieve the state-of-the-art performance. The automatic interpretation approach will simplify and expedite the conventional process of generating radiology reports and better assist human experts in decision making. As a valuable added benefit, uncertain radiographic observations are extracted and visualized by our model because it is important to direct more expert attention to such uncertainties for further analysis in practice.

Acknowledgment. This work is supported in part by NSF through award IIS-1722847, NIH through the Morris K. Udall Center of Excellence in Parkinson's Disease Research, and our corporate sponsor.

References

1. Demner-Fushman, D., et al.: Preparing a collection of radiology examinations for distribution and retrieval. JAMIA **23**(2), 304–310 (2016)
2. Denkowski, M., Lavie, A.: Meteor universal: language specific translation evaluation for any target language. In: Proceedings of the Ninth Workshop on Statistical Machine Translation, pp. 376–380 (2014)
3. Feng, Y., Ma, L., Liu, W., Luo, J.: Unsupervised image captioning. In: Proceedings of the IEEE Conference on Computer Vision and Pattern Recognition, pp. 4125–4134 (2019)
4. He, K., Zhang, X., Ren, S., Sun, J.: Deep residual learning for image recognition. In: Proceedings of the IEEE Conference on Computer Vision and Pattern Recognition, pp. 770–778 (2016)
5. Irvin, J., et al.: CheXpert: a large chest radiograph dataset with uncertainty labels and expert comparison. arXiv:1901.07031 (2019)
6. Jing, B., Xie, P., Xing, E.P.: On the automatic generation of medical imaging reports. In: Proceedings of the 56th Annual Meeting of the Association for Computational Linguistics, ACL 2018, Melbourne, Australia, pp. 2577–2586 (2018)
7. Li, C.Y., Liang, X., Hu, Z., Xing, E.P.: Knowledge-driven encode, retrieve, paraphrase for medical image report generation. arxiv:1903.10122 (2019)
8. Lin, C.Y.: Rouge: a package for automatic evaluation of summaries. In: Proceedings of the ACL-04 Workshop, pp. 74–81. Association for Computational Linguistics, Barcelona, July 2004
9. Papineni, K., Roukos, S., Ward, T., Zhu, W.J.: Bleu: a method for automatic evaluation of machine translation. In: Proceedings of the 40th Annual Meeting on Association for Computational Linguistics, pp. 311–318 (2002)
10. Selvaraju, R.R., Cogswell, M., Das, A., Vedantam, R., Parikh, D., Batra, D.: Grad-CAM: visual explanations from deep networks via gradient-based localization. In: Proceedings of the IEEE International Conference on Computer Vision, pp. 618–626 (2017)
11. Vinyals, O., Toshev, A., Bengio, S., Erhan, D.: Show and tell: a neural image caption generator. arxiv:1411.4555 (2015)
12. Wang, X., Peng, Y., Lu, L., Lu, Z., Bagheri, M., Summers, R.M.: ChestX-ray8: hospital-scale chest x-ray database and benchmarks on weakly-supervised classification and localization of common thorax diseases. In: Proceedings of the IEEE Conference on Computer Vision and Pattern Recognition, pp. 2097–2106 (2017)
13. Xu, K., et al.: Show, attend and tell: Neural image caption generation with visual attention. arxiv:1502.03044 (2015)
14. Xue, Y., et al.: Multimodal recurrent model with attention for automated radiology report generation. In: Frangi, A.F., Schnabel, J.A., Davatzikos, C., Alberola-López, C., Fichtinger, G. (eds.) MICCAI 2018. LNCS, vol. 11070, pp. 457–466. Springer, Cham (2018). https://doi.org/10.1007/978-3-030-00928-1_52

Multi-label Thoracic Disease Image Classification with Cross-Attention Networks

Congbo Ma[1,2], Hu Wang[1,3(✉)], and Steven C. H. Hoi[1,4]

[1] Singapore Management University, Singapore, Singapore
[2] South China University of Technology, Guangzhou, China
[3] The University of Adelaide, Adelaide, Australia
hu.wang@adelaide.edu.au
[4] Salesforce Research Asia, Singapore, Singapore

Abstract. Automated disease classification of radiology images has been emerging as a promising technique to support clinical diagnosis and treatment planning. Unlike generic image classification tasks, a real-world radiology image classification task is significantly more challenging as it is far more expensive to collect the training data where the labeled data is in nature multi-label; and more seriously samples from easy classes often dominate; training data is highly class-imbalanced problem exists in practice as well. To overcome these challenges, in this paper, we propose a novel scheme of Cross-Attention Networks (CAN) for automated thoracic disease classification from chest x-ray images, which can effectively excavate more meaningful representation from data to boost the performance through cross-attention by only image-level annotations. We also design a new loss function that beyond cross entropy loss to help cross-attention process and is able to overcome the imbalance between classes and easy-dominated samples within each class. The proposed method achieves state-of-the-art results.

Keywords: Multi-label · Imbalanced · Medical image classification · Cross-Attention Networks

1 Introduction

Chest diseases are constantly a big threat to people's health. Early diagnosis and treatment of chest diseases are very important. Computer aided x-ray analysis is an effective way to diagnose chest diseases. Wang et al. [1] constructed one of the largest public Chest X-Ray14 datasets. After that, Rajpurkar et al. [2] proposed a 121 layers convolutional neural network trained on Chest X-Ray14 dataset. Later on, Li et al. [4] proposed a unified structure that can perform disease identification and localization simultaneously. They used both normal labelled x-ray images and those with disease location annotations. However, annotated data are quite expensive to acquire and heavily dependent on expert

© Springer Nature Switzerland AG 2019
D. Shen et al. (Eds.): MICCAI 2019, LNCS 11769, pp. 730–738, 2019.
https://doi.org/10.1007/978-3-030-32226-7_81

experience. Recently, a large-scale chest x-ray dataset CheXpert [10] came out. For chest x-ray image processing, data is usually multi-labeled and for each label, positive-negative samples are often imbalanced and easy samples are usually in a dominant position, which usually result in poor performance. The general training data number upsampling or downsampling approach and cross entropy loss may not be an ideal solution for multi-label imbalance classification problem.

To this end, we propose Cross-Attention Networks with a new loss function to tackle imbalanced multi-label x-ray chest diseases classification from two different angles: (1) From image processing angle, we design a flexible end-to-end training Cross-Attention Network architecture which can effectively excavate more meaningful representation with only image-level annotations. By using hadamard product of two feature maps, the proposed structure could effectively eliminate attention noises. (2) From a learning and optimization perspective, we proposed a new loss function which consists of an attention loss that could facilitate the model to learn better representations and a multi-label balance loss to reduce imbalance between positive and negative classes within each disease and dominated easy samples. We have also used image-level supervised localization to validate our model which is able to localize at high risk pathogenic areas in a better manner. We make thorough experiments on Chest X-Ray14 and CheXpert datasets to evaluate the effectiveness of our different proposed components. Our method achieves the state-of-the-art results.

2   Model

2.1   Cross-Attention Networks

Feature Extraction Networks. After raw data pre-processing, the images are pumped into two feature extraction networks and gone through convolutional layers which are worked as feature extractors. Our proposed cross-attention method is flexible and the two networks can be easily substituted by other backbone networks. Different from standard CNNs, instead of pushing extracted features into activation layers and global average pooling layers, we keep these abstract image-level features for later use.

Cross-Attention Model. We proposed a new cross-attention model that two networks have attention on each other, which could generate more meaningful representations. In Fig. 1, after we get the features by pumping images into two networks which have different initialization or structures, the two feature maps will go through two ReLU layers respectively to ensure that negative activation values will not interfere the cross-attention features. Then these feature maps will be inputted to a transition layer to transform two groups of features into the same shape. Later on, instead of outer-producing two large tensors as self-attention [5] methods by building attention for each pair of data point, we used element-wise hadamard product to get cross-attention feature maps. Cross-attention structure enables networks to get attention on each other and eliminate noises, which means the Cross-Attention Networks have the ability to only focus on the areas

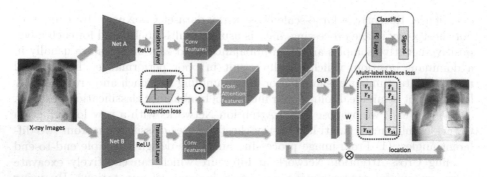

Fig. 1. The proposed Cross-Attention Networks. (1) Data are inputted through ReLU layers to eliminate the interference of negative activated values; (2) Transition layers play the role to transform two groups of feature maps into the same dimension; (3) The element-wise hadamard product is used to get cross-attention feature maps which urges networks to only focus on the area that have high pathogenic probabilities; (4) Dashed boxes represent attention loss and multi-label balance loss.

that have high pathogenic chances. Then the cross-attention feature maps will be concatenated with two output tensors.

$$Feature_{all\_cat} = Concat(F_{CA}, F_A, F_B), where \ F_{CA} = F_A \odot F_B$$

where F_A, F_B represents the feature maps of Network A and Network B, F_{CA} represents cross-attention feature maps. $Concat()$ function represents concatenate function. By using hadamard product, the cross-attention feature maps F_{CA} would be activated on those areas that only if the two groups of feature maps F_A and F_B are both activated, which eliminate the randomness of outliers. When the loss is back propagated, two networks affect each others' gradient flows which also enable two networks update in a more collaborative way.

Transition Layers and Classifier. The transition layers are to transform two groups of feature maps into the same dimension. We use $tran_N = Min(C_A, C_B)$ number of $1 * 1$ convolutional kernels to transform these two group of feature maps into the same shape. where C_A and C_B denote the channel numbers of different feature maps. By using transition layers, we ensure the dimension of two feature maps are the same and also add further non-linearity to our cross-attention model.

In Fig. 1, after getting the all concatenated cross-attention feature maps, we input these feature maps into a global average pooling layer and then the classifier. Our model is designed to have different binary classification for different labels. For each label, the disease probability score is calculated through a sigmoid function. So our classifier consists of a fully connected layer and a sigmoid layer to predict the probability of images which may have thoracic diseases.

2.2   Loss Design

Attention Loss. In order to further excavate more meaningful features in proposed cross-attention model, we define a new attention loss. In Fig. 1, we first fetch all feature maps from the last block before the global average pooling of two networks. Each pixel in these feature maps encodes different spatial information of the original image. Then we channel-wise sum up these features maps to form a pathogenic attention map. Different feature maps within one network have different activation areas, however, majority of these features would concentrate on the "right" areas. By getting the summation of these feature maps within one network, we would coarsely get a pathogenic attention map.

By feeding through a resize layer, we get two same size $1 * H' * W'$ pathogenic attention maps from two networks, where H' and W' represents the height and width of each feature map. After that, we normalized these two pathogenic attention maps by dividing the max value of each attention map to ensure each pixel has the same range of values. Then we calculate the L2 loss of the two pathogenic attention maps. Through attention loss, we set a constraint to urge two networks to find mutual pathogenic areas which would smooth the cross-attention process. The formulation of attention loss is given as below:

$$L_{att} = ||norm(\sum\nolimits_{n=1}^{N} f_n) - norm(\sum\nolimits_{m=1}^{M} f_m)||_2$$

where N and M denote the total size of feature channels within one network. n and m represent the index of each feature map. f_n and f_m are different feature maps from two networks respectively.

Multi-label Balance Loss. Poor performance can be easily caused by imbalance between classes, which is not ideal for standard cross entropy loss to solve. And easy-dominated samples hamper models to learning genuine discriminated features. Inspired by Lin et al. [3], we designed a loss that extends the focal loss to multi-label setting with balance factors. To our best of knowledge, it is the first work to do that. Through this loss, our model can not only handle the imbalance between positive-negative samples within each disease, but also excavate more meaningful representation out of dominated easy samples. We sum up the balance loss from each disease to represent multi-label balance loss.

$$L_{bal} = \sum\nolimits_{l=1}^{L} -w_{l-} \cdot [1 - p_l(Y = 0|X)]^{\gamma}(1 - y)logp_l(Y = 0|X) + \\ - w_{l+} \cdot [1 - p_l(Y = 1|X)]^{\gamma}ylogp_l(Y = 1|X)$$

where L is the total number of multiple labels and l means each label of different type of diseases. $w_{l+} = \frac{|N_l|}{|P_l| + |N_l|}$ and $w_{l-} = \frac{|P_l|}{|P_l| + |N_l|}$, which means balance factor to eliminate positive-negative sample imbalance between each binary classes. P_l and N_l represent numbers of positive and negative samples of a certain disease. Parameter γ controls the curvature and shape of the multi-label balance loss, which may have better performance to mine "hard" examples to contribute more to the model training in some γ settings, especially when "easy" examples dominate the dataset greatly.

Cross-Attention Loss Function. The cross-attention loss function is a combined loss function which is:

$$L = \alpha L_{att} + L_{bal}.$$

where α represents the trade-off factor between attention loss and multi-label balance loss. The attention loss could force the model to focus on pathogenic areas more accurately. Multi-label balance loss helps the model eliminate positive-negative sample imbalance problem and easy sample dominated problem within each disease.

3   Experiments

3.1   Experiments on Chest X-Ray14 Dataset

Experimental Settings. We validate our proposed Cross-Attention Networks on Chest X-Ray14 dataset [1] and follow the official train-val and test data split to keep fair comparison. We further split the official train-val set into 78485 images for training and 8039 images for validation and ensure no patient overlap among these three sets. We downscale input images to the size of 256 * 256 and random crop to 224 * 224 with the batch-size of 96 and initial learning rate of 0.001. We set the dropout rate of last fully connected layer to 0.2 and loss trade-off factor to 0.01. In the multi-label balance loss, we empirically set γ to 2. All experiments are evaluated in terms of AUROC values.

Model Comparison. The quantitative performance of models comparison is demonstrated in Table 1. CAN_1 represents the Cross-Attention Networks $model_1$ with densenet121 and densenet169 as its backbone networks and CAN_2 means the Cross-Attention Networks $model_2$ with two densenet121. The two networks within our model are initialized with different weights which are warmed up at the dataset. Since the experiments of Li et al. [4] is not done on the official split [1] and they leverage extra location labels to train, in order to have a fair comparison, their results will not participate in best result comparison in each row (marked in bold font).

From Table 2, the cross-attention model achieved the best result in terms of average AUROC scores for most individual disease cases. The improvements are remarkable especially for those diseases with extremely scarce positive samples. For example, "Hernia" only has 227 images (%0.202) and "Fibrosis" only contains 1686 images (%1.504) in the dataset, the proposed CAN_2 model obtained 0.932 and 0.827 in terms of the AUROC score respectively, which is much better than its competitors. This is because our cross-attention model with the newly designed cross-attention loss function penalizes those hard examples and can have better differentiate between positive/negative in a good manner.

Table 1. Results comparison between different methods on Chest X-Ray14 Dataset

Diseases	Wang etc. [1]	Yao etc. [6]	CheXNet [2]	Li etc. [4]*	Guendel etc. [7]	Xia etc. [8]	CAN$_1$	CAN$_2$
Split by Wang	Yes	Yes	Yes	No	Yes	Yes	Yes	Yes
Image resize	256 * 256	256 * 256	256 * 256	512 * 512	256 * 256	256 * 256	256 * 256	256 * 256
Atelectasis	0.773	0.733	0.759	0.800	0.767	0.743	0.772	**0.777**
Cardiomegaly	0.854	0.856	0.871	0.870	0.883	0.875	0.894	**0.894**
Effusion	**0.861**	0.806	0.821	0.870	0.828	0.811	0.828	0.829
Infiltration	0.636	0.673	0.700	0.700	**0.709**	0.677	0.703	0.696
Mass	0.761	0.718	0.810	0.830	0.821	0.783	0.830	**0.838**
Nodule	0.664	**0.777**	0.759	0.750	0.758	0.698	0.762	0.771
Pneumonia	0.664	0.684	0.718	0.670	**0.731**	0.696	0.721	0.722
Pneumothorax	0.799	0.805	0.848	0.870	0.846	0.810	0.856	**0.862**
Consolidation	**0.770**	0.711	0.741	0.800	0.745	0.726	0.756	0.750
Edema	**0.861**	0.806	0.844	0.880	0.835	0.833	0.846	0.846
Emphysema	0.736	0.842	0.891	0.910	0.895	0.822	0.892	**0.908**
Fibrosis	0.739	0.743	0.810	0.780	0.818	0.804	0.824	**0.827**
PT	0.749	0.724	0.768	0.790	0.761	0.751	0.773	**0.779**
Hernia	0.746	0.775	0.867	0.770	0.896	0.900	0.932	**0.934**
Average	0.758	0.761	0.801	0.806	0.807	0.781	0.814	**0.817**

Ablation Study. To evaluate the effectiveness of our different proposed components, we also implement them separately in ablation study to monitor how they influence the performance. In Table 3, "121" and "169" represent Densenet121 and Densenet169. "had" means element-wise hadamard product cross-attention. L_{bce}, "L_{bal}" and "L_{att}" are binary cross entropy loss, multi-label balance loss and attention loss. "all_cat" is the operation to get all concatenated cross-attention feature maps. In order to have a fair comparison, we have not only done the experiments to compare with existing methods, but also compared with different feature aggregation methods with exact parameter numbers. "add" and "max" means element-wise addition or maximum operation between two feature maps respectively, and these two methods have the same parameters with our proposed cross-attention networks.

Table 2. Results comparison between different methods

Methods		Methods	
121+L_{bce}	0.801	121+169(add+all_cat)+L_{bal}+L_{att}	0.810
121+L_{bal}	0.806	121+169(max+all_cat)+L_{bal}+L_{att}	0.810
169+L_{bal}	0.806	121+169(had)+L_{bal}+L_{att}	0.811
121+169(had)+L_{bal}	0.809	Cross-attention $model_1$(CAN$_1$)	0.814
121+169(had+all_cat)+L_{bal}	0.810	Cross-attention $model_2$(CAN$_2$)	**0.817**

From Table 2, we found that our CAN model boosts the performance in such imbalanced dataset. By using "hadamard" produce of two feature maps, the average AUROC score increases from 0.806 to 0.809. Because the randomness of "poor" activation and outliers are eliminated. Also, the model can be updated through back propagating gradients of each other in a more collaborative way; however, "add" and "max" operations do not have this attribute, so even with all concatenate feature maps and cross-attention loss function, the results are both stagnated at 0.810. With the help of proposed attention loss, the AUROC score is lifted to 0.811. Because attention loss drags the attention of two networks closer which would facilitate cross-attention process. Our CAN model achieves AUROC of 0.814 and 0.817, the new state-of-the-art results.

Image-Level Supervised Disease Localization. To better understand our model, disease localization heat maps are generated by only image-level supervised labels [9]. Since we used Global Average Pooling as our last pooling layer, we directly sum up the multiplication of weights and feature maps between pooling layer and fully connected layer to localize.

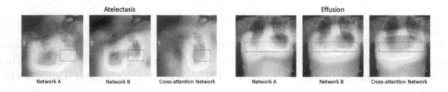

Fig. 2. The results of the localization of chest diseases.

In Fig. 2, the heat maps localize on high-probability disease areas and the blue bounding boxes indicate the ground-truth location of the diseases. Our proposed Cross-Attention Networks provide better performance to focus on high-probability disease areas in a better manner than using the networks separately. This means that Cross-Attention Networks enable model updates in a collaborative way and could have better feature representations.

3.2 Experiments on CheXpert Dataset

Experimental Settings. We also validate our proposed Cross-Attention Networks on newly released dataset CheXpert [10] with "Frontal views" and "Lateral views", and keep the exact same settings of compared methods and our method throughout all experiments. In the CheXpert experiments, in order to have enough data for testing, we split 222914 images for training and the other 734 images for testing, and we further ensure no patient overlap among them.

Model Comparison. In our experiments, we keep the consistent experimental settings by only using U(uncertain)-Ones introduced by the CheXpert paper [10]—mapping all instances of the uncertain label to 1, and we test all models on 14 labels by either just using "Frontal views" or treating "Frontal views" and "Lateral views" equally, which means we do not select the best uncertainty approach for each disease and do not use maximum probability of the observations across the views or other bells and whistles. We further compare the results obtained by "Add" and "Max" operations. Table 3 shows the experimental results comparison on 14 labels classification tasks.

From Table 3, We can find that the cross-attention model achieved the best AUROC scores for most individual disease cases in whether "Frontal Views Only" or "Frontal + Lateral Views" setting.

Table 3. Results comparison on 14 labels classification tasks on CheXpert dataset

Experiments	Frontal views only				Frontal + Lateral (Equally)			
Labels	CheXNet	Add	Max	CAN	CheXNet	Add	Max	CAN
Atelectasis	0.659	**0.683**	0.697	0.667	0.707	0.678	0.691	**0.713**
Cardiomegaly	0.775	**0.781**	0.760	0.773	0.775	0.777	0.757	**0.790**
Consolidation	0.702	**0.735**	0.729	0.732	0.755	0.746	0.730	**0.757**
Edema	0.827	**0.846**	0.843	0.840	0.863	0.858	**0.867**	0.861
Enlarged Cardio	0.551	0.505	0.518	**0.552**	0.531	0.491	**0.568**	0.555
Fracture	0.616	**0.732**	0.710	0.722	0.588	0.638	0.608	**0.735**
Lung Lesion	0.704	0.775	**0.831**	0.757	0.710	0.778	0.741	**0.805**
Lung Opacity	0.767	0.741	0.768	**0.788**	0.784	0.764	0.770	0.783
No Finding	0.887	0.879	0.883	**0.893**	0.872	0.865	0.865	0.859
Pleural Effusion	0.860	0.887	0.891	**0.892**	0.874	0.887	0.881	**0.892**
Pleural Other	0.607	0.699	0.647	**0.711**	0.710	**0.718**	0.710	0.680
Pneumonia	0.641	0.674	0.671	**0.710**	0.535	0.601	0.647	**0.666**
Pneumothorax	0.807	0.812	0.823	**0.824**	0.842	0.826	0.809	0.836
Support Devices	0.869	0.882	0.877	**0.889**	0.899	0.879	0.879	**0.913**
Average	0.734	0.759	0.760	**0.768**	0.746	0.750	0.752	**0.775**

4 Conclusion

This paper proposed an end-to-end trainable Cross-Attention Networks (CAN) scheme for multi-label x-ray chest diseases classification. The Cross-Attention Networks not only utilize the attention loss for better attention at the regions of interest, but also overcome the positive-negative sample imbalance and easy sample dominated problems with multi-label balanced loss. Cross-Attention Networks can effectively excavate meaningful representation from data by having attention on each other and updating models in a more collaborative way. Quantitative and qualitative results demonstrate the state-of-the-art performance of our method.

Acknowledgement. Most of this work were done when the authors worked at Singapore Management University.

References

1. Wang, X., Peng, Y., Lu, L., Lu, Z., Bagheri, M., Summers, R.M.: ChestX-ray8: hospital-scale chest X-ray database and benchmarks on weakly-supervised classification and localization of common thorax diseases. In: Proceedings of the IEEE Conference on Computer Vision and Pattern Recognition, pp. 2097–2106 (2017)
2. Rajpurkar, P., et al.: CheXNet: radiologist-level pneumonia detection on chest X-rays with deep learning. arXiv preprint arXiv:1711.05225 (2017)
3. Lin, T.Y., Goyal, P., Girshick, R., He, K., Dollár, P.: Focal loss for dense object detection. In: Proceedings of the IEEE International Conference on Computer Vision, pp. 2980–2988 (2017)
4. Li, Z., et al.: Thoracic disease identification and localization with limited supervision. In: Proceedings of the IEEE Conference on Computer Vision and Pattern Recognition, pp. 8290–8299 (2018)
5. Vaswani, A., et al.: Attention is all you need. In: Advances in Neural Information Processing Systems, pp. 5998–6008 (2017)
6. Yao, L., Poblenz, E., Dagunts, D., Covington, B., Bernard, D., Lyman, K.: Learning to diagnose from scratch by exploiting dependencies among labels. arXiv preprint arXiv:1710.10501 (2017)
7. Guendel, S., et al.: Learning to recognize abnormalities in chest X-rays with location-aware dense networks. arXiv preprint arXiv:1803.04565 (2018)
8. Wang, H., Xia, Y.: ChestNet: a deep neural network for classification of thoracic diseases on chest radiography. arXiv preprint arXiv:1807.03058 (2018)
9. Zhou, B., Khosla, A., Lapedriza, A., Oliva, A., Torralba, A.: Learning deep features for discriminative localization. In: Proceedings of the IEEE Conference on Computer Vision and Pattern Recognition, pp. 2921–2929 (2016)
10. Irvin, J., et al.: CheXpert: a large chest radiograph dataset with uncertainty labels and expert comparison. In: Thirty-Third AAAI Conference on Artificial Intelligence, January 2019

InfoMask: Masked Variational Latent Representation to Localize Chest Disease

Saeid Asgari Taghanaki[1,2,3]($\boxtimes$), Mohammad Havaei[2], Tess Berthier[2],
Francis Dutil[2], Lisa Di Jorio[2], Ghassan Hamarneh[3], and Yoshua Bengio[1]

[1] MILA, Université de Montréal, Montreal, Canada
[2] Imagia Inc., Montreal, Canada
[3] School of Computing Science, Simon Fraser University, Burnaby, Canada
sasgarit@sfu.ca

Abstract. The scarcity of richly annotated medical images is limiting supervised deep learning based solutions to medical image analysis tasks, such as localizing discriminatory radiomic disease signatures.
Therefore, it is desirable to leverage unsupervised and weakly supervised models. Most recent weakly supervised localization methods apply
attention maps or region proposals in a multiple instance learning formulation. While attention maps can be noisy, leading to erroneously
highlighted regions, it is not simple to decide on an optimal window/bag
size for multiple instance learning approaches. In this paper, we propose
a learned spatial masking mechanism to filter out irrelevant background
signals from attention maps. The proposed method minimizes mutual
information between a masked variational representation and the input
while maximizing the information between the masked representation
and class labels. This results in more accurate localization of discriminatory regions. We tested the proposed model on the ChestX-ray8 dataset
to localize pneumonia from chest X-ray images without using any pixel-
level or bounding-box annotations.

Keywords: Disease localization · Variational representation · Mutual
information

1 Introduction

Around 50,000 deaths attributed to pneumonia are reported every year in the
US alone [1]. Chest X-rays are currently the most frequently adopted imaging
modality for detecting pneumonia [21]. The large increase in imaging studies,
scarcity of radiologists and associated expense and intra-/inter-rater variability,
has resulted in an acceleration in the development and adoption of automated
image-based disease classification methods. In the last decade, deep learning
methods have resulted in great successes in classification of natural and medical images. Locating discriminatory regions in images, along with the predicted
class, renders deep models' decisions more interpretable and trustworthy. Localization of disease-indicator regions (i.e., radiomic biosignatures) is particularly

© Springer Nature Switzerland AG 2019
D. Shen et al. (Eds.): MICCAI 2019, LNCS 11769, pp. 739–747, 2019.
https://doi.org/10.1007/978-3-030-32226-7_82

important for medical applications since it reveals whether the machine diagnosis was based on the presence or absence of disease and not biased towards some unique yet unintuitive and unrelated pattern that happens to be exhibited among the training examples.

1.1 Related Work

The past few years have witnessed numerous advances in deep learning methods for localizing objects and detecting discriminatory regions in images.

Multiple Instance Learning and Region-Based Methods. Bency et al. [4] and Teh et al. [15] applied region-proposal and beam search based methods to localize objects from natural (i.e., non-medical) images. Training such hybrid localization-classification models requires large amounts of bounding-box level image annotations, which can suffer from rater-variability and can be prohibitively expensive or time consuming. Several existing methods [5,7,13,14,17] formulate the weakly-supervised localization as a multiple instance learning (MIL) problem. However, like for region-proposal based methods, it is difficult to find an optimal window size.

Attention/Activation Based Methods. Similarly to previous works [8, 18,22], Wei et al. [20] proposed an activation map based framework to produce tight bounding boxes around objects. However, in the context of object localization, there might be erroneously detected regions (false positives) or regions/activations which spread over unrealistically wide ranges. This is the case because saliency maps [11] are usually noisy.

Several works have attempted to smooth or regularize the saliency or attention maps [12] and prevent important features from being neglected due to saturation [3,10]. To produce class-discriminative 'explanation maps', the gradient-weighted class activation mapping method GradCAM [9] was used to capture the importance of a particular features of a target class. However, GradCAM and similar approaches are applied *after* a model is trained, i.e., there is no *explicit* spatial enforcement during training and GradCAM requires class labels during inference. To remove dependency on class labels during test, Fan et al. [6], trained a masking mechanism simultaneously with a classification network to localize objects. However, their masking mechanism is based on super-pixels which might miss fine details. Zolna et al. [23] reformulated the same problem as a min-max game. It is not clear to us how to weigh the regularization term in their proposed loss function and we have concerns about scalability of the method, as it needs to preserve many copies of the model with different parameters to produce different masks using each set of parameters. In this paper, instead of keeping different parameters of a model, we propose to perform variational online mask sampling from a normal distribution using a single model.

1.2 Contribution

The focus of the current study is to develop a method to localize radiologic presentations of pneumonia in unseen chest X-ray images while training on data with only image-level labels. The key idea of the proposed approach is to learn a low-dimensional latent parametric probability distribution (regularized by Kullback-Leibler divergence from a standard normal distribution) that encodes the input data and be not only discriminative but also spatially-selective to disregard irrelevant background from input images. To this end, we propose InfoMask, a variational model with a learnt attention mechanism and a sparsity-promoting masking operation.

In this paper we make the following contributions: (a) we propose to produce online variational masks during training without the need for class labels during inference; (b) we propose a weakly supervised localization method without requiring any choice of window/bag size (which is necessary in competing multiple instance learning formulations); (c) we introduce a masking mechanism applied to the latent variational representation to filter non-discriminatory information; and (d) we propose minimizing mutual information between the input and latent variational attention maps and increasing the mutual information between the masked latent representation and class labels.

2 Method

Given a training set of input images $\mathbf{x}$ and corresponding image-level labels y, our goal is to learn the parameters $\boldsymbol{\theta}$ of a class-predictive model $\hat{y} = g(\mathbf{x}; \boldsymbol{\theta})$ that not only has high classification accuracy but also localizes the discriminative regions with minimal inclusion of irrelevant pixels. The localization is represented via a binary mask M and $\boldsymbol{\theta}$ is learnt by maximizing $p(y|\boldsymbol{x}, M; \boldsymbol{\theta})$.

To this end, InfoMask learns to encode a bottleneck random variable Z that (i) captures minimal information about the input random variable X, hence minimizes the encoding of irrelevant information in the input, and (ii) holds maximal information about the distribution of the target label variable Y. Consequently, inspired by Alemi et al. [2] and the information bottleneck [16], we aim at maximizing

$$J(\boldsymbol{\theta}) = I(\boldsymbol{Z}, Y; \boldsymbol{\theta}) - \alpha I(\boldsymbol{Z}, \mathbf{X}; \boldsymbol{\theta}) \tag{1}$$

where $I(A, B)$ is the mutual information between random variables A and B, and α is a scalar weight.

We model $z \sim \mathcal{N}(\boldsymbol{\mu}_z, \boldsymbol{\sigma}_z)$ and learn to generate its mean and variance using convolutional layers, i.e., $\boldsymbol{\mu}_z = f_e^{\mu}(\boldsymbol{x})$ and $\boldsymbol{\sigma}_z = f_e^{\sigma}(\boldsymbol{x})$, and rewrite $I(\boldsymbol{Z}, Y; \boldsymbol{\theta})$ (and similarly $I(\boldsymbol{Z}, \mathbf{X}; \boldsymbol{\theta})$), for each element of $\boldsymbol{Z}$, as:

$$I(\boldsymbol{Z}, Y; \boldsymbol{\theta}, \boldsymbol{\mu}_z, \boldsymbol{\sigma}_z) = \int p(z, y; \boldsymbol{\theta}, \boldsymbol{\mu}_z, \boldsymbol{\sigma}_z) \log \frac{p(z, y; \boldsymbol{\theta}, \boldsymbol{\mu}_z, \boldsymbol{\sigma}_z)}{p(z; \boldsymbol{\theta}, \boldsymbol{\mu}_z, \boldsymbol{\sigma}_z) p(y; \boldsymbol{\theta})} dx dy \tag{2}$$

To sample $\boldsymbol{Z}$, we apply the reparameterization trick and write $z = f(\boldsymbol{x}, \epsilon) = \mu_z + \sigma_z \epsilon = a_e^\mu(\boldsymbol{x}) + a_e^\sigma(\boldsymbol{x})\epsilon$, where a_e is a deterministic function which outputs both μ and σ and $\epsilon \sim \mathcal{N}(0,1)$. We regularize the distribution by penalizing the Kullback-Leibler (KL) divergence from a standard normal distribution. The final loss function which we aim to minimize is given by

$$L = \frac{1}{N} \sum_{n=1}^{N} \mathbb{E}_{\epsilon \sim p(\epsilon)} \left[-\log q\left(y_n | a\left(\boldsymbol{x}_n, \epsilon\right)\right)\right] + \alpha \mathrm{KL}[p(\boldsymbol{Z}|\boldsymbol{x}_n), r(\boldsymbol{Z})] \qquad (3)$$

where N is the number of training examples, $q(.)$ is the variational approximation function, and $r(\boldsymbol{Z})$ is variational approximation. In our case, $\boldsymbol{Z}$ is not computed directly from the input but rather by sampling an attention map $\boldsymbol{A}$ from which μ_z and σ_z are derived. To *explicitly* enforce the model to generate more focused attention maps, we apply the following masking function $\boldsymbol{M}$ with threshold τ that localizes the discriminative areas of $\boldsymbol{Z}$.

$$\boldsymbol{M} = R\left(\tilde{z} - \tau\right) \quad \text{where} \quad \tilde{z} = (1 + \exp\left(-z\right))^{-1} \qquad (4)$$

where R is a ReLU function with upper bound of 1, i.e., $R(v) = \max(0, \min(v, 1))$. The block diagram of the proposed method is shown in Fig. 1.

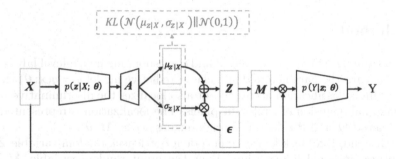

Fig. 1. Architecture and components of the proposed model. The input $\boldsymbol{X}$ is encoded via $p(z|X; \boldsymbol{\theta})$. $\boldsymbol{A}$ refers to an attention map computed from the last layer of the encoder using 1×1 convolution and ReLU. Note that $\boldsymbol{A}$ is upsampled to the size of $\boldsymbol{X}$. $\boldsymbol{M}$ is the masked latent matrix. $\boldsymbol{X}$, $\boldsymbol{A}$, μ, σ, $\boldsymbol{Z}$, and ϵ are of size $W \times H$.

3 Data

For evaluation, we used the NIH ChestX-ray8 Dataset [19], which comprises of 112,120 X-ray images from 30,805 unique patients with corresponding disease labels. We used 20547, 2568, and 2569 with pneumonia images as train, validation, and test sets, respectively. For training and to evaluate the test classification accuracy, we only used image-level labels. To evaluate the localization performance on test images, we used ground truth bounding boxes manually placed around the diseased areas.

4   Experiments and Results

We adopt a simple architecture as a baseline, i.e., an encoder $(p(z|X;\theta))$ of the form [conv(64, 3 × 3, relu), conv(64, 3 × 3, relu), maxpooling(2 × 2), conv(128, 3 × 3, relu), conv(128, 3 × 3, relu), maxpooling(2 × 2), conv(256, 3 × 3, relu), conv(16, 3×3, relu)] and a classification block $(p(Y|z;\theta))$ of [conv(128, 3×3, relu), maxpooling(2 × 2), conv(64, 3 × 3, relu), conv(64, 3 × 3, relu) maxpooling(2 × 2), global average pooling, softmax].

We then compare our proposed InfoMask to four competing disease localization methods: (i) GradCAM, gradient-weighted class activation mapping + baseline, i.e., during inference, we replace M in Fig. 1 with GradCAM; (ii) FeatureMask, masking the latent representation without KL divergence regularization + baseline; (iii) RegL1, L1 regularization over the generated masks instead of KL regularization; (iv) CheXCAM, GradCAM applied to the last layer of CheXNet [8]. Even though each patient could have multiple disease classes at the same time, we focus only on pneumonia disease detection (vs. normal) to analyze whether our method is able to only localize target regions in a complex environment where other diseases might also be present. Note that the results (Table 1 and Figs. 2, 3, and 4) reported next are based on the thresholded masks using the best threshold value, i.e., optimized, for each method, to minimize localization error over the validation set. To select the best epoch based on a validation set we first select N checkpoints which produce highest classification accuracy and then select the epoch with the highest localization score among them. As the detected thresholded masks could potentially have largely diverse patterns (e.g., from sparse disjoint localizations scattered over the whole image to large connected components, to anything in between), computing a single representative bounding box, as is provided by ground truth bounding box annotations, is not straightforward. Therefore, we replace the intersection over union (IoU) quality metric, commonly used for evaluating bounding box predictions, with a proposed intersection over predicted area (IoP), which reflects

Table 1. Disease localization performance evaluation of the proposed InfoMask vs. competing methods. IoP, FPR, and FNR represent the localization performance while Acc. and AUC show the classification performance.

	IoP	FPR	FNR	Acc	AUC
GradCAM	$0.12 \pm 3.0e{-}04$	$0.196 \pm 2.0e{-}04$	$0.20 \pm 2.0e{-}04$	0.8221	0.8333
FeatureMask	$0.19 \pm 2.0e{-}04$	$0.095 \pm 4.7e{-}05$	$0.81 \pm 2.0e{-}04$	0.8236	0.8375
RegL1	$0.11 \pm 2.0e{-}04$	$0.010 \pm 6.5e{-}06$	$0.99 \pm 3.7e{-}05$	0.8170	0.8306
CheXCAM	$0.34 \pm 5.0e{-}04$	$0.077 \pm 7.0e{-}05$	$0.71 \pm 4.0e{-}04$	0.8400	0.8644
InfoMask	$0.44 \pm 5.0e{-}04$	$0.025 \pm 3.6e{-}05$	$0.80 \pm 3.0e{-}04$	0.8248	0.8251

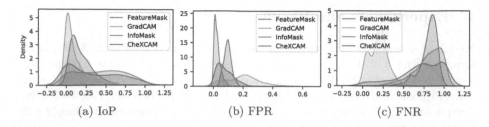

(a) IoP   (b) FPR   (c) FNR

Fig. 2. Kernel density estimation of different measures for disease localization

what percentage of the predicted area is inside the ground truth bounding box. As a small predicted areas inside the box can lead to a high score, we also compute false positive and negative rates, FPR and FNR respectively to measure over- and under-predicted areas. As reported in Table 1, the proposed InfoMask outperforms the competing methods by a large margin on IoP (at least 10% better), and obtains the second best FPR (only 1.5% higher than the lowest FPR). Examining the FPR values, it can be inferred that GradCAM tends to highlight larger areas of the input outside of the ground truth bounding boxes. Form the FNR column, we note that RegL1 generates smaller areas inside the boxes. Although the focus of the current study is not to improve classification accuracy, our proposed method achieves only slightly smaller classification accuracy (<2%) but with only 10% (7,000,000 vs. 700,000) of the parameters of CheXNet. The kernel density estimation plots in Fig. 2 support the quantitative results for the test images. Note how InfoMask obtains higher densities at larger IoP values (note: green curve in (a) for IoP $\in [0.5, 1]$), smaller FPR density (green peak in (b) for FPR $\in [0, 0.1]$) and in second best (behind CheXCAM) for FNR values. For a better interpretation of Table 1, we visualized a few samples of the

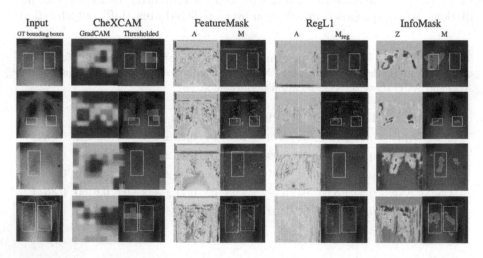

Fig. 3. Examples of pneumonia localization for various methods. GT bounding boxes shown in yellow. (Color figure online)

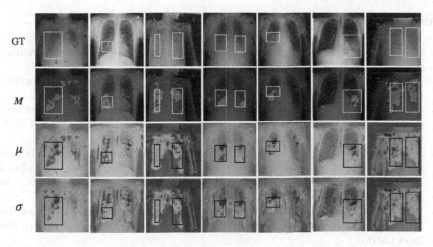

Fig. 4. A few localization samples of InfoMask with mean (μ) and variance (σ) maps.

attention maps and masked ones in Fig. 3 along with the ground truth (GT) bounding boxes in yellow. In Fig. 4, we visualized a few mean and variance samples computed for test images. As shown, there is less variance in the areas where the model is confident about absence of disease signs. As visualized InfoMask was able to localize pneumonia from images with different intensity distributions without using any bounding-box level annotation. As can be seen, FeatureMask and RegL1 produce scattered attention maps that cover only small portions of the GT bounding boxes. Among all, the proposed InfoMask generates contiguous attention areas with most agreement with ground truth boxes.

5   Conclusion

We proposed InfoMask, a method to localize disease-discriminatory regions trained with only image-level labels. Owing to the regularized variational latent representation with an attention mechanism, InfoMask generates contiguous and focused localization masks with higher agreement with ground truth annotations than competing methods (e.g., widely used GradCAM) without resorting to any bounding-box level annotations. A direction for future work aims at improving both classification and localization objectives by using stronger classification backbone models.

Acknowledgement. We thank Joseph Paul Cohen for his insightful discussions and comments.

References

1. Centers for disease control and prevention. https://www.cdc.gov/pneumonia/prevention.html. Accessed 25 Mar 2019
2. Alemi, A.A., Fischer, I., Dillon, J.V., Murphy, K.: Deep variational information bottleneck. arXiv preprint arXiv:1612.00410 (2016)
3. Ancona, M., Ceolini, E., Öztireli, C., Gross, M.: Towards better understanding of gradient-based attribution methods for deep neural networks. In: ICLR 2018 (2018)
4. Bency, A.J., Kwon, H., Lee, H., Karthikeyan, S., Manjunath, B.S.: Weakly supervised localization using deep feature maps. In: Leibe, B., Matas, J., Sebe, N., Welling, M. (eds.) ECCV 2016. LNCS, vol. 9905, pp. 714–731. Springer, Cham (2016). https://doi.org/10.1007/978-3-319-46448-0_43
5. Bilen, H., Vedaldi, A.: Weakly supervised deep detection networks. In: Proceedings of the IEEE Conference on Computer Vision and Pattern Recognition, pp. 2846–2854 (2016)
6. Fan, L.: Adversarial localization network. In: NIPS 2017 Workshop on Learning with Limited Labeled Data (2017)
7. Kumar, M.P., Packer, B., Koller, D.: Self-paced learning for latent variable models. In: Advances in Neural Information Processing Systems, pp. 1189–1197 (2010)
8. Rajpurkar, P., et al.: CheXNet: radiologist-level pneumonia detection on chest X-rays with deep learning. arXiv preprint arXiv:1711.05225 (2017)
9. Selvaraju, R.R., Cogswell, M., Das, A., Vedantam, R., Parikh, D., Batra, D.: Grad-CAM: why did you say that? Visual explanations from deep networks via gradient-based localization. CoRR abs/1610.02391 (2016)
10. Shrikumar, A., Greenside, P., Kundaje, A.: Learning important features through propagating activation differences. In: Proceedings of the 34th International Conference on Machine Learning, vol. 70, pp. 3145–3153. JMLR. org (2017)
11. Simonyan, K., Vedaldi, A., Zisserman, A.: Deep inside convolutional networks: visualising image classification models and saliency maps. arXiv preprint arXiv:1312.6034 (2013)
12. Smilkov, D., Thorat, N., Kim, B., Viégas, F., Wattenberg, M.: SmoothGrad: removing noise by adding noise. arXiv preprint arXiv:1706.03825 (2017)
13. Song, H.O., Girshick, R., Jegelka, S., Mairal, J., Harchaoui, Z., Darrell, T.: On learning to localize objects with minimal supervision. arXiv preprint arXiv:1403.1024 (2014)
14. Song, H.O., Lee, Y.J., Jegelka, S., Darrell, T.: Weakly-supervised discovery of visual pattern configurations. In: Advances in Neural Information Processing Systems, pp. 1637–1645 (2014)
15. Teh, E.W., Rochan, M., Wang, Y.: Attention networks for weakly supervised object localization. In: BMVC, pp. 1–11 (2016)
16. Tishby, N., Pereira, F.C., Bialek, W.: The information bottleneck method. In: The 37th Annual Allerton Conference on Communications, Control, and Computing, pp. 368–377 (1999)
17. Wang, C., Ren, W., Huang, K., Tan, T.: Weakly supervised object localization with latent category learning. In: Fleet, D., Pajdla, T., Schiele, B., Tuytelaars, T. (eds.) ECCV 2014. LNCS, vol. 8694, pp. 431–445. Springer, Cham (2014). https://doi.org/10.1007/978-3-319-10599-4_28
18. Wang, X., et al.: Weakly supervised learning for whole slide lung cancer image classification. Med. Imaging Deep Learn. (2018)

19. Wang, X., Peng, Y., Lu, L., Lu, Z., Bagheri, M., Summers, R.M.: ChestX-ray8: hospital-scale chest X-ray database and benchmarks on weakly-supervised classification and localization of common thorax diseases. In: Proceedings of the IEEE Conference on Vision and Pattern Recognition, pp. 2097–2106 (2017)
20. Wei, Y., et al.: TS2C: tight box mining with surrounding segmentation context for weakly supervised object detection. In: Proceedings of the European Conference on Computer Vision (ECCV), pp. 434–450 (2018)
21. WHO: Standardization of interpretation of chest radiographs for the diagnosis of pneumonia in children
22. Yan, C., Yao, J., Li, R., Xu, Z., Huang, J.: Weakly supervised deep learning for thoracic disease classification and localization on chest X-rays. In: Proceedings of the 2018 ACM International Conference on Bioinformatics, Computational Biology, and Health Informatics, pp. 103–110. ACM (2018)
23. Zolna, K., Geras, K.J., Cho, K.: Classifier-agnostic saliency map extraction. arXiv preprint arXiv:1805.08249 (2018)

Longitudinal Change Detection on Chest X-rays Using Geometric Correlation Maps

Dong Yul Oh[1], Jihang Kim[2], and Kyong Joon Lee[2(✉)]

[1] Interdisciplinary Program in Bioengineering, Seoul National University, Seoul,
Korea
dongyul.oh@snu.ac.kr
[2] Department of Radiology, Seoul National University Bundang Hospital,
Seongnam-si, Korea
{jihangkim,kjoon}@snubh.org

Abstract. The diagnostic decision for chest X-ray image generally considers a probable change in a lesion, compared to the previous examination. We propose a novel algorithm to detect the change in longitudinal chest X-ray images. We extract feature maps from a pair of input images through two streams of convolutional neural networks. Next we generate the geometric correlation map computing matching scores for every possible match of local descriptors in two feature maps. This correlation map is fed into a binary classifier to detect specific patterns of the map representing the change in the lesion. Since no public dataset offers proper information to train the proposed network, we also build our own dataset by analyzing reports in examinations at a tertiary hospital. Experimental results show our approach outperforms previous methods in quantitative comparison. We also provide various case examples visualizing the effect of the proposed geometric correlation map.

Keywords: Chest X-ray · Longitudinal analysis · Change detection · Geometric correlation · Neural network

1 Introduction

Chest X-ray (CXR) is the most commonly used radiological examination detecting a wide range of pulmonary diseases, such as pneumonia, tuberculosis, pleural effusion, pneumothorax, cardiomegaly, and lung cancer. Thanks to its short scan time and the low cost, most of the diagnostic routines include CXR as a basic screening tool, producing a massive amount of images to be read by radiologists.

The worldwide shortage of skilled radiologists has led to rising demand for a computer-aided detection system for CXR. Several algorithms using neural

Electronic supplementary material The online version of this chapter (https://doi.org/10.1007/978-3-030-32226-7_83) contains supplementary material, which is available to authorized users.

networks have recently been proposed to demonstrate diagnostic performance close to the radiologist-level [5,7,8]. However, those methods provide analysis for a limited set of disease classes with a cross-sectional single input image, while the radiologists make diagnostic decisions for every possible disease; and it is usually based on the longitudinal analysis that takes into account probable *changes* in the lesion, compared to the previous examination.

The longitudinal change in a lesion often plays a decisive role in diagnosis. If a mid-size lung nodule remains unchanged for a while, a routine follow-up will be recommended. But if the nodule suddenly appears or rapidly grows, we may need additional computed tomography examinations for careful management. In this regard, many radiologic reports include comments clarifying the changes, *e.g.*, *"no change since last study"*.

Despite this clinical significance, relatively little research has been introduced to exploit the longitudinal analysis. In [11], the modified Long Short-Term Memory (LSTM) algorithm decodes the pattern in sequential examinations to classify the disease in the latest examination. The goal of this method is, however, improving the accuracy of classification rather than detecting the change. A solution to find the change was proposed in [13] by categorizing each image in the longitudinal image sequence. The focus here is on the change in disease class, but clinically important is the change in lesion on subsequent examinations, regardless of the disease class.

This work aims to detect the longitudinal change in a lesion given two consecutive images of a patient. We investigate a large collection of reports attached to CXR examinations at a tertiary referral hospital and build our own dataset for training and testing. We then propose a novel neural network architecture that generates a map describing the geometric correlation between images and detects specific patterns of the map indicating the change.

2 Dataset

To the best of our knowledge, none of the public datasets for CXR provides sufficient information to train a neural network detecting longitudinal change. Two well-known public datasets, the ChestX-ray14 [16] and the CheXpert [2] contain 112,120 and 224,316 CXR images tagged with 14 disease classes, but they do not present information whether the lesion of the disease is changing over time. Other datasets introduced in [3] neither provide the information nor contain sufficient images for training.

Addressing this challenge, we built our own dataset based on the CXR images stored in a tertiary hospital. The institutional review board waived informed consent due to the retrospective study design and the use of anonymized patient data. We found more than 1.8 million images taken from 2003 to 2017, together with available reports confirmed by board-certified radiologists in the routine practice.

We analyzed the reports to find out examinations including longitudinal diagnostic decision. As some sentences repeatedly appear in the reports, we first decomposed all the report text into sentences. We then counted the frequency of each sentence in every report, ignoring minor variations like spaces, punctuation or line breaks. In total 252,209 such unique sentences, only 590 sentences (0.2%) have presented in reports more than 50 times. Interestingly, the number of reports containing those sentences was 1.4 million, exceeding 77% of all reports. The most frequently used sentence was *"no active lesion in the lung"* presented in more than 470,000 reports. Through a full survey of 590 sentences, we accepted 193 sentences that explicitly describe changes in the lesion by time-related keywords (such as aggravation, increment, disappear, decrease, stable.) We understand the rest of 252,016 sentences (including 397 high-frequency sentences) may also contain some indication of the changes, but we leave this issue for the future work, *e.g.*, employing natural language processing.

We divided the 193 sentences into two classes: 155 sentences for the change (shown in 18,911 reports;) and 38 sentences for the no-change (shown in 302,456 reports.) Several examples for the most frequent sentences in each class are demonstrated as follows: *"decreased amount of bilateral pleural effusion"*; *"improving pulmonary edema"*; *"mild improvement of consolidation in both lungs"* for the change class and *"no interval change since last study"*; *"no change of stable tuberculosis"*; *"emphysema, no interval change"* for the no-change class. Finally, we randomly selected examinations for each class and found corresponding previous examinations to create image pairs with at least 30 days interval: 1,751 pairs for the change class and 3,721 pairs for the no-change class, yielding total 5,472 pairs (10,944 images) finally included in our dataset. The classes of diseases shown in our dataset includes pleural effusion, pulmonary edema, pneumothorax, pleural thickening, haziness and so on.

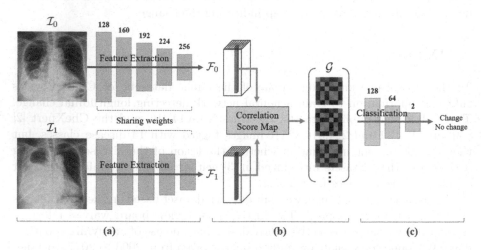

Fig. 1. Overall architecture. (a) Two streams of convolutional neural networks yield a pair of feature maps consisting of local descriptors. (b) Geometric correlation map: a set of score maps for every possible match of local descriptors between the two feature maps. (c) Binary classifier to detect specific patterns for the geometric correlation map.

3   Method

We design a novel neural network model to tackle the change detection. The overall architecture of our approach is outlined in Fig. 1. Given a pair of input images $(\mathcal{I}_0, \mathcal{I}_1)$ representing CXR images for previous and current examinations, we formulate the longitudinal change detection as a binary classification problem: change vs. no-change. We first extract features from both input images through two streams of convolutional neural networks, producing a pair of feature maps $(\mathcal{F}_0, \mathcal{F}_1)$ where $\mathcal{F}_{\{0,1\}} \in \mathbb{R}^{h \times w \times d}$ with $h, w, d \in \mathbb{N}$. These feature maps can be interpreted as a set of d-dimensional local descriptors defined on each pixel of $h \times w$ resolution image. Next, we apply a correlation score calculator for every possible match of local descriptors between two feature maps. That is, each descriptor in one feature map yields matching scores with every descriptor in another feature map. This operation generates a set of score maps which we called as *geometric correlation map*. In the final step, this correlation map is provided as an input to a binary classifier and we train the classifier to determine whether the map indicates a certain change between the input images. The following subsections describe the details of each step.

Two-Stream Feature Extraction

To extract feature maps from the input image pair, we adopt squeeze and excitation network (SENet) [1] that has been showing the state-of-the-art performance in many computer vision problems [14,15]. The network consists of attention blocks consisting of two modules: squeeze module that summarizes local information; and excitation module that scales the importance based on the local information.

Of note, the two networks are identical (*i.e.*, sharing weights) so that visually similar image patches can produce highly correlated descriptors. We implement five attention blocks with 128, 160, 192, 224 and 256 channels. The max pooling (2×2) is applied at the end of each layer.

Normalized Geometric Correlation Map

Next, we generate a matching pattern of the extracted two feature maps. We measure how strong a local descriptor in one feature map correlates with a local descriptor in the other feature map [9,10]. Since we cannot expect the two feature maps are originally aligned (due to patient posture, scan angle, etc.), we compute the correlation scores for every possible pairing of descriptors. A descriptor in $\mathcal{F}_0$ indexed by (i, j) yields a score map $\mathcal{S}^{i,j} \in \mathbb{R}^{h \times w}$ as it matches with every descriptors in $\mathcal{F}_1$; that is,

$$\mathcal{S}^{i,j}(p, q) = \tau(\mathcal{F}_0(i, j), \mathcal{F}_1(p, q)),$$

where τ is the correlation score function accepting two descriptor vectors as input arguments. Iterating all possible (i, j), we finally obtain a stack of $h \times w$ score maps that comprise the geometric correlation map $\mathcal{G}$, such that,

$$\mathcal{G} = \{\mathcal{S}^{1,1}, \mathcal{S}^{1,2}, ..., \mathcal{S}^{h,w}\}.$$

For the correlation score function τ, we employ a simple-yet-powerful calculator based on an inner product. If both descriptor vectors indicate a similar direction in d-dimensional space, they are highly correlated and the score converges to one; otherwise, it converges to zero. We additionally apply normalization and zero-out negative values, and finally define:

$$\tau(v_1, v_2) = max(0, \frac{v_1 \cdot v_2}{\|v_1\|\|v_2\|}).$$

Binary Classifier

The geometric correlation map is expected to show specific patterns according to the longitudinal change. Figure 2 visualizes the map in 3-dimensional space as a stack of score maps. The blank spaces in the map indicate no positive correlation while the vivid blue color means a strong correlation. In case the input images do not contain the change (first two rows), the correlation map seems to show high scores along the diagonal line. Otherwise (last two rows), the map tends to present relatively distracted scores.

We attach a binary classifier designed to detect such patterns. We employ a fully convolutional network (FCN) [6] composed of three convolutional layers without padding, and stride equal to one.

4 Experiment

We randomly split total 5,472 image pairs in our dataset into three sets for training (4,370), validation (551), and test (551). The proposed network is trained from scratch in end-to-end manner. Evaluation is conducted on the test set only. All images are normalized and resized to 256×256. The algorithm parameters are empirically fixed as $h = 8$, $w = 8$ and $d = 256$ throughout the experiments.

We compare our technique with recent longitudinal analysis methods. We first construct a baseline method using single stream network: passing the input image pair as a two-channel image, directly followed by FCN without any matching module. To show the effect of the geometric correlation map, we implement another method replacing the map module with channel-wise concatenation [12]. We also reproduce a method based on t-LSTM [11], modified to predict the presence of change instead of disease class.

Table 1 shows the performance comparison evaluated by the area under the ROC curve (AUC) with 95% confidence interval. The baseline method with single stream presents the lowest performance, as it does not contain any explicit design for image matching. The modified LSTM [11] provides almost the same

Table 1. Comparison of area under the ROC curve.

Model	AUC (95% CI)
Two channel (baseline)	0.77 (0.72−0.81)
Two stream + t-LSTM [11]	0.78 (0.72−0.81)
Two stream + channel-wise concatenation [12]	0.82 (0.78−0.86)
Two stream + geometric correlation map (ours)	0.89 (0.86−0.92)

AUC as the baseline method. This is probably because the sequence of two feature maps is too short for the LSTM algorithm, but we rarely consider more than two previous examinations in the routine practice. Channel-wise concatenation [12] shows substantial enhancement compared to the baseline. Separate feature maps through the two identical network streams may give an implicit matching effect even with the simple concatenation strategy. Finally the proposed approach with the geometric correlation map yields outstanding performance with $AUC = 0.89$ (sensitivity $= 0.83$ and specificity $= 0.82$ on Youden's Index) as it employs a proper algorithm to tackle image matching.

Figure 2 shows examples of the geometric correlation map generated by our algorithm. The first and second columns present the input images for previous and current examinations respectively. The lesion in each image is located by the red box. The third column visualize the geometric correlation maps. As mentioned earlier, the maps seem to show specific patterns according to the longitudinal change: concentrated (first two rows, change) vs. distracted (last two rows, no-change). Detailed description is provided for each case with the actual reporting sentences: The first row presents images for the normal chest with *"no significant interval change since last study"*. The case in the second contains *"pulmonary TB (tuberculosis), stable state."* We add the third row to show *"improving state of consolidation"* in the sequential examinations. In the last row, *"increased amount of left pleural effusion"* is demonstrated as the lesion is shown to be aggravated in the current image.

5 Discussion

We present a novel approach to detect the change in a lesion in two longitudinal CXR examinations of a patient. Our method is not limited by pre-defined classes of disease but is designed to sense any substantial changes in the consecutive image pair. This property is an important factor for building a *triage* system to help radiologists with massive CXR reading assignments.

In future work, we will try to improve the detection performance through several approaches: First, we plan to apply a spatial regularization prior to correlation matching. As our current algorithm theoretically allow infeasible twisted matching, we expect the regularization constraint can improve registration quality and help to detect subtle or smaller changes. Next, we hope to enrich our

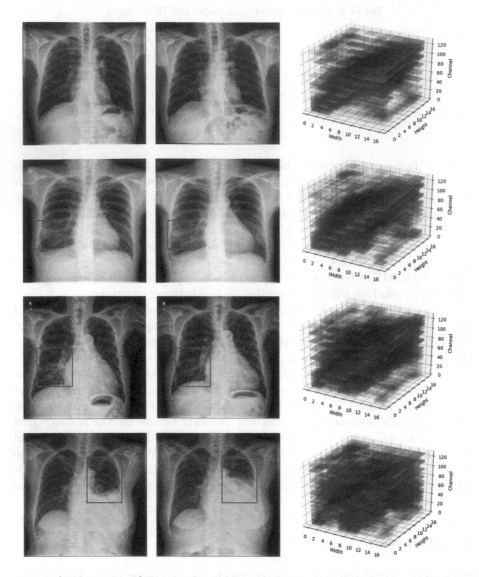

Fig. 2. (Column 1, 2) Images for previous and current examinations. The red box locates the lesion in each image. **(Column 3)** Geometric correlation map visualized by stacked score maps. The blank space indicates no positive correlation while the vivid blue color means a strong correlation. In case the images do not contain the change, the correlation map shows high scores along the diagonal line. Otherwise, the map presents relatively distracted scores. **(Row 1)** Normal chest with *"no significant interval change since last study"*. **(Row 2)** *"pulmonary TB (tuberculosis), stable state"* **(Row 3)** *"improving state of consolidation"*. **(Row 4)** *"increased amount of pleural effusion, left"*. The pleural effusion is shown to be aggravated in the current image. (Color figure online)

database in general. The labeling accuracy can be improved by more sophisticated natural language analysis tools [4]. The number of cases can increase through multi-center study. We also plan to open the database to the public, prepared with a larger size of samples and more accurate labels.

Acknowledgement. This work was supported by the Industrial Strategic technology development program (10072064) funded by the Ministry of Trade, Industry and Energy (MI, Korea) and by grant (no. 13-2019-006) from the SNUBH Research Fund.

References

1. Hu, J., Shen, L., Sun, G.: Squeeze-and-excitation networks. In: The IEEE Conference on Computer Vision and Pattern Recognition (CVPR), June 2018
2. Irvin, J., et al.: CheXpert: a large chest radiograph dataset with uncertainty labels and expert comparison. arXiv preprint arXiv:1901.07031 (2019)
3. Jaeger, S., Candemir, S., Antani, S., Wáng, Y.X.J., Lu, P.X., Thoma, G.: Two public chest X-ray datasets for computer-aided screening of pulmonary diseases. Quant. Imaging Med. Surg. **4**(6), 475 (2014)
4. Joulin, A., Grave, E., Bojanowski, P., Mikolov, T.: Bag of tricks for efficient text classification. In: Proceedings of the 15th Conference of the European Chapter of the Association for Computational Linguistics: Volume 2, Short Papers, pp. 427–431. Association for Computational Linguistics, April 2017
5. Lakhani, P., Sundaram, B.: Deep learning at chest radiography: automated classification of pulmonary tuberculosis by using convolutional neural networks. Radiology **284**(2), 574–582 (2017)
6. Long, J., Shelhamer, E., Darrell, T.: Fully convolutional networks for semantic segmentation. In: Proceedings of the IEEE Conference on Computer Vision and Pattern Recognition, pp. 3431–3440 (2015)
7. Nam, J.G., et al.: Development and validation of deep learning-based automatic detection algorithm for malignant pulmonary nodules on chest radiographs. Radiology 180237 (2018)
8. Rajpurkar, P., et al.: CheXnet: radiologist-level pneumonia detection on chest X-rays with deep learning. arXiv preprint arXiv:1711.05225 (2017)
9. Rocco, I., Arandjelovic, R., Sivic, J.: Convolutional neural network architecture for geometric matching. In: Proceedings of the CVPR, vol. 2 (2017)
10. Rocco, I., Arandjelovic, R., Sivic, J.: End-to-end weakly-supervised semantic alignment. In: Proceedings of the CVPR (2018)
11. Santeramo, R., Withey, S., Montana, G.: Longitudinal detection of radiological abnormalities with time-modulated LSTM. In: Stoyanov, D., et al. (eds.) DLMIA/ML-CDS -2018. LNCS, vol. 11045, pp. 326–333. Springer, Cham (2018). https://doi.org/10.1007/978-3-030-00889-5_37
12. Setio, A.A.A., et al.: Pulmonary nodule detection in CT images: false positive reduction using multi-view convolutional networks. IEEE Trans. Med. Imaging **35**(5), 1160–1169 (2016)
13. Singh, R., et al.: Deep learning in chest radiography: detection of findings and presence of change. PloS One **13**(10), e0204155 (2018)
14. Wang, F., et al.: Residual attention network for image classification. arXiv preprint arXiv:1704.06904 (2017)

15. Wang, X., Girshick, R., Gupta, A., He, K.: Non-local neural networks. In: The IEEE Conference on Computer Vision and Pattern Recognition (CVPR), vol. 1, p. 4 (2018)
16. Wang, X., Peng, Y., Lu, L., Lu, Z., Bagheri, M., Summers, R.M.: ChestX-ray8: hospital-scale chest X-ray database and benchmarks on weakly-supervised classification and localization of common thorax diseases. In: Proceedings of the IEEE Conference on Computer Vision and Pattern Recognition, pp. 2097–2106 (2017)

Adversarial Pulmonary Pathology Translation for Pairwise Chest X-Ray Data Augmentation

Yunyan Xing[1]([✉]), Zongyuan Ge[1]([✉]), Rui Zeng[1], Dwarikanath Mahapatra[2], Jarrel Seah[1], Meng Law[1], and Tom Drummond[1]

[1] Monash University, Melbourne, Australia
{yunyan.xing,zongyuan.ge}@monash.edu
[2] IBM Research, Melbourne, Australia

Abstract. Recent works show that Generative Adversarial Networks (GANs) can be successfully applied to chest X-ray data augmentation for lung disease recognition. However, the implausible and distorted pathology features generated from the less than perfect generator may lead to wrong clinical decisions. Why not keep the original pathology region? We proposed a novel approach that allows our generative model to generate high quality plausible images that contain undistorted pathology areas. The main idea is to design a training scheme based on an image-to-image translation network to introduce variations of new lung features around the pathology ground-truth area. Moreover, our model is able to leverage both annotated disease images and unannotated healthy lung images for the purpose of generation. We demonstrate the effectiveness of our model on two tasks: (i) we invite certified radiologists to assess the quality of the generated synthetic images against real and other state-of-the-art generative models, and (ii) data augmentation to improve the performance of disease localisation.

1 Introduction

Chest X-ray images are the most commonly used method for lung disease diagnosis. Nowadays, deep learning neural network models are available for investigation of classification, segmentation and other problems in medical imaging [3,4,12]. With the rapid growth in the number of X-ray images needed to be reviewed by radiologists in the hospital, building deep learning models as

This research was supported by the Australian Research Council Centre of Excellence for Robotic Vision (project number CE140100016).
Y. Xing and Z. Ge—Equal contribution authors.

Electronic supplementary material The online version of this chapter (https://doi.org/10.1007/978-3-030-32226-7_84) contains supplementary material, which is available to authorized users.

computer-aided diagnosis tools that quickly and accurately detect the pathology area can help reduce the workload of radiologists. Training a robust deep learning model requires a large number of high quality samples with accurate pathology information. However, it is difficult to obtain enough medical images because many diseases are rare.

Generative Adversarial Networks (GANs) [6] have become a new technique to perform data augmentation. Compared with the traditional mathematical data augmentation methods, such as rotations, translations, reflections and adding Gaussian noise [9], the advantage of GANs is that the models can generate new synthetic data with much larger diversity. Various GAN models have been proposed to generate synthetic images for data augmentation. Image-to-image translation models such as StarGAN [1] and CycleGAN [14] have been applied on CelebA [10] to generate new face images. DCGAN [11] has been applied in the chest X-ray imaging domain to perform data augmentation, showing improvement in disease classification accuracy [5,12].

Although the discussed data augmentation methods can improve recognition performance for some tasks, it is difficult to explain whether the augmented images benefit the model regularisation or discrimination. This is because medical images generated by DCGAN do not look visually plausible and vital disease features are missing. This would not be an issue for a general dataset such as ImageNet [2] or a face dataset such as CelebA, because deep learning models can make correct decisions based on the overall and contextual features. However, in the medical domain, clear and distinguishable biomarkers and pathological evidence are crucial to driving clinical decisions. To the best of our knowledge, none of the aforementioned GAN models can fully retain undistorted pathology areas for newly generated images.

To address the above issues, we employ an idea similar to image inpainting by generating regions around the undistorted pathology area with a pairwise image-to-image translation (Pix2Pix) model [8]. We leverage the limited number of bounding box labelled pathology data and unlabelled healthy data from the NIH Chest X-ray dataset [13] to create a set of artificial paired training images to fit into the training process of the Pix2Pix model. Our proposed approach is shown in Fig. 1. The generated chest X-ray images from our proposed method contain visually plausible lung structures and pathology evidence. We validate and show the superior performance of our model through two experiments: (i) a radiologist assessment test and (ii) data augmentation for lung disease localisation.

2   Methodology

2.1   Image-to-Image Translation with GANs

Recent work in generative adversarial networks (GANs) have achieved impressive results on image generation by using image-to-image translation [1,8]. Image-to-image translation learns a mapping from an input image x to a target output image y. Our target is to generate new disease training samples $\tilde{x}$ stemming from the original samples x via the image-to-image translation framework. In this work, we use Pix2Pix GAN as our main image generation framework.

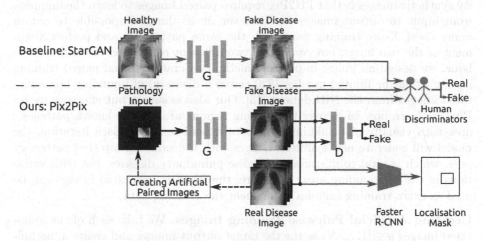

Fig. 1. The black arrows indicate the training process: for StarGAN (top), which is our baseline, the generator is given unpaired chest X-ray images to perform healthy image to diseased image translation. For our proposed Pix2Pix model (bottom), the generator is given an input image with the masked pathology area and is trained to produce a complete X-ray image with the surrounding lung details. The red arrows indicate the evaluation process: we invite two radiologists to act as 'human discriminators' to assess the quality of our synthetic images. We also use a Faster R-CNN model to measure the performance of our approach on data augmentation for disease localisation. (Color figure online)

Pix2Pix GAN Loss. The loss function for Pix2Pix consists of two parts. The first part is the adversarial loss, which is for the discriminator D to ensure the synthetic image $\tilde{x} = G(x)$ generated by the generator can be distinguished from the original target real image y. Further, the generator G is trained to minimise the adversarial loss to make the synthetic image more plausible. Therefore, D and G update iteratively against each other with the following objective function:

$$L_{GAN}(G, D) = \mathbb{E}_{x,y}[\log D(x, y)] + \mathbb{E}_x[\log(1 - D(x, G(x)))], \tag{1}$$

where G is trying to minimise this objective against D, which tries to maximise it. [8]. In addition, the Pix2Pix model includes a traditional construction loss, L1 distance, to ensure the quality of generated synthetic images:

$$L_{L1}(G) = \mathbb{E}_{x,y}[\||y - G(x)\||_1]. \tag{2}$$

Therefore, the full objective function for Pix2Pix is:

$$G^*, D^* = \arg \min_G \max_D L_{GAN}(G, D) + \lambda L_{L1}(G). \tag{3}$$

2.2 Pulmonary Pathology Data Augmentation

The key feature that makes the Pix2Pix model powerful in generating high quality synthetic images is that Pix2Pix requires paired images to learn the mapping from input to output images [8]. However, it is almost impossible to obtain many chest X-ray training pairs with the same patient ID and perfect alignment of the two lungs, but containing two different conditions. To address this issue, we design an image in-painting method to craft artificial paired training images using the limited number (820 across 6 diseases) of bounding box annotated images from the NIH dataset [13]. Our idea is simple but effective: we let Pix2Pix learn how to recover the missing regions around the known pathology area with visually plausible image structures and textures. Each iteration, the model will generate new synthetic images with the same undistorted pathology area, which is vital to diagnose or localise pulmonary diseases, but with variations in the surrounding area. Therefore, the Pix2Pix generated images can be used as extra training samples to augment the training data.

Creating Artificial Pairwise Training Images. We take each of the annotated images $y \in [1, ..., N]$ as the the target output images and create a 'pathology area only' image x with binary image mask m. Input image x is constructed from the raw images as $x \leftarrow y \odot m$. Mask m replaces the area outside the bounding box with zero values, keeping the area inside the mask unchanged. We use this 'pathology area only' image x and the corresponding original image y to create a training pair (x, y). This allows us to perform image-to-image translation on the pairwise images.

Training Pix2Pix with Artificial Training Pairs. During training, we pre-process the data to prepare training pairs (x, y). Generator G takes x as input, and outputs predicted image $x' = G(x)$ with the same size as the input. Combining image x' with the input image x, we get the new output $\tilde{x} \leftarrow x + G(x) \odot (1 - m)$. Then we train the discriminator with the adversarial loss to try to distinguish between the generated image $\tilde{x}$ and the real image y. We step the gradient descent algorithm on the discriminator and generator alternatively. The training procedure is shown in Algorithm 1. This training scheme means that the vital pulmonary pathology features from the original image bounding box are undistorted and well-retained in the generated synthetic images. This lowers the difficulty of the generator training. After employing our training technique, the generator only needs to learn how to reconstruct the surrounding lung features outside of the pathology area.

Adding Unannotated Healthy Samples. The primary goal of our Pix2Pix model is to retain undistorted pathology area and to train the generative model only to learn how to generate the lung features. To further extend the number of training samples, we discover that adding normal healthy lung X-ray images with random cropping areas into the training set can increase the quality of the synthetic images. By following the same training procedure in Algorithm 1, we add an extra 2,000 healthy lung X-ray images $\hat{y}$ and randomly generate masks

Algorithm 1. Training of pulmonary pathology data augmentation.

1: **while** G has not converged **do**
2:    **for** $i = 1, ... N$ **do**
3:        Sample target images y_i from the data with bounding box annotation;
4:        Extract masks m_i for y_i according to annotations;
5:        Construct inputs $x_i \leftarrow y_i \odot m_i$;
6:        Craft training pairs (x_i, y_i);
7:        Get predictions $\tilde{x}_i \leftarrow x_i + G(x_i) \odot (1 - m_i)$;
8:        Calculate gradients for G and D;
9:        Update G, D;

$\hat{m}$ with reasonable size. Healthy pairwise images $(\hat{x} \leftarrow \hat{y} \odot \hat{m}, \hat{y})$ are sampled along with disease images in Line 3 of Algorithm 1.

| Real | StarGAN | Pix2Pix | Pix2Pix-N |

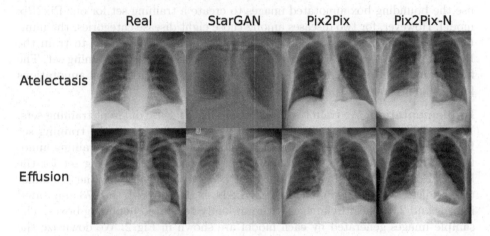

Fig. 2. Samples of real images and synthetic images generated by StarGAN and our models (Pix2Pix and Pix2Pix-N).

Comparing with StarGAN. In this paper, we compare our proposed generative method to another image-to-image translation GAN, StarGAN [1], which is based on CycleGAN [14]. The main advantage of either CycleGAN or StarGAN is that they can be trained using unpaired images. Bounding box annotations are not required to translate an image with a given disease label into other disease labels. The unique features belonging to a certain category are supposed to be learned implicitly during model training. Since the generator G and discriminator D are less than perfect, the structure and texture information of some pulmonary disease translations are not always correct, especially for diseases that have high intra-class variations, such as Pneumonia. This approach works well on tasks such as face generation; people are capable of recognising the identity in the generated image even with some misleading contents. However, this may lead to a catastrophic outcome when a deadly disease can not be recognised because of blurry or inaccurate generated pathology evidences. This is the reason we propose the generating mechanism to keep the most vital pathology information undistorted. The pairwise training requirement of PixPix guarantees the 'upper bound' that CycleGAN can achieve [14]. The training and evaluation procedures for our Pix2Pix model are shown in Fig. 1.

3   Experiments

Dataset. We use the NIH Chest X-ray dataset [13], which is by far the largest publicly available chest X-ray dataset. It consists of 112,120 frontal-view chest X-ray images with 14 disease categories and the healthy category. Each image is labelled with one or multiple diseases. The dataset also contains 984 bounding box annotations for 880 images corresponding to eight disease categories. We use the bounding box annotated images to create a training set for our Pix2Pix model. However, for two diseases among those eight disease categories, the number of bounding box annotations is too little and is not sufficient to train the Pix2Pix model. As such, we remove those two diseases from our training set. The final training set we use for our model contains 820 bounding box annotations for 741 images over six pathologies.

Implementation. We train two Pix2Pix models that use different training sets. We use 70% of the original 820 bounding box annotations as the training set for our Pix2Pix models and localisation model, amounting to 573 training annotations. The remaining 30% of annotations are used as the testing set for the localisation model. Our first model, **Pix2Pix**, is trained with only the 573 annotated images. Our second model, **Pix2Pix-N**, is trained with the 573 annotated images and 2,000 healthy images with randomly generated bounding boxes. The sample images generated by each model are shown in Fig. 2. We downsize the original images from 1024×1024 to 256×256 for fast processing. We also apply mathematical transformations, including rotations, reflections and cropping, to add variation into the network.

3.1   Qualitative Analysis

We invite two clinicians, R1 and R2[1] to verify the quality of the synthetic images generated by our proposed models. To compare the performance of our Pix2Pix models to other generative models, we use StarGAN as a baseline. We provide the radiologists with a verification set contains six pathologies with 100 images each. The verification set is comprised of 150 real images from the NIH dataset and

---

[1] R1 is a certified radiologist with 10 years of experience. R2 is a radiology registrar who also has two years of experience with deep learning. To ensure fairness, all of the real and generated images are cropped to remove most of the artefacts and downsized to 224×224. The radiologists are not aware of the disease prevalence or the proportion of real and fake images in the test set. The radiologists are asked to work independently to distinguish whether each image is real or fake.

three sets of 150 images generated by each of the generative models (**StarGAN**, **Pix2Pix** and **Pix2Pix-N**).

Figure 2 shows qualitative illustrations and Table 1 shows the number of images that the radiologists identify as real from each source. From Table 1, we observe that both R1 and R2 are good at picking real chest X-ray images. It is found that either Pix2Pix or Pix2Pix-N surpasses StarGAN by a large margin (15|0 vs. 108|45). This shows: (1) the merits of keeping undistorted pathology information, and (2) Pix2Pix based models produce plausible reconstructions of the surrounding lung features. Pix2Pix-N performs better than Pix2Pix, showing the necessity to include more healthy images for model generalisation. Finally, R2 is better than R1 at recognising the generated images as fake. This is likely because R2 has two years of research experience with GANs and is good at recognising GAN artefacts.

Table 1. Radiologist assessment results. The two values for each element are the number of images predicted as real by R1|R2, respectively. For the generative models (StarGAN, Pix2Pix and Pix2Pix-N), larger values indicate better performance.

Pathology	Real data	StarGAN	Pix2Pix	Pix2Pix-N
Atelectasis	25|25	2|0	12|2	19|6
Cardiomegaly	25|25	2|0	18|4	21|8
Effusion	25|24	5|0	11|3	17|6
Infiltration	25|25	6|0	11|3	18|10
Pneumonia	25|25	0|0	14|4	19|11
Pneumothorax	25|25	0|0	13|2	14|4
Total	150|149	15|0	79|18	108|45

3.2   Disease Localisation

In this section, we investigate the effectiveness of synthetic images generated by our proposed model on the task of pathology localisation. A Faster-RCNN [7] built on InceptionV2-ResNet is used as the detection model. We train the detection model using three different dataset augmentation protocols: original (**Ori**), **Ori+Pix2Pix**, and **Ori+Pix2Pix-N**. Ori uses the original images (573 in total) from the NIH dataset. Ori+Pix2Pix contains all real images and 688 synthetic images obtained from our Pix2Pix model. Ori+Pix2Pix-N is composed of all real images and 688 synthetic images obtained from our Pix2Pix-N model. For fair comparison, all protocols use the same parameters to perform the Faster-RCNN training. Specifically, all datasets are resized to 256×256 without any further augmentation. The learning rate is 0.0003 and the batch size for each training step is 2. The evaluation dataset consists of 247 real images. To clearly observe the trends of the performance of each dataset, correct location (CL) accuracy computed at an intersection over union (IoU) of 0.1 is chosen as the evaluation metric, as per [13]. To reduce the chance of performance oscillation, the results reported at a given training step s are selected from the best model in a step range $[s - 500, s + 500]$.

Table 2. Disease Localisation results of Ori, Ori+Pix2Pix, Ori+Pix2Pix-N datasets. $CL@_s^{0.1}$ is the best correct location accuracy computed at an IoU of 0.1 and selected from $[s - 500, s + 500]$ steps.

Pathology	Ori			Ori+Pix2Pix			Ori+Pix2Pix-N		
	$CL@_{5k}^{0.1}$	$CL@_{10k}^{0.1}$	$CL@_{15k}^{0.1}$	$CL@_{5k}^{0.1}$	$CL@_{10k}^{0.1}$	$CL@_{15k}^{0.1}$	$CL@_{5k}^{0.1}$	$CL@_{10k}^{0.1}$	$CL@_{15k}^{0.1}$
Atelectasis	0	0	0.018	0	0	0	0	0.018	0.111
Cardiomegaly	0.636	0.818	0.818	0.613	0.750	0.681	**0.636**	**0.840**	**0.863**
Effusion	0.173	0.217	0.304	0.173	0.195	0.130	**0.239**	**0.282**	**0.326**
Infiltration	0.378	0.432	0.459	0.297	0.351	0.324	**0.405**	**0.513**	**0.594**
Pneumonia	**0.333**	0.305	0.305	0.194	0.250	0.277	0.166	**0.361**	**0.527**
Pneumothorax	0.031	0.033	0.066	0	0	0.033	**0.033**	**0.033**	**0.100**
Total	**0.259**	0.301	0.328	0.213	0.234	0.233	0.235	**0.323**	**0.405**

Table 2 shows the disease localisation performance. The synthetic augmentation protocol **Ori+Pix2Pix-N** performs the best among all three datasets in terms of model performance and convergence. It significantly improves the disease localisation accuracy and convergence speed of the Faster-RCNN model. We conjecture that images generated from pathology annotated images and healthy images explicitly carry useful pathology information from the real data distribution, which is crucial for deep model localisation training. The **Ori+Pix2Pix** performed the worst among three training strategies. This is probably because synthetic disease images overfit the model training and increase the data bias.

4   Conclusion

In this paper, we proposed a model to perform data augmentation on pairwise chest X-ray images by using an image-to-image translation model (Pix2Pix). Our approach is able to generate high quality and plausible synthetic images with undistorted pathology areas, which is crucial for disease diagnosis and pathology area localisation. Our experimental results show that the synthetic images generated by our model are of a greater quality than those generated by Star-GAN and can significantly improve the performance of a deep learning disease localisation model on unseen data.

References

1. Choi, Y., Choi, M., Kim, M., Ha, J.W., Kim, S., Choo, J.: StarGAN: unified generative adversarial networks for multi-domain image-to-image translation. In: CVPR (2018)
2. Deng, J., Dong, W., Socher, R., Li, L.J., Li, K., Fei-Fei, L.: ImageNet: a large-scale hierarchical image database. In: CVPR (2009)
3. Eaton-Rosen, Z., Bragman, F., Ourselin, S., Cardoso, M.J.: Improving data augmentation for medical image segmentation. In: MIDL (2018)
4. Esteva, A., et al.: Dermatologist-level classification of skin cancer with deep neural networks. Nature **542**(7639), 115 (2017)
5. Frid-Adar, M., Klang, E., Amitai, M., Goldberger, J., Greenspan, H.: Synthetic data augmentation using GAN for improved liver lesion classification. In: ISBI (2018)
6. Goodfellow, I., et al.: Generative adversarial nets. In: NIPS (2014)
7. He, K., Gkioxari, G., Dollár, P., Girshick, R.: Mask R-CNN. In: ICCV (2017)
8. Isola, P., Zhu, J.Y., Zhou, T., Efros, A.A.: Image-to-image translation with conditional adversarial networks. In: CVPR (2017)
9. Krizhevsky, A., Sutskever, I., Hinton, G.E.: Imagenet classification with deep convolutional neural networks. In: NIPS (2012)
10. Liu, Z., Luo, P., Wang, X., Tang, X.: Deep learning face attributes in the wild. In: ICCV (2015)
11. Radford, A., Metz, L., Chintala, S.: Unsupervised representation learning with deep convolutional generative adversarial networks. arXiv preprint arXiv:1511.06434 (2015)
12. Salehinejad, H., Valaee, S., Dowdell, T., Colak, E., Barfett, J.: Generalization of deep neural networks for chest pathology classification in x-rays using generative adversarial networks. In: ICASSP (2018)
13. Wang, X., Peng, Y., Lu, L., Lu, Z., Bagheri, M., Summers, R.M.: Chestx-ray8: hospital-scale chest x-ray database and benchmarks on weakly-supervised classification and localization of common thorax diseases. In: CVPR (2017)
14. Zhu, J.Y., Park, T., Isola, P., Efros, A.A.: Unpaired image-to-image translation using cycle-consistent adversarial networks. In: ICCV (2017)

Semi-supervised Learning by Disentangling and Self-ensembling over Stochastic Latent Space

Prashnna Kumar Gyawali, Zhiyuan Li$^{(\boxtimes)}$, Sandesh Ghimire, and Linwei Wang

Rochester Institute of Technology, Rochester, NY, USA
{pkg2182,zl7904,sg9872,lxwast}@rit.edu

Abstract. The success of deep learning in medical imaging is mostly achieved at the cost of a large labeled data set. Semi-supervised learning (SSL) provides a promising solution by leveraging the structure of unlabeled data to improve learning from a small set of labeled data. Self-ensembling is a simple approach used in SSL to encourage consensus among ensemble predictions of unknown labels, improving generalization of the model by making it more insensitive to the latent space. Currently, such an ensemble is obtained by randomization such as dropout regularization and random data augmentation. In this work, we hypothesize – from the generalization perspective – that self-ensembling can be improved by exploiting the stochasticity of a disentangled latent space. To this end, we present a stacked SSL model that utilizes unsupervised disentangled representation learning as the stochastic embedding for self-ensembling. We evaluate the presented model for multi-label classification using chest X-ray images, demonstrating its improved performance over related SSL models as well as the interpretability of its disentangled representations.

Keywords: Semi-supervised learning · Self-ensembling · Disentangled representation learning

1 Introduction

While deep learning has seen tremendous successes in a variety of medical image analysis problems [9], many of these successes are achieved at the cost of a large labeled data set. Labeling a large collection of data however requires substantial human and financial resources, creating a primary hurdle to the wide-spread adoption of deep learning in clinical practice [9]. Semi-supervised learning (SSL) provides a promising solution by leveraging the structure of unlabeled data to improve the learning from a small set of labeled data [6,8].

Among existing SSL methods, self-ensembling is a simple approach that encourages consensus among ensemble predictions of unknown labels [8]. Such

---

P. K. Gyawali and Z. Li—Both authors contributed equally to this work.

© Springer Nature Switzerland AG 2019
D. Shen et al. (Eds.): MICCAI 2019, LNCS 11769, pp. 766–774, 2019.
https://doi.org/10.1007/978-3-030-32226-7_85

ensemble predictions can be formed by randomization such as network regularization (*e.g.*, dropout) and random input augmentation [8]. As later rationalized in [5], based on the analytical learning theory, these randomization techniques are critical as they improve the generalization of the model by making it more *insensitive* to the latent space. From this theoretical perspective, it is natural to hypothesize that the design of this randomization will benefit from the knowledge of the latent space, especially its stochasticity. This however is not considered in existing works. The input augmentation functions, for instance, are typically hand-crafted considering random translations or rotations of images [8], with little consideration to the distribution of latent variables.

In parallel, advances in representation learning – especially that of the variational auto-encoder (VAE) – has allowed us to infer posterior distributions of the latent variables in an unsupervised manner [7]. In the classic semi-supervised deep generative model presented in [6], it has also been shown that such an unsupervised embedding can largely facilitate the subsequent SSL training by providing a disentangled and thereby more separable latent space [6].

In this paper, drawing on the analytical learning theory [5], we rationalize that (1) disentangling and (2) self-ensembling over the stochastic latent space will improve the generalization ability of the model. Based on this rationale, we investigate using unsupervised disentangled representation learning as the stochastic input embedding in self-ensembling. The presented SSL model consists of a VAE-based unsupervised embedding of the data, followed by a semi-supervised self-ensembling network utilizing the stochastic embedding as the inherent random augmentation of the inputs. We evaluate the presented SSL model on the recently open-sourced Chexpert data set for *multi-label* classification of thoracic disease using chest X-rays [4]. To demonstrate the benefits gained by exploiting the stochastic latent space in self-ensembling, we compare the performance of the presented method with the standard self-ensembling method considering different image-level input augmentation methods [8], VAE-based embedding with and without a subsequent deep generative SSL [6], along with a generative adversarial network (GAN)-based SSL [11]. We further qualitatively demonstrate the disentangled representation obtained via unsupervised embedding, and discuss its use for data analysis and model interpretability.

2   Related Work

This work is mostly related to two lines of research: (1) SSL based on regularization with random transformations, and (2) disentangled representation learning and its use in SSL. In the former, consistency-based regularization is applied on ensemble predictions obtained by randomization techniques such as random data augmentation, dropout, and random max-pooling [8]. This randomization was empirically shown to improve the generalization and stability of the SSL model, while its theoretical basis was recently shown to be related to the reduction of model sensitivity to the latent space [3,5]. Motivated by this theory, in this work, we attempt to utilize the knowledge about the stochastic latent space – obtained in unsupervised learning – in this randomization process.

In the latter representation learning, deep neural networks have been combined with variational inference to jointly realize generative modeling of unlabeled data and posterior inference of latent variables [7]. Furthermore, the learned latent representations are encouraged to be semantically interpretable and mutually invariant, which is empirically shown to be useful for the downstream tasks [6]. For instance, an unsupervised VAE was used to provide a disentangled embedding (M1) for a subsequent VAE-based semi-supervised model (M2), commonly known as the M1+M2 model [6]. In this work, we make the first attempt to use the analytical learning theory to support the effect a disentangled embedding can have on the generalization ability of a model. Furthermore, we improve the M1+M2 model by replacing M2 with a self-ensembling SSL network, taking VAE's ability to model stochastic latent space to support self-ensembling.

Besides the approaches discussed above, there is also an active line of research in GAN-based SSL methods [10,11]. The general idea is to add a classification objective to the original mini-max game and increases the capacity of the discriminator to associate the inputs to the corresponding labels. The presented work differs from this line of research by the emphasis on obtaining, regularizing, and interpreting the latent representations in SSL.

An increased interest in SSL has also been seen in medical image analysis. The use of an unsupervised representation learning for better generalization has been investigated for the task of myocardial segmentation [2]. In [10], SSL was used in a similar X-ray data set, although the scope was limited to binary classifications between normal and abnormal categories. To our knowledge, we present the first multi-label SSL that investigates disentangled learning and self-ensembling of stochastic latent space in medical image classification.

3   Model

We consider training data $\mathcal{D} = \mathcal{D}_l \cup \mathcal{D}_u$, where $\mathcal{D}_l = \{\mathbf{x}_i, \mathbf{y}_i\}_{i=1}^{N_l}$ is the labeled set and $\mathcal{D}_u = \{\mathbf{x}_j\}_{j=1}^{N_u}$ the unlabeled set. As outlined in Fig. 1, a stochastic latent space will be learned in an unsupervised and disentangled manner (Sect. 3.1), which will then be regularized via self-ensembling for SSL (Sect. 3.2).

3.1   Unsupervised and Disentangled Learning of Stochastic Latent Space

To disentangle and obtain the posterior distribution in the latent space, we first utilize a VAE for unsupervised learning of the generative factors in the data. We assume data $\mathbf{x}$ to be generated by a likelihood $p_\theta(\mathbf{x}|\mathbf{z})$, involving a latent variable $\mathbf{z}$ with a certain prior distribution $p(\mathbf{z})$. Given the intractability of exact posterior inference, a distribution $q_\phi(\mathbf{z}|\mathbf{x})$ is introduced to approximate the true posterior $p(\mathbf{z}|\mathbf{x})$ using variational inference [7]. Both the approximated posterior $q_\phi(\mathbf{z}|\mathbf{x})$ and the likelihood $p_\theta(\mathbf{x}|\mathbf{z})$ are parameterized by deep neural networks.

The VAE is trained by maximizing the variational evidence lower bound of the marginal likelihood of the training data with respect to parameters θ and ϕ:

$$\log p(\mathbf{x}) \geq \mathcal{L} = \mathbb{E}_{q_\phi(\mathbf{z}|\mathbf{x})}[\log p_\theta(\mathbf{x}|\mathbf{z})] - KL(q_\phi(\mathbf{z}|\mathbf{x})||p(\mathbf{z})) \qquad (1)$$

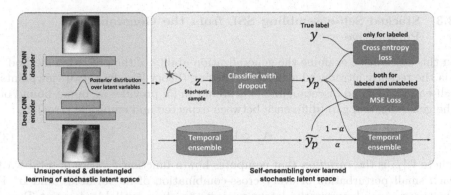

Fig. 1. Schematic diagram of the presented model.

where the first term can be interpreted as minimizing the reconstruction error, and the second term regularizes the learned posterior density $q_\phi(\mathbf{z}|\mathbf{x})$ by a prior $p(\mathbf{z})$ via the Kullback-Leibler (KL) divergence measure. We set the prior $p(\mathbf{z})$ to be an isotropic Gaussian which, through mutually independent latent dimensions, encourages disentangled latent representations in $q_\phi(\mathbf{z}|\mathbf{x})$ [7].

3.2   Regularizing the Stochastic Latent Space via Self-ensemble SSL

The unsupervised VAE embedding is then used as the input to a self-ensembling SSL model which, on unsupervised targets, applies coherence-based regularization to form consensus among ensemble predictions. For each training sample $\mathbf{x}^{(i)}$, its ensemble predictions are obtained from three sources:

1. Sampling from VAE-learned posterior density $q(\mathbf{z}^{(i)}|\mathbf{x}^{(i)})$. This utilizes a distribution learned from unlabeled data to replace the commonly-used hand-crafted augmentation functions to perturb $\mathbf{x}^{(i)}$ [8].
2. Network dropout that randomly neglects some units and utilizes a subnetwork during training.
3. Temporal ensemble [8] achieved by accumulating the predicted label $\mathbf{y}_p$ after every training epoch into an ensemble output $\tilde{\mathbf{y}}_p$ by $\tilde{\mathbf{y}}_p \leftarrow \alpha\tilde{\mathbf{y}}_p + (1-\alpha)\mathbf{y}_p$, where α controls how far the ensemble reaches into training history.

Given each pair of ensemble predictions $\mathbf{y}_p$ and $\tilde{\mathbf{y}}_p$, the network is trained, in each batch B, with the objective of minimizing the ensemble loss $\mathcal{L}^e$:

$$\mathcal{L}^e = \underbrace{\frac{1}{|B|} \sum_{n \sim (B \cap \mathcal{D}_l)} \sum_{l=1}^{L} \left[-y_{n,l} \log f(y_{n,p}|q(\mathbf{z}|\mathbf{x})) \right]}_{\text{only for labeled}} + \underbrace{\zeta \cdot \frac{1}{|B|} \sum_{n \sim B} \left\| \mathbf{y}_p - \tilde{\mathbf{y}}_p \right\|^2}_{\text{both for labeled and unlabeled}} \quad (2)$$

where the first term corresponds to the standard cross entropy loss and is evaluated for labeled data. The second term is evaluated for all data, encouraging consensus among ensemble predictions via mean squared loss. A ramp-up weighted function, starting from zero, is used for ζ as described in [8].

3.3   Stacked Self-ensembling SSL from the Generalization Perspective

In this section, we examine the generalization ability of the presented method – via the recently introduced analytical learning theory [5] – from two viewpoints: self-ensembling and disentangling. Theorem 1 in [5] provides an upper bound on the generalization gap (difference between expected and empirical error) Δ_g:

$$\Delta_g \leq V[f] \cdot \mathbb{D}^* \tag{3}$$

where $V[f]$ is the *variation* that computes how a function f varies in total w.r.t each small perturbation of every cross-combination of its variables, and $\mathbb{D}^*$ is the *discrepancy* between the latent projections of an available data set $\mathcal{D}$ and true data distribution. In our case, f is the composition of the loss function ℓ of coherence-based regularization and the mapping function f_y between stochastic latent sample $\mathbf{z}$ and the prediction $\mathbf{y}_p$, *i.e.*, $f = \ell \circ f_y$. Here, we rationalize how the presented method decreases the generalization gap by decreasing $V[f_y]$.

Self-ensembling: The second regularization term in (2) can be re-written over the input samples drawn from the posterior density $q(\mathbf{z}|\mathbf{x})$ from VAE embedding:

$$\ell = \int_{\mathbf{z_1}, \mathbf{z_2}} \left\| f_y(\mathbf{z_1}) - f_y(\mathbf{z_2}) \right\|^2 dP(\mathbf{z_1}, \mathbf{z_2}|\mathbf{x})$$

where $P(\mathbf{z_1}, \mathbf{z_2}|\mathbf{x}) = q(\mathbf{z_1}|\mathbf{x})q(\mathbf{z_2}|\mathbf{x})$. Minimizing this loss explicitly requires f_y to be more insensitive over the space of $\mathbf{z}$ which implicitly minimizes $V[f_y]$ and thus the bound on the generalization gap.

Disentangling: Given representation $(\mathbf{z}_y, \mathbf{z}_o)$ where $\mathbf{z}_y$ and $\mathbf{z}_o$ are respectively the latent variables related and unrelated to $\mathbf{y}$. Based on [5], the *variation* $V[f_y]$ is minimal when the mapping f_y from latent space $(\mathbf{z}_y, \mathbf{z}_o)$ is invariant over $\mathbf{z}_o$. A disentangled latent space by design thereby reduces the generalization gap.

4   Experiments

Data and Model Architecture: We evaluated the presented model on the recently open-sourced Chexpert data set that has strong reference standards compared to other similar large-scale chest X-ray data set [4]. It consists of 224,316 chest radiographs from 65,240 patients, with labels for 14 pathology categories extracted from radiology reports. Given uncertainty labels provided for all images, we first removed all uncertain samples from the data set. We also removed all lateral-view samples. Small labeled training sets were then created by balancing among each disease category, ranging from 100 to 500 samples per category. Another 5000 and 50000 samples were randomly selected as the validation and test sets, while the rest were used as unlabeled training data. All images were re-sized to 128×128 in dimension.

The encoder of the VAE had five convolutional layers followed by three fully-connected (FC) layers. The output of the last FC layer was divided into the mean and log variance of the posterior distribution of the latent variables. The decoder is symmetrical to the encoder, with two FC layers followed by five transposed convolutional layers. ReLU activation was used for all the layers, except the last encoder layer that has no activation and the last decoder layer that used sigmoid activation. The self-ensembling network consisted of three FC layers with dropout layers ($p = 0.5$) in between. ReLU activation was used for the first two FC layers, and sigmoid activation for the last one. We use the Adam optimizer throughout all our experiments.

Table 1. Mean AUROC for multi-label classification for 14 pathology categories. trained with a fixed number of unlabeled data and a varying number of labeled data.

Model	Size of labeled data set (k)				
	100	200	300	400	500
VAE embedding	0.5853	0.6119	0.6331	0.6416	0.6556
VAE embedding + SSL (M1 + M2)	0.6080	0.6272	0.6340	0.6390	0.6491
Image-space self-ensemble (with noise)	0.6012	0.6277	0.6444	0.6550	0.6626
Image-space self-ensemble (with augmentation)	0.6089	0.6301	0.6423	0.6530	0.6617
ACGAN	0.5865	0.6036	0.6064	0.6284	0.6372
Latent-space self-ensemble (presented)	**0.6200**	**0.6386**	**0.6484**	**0.6637**	**0.6697**

4.1 Multi-label Semi-supervised Classification

We quantitatively evaluated the SSL performance of the presented model in comparison to existing models as summarized in Table 1. We first trained a classifier (with the same architecture as the self-ensembling network) using the unsupervised VAE embedding on labeled training data (*VAE embedding*). We then considered two most-related models to the presented work: (1) the M1+M2 SSL model where the unsupervised VAE embedding was used to support a subsequent VAE-based SSL model (*VAE embedding + SSL*) [6], and (2) the self-ensembling SSL (with the same architecture as the VAE encoder followed by self-ensemling in the stacked model) with two different types of image-level augmentation: adding Gaussian noises (with $std = 0.15$) or random translation and rotation (maximum 12 pixels and 10°) to the images (*image-space self-ensembling*) [8]. To demonstrate how the presented work relates to GAN-based SSL methods, we also added a comparison to ACGAN [11] that was shown to generate globally coherent and discriminative samples assisting in SSL.

We tested all models on a varying number of labeled training data whilst keeping the number of unlabeled data fixed. Each model was tested on 10 different testing sets (5000 samples each). As shown, the three self-ensembling methods in general achieved better performance. Among the three self-ensembling methods, all the standard deviation is less than 0.008, and the improvement of the presented method over the two baseline self-ensembling methods is statistical significant ($p < 0.05$). This verified our hypothesis that, in comparison to

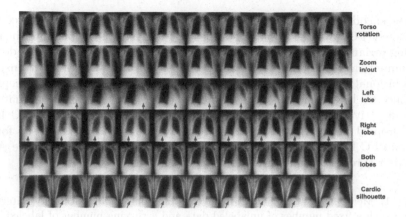

Fig. 2. Images generated by traversing over the [−3, 3] range of a specific latent dimension, based on latent values inferred from a different seed image for each row.

ad-hoc image-level augmentations, utilizing the stochasticity of the latent space can improve the performance of self-ensembling.

It was surprising that ACGAN performed worse (except $k = 100$) than VAE embedding. We speculated that, unlike natural images where ACGAN has seen superior performance, disease-related factors in X-ray images may be more difficult to capture among other disease-irrelevant factors (see Sect. 5).

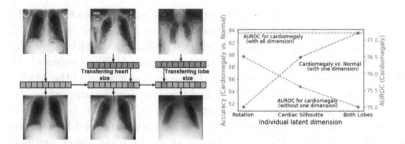

Fig. 3. [Best viewed in color] Left: demonstration of feature transfer by exchanging specific latent units. Top row: original images. Bottom row: reconstructed with original or exchanged latent codes. Right: Discriminative power of individual latent dimensions.

4.2   Interpreting the Disentangled Latent Representations

We then qualitatively evaluated the stochastic latent variables learned from the VAE. As shown in Fig. 2, as we traversed along a particular latent dimension and kept the others fixed, we were able to generate images reflecting changes in a particular semantic factor. With this knowledge, in Fig. 3 (left), we demonstrated that it is possible to transfer specific features (such as heart size and lobe size) between X-ray images by swapping the corresponding latent units.

In an attempt to quantify how these unsupervised disentangled representations may affect downstream classification tasks, we considered the pathology of cardiomegaly as an example which is reflected as changes in heart-chest ratio in X-ray images [1]. We built a binary classifier between the category of cardiomegaly and no-finding, *considering only one of the learned latent units at a time*. We randomly sampled respectively 500, 1000 and 2000 images that had either cardiomegaly or no-finding labels for training, validation, and testing. As shown in Fig. 3 (right: red curve), the more a specific unit captured the heart-chest ratio, the more discriminative it was for detecting cardiomegaly. We also re-trained the presented model (for k = 500) by removing one latent unit at a time, and evaluated the resulting AUROC for cardiomegaly. Similarly (Fig. 3 (right: blue curve)), the more a specific unit captured the heart-chest ratio, the larger its removal caused the drop in AUROC. These results suggest that improved disentangling in the latent representations may facilitate down-stream classification tasks as well as increase the interpretability of the results.

5   Conclusions and Discussion

We presented a stacked SSL method that uses unsupervised disentangling of the stochastic latent space as the input randomization in self-ensembling. From the analytical learning theory, we rationalized the effect of disentangling and self-ensembling over the latent space on the generalizability of the model. Empirically, we demonstrated both the quantitative improvement of the presented model in SSL and the interpretability of its disentangled representations.

We noted that, compared to many visual benchmark data sets, disease-specific factors in medical images may be buried by other more significant factors of variations in terms of contribution to pixel reconstruction or image distribution (*e.g.*, heart-chest ratio *vs.* torso shape). For instance, we attempted to remove the inactive dimensions (defined as $A_u < 10^{-2}$ where $A_u = Cov_x(\mathbb{E}_{u \sim q(u|x)}[u])$ for each dimension u in $\mathbf{z}$) from VAE embedding, a strategy shown to improve the performance of the M1+M2 model in visual benchmarks [6]. The mean AUROC of the presented model, however, decreased around 2% to 0.658 (for $k = 500$). This, we believe, may explain the relatively limited progress of unsupervised representation learning in medical images despite its recent traction in other visual domains, a pressing challenge to be resolved in order to leverage unlabeled data in a field where image labeling is especially costly and difficult. For future work, we plan to improve two-stage training strategy and disentangling by hierarchical generative models.

Acknowledgement. This work is supported by NSF CAREER ACI-1350374 and NIH NHLBI R15HL140500.

References

1. Battler, A., et al.: The initial chest x-ray in acute myocardial infarction. Prediction of early and late mortality and survival. Circulation **61**(5), 1004–1009 (1980)
2. Chartsias, A., et al.: Factorised spatial representation learning: application in semi-supervised myocardial segmentation. In: Frangi, A.F., Schnabel, J.A., Davatzikos, C., Alberola-López, C., Fichtinger, G. (eds.) MICCAI 2018. LNCS, vol. 11071, pp. 490–498. Springer, Cham (2018). https://doi.org/10.1007/978-3-030-00934-2_55
3. Ghimire, S., Gyawali, P.K., Dhamala, J., Sapp, J.L., Horacek, M., Wang, L.: Improving generalization of deep networks for inverse reconstruction of image sequences. In: Chung, A.C.S., Gee, J.C., Yushkevich, P.A., Bao, S. (eds.) IPMI 2019. LNCS, vol. 11492, pp. 153–166. Springer, Cham (2019). https://doi.org/10.1007/978-3-030-20351-1_12
4. Irvin, J., et al.: CheXpert: a large chest radiograph dataset with uncertainty labels and expert comparison. In: AAAI (2019)
5. Kawaguchi, K., Bengio, Y., Verma, V., Kaelbling, L.P.: Generalization in machine learning via analytical learning theory. arXiv preprint arXiv:1802.07426 (2018)
6. Kingma, D.P., Mohamed, S., Rezende, D.J., Welling, M.: Semi-supervised learning with deep generative models. In: NeurIPS (2014)
7. Kingma, D.P., Welling, M.: Auto-encoding variational bayes. In: ICLR (2013)
8. Laine, S., Aila, T.: Temporal ensembling for semi-supervised learning. In: ICLR (2017)
9. Litjens, G., et al.: A survey on deep learning in medical image analysis. Med. Image Anal. **42**, 60–88 (2017)
10. Madani, A., Moradi, M., Karargyris, A., Syeda-Mahmood, T.: Semi-supervised learning with generative adversarial networks for chest x-ray classification with ability of data domain adaptation. In: ISBI (2018)
11. Odena, A., Olah, C., Shlens, J.: Conditional image synthesis with auxiliary classifier GANs. In: ICML (2017)

An Automated Cobb Angle Estimation Method Using Convolutional Neural Network with Area Limitation

Kailai Zhang[1], Nanfang Xu[3], Guosheng Yang[4], Ji Wu[1,2(✉)], and Xiangling Fu[4]

[1] Department of Electronic Engineering, Tsinghua University, Beijing, China
wuji_ee@mail.tsinghua.edu.cn
[2] Institute for Precision Medicine, Tsinghua University, Beijing, China
[3] Peking University Third Hospital, Beijing, China
[4] School of Software Engineering, Beijing University of Posts and
Telecommunications, Beijing, China

Abstract. Cobb angle measurement is the gold standard for the idiopathic scoliosis assessment, and the measurement result is very important for the surgical planning and medical curing. Currently, the Cobb angle is measured manually by physicians. They find the four landmarks on each vertebra and calculate the Cobb angle by rules, which is time-consuming and unreliable. In this paper, we apply the convolutional neural network (CNN) to find the landmarks automatically based on anterior-posterior view X-rays, then output the Cobb angle results. The X-rays always have too much noise, which has a strong influence on the landmark estimation. Addressing this problem, we first detect each vertebra bounding box to provide an area limitation. Then we use the CNN with an enhancement module to find the landmarks on detected vertebra bounding boxes, which can remove the noise in the background. Our experiment results show that our two-stage framework achieves precise landmark location and small error on Cobb angle estimation. Therefore our method can provide reliable assistance for the physicians.

Keywords: Cobb angle · Convolutional neural network · Area limitation

1 Introduction

Idiopathic scoliosis is the most common type of spinal deformity [1] and is typically found in adolescents. Scoliosis in adolescents may progress during their growth period, and it can cause further deterioration of spinal imbalance, back pain, neurological deficits, and even cardiopulmonary compromise. Therefore, early detection and regular monitoring of curve progression are very important. Cobb angle [2], defined as the angle between the most tilted vertebras in anterior-posterior view X-rays, is the gold standard for assessment of curve severity and

© Springer Nature Switzerland AG 2019
D. Shen et al. (Eds.): MICCAI 2019, LNCS 11769, pp. 775–783, 2019.
https://doi.org/10.1007/978-3-030-32226-7_86

plays an important role in making surgical decision of each patient. In clinical practice, there are five lumbar vertebras and twelve thoracic vertebras in each X-ray for assessment. The physicians first find four landmarks and draw a quadrilateral accordingly on each vertebra (Fig. 1), then observe the most tilted position and extend the straight line from the edge of relevant quadrilaterals to get the Cobb angle. For manual measurement, the landmarks are determined by subjective judgement, which leads to large inter-rater variation, and the measurement takes a long time because some trials are required to get the final results. In order to reduce the variability of Cobb angle measurement and improve clinical efficiency, in this paper, we propose an automated Cobb angle estimation framework, which can provide reliable assistance for the physicians.

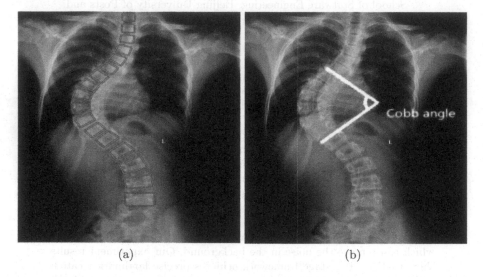

(a)   (b)

Fig. 1. (a) The vertebras labeled by physicians, four landmarks are connected to a quadrilateral on each vertebra. (b) The anterior-posterior view X-ray with Cobb angle.

Previous attempts on automated Cobb angle estimation can be divided to indirect estimation and direct estimation according to their respective methodology. The indirect estimation methods are based on vertebra location and segmentation. Such as [3] uses the snake model to segment the vertebras. [4] applies the particle model to determine the curvature on radiographical spinal images. After the segmentation, these methods attempt to fit straight lines based on the segmentation result or contour of each vertebra, and calculate the Cobb angle based on each pair of lines. The direct estimation methods aim to directly find all the landmarks of vertebras on the whole image, which is just like the manual measurement of physicians. Such as [5] uses the structured multi-output regression to predict the landmarks. [6] uses a special Boost-net to transform the feature space and finds the landmarks. [7] considers the relationship of adjacent vertebras, then uses a MVC-net to detect all the landmarks. After landmark prediction, the Cobb angle result can be obtained by rules.

The indirect and direct estimation methods have their own advantages and disadvantages. In indirect estimation methods, the whole vertebra area is large and robust against the noise, so that it can always be located and segmented. However, for each vertebra, the straight line fitting is sensitive to the segmentation result. Even a small change of segmentation result can lead to great change of the straight line, which may cause large error on Cobb angle measurement. In direct estimation methods, once the landmarks are predicted, the Cobb angle can be directly obtained by rules. However, a single landmark is less robust than a vertebra area, which can be severely influenced by the noise in the background, and lead to large deviation of Cobb angle.

The instinctive thought is to take advantages in both methods. Based on this motivation, we design a two-stage framework for the Cobb angle measurement. In last few years, the deep learning techniques especially the CNN methods have been developed rapidly, such as Resnet [8] and U-net [9] have reached high performance in medical image applications. Therefore we use CNN methods in our task. We first detect each vertebra in original X-ray and get the vertebra bounding box sequence. The bounding boxes provide the local vertebra areas, which are used as the area limitation for the landmark estimation. We design a CNN with an unsupervised enhancement module to predict four landmarks on each local vertebra area, which can remove the noise in the background. Finally we calculate the Cobb angle by rules. Compared to the indirect estimation and direct estimation methods, the experiment results[1] show that our hybrid method achieves much more precise landmark location and smaller error on Cobb angle. Therefore it can provide reliable diagnostic support for the physicians.

2   Methods

2.1   System Framework

Given an anterior-posterior view X-ray, our system can output the four landmarks of each vertebra and Cobb angle. The system framework is shown in Fig. 2. Our system takes advantages of the indirect and direct estimation methods to get better performance. The input X-ray is first sent to a vertebra detection network. It outputs the filtered vertebra boxes sequence, which provides the area limitation for the landmark estimation. Then each local vertebra area in the sequence is sent to the landmark estimation network to get four landmarks. Based on the vertebra sequence with landmarks, we can calculate the Cobb angle by rules. More details are explained in the following sections.

[1] This work is supported by the National Key Research and Development Program of China (No. 2018YFC0116800).

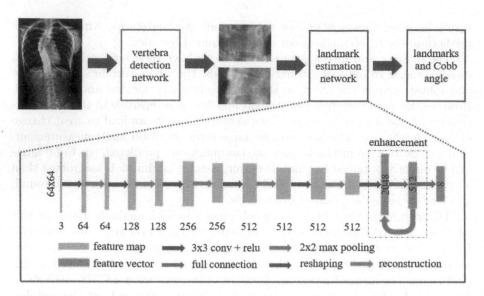

Fig. 2. Our two-stage system framework. The structure of landmark estimation network is shown above, and the number of channels is under each feature map.

2.2 Vertebra Detection Network

The vertebra detection network is used to find the boundary of each vertebra from the original X-rays. Since the missing vertebra bounding boxes will never be found in the following steps, the accurate detection of bounding boxes is required for the landmark estimation. The Mask R-CNN [10] is the state of the art method for object detection and segmentation, which performance is even better than the Faster R-CNN [11]. For these reasons, we adopt the Mask R-CNN structure as our vertebra detection network. For network training, we connect four labeled landmarks to get each vertebra area and generate the mask with pixel information, then we use the mask to train the network.

The vertebra detection network outputs all the vertebra bounding boxes $[x_{lt}, y_{lt}, x_{rb}, y_{rb}]$ for each X-ray, which represents the x-coordinate and y-coordinate of the left top and right bottom vertex of a bounding box. We use a filter to remove the wrong detection results. The center point of a bounding box can be calculated as $[x_c, y_c] = [\frac{x_{lt}+x_{rb}}{2}, \frac{y_{lt}+y_{rb}}{2}]$. We order the bounding box sequence from the top to bottom according to y_c. The distance of the adjacent center points $[x_{c1}, y_{c1}], [x_{c2}, y_{c2}]$ are calculated by $d = \sqrt{(x_{c1} - x_{c2})^2 + (y_{c1} - y_{c2})^2}$. If the two distances of one center point and its neighbors are both larger than a threshold D, then this center point is an outlier and the relevant bounding box is removed. After the refinement, we can get the filtered vertebra bounding box sequence for the landmark estimation.

2.3   Landmark Estimation Network

The landmark estimation network (LE-NET) we design is shown in Fig. 2. The local vertebra area is firstly extracted from original X-rays according to the relevant bounding box $[x_{lt}, y_{lt}, x_{rb}, y_{rb}]$, which provides the area limitation. The LE-NET receives the local vertebra area and resizes it to 64×64. It outputs a 8-dimension vector T after the convolution, max pooling and full connection. An extra enhancement module is inserted into LE-NET: we use the full connection operation to reconstruct the 2048-dimension feature vector based on the 512-dimension feature vector. An unsupervised mean square loss is used to minimize the difference between the original and reconstructed 2048-dimension feature vector, so that the 512-dimension vector is forced to be a compression representation of the 2048-dimension vector, which can provide better features for the landmark prediction. In order to deal with different resolution of detected bounding boxes, we use the normalized coordinate in $[0, 1]$ rather than the absolute coordinate to predict the landmarks. To achieve this goal, a sigmoid function is used to transfer T to the final prediction vector $pre = \frac{1}{e^{-T}+1}$, which includes the normalized x-coordinate and y-coordinate of four landmarks.

For network training, we extract the bounding boxes which include the four groundtruth landmarks of each vertebra, then randomly enlarge the bounding boxes to get the training data. Assuming that the height and width of an enlarged bounding box are $[h, w]$ (it will be resized to 64×64 before training), we first transform the absolute coordinate of the relevant four landmarks in original X-ray to the local bounding box, then the absolute coordinate vector $[x_1, y_1, x_2, y_2, x_3, y_3, x_4, y_4]$ in the bounding box can be transformed to normalized coordinate vector $gt = [\frac{x_1}{w}, \frac{y_1}{h}, \frac{x_2}{w}, \frac{y_2}{h}, \frac{x_3}{w}, \frac{y_3}{h}, \frac{x_4}{w}, \frac{y_4}{h}]$, which is used as the label of training data. Therefore the loss function can be defined as

$$loss = \sum_{i=1}^{8} (gt(i) - pre(i))^2 + \lambda \sum_{j=1}^{2048} (O(j) - R(j))^2 \qquad (1)$$

Where the O and R represent the original and reconstructed 2048-dimension vector respectively. λ is the weight of reconstruction error. We use formula 1 to train the LE-NET. When we predict the landmarks in bounding box $[x_{lt}, y_{lt}, x_{rb}, y_{rb}]$ output by vertebra detection network, once we get the predict vector $pre = [x_1^p, y_1^p, x_2^p, y_2^p, x_3^p, y_3^p, x_4^p, y_4^p]$, we can transform the normalized coordinate of four landmarks to absolute coordinate in original X-ray by using

$$x_i^a = x_i^p * (x_{rb} - x_{lt}) + x_{lt} \quad y_i^a = y_i^p * (y_{rb} - y_{lt}) + y_{lt} (i = 1, 2, 3, 4) \qquad (2)$$

Since we have ordered the vertebra bounding boxes, after we get the absolute coordinate of all the landmarks, we connect two top landmarks and two bottom landmarks, and get the slope of two straight lines on each vertebra. We calculate the angle for each two vertebras, by choosing the bottom line on the top vertebra and the top line on the bottom vertebra (Fig. 1). The largest angle from all the results is chosen as the final Cobb angle result.

3   Experiments

3.1   Dataset Description and Parameters Setting

For our experiments, the experiment environment is running on ubuntu 14.04 with gpu 1080Ti, and the relevant software is python with tensorflow. The dataset of anterior-posterior view X-rays provided by a local hospital has 1200 images in total and the size of each X-ray (Fig. 1) is 491 × 957. For all the images, four landmarks of each vertebra and the Cobb angle are labeled by five professional physicians with cross validation. Therefore the labeling results are thought as the gold standard in our experiments.

The stochastic gradient descent (SGD) optimizer with momentum is used for both networks in our system framework. The X-rays are randomly divided to training set, validation set and test set. The scale is set to 7:2:1. For vertebra detection network, the initial learning rate and momentum are set to 0.001 and 0.9. The batch size is set to 4 and the number of training epoches is set to 60. The threshold D is set to 50 pixels according to the size of X-rays. For LE-NET, the λ in formula 1 is set to 0.01. The initial learning rate and momentum are set to 0.0001 and 0.9. The batch size is set to 32 and the number of training epoches is set to 100. For both two networks, the training step is repeated for 10 times, and the average performance is considered.

3.2   Evaluation and Discussion

We evaluate the vertebra location performance of vertebra detection network. The groundtruth bounding boxes are generated from four labeled landmarks. We calculate the precision, recall and Fscore of the predicted bounding boxes. A predicted box is regarded as a correct one if its intersection over union (IOU) with a groundtruth box is larger than 0.5. The results are shown in Table 1.

Table 1. The location performance of vertebra detection network.

Location performance	Precision	Recall	Fscore
Without filter	0.960 ± 0.009	0.973 ± 0.006	0.966 ± 0.008
With filter	$\mathbf{0.974 \pm 0.013}$	$\mathbf{0.973 \pm 0.006}$	$\mathbf{0.973 \pm 0.010}$

From the results, the vertebra detection network achieves very high performance. This is because a vertebra area is large and robust against noise, which can be easily located by Mask R-CNN. With the filter, some wrong boxes are removed and the precision increases. The bounding boxes can be sent to the LE-NET based on the high performance of vertebra location. For landmark estimation, we compare the visualized results of our two-stage framework and the direct use of LE-NET on whole X-rays. An example is shown in Fig. 3.

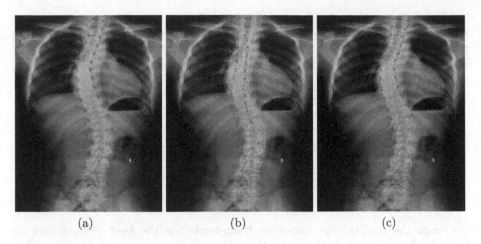

(a)   (b)   (c)

Fig. 3. (a) The groundtruth landmarks. (b) The landmarks predicted by the direct use of LE-NET on the whole X-ray. (3) The landmarks predicted by our two-stage framework.

From Fig. 3, the landmarks obtained by the direct use of LE-NET have large deviation from the groundtruth. Compared to the vertebra area, the single landmark is easier to be effected by the noise in background. By using the area limitation, the background is removed so that the landmarks can be predicted much more precisely. The scaled mean absolute error (MAE) metric is used to evaluate the deviation of landmarks:

$$scaled\ MAE = \frac{1}{N}\sum_{i=1}^{N} mean(|gt_i^l - pre_i^l|) \tag{3}$$

Where N is the number of vertebras and $mean()$ is the element-wise arithmetic mean of vector. gt_i^l and pre_i^l represent the normalized coordinate of groundtruth vector and prediction vector of four landmarks. For Cobb angle evaluation, two widely used evaluation metrics are the circular mean absolute error (CMAE) and symmetric mean absolute error (SMAPE), which are defined as

$$CMAE = \frac{1}{M}\sum_{i=1}^{M}|gt_i^a - pre_i^a| \quad SMAPE = \frac{1}{M}\sum_{i=1}^{M}\frac{|gt_i^a - pre_i^a|}{gt_i^a + pre_i^a} \times 100\% \tag{4}$$

Where gt_i^a and pre_i^a represent groundtruth and system output Cobb angle respectively. M is the number of images. We compare our two-stage framework with both the indirect and direct estimation methods. Since the Mask R-CNN can also output the segmentation results for each vertebra bounding box, it can be used in the indirect estimation method. We also use several straight line fitting methods based on the segmentation results of Mask R-CNN. Some previous works such as the snake model in [3], the Boost-net in [6] and the MVC-net in [7] are also considered for the comparison. The results are shown in Table 2.

Table 2. Comparison of different methods for landmark location and Cobb angle measurement. The hough transformation (HT), canny operator (CA) and least square method (LS) are used in the indirect estimation methods.

		Scaled MAE	CMAE (deg)	SMAPE (%)
Indirect estimation	Snake+HT [3]	–	10.73 ± 6.35	31.44 ± 9.63
	Mask R-CNN+CA	–	4.95 ± 1.85	15.92 ± 6.41
	Mask R-CNN+LS	–	5.52 ± 2.67	26.44 ± 11.55
Direct estimation	Boost-net [6]	0.0189 ± 0.0009	7.13 ± 4.06	20.95 ± 7.30
	MVC-net [7]	0.0161 ± 0.0012	8.28 ± 4.77	20.38 ± 8.40
	LE-NET	0.0198 ± 0.0007	8.80 ± 5.27	26.53 ± 8.49
Our framework	Without enhancement	0.0039 ± 0.0004	3.51 ± 1.90	10.14 ± 4.81
	With enhancement	$\mathbf{0.0037 \pm 0.0003}$	$\mathbf{3.29 \pm 1.48}$	$\mathbf{9.52 \pm 4.67}$

From the results, our two-stage framework has the best performance on both landmarks and Cobb angle. With the enhancement module, the performance achieves further improvement, because the output feature vector is more representative for the original bounding box. For indirect estimation methods, although the vertebra area can be located, the slope of the fitted straight line is sensitive to the segmentation results. The wrong segmentation of a small area can lead to large error of Cobb angle. Our method uses the vertebra bounding boxes rather than directly use the segmentation results, which can avoid this problem. For direct estimation methods, there is a large deviation of landmarks in these methods, because the landmarks are influenced by the noise in the background, which causes large landmarks prediction error and severely effects the Cobb angle result. In fact, the location of four landmarks depends on the vertebra itself, which does not need the global information. The background only makes distraction to the landmark estimation. By using the local vertebra areas, our framework removes the background to avoid this problem. Our method takes advantages in both indirect and direct estimation methods, which achieves much more precise landmark location and smaller error on Cobb angle estimation.

4   Conclusion

In this paper, we propose an automated Cobb angle estimation method, which can provide efficient and reliable assistance for the physicians. The landmark location is very important for the Cobb measurement, and it is effected by the noise in X-rays. We design a two-stage framework to do the landmark estimation with area limitation, which takes advantages of indirect and direct estimation methods. Our method achieves more precise landmark location and smaller error on Cobb angle than the previous works. In the future work, we will continue to improve the performance of landmark estimation and Cobb angle measurement.

References

1. Glassman, S., Bridwell, K., Berven, S., Horton, W., Schwab, F.: The impact of positive sagittal balance in adult spinal deformity. Spine J. 4(5–supp–S), S113–S114 (2004). P90
2. Cobb, J.: Outline for the study of scoliosis. Instr. Course Lect. **5**, 261–275 (1948)
3. Anitha, H., Prabhu, G.K.: Automatic quantification of spinal curvature in scoliotic radiograph using image processing. J. Med. Syst. **36**(3), 1943–1951 (2012)
4. Sardjono, T.A., et al.: Automatic cobb angle determination from radiographic images. Spine **38**(20), E1256–E1262 (2013)
5. Sun, H., Zhen, X., Bailey, C., Rasoulinejad, P., Yin, Y., Li, S.: Direct estimation of spinal cobb angles by structured multi-output regression. In: Niethammer, M., et al. (eds.) IPMI 2017. LNCS, vol. 10265, pp. 529–540. Springer, Cham (2017). https://doi.org/10.1007/978-3-319-59050-9_42
6. Wu, H., Bailey, C., Rasoulinejad, P., Li, S.: Automatic landmark estimation for adolescent idiopathic scoliosis assessment using BoostNet. In: Descoteaux, M., Maier-Hein, L., Franz, A., Jannin, P., Collins, D.L., Duchesne, S. (eds.) MICCAI 2017. LNCS, vol. 10433, pp. 127–135. Springer, Cham (2017). https://doi.org/10.1007/978-3-319-66182-7_15
7. Wu, H., Bailey, C., Rasoulinejad, P., Li, S.: Automated comprehensive adolescent idiopathic scoliosis assessment using MVC-Net. Med. Image Anal. **48**, 1–11 (2018)
8. He, K., Zhang, X., Ren, S., Sun, J.: Deep residual learning for image recognition. In: Proceedings of the IEEE Conference on Computer Vision and Pattern Recognition, pp. 770–778 (2016)
9. Ronneberger, O., Fischer, P., Brox, T.: U-Net: convolutional networks for biomedical image segmentation. In: Navab, N., Hornegger, J., Wells, W.M., Frangi, A.F. (eds.) MICCAI 2015. LNCS, vol. 9351, pp. 234–241. Springer, Cham (2015). https://doi.org/10.1007/978-3-319-24574-4_28
10. He, K., Gkioxari, G., Dollár, P., Girshick, R.: Mask R-CNN. In: Proceedings of the IEEE International Conference on Computer Vision, pp. 2961–2969 (2017)
11. Ren, S., He, K., Girshick, R., Sun, J.: Faster R-CNN: towards real-time object detection with region proposal networks. IEEE Trans. Pattern Anal. Mach. Intell. **39**(6), 1137–1149 (2017)

Endotracheal Tube Detection and Segmentation in Chest Radiographs Using Synthetic Data

Maayan Frid-Adar[1]([⊠])(iD), Rula Amer[1](iD), and Hayit Greenspan[1,2](iD)

[1] RADLogics Ltd., Tel-Aviv, Israel
{maayan,rula,hayit}@radlogics.com
[2] Department of Biomedical Engineering,
Tel Aviv University, Tel Aviv, Israel
hayit@eng.tau.ac.il

Abstract. Chest radiographs are frequently used to verify the correct intubation of patients in the emergency room. Fast and accurate identification and localization of the endotracheal (ET) tube is critical for the patient. In this study we propose a novel automated deep learning scheme for accurate detection and segmentation of the ET tubes. Development of automatic systems using deep learning networks for classification and segmentation require large annotated data which is not always available. Here we present an approach for synthesizing ET tubes in real X-ray images. We suggest a method for training the network, first with synthetic data and then with real X-ray images in a fine-tuning phase, which allows the network to train on thousands of cases without annotating any data. The proposed method was tested on 477 real chest radiographs from a public dataset and reached AUC of 0.99 in classifying the presence vs. absence of the ET tube, along with outputting high quality ET tube segmentation maps.

Keywords: ET tube · Chest radiographs · Deep learning · CNN · Classification · Segmentation

1 Introduction

The American College of Radiology recommends acquisition of chest radiographs following intubation, to ensure proper positioning of inserted tubes, for patients in the Intensive Care Unit (ICU) [1]. This is justified by studies, such as [2], which show that following intubation, physical examination identified tube malposition in only 2% to 5% of patients, whereas the radiograph revealed suboptimal positioning in 10% to 25%. The ideal endotracheal (ET) tube position is in the mid trachea if the patient head is in the neutral position. Malposition of the ET tube can cause serious complications if not detected, especially where the tube is too low and selective bronchial intubation occurs. Such complications include

© Springer Nature Switzerland AG 2019
D. Shen et al. (Eds.): MICCAI 2019, LNCS 11769, pp. 784–792, 2019.
https://doi.org/10.1007/978-3-030-32226-7_87

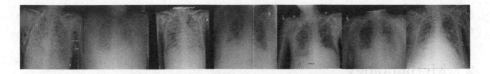

Fig. 1. Examples from the NIH public dataset [6]

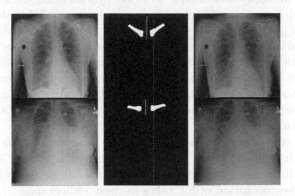

Fig. 2. Original X-ray images (left column), clavicles segmentation and synthesized ET tube (middle column) and Synthesized ET tubes blended into the original X-ray (right column)

a segmental or complete collapse of the contralateral lung, pneumothorax and atelectasis [2].

Using the acquired radiographs, Computer-Aided Detection (CAD) systems can assist physicians in automatic detection of the ET tubes. Previous studies used classical approaches to determine seed points followed by a line tracking algorithms [3,4]. A more recent study used a convolutional neural network (CNN) classification system for the presence or absence identification of the ET tube, with reported area under curve (AUC) of 0.99; and a second classification network for identification of low vs normal positioning of the ET tube, with AUC of 0.81 [5]. The above studies used private datasets of portable chest X ray images with a relatively small amount of cases: 64 [3] and 87 [4] were used for the classical approaches; 300 cases were used for the CNN based solution [5].

Collecting and labeling chest radiographs for presence of ET tubes requires collaboration with hospitals and data extraction methods. For the ET tube detection and ET tube segmentation annotation, expert physicians are needed. In this paper, we present an innovative solution for the task of detection and segmentation of ET tubes in chest radiographs, in the *scenario of limited expert labeled data*: We use a *public dataset of chest radiographs* [6] which allows us to collect a large data of normal and ET tube examples required for training a deep learning network. We then *synthesize ET tubes* on top of the X-ray images to generate ground truth data for the ET tube segmentation. Finally, we present a combined CNN for ET tube detection and segmentation in chest radiographs showing promising results.

2   Methodology

In this study, we apply a technique to insert synthetic ET tubes as an overlay to the original X-ray images taken from a publicly available dataset of chest radiographs [6] (hereon will be called the NIH dataset). This dataset contains over 100,000 frontal view images, many of them coming from ICU patients. While annotations are provided for 14 lung diseases, no annotations exist for the presence of ET tubes (or other tubes). A few sample images from the NIH dataset are shown in Fig. 1 - the cases have high variability and many have poor image quality. We only used cases in Anterior-Posterior (AP) positioning to simulate intubated patients.

In the first step of our proposed solution, we propose a technique to generate new images with ground truth ET tube segmentation masks. The new image set we form will be used in a follow-up step, for training a combined CNN for detection and segmentation of ET tubes in chest radiographs.

2.1   Generating Synthetic Data

Generating the synthetic ET tubes over real X-ray images includes the following main steps as shown in Fig. 2: (a) Selection of cases from the NIH dataset that do not contain ET tubes but may include other tubes (such as nasogastric (NG) tube, drainage tubes, catheters); (b) Segmentation of the clavicles in order to localize the synthetic ET tube in the trachea area; (c) Blending of generated synthetic ET tubes onto real X-ray images.

Clavicles Segmentation: ET tubes are inserted into the trachea to allow artificial ventilation of the lungs. X-ray images are mostly aligned with the trachea located between the clavicles. Therefore, correct segmentation of the clavicles assists in placing the synthetic ET tube in the trachea area. In [7] a methodology for organ segmentation within Chest radiographs was presented, and shown to outperform alternate schemes, when tested on a common benchmark of 247 chest radiographs from the JSRT dataset, with ground-truth segmentation masks from the SCR dataset [8]. The architecture proposed is based on a modified U-Net based architecture, in which pre-trained encoder weights were used, based on VGG16. In the current work, we use a similar scheme: For training we input 224×224 images, each normalized by its mean and standard deviation. We train the single-class segmentation model using Dice loss and threshold the output score maps to generate binary segmentation masks of the clavicles structure. This model gives us Dice coefficient score of 93.1% and Mean average contour distance of 0.871 mm.

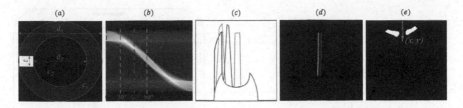

Fig. 3. Realistic ET tubes generation: (a) ET tube cross profile; (b) 2D projection of the tube; (c) sampled profile at different angles; (d) ET tube profile drawing; (e) drawing the ET tube relative to the location of the clavicles (using middle point x and lower point y)

Realistic ET Tubes Generation: We present next our methodology for generating synthetic ET tubes for adult X-ray images. In our solution, we were inspired by the work of Yi et al. [9] that generated synthetic catheters on pediatric X-ray images. Figure 3 depicts the ET tube generation steps: First, we created a 2D simulation of the ET tube, as a hollow tabular object with a rectangular marker made of a radiopaque material. The tube and the marker are made from different materials and therefore have different attenuation components ($c1$ and $c2$). The tube outer and inner width, $d1$ and $d2$, were chosen to fit an adult ET tube with strip thickness t. We defined $\{c1, c2, d1, d2, t\} = \{0.1, 1, 160, 100, 20\}$. All the parameters above were selected based on true physical properties of ET tubes or based on [9].

In order to simulate the ET tube from different rotations, we projected the 2D profile using a Radon transform and sampled the projection at $0°$, $30°$, $60°$, $90°$. For each synthetic ET tube we selected one of the four profiles and sampled the values of 15 pixels for drawing the tube.

The trace of the ET tube was simulated over the trachea area using the clavicles segmentation. We extracted the middle point x between the clavicles and the lowest point y. Then, we randomly selected 4 points with x offset of $[-2, 2]$ pixels and y-axis samples starting from 0 to y+offset of $[0, 30]$ pixels. The random points compose a line using B-spline interpolation. Finally, we draw the tube sampled profile over the line.

The last step for creating a realistic X-ray with an ET tube is to merge the synthetic tube with the real X-ray image. We selected AP X-ray images from the NIH dataset that do not contain ET tubes and blended the random synthetic ET tubes into the images. We used a simple blending with random weights in the range of $[0.1, 0.2]$.

2.2   Detection and Segmentation CNN

We propose a combined CNN architecture for ET tube detection and segmentation in chest radiographs, ETT-Net, as depicted in Fig. 4. The architecture is built from a VGG16 style encoder followed by two paths: One is a decoder that continues the U-Net shape for addressing the ET tube segmentation task; The

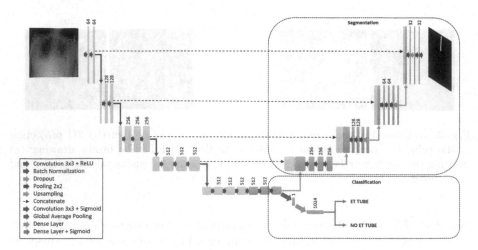

Fig. 4. ETT-Net: the proposed architecture for detection and segmentation of ET tubes

other path summarizes the features extracted at the end of the encoder using a global pooling layer followed by two dense layers and a sigmoid, for addressing the ET tube classification task. We used pre-trained VGG16 weights as initialization for the encoder. The two paths of the network are trained simultaneously for both the classification task and the segmentation task using a combined weighted Binary Cross-Entropy (BCE) loss and a Dice (D) loss as follows:

$$\mathcal{L} = BCE(\hat{L}, L) + \lambda D(\hat{S}, S) \tag{1}$$

where L and $\hat{L}$ are the classification output label and the ground truth label, respectively; S and $\hat{S}$ are the segmentation output mask and the ground truth mask, respectively. λ is the weight to balance between the loss components and was chosen (empirically) as 0.1.

The network inputs X-ray image of size 224×224 pixels duplicated 3 times (to fit the pre-trained encoder), the corresponding ET tube segmentation mask and a binary label for the presence or absence of ET tube. The input images are preprocessed with contrast limited adaptive histogram equalization (CLAHE) and normalized by their mean and standard deviation. The segmentation masks can be a blank "all zero" image where no ET tube is present or a binary segmentation mask of the ET tube. For the training we augmented the data using horizontal flipping and small rotations of $\pm 10°$.

3   Experiments and Results

3.1   Two Phase Training

In order to train our suggested CNN using the synthesized data and still benefit from the existence of hundreds of X-ray images containing ET tube in the public

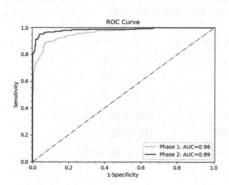

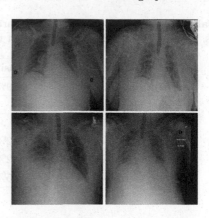

Fig. 5. ROC curve after the two phases of training

Fig. 6. Cases correctly classified with ET tube and their corresponding segmentation as overlay (in green color) (Color figure online)

dataset, we used a two phase training methodology. First, we trained the CNN using the generated data as explained in Sect. 2.1. Then, we used all the AP cases from the NIH dataset for inference: We extracted real cases to fine-tune the network to improve the classification and segmentation performance on real chest radiographs data. In both training phases, we trained the network for 50 epochs using an Adam optimizer with default parameters.

The data for the first training phase includes 1669 X-ray images: 869 synthetic examples with ET tube and 800 without. The segmentation masks of the positive cases were obtained using a simple binary threshold of the synthetic tube before the blending operation. For the second phase, we used all NIH dataset AP cases and set conditions on the classification and segmentation outputs of the model: Images with classification prob. higher than 0.8 and non zero segmentation map were selected as positive examples; Images with classification prob. lower than 0.01 and a zero segmentation map were selected as negative examples. These conditions resulted in 3972 positive X-ray images with ET tube, and 36557 X-ray images without ET tube. Overall, after balancing the data, we trained the second phase using 7944 real chest radiographs.

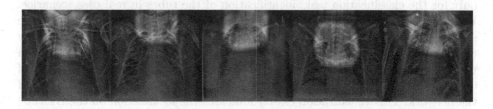

Fig. 7. Heatmap examples using ET tube classification CNN

Table 1. Comparison to state-of-the-art methods for classification between presence vs. absence of ET tube; "-" means that the score was not reported

	AUC	Sensitivity, Specificity	Testing size [pos, neg]
Ramakrishna et al. [3]	-	92.9%, 97.2%	64 [28, 36]
Chen et al. [4]	0.95	-	87 [44, 43]
Lakhani et al. [5]	0.99	-	60 [30, 30]
DenseNet	0.97	89.2%, 93.0%	479 [232, 247]
ETT-Net - phase1	0.96	89.2%, 93.0%	479 [232, 247]
ETT-Net - phase2	0.99	95.5%, 96.5%	479 [232, 247]

3.2   Test Set

The test set includes 479 real chest radiographs from the NIH dataset that were collected manually one time during the development and entirely independent from all training data. All cases are in AP view position, 232 cases with ET tube and 247 without ET tube. After collecting the cases, we verified that the label for each case is consistent with the presence of an ET tube. It is important to note that as we didn't use manual annotations for the segmentation of the tube, the ground truth segmentation maps are not pixel-wise accurate; still, they represent an expected range for the ET tube position in the images. The classification accuracy is an quantitative measure we can use. Thus, we tested our model using the AUC for the classification accuracy. The segmentation output was examined qualitatively.

3.3   Results

Training the combined model for classification and segmentation of ET tubes on synthetic X-ray images, we reached an AUC of 0.962 in classification accuracy. Using fine-tuning on real X-ray images, the accuracy improved to an AUC of 0.987 with both sensitivity and specificity over 95% (Fig. 5). Figure 6 shows real chest radiographs from the test set that were classified correctly for presence of ET tube and their output segmentation maps.

We conducted an additional experiment using a different CNN architecture only for the classification task: identification of the tubes in real case scenarios. We trained a DenseNet [10] architecture with the same dataset we used in the second phase of the combined model - real cases with and without ET tube ($n = 7944$) for 50 epochs and Adam optimizer. Training only for classification using a large real training data, we reached a high accuracy with an AUC of 0.975. Figure 7 shows a heatmap visualization of the last convolutional layer of the network. This visualization clearly indicates the localization on the ET tube area.

Table 1 compares state-of-the-art methods for the classification of presence or absent ET tube to our methods - results after the first phase of training using the ETT-Net model, Second phase results of the final model after fine-tuning with real examples and the only classification method using DenseNet. The table shows the amount of testing images used for testing each method, with separation for cases with ET tube (pos) and without (neg). Our best model, ETT-Net - Phase2, reached high performance with a test set size of one magnitude more than state-of-the-art methods. In addition our model was trained and tested using free public dataset (of real ICU patients) without the need for manual annotations, in contrast with the other methods were the cases were hand picked and annotated.

4   Conclusion

In this work, we proposed an approach for training a combined deep learning network for the tasks of detection and segmentation of the ET tube in adult chest radiographs without collecting and annotating data. We used a public dataset of X-ray images and synthesized realistic ET tubes blended into those images. We used the synthetic data as a first phase of training our model. Collecting real X-ray cases using the trained model, we continued to a second phase of training. Both stages are trained using the ETT-Net - a combined CNN architecture for ET tube detection and segmentation in chest radiographs. The combined model achieved a very high accuracy for the presence of ET tube in real ICU patients (0.99 AUC) using a test set which is ten times larger compared to previous studies and also outputs high quality segmentation maps that can assist in detection of the misplacement of the tubes. We also showed accurate results (0.97 AUC) using a CNN for classification only where the synthetic cases are used only for retrieval of real cases from the public dataset. Future work can include exploring a similar method for other tube types and combining them together in a multi-class detection and segmentation method. The ideas presented in our paper for synthesizing data over public dataset images, can be used in other medical imaging domains (for example generating tumors over healthy patients in X-ray or CT studies).

References

1. Godoy, M.C., Leitman, B.S., de Groot, P.M., Vlahos, I., Naidich, D.P.: Chest radiography in the ICU: part 1, evaluation of airway, enteric, and pleural tubes. Am. J. Roentgenol. **198**(3), 563–571 (2012)
2. Trotman-Dickenson, B.: Radiology in the intensive care unit (part i). J. Intensive Care Med. **18**(4), 198–210 (2003)
3. Ramakrishna, B., Brown, M., Goldin, J., Cagnon, C., Enzmann, D.: An improved automatic computer aided tube detection and labeling system on chest radiographs. In: Medical Imaging 2012: Computer-Aided Diagnosis, vol. 8315, p. 83150R. International Society for Optics and Photonics (2012)
4. Chen, S., Zhang, M., Yao, L., Xu, W.: Endotracheal tubes positioning detection in adult portable chest radiography for intensive care unit. Int. J. Comput. Assist. Radiol. Surg. **11**(11), 2049–2057 (2016)

792   M. Frid-Adar et al.

5. Lakhani, P.: Deep convolutional neural networks for endotracheal tube position and x-ray image classification: challenges and opportunities. J. Digital Imaging **30**(4), 460–468 (2017). https://doi.org/10.10007/s10278-017-9980-77
6. Wang, X., Peng, Y., Lu, L., Lu, Z., Bagheri, M., Summers, R.M.: Chestx-ray8: hospital-scale chest x-ray database and benchmarks on weakly-supervised classification and localization of common thorax diseases. In: IEEE Conference on Computer Vision and Pattern Recognition (2017)
7. Frid-Adar, M., Ben-Cohen, A., Amer, R., Greenspan, H.: Improving the segmentation of anatomical structures in chest radiographs using U-Net with an imagenet pre-trained encoder. In: Stoyanov, D., et al. (eds.) RAMBO/BIA/TIA -2018. LNCS, vol. 11040, pp. 159–168. Springer, Cham (2018). https://doi.org/10.1007/978-3-030-00946-5_17
8. Ginneken, B.V., Stegmann, M.B., Loog, M.: Segmentation of anatomical structures in chest radiographs using supervised methods: a comparative study on a public database. Med. Image Anal. **10**(1), 19–40 (2006)
9. Yi, X., Adams, S., Babyn, P., Elnajmi, A.: Automatic catheter detection in pediatric x-ray images using a scale-recurrent network and synthetic data. CoRR (2018). http://arxiv.org/abs/1806.00921
10. Huang, G., Liu, Z., Weinberger, K.Q.: Densely connected convolutional networks. CoRR (2016). http://arxiv.org/abs/1608.069936

Learning Interpretable Features
via Adversarially Robust Optimization

Ashkan Khakzar[1]([✉]), Shadi Albarqouni[1], and Nassir Navab[1,2]

[1] Technical University of Munich, Munich, Germany
ashkan.khakzar@tum.de
[2] Johns Hopkins University, Baltimore, MD, USA

Abstract. Neural networks are proven to be remarkably successful for classification and diagnosis in medical applications. However, the ambiguity in the decision-making process and the interpretability of the learned features is a matter of concern. In this work, we propose a method for improving the feature interpretability of neural network classifiers. Initially, we propose a baseline convolutional neural network with state of the art performance in terms of accuracy and weakly supervised localization. Subsequently, the loss is modified to integrate robustness to adversarial examples into the training process. In this work, feature interpretability is quantified via evaluating the weakly supervised localization using the ground truth bounding boxes. Interpretability is also visually assessed using class activation maps and saliency maps. The method is applied to NIH ChestX-ray14, the largest publicly available chest x-rays dataset. We demonstrate that the adversarially robust optimization paradigm improves feature interpretability both quantitatively and visually.

Keywords: Interpretability · Medical imaging · Adversarial training

1 Introduction

Deep learning methods have shown great promise in medical diagnosis [3]. Specifically, after the release of NIH ChestX-ray dataset, deep learning based methods achieved high performances on chest x-ray classification hitherto unprecedented on large scale [5,8,11,12]. Despite these promising accomplishments, the previously proposed methods for chest x-ray classification do not show adequate feature interpretability, while similar methods achieve higher feature interpretability on computer vision datasets [13]. Feature interpretability is critical in the clinical setting, as it helps explain why a diagnostic decision is made by the classifier [1,7]. Therefore it is also critical that the methods proposed for medical image diagnosis achieve high scores in interpretability metrics.

Several works consider interpretability of neural network classifiers. Rajpurkar et al. [8] propose a classification model for Pneumonia detection on NIH ChestX-ray14 dataset and visualize Class Activation Maps (CAMs) [13]

© Springer Nature Switzerland AG 2019
D. Shen et al. (Eds.): MICCAI 2019, LNCS 11769, pp. 793–800, 2019.
https://doi.org/10.1007/978-3-030-32226-7_88

to show interpretability of features used for Pneumonia prediction. They also propose a multi-label classification model with high classification accuracy for all classes in the dataset, however do not evaluate its interpretability. Wang et al. [11] propose a unified weakly supervised multi-label image classification and disease localization framework. The localization, which is based on CAMs, serves as a metric for evaluating the interpretability of the features. Their proposed weighted cross entropy scheme enforces the model to learn interpretable features in the highly imbalanced (in terms of positive and negative examples) NIH ChestX-ray dataset. However, the localization results do not keep pace with the classification results. Li et al. [5] improve the localization on the same dataset significantly by incorporating the annotated bounding boxes into training. Although this is an intuitive method to enforce the model to learn explainable features, lack of annotated data hinders the use of this approach. Biffi et al. [1] propose a method based on convolutional generative neural networks for designing models with interpretable features and the method is applied to the classification of cardiovascular diseases. The method enforces interpretability by design and limits the architecture of the neural network to only generative ones. Therefore, an approach that would enforce interpretability on all high performing models (and not just a specific architecture) is appreciated.

It is postulated that feature representations learned using robust training capture salient data characteristics [10]. Adversarially robust optimization is introduced as a method for robustness against adversarial examples in [2,6]. In this work, we improve the interpretability of the state of the art neural network classifiers via adversarially robust optimization. The work tries to steer the models toward learning features that are more semantically relevant to the pathologies in the classification problem. Initially, we propose a baseline neural network classifier based on the state of the art. Then we modify its loss to adversarially robust loss and measure the improvement in terms of interpretability and classification accuracy. To evaluate the feature interpretability of the proposed solution, its localization accuracy is measured. Moreover, CAMs and saliency maps [9] are presented for visual evaluation.

2   Methodology

2.1   Baseline Model

Given a database $X = \{x^{(1)}, ..., x^{(N)}\}$ of N X-ray images, and their corresponding labels $Y = \{y^{(1)}, ..., y^{(N))}\}$, where $y = [y_1, ..., y_j, ..., y_C]$ and $y_j \in \{0, 1\}$ with C being the number of classes, our aim is to train a model $\hat{y} = f_\theta(x)$, where $\hat{y}$ is the predicated label and θ denotes the parameters of the model. The loss to be minimized is binary cross entropy loss, and for each input example x is defined as:

$$\mathcal{L}(f_\theta(x), y) = -\sum_j \beta y_j \log(\hat{y}_j) + (1 - y_j) \log(1 - \hat{y}_j) \tag{1}$$

where β is a weighting factor to balance the positive labels, and defined as the ratio of the number of negative labels to the number of positive labels in a batch.

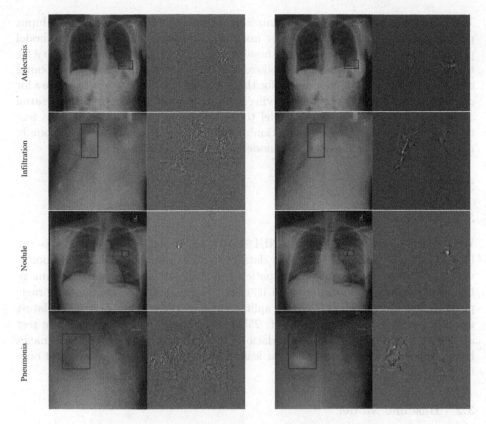

Fig. 1. Visualization of CAMs (overlayed on the input image) and saliency maps. (Left) our proposed baseline. (Right) our adversarially robust optimization method ($\epsilon = 0.005$). Blue boxes are ground truth annotation. (Images are best seen in electronic form) (Color figure online)

2.2 Adversarially Robust Optimization

This work aims at improving the learned feature representations of neural network classifiers through training models that are robust against adversarial examples. We view adversarial examples and robustness from the perspective of optimization. Given the loss formulated in Eq. 1, adversarial examples are perturbed inputs that try to maximize the loss

$$\max_{\delta \in \Delta} \mathcal{L}(f_\theta(x + \delta), y) \tag{2}$$

where δ is the perturbation and Δ defines the allowed perturbation [2]. In order to make models robust against these adversarial examples, the loss is modified to a min-max problem so that it incorporates robustness as an objective [6]:

$$\min_\theta \max_{\delta \in \Delta} \mathcal{L}(f_\theta(x + \delta), y) \tag{3}$$

The approach for solving the optimization problem is to repeatedly find input perturbations δ by solving the inner maximization, and then update the model parameters θ to reduce the loss on these perturbed inputs. It is not necessary for the inner maximization to be solved exactly, and an approximate lower bound could lead to a reasonable solution for the min-max problem [6]. Our purpose for robust optimization is not only having a high performance against adversarial attacks, but also steering the model towards learning more interpretable features. We choose a Δ and optimization method for Eq. 2 that is computationally reasonable, and we show that the model still learns robust features.

3   Experiments

3.1   Dataset

We evaluate our method on the NIH chestX-ray14 dataset [11], which is the largest publicly available chest x-ray dataset to date and includes 112,120 frontal-view X-ray images of 30,805 unique patients in 1024×1024 resolution. Each image has fourteen labels associated with it, each corresponding to common thoracic pathologies. We use the train/test split provided with the dataset in its latest update, i.e. from the entire dataset, 25596 images are in the test set. The rest are split to training (90%) and validation (10%) sets. In the test set, 880 images have bounding box annotations of at least one pathology. Annotations exist only for 8 out of 14 pathologies.

3.2   Baseline Model

In previous works [5, 8, 11], the feature maps of the last layer are of low resolution and they are used for generating the CAMs. These Low-resolution CAMs are not able to localize pathologies such as Nodule that are small in size. Hence, it is intuitive to modify the CNN to have larger feature maps in the last layer. Therefore we adopt a densely connected convolutional neural network [4], DenseNet-121, and remove the dense-blocks 3 and 4 and their corresponding transition layers (2 and 3) in order to get higher resolution feature maps in the last layer. The aforementioned neural network serves as our baseline model and its classification accuracy and interpretability evaluation are depicted in Figs. 2 and 3 respectively.

In all our experiments, the networks are trained using stochastic gradient descent with a learning rate of 0.01 and a momentum of 0.9. We use a batch size of 32 and do not use weight decay and dropout. The training is continued until the validation loss (Eq. 1) diverges, and the model with the smallest validation loss is used.

3.3   Interpretability Evaluation

Weakly-supervised localization accuracy is measured for each classification model and is used as a proxy for evaluating interpretability of the classification model. Localization is evaluated using intersection over union (IoU) between the thresholded CAM and the bounding box. The localization is correct when the IoU is greater than a certain threshold T(IoU). Localization accuracy is calculated for several values of T(IoU).

We do not generate bounding boxes from the thresholded CAMs and follow the same approach proposed by Li et al. [5], where the feature maps are directly evaluated using IoU metric without any bounding box generation. First, we upsample the CAMs via bilinear interpolation to the input image size that is 224×224 and then scale their values to a range (we used [0 255]) and subsequently threshold them by value. The method does not depend on further post-processing and bounding box generation approaches, thus directly evaluates the feature maps. We choose the thresholding value differently for each class based on its resulting localization performance on a validation set. The validation set is selected from the annotated images (from 880 images) in the test set. 20% (of 880 images) is chosen for finding the thresholding value and we perform 5-fold cross validation for correct evaluation.

3.4 Adversarially Robust Optimization

The min-max optimization in Eq. 3 is solved iteratively by solving the inner maximization and then the outer minimization, hence a method that requires several update steps for solving the inner maximization makes the solution computationally expensive. Many methods have been proposed in the literature for finding approximate solutions to the inner maximization problem. We use the FGSM [2] method as it requires only one update step for finding a local maxima.

If we start solving the min-max problem (Eq. 3) from a network not yet trained on the dataset, the adversarial examples make it hard for the network to learn the features of the dataset. Therefore, we initially train the network without adversarial loss, and after convergence, we continue training with the adversarial loss in Eq. 3. We observed that it is also helpful for training convergence, not to perturb all examples during training. Hence we only perturb half [10] of the input examples in each epoch during training with the adversarial loss (Eq. 3).

The amount of perturbation δ allowed for the FGSM method is defined by ϵ. FGSM finds a local maxima in Eq. 2 limited by the allowed perturbation set $\Delta = l_\infty$. Several values for ϵ are chosen in the experiments in order to see the effect of the amount of perturbation during training on the learned features of the network Fig. 4). As can be seen in Fig. 4, $\epsilon = 0.005$ results in more interpretable saliency maps, hence for quantitative analysis and comparison of the robust model with the baseline we use $\epsilon = 0.005$.

4   Results and Discussion

In this section and the Figs. 2 and 3 we refer to the work of Wang et al. [11] as NIH method, Rajpurkar et al. [8] as CheXNet, Li. et al. [5] as Supervised and our method that is based on adversarially robust optimization as Robust method.

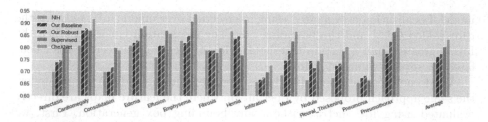

Fig. 2. Classification accuracies (AUC of ROC curve) for our proposed models and state of the art.

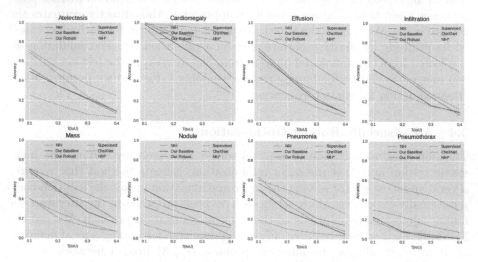

Fig. 3. Localization accuracy of state of the art models (dashed lines) [5,8,11] and our proposed models (Baseline and Robust). The horizontal axis represents the T(IoU) used for computing the localization accuracy

4.1 Baseline Model vs. State of the Art

CheXNet method achieves the highest AUC (Fig. 2). However, it has the lowest localization accuracy (Fig. 3), indicating that the model's learned features do not align well with the pathologies. The high AUC and lack of interpretable features of CheXNet can be attributed to its unweighted binary cross entropy loss where the imbalance between positive and negative examples is ignored.

The Supervised method uses 80% of annotated images during training, hence it achieves the highest localization accuracy. We report it as an upper bound for the localization accuracy, and it cannot be fairly compared with other methods since they are only trained on labels. However, our baseline surpasses the Supervised method in Nodule localization as it generates higher resolution CAMs.

For localization accuracy, NIH uses a different evaluation method than ours (Sect. 3.3). NIH method uses an ad-hoc CAM thresholding and bounding box generation approach. Therefore, in order to compare our baseline fairly with

NIH, we implemented NIH (using ResNet50 without transition layer) method and evaluated it using the procedure in Sect. 3.3, which is shown as NIH* in Fig. 3.

4.2   Robust Model vs. Baseline

Quantitative Evaluation: Our Robust model (trained with $\epsilon = 0.005$) shows improvement in localization accuracy for Cardiomegaly, Pneumonia, and Infiltration, yields lower accuracy for the Nodule class and comparable (still higher) results for the rest. Nevertheless, while quantitative results provide a means for measuring feature interpretability of the model on the entire test set, visually explainable features may still be essential for the clinical community.

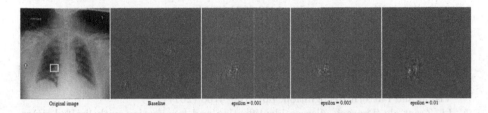

Original image   Baseline   epsilon = 0.001   epsilon = 0.005   epsilon = 0.01

Fig. 4. Effect of increasing the perturbation δ ($\delta = |\epsilon|$) used in our robust method on saliency maps. The blue box denotes the ground truth bounding box for Mass. (Images are best seen in electronic form) (Color figure online)

Visual Evaluation: The robust model yields significantly more interpretable gradients with respect to the input image as seen in saliency maps in Fig. 1. These are vanilla saliency maps [9], the gradients are only clipped by three standard deviations and scaled to [0 1] and no further processing (e.g. smoothing) is performed. The effect of increasing the amount of perturbation ϵ during adversarial robust optimization on visual interpretability is presented in Fig. 4. It can be seen that increasing the amount of perturbation during training steers the model toward focusing on the most salient feature of the image. It is also interesting in future research to study the effects of other perturbation sets Δ such as rotations on feature interpretability.

5   Conclusion

In this work, we demonstrated that adversarially robust optimization improves the feature interpretability of neural network classifiers both quantitatively and visually. Saliency maps of our adversarially trained models show significantly more interpretable features. The method does not have any dependency on the neural network architecture and the dataset. We also demonstrated that evaluating the model only using classification accuracy is not reliable since the high accuracy of a model could be due to its reliance on features that are not relevant to the pathologies.

Acknowledgement. We would like to thank Siemens Healthineers for their financial support.

References

1. Biffi, C., et al.: Learning interpretable anatomical features through deep generative models: application to cardiac remodeling. In: Frangi, A.F., Schnabel, J.A., Davatzikos, C., Alberola-López, C., Fichtinger, G. (eds.) MICCAI 2018. LNCS, vol. 11071, pp. 464–471. Springer, Cham (2018). https://doi.org/10.1007/978-3-030-00934-2_52
2. Goodfellow, I.J., Shlens, J., Szegedy, C.: Explaining and harnessing adversarial examples. arXiv preprint arXiv:1412.6572 (2014)
3. Greenspan, H., Van Ginneken, B., Summers, R.M.: Guest editorial deep learning in medical imaging: overview and future promise of an exciting new technique. IEEE Trans. Med. Imaging **35**(5), 1153–1159 (2016)
4. Huang, G., Liu, Z., Van Der Maaten, L., Weinberger, K.Q.: Densely connected convolutional networks. In: Proceedings of the IEEE Conference on Computer Vision and Pattern Recognition, pp. 4700–4708 (2017)
5. Li, Z., et al.: Thoracic disease identification and localization with limited supervision. In: Proceedings of the IEEE Conference on Computer Vision and Pattern Recognition, pp. 8290–8299 (2018)
6. Madry, A., Makelov, A., Schmidt, L., Tsipras, D., Vladu, A.: Towards deep learning models resistant to adversarial attacks. arXiv preprint arXiv:1706.06083 (2017)
7. Miotto, R., Wang, F., Wang, S., Jiang, X., Dudley, J.T.: Deep learning for healthcare: review, opportunities and challenges. Briefings Bioinf. **19**(6), 1236–1246 (2017)
8. Rajpurkar, P., et al.: CheXNet: radiologist-level pneumonia detection on chest x-rays with deep learning. arXiv preprint arXiv:1711.05225 (2017)
9. Simonyan, K., Vedaldi, A., Zisserman, A.: Deep inside convolutional networks: visualising image classification models and saliency maps. arXiv preprint arXiv:1312.6034 (2013)
10. Tsipras, D., Santurkar, S., Engstrom, L., Turner, A., Madry, A.: Robustness may be at odds with accuracy. arXiv preprint arXiv:1805.12152 (2018)
11. Wang, X., Peng, Y., Lu, L., Lu, Z., Bagheri, M., Summers, R.M.: ChestX-ray8: hospital-scale chest x-ray database and benchmarks on weakly-supervised classification and localization of common thorax diseases. In: Proceedings of the IEEE Conference on Computer Vision and Pattern Recognition, pp. 2097–2106 (2017)
12. Yao, L., Poblenz, E., Dagunts, D., Covington, B., Bernard, D., Lyman, K.: Learning to diagnose from scratch by exploiting dependencies among labels. arXiv preprint arXiv:1710.10501 (2017)
13. Zhou, B., Khosla, A., Lapedriza, A., Oliva, A., Torralba, A.: Learning deep features for discriminative localization. In: Proceedings of the IEEE Conference on Computer Vision and Pattern Recognition, pp. 2921–2929 (2016)

Synthesize Mammogram from Digital Breast Tomosynthesis with Gradient Guided cGANs

Gongfa Jiang[1], Yao Lu[1,2(✉)], Jun Wei[3], and Yuesheng Xu[4]

[1] Sun Yat-sen University, Guangzhou, China
jianggfa@mail2.sysu.edu.cn, luyao23@mail.sysu.edu.cn
[2] Key Laboratory of Machine Intelligence and Advanced Computing,
Ministry of Education, Guangzhou, China
[3] Perception Vision Medical Technologies LTD. Co., Guangzhou, China
weijun@pvmedtech.com
[4] Old Dominion University, Norfolk, USA
y1xu@odu.edu

Abstract. Compared to mammographic screening, digital breast tomosynthesis (DBT) as an adjunct to full-field digital mammography (FFDM) so called combo-mode has been shown to improve sensitivity and reduce false positive rates in breast cancer detection. However, combo-mode screening increases the radiation dose to the patient. In this study, our purpose is to develop a new approach to synthesize photo realistic digital mammogram (SDM) from reconstructed DBT volume to replace adjunct FFDM which in turn will reduce the radiation dose to the patient during breast cancer screening. A deep convolutional neural network (DCNN) is used to synthesize SDM from DBT with FFDM as ground truth during the training. When training our DCNN, a traditional mean squared error (MSE) loss is avoided due to over-smoothing problem. Instead, we propose a gradient guided cGANs (GGGAN) training method to retain subtle tissue structures and microcalcifications (MCs) in the SDM during the DCNN training. The contrast-to-noise ratio (CNR) and the full width at half maximum (FWHM) of the line profiles are used as image quality measures for quantitative comparison. In additional, a human observer perceptual experiment is conducted to qualitatively compare FFDM to SDM of the same patient. The results indicate that SDM has comparable perceptual image quality to FFDM both quantitatively and qualitatively.

Keywords: FFDM · DBT · Image synthesis · Deep learning

Electronic supplementary material The online version of this chapter (https://doi.org/10.1007/978-3-030-32226-7_89) contains supplementary material, which is available to authorized users.

© Springer Nature Switzerland AG 2019
D. Shen et al. (Eds.): MICCAI 2019, LNCS 11769, pp. 801–809, 2019.
https://doi.org/10.1007/978-3-030-32226-7_89

1   Introduction

Breast cancer remains one of the leading causes of death among women worldwide. Digital breast tomosynthesis (DBT) gradually replaces mammography as early screening tool in some advanced countries. Several large scale clinical studies indicate that false positive rate is lower and cancer detection rate is higher with DBT+FFDM screening so called combo-mode compared to those with FFDM screening alone [1]. However, combo-mode nearly doubles the radiation dose of FFDM alone [2] to the patient in each exam while more radiation exposure increases risk of radiation-induced breast cancer [3]. With the improved public awareness of radiation harm, there is a sense of urgency to address the issue of combo-mode.

One of the solutions to reduce the radiation dose during DBT screening is to synthetically reconstruct a 2D FFDM-like mammogram, called synthesized digital mammgoram (SDM) here on, from DBT volume to replace the FFDM [4], thereby reducing the radiation dose while maintaining the detection performance of DBT to be similar to DBT+FFDM [5]. In this work, we investigate a deep convolutional neural network (DCNN) approach to generate SDM from DBT by directly approaching the original FFDM. One potential problem is that commonly used mean squared error (MSE) objective function during the training produces overly smoothed image [6], which may not be suitable in SDM since the parenchymal information is important for breast cancer grading. We use a state-of-the-art conditional generative adversarial networks (cGANs) based method pix2pixHD [7] (called cGANs here on), in which a discriminator is trained to differentiate SDM from FFDM in the form of dissimilar patterns measured by adversarial loss and feature matching loss, and a generator is trained to minimize the dissimilarity in order to produce a sharper image. Another potential problem is that high frequency details such as microcalcifications (MCs) and subtle tissue structures may still be weaken by cGANs due to relatively smaller size compared to parenchymal texture. To retain those high frequency details, we newly propose a gradient guided cGANs (GGGAN) method which using the gradient of SDM and FFDM as additional input to discriminator. Some previous work [8,9] also used gradient information coupled with the GAN network for medical imaging.

2   Method

2.1   Training Methods

We denote training dataset by $\mathbf{S} = \{(\mathbf{x}_i, \mathbf{y}_i)|1 \leq i \leq M\}$, where $\mathbf{x}_i, \mathbf{y}_i$ is the ith pair of DBT and FFDM in $\mathbf{S}$, and M is the number of pairs in $\mathbf{S}$. The training objective is to obtain a generator DCNN, denoted by G, which can reconstruct a $\hat{\mathbf{y}} = G(\mathbf{x})$ as SDM. During the training of G, the difference between each output $\hat{\mathbf{y}}_i = G(\mathbf{x}_i)$ and the target FFDM $\mathbf{y}_i$ is measured and used to guide the optimization of G's parameters. We compare three training methods: MSE, cGANs and GGGAN detailed below:

Mean Squared Error. The MSE loss function is the empirical expectation of squared l_2-norm of difference between prediction $\hat{\mathbf{y}}$ and target $\mathbf{y}$:

$$\mathcal{L}_{MSE}(G) = \frac{1}{M} \sum_{i=1}^{M} \|\mathbf{y}_i - \hat{\mathbf{y}}_i\|_2^2, \tag{1}$$

where $\|\cdot\|_2^2$ is squared l_2-norm.

Conditional GANs. In cGANs, a discriminator D is trained to differentiate output $\hat{\mathbf{y}}_i$ from the target $\mathbf{y}_i$ with input $\mathbf{x}_i$ as condition. Given a trained discriminator D, the adversarial loss and feature matching loss are given by:

$$\mathcal{L}_{Adver}(G) = \frac{1}{M} \sum_{i=1}^{M} \|\mathbf{1} - D(\mathbf{x}_i, \hat{\mathbf{y}}_i)\|_2^2, \tag{2}$$

$$\mathcal{L}_{FM}(G) = \frac{1}{MT} \sum_{i=1}^{M} \sum_{j=1}^{T} \frac{1}{N_j} \left\| D^j(\mathbf{x}_i, \mathbf{y}_i) - D^j(\mathbf{x}_i, \hat{\mathbf{y}}_i) \right\|_1, \tag{3}$$

$$\mathcal{L}_{cGANs}(G) = \mathcal{L}_{Adver}(G) + \lambda_{FM}\mathcal{L}_{FM}(G), \tag{4}$$

where λ_{FM} is a weighting factor to balance between adversarial loss and feature matching loss, $\mathbf{1}$ is "ones" vector and has the same size as $D(\cdot)$, $D^j(\cdot)$ is the feature of jth layers of $D(\cdot)$, T is the total number of layers, N_j is the number of elements of the feature in jth layer and $\|\cdot\|_1$ is l_1-norm. The loss function used to train D is given by:

$$\mathcal{L}_{cGANs}(D) = \frac{1}{M} \sum_{i=1}^{M} \left(\|\mathbf{1} - D(\mathbf{x}_i, \mathbf{y}_i)\|_2^2 + \|\mathbf{0} - D(\mathbf{x}_i, \hat{\mathbf{y}}_i)\|_2^2 \right), \tag{5}$$

where $\mathbf{0}$ is "zeroes" vector and has the same size as $D(\cdot)$.

Gradient Guided cGANs. We use gradient of $\hat{\mathbf{y}}_i$ and $\mathbf{y}_i$ as additional input to D in cGANs. Gradient feature is extracted by a convolution layer, in which kernel weights are initialized by Sobel operators and fixed. We use Sobel operators with four directions: vertical, horizontal, and two diagonal directions. In addition, dilated convolution [10] with dilation rate of 1, 3 and 5 is used to enlarge the receptive field of the Sobel convolution layer and capture bigger edges in image. The gradient feature with 4×3 channels is obtained and concatenated with SDM/FFDM as multichannel image input for discriminator D.

2.2   Proposed Synthesizing Framework

For proposed generator DCNN, we use a U-Net consisted of a encoder to extracte multi-scale features from different scales of input and a decoder to derive a SDM by fusing extracted multi-scale features (Fig. 1). See supplementary material for more details of network architecture of generator and discriminator.

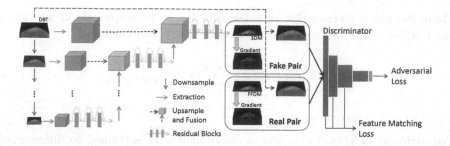

Fig. 1. The overall framework of the proposed method. For discriminator, DBT, SDM and gradient feature compose fake pair, while DBT, FFDM and gradient feature compose real pair. Those pairs are used to train the discriminator. In generator DCNN, multi-scale features are extracted from DBTs with different size, and then are sequentially upsampled and fused to derive SDM. Best viewed in color. (Color figure online)

Similar to [7], we train three discriminators with identical architecture simultaneously to handle multi-scale structures in SDM/FFDM. For the first discriminator, it takes original SDM/FFDM and DBT as inputs while the other two discriminators have down sampled SDM/FFDM and DBT of a factor of 2 and 4 as input.

2.3 SWGC for 3D Information in DBT

In this work, we use group convolution [11] to explicitly extract 3D structural information in DBT. In group convolution, input slices/channels are divided into several groups (empirically set to 32 in this work), and convolutions are applied separately for each group. Output features are concatenated in original group order to keep 3D information in input (Fig. 2). We propose a shared weight group convolution (SWGC) structure with the assumption that feature extraction process should be identical for individual groups. In SWGC, weights of convolution kernel of individual groups are shared (Fig. 2).

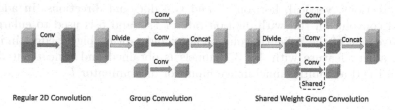

Fig. 2. Cubes with different colors indicate DBT slices/features of different groups. Note that regular 2D convolution cannot keep 3D information in input. Best viewed in color. (Color figure online)

We assume that 3D structural feature repetition and sharing properties also exists in feature upsampling and fusion processes. We use SWGC for upsampling and fusion to keep 3D structural information along the feature flow in generator.

3 Experiments

3.1 Data Preprocessing and Experimental Conditions

We retrospectively collected 1077 pairs of DBTs and FFDMs from breast cancer patients. We randomly split the whole set into training set of 977 cases and test set of 100. DBTs are padded with all zero slice on one side until each DBT has 96 slices. The grey level values of DBTs and FFDMs are normalized to range from −1 to 1. Then DBTs and corresponding FFDMs are cut into patches at 512×512 resolution without overlapping. The patches with high percentage of background in training dataset are discarded for better training convergency. This results a total of 33431 patches in the training dataset and 2921 patches in the test dataset. Horizontal flip augmentation is used for all patches and vertical flip augmentation is used for patches from CC-view mammogram. We empirically set number of layers $T = 3$, $\lambda_{FM} = 10$, which is the same as in [7]. Adam solver with a learning rate of 1×10^{-4} is used. We set batch size to 1

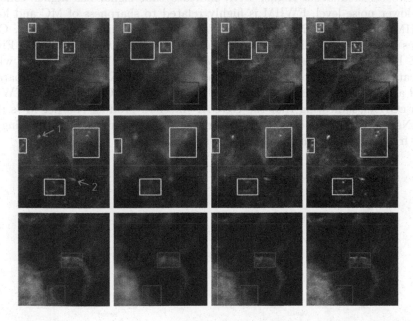

Fig. 3. From left to right are target FFDM, MSE, cGANs, and GGGAN. Rectangles outline sharp edges (green) and MCs (red) missed out by MSE and cGANs while maintained in GGGAN. Two MCs pointed by yellow arrows in FFDM of row 2 are selected for quantitative sharpness comparison. Best viewed on screen with zoom in. (Color figure online)

due to the limitation of GPU memory and train for 6 epochs (about 200,000 iterations). Training takes 80 h on an NVIDIA TitanX GPU.

3.2 Synthesis Results

Three generators are trained with MSE, cGANs and GGGAN respectively. We show some representative visual results produced by the three methods in Fig. 3. Visual comparison of the images shows that cGANs and GGGAN significantly alleviated the overly smoothness problem of MSE. ROIs in Fig. 3 highlight the MCs and sharp edges which are missed out by MSE and cGANs while maintained by GGGAN. The capability of GGGAN to retain MCs and sharp edges indicates effective guidance by gradient attention for the discriminator to focus more on high frequency components.

3.3 Quantitative Evaluation

The three methods are quantitatively compared in terms of the signal quality and sharpness by CNR and FWHM. Two MCs which appear in SDMs of all three methods are selected for quantitative comparison (pointed by yellow arrows in FFDM of row 2 in Fig. 3). See supplementary material for line profiles of the two selected MCs. Higher CNR indicate that signal has higher contrast and lower noise level. FWHM is highly related to sharpness of MC and lower FWHM indicate that MC has lower standard deviation and is sharper. CNR values and FWHM of line profiles of the two selected MCs are shown in Fig. 4. MSE has lowest CNR and highest FWHM among the three methods, which indicate that MSE produces most smooth MCs. cGANs achieves comparable CNR and FWHM to FFDM, while GGGAN have higher CNR and lower FWHM than cGANs, indicating that the GGGAN method produce sharper MCs than cGANs and FFDM. The proposed gradient attention is succeed in enhancing the high frequency components such as MCs in SDM.

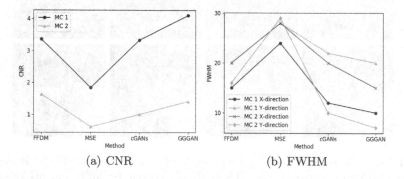

(a) CNR   (b) FWHM

Fig. 4. CNR values and FWHM of line profiles of the two selected MCs. Higher CNR value and lower FWHM are better.

The three methods are also quantitatively compared using peak-to-noise ratio (PSNR) and structural similarity (SSIM). The result on test dataset is in Table 1. MSE achieves higher PSNR and SSIM than cGANs and GGGAN. This result is consistent with results in [12], in which low dose CT denoising network trained with MSE loss outperforms GAN based methods in terms of PSNR and SSIM while inferior in terms of other metrics. This may indicate that PSNR and SSIM are not sufficient in evaluating image quality [12].

Table 1. PSNR and SSIM (mean ± standard deviation) of MSE, cGANs, GGGAN.

	PSNR	SSIM
MSE	**26.70 ± 4.08**	**0.708 ± 0.160**
cGANs	25.46 ± 3.98	0.622 ± 0.200
GGGAN	25.77 ± 4.05	0.629 ± 0.196

To evaluate the effectiveness of the proposed gradient attention on improvement on subjective perceptual image quality by producing high frequency components, we design a perceptual ranking experiment on FFDM and SDMs from generators trained with cGANs and GGGAN, with three radiologists as human observers. Totally 1000 pairwise comparisons are randomly selected from the test dataset for each radiologists, and both left-right order and the order of pairs are randomized. Pairwise ranking results are listed in Tables 2 and 3. In Table 2, when compared to FFDM, 5%–10% more SDMs from GGGAN is comparable than cGANs do. In Table 3, when directly compared to cGANs, 13.5%–47.6% more SDMs from GGGAN are better. The results indicate that GGGAN produces more SDM with comparable perceptual image quality to FFDM, and outperforms cGANs without gradient attention.

Table 2. Percentage of SDMs from cGANs and GGGAN which have better, worse or equal image quality when compared to FFDM ranked by each radiologist.

	Radiologist 1			Radiologist 2			Radiologist 3		
	Better	Worse	Equal	Better	Worse	Equal	Better	Worse	Equal
cGANs	11.2%	74.5%	14.3%	4.0%	90.9%	5.1%	21.9%	66.8%	11.3%
GGGAN	**16.1%**	**64.0%**	**19.9%**	**7.1%**	**85.9%**	**7.0%**	18.7%	**62.0%**	**19.3%**

3.4   Effectiveness of SWGC

The importance of SWGC is also studied by comparing generator DCNN using regular 2D convolution, group convolution and SWGC. The three generator

Table 3. Percentage of SDMs from GGGAN which have better, worse or equal image quality when compared to cGANs ranked by each radiologist.

	GGGAN	cGANs	Equal
Radiologist 1	**53.9%**	17.0%	29.1%
Radiologist 2	**63.2%**	15.6%	21.2%
Radiologist 3	**42.9%**	29.4%	27.7%

DCNN models are all trained with GGGAN. A representative visual result is provided in Fig. 5. The visual result indicate that generator using SWGC derive SDM with shaper edges and less smooth textures than using group convolution, and avoid artifacts that occur to generator using regular 2D convolution.

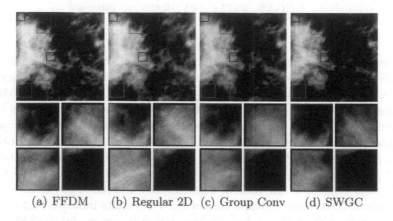

(a) FFDM   (b) Regular 2D (c) Group Conv   (d) SWGC

Fig. 5. Four zoomed-in regions of a mass are provided. Regular 2D convolution results in artifact (bottom left zoomed-in region) which dose not exists in FFDM. Overly smoothed edges and textures (the other three zoomed-in regions) on SDM from 2D convolution and group convolution, on which SWGC shows better performance. Best viewed in color. (Color figure online)

4 Conclusion and Discussion

In this work, we have presented a DCNN that extract multi-scale and 3D structural information in DBT to generate SDM. During the training, we adopt a cGANs to overcome the smoothness of MSE loss function. Moreover, we propose a gradient guided cGANs training method and result the SDM with enhanced high frequency components such as sharp edges and MCs and comparable image quality as FFDM both quantitatively and qualitatively. In the future work, we may introduce other features derived from supervised learning methods, like perceptual loss used in computer vision field, or use GAN with higher performance such as WGAN-GP, to further improve image quality. Combination of MSE and GAN method and the validation work is also scheduled for future work.

References

1. Hodgson, R., et al.: Systematic review of 3D mammography for breast cancer screening. Breast **27**, 52–61 (2016)
2. Svahn, T., et al.: Review of radiation dose estimates in digital breast tomosynthesis relative to those in two-view full-field digital mammography. Breast **24**(2), 93–99 (2015)
3. Miglioretti, D.L., et al.: Radiation-induced breast cancer incidence and mortality from digital mammography screening: a modeling study. Ann. internal Med. **164**(4), 205–214 (2016)
4. Wei, J., et al.: Synthesizing mammogram from digital breast tomosynthesis. Phys. Med. Biol. **64**(4), 045011 (2019)
5. Zuckerman, S.P., et al.: Implementation of synthesized two-dimensional mammography in a population-based digital breast tomosynthesis screening program. Radiology **281**(3), 730–736 (2016)
6. Ledig, C., et al.: Photo-realistic single image super-resolution using a generative adversarial network. In: Proceedings of the IEEE Conference on Computer Vision and Pattern Recognition, vol. 2, p. 4 (2017)
7. Wang, T.C., et al.: High-resolution image synthesis and semantic manipulation with conditional GANs. arXiv preprint arXiv:1711.11585 (2017)
8. Shan, H., et al.: Can deep learning outperform modern commercial CT image reconstruction methods? arXiv preprint arXiv:1811.03691 (2018)
9. Yu, B., et al.: Ea-GANs: edge-aware generative adversarial networks for cross-modality MR image synthesis. IEEE Trans. Med. Imaging **38**(7), 1750–1762 (2019)
10. Chen, L.C., et al.: Rethinking atrous convolution for semantic image segmentation. arXiv preprint arXiv:1706.05587 (2017)
11. Ioannou, Y., et al.: Deep roots: improving CNN efficiency with hierarchical filter groups. In: Proceedings of the IEEE Conference on Computer Vision and Pattern Recognition, pp. 1231–1240 (2017)
12. Yang, Q., et al.: Low-dose CT image denoising using a generative adversarial network with Wasserstein distance and perceptual loss. IEEE Trans. Med. Imaging **37**(6), 1348–1357 (2018)

Semi-supervised Medical Image Segmentation via Learning Consistency Under Transformations

Gerda Bortsova[1]([✉]), Florian Dubost[1], Laurens Hogeweg[2],
Ioannis Katramados[2], and Marleen de Bruijne[1,3]

[1] Biomedical Imaging Group Rotterdam,
Department of Radiology and Nuclear Medicine, Erasmus MC,
Rotterdam, The Netherlands
gerdabortsova@gmail.com
[2] COSMONiO, Groningen, The Netherlands
[3] Department of Computer Science, University of Copenhagen,
Copenhagen, Denmark

Abstract. The scarcity of labeled data often limits the application of supervised deep learning techniques for medical image segmentation. This has motivated the development of semi-supervised techniques that learn from a mixture of labeled and unlabeled images. In this paper, we propose a novel semi-supervised method that, in addition to supervised learning on labeled training images, learns to predict segmentations consistent under a given class of transformations on both labeled and unlabeled images. More specifically, in this work we explore learning equivariance to elastic deformations. We implement this through: (1) a Siamese architecture with two identical branches, each of which receives a differently transformed image, and (2) a composite loss function with a supervised segmentation loss term and an unsupervised term that encourages segmentation consistency between the predictions of the two branches. We evaluate the method on a public dataset of chest radiographs with segmentations of anatomical structures using 5-fold cross-validation. The proposed method reaches significantly higher segmentation accuracy compared to supervised learning. This is due to learning transformation consistency on both labeled and unlabeled images, with the latter contributing the most. We achieve the performance comparable to state-of-the-art chest X-ray segmentation methods while using substantially fewer labeled images.

Keywords: Semi-supervised learning · Segmentation · Chest X-ray

1 Introduction

Supervised deep learning algorithms often require numerous labeled examples for training to yield satisfactory performance. In the domain of medical imaging, however, labeled data is often very scarce, which is especially true for dense labels

© Springer Nature Switzerland AG 2019
D. Shen et al. (Eds.): MICCAI 2019, LNCS 11769, pp. 810–818, 2019.
https://doi.org/10.1007/978-3-030-32226-7_90

such as segmentations, as they are particularly costly to produce. On the other hand, for many medical image analysis tasks, unlabeled data coming from the same or similar distribution as the labeled data is available in abundance. This motivates the development of semi-supervised algorithms.

Many ideas have been proposed for improving performance of deep learning algorithms for medical image analysis through utilizing unlabeled data [2]. Self-supervised approaches learn to perform an auxiliary task related to the target prediction task on unlabeled data, examples including image colorization [12] and predicting one image modality from another [5]. Auxiliary manifold embedding [1] learns to place unlabeled examples far or close in the feature space with respect to each other and to labeled examples according to prior adjacency information. Self-ensembling approaches learn from synthetic labels on unlabeled data, which are constructed using past iterations of the same network [7,9].

In this paper, we propose an approach in which we learn consistency under transformations on both labeled and unlabeled data, in addition to supervised learning from labeled data. We implement this consistency learning through a Siamese architecture trained end-to-end. The network has two identical branches each of which receives differently transformed versions of the same images as inputs and is supervised to output segmentations consistent with the other branch, in addition to learning from labeled images in a supervised fashion. Combining supervised and unsupervised consistency learning in the network is achieved by a composite objective consisting of two respective terms. This idea was already explored before and applied to the prediction of image-level labels: image classification [10,13] and landmark coordinate regression [6]. We extend this method so that it can be applied efficiently to learning to predict pixel-level labels consistent under spatial transformations of images. This entails including a special differentiable layer into the Siamese architecture that transforms the pixel-wise predictions of one of the branches so as to align it with the predictions of the second branch and consequently allow their pixel-wise comparison in the consistency loss term. Self-ensembling approaches [7,9] are similar to the proposed approach in that they use a transformation consistency prior: they construct their synthetic labels on unlabeled data using predictions on differently transformed inputs. Unlike these methods, the proposed Siamese approach does not train the network to fit specific targets on unlabeled images (i.e. the synthetic labels), which are unknown and cannot be reliably estimated; it only encourages the outputs to have the desired transformation consistency property.

We evaluate our method on the JSRT chest X-ray dataset [15,16]. In this paper, we focus on learning equivariance to elastic deformations, although our method can be readily applied to a broader class of transformations. Through our experiments, we evaluate: (1) the contribution of learning this equivariance on labeled data (i.e. as a regularization in supervised-only learning) to the segmentation performance; (2) the contribution of adding different amounts of unlabeled data into the equivariance learning; (3) how these contributions vary with the size of the labeled portion of the training set. We compare the proposed method

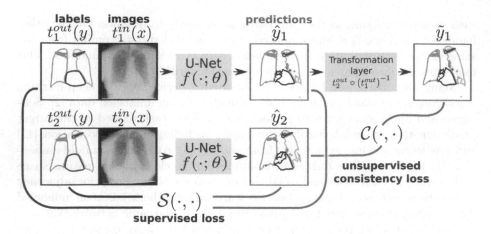

Fig. 1. The proposed network. The inputs are mixed batches of labeled and unlabeled images. Every image x is transformed by two random mappings t_1^{in} and t_2^{in}. The label y, if available, is transformed by t_1^{out} and t_2^{out}. $t_1^{in}(x)$ and $t_2^{in}(x)$ are fed to the two identical branches of the network. The output of one of the branches is transformed by a differentiable layer for comparison with the output of the second branch in the consistency loss $\mathcal{C}$. The network is trained end-to-end using a combination of $\mathcal{C}$ and a supervised loss $\mathcal{S}$ (defined only on labeled images) as specified by Eq. 1.

trained in the small data (20 labeled images) and full supervision regimes with state-of-the-art methods [3,4,8,14] and the inter-observer agreement [16].

2 Method

Let $\mathcal{X}_l$ be a set of training examples with corresponding ground truth labels $\mathcal{Y}$ and $\mathcal{X}_u$ be a set of unlabeled examples. Let $\mathcal{T}$ be a distribution of tuples of mappings such that for a tuple $(t^{in}, t^{out}) =: t \sim \mathcal{T}$ applying transformation t^{in} to any image $x \in \mathcal{X} := \mathcal{X}_u \cup \mathcal{X}_l$ would result in the corresponding label y being transformed into $t^{out}(y)$ and t^{out} is invertible. Let $\mathcal{X}_l^{\mathcal{T}}$ be a set of all images from $\mathcal{X}_l$ with corresponding labels, augmented by examples $(t^{in}(x), t^{out}(y))$. We would like to find parameters θ of a network f that optimize the following objective:

$$\min \mathcal{L}_{sup}^{\mathcal{T}}(\theta) + \lambda \mathcal{L}_{cons}^{\mathcal{T}}(\theta)$$

with $\mathcal{L}_{sup}^{\mathcal{T}}(\theta) = 1/|\mathcal{X}_l^{\mathcal{T}}|(\sum_{(x,y) \in \mathcal{X}_l^{\mathcal{T}}} \mathcal{S}(y, f(x; \theta)))$ being a regular supervised loss (using $\mathcal{T}$ as a data augmentation strategy and $\mathcal{S}$ as an image-wise loss) and $\mathcal{L}_{cons}^{\mathcal{T}}(\theta)$ being an unsupervised consistency loss defined as:

$$\mathcal{L}_{cons}^{\mathcal{T}}(\theta) = \frac{1}{|\mathcal{X}|} \sum_{x \in \mathcal{X}} \mathbb{E}_{t_1, t_2 \sim \mathcal{T}} \left[\mathcal{C}\Big((t_2^{out} \circ (t_1^{out})^{-1})(f(t_1^{in}(x); \theta)), f(t_2^{in}(x); \theta) \Big) \right]$$

$\mathcal{L}_{cons}^{\mathcal{T}}(\theta)$ encourages the selection of θ that maximizes consistency of network predictions under transformations $\mathcal{T}$ on $\mathcal{X}$ as measured by image-wise loss $\mathcal{C}$.

We approximate minimization of this objective by a mini-batch training scheme in which we sample a set of labeled examples $\mathcal{B}_l$, a set of unlabeled examples $\mathcal{B}_u$ and two transforms $t_1, t_2 \sim \mathcal{T}$ for every example. A member of a batch $\mathcal{B}$ thus is a tuple (x, t_1, t_2) with or without ground truth label y. The mini-batch objective is:

$$\mathcal{L}^{\mathcal{T},\mathcal{B}}(\theta) = \frac{1}{2|\mathcal{B}_l|} \sum_{(x,y,t_1,t_2)\in\mathcal{B}_l} \Big(\mathcal{S}\big(t_1^{out}(y), f(t_1^{in}(x);\theta)\big) + \mathcal{S}\big(t_2^{out}(y), f(t_2^{in}(x);\theta)\big) \Big) +$$
$$\frac{\lambda}{|\mathcal{B}|} \sum_{(x,t_1,t_2)\in\mathcal{B}} \mathcal{C}\big((t_2^{out} \circ (t_1^{out})^{-1})(f(t_1^{in}(x);\theta)), f(t_2^{in}(x);\theta)\big) \quad (1)$$

The first sum approximates $\mathcal{L}_{sup}^{\mathcal{T}}(\theta)$ and the second approximates $\mathcal{L}_{cons}^{\mathcal{T}}(\theta)$. In the rest of the paper we will abuse notations $\mathcal{L}_{sup}^{\mathcal{T}}$ and $\mathcal{L}_{sup}^{\mathcal{T}}$ to refer to the first and the second sums in Eq. 1, respectively.

The overview of the network implementing this scheme is shown in Fig. 1. The architecture has two branches with shared weights θ. For every example $(x, t_1, t_2) \in \mathcal{B}$, we feed two differently deformed versions of x ($t_1^{in}(x)$ and $t_2^{in}(x)$) to the two branches of the network. The output of the first branch, $\hat{y}_1 := f(t_1^{in}(x); \theta)$, is transformed by $t_2^{out} \circ (t_1^{out})^{-1}$ using a custom differentiable layer so as to align it with the prediction of the second branch $\hat{y}_2 := f(t_2^{in}(x); \theta)$ for pixel-wise comparison by the consistency term $\mathcal{C}$. In addition to $\mathcal{C}$, if x happens to be labeled, the supervised loss $\mathcal{S}$ is applied to both $\hat{y}_1$ and $\hat{y}_2$. The network is thus trained end-to-end using Eq. 1 as a composite loss.

Note that since our transformation layer is differentiable, the gradient can flow through both branches. If the layer did not let the gradient through, training the network would be equivalent to applying the network to $t_1^{in}(x)$ and using $\tilde{y}_1 := (t_2^{out} \circ (t_1^{out})^{-1})(\hat{y}_1)$ as a target for $t_2^{in}(x)$ (such approach was adopted by [7]). In this case, the network is forced to update the prediction for $t_2^{in}(x)$ to be more similar to $\tilde{y}_1$, even if $\tilde{y}_1$ is incorrect. In the case of a differentiable layer, the network has the freedom to update its predictions in any way that optimizes $\mathcal{C}$, which includes changing the prediction for $t_1^{in}(x)$ to be more consistent with that for $t_2^{in}(x)$, the other way around or changing both of them in the same direction. In other words, the proposed methodology encourages predictions to have the desired property of transformation consistency without encouraging any specific predictions for unlabeled images, which might otherwise introduce a bias when the targets for these images cannot be reliably inferred.

In this work, we use elastic deformations as the event space for $\mathcal{T}$. Our transformation layer, in addition to the predicted segmentation, takes as its inputs deformation fields specifying forward and backward transformations $t_2^{out} \circ (t_1^{out})^{-1}$ and $t_1^{out} \circ (t_2^{out})^{-1}$. The latter is necessary for backpropagating the gradients through the layer:

$$\frac{\partial \mathcal{C}(\hat{y}_1, \hat{y}_2)}{\partial \hat{y}_1}\Big) = (t_1^{out} \circ (t_2^{out})^{-1})\Big(\frac{\partial \mathcal{C}(\tilde{y}_1, \hat{y}_2)}{\partial \tilde{y}_1}\Big)$$

In principle, any transformations t^{in} and t^{out} could be implemented, as long as the inverse $(t^{out})^{-1}$ can be computed.

3   Experiments

Dataset and Validation. We used the Japanese Society of Radiological Technology (JSRT) dataset [15], which contains 247 posterior-anterior chest radiographs with a resolution 2048×2048, 0.175 mm pixel size and 12-bit depth. Segmentations of the left and right lung fields, left and right clavicles and the heart were made available by [16]. We created five splits of the dataset by choosing images with either even or odd IDs as the test set ($|\mathcal{X}^{\text{test}}| = 123$ or 124) as prescribed by [16] and randomly splitting the rest into the training ($|\mathcal{X}^{\text{train}}| = 100$) and validation portions. For every split, we sampled subsets $\mathcal{X}_l^{\text{train}}$ of 5, 10, 25 and 50 examples (with larger subsets containing smaller ones) from $\mathcal{X}^{\text{train}}$ to be used as labeled portions of the training set. The rest of the images from $\mathcal{X}^{\text{train}}$ were assigned to the unlabeled portion of the training set $\mathcal{X}_u^{\text{train}}$, to be used by the proposed semi-supervised algorithm.

Implementation Details. We used a U-Net-like architecture [11] as the basis for the Siamese network. For every cross-validation (CV) split and labeled-unlabeled training set split, we first trained a network using $\mathcal{L}_{sup}^{\mathcal{T}}$ loss (i.e. in a purely supervised way). We used this network as a basis for fine-tuning four different networks: two supervised and two semi-supervised. The two supervised networks were fine-tuned using $\mathcal{L}_{sup}^{\mathcal{T}}$ or $\mathcal{L}_{sup}^{\mathcal{T}} + \lambda\mathcal{L}_{cons}^{\mathcal{T}}$. We refer to them as "the baseline" and the supervised transformation-consistent network or $SupTC$, respectively. The semi-supervised networks were fine-tuned using $\mathcal{L}_{sup}^{\mathcal{T}} + \lambda\mathcal{L}_{cons}^{\mathcal{T}}$, with batches containing equal numbers of labeled and unlabeled examples. (The total batch size was the same as in the supervised cases.) One of the semi-supervised networks only used unlabeled images from the training set $\mathcal{X}_u^{\text{train}}$ (we dubbed it $SemiTC$), while the other one additionally used images from the corresponding validation and test sets as unlabeled ($SemiTC+$). We used intersection over union (IOU) averaged over six classes (the five structures and the background) as both supervised and unsupervised loss terms: $\mathcal{S}(y, \hat{y}) = \mathcal{C}(y, \hat{y}) = 1/6 \sum_c (\sum_i y_c^{(i)} \hat{y}_c^{(i)} / (\sum_i y_c^{(i)} + (1 - y_c^{(i)}) \hat{y}_c^{(i)}))$. The weight λ of the consistency term was arbitrarily set to 1, giving the supervised and consistency terms equal importance. Adadelta optimizer was used for both training and fine-tuning. The images and segmentation maps were subsampled to a resolution of 512×512 for training. The deformation fields for elastic deformations were created by randomly sampling two-dimensional displacement maps from a uniform distribution $\mathcal{U}(-1000, 1000)$ and smoothing them with a Gaussian filter with the standard deviation of 100 pixels. Spline interpolation was applied to images and nearest neighbor interpolation was applied to labels and predictions. To reduce computational time, probability distribution $\mathcal{T}$ was specified as drawing an identity transform ($\text{id}_{\mathcal{X}}, \text{id}_{y \cup \hat{y}}$) or a random elastic deformation (t^{in}, t^{out}) (specified by a deformation field sampled as described above) with 50% chance.

Table 1. Means and standard deviations of mIOU over the five test sets corresponding to different versions of the method (rows) and labeled training set sizes (columns). These versions are: the proposed architecture trained with $\mathcal{L}_{sup}^{\mathcal{T}}$ only, the consistency-regularized version of the latter ($SupTC$), and the proposed semi-supervised method using either only unlabeled examples from the training set ($SemiTC$) or additionally validation and test set as unlabeled examples ($SemiTC+$). Note that with the largest training set size $SupTC$ is equivalent to $SemiTC$, since all labels are available.

Methods	Loss	$\mathcal{X}_u$	5	10	25	50	100
Baseline	$\mathcal{L}_{sup}^{\mathcal{T}}$	$\varnothing$	74.2 ± 3.8	82.8 ± 1.3	87.5 ± 0.4	89.0 ± 0.3	90.6 ± 0.2
$SupTC$	$\mathcal{L}_{sup}^{\mathcal{T}}+\mathcal{L}_{cons}^{\mathcal{T}}$	$\varnothing$	76.4 ± 3.8	83.6 ± 1.4	87.8 ± 0.4	89.5 ± 0.2	90.9 ± 0.3
$SemiTC$		$\mathcal{X}_u^{train}$	85.4 ± 1.0	86.9 ± 1.4	88.7 ± 1.0	89.7 ± 0.2	–
$SemiTC+$		$\mathcal{X}_u^{train} \cup \mathcal{X}^{val+test}$	85.0 ± 2.8	87.9 ± 0.8	89.7 ± 0.4	90.5 ± 0.3	91.1 ± 0.1

The transformation layer was implemented in Tensorflow, which allows implementing operations with custom gradients. Gradient backpropagation through the layer was implemented by copying gradients with respect to the layer output pixels to the positions where those pixels' values came from in the forward pass, which is elastic deformation with nearest neighbor interpolation. Pixel values that are not copied in the forward pass receive no gradient.

4 Results and Discussion

Table 1 compares the four versions of the proposed network. The metric used is IOU averaged over the five anatomical structures (mIOU).

The consistency term $\mathcal{L}_{cons}^{\mathcal{T}}$ improved the performance even when all training images were labeled. Although this improvement was modest, it was very reliable: $\mathcal{L}_{cons}^{\mathcal{T}}$ improved mIOU in 24 experiments out of 25 (5 CV splits × 5 training set sizes). Interestingly, $SupTC$ networks achieved similar or higher supervised training loss $\mathcal{L}_{sup}^{\mathcal{T}}$ most of the time, while expectedly having lower consistency loss $\mathcal{L}_{cons}^{\mathcal{T}}$ and lower total loss $\mathcal{L}_{sup}^{\mathcal{T}} + \mathcal{L}_{cons}^{\mathcal{T}}$, compared to their non-consistency-regularized counterparts. This rules out a hypothesis that the consistency term merely helps the network to converge to a lower $\mathcal{L}_{sup}^{\mathcal{T}}$ (e.g. because of an increase in the learning rate). We believe that this performance gain can be explained by that image-to-segmentation mappings that are more consistent under elastic deformations are more likely to be correct even if the resulting segmentations of training images fit less to the ground truth (which might be wrong or ill-defined).

The proposed semi-supervised approach $SemiTC$ outperformed the supervised $SupTC$ substantially when the size of the labeled training set was small (5 or 10 images). This improvement was also very consistent: $SemiTC$ was better than $SupTC$ in all five CV splits. For larger training set sizes, the improvement was more modest but still consistent (at least 4 out of 5 CV splits). With $SemiTC+$, which added validation and test images to the pool of unlabeled images for training, we achieved an additional small but consistent improvement (in 20 experiments out of 25). The comparison of the performance gains

Table 2. The comparison of the inter-observer agreement, state-of-the-art techniques, our baseline and *SemiTC+* trained on 20 or 124(123) labeled images. The metrics reported are means and standard deviations of per-structure IOU and mean absolute contour distance (MACD) averaged over CV splits. Dai et al. [3] and Novikov et al. [8] did not report MACD.

	Methods	$|\mathcal{X}_l^{train+val}|$	$|\mathcal{X}_u^{train}|$	Lungs	Heart	Clavicles
IOU, %	Human [16]			94.6 ± 1.8	87.8 ± 5.4	89.6 ± 3.7
	Dai et al. [3]	209		94.7 ± 0.4	86.6 ± 1.2	
	Novikov et al. [8]	165		94.8	87.8	**85.9**
	Frid-Adar et al. [4]	124(123)		**96.1 ± 1.4**	**90.6 ± 3.8**	85.5 ± 4.5
	Supervised baseline	20		93.3 ± 3.4	81.7 ± 13.1	75.7 ± 12.4
	SemiTC+	20	237	94.5 ± 2.1	85.2 ± 9.4	83.3 ± 6.6
	Supervised baseline	124(123)		95.3 ± 2.3	**88.8 ± 5.2**	87.3 ± 4.6
	SemiTC+	124(123)	147	**95.5 ± 1.9**	**88.8 ± 4.9**	**88.1 ± 4.4**
MACD, mm	Human [16]			1.64 ± 0.69	3.78 ± 1.82	0.68 ± 0.26
	Frid-Adar et al. [4]	124(123)		1.02 ± 0.56	2.54 ± 1.13	0.85 ± 0.32
	Supervised baseline	20		1.67 ± 0.99	5.56 ± 4.41	1.93 ± 2.42
	SemiTC+	20	237	1.35 ± 0.58	4.51 ± 3.20	1.16 ± 0.57
	Supervised baseline	124(123)		1.17 ± 0.70	**3.36 ± 1.61**	0.87 ± 0.39
	SemiTC+	124(123)	147	**1.10 ± 0.57**	3.37 ± 1.58	**0.81 ± 0.32**

achieved by adding $\mathcal{L}_{cons}^{\mathcal{T}}$ to the loss (i.e. the improvement of *SupTC* over the baseline) and introducing unlabeled images to the training (i.e. the improvement of *SemiTC* and *SemiTC+* over *SupTC*) suggests that the latter is mainly responsible for the superior performance of the proposed method compared to the baseline.

The proposed method substantially outperformed MS-Net [14], the only weakly supervised method evaluated on JSRT that is known to us. MS-Net achieved 67% and 81% mIOU (extracted from Fig. 4 in [14]) when trained in 20% and 100% strong supervision (124(123) labeled training images) modes, respectively. (In the former case, bounding boxes and landmarks were used as labels for the remaining 80% of the images.) *SemiTC* reached $87 \pm 1.5\%$ mIOU in <20% supervision mode (10 labeled images for training and 10 for validation).

Table 2 compares our baseline network and the proposed *SemiTC+* with the inter-observer agreement [16] and state-of-the-art chest X-ray segmentation methods [3,4,8]. All these methods are based on fully convolutional networks and are trained in a supervised way using at least 124(123) labeled images from the JSRT dataset. For these comparisons, we post-processed all predicted segmentations as described in [4] (small objects removal, hole filling).

Both our baseline and *SemiTC+* trained using 124(123) labeled images outperformed Dai et al. [3] and Novikov et al. [8] in segmentation of all structures (without post-processing as well). Both methods performed similarly to the method of Frid-Adar et al. [4], with the heart segmentation being slightly worse and clavicle segmentation being slightly better. (Note that the network of Frid-Adar et al. [4] benefited from pre-training on ImageNet.) We reached human-level performance in lung and heart segmentation and approached it closely in clavicle segmentation, unlike all other methods, which had a larger gap between their performance and the observers' for clavicle segmentation.

SemiTC+ trained only on 20 images (10 for training and 10 for validation) reached human-level performance in lung segmentation and was only slightly worse than the observers in heart segmentation (2.6% lower IOU). Its clavicle segmentation performance was substantially worse than human, but was only slightly worse than the automatic methods [4,8] trained using the fully labeled dataset (2.6% and 2.2% lower IOU, respectively). This could not be achieved by purely supervised training with the small labeled set, which was substantially worse in segmentation of all structures.

5   Conclusion

We proposed a novel semi-supervised segmentation method that learns consistency under transformations. The evaluation on a public chest X-ray dataset showed that the proposed consistency regularization improved the segmentation performance both when all training data was labeled and when additional unlabeled data was used for training. We achieved the performance comparable to the state-of-the-art while using more than five times fewer labeled images.

Acknowledgments. This research is part of the research project Deep Learning for Medical Image Analysis (DLMedIA) with project number P15-26, funded by the Netherlands Organisation for Scientific Research (NWO). The computations were carried out on the Dutch national e-infrastructure with the support of SURF Cooperative.

References

1. Baur, C., Albarqouni, S., Navab, N.: Semi-supervised deep learning for fully convolutional networks. In: Descoteaux, M., Maier-Hein, L., Franz, A., Jannin, P., Collins, D.L., Duchesne, S. (eds.) MICCAI 2017. LNCS, vol. 10435, pp. 311–319. Springer, Cham (2017). https://doi.org/10.1007/978-3-319-66179-7_36
2. Cheplygina, V., de Bruijne, M., Pluim, J.P.: Not-so-supervised: a survey of semi-supervised, multi-instance, and transfer learning in medical image analysis. Med. Image Anal. **54**, 280–296 (2019)
3. Dai, W., Dong, N., Wang, Z., Liang, X., Zhang, H., Xing, E.P.: SCAN: structure correcting adversarial network for organ segmentation in chest X-rays. In: Stoyanov, D., et al. (eds.) DLMIA/ML-CDS-2018. LNCS, vol. 11045, pp. 263–273. Springer, Cham (2018). https://doi.org/10.1007/978-3-030-00889-5_30
4. Frid-Adar, M., Ben-Cohen, A., Amer, R., Greenspan, H.: Improving the segmentation of anatomical structures in chest radiographs using U-Net with an ImageNet pre-trained encoder. In: Stoyanov, D., et al. (eds.) RAMBO/BIA/TIA -2018. LNCS, vol. 11040, pp. 159–168. Springer, Cham (2018). https://doi.org/10.1007/978-3-030-00946-5_17

5. Hervella, Á.S., Rouco, J., Novo, J., Ortega, M.: Retinal image understanding emerges from self-supervised multimodal reconstruction. In: Frangi, A.F., Schnabel, J.A., Davatzikos, C., Alberola-López, C., Fichtinger, G. (eds.) MICCAI 2018. LNCS, vol. 11070, pp. 321–328. Springer, Cham (2018). https://doi.org/10.1007/978-3-030-00928-1_37

6. Honari, S., Molchanov, P., Tyree, S., Vincent, P., Pal, C., Kautz, J.: Improving landmark localization with semi-supervised learning. In: CVPR, pp. 1546–1555 (2018)

7. Li, X., Yu, L., Chen, H., Fu, C.W., Heng, P.A.: Semi-supervised skin lesion segmentation via transformation consistent self-ensembling model. In: BMVC (2018)

8. Novikov, A.A., Lenis, D., Major, D., Hladuvka, J., Wimmer, M., Buehler, K.: Fully convolutional architectures for multiclass segmentation in chest radiographs. TMI 37(8), 1865–1876 (2018)

9. Perone, C.S., Cohen-Adad, J.: Deep semi-supervised segmentation with weight-averaged consistency targets. In: Stoyanov, D., et al. (eds.) DLMIA/ML-CDS - 2018. LNCS, vol. 11045, pp. 12–19. Springer, Cham (2018). https://doi.org/10.1007/978-3-030-00889-5_2

10. Rasmus, A., Berglund, M., Honkala, M., Valpola, H., Raiko, T.: Semi-supervised learning with ladder networks. In: NIPS, pp. 3546–3554 (2015)

11. Ronneberger, O., Fischer, P., Brox, T.: U-Net: convolutional networks for biomedical image segmentation. In: Navab, N., Hornegger, J., Wells, W.M., Frangi, A.F. (eds.) MICCAI 2015. LNCS, vol. 9351, pp. 234–241. Springer, Cham (2015). https://doi.org/10.1007/978-3-319-24574-4_28

12. Ross, T., et al.: Exploiting the potential of unlabeled endoscopic video data with self-supervised learning. IJCARS 13, 925–933 (2018)

13. Sajjadi, M., Javanmardi, M., Tasdizen, T.: Regularization with stochastic transformations and perturbations for deep semi-supervised learning. In: NIPS, pp. 1163–1171 (2016)

14. Shah, M.P., Merchant, S.N., Awate, S.P.: MS-Net: mixed-supervision fully-convolutional networks for full-resolution segmentation. In: Frangi, A.F., Schnabel, J.A., Davatzikos, C., Alberola-López, C., Fichtinger, G. (eds.) MICCAI 2018. LNCS, vol. 11073, pp. 379–387. Springer, Cham (2018). https://doi.org/10.1007/978-3-030-00937-3_44

15. Shiraishi, J., et al.: Development of a digital image database for chest radiographs with and without a lung nodule: receiver operating characteristic analysis of radiologists' detection of pulmonary nodules. Am. J. Roentgenol. 174(1), 71–74 (2000)

16. Van Ginneken, B., Stegmann, M.B., Loog, M.: Segmentation of anatomical structures in chest radiographs using supervised methods: a comparative study on a public database. MedIA 10(1), 19–40 (2006)

Improved Inference via Deep Input Transfer

Saeid Asgari Taghanaki(✉) ⓘ, Kumar Abhishek ⓘ, and Ghassan Hamarneh ⓘ

School of Computing Science, Simon Fraser University, Burnaby, Canada
{sasgarit,kabhishe,hamarneh}@sfu.ca

Abstract. Although numerous improvements have been made in the field of image segmentation using convolutional neural networks, the majority of these improvements rely on training with larger datasets, model architecture modifications, novel loss functions, and better optimizers. In this paper, we propose a new segmentation performance boosting paradigm that relies on optimally modifying the network's input instead of the network itself. In particular, we leverage the gradients of a trained segmentation network with respect to the input to transfer it to a space where the segmentation accuracy improves. We test the proposed method on three publicly available medical image segmentation datasets: the ISIC 2017 Skin Lesion Segmentation dataset, the Shenzhen Chest X-Ray dataset, and the CVC-ColonDB dataset, for which our method achieves improvements of 5.8%, 0.5%, and 4.8% in the average Dice scores, respectively.

Keywords: Semantic image segmentation · Convolutional neural networks · Gradient-based image enhancement

1 Introduction

Recently, there have been considerable advancements in semantic image segmentation using convolutional neural networks (CNNs), which have been applied to interpretation tasks on both natural and medical images [13]. The improvements are mostly attributed to exploring new neural architectures (with varying depths, widths, and connectivity or topology), designing new types of components or layers, adopting new loss functions, and training on larger datasets (via augmentation or acquisition). As one of the first high impact CNN-based segmentation models, Long et al. [14] proposed fully convolutional networks for pixel-wise labeling. Next, encoder-decoder (and similarly convolution-deconvolution) segmentation networks were introduced [1]. Soon after, Ronneberger et al. [18] showed that adding skip connections to the segmentation network improves model accuracy and addresses vanishing gradients. More recent advancements include densely connected CNN architectures [10], learnable skip connections [21], hybrid object detection-segmentation [9], and a new encoder-decoder architecture with atrous separable convolution [5].

© Springer Nature Switzerland AG 2019
D. Shen et al. (Eds.): MICCAI 2019, LNCS 11769, pp. 819–827, 2019.
https://doi.org/10.1007/978-3-030-32226-7_91

Designing new loss functions also resulted in improvements in subsequent inference-time segmentation accuracy, e.g., optimizing various segmentation prediction metrics, such as the intersection over union [3] and the Dice score [15], controlling the level of false positives and negatives [22,23], and adding regularizers to loss functions to encode geometrical and topological shape priors [2,16].

Some previous works resorted to modifying the input image to improve the segmentation results. These modifications included applying conventional image normalization techniques prior to feeding the image to a segmentation network, e.g., Haematoxylin and Eosin pre-processing [7], edge-preserving smoothing [17], and whitening transformation [11]. Other works generated variants of the input image to augment the training data by applying radiometric and spatial image transformations, e.g., rotation, color shifting/normalization, and elastic deformation [19]. The shortcoming of such pre-processing methods is that they are not explicitly optimized to improve a specific task e.g., segmentation or classification. To the best of our knowledge, no previous work has optimized the manipulation of the input image in order to improve segmentation accuracy of a trained network. Recently, Drozdzal et al. [8] showed that attaching a pre-processing module at the beginning of a segmentation network improves the network performance. However, we argue that adding a pre-processor without any other explicit constraint(s) amounts to adding (or prefixing) more layers, i.e., essentially making the model deeper. Inspired by adversarial perturbations [12,24], in this paper, we choose to optimally modify the input image prior to feed-forward inference. Our input-transformation is carried out via a novel gradient based method that leverages the computational processes of any trained segmentation network. After calculating these optimal transformations on training data, we then learn an image-to-image translation network that estimates an image modification mapping for novel *test* images. Note that our input transformation is *not* a data-augmentation method (albeit data augmentation may still be performed independently of our method), rather, we learn (from training data) a translation network that will pre-process novel input at inference time.

In this paper, we make the following contributions: (a) we introduce the first iterative gradient-based input pre-processing method, (b) we adopt an explicit objective to effectuate the purpose of the pre-processor, and (c) we show how targeted gradient-based adversarial perturbation methods can be leveraged for a better segmentation performance.

2   Method

Segmenting an input image $\mathbf{I}$ of size $n \times m$ assigns a label $l_i \in \mathcal{C} = \{0, 1, \cdots, L-1\}$ to the each pixel in $\mathbf{I}$, where L is the number of classes. Given a segmentation network with parameters Θ, let $f(\mathbf{I}; \Theta)$ denote the pixel-wise activation for $\mathbf{I}$ before the softmax normalization (denoted by $\xi_{\mathcal{C}}$), and let $\hat{\mathcal{S}} \in \mathbb{R}^{n \times m \times L}$ represent the segmented image as,

$$\xi_{\mathcal{C}}\left(f(1 - \mathcal{S}(\mathbf{I} + \mathbf{\Delta_I}); \Theta)\right) = \hat{\mathcal{S}}. \tag{1}$$

Let $\mathcal{S} \in \mathbb{R}^{n \times m \times L}$ denote the ground truth segmentation for $\mathbf{I}$. For a perfect segmentation, $\hat{\mathcal{S}} = \mathcal{S}$. Our goal is to introduce a perturbation $\boldsymbol{\Delta_I}$ to $\mathbf{I}$, such that the segmentation output of the modified image $\mathbf{I} + \boldsymbol{\Delta_I}$ is equal to the ground truth, i.e.,

$$\xi_{\mathcal{C}}\left(f(\mathcal{S}(\mathbf{I} + \boldsymbol{\Delta_I}); \boldsymbol{\Theta})\right) = \mathcal{S} \tag{2}$$

Let $f_{\hat{\mathcal{S}}}(\mathbf{I}; \boldsymbol{\Theta})$ and $f_{\mathcal{S}}(\mathbf{I}; \boldsymbol{\Theta})$ represent the pixel-wise activations corresponding to the segmentation outputs $\hat{\mathcal{S}}$ and $\mathcal{S}$ respectively. We apply a gradient descent algorithm for estimating the perturbation $\boldsymbol{\Delta_I}$ to be added to $\mathbf{I}$. The objective function $\mathcal{G}$ for this can be written as

$$\mathcal{G}(\mathbf{I}, \hat{\mathcal{S}}, \mathcal{S}, \boldsymbol{\Theta}) = f_{\hat{\mathcal{S}}}(\mathbf{I} + \boldsymbol{\Delta_I}, \boldsymbol{\Theta}) - f_{\mathcal{S}}(\mathbf{I} + \boldsymbol{\Delta_I}, \boldsymbol{\Theta}). \tag{3}$$

Starting with the original image $\mathbf{I}$, we iteratively compute the gradient of the loss $\mathcal{G}(\mathbf{I}, \hat{\mathcal{S}}, \mathcal{S}, \boldsymbol{\Theta})$ with respect to $\mathbf{I} + \boldsymbol{\delta}_{\mathbf{I}}'^{(k)}$ and add it to the image. Note that $\boldsymbol{\delta}_{\mathbf{I}}'^{(k)}$ is zero for the first iteration. Let $\mathbf{I}^{(k)}$ denote the perturbed image after the kth iteration of gradient descent. For the kth iteration, we have

$$\mathbf{I}^{(k+1)} = \mathbf{I}^{(k)} + \gamma\, \boldsymbol{\delta}_{\mathbf{I}}'^{(k)} \tag{4}$$

where γ is a scaling constant, and $\boldsymbol{\delta}_{\mathbf{I}}'^{(k)}$ is the gradient obtained for the kth iteration calculated by gradient descent update as

$$\begin{aligned}
\boldsymbol{\delta}_{\mathbf{I}}^{(k)} &= \nabla \mathcal{G}(\mathbf{I}, \hat{\mathcal{S}}, \mathcal{S}, \boldsymbol{\Theta}) \\
&= \nabla_{\mathbf{I}^{(k)}} f_{\hat{\mathcal{S}}}(\mathbf{I} + \boldsymbol{\Delta_I}, \boldsymbol{\Theta}) - \nabla_{\mathbf{I}^{(k)}} f_{\mathcal{S}}(\mathbf{I} + \boldsymbol{\Delta_I}, \boldsymbol{\Theta})
\end{aligned} \tag{5}$$

and then normalized using its L_∞ norm for numerical stability as

$$\boldsymbol{\delta}_{\mathbf{I}}'^{(k)} = \frac{\boldsymbol{\delta}_{\mathbf{I}}^{(k)}}{\|\boldsymbol{\delta}_{\mathbf{I}}^{(k)}\|_\infty}. \tag{6}$$

The algorithm terminates if the segmentation of the modified image is equal (or close enough within an error margin) to the ground truth, or it reaches a certain maximum number of iterations K. The total perturbation for image $\mathbf{I}$ is then calculated as the sum of the individual perturbations, i.e., $\boldsymbol{\Delta_I} = \sum_k \boldsymbol{\delta}_{\mathbf{I}}'^{(k)}$. The segmentation output of this perturbed image $\mathbf{X} + \boldsymbol{\Delta_I}$ is denoted by $\mathcal{S}^*$.

The calculation of $\boldsymbol{\Delta_I}$ requires knowledge of the ground truth segmentation mask and thus is only available for the training data. To test the hypothesis that the proposed gradient-based method improves the segmentation performance, we perturb the test images with their corresponding ground truths, and we obtain an almost perfect segmentation (Dice score ~ 1.0). However, since the ground truth segmentation masks for test images are not available in practice, we propose to reconstruct an estimate of the perturbed test images. In particular, given pairs of training images and their corresponding perturbations, $\{(\mathbf{I}_{train}, \mathbf{I}_{train} + \boldsymbol{\Delta}_{\mathbf{I}_{train}})\}$, we train a deep model to learn $\boldsymbol{\Phi} : \mathbf{I}_{train} \rightarrow \mathbf{I}_{train} + \boldsymbol{\Delta}_{\mathbf{I}_{train}}$. Subsequently, we apply the learned $\boldsymbol{\Phi}$ to the test data to obtain the reconstruction $\mathbf{I}_{test} \rightarrow \mathbf{I}_{test} + \boldsymbol{\Delta}_{\mathbf{I}_{test}}$. To learn the transformation function $\boldsymbol{\Phi}(\cdot)$, an image-to-image translation network can be used. Figure 1 shows an overview of the proposed method.

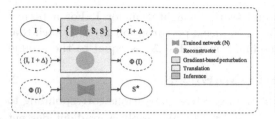 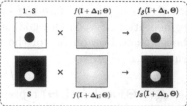

Fig. 1. Left: Passing image $\mathbf{I}$ through the trained network N generates sub-optimal output $\hat{S}$. Gradient perturbation module (top) calculates perturbation $\boldsymbol{\Delta}$ on $\mathbf{I}$, such that passing $\mathbf{I} + \boldsymbol{\Delta}$ through N yields results closer to ground truth S. Translation network (middle) is trained to learn mapping $\boldsymbol{\Phi} : \mathbf{I} \rightarrow \mathbf{I} + \boldsymbol{\Delta}$. Test images are first transformed via $\boldsymbol{\Phi}$ before feeding them into N (bottom), which results in an improved segmentation output S^*. Right: Reducing the logits of background and increasing that of foreground.

3   Implementation Details and Data

3.1   Models

As the goal of this work is to demonstrate the effectiveness of the proposed gradient-based perturbation, we use a state-of-the-art baseline segmentation network i.e., the U-Net [18] and optimize it using Adadelta with a batch size of 64. To learn the transformations made by the proposed gradient-based perturbation method (GP) from the training data as discussed in Sect. 2, we use two image-to-image translation networks: Cycle-GAN (cG) [25] and the hundred-layers Tiramisu segmentation network (T) [10]. We modify the latter as an image-to-image translation network and replace the original Tiramisu network's loss function with a loss function consisting of two terms: a Structural Similarity Index Measure (SSIM) term and a mean absolute error (L1 loss) term:

$$\mathcal{L} = \sum_{\mathbf{I}_{train}} \left[(1 - \mathcal{SSIM}(\mathbf{I}, \mathbf{I} + \boldsymbol{\Delta})) + \lambda \, \|\mathbf{I}, \mathbf{I} + \boldsymbol{\Delta}\|_1 \right] \qquad (7)$$

where $\mathcal{SSIM}(\mathbf{I}, \mathbf{I} + \boldsymbol{\Delta})$ is the SSIM calculated between $\mathbf{I}$ and $\mathbf{I} + \boldsymbol{\Delta}$, and λ is a scaling constant. The SSIM loss captures the finer perceptual details to which the human visual system is sensitive, such as contrast, luminance, and structure for which the L1 loss fails. When reporting results, we use the following abbreviations (i) ORIG: the original U-Net; (ii) GP$_{cG}$: the proposed GP ($\gamma = 1.0$) + Cycle-GAN for reconstructing the test image perturbation; (iii) GP$_T$: GP ($\gamma = 0.1$) + Tiramisu reconstruction with L1 loss; and (iv) GP$_{Ts}$: GP ($\gamma = 1.0$) + Tiramisu reconstruction with SSIM loss (s; Eq. 7). We choose the maximum possible value of $\gamma = 1.0$ in Eq. 4 for GP$_{Ts}$ and GP$_{cG}$ methods to maximally perturb images with the goal of highest possible segmentation performance, and run the optimization for $K = 100$ iterations. Because the perturbations can have negative values, we use a linear activation function for the last layer in all the aforementioned image-to-image translation networks.

3.2   Data

We use three datasets to evaluate our method. (a) The ISIC 2017 Skin Lesion Segmentation Dataset [6], hereafter referred to as SKIN, consists of 2000 skin lesion images for training and 600 test images. For all the images, the lesions have been manually annotated by expert dermatologists for normal skin and other miscellaneous structures. (b) The Shenzhen Chest X-Ray Dataset [20], hereafter referred to as LUNG, consists of 662 frontal chest X-Ray images, out of which 336 are cases with manifestations of tuberculosis and the remaining 326 are healthy. The corresponding ground truth masks contain manually traced out boundaries for the left and the right lungs. (c) The CVC-ColonDB [4], hereafter referred to as COLON, is a database of frames along with the corresponding annotated polyp masks extracted from colonoscopy videos. The dataset consists of 300 training images and 50 test images.

4   Results and Discussion

To test the effectiveness of the proposed transformation method, in this section, we present both quantitative and qualitative results on the three aforementioned datasets. We start with SKIN and the different derivatives of the proposed gradient-based perturbation method as discussed in Sect. 3.1, i.e., GP_{cG}, GP_T, and GP_{Ts} and compare them to ORIG. As shown in Fig. 2, the proposed method (i.e., GP_{Ts}) produces the closest segmentation mask to the ground truth (GT) compared to other methods. Looking at the second row of Fig. 2, GP_{Ts} perturbs the pixel values in a band surrounding the lesion, enhancing its contrast, making it more distinguishable from the background, thereby boosting the segmentation network's result, especially around the critical lesion boundary pixels. In Fig. 2, we show qualitative results for SKIN obtained with U-Net. As shown, all the gradient-based perturbation methods outperform ORIG, with the proposed GP_{Ts} method achieving a significant improvement of the mean Dice score by 5.8% compared to ORIG.

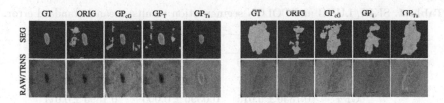

Fig. 2. Segmentation results on 2 sample images from SKIN. The top row shows the segmentation masks overlaid on top of the image, while the bottom row shows the original images (RAW) in the first two columns and the transformed images (TRNS) in the next three columns.

Moreover, a visual inspection of the ORIG and the GP_{Ts} results (Fig. 2, right) shows that the latter is more adept at rejecting false negative pixels, which is also supported by the results from Fig. 3 where GP_{Ts} improves the False Negative Rate (FNR) by a considerably large amount (5.87%). Next, we pick the best-performing method from SKIN experiments, i.e., GP_{Ts}, and evaluate its performance on the remaining two datasets: COLON and LUNG. Figure 3 shows the qualitative results obtained for ORIG and GP_{Ts} applied to three sample images from LUNG and COLON. As can be seen from the results, GP_{Ts} obtains segmentation results much closer (i.e., smoother with no perforated or disconnected blobs) to the ground truth segmentation (GT). This is also validated by the quantitative results reported in Table 1 where GP_{Ts} outperforms ORIG in all the three metrics - Dice score, FPR, and FNR, obtaining 4.8% and 0.5% improvements in the mean Dice score for COLON and LUNG, respectively. To further capture the improvement in segmentation performance, we plot the Gaussian kernel density estimates to estimate the probability density functions

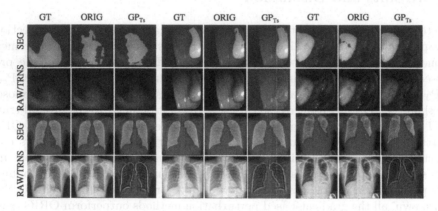

Fig. 3. Sample segmentation and transformed results for the COLON (rows 1 and 2) and LUNG (rows 3 and 4) datasets. RAW and TRNS refer to normal and transformed images, respectively.

Table 1. SKIN, LUNG and COLON segmentation results; mean ± standard error.

Data	Method	Dice	FPR	FNR
SKIN	ORIG	0.7743 ± 0.020	0.0327 ± 0.005	0.1905 ± 0.022
	GP_{cG}	0.7928 ± 0.017	$\mathbf{0.0281 \pm 0.002}$	0.1759 ± 0.014
	GP_T	0.7836 ± 0.015	0.0396 ± 0.005	0.1595 ± 0.017
	GP_{Ts}	$\mathbf{0.8190 \pm 0.015}$	0.0399 ± 0.006	$\mathbf{0.1318 \pm 0.014}$
LUNG	ORIG	0.9527 ± 0.003	0.0133 ± 0.0010	0.0504 ± 0.005
	GP_{Ts}	$\mathbf{0.9578 \pm 0.003}$	$\mathbf{0.0126 \pm 0.0007}$	$\mathbf{0.0441 \pm 0.005}$
COLON	ORIG	0.7384 ± 0.040	0.0115 ± 0.0030	0.2799 ± 0.042
	GP_{Ts}	$\mathbf{0.7737 \pm 0.033}$	$\mathbf{0.0099 \pm 0.0020}$	$\mathbf{0.2235 \pm 0.038}$

of Dice score, FPR, and FNR for the three datasets. The plots in Fig. 4 support the quantitative results with higher peaks (which correspond to higher densities) at larger Dice values for GP_{Ts} as compared to ORIG for all three datasets. Next, we look at range of the three metrics, and observe that they are in general more restricted to higher values for Dice score and lower values for FPR and FNR for GP_{Ts} than ORIG. Although we achieve up to $\sim 5\%$ improvement in Dice score, it is important to note that a much larger possible improvement is lost during the reconstruction phase. For example, for SKIN, when we perturb the test images with their corresponding ground truths as described in Sect. 2, we obtain almost perfect segmentation results i.e. Dice ~ 1.0 (we emphasize that the performance improvement is solely from the perturbation and not from the image-to-image translation components), but the best results we obtain through reconstruction are far lesser. A SSIM of 0.32 ± 0.009 between the GP and the GP_{Ts} images supports our hypothesis that a lot of information is lost in the reconstruction phase. Since training our input-perturbing mechanism requires gradients from an already-trained segmentation network, along with pixel-level class labels, training our perturbation module and training the segmentation network cannot be done simultaneously. In our next experiment, we set out to demonstrate that using (i) our pre-trained perturbation network as a pre-processor to a segmentation network leads to better results than (ii) an end-to-end training of the pre-processor network serially connected to the segmentation network. In other words, we compare the segmentation performance when training the pre-processor with (i) vs. without (ii) the proposed gradient based constraint. We find that the proposed method (i) achieves a higher Dice score of 0.8190 compared to 0.8019 using (ii).

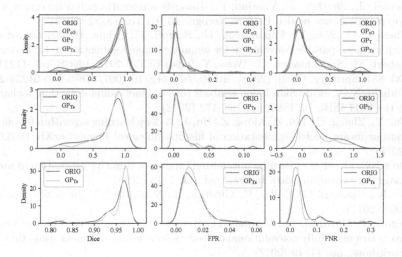

Fig. 4. Kernel density estimation; 1st row: SKIN; 2nd row: COLON; 3rd row: LUNG.

5 Conclusion

We proposed a novel input image transformation optimized for improved segmentation. A network gradient-based method calculates signed input perturbations on training images, which are then used to train deep networks to infer test image transformations. Our evaluations showed that the proposed approach can improve the performance of baseline methods for a variety of medical imaging modalities. A direction for future work includes focusing on improving the translation step of the proposed method. Moreover, the proposed method can be extended to other tasks such as image classification and object detection.

Acknowledgement. Partial funding for this project is provided by the Natural Sciences and Engineering Research Council of Canada (NSERC). The authors are grateful to the NVIDIA Corporation for donating Titan X GPUs and to Compute Canada for HPC resources used in this research.

References

1. Badrinarayanan, V., Kendall, A., Cipolla, R.: SegNet: a deep convolutional encoder-decoder architecture for image segmentation. arXiv:1511.00561 (2015)
2. BenTaieb, A., Hamarneh, G.: Topology aware fully convolutional networks for histology gland segmentation. In: Ourselin, S., Joskowicz, L., Sabuncu, M.R., Unal, G., Wells, W. (eds.) MICCAI 2016. LNCS, vol. 9901, pp. 460–468. Springer, Cham (2016). https://doi.org/10.1007/978-3-319-46723-8_53
3. Berman, M., Rannen Triki, A., Blaschko, M.B.: The Lovász-Softmax loss: a tractable surrogate for the optimization of the intersection-over-union measure in neural networks. In: CVPR, pp. 4413–4421 (2018)
4. Bernal, J., Sánchez, J., Vilarino, F.: Towards automatic polyp detection with a polyp appearance model. Pattern Recogn. **45**(9), 3166–3182 (2012)
5. Chen, L.-C., Zhu, Y., Papandreou, G., Schroff, F., Adam, H.: Encoder-decoder with atrous separable convolution for semantic image segmentation. In: Ferrari, V., Hebert, M., Sminchisescu, C., Weiss, Y. (eds.) ECCV 2018. LNCS, vol. 11211, pp. 833–851. Springer, Cham (2018). https://doi.org/10.1007/978-3-030-01234-2_49
6. Codella, N.C., et al.: Skin lesion analysis towards melanoma detection: a challenge at the 2017 ISBI. In: ISBI, pp. 168–172 (2018)
7. Cui, Y., Zhang, G., Liu, Z., Xiong, Z., Hu, J.: A deep learning algorithm for one-step contour aware nuclei segmentation of histopathological images. arXiv:1803.02786 (2018)
8. Drozdzal, M., et al.: Learning normalized inputs for iterative estimation in medical image segmentation. Med. Image Anal. **44**, 1–13 (2018)
9. He, K., Gkioxari, G., Dollár, P., Girshick, R.: Mask R-CNN. In: ICCV, pp. 2961–2969 (2017)
10. Jégou, S., Drozdzal, M., Vazquez, D., Romero, A., Bengio, Y.: The one hundred layers tiramisu: fully convolutional densenets for semantic segmentation. In: CVPR Workshops, pp. 11–19 (2017)
11. Kannan, S., et al.: Segmentation of glomeruli within trichrome images using deep learning. Kidney Int. Rep. **4**(7), 955–962 (2019)
12. Kurakin, A., Goodfellow, I., Bengio, S.: Adversarial examples in the physical world. arXiv:1607.02533 (2016)

13. Litjens, G., et al.: A survey on deep learning in medical image analysis. Med. Image Anal. **42**, 60–88 (2017)
14. Long, J., Shelhamer, E., Darrell, T.: Fully convolutional networks for semantic segmentation. In: CVPR, pp. 3431–3440 (2015)
15. Milletari, F., Navab, N., Ahmadi, S.A.: V-net: fully convolutional neural networks for volumetric medical image segmentation. In: 3DV, pp. 565–571 (2016)
16. Mirikharaji, Z., Hamarneh, G.: Star shape prior in fully convolutional networks for skin lesion segmentation. In: Frangi, A.F., Schnabel, J.A., Davatzikos, C., Alberola-López, C., Fichtinger, G. (eds.) MICCAI 2018. LNCS, vol. 11073, pp. 737–745. Springer, Cham (2018). https://doi.org/10.1007/978-3-030-00937-3_84
17. Pal, C., Chakrabarti, A., Ghosh, R.: A brief survey of recent edge-preserving smoothing algorithms on digital images. arXiv:1503.07297 (2015)
18. Ronneberger, O., Fischer, P., Brox, T.: U-Net: convolutional networks for biomedical image segmentation. In: Navab, N., Hornegger, J., Wells, W.M., Frangi, A.F. (eds.) MICCAI 2015. LNCS, vol. 9351, pp. 234–241. Springer, Cham (2015). https://doi.org/10.1007/978-3-319-24574-4_28
19. Shen, X., et al.: Automatic portrait segmentation for image stylization. Comput. Graph. Forum **35**, 93–102 (2016)
20. Stirenko, S., et al.: Chest X-ray analysis of tuberculosis by deep learning with segmentation and augmentation. In: 2018 IEEE 38th International Conference on Electronics and Nanotechnology (ELNANO), pp. 422–428 (2018)
21. Taghanaki, S.A., et al.: Select, attend, and transfer: light, learnable skip connections. arXiv:1804.05181 (2018)
22. Taghanaki, S.A., et al.: Combo loss: handling input and output imbalance in multi-organ segmentation. Comput. Med. Imaging Graph. **75**, 24–33 (2019)
23. Wong, K.C.L., Moradi, M., Tang, H., Syeda-Mahmood, T.: 3D segmentation with exponential logarithmic loss for highly unbalanced object sizes. In: Frangi, A.F., Schnabel, J.A., Davatzikos, C., Alberola-López, C., Fichtinger, G. (eds.) MICCAI 2018. LNCS, vol. 11072, pp. 612–619. Springer, Cham (2018). https://doi.org/10.1007/978-3-030-00931-1_70
24. Xie, C., Wang, J., Zhang, Z., Zhou, Y., Xie, L., Yuille, A.: Adversarial examples for semantic segmentation and object detection. In: ICCV, pp. 1369–1378 (2017)
25. Zhu, J.Y., Park, T., Isola, P., Efros, A.A.: Unpaired image-to-image translation using cycle-consistent adversarial networks. In: CVPR, pp. 2223–2232 (2017)

Neural Architecture Search for Adversarial Medical Image Segmentation

Nanqing Dong[1,2]([⊠]), Min Xu[1,3], Xiaodan Liang[1,4], Yiliang Jiang[5], Wei Dai[6], and Eric Xing[1]

[1] Petuum, Inc., Pittsburgh, USA
[2] University of Oxford, Oxford, UK
nanqing.dong@keble.ox.ac.uk
[3] Carnegie Mellon University, Pittsburgh, USA
[4] Sun Yat-sen University, Guangzhou, China
[5] New York University, New York City, USA
[6] Apple Inc., Seattle, USA

Abstract. Adversarial training has led to breakthroughs in many medical image segmentation tasks. The network architecture design of the adversarial networks needs to leverage human expertise. Despite the fact that discriminator plays an important role in the training process, it is still unclear how to design an optimal discriminator. In this work, we propose a neural architecture search framework for adversarial medical image segmentation. We automate the process of neural architecture design for the discriminator with continuous relaxation and gradient-based optimization. We empirically analyze and evaluate the proposed framework in the task of chest organ segmentation and explore the potential of automated machine learning in medical applications. We further release a benchmark dataset for chest organ segmentation.

Keywords: Neural architecture search · Adversarial networks · Medical image segmentation

1 Introduction

Inspired by the *generative adversarial networks* (GANs) [4], adversarial training for semantic segmentation was first proposed in [9], where an auxiliary discriminator is introduced to distinguish between the ground truth, and the segmentation output and the segmentation network is trained to fool the discriminator. A recent cognitive study implies that *convolutional neural networks* (CNNs) are more sensitive to the local texture of an object than the global shape [1]. A well-designed discriminator is expected to learn high-order statistics of the objects [3], which is a complement to a stand-alone segmentation network. Compared with general objects, organs, anatomies, and tissues usually share similar representation among different patients, which controls the variance of the high-order statistics. For medical images, the segmentation network is expected to converge faster and output realistic and robust prediction under adversarial training [2].

© Springer Nature Switzerland AG 2019
D. Shen et al. (Eds.): MICCAI 2019, LNCS 11769, pp. 828–836, 2019.
https://doi.org/10.1007/978-3-030-32226-7_92

Adversarial training has achieved state-of-the-art performance in many medical image segmentation tasks [3,5,10], but it is still unclear how to design adversarial networks. While a bad segmentation network can hinder the performance, a bad discriminator can sabotage the whole machine learning system. Human expertise and intuition still play important roles in designing the discriminator. Fueled by the advances in both deep learning and computer hardware, there is a growing interest in the study of *neural architecture search* (NAS), which automates the manual process of architecture design. Even though the models discovered by NAS have outperformed human-invented models in image classification and language modeling tasks [7,11,15,16], NAS for adversarial networks and semantic segmentation is still underdeveloped. In addition, the underlying idea of NAS is that each dataset has a unique best-performing architecture. In the medical domain, data scarcity has been a long-standing challenge. The pixel-level ground truth requires manual annotation by the clinical professionals, which is often expensive to acquire. It is natural to leverage limited data by deploying an efficient model. An algorithmic solution to automated architecture design in adversarial training is desired by both the machine learning community and the medical image computing community.

In this work, we propose a NAS framework for adversarial medical image segmentation. The proposed framework will automatically find the architecture of a discriminator based on a segmentation network backbone. The automatically designed discriminator will improve the performance of the segmentation network through adversarial training. There are previous studies on NAS using reinforcement learning [11,15,16] or evolutionary algorithm [14]. These methods require a huge amount of computational power when searching over the discrete domain, which is impractical in adversarial training. We develop our method based on *differentiable architecture search* [7], which relaxes the search space from discrete to continuous and can be optimized through gradient descent. Compared with a single end-to-end network in [7], we take the mutual effect between two adversarial networks into consideration during the alternative optimization process. To the best of our knowledge, this is the first study on NAS in adversarial training and the first application of NAS in the medical domain. Adversarial training is a complex non-convex optimization problem. Currently, we cannot mathematically prove that the proposed method can find the best architecture of the discriminator. Here, we treat this as a black-box optimization problem and approximate the optimal solution numerically. We empirically analyze and evaluate the proposed method in the task of chest organ segmentation on two datasets. We choose chest organ segmentation because it is a representative task in medical image segmentation that can be solved by adversarial training. Besides, chest organ segmentation has less computational cost than other complicated tasks, which allows for fast prototyping under limited computational power. The experiments show that our method can automate the process of architecture design in adversarial training and achieve comparable performance. The framework can be further extended to more complicated medical image segmentation tasks.

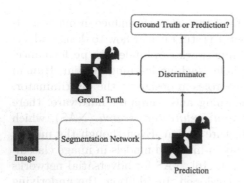

Ground Truth or Prediction?

Discriminator

Ground Truth

Image

Segmentation Network

Prediction

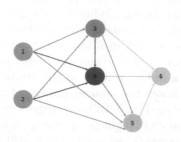

Fig. 1. Adversarial semantic segmentation for chest organs.

Fig. 2. An example of topological graph when $B = 6$. Green nodes are the input nodes and red node is the output node. (Color figure online)

2 Method

In standard adversarial training for semantic segmentation, there is one segmentation network S and one discriminator D. S is a *fully convolutional network* (FCN) [8], which is parameterized as f_θ, and D is a CNN for binary classification, which is parameterized as g_ϕ. S is trained to output prediction realistic enough to confuse D, which in turn tries to discriminate the prediction from ground truth. A pipeline for chest organ segmentation is shown in Fig. 1. Let x denote the input image and y denote the corresponding ground truth. S and D are optimized alternatively. Given ϕ fixed, θ is updated by minimizing

$$\mathcal{L}(\theta) = \mathcal{L}_{seg}(f_\theta(x), y) - \lambda_{adv} \log g_\phi(f_\theta(x)), \tag{1}$$

where $\mathcal{L}_{seg}$ is the softmax cross-entropy and λ_{adv} controls the weight of adversarial loss. Given θ fixed, ϕ is updated by minimizing

$$\mathcal{L}(\phi) = -\log g_\phi(y) - \log(1 - g_\phi(f_\theta(x))). \tag{2}$$

2.1 Problem Formulation

The focus of this work is to study how to automatically design the architecture of D. The intuition behind is that, given a dataset, for $\forall S \in \{\mathcal{S}\}$, $\exists D \in \{\mathcal{D}\}$, where (S, D) can have optimal performance under adversarial training. Here, to study the behavior of D alone, we fix the architecture of S. Assume the architecture of D can be parameterized as α by treating the architecture as a hyperparameter [7]. So D can be represented as $g_{\alpha,\phi}$. The goal is to jointly learn (α, θ, ϕ). To easily understand the relationships among (α, θ, ϕ), we decompose the problem into two stages. If we feed D with inputs independent of S, the problem becomes a standard NAS for CNN. For an isolated D, ϕ is associated with α. Then, by taking (α, ϕ) as a whole, S and D have mutual effects during the adversarial training, as stated in Eqs. 1 and 2. Note, the relationship here does not imply any statistical dependency.

Here, we propose our method. We transform the problem into a bilevel optimization problem [7]. Given α fixed, the problem becomes a standard adversarial training, where we already know how to jointly optimize (θ, ϕ). Given (θ, ϕ) fixed, we can then optimize α, if the parameterization of α can be independent of ϕ. As a standard practice in NAS [7,11,15,16], the training data is split into *train* and *val*. *train* is used to learn the weights and *val* is used to meta-learn the architecture. Let $\mathcal{J}$ denote certain joint optimization objective in adversarial training in Eqs. 1 and 2. Assume $\mathcal{J}$ can be minimized to provide the best segmentation performance, the optimization goal for architecture search is to find α^* that minimizes $\mathcal{J}_{val}(\alpha^*, \theta^*, \phi^*)$, where the (θ^*, ϕ^*) are obtained by minimizing $\mathcal{J}_{train}(\alpha^*, \theta, \phi)$. Analogous to [7], we have

$$\min_{\alpha} \mathcal{J}_{val}(\alpha, \theta^*, \phi^*), \tag{3}$$

$$\text{where } \theta^*, \phi^* = \operatorname*{argmin}_{\theta, \phi} \mathcal{J}_{train}(\alpha, \theta, \phi). \tag{4}$$

2.2 Neural Architecture Search Setting

It is impractical to search the model architecture starting from scratch, which can take more than 2000 GPU days for a simple classification task [15]. Here, we follow the basic setting of NAS introduced by [7,11,16]. We restrict the search space by searching the architecture of the computation *cell*. The cell is the basic unit, which can be stacked multiple times to form a CNN. A cell can be viewed as a directed acyclic graph which consists of B ordered nodes. The goal is to search the topology of the cell. Each node (vertex) v^i is a feature map and each directed edge (i, j) is certain operation $e^{(i,j)}$ applied to v^i. Each cell has two input nodes and one output node. The input nodes are the output nodes of two previous cells and the output node concatenates all intermediate nodes within the cell. The intermediate node takes the sum over all previous nodes.

$$v^j = \sum_{i<j} e^{(i,j)}(v^i) \tag{5}$$

An example topology is illustrated in Fig. 2.

As discussed in Sect. 2.1, the parameterization of α is required to be independent of ϕ. We adopt *continuous relaxation* proposed by [7]. Let $\mathcal{E}$ denote the set of all possible operations for certain e. The possible operations are mixed through a softmax function. α is now related to a probability distribution over all operations, where each operation has its own weights.

$$\bar{e}^{(i,j)}(v^i) = \sum_{e \in \mathcal{E}} \frac{\exp(\alpha_e^{(i,j)})}{\sum_{e' \in \mathcal{E}} \exp(\exp(\alpha_{e'}^{(i,j)}))} e^{(i,j)}(v^i) \tag{6}$$

Algorithm 1: Neural Architecture Search for Discriminator in Adversarial Training

---

Initialize (α, θ, ϕ)
while *not converged* **do**
    | Update α by descending $\nabla_\alpha \mathcal{J}_{val}(\alpha, \theta^*, \phi^*)$
    | Update (θ, ϕ) by descending $\nabla_{\theta,\phi} \mathcal{J}_{train}(\alpha, \theta, \phi)$
end
Derive the final architecture.

A discrete architecture can be decoded after α is learned. For each (i, j), only one operation is derived.

$$e^{(i,j)} = \underset{e \in \mathcal{E}}{\operatorname{argmax}} \, \alpha_e^{(i,j)} \tag{7}$$

For node v^j, top-k $(0 < k \leq j)$ most likely operations are retained from all previous nodes $\{v^i | i < j\}$. The probability of $e^{(i,j)}$ is just the weight of this operation ($\frac{\exp(\alpha_e^{(i,j)})}{\sum_{e' \in \mathcal{E}} \exp(\exp(\alpha_{e'}^{(i,j)}))}$) in Eq. 6. The probabilities over all possible i are calculated and the highest k nodes are chosen.

2.3 Optimization

With the continuous relaxation of α in Sect. 2.2, the architecture search can be achieved through gradient-based optimization. It is difficult to get a closed form solution to Eqs. 3 and 4. Instead, we use an iterative approach to approximate the architecture gradient $\nabla_\alpha \mathcal{J}_{val}(\alpha, \theta^*, \phi^*)$, where

$$\mathcal{J}_{val}(\alpha, \theta^*, \phi^*) = -\log g_{\alpha,\phi^*}(y) - \log(1 - g_{\alpha,\phi^*}(f_{\theta^*}(x))). \tag{8}$$

To optimize α, we approximate (θ^*, ϕ^*) by updating (θ, ϕ) with a single step on *train* [7]. So the optimization of α takes both (θ, ϕ) into consideration.

$$\begin{aligned} \theta^* &\approx \theta - \eta \nabla_\theta \mathcal{L}_{train}(\theta, \alpha) \\ \phi^* &\approx \phi - \eta \nabla_\phi \mathcal{L}_{train}(\phi, \alpha) \end{aligned} \tag{9}$$

Given α fixed, the optimization of (θ, ϕ) is to minimize $\mathcal{J}_{train}(\alpha, \theta, \phi)$ by Eqs. 1 and 2. We use the finite difference approximation in calculating the Hessian matrix in Eq. 9 suggested by [7]. The training procedure is outlined in Algorithm 1.

3 Experiments

3.1 Datasets

JSRT. JSRT is a classic dataset for lung nodule study released by the Japanese Society of Radiological Technology [13]. JSRT contains 247 chest X-ray images

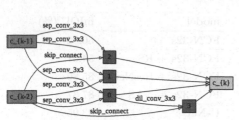
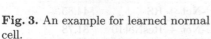

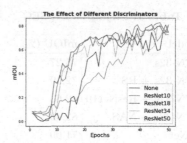

Fig. 3. An example for learned normal cell.

Fig. 4. *None* means FCN-32s without adversarial training.

(CXRs) with pixel-wise ground truth labels of left lung, right lung and heart. Each CXR has a fixed resolution of 2048×2048 and was taken by the same machine under the same imaging protocols.

CX-SEG. CX-SEG is a new benchmark dataset for chest organ segmentation, which contains 259 CXRs with pixel-wise ground truth labels of left lung, right lung and heart. The annotation was conducted by 3 licensed radiologists. The CXRs were collected from multiple hospitals and various patient groups with different machines and imaging protocols. Compared with JSRT, CX-SEG shows large variation in terms of data sources, contrast, color and resolution, which can be used to test the robustness of the model. The CX-SEG is released for academic purpose.

3.2 Implementation

The proposed method is implemented in PyTorch based on the source code of [7]. We use the same search space for the set of possible operations $\mathcal{E}$ defined in [7,16]. Two types of cells searched are *normal* cell and *reduction* cell. The reduction cell will downsample the resolution by using a stride 2 in the operations(edges) adjacent to the input nodes. For each cell, we set $B = 7$ and $k = 2$, which means 2 input nodes, 4 intermediate nodes, and 1 output node. An example of a learned normal cell is showed in Fig. 3. When designing the architecture of the discriminator, the stacked cells are the main body. In this study, we have four building blocks in the main body. In the first three building blocks, each normal cell is followed by a reduction cell, while there is only one normal cell in the last building block. We also add a pre-defined head and bottom to form a complete classification network. The head is one 3×3 convolutional layer and one 2×2 max pooling layer. The bottom is 1 fully-connected layer for binary classification.

We use a constant learning rate 10^{-4} and $\lambda_{adv} = 0.01$ in all experiments. Two classic segmentation networks are chosen as backbones, which are FCN-32s [8] and U-Net [12]. The images and ground truth labels are resized to 512×512. For each dataset, 50 images are randomly selected as the training data and the

834   N. Dong et al.

<table>
<tr><td colspan="2">Table 1. Results on CX-SEG</td></tr>
</table>

Model	mIOU (%)
FCN-32s	75.27
FCN-32s + RS	72.69
FCN-32s + ResNet10	82.66
FCN-32s + NAS	82.43
U-Net	71.09
U-Net + RS	68.59
U-Net + ResNet10	79.32
U-Net + NAS	81.86

Table 2. Results on JSRT

model	mIOU (%)
FCN-32s	50.82
FCN-32s + RS	54.61
FCN-32s + ResNet10	85.86
FCN-32s + NAS	87.37
U-Net	43.95
U-Net + RS	44.85
U-Net + ResNet10	81.78
U-Net + NAS	83.78

rest as the test data. We split the data this way to simulate a dataset with limited supervision and to maximally highlight the influence of the different discriminators. There is no normalization or data augmentation on the training data. We use mean Intersection-Over-Union (mIOU) as the evaluation metric. The training data is further split into *train* and *val* by half. We use two GTX Titan X GPUs in this study. Each search takes at least 3 days. After the search is done, the learned model is trained on the whole training data for 50 epochs to give the final performance.

3.3   Evaluation

First, we use FCN-32s as the segmentation network and ResNet [6] as the discriminator. Intuitively, we illustrate the effect of the discriminator's architecture on the segmentation performance. The test results are presented in Fig. 4. Adversarial training with ResNet10 and ResNet18 outperform FCN-32s in both performance and convergence, while ResNet50 can only achieve a comparable result as non-adversarial training with poor convergence speed. ResNet10 is a variant of ResNet18 with only 4 residual blocks. Note, ResNets are already well-designed networks with guaranteed convergence. Poorly-designed discriminators cannot even guarantee convergence.

We use the proposed method to automatically design the discriminators for FCN-32s and U-Net in adversarial training. To fairly assess the proposed method, for each backbone network, we compare the NAS result with the segmentation network without adversarial training, adversarial training with the discriminator generated by *random search* (RS) and adversarial training with a well-designed discriminator. For the experiments of each backbone network, the segmentation networks share the same randomly initilized weights. For RS, we randomly initiate α 10 times to generate 10 different discriminators. We report the mean mIOU for 10 runs. We choose ResNet10 as the discriminator according to the test results in the last experiment. The results on CX-SEG and JSRT are presented in Tables 1 and 2. Adversarial training improves the performance of the segmentation network by a large margin. The discriminator designed by NAS can

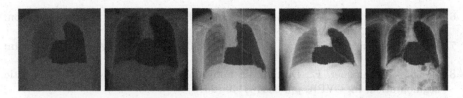

Fig. 5. Visualization of the chest organ segmentation on CX-SEG data.

achieve comparable even better results than the manually-designed discriminator. We conclude that the proposed method can be used to automatically design the architecture of the discriminator in adversarial training with limited human intervention. Qualitative results on CX-SEG can be seen in Fig. 5. We also want to point out that adversarial training often suffers from instability, which may also happen in our experiments. So the results maybe only the sub-optimal. We leave the theoretical discussion in future work.

4 Conclusions

In this paper, we present an approach to automatically design the architecture for the discriminator in adversarial training. We evaluate the proposed method with extensive experiments. This is the first study on neural architecture search in adversarial training while we admit that the proposed method requires further theoretical justification and still has a few limitations in both algorithmic and engineering perspective. In future work, we will optimize the memory storage mechanism and make the algorithm more efficient. It will also be interesting to incorporate the depth of the discriminator into the search space or jointly search for the architectures of both segmentation network and discriminator.

References

1. Baker, N., Lu, H., Erlikhman, G., Kellman, P.J.: Deep convolutional networks do not classify based on global object shape. PLoS Comput. Biol. **14**(12), c1006613 (2018)
2. Dai, W., Dong, N., Wang, Z., Liang, X., Zhang, H., Xing, E.P.: SCAN: structure correcting adversarial network for organ segmentation in chest X-rays. In: Stoyanov, D., et al. (eds.) DLMIA/ML-CDS -2018. LNCS, vol. 11045, pp. 263–273. Springer, Cham (2018). https://doi.org/10.1007/978-3-030-00889-5_30
3. Dong, N., Kampffmeyer, M., Liang, X., Wang, Z., Dai, W., Xing, E.: Unsupervised domain adaptation for automatic estimation of cardiothoracic ratio. In: Frangi, A.F., Schnabel, J.A., Davatzikos, C., Alberola-López, C., Fichtinger, G. (eds.) MICCAI 2018. LNCS, vol. 11071, pp. 544–552. Springer, Cham (2018). https://doi.org/10.1007/978-3-030-00934-2_61
4. Goodfellow, I., et al.: Generative adversarial nets. In: NIPS, pp. 2672–2680 (2014)
5. Han, Z., Wei, B., Mercado, A., Leung, S., Li, S.: Spine-GAN: semantic segmentation of multiple spinal structures. Med. Image Anal. **50**, 23–35 (2018)

6. He, K., Zhang, X., Ren, S., Sun, J.: Deep residual learning for image recognition. In: CVPR, pp. 770–778 (2016)
7. Liu, H., Simonyan, K., Yang, Y.: DARTS: differentiable architecture search. In: ICLR (2019)
8. Long, J., Shelhamer, E., Darrell, T.: Fully convolutional networks for semantic segmentation. In: CVPR, pp. 3431–3440 (2015)
9. Luc, P., Couprie, C., Chintala, S., Verbeek, J.: Semantic segmentation using adversarial networks. In: NIPS Adversarial Training Workshop (2016)
10. Moeskops, P., Veta, M., Lafarge, M.W., Eppenhof, K.A.J., Pluim, J.P.W.: Adversarial training and dilated convolutions for brain MRI segmentation. In: Cardoso, M.J., et al. (eds.) DLMIA/ML-CDS -2017. LNCS, vol. 10553, pp. 56–64. Springer, Cham (2017). https://doi.org/10.1007/978-3-319-67558-9_7
11. Pham, H., Guan, M.Y., Zoph, B., Le, Q.V., Dean, J.: Efficient neural architecture search via parameter sharing. In: ICML, pp. 4092–4101 (2018)
12. Ronneberger, O., Fischer, P., Brox, T.: U-Net: convolutional networks for biomedical image segmentation. In: Navab, N., Hornegger, J., Wells, W.M., Frangi, A.F. (eds.) MICCAI 2015. LNCS, vol. 9351, pp. 234–241. Springer, Cham (2015). https://doi.org/10.1007/978-3-319-24574-4_28
13. Shiraishi, J., et al.: Development of a digital image database for chest radiographs with and without a lung nodule: receiver operating characteristic analysis of radiologists' detection of pulmonary nodules. Am. J. Roentgenol. **174**(1), 71–74 (2000)
14. Xie, L., Yuille, A.: Genetic CNN. In: ICCV, pp. 1379–1388 (2017)
15. Zoph, B., Le, Q.V.: Neural architecture search with reinforcement learning. In: ICLR (2017)
16. Zoph, B., Vasudevan, V., Shlens, J., Le, Q.V.: Learning transferable architectures for scalable image recognition. In: CVPR, pp. 8697–8710 (2018)

MeshSNet: Deep Multi-scale Mesh Feature Learning for End-to-End Tooth Labeling on 3D Dental Surfaces

Chunfeng Lian[1], Li Wang[1](✉), Tai-Hsien Wu[2], Mingxia Liu[1](✉),
Francisca Durán[2], Ching-Chang Ko[3], and Dinggang Shen[1](✉)

[1] Department of Radiology and BRIC,
University of North Carolina at Chapel Hill, Chapel Hill, NC 27599, USA
{li_wang,mxliu,dgshen}@med.unc.edu
[2] Department of Oral and Craniofacial Health Sciences,
University of North Carolina at Chapel Hill, Chapel Hill, NC 27516, USA
[3] Department of Orthodontics, University of North Carolina at Chapel Hill,
Chapel Hill, NC 27516, USA

Abstract. Accurate tooth labeling on 3D dental surfaces is a vital task in computer-aided orthodontic treatment planning. Existing automated or semi-automated methods usually require human interactions, which is time-consuming. Also, they typically use simple geometric properties as the criteria for segmentation, which cannot well handle the high variation of tooth appearance across different patients. Recently, several pioneering deep neural networks (e.g., PointNet) have been proposed in the computer vision and computer graphics communities to efficiently segment 3D shapes in an end-to-end manner. However, these methods do not perform well in our specific task of tooth labeling, especially considering that they cannot explicitly model fine-grained local geometric context of teeth (although only a small portion of dental surfaces but with different shapes and appearances). In this paper, we propose a specific deep neural network (called *MeshSNet*) for end-to-end tooth segmentation on 3D dental surfaces captured by advanced intraoral scanners. Using directly raw mesh data as input, our MeshSNet adopts novel graph-constrained learning modules to hierarchically extract multi-scale contextual features, and then densely integrates local-to-global geometric features to comprehensively characterize mesh cells for the segmentation task. We evaluated our proposed method on an in-house clinic dataset via 3-fold cross-validation. The experimental results demonstrate the superior performance of our MeshSNet method, compared with the state-of-the-art deep learning methods for 3D shape segmentation.

1 Introduction

As a fundamental part of computer-aided-design (CAD) systems for orthodontic treatment planning, accurate tooth segmentation/partition from digitalized dental surface model is a precondition for the analyses and rearrangements of tooth

© Springer Nature Switzerland AG 2019
D. Shen et al. (Eds.): MICCAI 2019, LNCS 11769, pp. 837–845, 2019.
https://doi.org/10.1007/978-3-030-32226-7_93

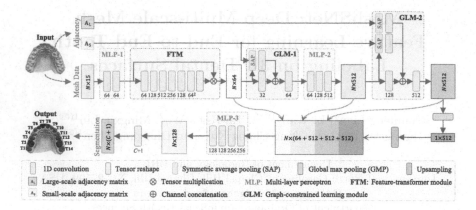

Fig. 1. Illustration of our MeshSNet model, a multi-scale deep neural network to learn high-level geometric features for end-to-end tooth segmentation on 3D dental surfaces.

positions [4]. In clinical orthodontic practice, 3D intraoral scanners (IOS) are becoming widespread for the direct reconstruction of the digital surface model of the dentogingival tissues [5]. Compared with conventional physical impressions, such direct digital impressions are more time-efficient and comfortable for patients, avoiding the potential risk of allergies caused by many constituents of physical impression materials [9]. Automatically segmenting teeth on 3D dental surface is a challenging task, primarily considering that tooth shapes vary dramatically across different subjects and also the patients' teeth usually have abnormal appearances (e.g., neighboring teeth are crowded and misaligned) [12]. The segmentation task becomes even more challenging on the raw dental surface acquired by IOS, since the non-tooth parts (e.g., gingival tissues) usually have significantly irregular shapes and the deep intraoral regions (e.g., the 2nd/3rd molars) may not be perfectly captured by the light source.

Conventional methods for automated or semi-automated tooth segmentation usually project 3D meshes onto 2D images [4] or directly separate 3D meshes according to some preselected geometric properties [14]. Although the ideas are direct and intuitive, most of these conventional methods require time-consuming human interactions, and their performance is sensitive to the variation of tooth appearances [12]. Learning-based shape/geometry analysis has been comprehensively studied in both computer vision and computer graphics communities, which is also potentially applicable to the specific task of tooth segmentation. For example, in [12], hand-crafted geometric features were predefined and reshaped as an image to train a multi-stage convolutional neural network (CNN) for labeling mesh cells on dental surfaces. However, such direct application of CNNs may lead to unstable segmentations, because it ignores the fact that the input geometric features are unordered, i.e., different organizations of them result in different "images". Another potential limitation is that this multi-stage CNN performs different steps independently, which may hamper its practical usage due to system complexity. Recently, a pioneering work of PointNet [7] was proposed for end-to-end 3D shape analysis. Using directly the *raw* geometric data (e.g., the coordinates and normal vectors of point clouds) as input, PointNet learns translation-invariant deep features for shape classification/segmentation, yielding state-of-the-art performance in terms of efficiency and accuracy. The major limitation of the original PointNet is that it ignores the local geometric context, while effectively modeling local structures has been proven to be critical for the success of deep neural networks in fine-grained segmentation tasks. Although some efforts [2,6,11] have been proposed to extend PointNet by including contextual information, they usually coarsely group points into several clusters according to their spatial relationship. Such coarse operations cannot perform well in our specific task of fine-grained tooth segmentation, especially considering that each tooth only takes a very small portion of the entire dental surface.

In this paper, we propose an *end-to-end* deep neural network (called Mesh-SNet) to learn directly high-level geometric features from the *raw dental mesh* data for automated tooth segmentation, with the schematic diagram shown in Fig. 1. Specifically, our MeshSNet method extends the state-of-the-art PointNet from three aspects: (1) We replace points with mesh cells as input, because mesh cells naturally unite topologically-linked points to show the local structure clearly [1]; (2) We propose *multi-scale graph-constrained learning modules* to explicitly model local geometric context and mimic hierarchical feature learning procedure of CNNs; and (3) We densely fuse cell-wise features, multi-scale contextual features, and translation-invariant holistic features for cell annotation.

2   Method

Input: The input $\mathbf{F}^0$ of our MeshSNet model are the raw mesh surface data with the size of $N \times 15$, where N is the number of mesh cells. Each cell is initially described by a 15-dimensional input. Specifically, apart from the coordinates of the three vertices (9 units) and the normal vector (3 units) of each cell, the relative position (3 units) of each cell with respect to the whole surface is also included to provide supplementary information.

MeshSNet Architecture: As shown in Fig. 1, our MeshSNet follows the architecture of PointNet and employs successive multi-layer perceptrons (MLPs) to extract increasingly higher-level geometric features. Similar to convolutional (Conv) layers in CNNs, the learnable parameters of each MLP in MeshSNet are shared across all input mesh cells. Also, in line with [7], the first MLP (i.e., MLP-1) in our MeshSNet is followed by a feature-transformer module (FTM), which maps all inputs into a canonical feature space to improve the robustness of learned feature representations with respect to potential geometric transformations of input surfaces. Denote $\mathbf{F}^1 \in \mathbb{R}^{N \times 64}$ as the features learned by MLP-1. The FTM predicts an 64×64 transformation matrix $\mathbf{T}$ from $\mathbf{F}^1$, and directly updates the feature matrix as $\hat{\mathbf{F}}^1 = \mathbf{F}^1\mathbf{T}$. Compared with the original PointNet architecture, the major innovations of our MeshSNet model include: **(1)** graph-constrained hierarchical learning of multi-scale local geometric features, and **(2)** dense fusion of local-to-global features for the segmentation task.

(1) Multi-scale graph-constrained learning: We propose a graph-constrained learning module (GLM) to explicitly capture local geometric context of the input surface. The GLMs (i.e., GLM-1 and GLM-2) are integrated at different stages along the forward path of MeshSNet (i.e., after both FTM and MLP-2), which mimic CNNs to gradually increase the receptive field for learning hierarchical multi-scale contextual features. Specifically, regarding each cell of a 3D mesh as the centroid, we define its neighborhood balls with two different radiuses, and the resulting $N \times N$ adjacency matrices (i.e., $\mathbf{A_S}$ and $\mathbf{A_L}$ for small and large balls, respectively) describe the graph connections between any two cells in the underlying Euclidean space. Based on $\mathbf{A_S}$, GLM-1 in our MeshSNet first applies a graph-based fusion operation (called *symmetric average pooling*, SAP) on $\hat{\mathbf{F}}^1$ (i.e., the output of FTM) to propagate the contextual information (provided by neighboring cells) onto each centroid cell. The resulting feature matrix $\tilde{\mathbf{F}}^1 \in \mathbb{R}^{N \times 64}$ encoding local geometric context has the form of

$$\tilde{\mathbf{F}}^1 = \left(\tilde{\mathbf{D}}_\mathbf{S}^{-\frac{1}{2}} \tilde{\mathbf{A}}_\mathbf{S} \tilde{\mathbf{D}}_\mathbf{S}^{-\frac{1}{2}} \right) \hat{\mathbf{F}}^1, \tag{1}$$

where $\tilde{\mathbf{A}}_\mathbf{S} = \mathbf{A_S} + \mathbf{I}$ can be regarded as an adjacency with self-loops, $\tilde{\mathbf{D}}_\mathbf{S}^{-\frac{1}{2}} \tilde{\mathbf{A}}_\mathbf{S} \tilde{\mathbf{D}}_\mathbf{S}^{-\frac{1}{2}}$ is the respective symmetric-normalized adjacency, and $\tilde{\mathbf{D}}_\mathbf{S}$ is the diagonal degree matrix. After SAP, both $\tilde{\mathbf{F}}^1$ and $\hat{\mathbf{F}}^1$ are further squeezed by shared-weights 1D Convs with 32 channels. The resulting feature matrices are then concatenated across channels, followed by the fusion by another 1D Conv with 64 channels. Notably, the complete operation of our GLM is in some sense an extension of graph convolutional network [3], e.g., the output $\mathbf{F}^{S1}$ of GLM-1 has the form of

$$\mathbf{F}^{S1} = \sigma\left(\left\{ \sigma(\hat{\mathbf{F}}^1 \mathbf{W}^1) \oplus \sigma(\tilde{\mathbf{F}}^1 \mathbf{W}^1) \right\} \mathbf{W}^2 \right), \tag{2}$$

where $\sigma(\tilde{\mathbf{F}}^1 \mathbf{W}^1) = \sigma(\tilde{\mathbf{D}}_\mathbf{S}^{-\frac{1}{2}} \tilde{\mathbf{A}}_\mathbf{S} \tilde{\mathbf{D}}_\mathbf{S}^{-\frac{1}{2}} \hat{\mathbf{F}}^1 \mathbf{W}^1)$ is similar to a graph Conv layer [3], $\sigma(\cdot)$ is the ReLU activation, $\oplus$ denotes channel-wise concatenation, and $\mathbf{W}^1$ and $\mathbf{W}^2$ are the learnable weights for 1D Convs with 32 and 64 channels, respectively.

Different from GLM-1, GLM-2 enlarges the receptive field and learns multi-scale contextual features. Specifically, based on Eq. (1), the $N \times 512$ feature matrix from MLP-2 (i.e., $\mathbf{F}^2$) is processed by two parallel SAPs in terms of $\mathbf{A_S}$ and $\mathbf{A_L}$, respectively. The resulting feature matrices and $\mathbf{F}^2$ are then squeezed by shared-weights 1D Convs with 128 channels, which are finally concatenated across channels and fused by another 1D Conv with 512 channels. Notably, although we empirically use only two GLMs in our current implementation, as a general architecture, our MeshSNet can integrate more GLMs along its forward path to learn more scales of contextual features according to task requirements.

(2) Dense fusion of local-to-global features: Following [7], we apply global max pooling (GMP) on the output of GLM-2 to produce the translation-invariant holistic features, aiming to encode the semantic information of the whole dental surface. Different from PointNet that inserts only skip connections between cell/point-wise and holistic features, we assume that the multi-scale contextual features (produced by intermediate GLMs) could provide additional information to comprehensively describe mesh cells. Correspondingly, we densely concatenate the local-to-global features from FTM, GLM-1, GLM-2 and (upsampled) GMP, followed by MLP-3 to yield a $N \times 128$ feature matrix. Based on this matrix, a 1D Conv layer with softmax activation is used to predict a $N \times (C+1)$ probability matrix, with each row denoting the probabilities of the respective cell belonging to specific categories (i.e., C teeth and gingiva).

Implementation and Data Augmentation: As shown in Fig. 1, our Mesh-SNet model consists of three MLPs (i.e., MLP-1, MLP-2, and MLP-3), one FTM, two GLMs (i.e., GLM-1 and GLM-2), and a final 1D Conv layer to output softmax segmentation probabilities. MLP-1 contains two 1D Convs, both with 64 channels. MLP-2 has three 1D Convs, each with 64, 128, and 512 channels, respectively. MLP-3 contains four 1D Convs, each with 256, 256, 128, and 128 channels, respectively. All 1D Convs in these MLPs and the GLMs are followed by batch normalization (BN) and ReLU activation. To learn the 64×64 feature transformation matrix $\mathbf{T}$ for $\mathbf{F}^1$ (i.e., the output of MLP-1), FTM employs six 1D Convs with 64, 128, 512, 256, 128, and 64^2 channels, respectively, where each of the first five layers is followed by BN and ReLU, while the last layer (without BN and ReLU) is followed by a tensor reshape operation.

Our MeshSNet was implemented using Python based on Keras. It was trained by minimizing the generalized Dice loss [10] using the AMSGrad variant [8] of the Adam optimizer (mini-batch size: 10; number of epochs: 200). To improve the generalization ability of trained networks, we augmented the training and validation sets by combining (1) random rotation, (2) random translation, and (3) random rescaling (e.g., zoom-in/out) of each 3D surface in reasonable ranges. After that, on each training/validation surface (with roughly 10,000 cells), we randomly sampled 50% cells from each tooth and then randomly sampled the remaining cells from the gingival as the network input (with 6,000 cells in total). Notably, the combination of all above operations could largely enrich the training set, and also mitigate the imbalanced learning challenge caused by the fact that each tooth only takes a very small part on the whole dental surface. After network training, we directly applied trained networks on unseen test surfaces to predict the corresponding segmentations. That is, in contrast to the training phase, our network can *directly process the whole dental surfaces with varying sizes in the test phase*, which should be a practically meaningful property in practice.

3   Experiments

Dataset and Experimental Setup: The raw dataset studied in this paper consists of 20 maxillary dental surfaces for different subjects acquired by an in-house 3D IOS. The original surfaces roughly contain 100, 000 mesh cells, which were downsampled to 10, 000 cells while preserving the original topologies. The ground-truth segmentations for $C = 14$ teeth (i.e., from the central incisor to the second molar on both left and right sides) were manually annotated by a dental resident (guided by experienced dentists) on downsampled surfaces.

We performed 3-fold cross-validation on this dataset. In each iteration, one surface was randomly selected from the training set for validation, and the resulting training and validation sets were then enlarged using the data augmentation protocol described in Sect. 2, by simulating 100 "new" surfaces for each training/validation surface. The training/validation inputs (size: $6,000 \times 15$) were then randomly sampled on each surface on-the-fly. Using the same experimental setup, loss function, and optimizer, we compared our **MeshSNet** method with the state-of-the-art **PointNet** approach [7]. For a more comprehensive evaluation, we also designed a dense variant of PointNet (called **PointNet-D**), in which intermediate features were concatenated with mesh-wise and holistic features for the segmentation task. To verify the effectiveness of two essential components (i.e., multi-scale graph-constrained learning and dense fusion of local-to-global features) of MeshSNet, we also compared MeshSNet with its two variants, called **MeshSNet-S** and **MeshSNet-F**, respectively. In MeshSNet-S, the A_L-related SAP and Conv layers were removed from GLM-2, and the respective network can only perform mono-scale local context modeling. In MeshSNet-F, we only fused the mesh-wise and holistic features for MLP-3, by removing the connections from GLM-1 and GLM-2. Based on the ground-truth annotations, the segmentation results were quantitatively evaluated by three metrics, i.e., Dice similarity coefficient (DSC), sensitivity (SEN), and positive prediction value (PPV).

Table 1. Segmentation results (mean ± standard deviation) for all teeth quantified under 3-fold cross-validation, where p indicates the p-value for the statistical significance comparison between our MeshSNet approach and each competing method.

Metric	PointNet	PointNet-D	MeshSNet-S	MeshSNet-F	MeshSNet
DSC	0.781 ± 0.134	0.806 ± 0.121	0.859 ± 0.134	0.894 ± 0.083	**0.938 ± 0.060**
	$p = 1.6e{-}10$	$p = 7.6e{-}8$	$p = 5.1e{-}4$	$p = 1.5e{-}3$	n/a
SEN	0.828 ± 0.167	0.867 ± 0.146	0.882 ± 0.151	0.903 ± 0.100	**0.946 ± 0.062**
	$p = 8.1e{-}7$	$p = 6.3e{-}5$	$p = 8.5e{-}3$	$p = 6.5e{-}3$	n/a
PPV	0.766 ± 0.163	0.772 ± 0.145	0.849 ± 0.141	0.893 ± 0.099	**0.934 ± 0.077**
	$p = 6.1e{-}9$	$p = 3.4e{-}7$	$p = 5.8e{-}4$	$p = 2.2e{-}2$	n/a

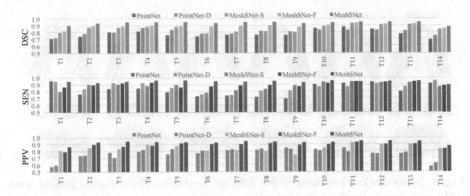

Fig. 2. Segmentation results for each of 14 teeth (i.e., T1–T14) quantified under 3-fold cross-validation, in terms of three evaluation metrics (i.e., DSC, SEN, and PPV).

Results: In terms of the three metrics, the overall segmentation results for all teeth are summarized in Table 1, and the specific segmentation results for each tooth are detailed in Fig. 2. From Table 1, we can have at least three observations. *First*, compared with the state-of-the-art PointNet method, our MeshSNet and its two variants (i.e., MeshSNet-S and MeshSNet-F) led to significantly better results. It suggests that our proposed method could effectively capture and leverage local geometric context to improve the segmentation performance. *Second*, our MeshSNet significantly outperformed its variant MeshSNet-S in terms of all metrics, which implies that explicitly learning multi-scale contextual features is desired for tooth segmentation on dental surfaces, considering that the density of mesh cells may vary across different surfaces and/or different positions. *Third*, our MeshSNet also yielded superior performance than its variant MeshSNet-F. This indicates that, compared with using solely the local and global features, the dense fusion of local-to-global (i.e., cell-wise, multi-scale contextual, and holistic) features could bring additional information for more accurate segmentation. By comparing PointNet-D with PointNet, one could see that the dense fusion strategy also boosts the performance of the original PointNet method.

The per-tooth segmentation results presented in Fig. 2 are consistent with the overall segmentation results summarized in Table 1. From Fig. 2, we can see that our MeshSNet yielded better DSC values than all other competing methods on all teeth (i.e., from T1 to T14), while its variants (i.e., MeshSNet-S and MeshSNet-F) outperformed the state-of-the-art PointNet and its variant (i.e., PointNet-D) on most teeth. These results further verify the effectiveness of our proposed method in the task of automated tooth segmentation on 3D dental surfaces. On the other hand, it is worth noting that, the improvement brought by our MeshSNet method is relatively more significant for the segmentation of *molars* (e.g., T1 and T14), compared with PointNet. For example, our MeshSNet improved the DSC from 0.711 to 0.900 (p-value $< 1e-4$), and improved the PPV from 0.575 to 0.867 (p-value $< 1e-6$) for segmenting T1. Note that segmenting molars is a very challenging task, because they locate at deep intraoral regions

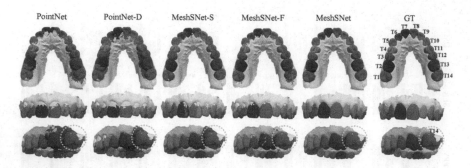

Fig. 3. Segmentations produced by five different methods and the manual ground-truth (GT) annotations for three representative examples.

and might not be completely captured by the light source. These results further suggest the robustness of our proposed method.

In Fig. 3, we visually compare the automated segmentations and ground-truth annotations for three representative examples. From Fig. 3, we can observe that our MeshSNet method has an overall better performance than other competing methods. For example, compared with PointNet and PointNet-D, MeshSNet effectively reduced false positives for segmenting molars (e.g., the first row of Fig. 3), and also reduced false negatives for segmenting central incisors (e.g., the second row of Fig. 3). Especially, our MeshSNet method can more precisely annotate molars that were not completely captured by IOS, which can be observed in green circles in the third row of Fig. 3. Both the visual evaluation in Fig. 3 and the quantitative evaluation in Table 1 and Fig. 2 suggest that our method is potentially useful in practice for automated tooth labeling on dental surfaces.

4 Conclusion

In this paper, we have proposed a deep neural network (called MeshSNet) for end-to-end 3D tooth segmentation on raw dental surfaces acquired by advanced intraoral scanners. Our MeshSNet method integrated novel graph-constrained learning modules to explicitly model the multi-scale local geometric context on mesh surface, and then employed a dense fusion strategy to effectively combine local-to-global features for the comprehensive description of mesh cells. Experimental results on an in-house clinical dataset have demonstrated the superior performance of our proposed method compared with the state-of-the-art deep learning methods for 3D shape segmentation. As the future work, we will integrate trainable post-processing modules (e.g., based on conditional random fields [13]) into our current model to further smooth the segmentations, e.g., by avoiding isolated false positives. In addition, our proposed method should be evaluated on more subjects to further verify its generalization capacity.

References

1. Feng, Y., et al.: MeshNet: mesh neural network for 3D shape representation. In: AAAI (2019)
2. Huang, Q., et al.: Recurrent slice networks for 3D segmentation of point clouds. In: CVPR, pp. 2626–2635 (2018)
3. Kipf, T.N., Welling, M.: Semi-supervised classification with graph convolutional networks. In: ICLR (2017)
4. Kondo, T., et al.: Tooth segmentation of dental study models using range images. IEEE Trans. Med. Imaging 23(3), 350–362 (2004)
5. Martin, C.B., et al.: Orthodontic scanners: what's available? J. Orthod. 42(2), 136–143 (2015)
6. Qi, C.R., et al.: PointNet++: deep hierarchical feature learning on point sets in a metric space. In: NeurIPS, pp. 5099–5108 (2017)
7. Qi, C.R., et al.: PointNet: deep learning on point sets for 3D classification and segmentation. In: CVPR, pp. 652–660 (2017)
8. Reddi, S.J., et al.: On the convergence of adam and beyond. In: ICLR (2018)
9. Roberta, T., et al.: Study of the potential cytotoxicity of dental impression materials. Toxicol. Vitro 17(5–6), 657–662 (2003)
10. Sudre, C.H., et al.: Generalised dice overlap as a deep learning loss function for highly unbalanced segmentations. In: DLMIA, pp. 240–248 (2017)
11. Wu, W., et al.: PointConv: deep convolutional networks on 3D point clouds. In: CVPR, pp. 9621–9630 (2019)
12. Xu, X., et al.: 3D tooth segmentation and labeling using deep convolutional neural networks. IEEE Trans. Vis. Comput. Graph. 25, 2336–2348 (2018)
13. Zheng, S., et al.: Conditional random fields as recurrent neural networks. In: CVPR, pp. 1529–1537 (2015)
14. Zou, B., et al.: Interactive tooth partition of dental mesh base on tooth-target harmonic field. Comput. Biol. Med. 56, 132–144 (2015)

Improving Robustness of Medical Image Diagnosis with Denoising Convolutional Neural Networks

Fei-Fei Xue[1,2], Jin Peng[1], Ruixuan Wang[1,2]([✉]), Qiong Zhang[1,3], and Wei-Shi Zheng[1,2]

[1] School of Data and Computer Science, Sun Yat-sen University, Guangzhou, China
wangruix5@mail.sysu.edu.cn
[2] Key Laboratory of Machine Intelligence and Advanced Computing,
MOE, Guangzhou, China
[3] Guangdong Key Laboratory of Information Security Technology,
Guangzhou, China

Abstract. Convolutional neural networks (CNNs) are vulnerable to adversarial noises, which may result in potentially disastrous consequences in safety or security sensitive systems. This paper proposes a novel mechanism to improve the robustness of medical image classification systems by bringing denoising ability to CNN classifiers with a naturally embedded auto-encoder and high-level feature invariance to general noises. This novel denoising mechanism can be adapted to many model architectures, and therefore can be easily combined with existing models and denoising mechanisms to further improve robustness of CNN classifiers. This proposed method has been confirmed by comprehensive evaluations with two medical image classification tasks.

Keywords: Robustness of CNN · Adversarial noises · Denoising CNN · Skin disease · Chest X-ray

1 Introduction

Convolutional neural networks (CNN) have been widely used in medical image analysis, such as automatic segmentation of tumor regions in MRI [13] and intelligent diagnosis of skin cancers [4]. However, the application of a medical analysis system would be limited if it is sensitive to various noises and varying environments. One way to critically evaluate the robustness of a medical image system is by adversarial attacks [14]. Specifically, clean images can be altered with imperceptible perturbations (called adversarial noises) to generate adversarial examples, and such adversarial examples can fool CNN classifiers to make incorrect predictions with high confidence. Recent studies on natural images clearly

---

F.-F. Xue and J. Peng—The authors contribute equally to this paper.

© Springer Nature Switzerland AG 2019
D. Shen et al. (Eds.): MICCAI 2019, LNCS 11769, pp. 846–854, 2019.
https://doi.org/10.1007/978-3-030-32226-7_94

demonstrate that CNN classifiers can be easily attacked and become completely crashed [8]. Adversarial attacks have also been performed on medical images [12], confirming the high sensitivity of CNN diagnosis systems to adversarial noises. Therefore, it is highly demanding to improve the robustness of intelligent diagnosis systems.

System robustness can be improved by providing the system with the ability of defending adversarial attacks. Multiple defense approaches have been proposed for this purpose. For example, adversarial training and its variants can improve system's defense ability simply by adding one or more types of adversarial examples into the training data during classifier training [5,8,15], while denoising approach pre-processes images often with certain type of auto-encoders, aiming to remove potential adversarial noises before inputting images to classifiers [1,10]. Adversarial training requires embedding adversarial attacking process into classifier training [5,8,15], and denoising approach often suffers from accuracy reduction in classifying clean images [1,10]. Another approach is to train a distillation network which can improve defense ability by effectively enlarging gaps between distributions of classes in the high-level semantic feature space [11].

While the attacking and defense studies of deep neural networks have been actively investigated on natural images in the past several years, few work has investigated the robustness of medical image analysis associated with its defense ability. This paper proposes a novel defense strategy to improve the robustness of intelligent diagnosis systems. Different from existing approaches, the proposed method directly improves network classifier's denoising ability with a naturally embedded auto-encoder and a semantic feature invariance strategy for general noises. This novel denoising mechanism can be adapted to many classifier architectures and is independent of any image pre-processing procedure. Therefore, it can be easily combined into the existing models and denoising mechanisms to further improve the robustness of network classifiers. Experiments on a skin image dataset and a chest X-ray dataset demonstrate that, it can always significantly improve the robustness of the classifiers via integrating the proposed denoising mechanism into the existing CNN classifiers, no matter whether the classifiers have employed other defense methods.

2 Methods

In adversarial attacks, image pixel values can be manipulated via small and carefully-crafted perturbations, such that the originally imperceptible adversarial noise can be progressively amplified over layers in deep neural networks, leading to incorrect classifications. Consider an image as a point in the original high-dimensional image space, and the re-ordered output of the last convolutional layer in a CNN classifier as a point in a low-dimensional high-level semantic feature space. For an original (clean) image which can be correctly classified by the neural network classifier, the corresponding adversarial example should be in a small hypersphere centered at the clean image in the image space, while the two images should be relatively far from each other in the high-level semantic feature space due to mis-classification of the adversarial example. To defend

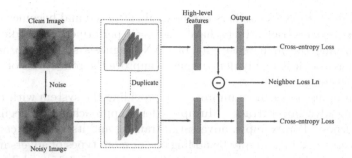

Fig. 1. Training a CNN classifier with an additional loss to emphasize similarity between noisy images and clean images in the semantic feature space. Each noisy image is generated by adding random noise to the corresponding clean image.

attacks from adversarial examples, one intuitive idea is to assure that the convolutional layers in the classifier can transform all neighboring points around each clean image to the same point in the semantic feature space as that of the clean image. The popular adversarial training, which adds adversarial examples to the training set, can be considered as one simplified implementation of this idea. Another idea is to remove (both general and adversarial) noises by projecting images to and then conducting reconstruction from a lower dimensional space, supposing that the clean images lie on a low-dimensional manifold while the noisy images are not. With this idea, auto-encoder has been applied to process images often before they are fed into the classifier. By combining the two ideas, but without using adversarial examples and the pre-processing procedure, we propose a novel plug-and-play mechanism to defend adversarial attacks, thus improving system robustness.

2.1 Transforming Neighboring Noisy Images to the Same Point

Because each adversarial example falls within a small neighborhood of the corresponding clean image in the image space, the classifier trained additionally with all the available noisy images, within the neighborhood of each training image, should become more robust to adversarial attacks, in the sense that all noisy images around a clean image would be projected to the same point in the semantic feature space. However in practice, it is infeasible to collect all such noisy images. Here by trying to project a small subset of general noisy images within the neighborhood of each clean image to the same point as that of the clean image in the semantic feature space, we expect adversarial examples within the neighborhood would be more likely projected to the same point as well. In this case, the adversarial examples would be more likely recognized as the same class of the clean image, thus improving robustness of the classifier.

Formally, for the i-th clean image x_i in the original training set, let us denote by x_i' a noisy image generated by adding uniform random noise $[-\sigma, \sigma]$ to each pixel of the clean image x_i, and $f(x_i)$ and $f(x_i')$ be the corresponding semantic feature vectors generated by the output of the final convolutional layer in the classifier. Then the objective of transforming neighboring noisy images to the same point in the semantic feature space can be formulated as an optimization problem, i.e., training the classifier (see Fig. 1) such that the following loss function L_n (called neighbor loss) is minimized:

$$L_n = \frac{1}{N} \sum_{i=1}^{N} \| f(x_i) - f(x_i') \|. \tag{1}$$

Note that x_i' can be randomly generated over training iterations such that multiple different noisy images are used for each clean image. Using random noise rather than adversarial noise during model training is one key difference between our approach and existing ones (e.g., [9]).

2.2 Embedded Auto-Encoder

The existing denoising approaches often employ a separate auto-encoder to remove potential adversarial noise from images before sending image data to the classifier. However, fine details in normal regions in the images could also be modified by the auto-encoder. Such change in normal regions actually causes new noises compared to the original clean images, and these new noises may be progressively amplified over layers in the classifier. Just as the adversarial noises, such new noises may also lead to mis-classification of the images, which actually has been observed in related studies [10] and in our experiments.

To avoid the downgraded classification performance on clean images and meanwhile make use of denoising ability from auto-encoder, we propose to embed the auto-encoder into the network classifier, where the encoder part shares low-to-middle convolutional layers of the classifier (Fig. 2 Left). Because the auto-encoder denoises images mainly by projecting them to a lower-dimensional space via the encoder part, sharing the encoder with the CNN classifier would naturally transfer the denoising competence to the classifier. Meanwhile, the classifier still uses original images rather than reconstructed images from the auto-encoder as input. This is clearly different from the existing approach which used a separate auto-encoder before the CNN classifier [9] (Fig. 2 Right).

Thus, for the clean image x_i and one corresponding noisy image x_i', with their reconstructed results $\hat{x}_i$ and $\hat{x}_i'$ from the embedded auto-encoder, the classifier can be trained to not only improve the classification performance, but also help improve the reconstruction performance of the embedded auto-encoder by additionally minimizing the reconstruction error L_a:

$$L_a = \frac{1}{N} \sum_{i=1}^{N} \{ \| x_i - \hat{x}_i \|_2 + \| x_i - \hat{x}_i' \|_2 \}. \tag{2}$$

Note that the target of the reconstructed noisy image $\hat{x}_i'$ is the clean image x_i. Similarly as in Eq. (1), multiple noisy x_i' can be randomly generated for each clean image.

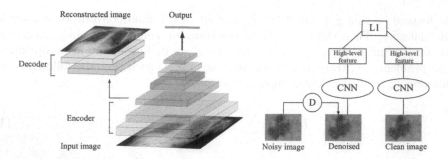

Fig. 2. The proposed embedded auto-encoder with a CNN network (Left) is different from the recently proposed high-level feature guided denoiser [9] (Right). D represents auto-encoder, and L1 represents L_1 distance.

Combining both ideas (Eqs. 1 and 2), a more robust classifier can be obtained by simultaneously training the classifier and the embedded auto-encoder, with the constraint to make clean and noisy images similar to each other in the semantic feature space, i.e., by minimizing the loss function L,

$$L = L_c + \lambda_n L_n + \lambda_a L_a. \tag{3}$$

Here L_c denotes the cross-entropy loss for the classifier itself to improve its classification performance on both clean and noisy images, λ_n and λ_a are hyper-parameters to respectively control the relative weights of loss terms L_n and L_a.

3   Experiments

3.1   Experimental Settings

The experiments were performed on two medical image datasets, the skin image dataset from ISIC2018 Challenge with 7 disease categories(SKIN4) [3], and the chest X-ray dataset with 3 categories[1]. To reduce the data imbalance between classes in the skin dataset, four classes (MEL, NV, BCC and BKL) in which the number of images exceeded 500 were selected and 1,500 images of NV class were randomly selected from 6,705, while keeping the other classes of data unchanged. The selected images were split to training set and test set with the rate around 5:1. For the chest X-ray dataset, we randomly split the raw training set to two parts, with 21,000 images as our training set and the left 6,000 images as test set. Also, to generate adversarial images for the evaluation of the proposed defense approach, different attacking methods, including the Fast Gradient Sign Method (FGSM) [5], the iterative FGSM (IFGSM) [7], and the Carlini and Wagner [2] method (C&W), were applied to four widely used network classifiers, including ResNet18 [6] and VGG-16. For each training sample, we generated two adversarial examples with the perturbation level ϵ in $\{4, 8\}$ for FGSM and

---

[1] https://www.kaggle.com/c/rsna-pneumonia-detection-challenge.

IFGSM. And for C&W, we set the searching times to 5 and the iteration times to 1000.

There are mainly two types adversarial attacks based on different assumptions on the knowledge of the target network, i.e., white-box and black-box attacks. In the black-box attack, an attacker can observes only the network's output information on some probed input information, which is more realistic and applicable. In comparison, in the white-box attack, an attacker has detailed information on the network architecture and model parameters. The evaluations here mainly focus on the defense of black-box attacks.

All the CNN classifiers used in experiments were optimized using SGD, with initial learning rate set 0.01, and weight decay set 0.0001. Each model was trained on a single GPU with batch size 64. The number of training epochs was set 80. Note that due to limited space, only part of the evaluation results were shown below, and the attacking model was ResNet18 unless otherwise mentioned.

Table 1. Classification accuracy on the adversarial examples generated from the SKIN4 test set. Rows 2 to 4 indicate the influence of neighbor loss and rows 5 to 7 represent the influence of reconstruction loss. Clean stands for original clean images. NA means no defense.

Defense		Clean	FGSM		IFGSM10		C&W
λ_n	λ_a		$\epsilon = 4$	$\epsilon = 8$	$\epsilon = 4$	$\epsilon = 8$	
NA	NA	84.28	19.27	21.99	3.78	3.78	1.54
0.1	-	81.32	41.84	30.97	49.29	30.61	16.31
1		**82.74**	**46.34**	**32.51**	**56.15**	**38.65**	**21.28**
10		64.78			-		
-	0.1	83.22	39.13	27.54	45.27	28.49	15.25
	1	82.62	41.02	29.20	53.43	33.57	19.39
	10	82.39	41.66	29.55	49.41	31.80	18.91
1	10	78.96	57.92	45.86	65.37	54.37	35.22

3.2 Evaluations on Skin Dataset

This section evaluates the effect of the proposed approach in improving robustness of a CNN classifier ResNet18 with ablation study on the skin dataset. Table 1 showed that when including the neighbor loss during training, with the embedded auto-encoded excluded, the trained classifiers (rows 2–4) performed significantly better than the classifier without any defense (first row), when attacked by different methods at different perturbation levels (ϵ). It also shows that with increasing weight λ_n of the neighbor loss, the defense performance increased accordingly. However, large λ_n (10.0) might lead to downgraded performance in classifying clean images. This is reasonable because larger λ_n would make the network pay less attention to the cross-entropy loss during training. As a trade-off, $\lambda_n = 1$ was chosen for subsequent tests on the skin dataset. Note that the decrease in classification accuracy on clean images is a common phenomenon in most defense methods (e.g., see [7,10]).

Similarly, by adding only the embedded auto-encoder to the classifiers, with the neighbor loss excluded during training, Table 1 (fifth row to second last row) showed the trained classifiers also performed significantly better than the classifier without any defense (first row) at various attacking scenarios. As a trade-off, $\lambda_a = 10$ was chosen for subsequent tests. Note that $\lambda_a = 100$ lead to downgraded performance in classifying clean images.

By combing both the neighbor loss and the embedded auto-encoder into the classifier, the trained classifier showed superior performance than all the above results (Table 1, last row), suggesting that the two proposed two ideas work together to further improve the robustness of the classifier. Similar results were obtained on the chest X-ray dataset (Table 2).

Table 2. Classification accuracy of the classifiers on the adversarial examples generated from the chest X-ray test set.

Defense		Clean	FGSM		IFGSM10		C&W
λ_n	λ_a		$\epsilon = 4$	$\epsilon = 8$	$\epsilon = 4$	$\epsilon = 8$	
NA	NA	76.00	20.86	20.91	28.21	16.13	12.39
1	0	75.27	68.48	63.07	71.84	68.68	60.29
0	10	74.85	67.66	62.04	70.66	68.34	57.74
1	10	73.97	71.21	68.66	72.35	70.79	60.87

Table 3. Classification accuracy of the architecture on the SKIN4 test set with modified model based on VGG16. The attacking model is ResNet18.

Defense		Clean	FGSM		IFGSM10		C&W
λ_n	λ_a		$\epsilon = 4$	$\epsilon = 8$	$\epsilon = 4$	$\epsilon = 8$	
NA	NA	84.28	38.77	28.25	50.71	29.08	15.60
1	0	82.74	68.68	58.75	74.00	69.50	50.12
0	10	82.39	66.55	56.03	73.05	67.85	44.21
1	10	78.96	70.21	64.18	74.00	70.45	54.73

3.3   Combinations with Different Model Structures

To show that our approach can work with different model structures, we combined our idea with another model VGG-16. Table 3 again showed that the proposed defense approach improved the robustness of the CNN classifier with a different structure, compared to the classifier without using defense (row with 'NA'). Combined with the evaluations on the ResNet18 structure above, it supports that the proposed approach helps improve robustness of multiple CNN model structures.

3.4   Combinations with Existing Defense Approaches

To show that our approach is complementary to existing defense approaches, we combined our approach with two existing approaches, the Reformer approach [10] and the HGD approach [9]. Table 4 clearly showed that when one or both of our ideas ($L_n, L_a, L_n + L_a$, corresponding to the neighbor loss, the embedded auto-encoder, or both) were combined with the existing two approaches, the combination further improved the robustness of the classifiers compared to the performance from the existing approaches alone.

Table 4. Classification accuracy when ours combined with existing approaches. The results are based on the SKIN4 test images. R denotes the Reformer approach.

Defense	FGSM		IFGSM10		C&W
	$\epsilon = 4$	$\epsilon = 8$	$\epsilon = 4$	$\epsilon = 8$	
NA	19.27	21.99	3.78	3.78	1.54
Reformer (Pixel-level Denoiser [10])					
R	30.16	27.44	18.64	14.41	9.71
$R + L_n$	48.37	36.85	58.17	42.14	26.06
$R + L_a$	42.71	31.28	53.47	33.49	25.46
$\mathbf{R} + L_n + L_a$	**59.17**	**46.48**	**69.66**	**55.54**	**44.71**
HGD* (High-level features Guided Denoiser [9])					
HGD*	41.80	36.97	42.49	26.01	22.73
HGD* + L_n	56.42	57.01	63.52	46.32	36.77
HGD* + L_a	51.14	47.41	58.18	41.34	31.59
HGD* + $L_n + L_a$	**64.13**	**51.83**	**70.52**	**58.67**	**49.55**

4 Conclusion

In this paper, we proposed a novel defense mechanism to improve robustness of medical image classification systems. This mechanism embeds an auto-encoder into the CNN structure and keeps high-level features invariant to general noises. It is complementary to existing defense approaches and therefore can be combined together to further improve the robustness of CNN classifiers.

Acknowledgement. This work is supported in part by the National Key Research and Development Plan (grant No. 2018YFC1315402) and by the Guangdong Key Research and Development Plan (grant No. 2019B020228001).

References

1. Akhtar, N., Liu, J., Mian, A.: Defense against universal adversarial perturbations. In: CVPR, pp. 3389–3398 (2018)
2. Carlini, N., Wagner, D.: Towards evaluating the robustness of neural networks. In: IEEE Symposium on Security and Privacy, pp. 39–57 (2017)
3. Codella, N.C.F., et al.: Skin lesion analysis toward melanoma detection: a challenge at the 2017 international symposium on biomedical imaging, hosted by the international skin imaging collaboration. In: ISBI, pp. 168–172 (2018)
4. Esteva, A., et al.: Dermatologist-level classification of skin cancer with deep neural networks. Nature **542**(7639), 115 (2017)
5. Goodfellow, I.J., Shlens, J., Szegedy, C.: Explaining and harnessing adversarial examples. In: ICLR (2015)
6. He, K., Zhang, X., Ren, S., Sun, J.: Deep residual learning for image recognition. In: CVPR, pp. 770–778 (2016)

7. Kurakin, A., Goodfellow, I., Bengio, S.: Adversarial examples in the physical world. arXiv:1607.02533 (2016)
8. Kurakin, A., Goodfellow, I.J., Bengio, S.: Adversarial machine learning at scale. CoRR: abs/1611.01236 (2016)
9. Liao, F., Liang, M., Dong, Y., Pang, T., Hu, X., Zhu, J.: Defense against adversarial attacks using high-level representation guided denoiser. In: CVPR, pp. 1778–1787 (2018)
10. Meng, D., Chen, H.: MagNet: a two-pronged defense against adversarial examples. In: ACM Conference on Computer and Communications Security, pp. 135–147 (2017)
11. Papernot, N., McDaniel, P., Wu, X., Jha, S., Swami, A.: Distillation as a defense to adversarial perturbations against deep neural networks. In: IEEE Symposium on Security and Privacy, pp. 582–597 (2016)
12. Paschali, M., Conjeti, S., Navarro, F., Navab, N.: Generalizability *vs.* robustness: investigating medical imaging networks using adversarial examples. In: Frangi, A.F., Schnabel, J.A., Davatzikos, C., Alberola-López, C., Fichtinger, G. (eds.) MICCAI 2018. LNCS, vol. 11070, pp. 493–501. Springer, Cham (2018). https://doi.org/10.1007/978-3-030-00928-1_56
13. Pereira, S., Pinto, A., Alves, V., Silva, C.A.: Brain tumor segmentation using convolutional neural networks in MRI images. IEEE Trans. Med. Imaging **35**(5), 1240–1251 (2016)
14. Szegedy, C., et al.: Intriguing properties of neural networks. In: ICLR (2014)
15. Tramèr, F., Kurakin, A., Papernot, N., Goodfellow, I., Boneh, D., McDaniel, P.: Ensemble adversarial training: attacks and defenses. arXiv:1705.07204 (2017)

Author Index